Diagnostic Procedures in
OPHTHALMOLOGY

Diagnostic Procedures in OPHTHALMOLOGY

Fourth Edition

Editors

HV Nema MS
Former Professor and Head
Department of Ophthalmology
Institute of Medical Sciences
Banaras Hindu University
Varanasi, Uttar Pradesh, India

Nitin Nema MS DNB
Professor
Department of Ophthalmology
Sri Aurobindo Institute of Medical Sciences
Indore, Madhya Pradesh, India

JAYPEE BROTHERS MEDICAL PUBLISHERS
The Health Sciences Publisher
New Delhi | London

Jaypee Brothers Medical Publishers (P) Ltd

Headquarters
Jaypee Brothers Medical Publishers (P) Ltd
EMCA House, 23/23-B
Ansari Road, Daryaganj
New Delhi 110 002, India
Landline: +91-11-23272143, +91-11-23272703
+91-11-23282021, +91-11-23245672
Email: jaypee@jaypeebrothers.com

Corporate Office
Jaypee Brothers Medical Publishers (P) Ltd
4838/24, Ansari Road, Daryaganj
New Delhi 110 002, India
Phone: +91-11-43574357
Fax: +91-11-43574314
Email: jaypee@jaypeebrothers.com

Overseas Office
JP Medical Ltd
83 Victoria Street, London
SW1H 0HW (UK)
Phone: +44 20 3170 8910
Fax: +44 (0)20 3008 6180
Email: info@jpmedpub.com

Website: www.jaypeebrothers.com
Website: www.jaypeedigital.com

Diagnostic Procedure in Ophthalmology

First Edition: 2002
Second Edition: 2009
Third Edition: 2014
Fourth Edition: **2023**
Reprint: **2024**

ISBN: 978-93-89776-99-7

Printed at: Sterling Graphics Pvt. Ltd. India.

Dedicated to

Ma

Contributors

A Narayanaswamy MS
Research Associate
Department of Glaucoma
Singapore Eye Hospital
Singapore

A Parivadhini MS
Consultant
Department of Glaucoma
Sankara Nethralaya
Chennai, Tamil Nadu, India

AK Grover MD FRCS
Chairman
Department of Ophthalmology
Sir Ganga Ram Hospital
New Delhi, India

Amrita Sawhney DNB MNAMS
Senior Resident
Department of Ophthalmology
Sir Ganga Ram Hospital
New Delhi, India

Anand Rajendran FRCS DNB
Professor and Senior Consultant
Vitreoretinal Services
Aravind Eye Hospital
Chennai, Tamil Nadu, India

Arijit Mitra MS
Consultant
Department of Glaucoma
Aravind Eye Hospital
Tirunelveli, Tamil Nadu, India

Arulmozhi Varman MS
Director
Uma Eye Clinic
Chennai, Tamil Nadu, India

Arup Chakrabarti MS
Director
Chakrabarti Eye Care Centre
Trivandrum, Kerala, India

Ashwin Shetty DOMS DNB
Narayana Nethralaya
Bengaluru, Karnataka, India

Chaitra Jayadev DO Ph D
Consultant Vitreoretina
Narayana Nethralaya
Bengaluru, Karnataka, India

Devendra Sood DO
Director
Eye-Q Institute of Glaucoma
New Delhi, India

Digvijay Singh MD
Dr Rajendra Prasad Centre for Ophthalmic Sciences
All India Institute of Medical Sciences
New Delhi, India

Francisco Arnalich Montiel MD
Vissum
Institute of Ophthalmology Alicante
Alicante, Spain

G Chandra Sekhar MS FRCS
Director
LV Prasad Eye Institute
Hyderabad, Telangana, India

Garima Tyagi B Opt
Optician
LV Prasad Eye Institute
Hyderabad, Telangana, India

George N Thomas MD MMed
Senior Resident
Department of Ophthalmology
National University Hospital
Singapore

Harinder Singh Sethi MS FRCS
Associate Professor
Vardhman Mahavir Medical College
New Delhi, India

Hima Pendharkar DMRD DNB (Radiodiagnosis) DM (Diagnosis & Interventional Neuroradiology)
Associate Professor
Department of Neuroimaging and Interventional Radiology
National Institute of Mental Health and Neurosciences
Bengaluru, Karnataka, India

Himanshu Shekhar MD
Senior Registrar
Dr Rajendra Prasad Centre for Ophthalmic Sciences
All India Institute of Medical Sciences
New Delhi, India

HV Nema MS
Former Professor and Head
Department of Ophthalmology
Institute of Medical Sciences
Banaras Hindu University
Varanasi, Uttar Pradesh, India

Jayamuruga Pandian Arunachalam PhD
Reader
Department of Genetics
Sankara Nethralaya
Chennai, Tamil Nadu, India

Jayesh Vazirani MS
Consultant
LV Prasad Eye Institute
Hyderabad, Telangana, India

Jeewan S Titiyal MD
Professor
Dr Rajendra Prasad Centre for Ophthalmic Sciences
All India Institute of Medical Sciences
New Delhi, India

Jorge L Alió y Sanz MD PhD
Director
Vissum, Institute of Ophthalmology Alicante
Alicante, Spain

Jorge L Alió Del Barrio MD PhD
Vissum Corporation, Alicante
Division of Ophthalmology
Universidad Miguel Hernández
Alicante, Spain

Joveeta Joseph PhD
Microbiologist
Jhaveri Microbiology Center
Brien Holden Eye Research Center
Kallam Anji Reddy Campus
LV Prasad Eye Institute
Hyderabad, Telangana, India

Jyotirmay Biswas MS FMRF FNAMS FIC (Path) FAICO
Director of Uvea and Head
Department of Ocular Pathology
Medical and Vision Research Foundations
Sankara Nethralaya
Chennai, Tamil Nadu, India

Kallakuri Sumasri B Opt
Optician
LV Prasad Eye Institute
Hyderabad, Telangana, India

L Vijaya MS
Deputy Director
Smt Jadhavbai Nathmal Singhvee Glaucoma Service
Sankara Nethralaya
Chennai, Tamil Nadu, India

Lingam Gopal MS FRCS
Senior Consultant
Medical Research Foundation
Sankara Nethralaya
Associate Professor, National University Hospital, Singapore

LS Mohan Ram D Opt BS
Optician
LV Prasad Eye Institute
Hyderabad, Telangana, India

Luci Kaweri MD
Consultant
Department of Cataract and Refractive Surgery
Narayana Nethralaya
Bengaluru, Karnataka, India

Mahesh Shanmugam MBBS DO FRCS(Ed) PhD FAICO
Head
Vitreo-Retina and Oncology Services
Sankara Eye Hospitals
Bengaluru, Karnatala, India

Manotosh Ray MD FRCS
Associate Consultant
National University Hospital
Singapore

Mayuresh Naik MS DNB
Senior Resident
Department of Ophthalmology
Vardhman Mahavir Medical College
New Delhi, India

Meena Chakrabarti MS
Senior Consultant
Chakrabarti Eye Care Centre
Trivandrum, Kerala, India

Mihir Kothari MS DNB FPOS FAICO Diploma in Pediatric Ophthalmology and Strabismus (USA)
Director
Ocular Motility Lab and Pediatric Low Vision Center
Jyotirmay Eye Clinic
Maharashtra, India

Mohammad Javed Ali MS FRCS
LV Prasad Eye Institute
Hyderabad, Telangana, India

Nagasamy Soumittra MSc PhD
Department of Genetics
Sankara Nethralaya
Chennai, Tamil Nadu, India

Navin Jayakumar MBBS DO FRCS(Ed)
Director
Darshan Eye Clinic
Consultant
Vasan Eye Care Hospitals
Chennai, Tamil Nadu, India

Nazneen Nazm MS DNB
Assistant Professor
ESI Medical College
Kolkata, West Bengal, India

Nikhil S Choudhari MS
Consultant
LV Prasad Eye Institute
Hyderabad, Telangana, India

Nitin Nema MS DNB
Professor
Department of Ophthalmology
Sri Aurobindo Institute of Medical Sciences
Indore, Madhya Pradesh, India

NR Rangaraj MS DO
Director
Premier Eye Care and Surgical Center
Chennai, Tamil Nadu, India

P Vijayalakshmi MS
Head
Department of Pediatric Ophthalmology
Aravind Eye Hospital and Postgraduate Institute of Ophthalmology
Madurai, Tamil Nadu, India

P Vrushali DNB
Aravind Eye Hospital and Postgraduate Institute of Ophthalmology
Madurai, Tamil Nadu, India

Parijat Chandra MD
Associate Professor
Dr Rajendra Prasad Centre for Ophthalmic Sciences
All India Institute of Medical Sciences
New Delhi, India

Pradeep Sagar MD (FVR)
Fellow in Vitreo-Retina and Ocular Oncology
Sankara Eye Hospital
Bengaluru, Karnataka, India

Pradeep Sharma MD
Professor
Department of Neuro-ophthalmology
Dr Rajendra Prasad Center for Ophthalmic Sciences
All India Institute of Medical Sciences
New Delhi, India

Pradeep Venkatesh MD
Professor
Department of Retina
Dr Rajendra Prasad Center for Visual Sciences
All India Institute of Medical Sciences
New Delhi, India

Pukhraj Rishi MD
Consultant
Department of Retina Services
Sankara Nethralaya
Chennai, Tamil Nadu, India

R Muralidhar MS
Consultant
Pediatric Ophthalmology
Aravind Eye Hospital and Postgraduate Institute of Ophthalmology
Madurai, Tamil Nadu, India

R Ramakrishnan MS
Chief Medical Officer
Aravind Eye Hospital
Tirunelveli, Tamil Nadu, India

Rajeev R Pappuru MS
Consultant
Department of Retina Services
LV Prasad Eye Institute
Hyderabad, Telangana, India

Rajesh Ramanjulu MD DNB FVR FAICO
Junior Consultant
Department of Vitreo-Retina and Ocular Oncology
Sankara Eye Hospital
Bengaluru, Karnataka, India

Rajesh Sinha MD FRCS
Professor
Dr Rajendra Prasad Centre for Ophthalmic Sciences
All India Institute of Medical Sciences
New Delhi, India

Rajni Sharma MD
Assistant Professor
Department of Pediatrics
Lady Hardinge Medical College
New Delhi, India

Rajul Parikh MS
Consultant
Shreeji Eye Clinic
Mumbai, Maharashtra, India

Rajvardhan Azad MD
Former Chief
Dr Rajendra Prasad Centre for Ophthalmic Sciences
All India Institute of Medical Sciences
New Delhi, India

Ranju Kharel (Sitaula) MD
Lecturer
Department of Ophthalmology
BP Koirala Lions Center for Ophthalmic Studies
Tribhuvan University, Institute of Medicine
Maharajgunj, Kathmandu, Nepal

RD Ravindran DNB
Professor and Chairman
Aravind Eye Hospital
Madurai, Tamil Nadu, India

Reesha KR
Sankara Nethralaya
Chennai, Tamil Nadu, India

Rituraj Baruah
Lady Hardinge Medical College
New Delhi, India

Rohit Shetty DNB FRCS PhD
Vice President
Narayana Nethralaya
Bengaluru, Karnataka, India

Rohit Agrawal MS
Fellow Vitreo-Retina
Narayana Nethralaya
Bengaluru, Karnataka, India

Ronnie Jacob George MS
Head
Department of Glaucoma Service
Sankara Nethralaya
Chennai, Tamil Nadu, India

Sadao Kanagami FOPS
Former Professor
Kitasato University School of Medicine
Teikyo, Japan

Santosh G Honavar MD FAMS
Director
Ophthalmic and Facial Plastic Surgery and Ocular Oncology
Center for Sight Super Specialty Eye Hospital
Hyderabad, Telangana, India
Director, Medical Services—CFS Group
Director, National Retinoblastoma Foundation

Santosh Gopikrishna Gadde DNB FVR
Consultant
(Vitreo-Retina)
Narayana Nethralaya
Bengaluru, Karnataka, India

Sarangapani Sripriya MSc PhD
Department of Genetics
Sankara Nethralaya
Chennai, Tamil Nadu, India

Savitri Sharma MD FAMS
Head
Jhaveri Microbiological Center
LV Prasad Eye Institute
Hyderabad, Telangana, India

Savleen Kaur MS
Senior Resident
Advanced Eye Center
Postgraduate Institute of Medical Education and Research
Chandigarh, India

Shaloo Bageja MS
Consultant
Department of Ophthalmology
Sir Ganga Ram Hospital
New Delhi, India

Shefali Parikh MS
Consultant
Shreeji Eye Clinic
Mumbai, Maharashtra, India

Shivcharan L Chandravanshi MS
Associate Professor
Department of Oculoplastic
SS Medical College
Rewa, Madhya Pradesh, India

Shubhra Goel DO DNB (Gold Medalist) MNAMS FMRF
Consultant
Department of Ophthalmic Facial Plastic and Cosmetic Surgery
Apollo Hospitals
Apollo Health City Complex
Hyderabad, Telangana, India

Siddharth Malaiya MS FLVPEI
Consultant
Cornea, Cataract, Refractive Services
ASG Eye Hospitals
Bhopal, Madhya Pradesh, India

Sneha Jay Shah DNB
LV Prasad Eye Institute
Hyderabad, Telangana, India

Sreedharan Athmanathan MD DNB
Senior Consultant Microbiologist
Rainbow Children's Hospital
Bengaluru, Karnataka, India

Sripathi Kamath MS
Fellow
LV Prasad Eye Institute
Hyderabad, Telangana, India

Su Xinyi MBBS PhD MMed
Eye Research Institute of Molecular and Cell Biology
Singapore and National University Hospital
Singapore

Subhadra Jalali MS
Head
Smt Kanuri Santhamma Retina-Vitreous Center
LV Prasad Eye Institute
Hyderabad, Telangana, India

Sudha Dhandayuthapani MSc
Department of Genetics
Sankara Nethralaya
Chennai, Tamil Nadu, India

Sushmita Kaushik MS
Professor
Department of Glaucoma
Advanced Eye Center
Postgraduate Institute of Medical Education and Research
Chandigarh, India

Tarun Sharma MD FRCS
Director, Retina Service
Sankara Nethralaya
Chennai, Tamil Nadu, India

Vinay PG MS
Assistant Professor
Department of Ophthalmology
Father Muller Medical College
Mangaluru, Karnataka, India

Virender Sangwan MS
Associate Director
LV Prasad Eye Institute
Hyderabad, Telangana, India

Vishal MY MS
Consultant
Department of Vitreo-Retinal Services
Aravind Eye Hospital
Madurai, Tamil Nadu, India

VSD Kiranmayi MS
Retina Fellow
Department of Vitreo-Retinal Service
Aravind Eye Hospital
Madurai, Tamil Nadu, India

Yog Raj Sharma MD
Former Professor and Head
Retina Unit
Dr Rajendra Prasad Centre for Ophthalmic Sciences
All India Institute of Medical Sciences
New Delhi, India

Preface to the Fourth Edition

The *Diagnostic Procedures in Ophthalmology* is a well-received book by readers. The book was translated in Spanish for the benefit of readers in the Spanish-speaking countries. Encouraged by the response of readers, the fourth edition is prepared. The book is further expanded by adding four more chapters—Fundus Autofluorescence Angiography, Optical Coherence Tomography Angiography in Retinal Diseases, Videonystagmography and Cerebral Angiography in Neuro-ophthalmology.

The book is a rich source of material for routine and advanced diagnostic procedures in diseases of the eye. The routine tests required for examination of the eye patients, including recording of visual acuity, color vision and color defects, slit-lamp examination, tonometry, gonioscopy, optic disc assessment, ophthalmoscopy, and perimetry are described in some detail.

Advanced procedures such as different types of angiography, ultrasonography, electrophysiological tests, corneal topography, anterior and posterior segments optical coherence tomography, and Pentagan are also described. A comprehensive evaluation of ptosis, proptosis, pupil, dry eye, and epiphora is presented. Diagnostic modalities of infectious keratitis, uveitis, strabismus, ocular motor nerve palsies, and intraocular malignancies are extensively covered. The chapter on Diagnostic Procedures for Genetically Transmitted Eye Diseases describes the molecular diagnostics and cytogenetics. In the present edition, most of the chapters are updated for the accurate and speedy diagnosis of eye diseases. All chapters are profusely illustrated.

Modern diagnostic procedures in ophthalmology have revolutionized the treatment of eye diseases. Early diagnosis is key to early treatment and a better prognosis. Hopefully, postgraduate students, residents and general ophthalmic practitioners will find the fourth edition of the book more useful for the preparation of their examination and in day-to-day clinical practice.

HV Nema
Nitin Nema

Preface to the First Edition

The word *diagnosis* comes from the Greek word *diagignoskein* meaning to distinguish or discern. Besides history and clinical examination of the patient, diagnostic tests are required to aid in making correct diagnosis of eye diseases. The role of diagnostic technology is not inferior to that of a clinician's acumen. A correct diagnostic report helps in differentiating functional from organic and idiopathic from non-idiopathic diseases. The number of diagnostic tests available to an ophthalmologist has increased significantly in the last two decades. Both selective and non-selective tests are presently used for the clinical and research purposes. Non-selective approach to testing is costly and does not provide useful information. In order to be useful, diagnostic tests have to be properly performed, accurately read, and correctly interpreted. The ordering oculist should always compare the results of test with the clinical features of the eye disease.

The main aim of the book—*Diagnostic Procedures in Ophthalmology* is to provide useful information on diagnostic tests, which an ophthalmologist intends to perform or order during his clinical practice. Some of the procedures described in the book, assessment of visual acuity, slit-lamp examination, tonometry, gonioscopy, perimetry, and ophthalmoscopy, are routine examinations. However, the technique of proper examination and interpretation of findings to arrive at a correct diagnosis must be known to the practicing ophthalmologist or optometrist.

Procedures such as ophthalmic photography, evaluation of optic nerve head, fundus fluorescein angiography, and indocyanine green angiography are invaluable because they not only help in the diagnosis and documentation but also help in monitoring the management of eye disease. Corneal topography gives useful data about corneal surface and curvature and contributes to the success of LASIK surgery to a great extent. The role of A-scan ultrasonography in the measurement of axial length of the eye and biometry cannot be overemphasized. B-scan ultrasonography is needed to explore the posterior segment of the eye when media are opaque or an orbital mass is suspected. Ultrasound biomicroscopy (UBM) and optical coherence tomography (OCT) are relatively new noninvasive tools to screen the eye at the microscopic level. UBM helps in understanding the pathogenesis of various forms of glaucoma and their management. OCT obtains a tomograph of the retina showing its microstructure incredibly similar to a histological section. It helps in the diagnosis and management of the macular and retinal diseases. Electrophysiological tests allow objective evaluation of visual system. They are used in determination of visual acuity in infants and in the diagnosis of the macular and optic nerve disorders. What diagnostic tests should be ordered in the evaluation of the patients with infective keratitis or uveitis? Chapters on Diagnostic Procedures in Infective Keratitis and Diagnostic Procedures in Uveitis provide an answer.

The experts who have credibility in their fields have contributed chapters to the book. Not only the procedures of diagnostic tests are described but to make the reader conversant, characteristic findings in the normal and the diseased eye are also highlighted with the help of illustrations.

The book should be of great help to the practicing ophthalmologists, resident ophthalmologists, optometrists and technicians as it provides instant access to the diagnostic procedures in ophthalmology.

We are indebted to all contributors for their excellent contributions in short time in spite of their busy schedule. Shri Jitendar P Vij deserves our sincere thanks for nice publication of the book.

HV Nema
Nitin Nema

Acknowledgments

We are indebted to all contributors of the book for writing their valuable chapters. A large majority of authors has updated their articles. Our special appreciation goes to Drs Anand Rajendran, Chaitra Jayadev, Hima Pendharkar, and Mihir Kothari for writing new chapters on a short notice.

Shri Jitendar P Vij (Group Chairman), Mr Ankit Vij (Managing Director), Ms Chetna Malhotra (Senior Director—Professional Publishing, Marketing and Business Development) of M/s Jaypee Brothers Medical Publishers (P) Ltd, New Delhi, India, deserve our sincere thanks for their keen interest in the publication of the fourth edition of the *Diagnostic Procedures in Ophthalmology*. We appreciate the hard work of Ms Kritika Dua (Senior Development Editor) for the production of the book.

Contents

CHAPTER

1 Assessment of Visual Acuity

Siddharth Malaiya, Nitin Nema

INTRODUCTION

Visual acuity (VA) is a measure of spatial resolution of the visual processing system. The minimum angle of resolution (MAR), that allows a human optical system to identify two points as different stimuli, is defined as the *threshold of resolution*. The MAR lies between 30 seconds and 1 minute of an arc. VA is reciprocal of the threshold of resolution.[1] It is the most important criterion for testing the functional integrity of the eye and visual pathway. It is maximum at fovea where photoreceptors (cones) are closely packed and highly differentiated.

HISTORY

In 1854, Eduard von Jaeger published a set of reading charts in German, French, and English languages to record the VA. Donders for the first time coined the term visual acuity to describe the sharpness of vision and defined it as a ratio of patient's VA and standard VA. Hermann Snellen published his classical chart for recording the VA in 1862. Unlike Jaeger, he did not use the fonts from printing house but designed special letters, based on 5 × 5 grid, which he called *optotypes*. An optotype is a symbol or letter, the recognition of a particular optotype amounts to definite level of VA.[2]

PRINCIPLE

The Snellen test types are constructed on the principle that two distant points can be visible as separate only when the minimum angle subtended by them at the nodal point of the eye is 1 minute. This forms the standard of normal VA. The VA depends upon the resolving power of the eye and varies with the wavelength of the light and size of the pupil. It is also known as *minimum resolvable acuity*. Other subdivisions of VA include *minimum visible*, which is the detection of mere presence of stimulus, and *minimum discriminable* (hyperacuity), the relative position of two or more visible features with respect to each other.[3]

The Snellen test types consist of letters arranged in lines **(Fig. 1)**. The size of the letters gradually diminishes from above downward. Each letter is so designed that it fits in a square, the sides of which are five times the breadth of the constituent lines. Therefore, at a given distance, the letter subtends an angle of 5 minutes at the nodal point of the eye **(Fig. 2)**. The top letter of the chart subtends a 5-minute angle at the nodal point of the observer's eye from a distance of 60 m. The letters in the subsequent lines subtend same angle, if they are 36 m, 24 m, 18 m, 12 m, 9 m, and 6 m away from the eye. The chart should be well-illuminated (20 foot-candles) for recording the vision correctly.

RECORDING OF DISTANT VISUAL ACUITY

For recording the VA, the patient should be seated at a distance of 6 m from the chart as the rays of light are practically parallel from this distance, and accommodation is negligible. When the space in the room is limited, the test types may be seen after being reflected from a plane mirror kept at a distance of 3 m from the patient. The patient is asked to read the test types after occluding one eye either by an occluder or by palm of the hand. The VA is expressed as a fraction, the numerator of which is the distance of the chart from the patient (6 m) and the denominator is the numerical number written underneath the line up to which the patient can read. For example, if a patient can read only the top letter, his VA is recorded as 6/60. When patient reads the second, third, fourth, fifth, sixth, and seventh lines, the VA of the patient is recorded as 6/36, 6/24, 6/18, 6/12, 6/9, and 6/6, respectively. When the unit of measurement is feet (as commonly done in US), VA is expressed as fraction 20/200, 20/125, 20/80, 20/40, 20/32, and 20/20.

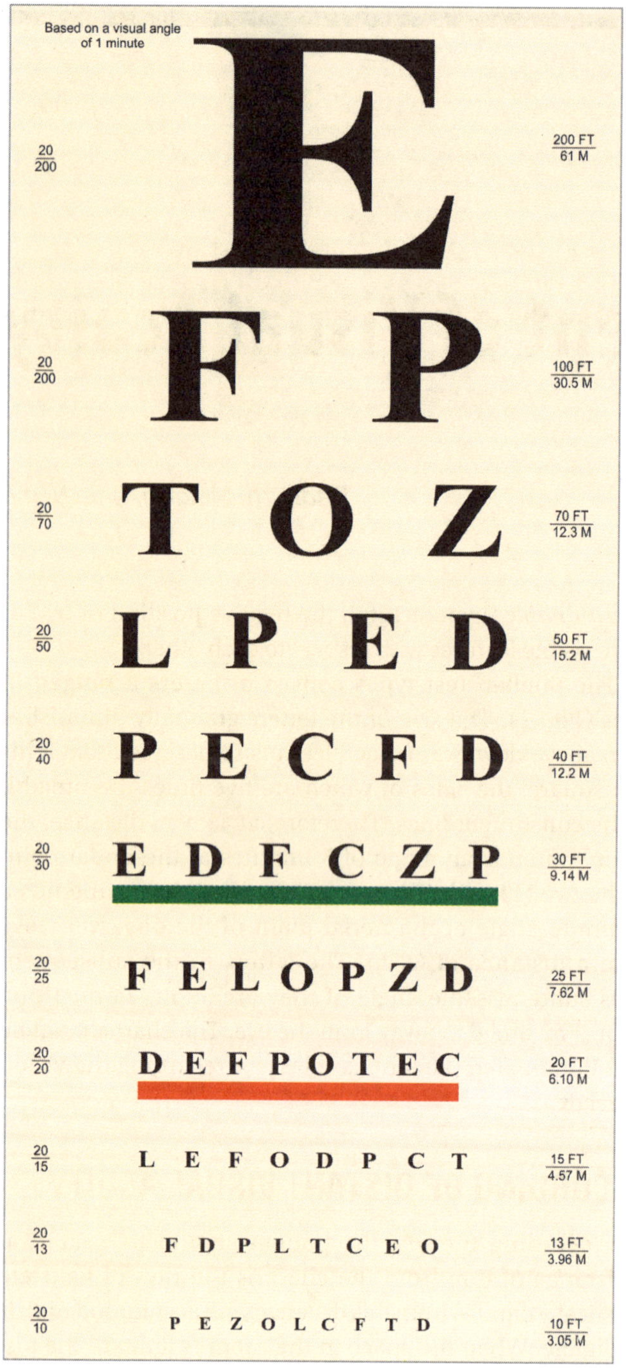

Fig. 1: Snellen chart.

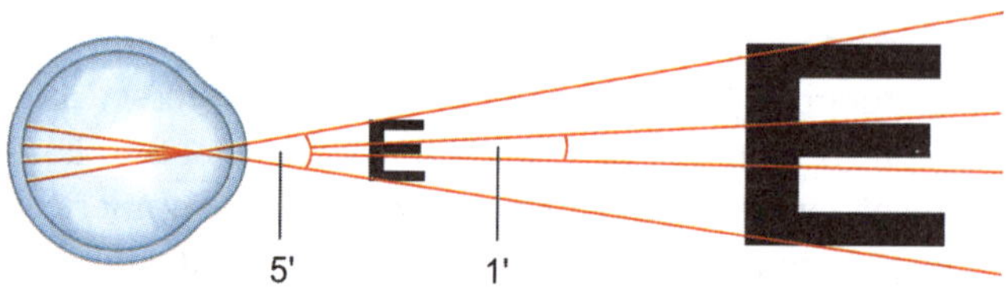

Fig. 2: The Snellen letters subtend 5 minutes of visual angle and each component subtends 1 minute of the angle.

Table 1: Visval acuity in feet, meters, decimal and logMAR.

VA in feet	*VA in meters*	*VA in decimal*	*VA in logMAR*
20/20	6/6	1.0	0.0
20/32	6/9.5	0.63	0.2
20/40	6/12	0.50	0.3
20/50	6/15	0.40	0.4
20/63	6/18	0.32	0.5
20/80	6/24	0.25	0.6
20/100	6/30	0.20	0.7
10/125	6/38	0.16	0.8
20/200	6/60	0.10	1.0
20/400	6/120	0.05	1.3

(VA: visual acuity; MAR: minimum angle of resolution)

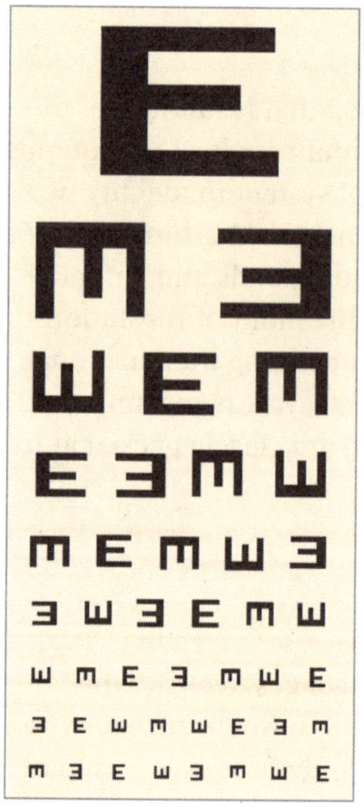

Fig. 3: E chart.

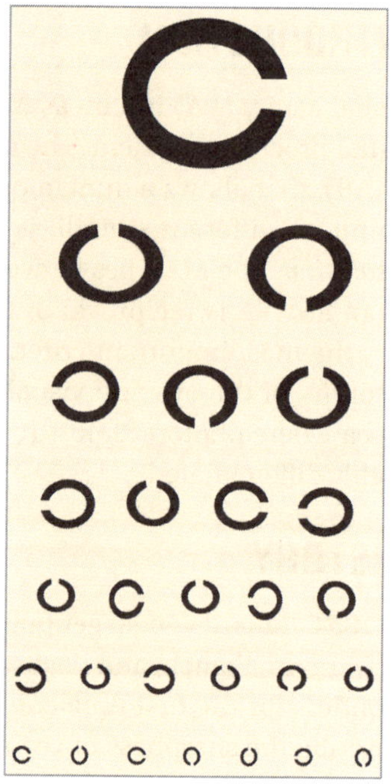

Fig. 4: Landolt chart.

Another commonly used scale is logMAR, which expresses the logarithm of minimum angle of resolution. VA scales in feet, meters, decimal, and logMAR are shown in **Table 1**.

Normally, a person can read the line marked 6 and the VA is expressed as 6/6 or 20/20. When the top letter cannot be read, the patient is asked to move toward the chart, and if he or she reads the top letter from 3 m distance, the VA is recorded as 3/60. If the patient cannot appreciate the top letter even from a distance of 1 m then the distance in feet or inches is recorded at which finger counting (FC) is possible. When the patient fails to count the fingers, he is asked to appreciate the movements of hand (HM). In absence of recognition of hand movements, perception of light (PL) should be tested. Projection of rays (PR) is checked in all quadrants of eye, by throwing penlight from superior, inferior, nasal, and temporal directions and response of subject is noted. The test is done in darkroom.[4] The examination should be repeated for the fellow eye.

In ill-literate persons "E" test types **(Fig. 3)** or Landolt broken rings **(Fig. 4)** should be used. The patient is directed

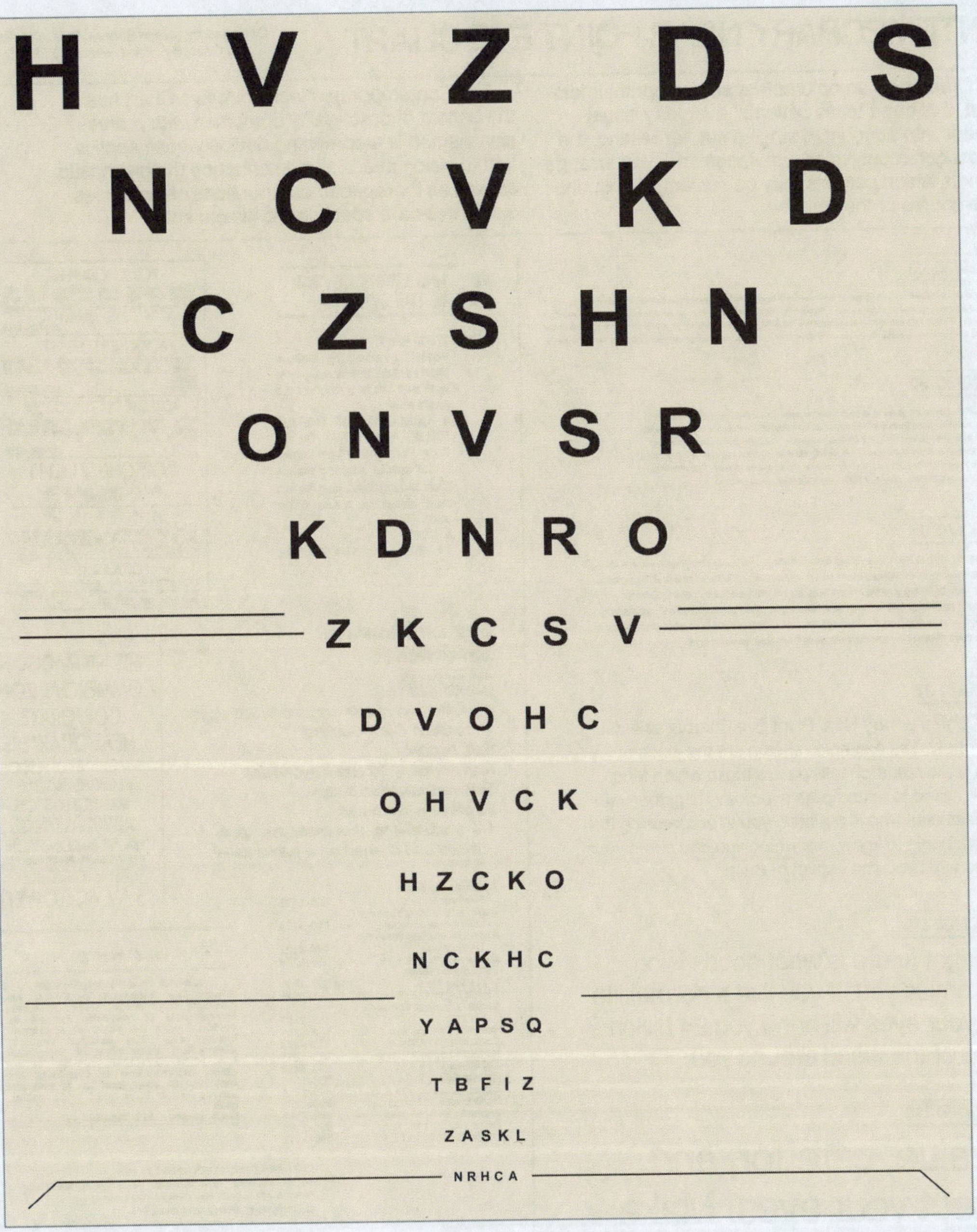

Fig. 5: Bailey-Lovie chart.

to point his finger in the same direction as bars of E or open end of C.

LogMAR Charts

The conventional Snellen charts are not accurate as there is no equal progression of size of letters from one line to another. There are some letters that can be recognized easily (letter L), while others are difficult (letter B) to recognize. Therefore, logMAR charts are developed. The chart has standard spacing between letters on each line and between lines of print. LogMAR charts have geometric progression of size of letters in each line by $\log_{10}10$. VA can be measured up to each letter and each letter amounts to 0.02 added to normal logMAR of Snellen's value for extra-read letters. Bailey-Lovie chart **(Fig. 5)** is a logMAR chart that contains 10 lines, and each line has five letters. These letters are structured in a ratio of 5:4. Early Treatment of Diabetic Retinopathy Study (ETDRS) also used this chart as these are more useful for recording VA in low vision patients. However, here the letters are structured in a ratio of 5:5.[5]

Normal Vision

Normal VA is often considered as 20/20 (in feet), 6/6 (in meters), 1.00 decimal, or 0.0 logMAR. The 20/20 standard should be considered as the lower limit of normal or as a screening cutoff. Normal acuity in healthy adults is one or two lines better than that. Average acuity in a population sample does not drop below the 20/20 level until the age of

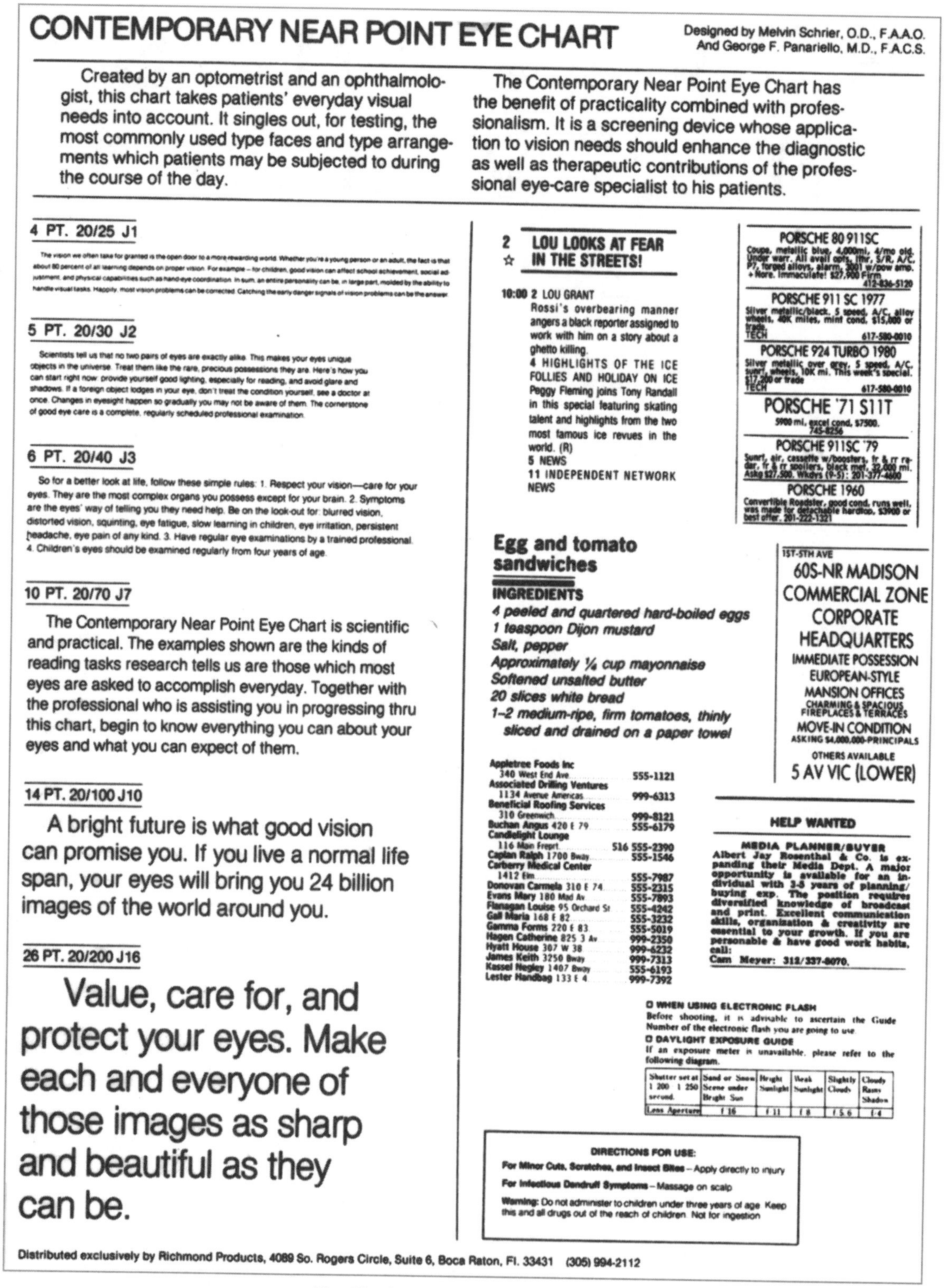

CONTEMPORARY NEAR POINT EYE CHART

Designed by Melvin Schrier, O.D., F.A.A.O.
And George F. Panariello, M.D., F.A.C.S.

Created by an optometrist and an ophthalmologist, this chart takes patients' everyday visual needs into account. It singles out, for testing, the most commonly used type faces and type arrangements which patients may be subjected to during the course of the day.

The Contemporary Near Point Eye Chart has the benefit of practicality combined with professionalism. It is a screening device whose application to vision needs should enhance the diagnostic as well as therapeutic contributions of the professional eye-care specialist to his patients.

4 PT. 20/25 J1

The vision we often take for granted is the open door to a more rewarding world. Whether you're a young person or an adult, the fact is that about 80 percent of all learning depends on proper vision. For example – for children, good vision can affect school achievement, social adjustment, and physical capabilities such as hand-eye coordination. In sum, an entire personality can be, in large part, molded by the ability to handle visual tasks. Happily, most vision problems can be corrected. Catching the early danger signals of vision problems can be the answer.

5 PT. 20/30 J2

Scientists tell us that no two pairs of eyes are exactly alike. This makes your eyes unique objects in the universe. Treat them like the rare, precious possessions they are. Here's how you can start right now: provide yourself good lighting, especially for reading, and avoid glare and shadows. If a foreign object lodges in your eye, don't treat the condition yourself, see a doctor at once. Changes in eyesight happen so gradually you may not be aware of them. The cornerstone of good eye care is a complete, regularly scheduled professional examination.

6 PT. 20/40 J3

So for a better look at life, follow these simple rules: 1. Respect your vision—care for your eyes. They are the most complex organs you possess except for your brain. 2. Symptoms are the eyes' way of telling you they need help. Be on the look-out for: blurred vision, distorted vision, squinting, eye fatigue, slow learning in children, eye irritation, persistent headache, eye pain of any kind. 3. Have regular eye examinations by a trained professional. 4. Children's eyes should be examined regularly from four years of age.

10 PT. 20/70 J7

The Contemporary Near Point Eye Chart is scientific and practical. The examples shown are the kinds of reading tasks research tells us are those which most eyes are asked to accomplish everyday. Together with the professional who is assisting you in progressing thru this chart, begin to know everything you can about your eyes and what you can expect of them.

14 PT. 20/100 J10

A bright future is what good vision can promise you. If you live a normal life span, your eyes will bring you 24 billion images of the world around you.

26 PT. 20/200 J16

Value, care for, and protect your eyes. Make each and everyone of those images as sharp and beautiful as they can be.

2 ☆ LOU LOOKS AT FEAR IN THE STREETS!

10:00 2 LOU GRANT
Rossi's overbearing manner angers a black reporter assigned to work with him on a story about a ghetto killing.
4 HIGHLIGHTS OF THE ICE FOLLIES AND HOLIDAY ON ICE
Peggy Fleming joins Tony Randall in this special featuring skating talent and highlights from the two most famous ice revues in the world. (R)
5 NEWS
11 INDEPENDENT NETWORK NEWS

PORSCHE 80 911SC
Coupe, metallic blue, 4,000mi, 4/mo old. Under warr. All avail opts, lthr, S/R, A/C, P7, forged alloys, alarm, 3001 w/pow amp. + More. Immaculate! $27,900 Firm. 412-836-5120

PORSCHE 911 SC 1977
Silver metallic/black, 5 speed, A/C, alloy wheels, 40K miles, mint cond. $15,000 or trade.
TECH 617-580-0010

PORSCHE 924 TURBO 1980
Silver metallic over grey, 5 speed, A/C, sunrf, wheels, 10K mi. This week's special. $17,200 or trade
TECH 617-580-0010

PORSCHE '71 S11T
5900 mi., excel cond. $7500. 745-8256

PORSCHE 911SC '79
Sunrf, air, cassette w/boosters, fr & rr radar, fr & rr spoilers, black met. 32,000 mi. Askg $27,500. Wkdys (9-5): 201-377-4600

PORSCHE 1960
Convertible Roadster, good cond. runs well, was made for detachable hardtop. $3900 or best offer. 201-222-1321

Egg and tomato sandwiches

INGREDIENTS

4 peeled and quartered hard-boiled eggs
1 teaspoon Dijon mustard
Salt, pepper
Approximately ¼ cup mayonnaise
Softened unsalted butter
20 slices white bread
1–2 medium-ripe, firm tomatoes, thinly sliced and drained on a paper towel

1ST-5TH AVE
60S-NR MADISON
COMMERCIAL ZONE
CORPORATE
HEADQUARTERS
IMMEDIATE POSSESSION
EUROPEAN-STYLE
MANSION OFFICES
CHARMING & SPACIOUS FIREPLACES & TERRACES
MOVE-IN CONDITION
ASKING $4,000,000-PRINCIPALS
OTHERS AVAILABLE
5 AV VIC (LOWER)

Appletree Foods Inc
340 West End Ave ... 555-1121
Associated Drilling Ventures
1134 Avenue Americas ... 999-6313
Beneficial Roofing Services
310 Greenwich ... 999-8121
Buchan Angus 420 E 79 ... 555-6179
Candlelight Lounge
116 Main Freprt ... 516 555-2390
Caplan Ralph 1700 Bway ... 555-1546
Carberry Medical Center
1412 Elm ... 555-7987
Donovan Carmela 310 E 74 ... 555-2315
Evans Mary 180 Mad Av ... 555-7893
Flanagan Louise 95 Orchard St ... 555-4242
Gall Maria 168 E 82 ... 555-3232
Gamma Forms 220 E 83 ... 555-5019
Hagen Catherine 825 3 Av ... 999-2350
Hyatt House 307 W 38 ... 999-6232
James Keith 3250 Bway ... 999-7313
Kassel Negley 1407 Bway ... 555-6193
Lester Handbag 133 E 4 ... 999-7392

HELP WANTED

MEDIA PLANNER/BUYER
Albert Jay Rosenthal & Co. is expanding their Media Dept. A major opportunity is available for an individual with 3-5 years of planning/buying exp. The position requires diversified knowledge of broadcast and print. Excellent communication skills, organization & creativity are essential to your growth. If you are personable & have good work habits, call:
Cam Meyer: 312/337-8070.

☐ WHEN USING ELECTRONIC FLASH
Before shooting, it is advisable to ascertain the Guide Number of the electronic flash you are going to use.
☐ DAYLIGHT EXPOSURE GUIDE
If an exposure meter is unavailable, please refer to the following diagram.

Shutter set at 1/200–1/250 second.	Sand or Snow Scene under Bright Sun	Bright Sunlight	Weak Sunlight	Slightly Cloudy	Cloudy Rainy Shadow
Lens Aperture	f 16	f 11	f 8	f 5.6	f 4

DIRECTIONS FOR USE:
For Minor Cuts, Scratches, and Insect Bites – Apply directly to injury
For Infectious Dandruff Symptoms – Massage on scalp
Warning: Do not administer to children under three years of age. Keep this and all drugs out of the reach of children. Not for ingestion

Distributed exclusively by Richmond Products, 4089 So. Rogers Circle, Suite 6, Boca Raton, Fl. 33431 (305) 994-2112

Fig. 6A: Jaeger type near vision chart.

60 years or 70 years. This explains the existence of the two lines smaller than 20/20: 20/15 and 20/10. *Super acuity* and *hyperacuity* are the terms used for vernier acuity that measures the ability to align two line segments. The vernier acuity is about 0.13 arc min, well below normal VA (which is about 0.6 arc min); therefore, it is presumed to be function of visual cortex rather than retina.

Near Visual Acuity

The near VA is usually tested with the help of Jaeger test types **(Fig. 6A)** or Roman test types. Roman test types are based on "point system" where one point equates to 1/72th of an inch (~0.353 mm). The size of optotypes is in multiple of this and Times Roman font is kept as standard.[6]

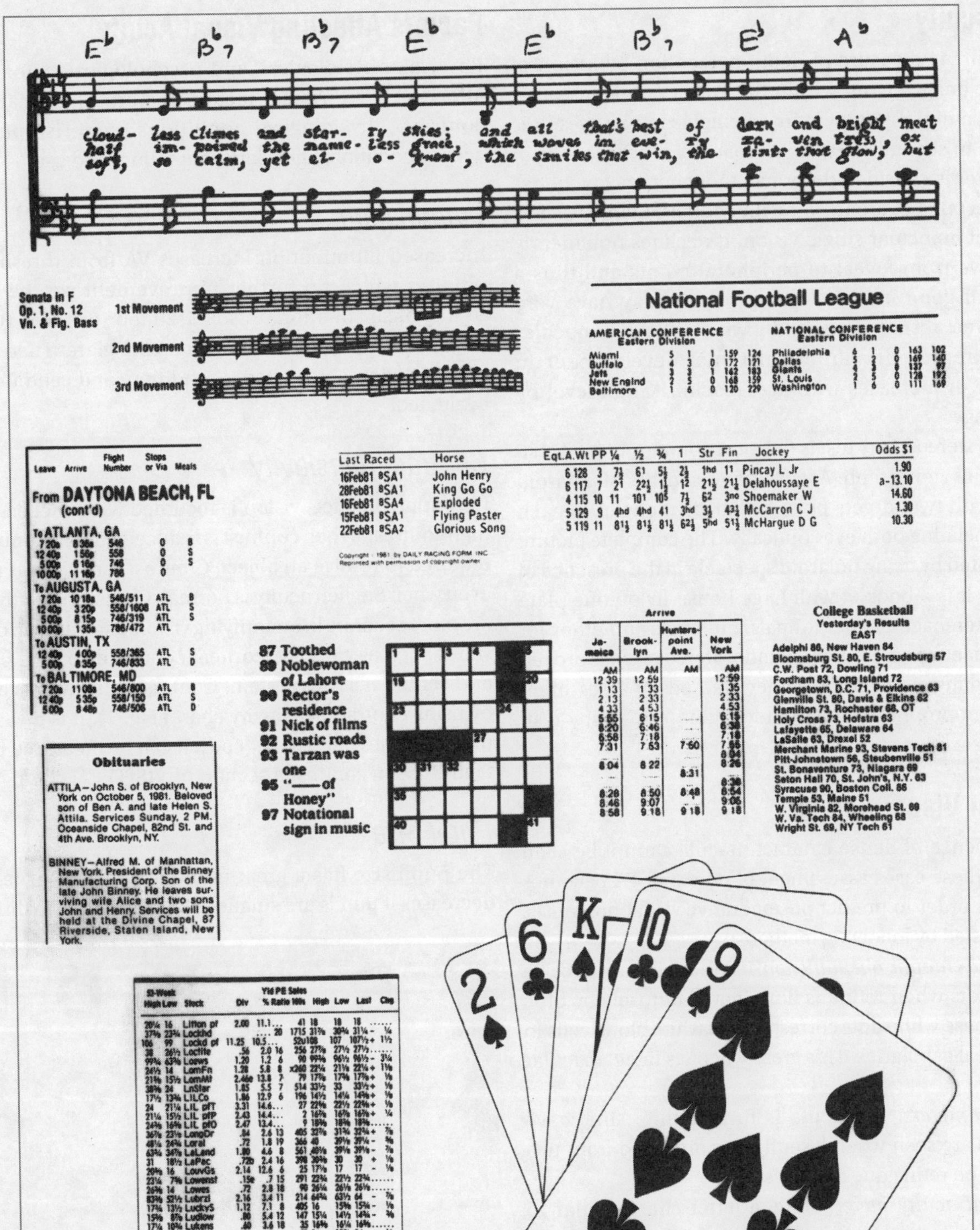

Fig. 6B: Mixed near vision chart showing music types, tables, crosswords, print types and playing cards.

The Snellen's notation maintaining the same visual angle may also serve the purpose. In Jaeger test types, a series of different sizes of print types are arranged in increasing order and arbitrarily marked 1, 2, 3, 4, 5, 6, and 7. Rosenbaum Pocker Vision Screener or Lebensohn charts can also be used. The near vision is also tested by music-types, numericals or tables **(Fig. 6B)**. It is usually tested in good illumination, preferably in daylight. The patient is asked to read the chart kept at a distance of 16 inches or 40 cm. Generally, a person with normal vision and accommodation reads the smallest types easily. If unable to read the smallest types on the chart, the smallest type, which the patient can read should be noted. Patients with high hyperopia, presbyopia, or anomalies of accommodation have defective near vision.

Stereoacuity

Stereoacuity is measure of depth perception by fusion of dissimilar images lying within the Panum's fusional area and stimulating disparate retinal elements in two eyes. It is measured in seconds of arc. Stereoacuity of 60 seconds of arc or better is considered normal, though it may be better than 15 seconds of arc in some individuals. Stereopsis is a function of binocular single vision. It declines nonlinearly as we move from foveal to peripheral points and thus a function of good macula.[7] Some people may have very poor or even absent stereoacuity with normal monocular acuity. It represents abnormal visual development in young age. It increases with age, reaching adult level by 7 years of age.[8]

Titmus stereoacuity test is the most commonly used test. It is a kind of vectograph. A vectograph consists of polaroid material with two targets polarized at right angles to each other dissociating both eyes optically. The complete picture is appreciated by using polaroid spectacle in the presence of stereopsis. It is a booklet with large house-fly on one plate for gross stereoacuity and animals and circles on other for finer stereoacuity assessment. Randot stereo test has proved better in younger age group. Other methods of assessment include synoptophore, TNO random dot test, Frisby test, and Lang test.[8]

Potential Visual Acuity

In the presence of dense cataract macula cannot be seen clearly. In these cases assessment of potential VA becomes essential in order to predict postoperative visual prognosis. It can be tested by following methods:

- *Blue field entoptic phenomenon*: It is the ability to perceive white dots when retina is illuminated diffusely by blue light. These white dots correspond to white blood cells in perifoveal capillaries. This grossly depicts intact macular function.
- *Interferometers*: If macula is functioning, sine wave gratings are seen when laser light is projected from two sources on retina due to interference.
- *Potential acuity meter*: Here, a letter chart similar to Snellen's VA chart is projected on the retina through the pupil and subject is asked to read it.[2]

Photostress Test

The patient's visual acuity is recorded on Snellen's chart after occluding other eye followed by exposure of macula to bright light of an ophthalmoscope for 10 seconds. The patient is asked to read the line just above the line of best acuity before light exposure, and recovery time is recorded. The normal recovery time is 45–60 seconds. Recovery time is prolonged in macular diseases.[5]

Factors Affecting Visual Acuity

Physical, physiological, and psychological factors usually affect VA.[9,10] Physical factors include illumination and contrast. Physiological conditions comprise pupil size, accommodation, light-dark adaptation, and age.

Illumination

Increased illumination increases VA from threshold to a point at which no further improvement can be elicited. In a clinical situation, this is 5–20 foot-candles. Beyond a certain point, illumination can create glare. Therefore, VA is recorded under photopic condition, and central vision is evaluated.

Contrast Sensitivity

In routine practice, vision is recorded with Snellen chart in high contrast. When contrast is reduced, more illumination is required to resolve an object. Contrast sensitivity is reduced even when Snellen acuity is normal. Contrast sensitivity tests are more accurate in quantifying vision, especially in diseased states such as cataract, corneal edema, disorders of retina, and central nervous system. Contrast sensitivity is assessed by using contrast sensitivity chart **(Fig. 7)**. It is measured in units of cycles per degree (cpd). It can be measured by using Pelli-Robson contrast test chart or VISITECH chart.

Pupil Size

The pupil size has a great influence on VA. Visual acuity decreases if pupils are smaller than 1 mm due to diffraction

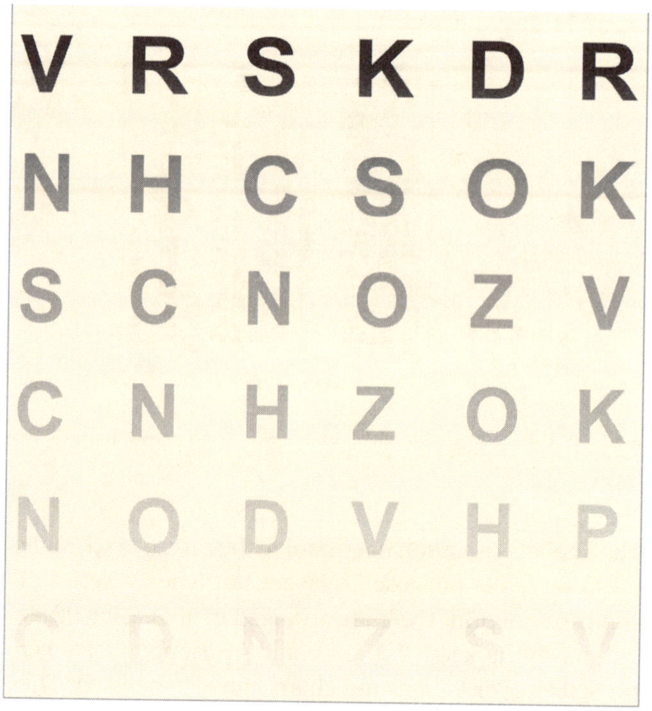

Fig. 7: Contrast sensitivity chart.

and reduced retinal illumination. Pupil diameter larger than 6 mm increases the spherical aberration and scattering of light, thereby reducing VA. Variation in pupil size changes acuity by altering illumination, depth of focus, and modifying the diameter of circle of blur on the retina.

Retinal Eccentricity

Visual acuity is maximum at the center of fovea. About 60% reduction in VA occurs just at 1° away from the center.[10] The reduction in VA is due to further separation of cones as the distance from the fovea increases.

Refractive Errors

Uncorrected refractive error affects the VA maximally and is a common cause of poor VA. A young hypermetropic patient can compensate the small error by accommodation. However, high refractive errors, especially hypermetropia and astigmatism, are known to cause amblyopia if not corrected.

Accommodation

Accommodation creates miosis which accounts for small hyperopic prescriptions being rejected for distance viewing in young individuals. Spasm of accommodation induces myopia and decreases VA.

Age

Normal VA depends on the integrity of the eye and visual pathway. It is seen that after the age of 40 years about 50% of eyes show aging changes and deterioration in vision.

Mental Status

The assessment of VA will not be correct if patient is feeling sleepy, intoxicated, or having a disease that can alter the patient's consciousness or his mental status.

Visual Acuity Assessment in Infants and Children

Visual acuity measurement should be performed at the earliest possible age that is practical (usually at approximately 3 years of age). Early detection and prompt treatment of ocular disorders in children are important to avoid permanent visual impairment. All infants who are premature or have family history of congenital cataract, metabolic or genetic diseases must be screened as early as possible. Children usually do not complain of visual deficit, therefore, first VA testing must be done in all children at the age of 3 years.

Accurate testing of VA is difficult in infants; sophisticated tests are used for recording the vision. Assessment of the VA (vision screening) represents one of the most sensitive techniques for the detection of eye abnormalities in children. The American Academy of Pediatrics Section on Ophthalmology,[11] in cooperation with the American Association for Pediatric Ophthalmology and Strabismus and the American Academy of Ophthalmology, has developed some guidelines to be followed by ophthalmologists and opticians for the assessment of VA in children.

Procedure for Testing Visual Acuity in Children

It is often helpful and convenient to explain the examination procedure to the parent of the child. The child should comfortably sit on the parent's lap. The cooperation of child can be enhanced by explaining and demonstrating the anticipated testing procedure. Before the measurement of VA, it is essential to examine both the eyes to exclude ocular structural abnormalities, such as cataract, corneal opacities, and ptosis, which are known to result in poor vision.

Vision in each eye should be tested separately; however, most children dislike occlusion of the one eye. Occlusion must be perfect and it should not allow peeking. Occluding patches are commercially available. They provide complete occlusion.

Visual Acuity Measurement at 0–3 Years of Age

Before the assessment of vision, it must be ensured that the child is awake and alert. Vision in children younger than 3 years is assessed by evaluating the child's ability to fix and follow objects.[12,13] Initially, it should be determined binocularly that both eyes fixate on an object, maintain fixation, and follow the object in all directions of gaze. Then it should be tested monocularly. If the eyes fail to perform these maneuvers, a significant bilateral eye or brain abnormality is suspected.[14-16] Aversion for uniocular occlusion suggests decreased VA in the unoccluded eye. Other signs of decreased VA are squint, nystagmus, and occulodigital sign, i.e. frequent rubbing of the diseased eye by child. Besides ocular motility, following procedures can roughly assess the vision in infants and preschool children:

- Optokinetic nystagmus
- Electroretinogram (ERG)
- Visual evoked potential
- Preferential looking test
- Flook's symbols or other picture matching charts
- Bruckner test.

Optokinetic Nystagmus Test

A rotating pediatric optokinetic nystagmus (OKN) drum with eight alternating black and white stripes is

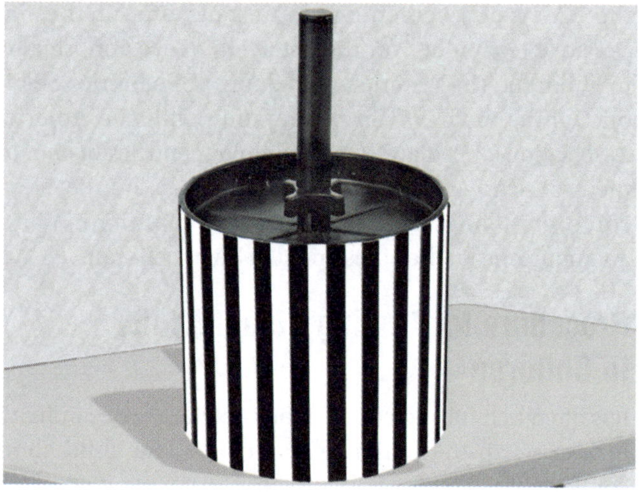

Fig. 8: Optokinetic nystagmus drum.

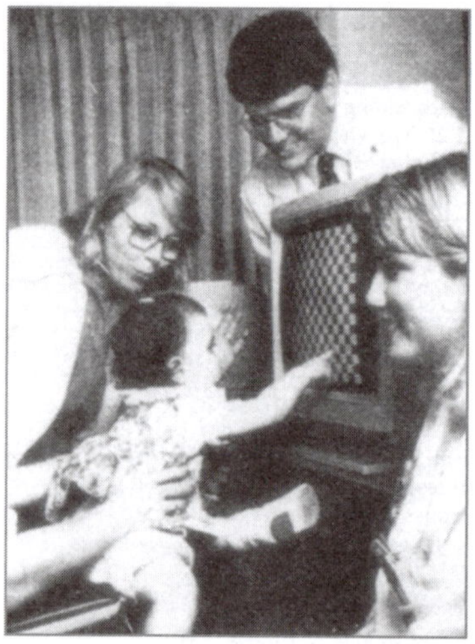

Fig. 9: Visual evoked potential testing.
Courtesy: Dr E Vaithalingam

used **(Fig. 8)**. Involuntary pursuit response to the stripes is observed. A positive nystagmus response indicates that the infant has at least counting fingers vision between 3 ft and 5 ft.

Similarly, horizontal eye movement can be stimulated by Catford drum where black dots of varying sizes oscillate against a white background and VA is graded accordingly ranging from 6/6 to 2/60. The test is performed from a distance of 60 cm.

The STYCAR (Screening Test for Young Children and Retards) rolling ball and Worth's ivory ball tests are done by rolling the balls across a well-illuminated contrasting floor at a distance of 3 m and pursuit eye movements of the child are observed.[2]

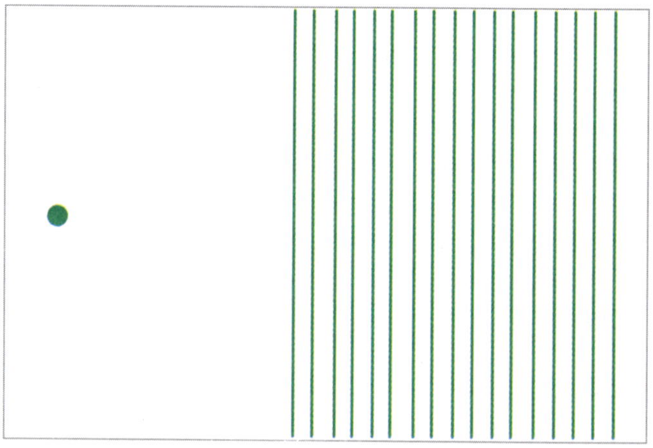

Fig. 10: Preferential looking test.

Electroretinogram

The electroretinogram (ERG) consists of three waves—an initial a-wave, large positive b-wave, and a mild deflected c-wave. Both cone (photopic) and rod (scotopic) responses are obtained. The b-wave response arises from the bipolar cells of retina and it is usually about 150 mV. In degenerative conditions of the retina-like retinitis pigmentosa and cone dystrophy, it is often subnormal or extinguished. Focal ERG provides information about macular function.

Visual Evoked Potential

The visual evoked potential (VEP) can be used to test the VA in infants **(Fig. 9)** and children especially in whom other vision tests, like the preferential looking test, are giving ambiguous and unreliable information. It measures the acuity by assessing the response of the brain to alternating black and white stripes or checkerboard patterns. The three metal electrodes on the head are placed and connected to a computer. The child is then positioned in front of a TV screen displaying alternating black and white checkerboard patterns. As the child views the stripes, a signal is relayed from the eyes to the brain (the visual cortex). This signal is detected by the electrodes. The vision of each eye is tested separately in VEP.

Preferential Looking Test

The preferential looking test (PLT) is used to test the VA in infants and young children who are unable to identify pictures or letters. The child is presented two types of fields, one with stripes and the other homogeneous **(Fig. 10)**. Both fields have same luminance. The location of the stripes is randomly alternated. Generally, infants and children prefer to look at more interesting stripes rather than looking at the blank field. The smallest stripe width that the child has preferred to see is considered to be his resolution threshold or visual acuity.

The visual development in a new born, when measured by PLT, is 20/600 at birth and 20/120 by 3 months. A modest improvement of 20/60 occurs by 12 months. VA becomes 6/6 by the age of 3–5 years. Modified version of PLT is Teller acuity test **(Fig. 11)** which employs the use of high contrast

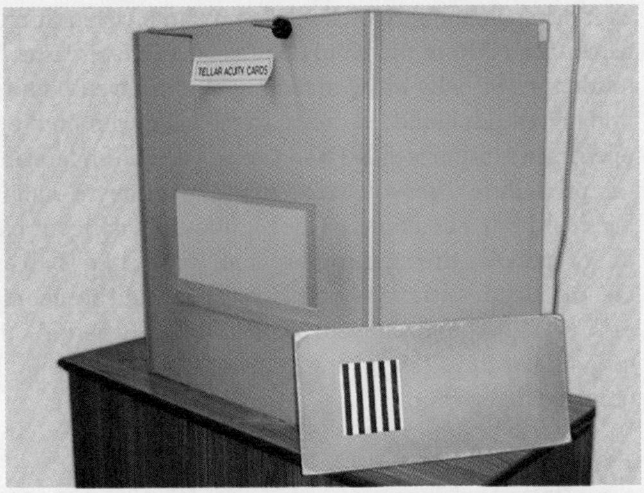

Fig. 11: Teller acuity chart.

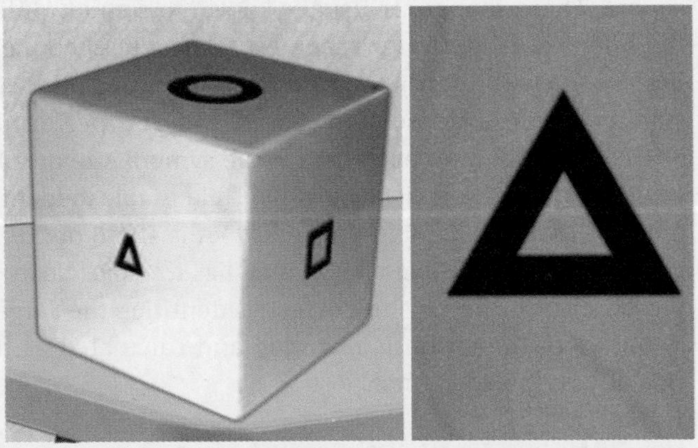

Fig. 12: Flook's symbols.

cards with black and white square wave gratings and cards with uniform gray field. Cardiff acuity is another test which is based on the principles of preferential looking and fading optotypes. Both these tests are designed for children younger than 3 years.

Studies on visual function maturity in young children are done on both VEP and PLT. The VA derived from both methods has slight differences. It was found that VEP is more useful for children <2 years of age and for age >2 years, PLT and VEP are equally good, however, VEP values correspond more closely to Snellen's acuity.[5]

Flook's Symbols

The Flook's test uses simple symbols such as squares, circles, and triangles **(Fig. 12)**. The child is shown a figure of circle or triangle from a distance of 3 m and asked to match it from the figures kept in front of him.

Matching toy test and other familiar picture tests are useful in assessing VA in children who are 2–3 years old. These tests include Kay picture test and Allen preschool test. STYCAR letter test uses five letters (H, O, T, V, X) which are first recognized by a growing child. Sheridan-Gardiner test uses seven letters (H, O, T, V, X, A, U) for matching.[2]

Bruckner Test

In 1962, Bruckner described "transillumination" test to assess small angle deviations and amblyopia in young uncooperative children. It is also helpful in diagnosing any opacities in refractive ocular media. The test is performed in a dark-room.

The light from direct ophthalmoscope is focused on each pupil individually approximately 12–18 inches away from the eye, and then both eyes are viewed simultaneously from a distance of about 3 ft (1 m). Corneal reflex position (Hirschberg test) and brightness difference in fundus glow from both eyes are recorded. Generally, a bright red reflex is seen in each eye.[17] In presence of squint the reflex is brighter in the deviated eye. The presence of black spots in the red reflex, or a white reflex is also indicative of ocular pathology. Photo screening examination[18,19] of pupils (size, shape, and reactions of both pupils), and binocular red reflex provide a wealth of information. The parents should be informed about the disability of the child who fails in vision screening test and recommended to consult a pediatric ophthalmologist trained in treating the condition.

Visual Acuity Measurement in Children Older than 3 Years of Age

Pictures instead of letters as optotype based on Snellen's principle are better in recording the VA in slightly older children.[5] Picture tests, like Lea symbols and Allen cards, are used for children between 2 years and 4 years of age. Wall charts, such as Snellen letters, Snellen numbers, the tumbling E test, and the HOTV test (a letter-matching test involving these four letters), can be used to measure VA in children older than 4 years.[16] The child should be seated at a distance of 3 m or 10 ft for most of these tests except for the Allen card test which is done at a farther distance.

Snellen Acuity Chart

While testing the child's right eye, occlude the left. If the child uses corrective eye glasses, the vision should be tested with them. Ask the child to read the chart. If he fails to recognize, then move him toward the chart to enable him to correctly identify at least two symbols. The child must correctly identify at least four of the six symbols in a line. Repeat the procedure covering the right eye.

Tumbling E

The tumbling E **(Fig. 13)** is used for children who do not cooperate in vision testing by letters and numbers. Ask the child to indicate the direction of tumbling E.

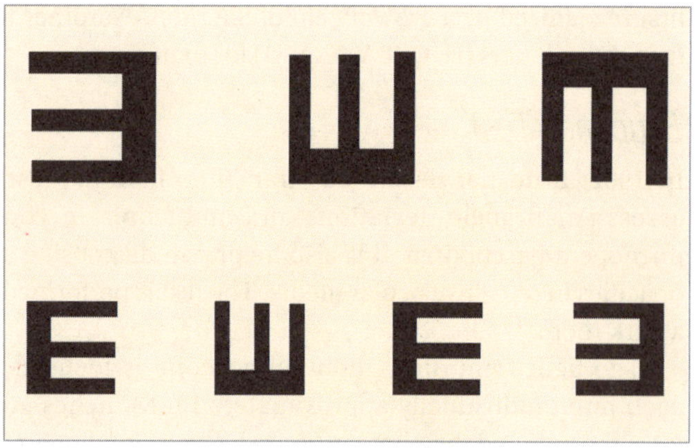

Fig. 13: Tumbling E chart.

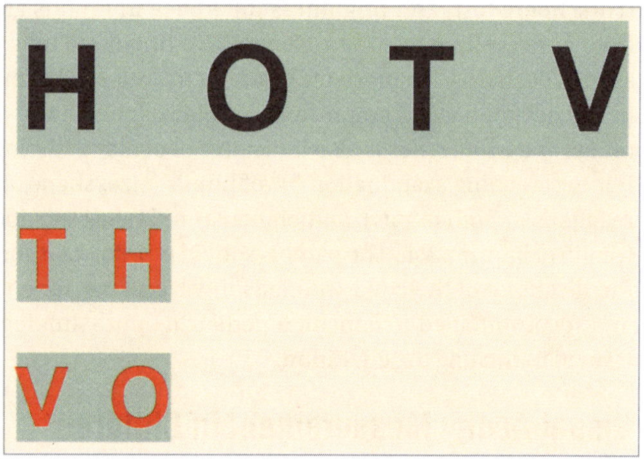

Fig. 14: HOTV test.

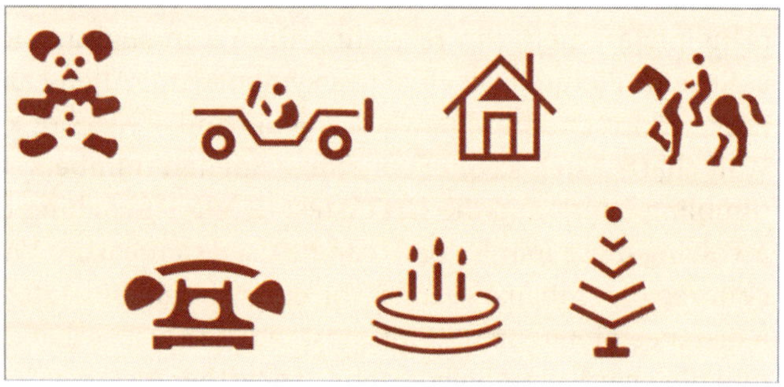

Fig. 15: Allen cards.

HOTV Test

HOTV test is an excellent test for 3–5 years old children who could not recognize alphabets. The test comprises a wall chart composed only of Hs, Os, Ts, and Vs **(Fig. 14)**. The child is provided a board on which the alphabets H, O, T, and V are written with bold letters. The examiner points to a letter on the wall chart, and asks the child to match the correct letter on the board.

Allen Cards

The Allen card test consists of four flash cards containing seven figures—a truck, a house, a birthday cake, a bear, a telephone, a horse, and a tree **(Fig. 15)**. When viewed at 20 ft distance, these figures represent 20/30 vision. It must be confirmed from the child before testing that he is going to identify verbally or by matching all the seven pictures. Initially, cards should be shown to the child with both eyes open from a distance of 2–3 ft and ensure that he understands the procedure. Present 1 or 2 figures and begin walking backward 2–3 ft at a time, as long as the child correctly calls out or matches the figures presented. If the child is able to identify pictures accurately at 15 ft, the VA would be recorded as 15/30. This is equivalent to 20/40 or 10/20. To perform this test, similar to HOTV testing, a matching panel should be provided to the child.

LH Symbols

The LH symbols are made up of flash cards. The flash cards of this picture test contain a house, an apple, a circle, and a square. These shapes are usually known to a child. Unlike the Allen cards, the LH symbol test (or Lea test) contains flash cards with more than one figure per card and with smaller figure sizes so that testing may be performed at 10 ft. Recorded on each card is the symbol size and VA value for 10 ft testing distance. If the child is able to identify the 10/15 symbol at 10 ft, the child's VA is 10/15 or 20/30. If testing is not possible at 10 ft, one has to move closer to the child until he or she correctly identifies the largest symbol, but the vision is recorded and calculated as the smallest symbol identified.

Near Vision in Children

Visually directed reaching is attained in infants between 3 and 5 months of age. Picking up of small pebbles or jemmies by 15 months or older child suggests VA of 6/24 or better. This rules out any significant visual deficit, though this can also be falsely due to high myopia.[2] Near VA in children can also be tested with the Allen picture cards or Lighthouse picture cards.

SUMMARY

Human vision is a multi-dimensional term with VA as the most important dimension which can be affected by various factors. Assessment of VA is the first and essential step in the examination of eye. Measurement of VA in infants and children needs a lot of time and patience. A little care in ensuring the proper environment for testing can significantly improve the accuracy. Snellen's charts are used universally for adults, but logMAR charts are considered better as there is linear progression in sizes and gaps between the optotypes.

Vision disorders have an impact on the quality of life of patients of all age groups. Reading charts or other near vision testing charts should be used as part of the routine assessment of the VA. Insufficient illumination, aging bulbs, soiled vision charts, small pupils, and nonstandardized charts should be avoided as they may lead to errors in the assessment of visual acuity.

REFERENCES

1. Sloan LL. Measurement of visual acuity: a critical review. AMA Arch Ophthalmol. 1951;45(6):704-25.
2. Elkington AR, Frank HJ, Greaney MJ. Clinical Optics, 3rd edition. Chapter 1. Great Britain: Wiley-Blackwell; 1999. pp. 12-6.
3. Hart WM. Adlers Physiology of the eye, 9th edition. Chapter 17. India: Harcourt Brace & Company Asia PTE; 1998. p. 535.
4. Sihota R, Tandon R. Parsons Diseases of the Eye, 21st edition. Chapter 18. New Delhi: Elsevier; 2011. p. 270.
5. Sihota R, Tandon R. Parsons Diseases of the Eye, 21st edition. Chapter 10. New Delhi: Elsevier; 2011. pp. 100-2.
6. Cambell FW, Green DG. Optical and retinal factors affecting visual resolution. J Physiol. 1965;181(3):576-93.
7. Fendick M, Westheimer G. Effects of practice and the separation of test targets on foveal and peripheral stereoacuity. Vision Res. 1983;23(2):145-50.
8. Cooper J, Feldman J, Medlin D. Comparing stereoscopic performance of children using the Titmus, TNO, and Randot stereo tests. J Am Optom Assoc. 1979;50(7):821-5.
9. Westheimer G. Visual acuity. In: Moses RA, Hart WM (Eds). Adlers Physiology of the Eye, 8th edition. St. Louis: Mosby; 1987. pp. 415-28.
10. Weymouth FW, Hines DC, Acres LH, et al. Visual acuity within the area centralis and its relation to eye movements and fixation. Am J Ophthalmol. 1928;11(12):947-60.
11. American Academy of Pediatrics. Section on Ophthalmology. Proposed Vision Screening Guidelines. AAP News. 1995; 11:25.
12. Recommendations for Preventive Pediatric Health Care. Committee on Practice and Ambulatory Medicine. Pediatrics. 1995;96(2 Pt 1):373-4.
13. Wasserman RC, Croft CA, Brotherton SE. Preschool vision screening in pediatric practice: A study from the Pediatric Research in Office Settings (PROS) Network. American Academy of Pediatrics. Pediatrics. 1992;89(5 Pt 1): 834-8.
14. Simons K. Preschool vision screening: rationale, methodology and outcome. Surv Ophthalmol. 1996;41(1):3-30.
15. American Academy of Ophthalmology. Amblyopia: Preferred Practice Pattern. San Francisco, CA: American Academy of Ophthalmology; 1997.
16. Hartmann EE, Dobson V, Hainline L, et al. Preschool vision screening: Summary of a task force report. Behalf of the Maternal and Child Health Bureau and the National Eye Institute Task Force on Vision Screening in the Preschool Child. Pediatrics. 2000;106(5):1105-16.
17. Tongue AC, Cibis GW. Brückner test. Ophthalmology. 1981;88(10):1041-4.
18. Ottar WI, Scott WE, Holgado SI. Photoscreening for amblyogenic factors. J Pediatr Ophthalmol Strabismus. 1995; 32(5):289-95.
19. Committee on Practice and Ambulatory Medicine and Section on Ophthalmology; American Academy of Pediatrics, Use of photoscreening for childrens vision screening. Pediatrics. 2002;109(3):524-5.

CHAPTER

2

Color Vision and Color Blindness

Harinder Singh Sethi, Mayuresh Naik

INTRODUCTION

Color vision examination is an essential part of screening before a person is taken up for a job. A person who has color vision defect may go through life quite unconscious of his color deficiency and without making any incriminating mistakes, differentiating objects by their size, shape, and luminosity, using all the time a complete color vocabulary based on his experience that teaches him that color terms are applied with great consistency to certain objects and to certain achromatic shades, until circumstances are arranged to eliminate these accessory aids and then he realizes that his sensations differ in some way from the normal. Various tests have been developed to enable screening of anomalous subjects with color deficiency from a much larger group of normal subjects.

COLOR VISION

Color is a sensation and not a physical attribute of an object. Color is what we see and is result of stimulation of retina by radiant energy in a small band of wavelengths of the electromagnetic spectrum usually considered to span about one octave, from 380 nm to 760 nm. There are three main characteristics of color, namely hue, saturation, and brightness. Hue is a function of wavelength. It depends on what the eye and brain perceive to be the predominant wavelength of the incoming light. An object's "hue" is its "color". Saturation refers to the richness of a hue as compared to a gray of the same brightness. Saturation is also known as "chroma". Brightness correlates to the ease with which a color is seen, other factors being equal. Brightness is characterized by an object's being dim or bright, dark or light.

The spectral wavelengths of different colors are as follows—violet 430 nm; blue 460 nm; green 520 nm; yellow 575 nm; orange 600 nm; and red 650 nm. The concept of white light is vague; most agreeable definition is, white surface is one which has spectral reflection factors independent of wavelength (in the visible spectrum) and greater than 70%.

FACTORS AFFECTING COLOR VISION

Crystalline Lens

The lens absorbs shorter wavelengths; in young, wavelengths of less than 400 nm and in old people up to 550 nm or 600 nm are absorbed by the lens resulting in defective color vision on shorter wavelength side.

Retinal Distribution of Color Vision

The center of the fovea (1/8°) is blue blind. Trichromatic vision extends 20°–30° from the point of fixation. Peripheral to this red-green becomes indistinguishable up to 70°–80° and in far peripheral retina all color sense is lost although cones are still found in this region. In the central 5°, macula contains carotenoid pigment, xanthophyll. The molecules of the pigment are arranged in such a way that they absorb blue light polarized in the radial direction. If one looks at a white card through linear polarizer, one will see two blue sectors separated by two yellow sectors; the figure is called Haidinger's brushes. Macular pigment may also be seen as in homogeneity in the field of blue or white light called Maxwell's spot.

Wavelength Discrimination

The normal observer is able to detect a difference between two spectral lights that differ by as little as 1 nm in wavelength in the regions of 490 nm and 585 nm. In the region of violet and red a difference of greater than 4 nm is necessary.

Hue, Saturation and Lightness

Hue is the extent to which the object is red, green, blue, or yellow. Saturation is the extent to which a color is strong or weak. Lightness is self-explanatory attribute, e.g. yellow by color is light.

ILLUMINATION

Illumination affects color vision of low illuminances; the errors increase due to poorer discrimination for most of the hue range while testing color vision. An illuminance of 400 lux (±100 lux) would be practical value for most clinical applications.

Bezold-Burcke Effect

von Bezold (1873) and Burcke (1878) discovered independently the phenomenon named after them, that variation of the luminance levels modifies hues.

Color Constancy: Aperture Colors and Surface Colors

Color constancy is a phenomenon in which color of the objects can be recognized unchanged in spite of possible differences in the illumination. Aperture colors are the colors that alter due to change in illumination. Surface colors do not vary with illumination. Extrafoveal vision favors the appearance of aperture colors and foveal vision that of surface colors.

Complementary Wavelengths

Complementary wavelengths are those which, when mixed in appropriate proportions, give white.

Simultaneous Color Contrast

Color contrast is visually demonstrated by observing the color of a spot in a surround. The general rule is that the color of the spot tends toward the complementary of the color of the surround.

Successive Color Contrast

Successive color contrast is more commonly described as colored after images, when one stares at a red spot for several seconds and then looks at a gray card. One sees a green spot on the card. The afterimage tends toward the complementary of the primary image (*Stiles-Crawford effect*). The light entering near the edge of the pupil is less effective than light entering at the center of the pupil because of the shape of the receptors and the fact that they are embedded in a medium of different refractive index. This effect is wavelength-dependent.

Color Triangle

Color triangle can be drawn to describe the trichromacy of color mixtures and is useful for deciding, which bands of wavelength are indistinguishable from each other. Three reference wavelengths are chosen, i.e. 450 nm, 520 nm, and 650 nm, and are placed at vertices of X, Y, and Z of a triangle; the position of other wavelengths is determined. A color triangle does not describe the color of a band of wavelengths unless other circumstances are defined.

THEORIES OF COLOR VISION

This is a complex topic as no theory explains the phenomenon of color vision fully. Few important theories are given here.

Young–Helmholtz Theory (Trichromatic Theory)

Young's concept is that there are three types of retinal receptors with different spectral sensitivities. Young's principal colors are red, green, and violet. Young's hypothesis was not followed up until it was revived by Helmholtz in 1852. The Young's theory may be summarized as follows:

- At some stage of visual receptor mechanism there are three different types of sensory apparatus—G1, G2, and G3. These receptors must be same for everyone but they may not be same at the fovea as at the periphery.
- Each of these receptors is characterized from the spectral point of view by particular function of wavelengths which may be denoted by G and the response G1 of a receptor for radiation with a spectral energy distribution $E\lambda$ may be supposed to have the form:

$$G1 = Sgi\ E\lambda\ d\lambda.$$

- Sensation of color is a function of the relative values of the three responses G1.
- Sensation of light is a function of a linear combination of the three responses.

Fundamental Sensations

By determining approximately the coordinate of the confusion points of dichromats Arthur Konig in 1893 established a system of fundamental sensations and identified red, green, and violet as fundamental colors. Blue was also identified as fundamental color in addition to red and green by Gothelin.

Granit's Theory of Color Vision

Granit divides retina into receptor units, each unit comprising groups of cones and rods, which are connected with a single ganglion cell or several ganglion cells, which synchronize their discharges. These units are classified as "dominators" or "modulators". The dominators, which are numerous, have a spectral sensitivity curve, which indicates that they are responsible for the sensations of luminosity. Modulators show a selective sensitivity, which makes them responsible for color discrimination. Granit's theory does not explain the fact of trichromatism.

Herring's Theory of Color Vision (Opponent Color Theory)

Herring assumed six distinct sensations arranged in three opposing pairs—white-black, yellow-blue, and red-green; he explains three pairs as being due to opposing actions of light on three substance of the retina, a catabolism producing warm sensation (white, yellow, and red) and an anabolism the cold ones. This theory is clearly a psychological concept and aims at explaining complex percepts than the intermediate effect of the stimuli.

ANATOMY OF COLOR VISION

The understanding of visual pathway is complex and not evident fully. There are two types of photoreceptors in the retina: rods and cones. Approximately, 120 million rods are responsible for night and peripheral vision. Rods contain a photopigment called rhodopsin, a chemical variant of vitamin A and a protein called *opsin* that serves at very low levels of illumination. Rods have their maximum density about 5° from the fovea and cannot distinguish one color from another. The fovea itself is essentially rod-free containing only cones. Approximately, 7 million cones are responsible for central and color vision. Cones have their maximum density within 2° of the center of the fovea. Both types of receptors diminish in number toward the retinal periphery.

Cones

In the retina, three types of cones responsible for the red, green, and blue sensations have been isolated. Three types of cone pigments in the human retina absorb photons with wavelengths between 400 nm and 700 nm. Color vision is mediated by these three cone photoreceptors referred to as long, middle, and short wavelength-sensitive (LWS, MWS, SWS) cones. The long wavelength-sensitive (LWS) cones (sometimes called "red" or "red-catching") contain a pigment called *erythrolabe*, which is best stimulated by a wavelength near 566 nm. Medium wavelength-sensitive (MWS) cones ("green" or "green-catching") contain the pigment chlorolabe, which has a maximal sensitivity to a wavelength near 543 nm. Short wavelength-sensitive (SWS) cones ("blue" or "blue-catching") contain cyanolabe, which have maximal sensitivity at 445 nm. The blue cones are absent in the center of the macula. Trichromatic vision perception occurs in central 30° field. It is not uncommon to hear the cones referred to as blue, green, and red cones, but such nomenclature is misleading because the LWS cones are more sensitive to blue lights than they are to red lights. The spectral sensitivities of the three cone pigments overlap somewhat. For example, light of 540 nm and 590 nm stimulate both green (MWS) and red (LWS) receptors yet we can easily distinguish between these two wavelengths as "green" and "yellow". If the human retina contains all three cone pigments in normal concentrations, and has normal retinal function, the subject is a trichromat. Any color the trichromat sees can be matched with a suitable mixture of red, green, and blue light.

Color-coded Cells

Two types of color-coded cells are found at peripheral levels (ganglion cells and lateral geniculate body) of the visual system and they have been named opponent color cells and double opponent color cells. More complex types are found at more central levels (striate cortex).

Opponent Color Cells

An opponent color cell is one that gives only polarity of response for some wavelengths and opposite polarity of response for other wavelengths. Opponent color cells are concerned with successive color contrast.

Double Opponent Color Cells

These are cells opponent for both color and space. The response may be onto red light, off to green light in the center of the receptive field and off to red light, onto green light in the periphery of the receptive field. Double opponent cells are concerned with simultaneous color contrast.

Simple, Complex, and Hypercomplex Cells

In rhesus monkey striate cortex, a variety of cells is specific for both color and orientation. They have been categorized as color-sensitive simple, complex, and hypercomplex cells. Simple cells have a bar-flank double opponent arrangement to their receptive fields. Complex color coded cells respond to color boundaries of the appropriate orientation and the response is independent of the part of the receptive field being stimulated. The edge of hypercomplex cells must be short.

Opponent color cells are found among ganglion cells of the retina and lateral geniculate body. Double opponent cells with center-surround or flank receptive fields are present in the input layer IV of the striate cortex. Complex and hypercomplex color coded cells are also found in the striate cortex in layers II, III, V and VI. Vaetichin in 1953 recorded a negative slow potential from fish retinae called "S-potential" of two types—L-type (luminosity type) and C-type (chromaticity type). Mitarai in 1961 regarded horizontal cells as responsible for S-potentials of L-type and Muller's fibers for those of C-type. The properties of S-potentials support the Herrings opponent color theory more than the trichromatic theory of Young.

ANOMALIES OF COLOR VISION

Deficiency of color vision was first described by Dalton in 1794, the founder of the atomic theory, who himself was color blind; hence, the term *Daltonism* was coined. The color deficiency is of two types:

1. Congenital, and
2. Acquired.

In clinical evaluation of color vision, it is important to distinguish between acquired and congenital defects.

Congenital versus Acquired Color Deficiencies

Congenital color vision deficiencies can be distinguished functionally from acquired deficiencies in a number of ways. Congenital deficiencies typically involve red-green confusions, whereas acquired deficiencies, more often than not, are a blue-yellow (*Köllner's rule*). Also, because some of the most common congenital defects are linked to the X-chromosome, they are more prevalent in males than females. Acquired defects, in contrast, are not related to gender except by gender differences to trauma or toxic exposure. Acquired color deficiencies are more likely to be asymmetric between the two eyes than are hereditary defects; they are also less likely to be stable with time. Congenital defects are usually easier to detect with standard clinical color vision tests, but some acquired ones can be more subtle and thus are difficult to diagnose. Finally, those with acquired color deficiencies are also more likely to display color-naming errors because, unlike those with congenital deficiencies, they lack the lifelong experience with defective color perception (CP).

Congenital Color Vision Deficiency

The color vision anomalies commonly being X-linked are relatively common (8%) in men and rare in women **(Fig. 1)**. Nearly all congenital color defects are due to absence or alteration of one of the pigments in photoreceptors. Congenital color deficits may be divided into classes according to whether the patients are red deficient (protans), green deficient (deuterans) or blue deficient (tritans). The term *anopia* is used for absolute deficiency and *anomaly* for relative deficiency **(Tables 1 and 2)**.

Anomalous trichromats are people who generally require three wavelengths to match another wavelength but do not accept the color matches made by normal people. Lord Rayleigh in 1881 discovered trichromacy. Anomalous trichromats have three classes of cones but one is abnormal. Protanomalous people lack the red receptors and instead they have two pigments both peaking in the range of the normal green. Similarly, the deuteranomalous people lack green receptors.

Dichromats require only two wavelengths to match another wavelength and will accept the color matches made by normal people. The dichromats have two classes of cone receptors with normal spectral sensitivity, the third class being absent. Measurements of their pigments can be made by reflection densitometer and cone processes isolated by colored backgrounds confirm the findings. Protanopes have normal green and blue cones, red cones being absent. Deuteranopes have normal red and blue cones and tritanopes normal red and green cones.

Protans color deficient subjects are easier to test and classify than deuterans and tritans because the red cone pigment is quite sensitive to green wavelengths and both red and green cone pigments are quite sensitive to blue wavelength covering the green and blue range, in deuterans and tritans, as the sensitivity of visual pigment does not fall off sharply on the short wavelength side of the peak.

Monochromatics can be blue cone monochromatics and rod monochromatics. Blue cone monochromatics have normal blue cone pigment but no red or green cone pigment. In rod monochromatism, only 500 nm pigment is present in the retina and all three cones pigments are absent.

Genetics of Congenital Color Deficiencies

The protans and deuterans are commonly sex-linked recessive. About 1% males are protanopes, 1% protanomalous, 1% deuteranopes, and 5% deuteranomalous. The incidence of color vision deficiency (CVD) (red-green) in females is 0.4%. The gene for tritans is autosomal

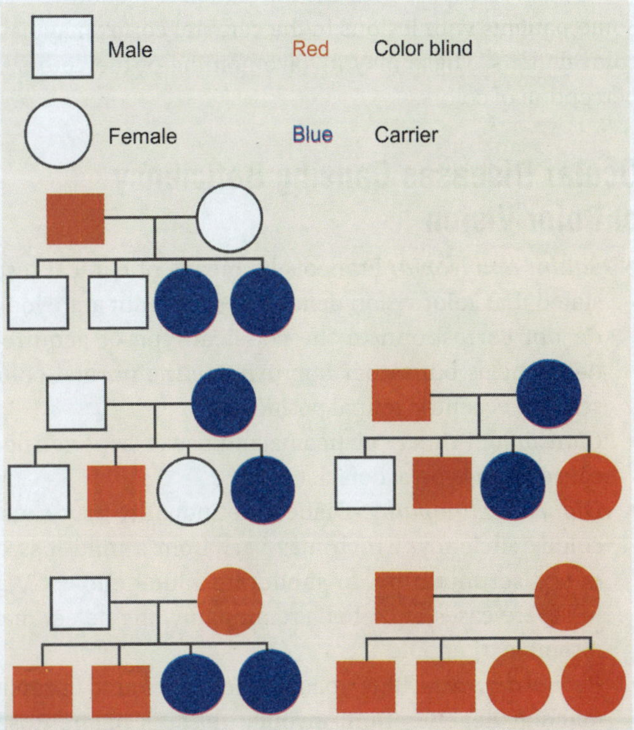

Fig. 1: Inheritance pattern of congenital color vision defects.

Table 1: Classification of color blindness.

Congenital: Males (8%), females (0.4%) classically X-linked recessive inheritance pattern, always bilateral

- *Achromatopsia*:
  - Cone monochromats
  - Rod monochromats
- *Dyschromatopsia dichromats*:
  - Deuteranopia
  - Protanopia
  - Tritanopia
- *Anomalous trichromats*:
  - Protanomaly
  - Deuteranomaly
  - Tritanomaly

Acquired:

Unilateral	Red-green defect Blue-yellow defect
Bilateral	Red-green defect Blue-yellow defect

Disease	**Acquired defect**
Glaucoma	Blue-yellow
Hypertensive retinopathy	Blue-yellow
Diabetic retinopathy	Blue-yellow
Age-related macular degeneration	Blue-yellow
Lesions of visual pathway	Red-green
Alcohol-nicotine	Red-green

Table 2: Various types of color deficiency.

	Red deficient	*Green deficient*	*Blue deficient*
Anomalous trichromats	Protanomaly	Deuteranomaly	Tritanomaly
Dichromats	Protanopia	Deuteranopia	Tritanopia
Monochromats	Rod monochromat	Blue monochromat	

Table 3: Drugs causing color deficiency.

Drugs	*Type of color deficiency*
Chloroquine, indomethacin, oral contraceptives, antihistaminics, estrogens, digitalis and butazolidin	Blue-yellow
Ethyl alcohol, ethambutol	Red-green
Tri- and bicyclic antidepressants	Mixed type

incompletely dominant. Rod monochromatism is very rare; occurs 1 in 30,000, autosomal recessive and thus an increased incidence is seen in consanguineous offsprings.

Acquired Deficiency of Color Vision

Koellner formulated that lesions in the outer layers of the retina give rise to a blue-yellow defect, while lesions in the inner layers of the retina and the optic nerve gives rise to red-green defect. However, the correlation is not always true. Some patients with lesions in the cerebral cortex may have color deficits. These may involve naming of the colors or perception of colors.

Ocular Diseases Causing Deficiency of Color Vision

- *Squint amblyopia:* Francois by means of clinical tests stated that color vision deficiencies in squint amblyopia do not correspond to the classical type of acquired deficiencies but rather approximate the normal color sense of eccentric retinal positions.
- *Glaucoma:* Primary glaucoma and ocular hypertension cause tritan-type of defect.
- *Diabetic retinopathy:* Diabetic retinopathy may cause color deficiency, which may vary from a mild loss of hue discrimination to moderate blue-yellow CVD. In severe cases of diabetic retinopathy, the defect may resemble tritanopia.
- *Retinal disorders:* Blue-yellow deficits are found in senile macular degeneration, myopia, retinitis pigmentosa, siderosis bulbi, and chorioretinitis.
- *Optic nerve disorders:* In one study, about 57% of patients with resolved optic neuritis were found to have color vision defects. Red-green defects have been found in cases of multiple sclerosis and optic atrophy. Tobacco amblyopia causes red-green defect.
- *Color vision after laser photocoagulation:* After argon-laser photocoagulation, there may be overall loss of hue discrimination and color deficiency, mostly of blue-yellow.

Drugs Causing Deficiency in Color Vision

Many drugs are known to cause deficiency of color vision. They can cause more than one type of color deficiency **(Table 3)**.

Systemic Disorders Causing Deficiency in Color Vision

Besides diabetes, a few systemic disorders are known to be associated with defective color vision. Following diseases may cause color deficiency:

- *Cardiovascular disease:* Patients with heart diseases have been found to have blue-yellow deficiency.
- *Turner's syndrome:* Red-green color deficiency was usually encountered in the syndrome.

COLOR VISION TESTING

The main objective for testing the color blindness is to determine the exact nature of the defect and whether the color deficiency is likely to be a source of danger to the community and/or to the individual, if given a particular job.

Types of Color Vision Tests

Color Confusion Tests

Pseudoisochromatic (PIC) plates are example of color confusion tests **(Figs. 2A to C)**. PIC tests are designed on the basis of the color confusions made by persons with color defects. In these, a symbol or figure in one color is placed on a background of another color so that the figure and background are isochromatic for the color-defective person. PIC tests are used primarily as screening tests to identify those with an inherited color defect, although some of the tests permit a diagnosis of type and severity. Because the inventory of PIC tests is extensive, only the more commonly used tests are described here.

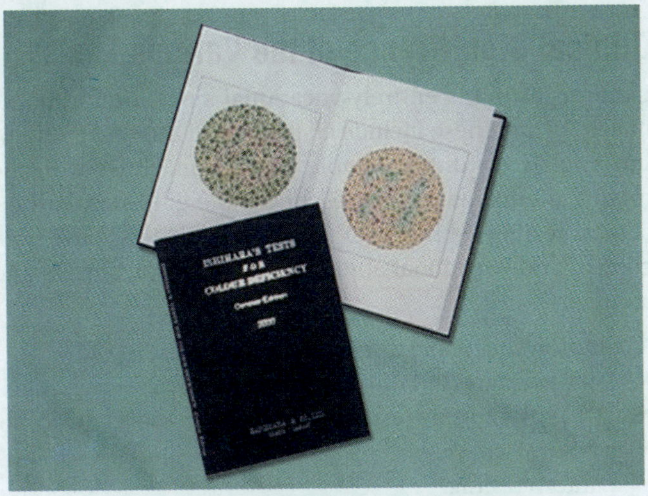

Fig. 2A: Ishihara pseudoisochromatic plates.

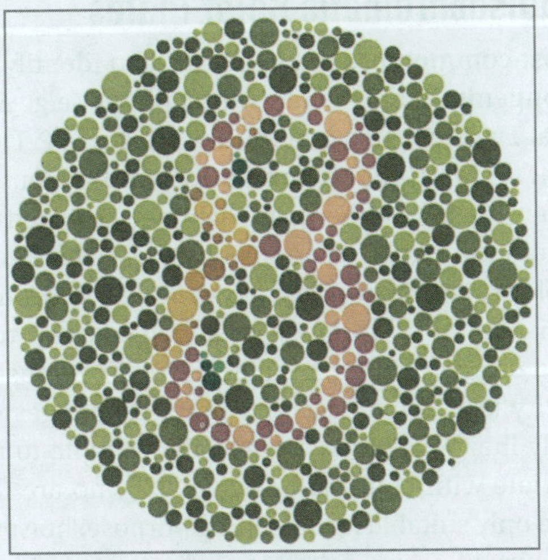

Fig. 2B: Transformation plate seen as "3" by patients with anomalous red-green color defect.

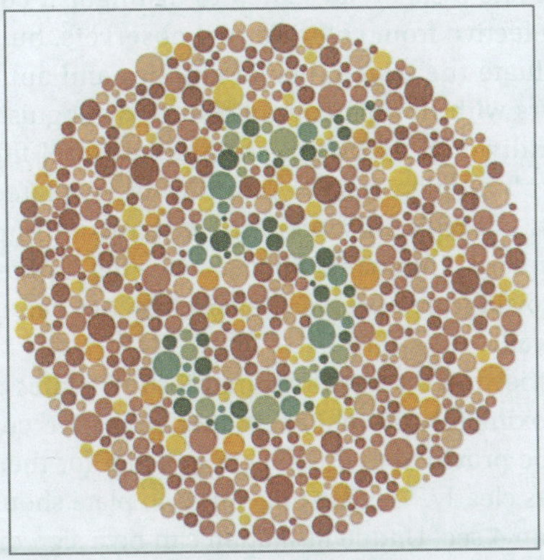

Fig. 2C: "Vanishing" or "disappearing" digit type.

The most widely used test, Ishihara PIC plates, is a screening test used to determine the presence of X-linked congenital (red/green) color deficiency. Most screening tests are designed to give a quick, accurate assessment of red/green deficiencies. The Ishihara test is not designed to detect tritan disorders or acquired color defects unless the optic neuropathy is severe.

Arrangement Tests

The arrangement tests require the observer to place colored samples in sequential order on the basis of hue, saturation, or lightness or to sort samples on the basis of similarity. One of the earliest tests of this nature that is still available but is rarely used today is the Holmgren Wool Test. In this matching test, 46 numerically coded comparison schemes of yarn are selected to match three test colors—yellow-green, pink, and dark red. The comparison schemes differ from the test schemes in being lighter or darker. The test is not accurate for screening or classification and is not recommended for clinical use. It is of historical significance as an early occupational test. The clinical arrangement tests that are in use today are colored papers mounted in black plastic caps. The caps are placed in order according to specific instructions, and the order is recorded as the sequence of numbers printed on the underside of the caps. Results are plotted on score forms for analysis and interpretation and quantitative scores computed. The tests are standardized for CIE standard illuminant C.

The Farnsworth-Munsell Dichotomous-15 (D-15) and the FM-100 test are examples of hue discrimination based on arrangement tests utilizing color chips mounted in a circular cap that subtend exactly 1.5° at a test distance of 50 cm. This ensures that the observations of the subject are made with the central rod-free retina. The D-15 contains 15 colored chips and the FM-100 contains 85 chips. The chips have identical brightness and saturation, and differ from one another Farnsworth-Munsell tests reveal the type of defect, but not the severity.

Color Matching Tests

The spectral anomaloscope and Pickford-Nicolson anomaloscope are used for color matching examinations. They can provide the examiner with information on the severity of a particular color vision defect. The Nagel anomaloscope is most widely used. It consists of a spectroscope in which two halves of a circular field are illuminated respectively by monochromatic yellow (589 nm) and a mixture of monochromatic red and green (670 nm and 546 nm, respectively). The observer is asked to match the two halves of the circle with the three primary colors available.

The most widely used color vision tests are the PIC plates and the D-15 panel due to their ease of use and relative low cost. The Nagel anomaloscope and FM-100 tests are usually only found in academic or research settings.

All color vision tests have specific requirements for lighting, viewing distance, and viewing time. It is important for the examiner to be familiar with the test requirements and score sheets before conducting a color vision test; otherwise the results may be inaccurate.

Lantern Tests

Lantern tests are used only for occupational purpose. Different types of lantern tests are in use in different countries. The Farnsworth Lantern (FALANT) is used in the United States by marine and aviation authorities; the Holmes Wright Type A is used in the United Kingdom by aviation authorities; and the Holmes Wright Type B is used in Australia, the United Kingdom and other Commonwealth countries by marine authorities. The Edridge-Green Lantern is included in the United States Coast Guard requirements, but it is surpassed by the FALANT. Electroretinography (ERG) and microspectrophotometry may be used in special circumstances.

Test Conditions

Lantern testing is performed after dark adaptation but all other tests require artificial daylight conditions. Light adaptation is critical for anomaloscopy and especially for 100 hue testing, but a color-neutral glare-free background and correct illumination are more important. Reliable results can be obtained with an artificial daylight source (such as a Macbeth Sol source) or fluorescent lighting with a color temperature between 5850° and 6850° Kelvin and good color rendering index (Ra over 90). If appropriate artificial light is not available then skylight is a good source. The illumination should be between 250 lux and 350 lux (approximately 1.5 m below twin fluorescent globe). A failed Ishihara test under incandescent lamp is a failure of the examiner to observe basic principles, not a failure of the subject. A pass on the other hand is still a pass and is statistically the more likely outcome.

The viewing geometry should be with the light 45° to the surface and the subject viewing the pages at 90° to the surface. Newly printed books sometimes have differential reflectance between pigments, so when tilted back and forth in the light by an anomalous observer they may provide luminance clues. Appropriate optical correction for the 65 cm viewing distance must be available if required. Experienced testers know that some people read the small identifying numbers on the bottom of each page and give a memorized response. Cheating can be prevented by covering these identifying numbers with a secret label.

Clinical Significance of the Various Tests

Lantern testing is entirely vocational since around 5% of males fail and these include all those with a severe anomaly but a relatively unpredictable group from those with the milder anomalies. Anomaloscopy is the gold standard for clinical testing, while the D-15 and FM-100 tests have both clinical and vocational applications (diamond sorters and croupiers).

A common vocational test battery should consist of:

- Ishihara plates 2–17 from the 38 plate series
- D-15 color sorting test (three or more crossover errors are a failure)
- Lantern testing.

Pseudoisochromatic Color Plates

The most common use of plate tests is to identify persons with congenital color defects. PIC plates (e.g. AO-HRR, Ishihara, Dvorine, Tokyo Medical College, SPP-1) provide efficient screening of congenital red-green defects (efficiency 90–95%). Other tests have been designed to detect achromatopsia (Sloan Achromatopsia test), to differentiate incomplete achromatopsia from complete achromatopsia (Berson blue cone monochromatism plates), to detect acquired defects (SPP-2), or to detect color confusion (City University test). Plate tests have the advantages of being relatively inexpensive, easily available, simple to use, and appropriate with children and persons who are illiterate. They are only suitable for screening purpose; however, they neither provide a quantitative evaluation of color vision nor distinguish the type and severity of the color vision defect. Plate tests are designed to distinguish congenital color-defective from color-normal observers, but they do not evaluate the wide range of abilities and aptitudes of observers with normal color vision to distinguish colors. Given individual differences in prereceptoral filters and normal photo pigment polymorphisms, no plate test can be 100% effective in screening. When used improperly (nonstandard illuminant, binocular viewing, colored lenses not removed from observer), their efficiency can diminish dramatically.

The viewing distance required for PIC plates is 75 cm or approximately 30 inches. Proper refractive correction should be provided to the patient in order for them to see the plates clearly. Viewing time for each plate should be no more than 4 sec. Undue hesitation can be a sign of a slight color deficiency.

Ishihara Pseudoisochromatic Plates (Confusion Charts)

The Ishihara color vision charts are developed by Shinobu Ishihara in 1917. This test is based on the principle of confusion of the pigment color in red-green color defectives **(Fig. 2B)**. There are three editions—A 16-plate series, 24-plate series, and a 38-plate series. The 10th edition of Ishihara has 38 plates. It is best to use the larger series because there are relatively few reliable plates in the smaller series. Both 24-set and 38-plate series set consist of two groups of plates—a group for those who are literate/numerate which starts from plate 1 at the front of the book and a group for illiterates/innumerate in which the colored pattern is a meandering path of connected dots between two X symbols. The second group is arranged so as to commence with the last page of the book and proceed in reverse order. The group of plates for innumerate are seldom used because they are not as easy or reliable to score, but they are based on the same colorimetric principles as the set for numerates. It is not necessary to use both types in the one subject. From a colorimetric perspective, there are four different types of test plate employed in both the 38- and 24-plate series preceded by a demonstration plate that is not for scoring. In the large series, plates 1 and 38 are both for demonstration only, while in the smaller series, plates 1 and 24 are for demonstration. If the subject fails viewing the demonstration plate, do not proceed with the test. The following description applies to the numerate plates in the 38-plate series. The different types of plates in the test are:

- *Transformation plates* **(Fig. 2B)**: Anomalous color observers give different responses to color normal observers. In these plates, one number is seen by a normal trichromat and another (different) number is seen by a color-deficient person. Those with true total color blindness cannot read any numeral. These are the plates numbered 2–9 inclusive.
- *Disappearing digit (vanishing) plates* **(Fig. 2C)**: The normal observer is meant to recognize the colored pattern. On these plates, a number can be seen by a normal trichromat but nothing can be seen by the color-deficient person. These are plates 10–17 inclusive in the 38-plate series.
- *Hidden digit plates:* The anomalous observer should see the pattern. The number on a hidden digit design cannot be seen by a normal trichromat but can be seen by most people with red/green deficiencies. Those people with total color blindness cannot see any numeral. These are plates 18–21 inclusive.
- *Qualitative plates:* These are intended to classify protan from deuteran and mild from severe anomalous CP. The plates are numbered 22–25.

Procedure of Testing

The plates are designed to be appreciated correctly in a room which is lit adequately by daylight. Introduction of direct sunlight or the use of electric light may produce some discrepancy in the results because of an alteration in the color values of the charts. It is suggested that when it is convenient only to use electric light, it should be adjusted as far as possible to resemble the effect of natural daylight. The plates are held 75 cm from the subject and tilted at right angles to the line of vision. A missed/misread plate must be reread (may be in a random order). The findings should be recorded on the Ishihara color vision test and interpretation marking chart **(Table 4)**.

A correct response to the Ishihara introductory plate is expected and demonstrates suitable visual acuity to perform the test and rules out malingering.

- Plates 1–25 have numerals and each answer should be given without more than 3 seconds of delay.

Table 4: The interpretation and marking of the Ishihara color vision test.

Number of plate	Normal person	Person with red-green deficiency				Person with total color blindness and weakness
1	12	12				12
2	8	3				x
3	6	5				x
4	29	70				x
5	57	35				x
6	5	2				x
7	3	5				x
8	15	17				x
9	74	21				x
10	2	x				x
11	6	x				x
12	97	x				x
13	45	x				x
14	5	x				x
15	7	x				x
16	16	x				x
17	73	x				x
18	x	5				x
19	x	2				x
20	x	45				x
21	x	73				x
		Protan		Deuteran		
		Strong	Mild	Strong	Mild	
22	26	6	(2)6	2	2(6)	
23	42	2	(4)2	4	4(2)	
24	35	5	(3)5	3	3(5)	
25	96	6	(9)6	9	9(6)	

- Plates 26–38 are tracings for use in illiterates, and windings lines between the two Xs are traced with a dry soft brush. Each tracing should take less than 10 seconds.

Each eye should be tested separately (as should be done for all color vision tests).

The recommendations of the test state that of the first 21 plates if 17 or more plates are read correctly by an individual his color sense should be regarded as normal. If 13 or less plates are correctly read then the person has a red-green color defect. It is rare to have persons who read 14–16 plates correctly.

Hardy, Rand, Rittler Plates

Hardy, Rand, Rittler (H-R-R) plates are another type of PIC plate test. This test is similar to the Ishihara test except that the H-R-R plates classify and quantify the type of color defect whether it is protan, deuteran, or tritan (blue/yellow). H-R-R plates have colored symbols/shapes rather than numbers. This makes H-R-R plates a good choice for children and illiterates. Since it is capable of detecting tritan disorders, this test is especially useful when an acquired color vision defect is suspected. Lighting, viewing distance, and viewing time are the same as when testing with Ishihara plates. The first four (non-numbered) plates of the H-R-R series are for demonstration only (similar to the Ishihara "12"). The first six (numbered) plates are screening plates. Color vision is deemed "normal" and no further testing needs to be done if the subject gives correct responses to the screening plates. If there is an incorrect response one or more of the screening plates, the examiner must follow the directions on the scoring sheet and show additional plates to the subject in order to specifically classify the color vision defect.

City University Color Vision Test (Fig. 3)

Fletcher developed the City University test. It consists of 10 black charts each of which has 5 color dots. One of the dots is located in the center being encircled with 4 other dots so that a subject has to match the central color dot with one of the 4 other dots.

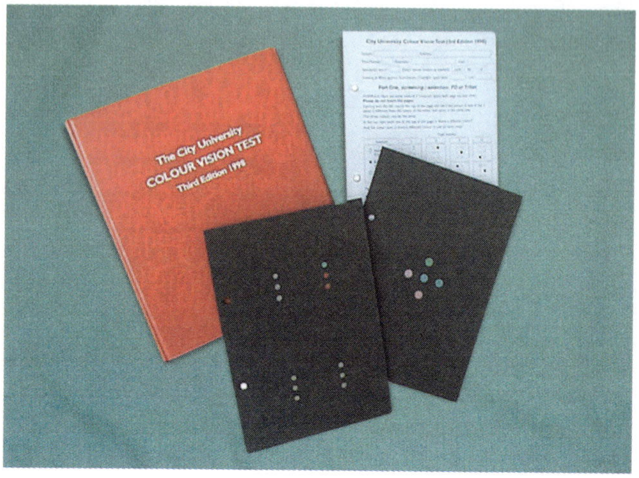

Fig. 3: City University test.

American Optical Company Plates

The American Optical Company (AOC) Plates, a screening test for protan and deutan defects, appears to be a composite of other tests. In addition to a demonstration plate, there are 14 test plates that include 6 transformation and 8 vanishing plates. The figures are single- and double-digit Arabic numerals. There are at least two different fonts used on different plates. Five or more errors on the 14 test plates constitute failure of the test. Plates with double-digit numbers are failed, if the response to either digit is incorrect.

Dvorine

The Dvorine is another widely used screening test for protan and deutan defects. The test booklet contains both PIC plates and a nomenclature test, which is a unique and valuable feature of this test. The plates are presented in two sections: (1) 15 plates with Arabic numerals and (2) 8 plates with wandering trails, with 1 demonstration plate in each section. Any symbol missed is an error. Three or more errors in the first section constitute a failure. The Dvorine Nomenclature Test is used to assess color-naming ability. There are eight disks (2.54 cm in diameter) of saturated color and eight disks of unsaturated or pastel colors, which include red, brown, orange, yellow, green, blue, purple, and gray. A rotatable wheel allows the presentation of one disk at a time. Color-naming aptitude adds another dimension to a color vision assessment, and the results are appreciated by patients and employers curious to know the impact of a color defect on the ability to name colors.

Tritan Plate

The tritan plate or F-2 is a single plate that Farnsworth designed to screen for tritan color defects. It is a good test and it can also be used for screening for red-green (protan-deutan) defects. The test is performed by a vanishing plate consisting of outlines of two interlocking squares with different chromaticities on a purple background. One square is purple-blue and vanishes for patients with the red-green defects; the other square is green-yellow and vanishes, or is seen less distinctly compared with the purple-blue square, for the tritan. Persons with normal color vision see both squares, but the green-yellow one is more distinct.

Arrangement Tests

Farnsworth-Munsell 100 Hue Test (Pigment Matching Test)

Farnsworth-Munsell test **(Fig. 4A)** is a psychotechnical test, which quantifies a person's ability to discriminate

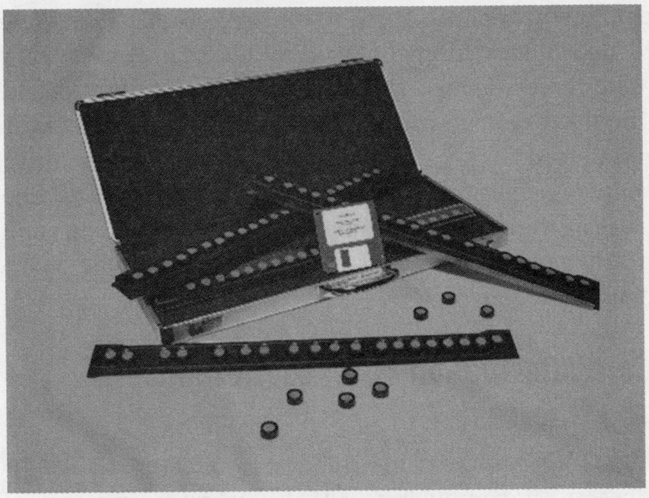

Fig. 4A: Farnsworth-Munsell 100 Hue test.

hues of pigment color. This simple and useful test consists of 85 colored chips that are designed to approximate the minimum difference between the hues that a normal observer can distinguish (1–4 nm). Color-deficient persons make characteristic errors in arranging the chips. The results are recorded on a circular graph. The greater the error arranging the chips, the farther the score is plotted from the center of the circle **(Fig. 4B)**. Automated score for FM 100 Hue test is also available.

The currently available standard version consists of 85 knobs with pigment-colored paper on top arranged in 4 horizontal panels. Each panel has 2 knobs fixed at its 2 ends. The subject is required to arrange the knobs in each panel in such a manner that the colors of the knobs appear to be changing gradually from one end of the panel to another.

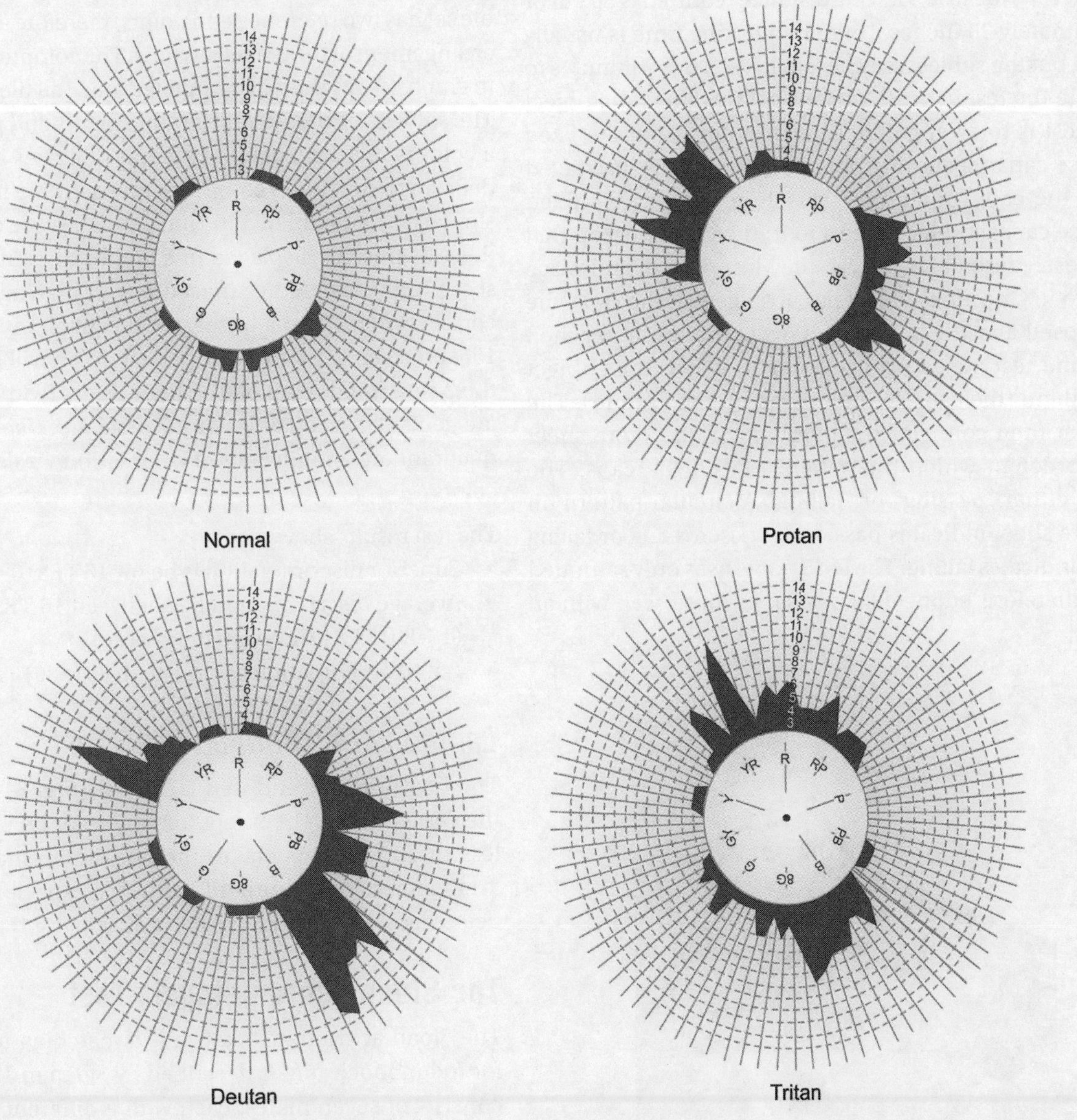

Fig. 4B: Farnsworth-Munsell 100 Hue test results from four subjects: Normal; Protan defects; Deutan defects; Tritan defects.

Generally, recommended time for arranging each panel is 2 minutes. The time spent on arranging each panel is recorded. Scores of a knob/cap is the sum of the differences between the number of that cap and the number of the caps adjacent to it on either side. Sum of the scores of the entire set of knob/caps goes to make the tile evaluation score (TES). Then, the scores of each knob are plotted on a circular graph. By plotting the scores in a graph, it is seen that characteristic patterns are obtained in specific defects **(Fig. 4B)**. The test is capable of detecting all types of color deficiencies. The test results show that:

- Average discrimination lies between 20 TES and 100 TES.
- Superior discrimination is below 20 TES.
- Low discrimination is more than 100 TES.

Farnsworth D-15 Test

The Farnsworth D-15 test **(Fig. 5)** consists of single box of 15-colored chips. The test can be carried out more rapidly than the 100 Hue test. Viewing distance required is 50 cm or approximately 20 inches. Unlimited testing time is usually allowed but the subject may be told he/she has 2 minutes to complete the test in order to prevent dawdling. The object of the test is to arrange the caps in order using the fixed reference cap as a starting point. The subject is instructed to take the cap, which most closely resembles the fixed reference cap, and place it next to it; then find the cap that most closely resembles the cap they just placed, and place it next to it. Once the subject has arranged all the caps, the lid is closed and the box flipped over. The examiner then scores the test based on the order in which the subject placed them (the caps are numbered on the bottom). The examiner then connects the numbers on the score sheet in the order in which the patient placed the caps. The score is either "passing" or "failing". A circular pattern on the score sheet indicates passing, a crisscrossing or lacing pattern indicates failing. The D-15 panel uses only saturated colors; therefore, subtle defects such as those seen with an anomalous trichromat may be missed. The D-15 is useful for detecting dichromacy, in particular, tritan defects, which are often associated with eye diseases and drug toxicity. The disadvantage with this test is that minor defects are not detected. Dichromatic subjects will generally form a series of parallel or crisscrossing lines with at least two lines crossing the chart in the same direction. The index line most nearly parallel to the crossover lines indicated the type of deficiency.

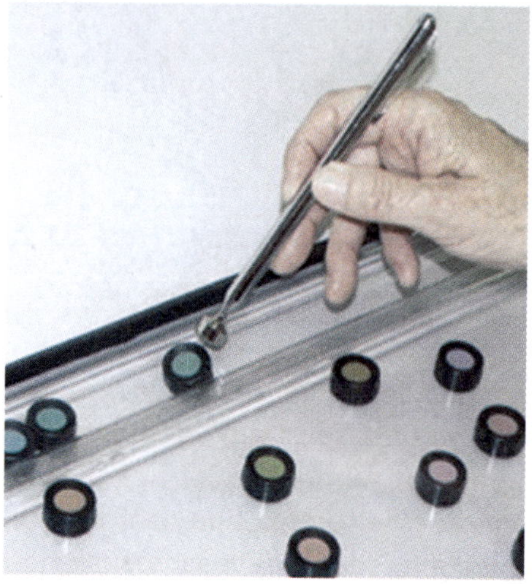

Fig. 5: Farnsworth D-15 color test kit.

Computer-based Farnsworth-Munsell 100 Hue Test

Computer-based FM 100 Hue test is based on the FM 100 Hue test. The computer-based FM 100 Hue is an effective and rapid method for detecting, classifying, and grading color vision anomalies. The subjects are required to arrange four sets of tiles on the basis of color, to the best of his or her ability. Tiles are dragged into place with the help of the mouse. Each tile set has two reference end points; therefore, only one valid arrangement of the tiles is possible. The computerized option to graph the results will be enabled, once all tiles are in place. The software scores the tile arrangements and plots them on a color wheel. The resultant graph indicates areas of color deficiency. Scoring is computed for each chip in the manner similar to manual FM 100 Hue test. TESs are obtained and these scores are displayed in a graphical manner. A higher score indicates greater inaccuracy in placing chips in the correct order. The major rings of the graph indicate 2, 5, 10, 15, and 20 error points. The perfect graph will be a circle on the 2 ring (total score of 0). Minor errors (within the 5 ring) are generally acceptable. Large imbalances/spikes toward a quadrant are an indicator of color vision weakness in those colors.

The test results show that:

- Superior discrimination is below 16 TES (0–16).
- Average discrimination lies between 16 TES and 80 TES (16–80) TES (Tile evaluation score).
- Low discrimination is more than 80 (>80) TES.

Lanthony Desaturated D-15 Test

The Lanthony desaturated D-15 test **(Fig. 6)** is similar to the Farnsworth D-15 except that the color on chips is much less saturated. This makes the hue circle smaller and the arrangement task more difficult. It is especially useful for detecting subtle acquired color deficiencies.

The Sloan Achromatopsia Test

The Sloan achromatopsia test is a matching test designed for rod monochromats described by Sloan in 1954. The test consists of seven plates, each with a different color—gray, red, yellow-red, yellow, green, purple-blue, and red-purple.

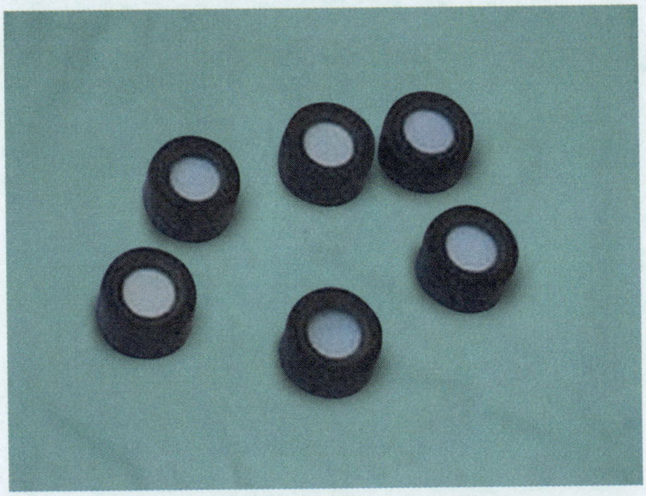

Fig. 6: Lanthony desaturated D-15.

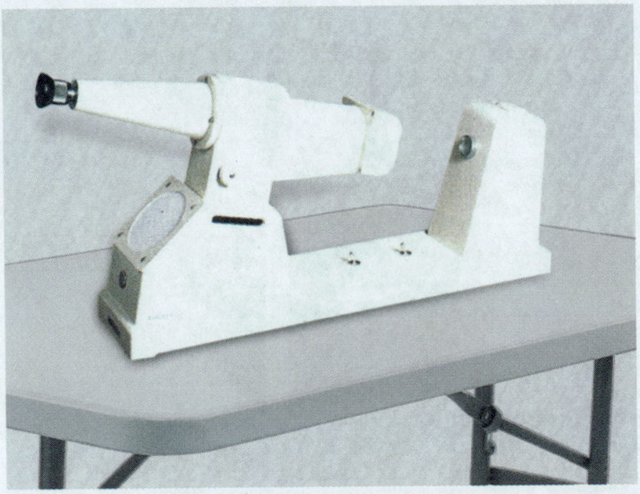

Fig. 7: Nagel's anomaloscope.

Each plate includes 17 rectangular strips forming a gray scale from dark to light in 0.5 steps of the Munsell value. In the center of each rectangle, is a colored disk that has the same Munsell value from one end of the gray scale to the other. The patient's task is to identify the rectangle that matches the lightness of the colored disk. This is a difficult task for persons with normal color vision because of the color difference, but it is readily and precisely accomplished by complete achromats, who see the colors as gray of different lightness. There are normative data for both persons with normal color vision and achromats.

Anomaloscopes

Anomaloscopes are instruments that assess the ability to make metameric matches. The results are used for definitive diagnosis and quantitative assessment of color vision status. Anomaloscopes are much more difficult to administer than PIC plates and arrangement tests. The first anomaloscope was designed by Nagel and is based on the color match known as the *Rayleigh equation,* that is, R + G = Y. Because of their relatively high price, anomaloscopes are rarely used in private practice.

Nagel's Anomaloscope (Spectral Matching Test)

Nagel (1970) constructed anomaloscope for studying the color vision defects. It is based on the color match known as the Rayleigh equation, that is red (R) + green (G) = yellow (Y). The Nagel anomaloscope **(Fig. 7)** assesses the observer's ability to make a specific color match. In anomaloscope, the observer is asked to match a mixture of red and green wavelengths to a yellow. This instrument consists of a source of white light, which is split into spectral colors by a prism. These colors are viewed through a telescope. The field of vision consists of a circle divided into two halves. The lower half projects a spectral Yellow (Sodium line) and this has to be matched by a mixture of Red (Lithium line) and Green (Thallium line) in the other half. The ratio of the two component lights can be controlled by (press) buttons on the base of the telescope on a scale of 0–73, where 0 is pure green and 73 is pure red. The readings are interpreted as follows—the red/green mix proportions can be expressed in the form of an anomaly quotient (AQ). Normal observers have AQ between 0.7 and 1.4; higher AQs indicate deuteranomaly (AQ usually >1.7), whereas lower AQs indicate protanomaly. A major advantage of the Nagel's anomaloscope is that it can distinguish between dichromatic and anomalous trichromatic vision by measuring the balance of red and green wavelengths in the mixture field.

Pickford-Nicolson Anomaloscope

The Pickford-Nicolson anomaloscope can be used for three different matches or colorimetric equations:

1. The Rayleigh equation (R + G = Y),
2. The Engelking equation (B + G = CY)
3. The Pickford-Lakowski equation (B + Y = W).

The matching field is presented on a screen for free viewing at a variety of distances, and there are no intervening optics between the patient and the matching field. The size of the field is changed by selecting different apertures—the largest is 2.54 cm (1 inch) in diameter and the smallest, 0.48 cm (3/16 inch). Different colors are obtained by inserting broadband filters. The Pickford-Lakowski equation is used to assess the consequence of senescent changes in the spectral transmission of the ocular media (yellowing of the lens), but it also has value in examining acquired color defects. The Engelking equation is used for diagnosis of the blue-yellow or tritan color defects. Individual variability in density of the macular pigment and lens pigmentation affects both the Engelking and Pickford-Lakowski equations and, accordingly, confounds the interpretation of an individual result.

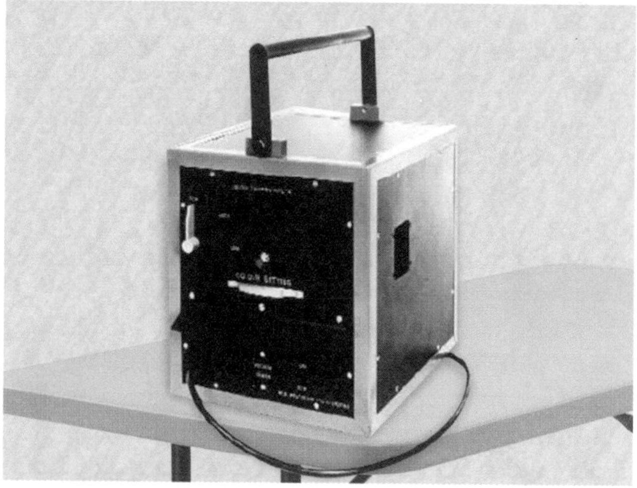

Fig. 8: Holmes Wright lantern.

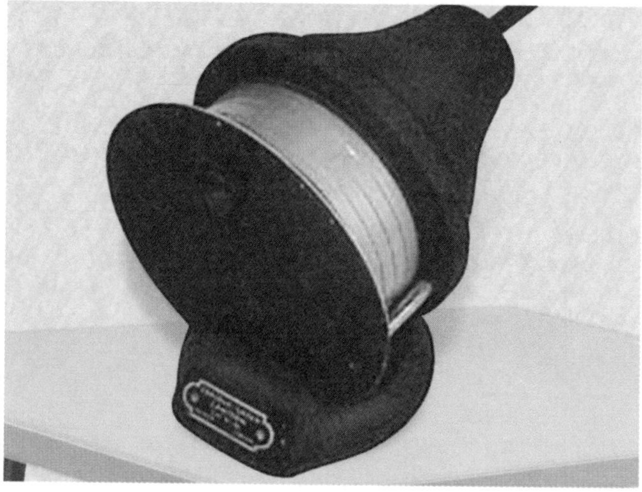

Fig. 9: Edridge-Green lantern.

Lantern Tests

In marine, rail, and airline transportation and in the armed forces, colored signals and navigational aids are extensively used. Lantern tests are performance-based, and they do not diagnose, classify, or grade the level of color vision defect. Rather, they attempt to determine whether the person is capable of performing the color signal recognition tasks with adequate proficiency to maintain safety standards. There are two types of lantern tests, those that use actual signal light filters and those that use simulations of signal lights.

Farnsworth Lantern Test

In the United States, the Farnsworth lantern is the standard lantern test and is comparable to the Holmes Wright lantern **(Fig. 8)**. It simulates marine signal lights under a variety of atmospheric conditions. Two lights are presented in a vertical display in any of the nine possible combinations of three colors—red, green, and white—in the two positions. A subject must average eight out of nine correct responses to pass the test. White lights are particularly problematic, especially for milder color defects. It is reported that the test is not representative of actual field conditions.

Edridge-Green Lantern Test

The Edridge-Green lantern **(Fig. 9)** is an instrument used for testing the ability of a person to recognize color of transmitted light. It was built to simulate the light of railway traffic signals, as they are visible from a distance. The apertures represent the equivalents of five and half-inch railway signals at 600 yards, 800 yards, and 1,000 yards, respectively when viewed from 20 ft distance. Usually two apertures 1.3 mm and 13 mm are used, set of filters showing signal red, yellow, green, and blue colors are shown, each color being shown twice for each aperture size.

The recommendations of the test state that a candidate should be rejected if he calls:

- Red as green
- Green as red
- White light as green or red or vice versa
- Red-green or White light as black.

Any candidate who makes any other errors should be tested with other test.

OTHER TESTS

Electroretinography

Use of electroretinography (ERG) in the modern era is more useful for detection of color vision deficiencies for two reasons: (1) new methods allow to separate and observe accurately the photopic and scotopic components of ERG with the possibility of better study of cone activity, and (2) with the use of computer averaging, picking up of oscillatory potentials is easier.

Microspectrophotometry

In spectrophotometry, an individual cone of a dissected retina is aligned under a small spot of light and its absorption is measured at various wavelengths. The most direct evidence of Young's trichromatic theory (three classes of cones) comes from spectrophotometry. The results of microspectrophotometry confirm three groupings with peak sensitivities at 437–458 nm, 520–542 nm, and 562–583 nm.

Color Vision Deficiencies and Everyday Life

Many tasks depend on our ability to discriminate color. Selecting products at the grocery store, matching paint colors or items of clothing, or connecting color coded wiring—all depend on efficient color vision. Color vision deficiencies can seriously affect an individual's ability to learn, to work at a chosen occupation, and move effectively in the world.

Young children are expected to learn color names early in their educational experience and color is frequently used to categorize educational materials. Good color vision is also important for students of art, chemistry, biology, geology, and geography. A child with deficient color vision will have disadvantage on such tasks as color naming, coding, and matching. Color vision testing should be done for all children as early as possible, and certainly prior to starting school.

If a color deficiency is present, the child's school, teacher, and parents should be informed so that methods of instruction can be modified to meet their visual needs. Teachers and parents can help the child in a number of different ways. First, images and utensils such as crayons, pencil crayons, and pens can be labeled with words or symbols. Second, discrimination between items of different color can be facilitated by the use of high luminance contrast. For example, it would be better to use white chalk on a black or green chalkboard or a dark marker on a white board than combinations that provide less luminance contrast. The level of luminance contrast in colored materials can be determined quite easily by making a black and white photocopy of them or by converting them to black and white on your computer. Third, children should be taught common objects by their usual color (e.g. bananas are normally yellow and the sky is blue). Occupations vary in their requirement of color identification. For some, good color judgment is desirable but not necessary. For others, knowledge of one's color vision is critical. Examples, where good color judgment can be critical for careers include a painter, safety officer, dermatologist, pharmacist, cartographer, coroner, chemist, buyer of textiles, food inspector, electrician, and marine navigator. CP failures in such jobs could be costly, even disastrous.

Professional/Legal Requirements for Color Vision

Testing candidates for CVD forms an intricate part of the legal battery of most preenrolment tests in any profession. Of all the available armamentarium for color vision tests, there is no general consensus on the ideal testing method; different testing methods predominate in different countries. In India we widely rely on the Ishihara charts even though for the Civil Services, we need the Edridge-Green lantern test in addition and the armed forces rely on the Martin lantern test. The Ishihara test is not only quick and easy but is also an excellent screening tool to detect those with red-green CVD. However, its ability to classify CVD and determine its severity is limited.

Both the Ishihara's plates and Edridge-Green lantern should be used for testing color vision. If the color vision testing with Ishihara plates show defective color vision, one may not need to do Edridge-Green lantern test. If the color vision testing with Ishihara plates show defective color vision, then we need to check the candidate with Edridge-Green lantern test. On the basis of Edridge-Green lantern test, the color vision is graded into higher and lower grade depending on the size of the aperture in the Edridge-Green lantern (1.3 mm vs 13 mm) as described below. The technical services category of Indian Civil Services, which include "Police service" requires higher grade of color vision. The United States Police service no longer implements a color vision standard though monochromats are barred. Those who fail initial color vision screening by Ishihara's PIC plates should be further evaluated by Nagel's anomaloscope or Farnsworth Panel D-15 test to include anomalous trichromats who are the most numerous among the CVD persons.

Organizations that require accurate recognition of colored signals (principally transport groups such as the Railways, Maritime, Naval, Civil Aviation Authority, and Air Force) entrust upon a standard lantern test which imitates actual signal systems simulating the workplace. The testing of color vision is hence compulsory. Satisfactory color vision constitutes recognition of signal red, green, and yellow colors with ease and without hesitation.

Since color judgment is an integral part of work in various professions, a screening test to establish color vision normality or deficiency should be undertaken as a part of vocational counseling while deciding one's career. An early diagnosis of CVD might facilitate for early modifications in choice and decisions of educational and life activities.

Grading Level of Color Perception

Color perception should be graded into higher and lower grades depending upon the size of the aperture in the lantern as described the **Table 5**.

Higher grade of CP is absolutely essential for all technical posts but persons with low grade of CP may be eligible for nontechnical posts only.

Color perception can be graded as follows:

- *CP-1*: Correct answers to the series of colors with smallest aperture of Martin lantern test at 6 m.

Table 5: Grading level of color perception.

Grade	*Higher grade of color perception*	*Lower grade of color perception*
Distant between the lamp and the candidate	16 ft	16 ft
Size of aperture	1.3 mm	13 mm
Size of aperture	5 seconds	5 seconds
Result	*Perceives all colors correctly*: High grade of color perception present	*Perceives all colors correctly*: Low grade of color perception present
	If any mistakes: High grade of color perception absent then check with 13 mm aperture	*Perceives no color correctly*: Color perception absent

- *CP-2*: Must pass the Ishihara PIC plates with no errors.
- *CP-3*: Should be able to recognize white, red, and green color signal correctly at a distance of 1.5 m using largest aperture or able to read requisite plates of Ishihara.
- *CP-4*: When mistakes are made with white, red or green colors in the tests described under CP-3.

Accepted level of CP is CP-3 or above for Army and CP-1 for Indian Air Force and Navy.

The possibility that persons who fail the lantern test as described above have no color vision is remote since total color blindness is extremely rare. This can be due to two reasons:

1. When total color blindness is due to rod monochromism, the visual acuity is poor and there is sensory nystagmus—rendering such a candidate unfit for technical posts. They may, however, be considered fit for those nontechnical posts where persons with visual disability can be employed.
2. When total color blindness is due to cone monochromism, the vision may be normal and they are fit for nontechnical posts.

Congenital Color Deficiency in Medical Profession

Often, ophthalmologists are faced with prevocational screening of medical students based on presence and severity of color deficit. Medical profession utilizes a number of descriptive terms like pallor, cyanosis, jaundice, altered blood, etc. Color vision thus forms an integral part of blood and urine test strips, histological specimens, fundus examination, etc. It, therefore, becomes not only advisable but in fact imperative that medical students and doctors be regularly screened for the deficiency and advised about it prior to career decisions. The effects of CVD on decision-making in general practice and other specialties need to be delved into more, so that alternative career choices can be made.

Enhancing Performance with Filters

The color performance of the patients with color deficiency can be sometimes enhanced using colored filters. By absorbing wavelengths selectively, these filters help the observer to differentiate stimuli based on their relative brightness. For example, a red object viewed through a green filter or a green object viewed through a red filter will appear much darker. For example, the X-chrom lens is a red contact lens worn on one eye that absorbs shorter wavelengths and passes longer ones. By comparing the relative brightness in eye with the X-chrom lens to that in the eye without it, a dichromat's ability to distinguish red from green can be enhanced. While such monocular comparisons may be useful in specific applications, the user remains a dichromat and is unlikely to find the approach practical for everyday use.

CONCLUSION

Ophthalmic personnel are frequently asked to perform color vision testing. Knowing whether a congenital or acquired defect is suspected can help determine, which color vision test should be administered. All color vision tests have specific requirements for lighting, viewing distance, viewing time, and scoring. It is important to be familiar with the various testing and scoring guidelines in order to provide the requesting doctor with accurate and useful information.

SUGGESTED READING

1. Alpern M, Mocller J. The red and green cone visual pigments of deuternomalous trichromacy. J Physiol. 1977;266(3):647-75.
2. Brown PK, Wald G. Visual pigments in single rods and cones of the human retina. Direct measurements reveal mechanisms of human night and color vision. Science. 1964;144(3614):45-52.
3. Chisholm CM. New vision standards for police constable recruits. Optom Pract. 2005;6:131-8.
4. Chrousos GA, Ross JL, Chrousos G, et al. Ocular findings in Turner syndrome: a perspective study. Ophthalmology. 1984;91(8):926-8.
5. Dada VK. Practical problems of colour vision defectives. Indian Practitioner. 1977;30:251-5.
6. Dalton J. Extraordinary facts relating to the vision of colours. Mem Manchester Lit Phil Soc. 1798;5(Pt 1):28-45.
7. Daw NW, Moses R. Colour vision: Adler's Physiology of the Eye, St Louis: Mosby:1981.
8. De valois RL, Abramov I, Jacobs GH. Analysis of response patterns of LGN cells. J Opt Soc Am. 1966;56:966.
9. Duke-Elder S. Colour vision. In: Kimpton H (Ed). System of Ophthalmology. Vol IV. Chapter 16. London; 1968. pp. 617-51.
10. Duke-Elder S. Congenital colour defects. In: Kimpton H (Ed). System of Ophthalmology. Vol III (Part 2). Chapter 14. London; 1964. pp. 661-8.
11. Duke-Elder S. Diagnostic methods: The colour sense. In: Kimpton H (Ed). System of Ophthalmology. London; C.V. Mosby Company; 1962. pp. 380-4.
12. Edridge-Green. Physiology of Vision. London; G. Bell and Sons, Ltd.; 1920.
13. Farnsworth D. Manual of the Farnsworth-Munsell 100-hue test for the Examination of Color Discrimination. Maryland: Munsell Color Company; 1949. pp. 1-7.
14. Farnsworth D. Protan, deutan and tritan. J Opt Soc Amer. 1943;33:568.
15. Farnsworth DR. Small-field Tritanopia. USN Submar Med Res Lab Rep No. 19. 1944.
16. Fleishman JA, Beck RW, Linares OA, et al. Deficits in visual function after resolution of optic neuritis. Ophthalmology. 1987;94(8):1029-35.
17. Francois J, Verriest G. Acquired diseases producing colour vision defects. Vision Res. 1961;1:201.

18. Francois J. La discrimination chromatique dans amblyopie strabique. Documents Ophthal. 1967;23:318.
19. Geddes. Prevalence of colour vision deficients. Br J Psychol. 1946;37:30.
20. Gouras P. Identification of cone mechanisms in monkey ganglion cells. J Physiol. 1968;199(3):533-47.
21. Grand YL. Light Colour and Vision. London: Chapman and Hall; 1957.
22. Hardy LH, Rand G, Rittler MC. The H-R-R polychromatic plates. I. A. test for the detection, classification, and estimation of the degree of defective color vision. AMA Arch Ophthalmol. 1954;51(2):216-28.
23. Hart WM Jr. Acquired dyschromatopsias. Surv Ophthalmol. 1987;32(1):10-31.
24. Hart WM Jr. Colour vision. In: Adler FH, Hart WM Jr (Eds). Adler's Physiology of the Eye: Clinical Application. Chapter 22. St. Louis Mosby Year Book; 1992. pp. 708-27.
25. Hering E. Zur Lehre vom Lichtsinne. Wien: Druck Und Verlag Von Carl Gerold's Sohn; 1878.
26. Holmgren. Holmgren's wool test. Ann Rep Smithsonian Inst. 1877;131.
27. Ishihara S. Test for Colour Blindness: Manual of Ishihara Plates, 1917, 5th edition and 14th edition. Tokyo: Kanehara Shuppan Co Ltd; 1925. p. 1959.
28. Kapoor G, Vats DP, Parihar JK. Development of computerized color vision testing as a replacement for Martin Lantern. Med J Armed Forces India. 2013;69(1):11-5.
29. Kinnear PR, Sahraie A. New Farnsworth-Munsell 100 hue test norms of normal observers for each year of age 5-22 and for age decades 30-70. Br J Ophthalmol. 2002;86(12):1408-11.
30. Ladd-Franklin. Tetrachromatic theory. Z Psychol Physiol Sinnes. 1893;4:211.
31. Maxwell C. Fundamental response curve of the cone pigment. Trans Roy Soc Edin. 1885;21(2):275.
32. Michael CR. Colour vision mechanisms in monkey striate cortex: simple cells with dual opponent-colour receptive fields. J Neurophysiol. 1978;41(5):1233-49.
33. Michael CR. Colour-sensitive complex cells in monkey striate cortex. J Neurophysiol. 1978;41(5):1250-66.
34. Michael CR. Colour-sensitive hypercouplex cells in monkey striate cortex. J Neurophysiol. 1979;42(3):726-44.
35. Miller SJ. Colour blindness or achromatopsia. In: Miller SJ (Ed). Parsons' Diseases of the Eye, 18th edition. Edinburgh: Churchill Livingstone; 1900. pp. 269-70.
36. Mitarai G. Glia-neuron interactions and adaptional mechanisms of the retina. In: Jung R, Kormaluber H (Eds). The Visual System: Neuroplysiology and Psychophysics. 1961.
37. Nakamura K, Okajima O, Nishio Y, et al. New color vision tests to evaluate faulty color recognition. Jpn J Ophthalmol. 2002;46(6):601-6.
38. Neitz J, Jacobs GH. Polymorphism in normal human color vision and its mechanism. Vision Res. 1990;30(4):621-36.
39. Newton I. Composition of white light. Phil Trans. 1672;6:3075.
40. Pearlman AL, Birch J, Meadows JC. Cerebral colour blindness: an acquired defect in hue discrimination. Annr Neurol. 1979;5(3):253-61.
41. Rushton WA. A cone pigment in the protanope. J Physiol. 1963;168:345-59.
42. Schubert HD, Atebara NH, Kaiser RS, et al. Basic and Clinical Science Course (BCSC): Retina and Vitreous. San Francisco, CA: American Academy of Ophthalmology; 2012-2013. pp. 48-9.
43. Spalding JA. Colour vision deficiency in the medical profession. Br J Gen Pract. 1999;49(443):469-75.
44. Swanson WH, Cohen JM. Color vision. Ophthalmol Clin North Am. 2003;16(2):179-203.
45. Taylor WO. Effects on employment of defects in colour vision. Br J Ophthalmol. 1971;55(11):753-60.
46. The Gazette of India. Extraordinary, Part 1. Sec. 1. p. 249.
47. Vola JL, Leprince G, Cornu L, et al. The 100 hue at mesopic level. Mod Probl Ophthalmol. 1978;19:67-70.
48. Wald G. Defective colour vision and its inheritance. Proc Nat Acad Sci USA. 1966;55(6):1347-63.
49. Wiesel TN, Hubel DH. Spatial and chromatic interactions in the lateral geniculate body of the rhesus monkey. J Neurophysiol. 1966;29(6):1115-56.
50. Young T. A course of lectures on natural physiology. Phil Trans. 1845;91:1801-7.

CHAPTER

3 Slit-lamp Examination

Arulmozhi Varman

INTRODUCTION

The slit lamp is an instrument consisting of a high intensity light source that can be focused to shine a thin beam of light into the eye. Today, the slit lamp is the most frequently used instrument for ocular examination by the ophthalmologist. It facilitates examination of the anterior segment which includes the eyelid, conjunctiva, sclera, cornea, iris, anterior chamber, crystalline lens, and also the anterior vitreous body. The binocular slit-lamp examination provides a stereoscopic magnified view of the eye structures in detail, enabling anatomical diagnoses to be made for a variety of eye conditions. Supplementary optical aids such as hand-held lenses are used in conjunction with the slit lamp to examine the retina and angle of anterior chamber which are not visible in the direct optical path. A number of accessories have been coupled with the slit lamp extending their range of application for measurement of intraocular pressure (IOP) and as a teaching aid. Slit-lamp photography enables documentation of findings thereby providing a convenient option for tracking the progression of disease in the eye.

HISTORY OF SLIT-LAMP DEVELOPMENT

The first slit lamp was developed by Allvar Gullstrand **(Fig. 1)** in 1911.

However, the instrument never received much acceptance and attention. In 1919, several improvements were made to the Gullstrand slit lamp by Vogt and Henker. In 1920, Koeppe tried to use the slit lamp for examination of the posterior segment of the eye by introducing contact lens examination of the fundus.

In 1926, the slit lamp underwent a landmark modification. The slit lamp was redesigned with a vertical arrangement of the projector, making it easier to handle. Soon Coomberg established the copivotal and isocentric relationship between the microscope and the slit illuminator.

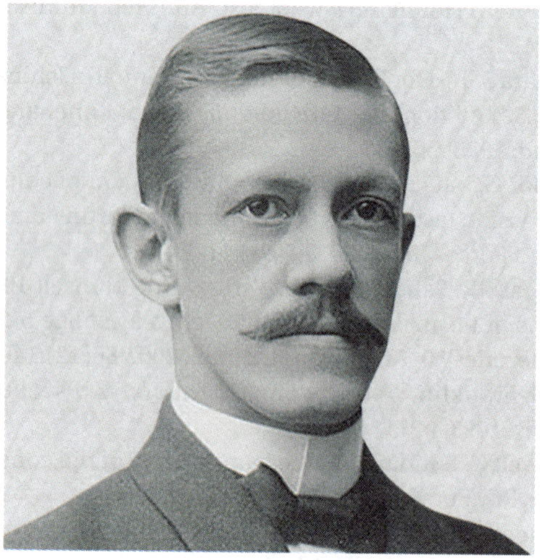

Fig. 1: Swedish Ophthalmologist Allvar Gullstrand.

For the first time, the axis through the patient's eye was fixed at a common swiveling axis for both slit lamp and the microscope. This was a fundamental principle that was adopted for every slit-lamp instrument developed thereafter. In 1927, stereo cameras were developed and added to the slit lamp by Hartinger. In 1930, Rudolf Theil further developed the slit lamp. Horizontal and vertical coordinate adjustments were performed with three control elements on the cross-slide stage. The common swivel axis for microscope and illumination system was connected to the cross-slide stage, which allowed it to be brought to any part of the eye to be examined. A further improvement was made in 1938 when a control lever or joystick was used for the first time to allow for horizontal movement. Following World War II, the slit lamp developed by Coomberg was modified again, and thereby the slit projector could be swiveled continuously across the front of the microscope. In 1950, Littmann redesigned the slit lamp by adopting the joystick control from the Goldmann instrument and the illumination path present in the Coomberg instrument, and adding the stereotelescope

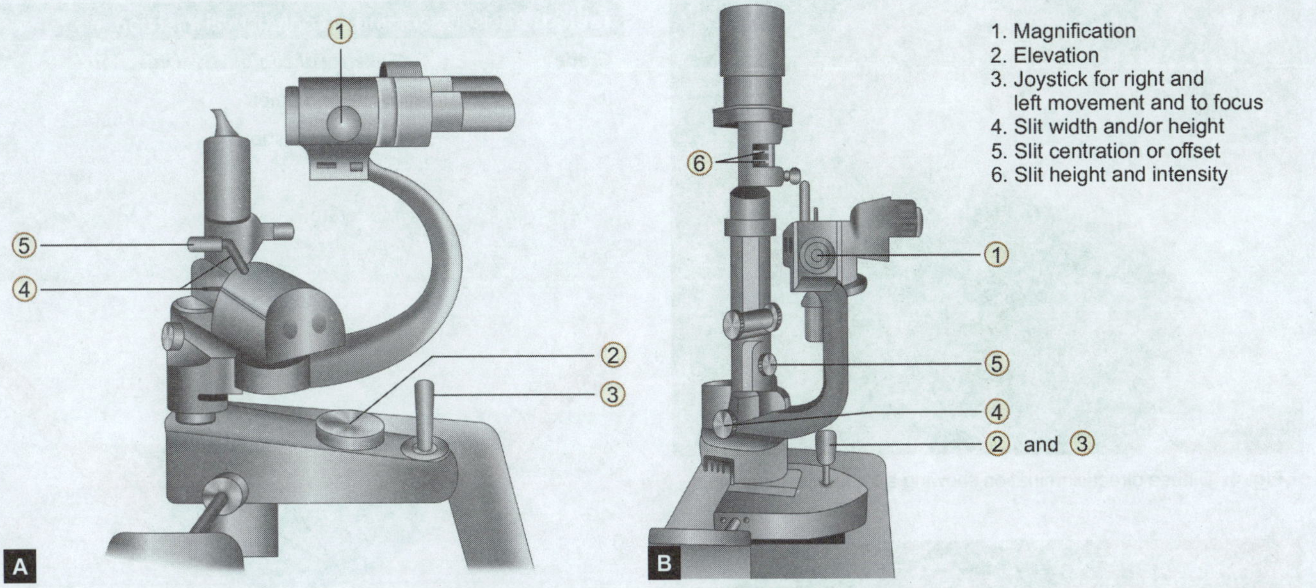

Figs. 2A and B: Parts of a slit lamp. (A) Zeiss type; (B) Haag-Streit type.

system with a common objective magnification changer. Later, halogen lamps replaced the old illumination systems to make them brighter and essentially of daylight quality. From 1994 onward, new slit lamps were introduced which took advantage of new technologies. The various parts of the slit lamp are given in **Figures 2A and B**.

TYPES OF ILLUMINATION USED IN SLIT-LAMP EXAMINATION

The slit lamp is mounted on a moveable stand. A joystick is used to move it right and left, as well as back and forth (focusing). The joystick or similar arrangement is used to raise or lower the slit lamp. The slit projector pivots around the microscope mount and can be swung 180° in front of the specimen. The beam can be projected tangential, perpendicular, or at any angle to the specimen. While performing an examination, the light should be moved frequently, as the different angles at which the light hits the cornea may make pathology more obvious.

Direct Illumination

Direct illumination can be diffuse direct illumination or direct focal illumination.

Diffuse direct or wide beam illumination **(Fig. 3)** has the light source wide open, and its main purpose is to illuminate as much of the eye and its adnexa as possible, for general survey and observation. It gives a good overall picture of the eye, but no fine details. This is especially useful when the media including the cornea is opaque and optical section images are difficult to obtain. In diffuse illumination, a wide beam of light with the slit fully opened is directed at the cornea or the area intended to be examined from an angle of approximately 30–50°. If needed, an attenuated illumination

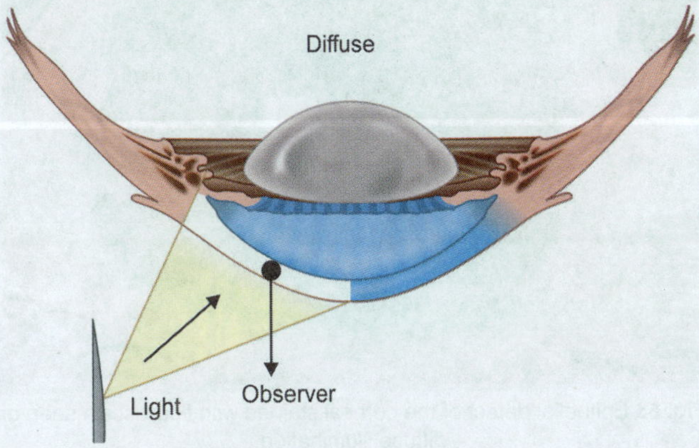

Fig. 3: Diffuse direct illumination.

is produced by inserting a ground glass screen or diffuser in the illuminating path. The microscope is positioned directly in front of the patient's eye at 0° and achromatic light is focused on the anterior of the cornea. Low to medium magnification (5–12×) is used which allows the observer to view a wide field. A higher magnification (30×) may be used for assessment of tear film. The findings elicited by diffuse direct illumination are investigated more thoroughly with other types of illumination.

Applications of Diffuse Direct Illumination

- *To view*:
  - The entire extent of a corneal scar or infiltrates and epithelial defects
  - The presence of Descemet's membrane folds
  - The presence of any invading blood vessels in the cornea
  - Corneal epithelial edema is seen as a hazy, gray, and granular appearance
  - Lids, eyelashes, caruncle, and scleral vessels

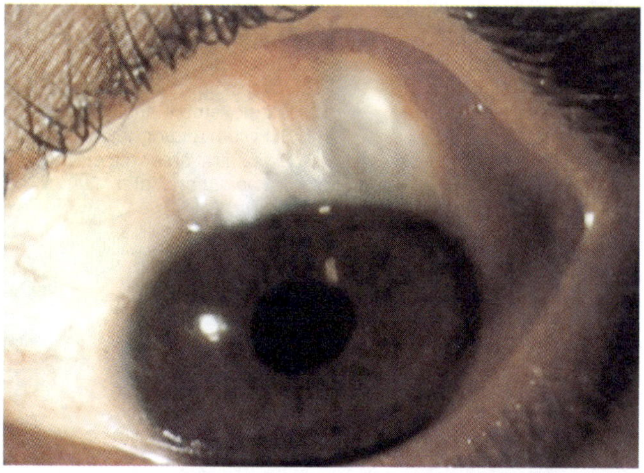

Fig. 4: Diffuse direct illumination showing a trabeculectomy bleb.

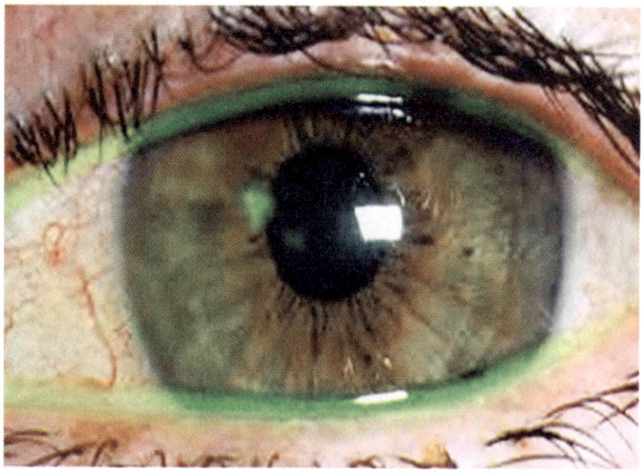

Fig. 5: Epithelial defect of the corneal stained with fluorescein seen on diffuse illumination.

- Trabeculectomy bleb
- Tear film.

Diffuse direct illumination can be used conjointly with cobalt blue filter or green (red-free) filter and in conjunction with various dyes to diagnose and evaluate various conditions in the eye **(Fig. 4)**.

- Cobalt blue filter and fluorescein sodium permit evaluation of corneal and conjunctival epithelium. Fluorescein sodium will stain the cornea and conjunctiva if the epithelium is compromised and this can be visualized in diffuse illumination with or without cobalt blue filter **(Fig. 5)**.
- With cobalt blue filter and fluorescein sodium, diffuse illumination permits evaluation of the position, movement, and bearing of contact lenses.
- With diffuse illumination, after instilling fluorescein sodium, we can assess the tear film break up time with the aid of cobalt blue filter.
- Rose Bengal staining with achromatic light will show pink staining of damaged epithelial cells as in cases of keratoconjunctivitis sicca.

Table 1: Abelson's grading of conjunctival injection.

Grade	*Severity of conjunctival injection*
0	White and quiet
½	Slight congestion
1–1+	Mild
2–2+	Moderate
3–3+	Severe

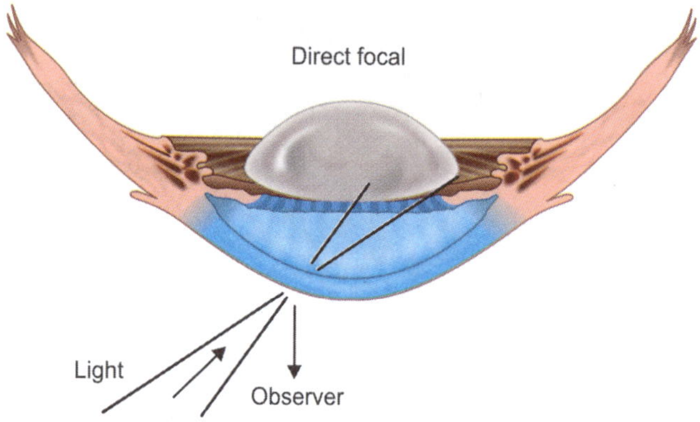

Fig. 6: Direct focal illumination.

Diffuse and wide beam illumination together with red-free (green) filter is helpful to view bulbar conjunctiva and episcleral blood vessels. With the aid of red-free filter, small retinal hemorrhages, aneurysms, and engorged blood vessels are readily seen. Conjunctival vessels are superficial and move with friction from the eyelid. Superficial episcleral vessels show minimal or no movement with the overlying conjunctiva. Deeper scleral injection appears darker and gives an overall purplish hue.

Abelson proposed a standardized grading system for judging different types of scleral and conjunctival injection **(Table 1)**.

Direct Focal Illumination

Direct focal illumination **(Fig. 6)** is the most frequently applied method of examination with the slit lamp. In this method, the axes of illuminating and viewing path intersect in the area to be examined, e.g. the individual corneal layers. Here, the biomicroscope should be directly in front of the patient's eye. The angle between illuminating and viewing path should be as large as possible (up to 90°), whereas the slit length should be kept small to minimize dazzling the patient. With a narrow slit (about 0.1–0.25 mm wide and 7–9 mm high) and a sufficiently small angular aperture, the illuminating beam takes the form of two knife blades placed edge to edge. Slit width and magnification may be varied depending on the object to be examined, with low magnification (7–10×) being most often used. The height of the coaxial beam can be adjusted to measure the horizontal and vertical size of the lesion. With this method, brilliant optical section images can be obtained from the cornea up to the posterior surface of the crystalline lens. To maintain a clear, distortion-free view, the illumination source is always moved to the opposite side when crossing the midline of the cornea about the center of the pupil.

With a narrow slit, the depth and position of different objects (e.g. the depth of penetration of foreign bodies, shape of the lens, etc.) can be resolved more easily. With a wider slit, their extension and shape are visible more clearly. It is, therefore, useful to vary the slit width during the examination. At the cornea, an optical section gives a luminous prismatic tissue section. The corneal epithelium is visible in a very thin precisely focused optical section as a thin blue streak right in front of the brighter Bowman's zone. The stroma appears as a gray granular area under low power and shows nerve fibers and arachnoid corpuscles under higher power.

Examination of the anterior chamber is performed with wider slit. At low magnification, the Tyndall light (Tyndall phenomenon in aqueous humor) is visible in front of the dark pupil. Cells in the aqueous humor, however, are visible only at higher magnifications. During observation it is important that the background always remains as dark as possible. The crystalline lens is particularly suited for viewing via an optical section where the various zones of the nucleus can be made visible with a narrow slit. For examination of the anterior segment of the vitreous body, it is advisable to use the smallest possible slit length to avoid dazzling of both patient and examiner. In these examinations, slit brightness should be high. The slit lamp is especially configured for observation with an optical section. As both microscope and illumination system are mechanically coupled, the slit image is always located in the focal plane and the center of the field of view of the microscope is independent of focusing and selected magnification.

Main Applications of Direct Focal Illumination

The features that are seen in diffuse illumination need to be studied in detail; e.g. assessment of cataract **(Fig. 7)**, corneal scars, nerves, vessels, etc. Direct focal illumination is useful in following conditions:

- For the determination of the stabilization axis of toric contact lenses.
- For delineating sections through the crystalline lens. Capsule, cortex, lens, and cataracts can be observed without any difficulty.
- Van Herick technique for grading the anterior chamber angle **(Table 2)** uses optical section placed near the limbus with the light source always at 60°. The biomicroscope is placed directly before the patient's eye. This technique allows us to judge the temporal and nasal angle **(Figs. 8 and 9)**.
- To discover thickening, thinning, and distortions in the corneal contour (e.g. keratoconus).
- To determine the depth of foreign bodies or opacities in the corneal layers. One way of describing depth is as a percentage of the total corneal thickness.

Table 2: Van Herick angle estimation method.

Angle grade	*Risk of angle closure*	*Cornea to angle ratio*
4	Wide open angle—incapable of closure. Iris to corneal angular separation is 35–40°	Anterior chamber depth (shadow) is equal to or greater than corneal thickness
3	Moderately open angle—incapable of closure. Iris to corneal angular separation is 20–35°	Anterior chamber depth (shadow) is between ¼ and ½ the corneal thickness
2	Moderately narrow angle—closure possible. Iris to corneal angular separation equals 20°	Anterior chamber depth (shadow) is equal to ¼ the corneal thickness
1	Extremely narrow angle—closure probable. Iris to corneal angular separation equals 10°	Anterior chamber depth (shadow) is equal to less than 1/4 the corneal thickness
0	Closed angle—closure is imminent. Iris to corneal angular separation equals 0°	Anterior chamber depth (shadow) is only a very narrow slit or no anterior chamber angle

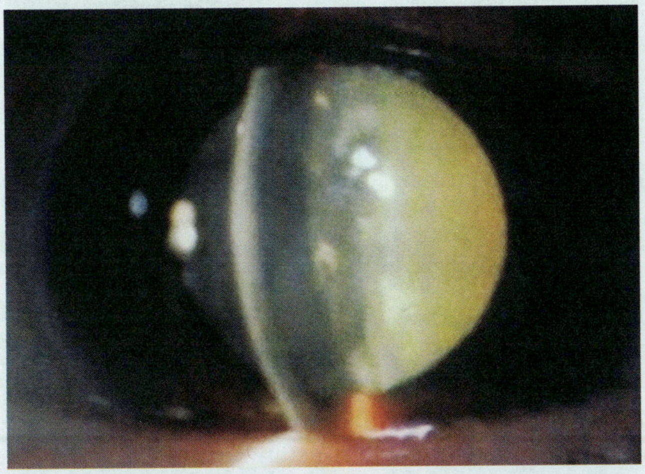

Fig. 7: Direct focal illumination showing an intumescent cataract.

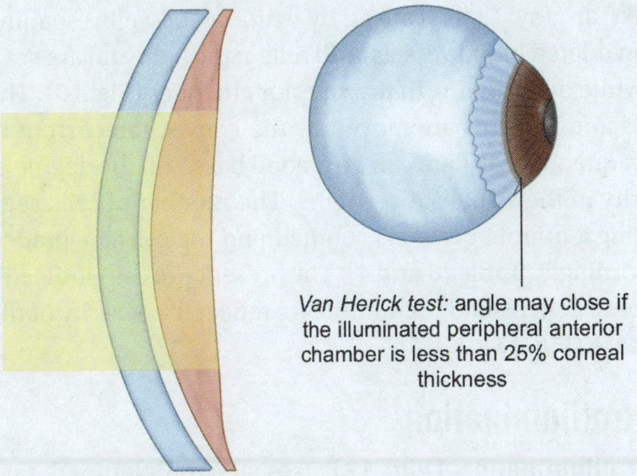

Fig. 8: Van Herick's method of angle estimation.

Fig. 9: Grade I Van Herick angle.

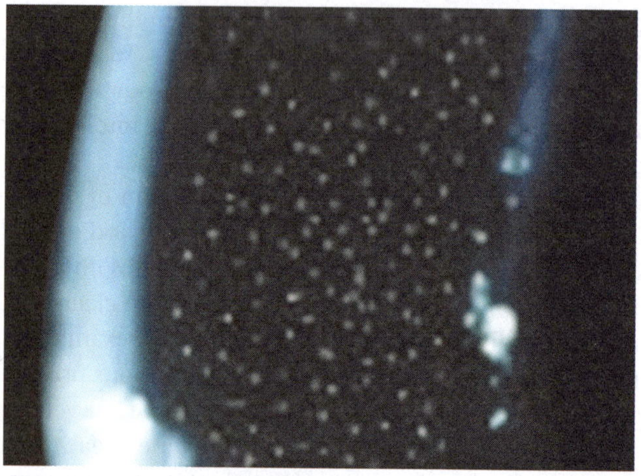

Fig. 10: Direct focal illumination showing cells in anterior chamber.

- Direct focal illumination is also used for examination of anterior chamber cells and flare, which however, must be performed either before dilatation or instillation of fluorescein for applanation tonometry. This is because dilatation and fluorescein used in applanation tonometry causes an increase in flare. This type of illumination helps to detect floating aqueous cells and flare by utilizing the principles of the Tyndall effect.

The traditional method for locating and grading cells and flare is to use a parallelepiped slit approximately 1 mm wide and 2 mm long with the maximal light intensity and magnification. The light source should be 45°–60° temporally and directed onto the pupil. The biomicroscope should be positioned directly in front of the patient's eye. The room should be dark, and the examiner should allow himself or herself a period of time for dark adaptation. The conical beam is focused between the cornea and the anterior lens surface and concentrated on the dark zone between the out of focus cornea and the lens. Examination should be done under high magnification. The zone between the out-of-focus cornea and the lens is normally optically empty and appears totally black. Flare (caused by proteins escaping from dilated vessels due to disruption of the blood-aqueous barrier) makes the normally optically empty zone appear milky or gray. Cells (caused by white blood cells escaping from dilated blood vessels) will reflect the light and are seen as white dots floating in the anterior chamber **(Fig. 10)**. The cells and proteins are moved by the convection current in the aqueous. The flare can be graded based on the degree of clarity in the visualization of iris. The number of cells seen during a minute period is counted and the cells are graded accordingly **(Tables 3 and 4)**. The presence of cells indicates disease activity and their numbers reflect the severity of the disease **(Fig. 11)**.

Table 3: Grading of anterior chamber flare.

Grade	Description
0	Nil
1+	Faint haze
2+	Moderate (iris and lens details clear)
3+	Marked (iris and lens details hazy)
4+	Dense haze (fibrin collection on the iris)

Table 4: Grading of anterior chamber cells.

Grade	Description
0	<1
0.5+	1–5
1+	6–15
2+	16–25
3+	26–50
4+	50

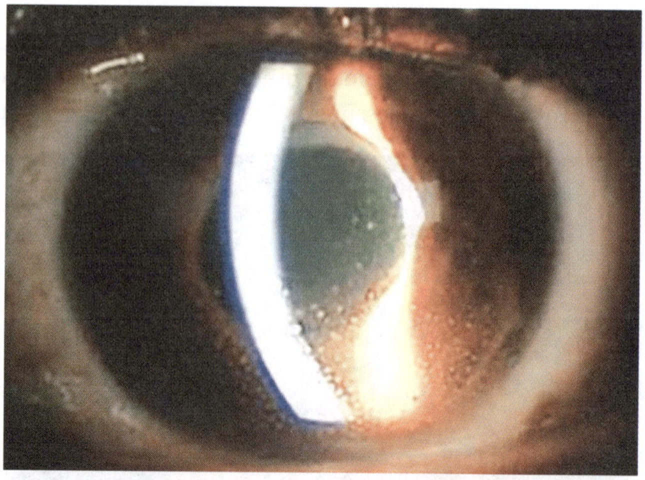

Fig. 11: Direct focal illumination showing keratic precipitates.

Retroillumination

Retroillumination **(Fig. 12)** uses a parallelepiped that bounces unfocused light off one structure while observing the backlighting of another. The beam of light from the light source is reflected off structure like the iris, crystalline lens, or the retina while the biomicroscope is focused on a

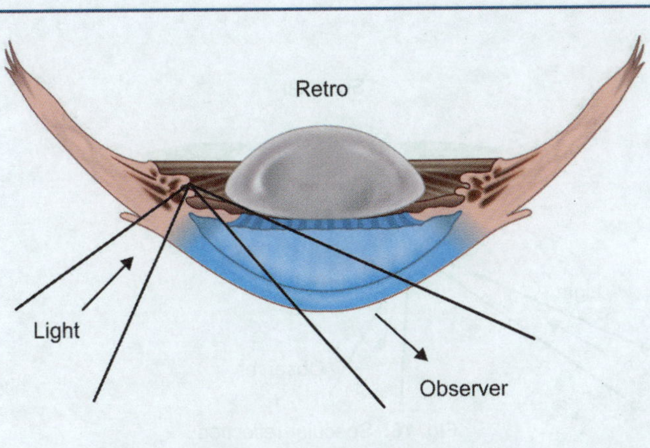

Fig. 12: Retroillumination.

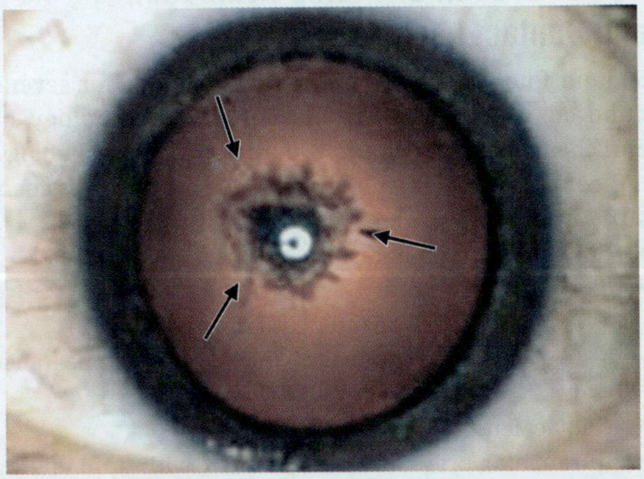

Fig. 13: Retroillumination showing posterior subcapsular cataract.

more anterior structure. In this method, low magnification (7–10×) is used. The slit width is 1–2 mm wide and 4–5 mm high with the biomicroscope and light source placed in direct alignment with each other. The slit is focused just off the edge of the iris and in front of the lens. In this way, defects or atrophy of the iris will be seen as an "orange" glow coming through the defect.

The most typical use of retroillumination is to study the cornea in the light reflected from the iris or fundus after pupil dilatation. This allows detection of fine epithelial and endothelial changes, such as epithelial edema, microcysts, vacuoles, keratic precipitates, corneal scars, and small blood vessels. Keratic precipitates (accumulation of white blood cells and fibrin) will appear white in direct illumination but dark by retroillumination. Similarly, changes in the lens, such as posterior subcapsular cataract posterior polar cataract **(Fig. 13)** are better appreciated in retroillumination. Features in retroillumination will either be opaque to light or scatter light. Features opaque to light appear dark against a light background (e.g. scars, pigments, and vessels containing blood) and those which scatter light appear lighter than the dark background (e.g. epithelial edema).

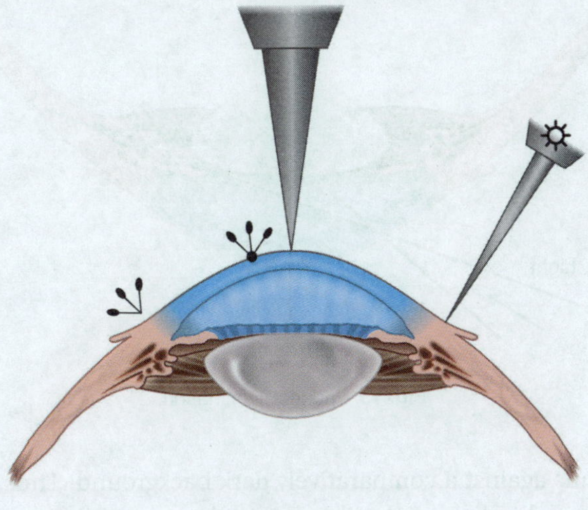

Fig. 14: Sclerotic scatter.

Sclerotic Scatter

In sclerotic scatter **(Fig. 14)**, a narrow light beam is directed onto the limbal region of the cornea at an extremely low angle of incidence, with a laterally decentered illuminating prism and centrally focused microscope. Adjustment must allow the light beam to transmit through the corneal parenchymal layers according to the principle of total internal reflection, allowing the interface with the cornea to be brightly illuminated and the limbus glows 360°. With a slit width of approximately 0.5 mm, maximum illumination and a low magnification (6–10×), the entire cornea can be seen at a glance. The slit illumination system is temporarily directed to the scleral region directly adjacent to the limbus. In its normal physiological state, the cornea is fully transparent and appears completely clear.

A corneal stromal lesion will become illuminated because of forward light scatter. This technique is especially useful to detect subtle stromal haze and cellular or lipid infiltration. The irregularities in the corneal structure due to inclusions, scars, opacities, foreign bodies, etc. cause light scatter allowing those disturbances to be located.

Indirect Illumination

With indirect illumination **(Fig. 15)**, light enters the eye through a narrow-to-medium slit (2–4 mm) to one side of the area to be examined. The biomicroscope is placed directly in front of the patient's eye, and the illumination light source is at about 45°. The axes of illuminating and viewing path do not intersect at the point of image focus. Here, the illuminating prism is decentered by rotating it about its vertical axis off the normal position. The beam is sharply focused on a given structure like the cornea. The light passes through the cornea and falls out of focus on the iris. The dark area just lateral or proximal to the beam is the indirect zone of illumination which one surveys through the biomicroscope. Observation

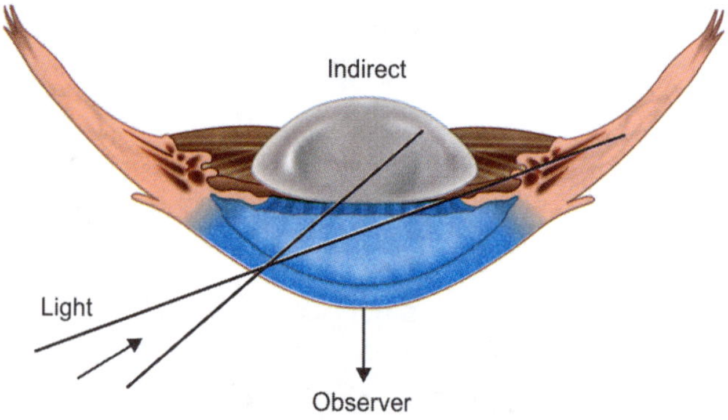

Fig. 15: Indirect illumination.

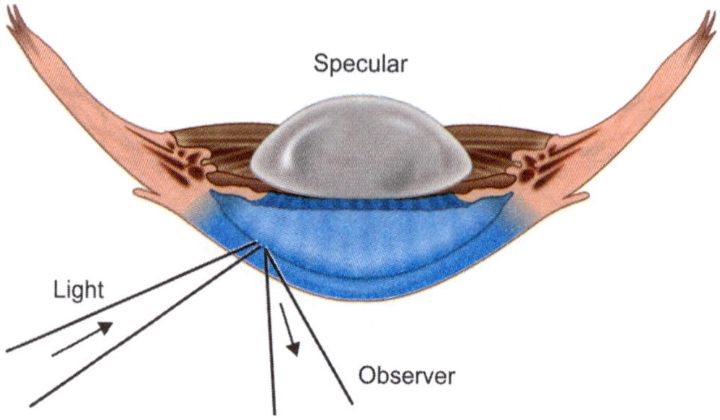

Fig. 16: Specular reflection.

is thus against a comparatively dark background. Thus, the reflected indirect light illuminates the area of the anterior chamber or cornea to be examined. This technique is very useful in detecting microcytic corneal edema, faint corneal infiltrates, and irregularities of the corneal epithelium and tear film.

Specular Reflection

The basic requirements for specular reflection are as follows:

- The angle between the illumination source and the biomicroscope is approximately 60°
- High illumination
- High magnification
- A parallelepiped beam of light
- Uniocular viewing.

The biomicroscope is directly placed in front of the patient's eye and the parallelepiped light source is placed 45–60°. A sharply focused parallelepiped of the cornea is obtained just off the limbus and it is advanced slowly across the cornea until a dazzling reflection of the filament is seen within the microscope. This reflection is seen only with uniocular viewing. Keeping the reflected light within the biomicroscope field of view, the focus is moved back toward the endothelial cells. There will be point where the two images of the filament are seen—one bright and the other ghost-like. Once these two images are seen, focus the biomicroscope on the latter, until a mosaic of hexagonal cells is seen.

Clinical Applications of Specular Reflection

Specular reflection visualizes:

- Abnormalities of the endothelium such as reduced cell density and guttata
- Irregularities of the anterior surface of the cornea
- Front and back surfaces of the crystalline lens
- Details of precorneal tear film, debris, and mucus **(Fig. 16)**.

Use of Dyes in Slit-lamp Evaluation and Contact Lens Fitting

Sodium fluorescein, a dye used in medicine for several hundred years was introduced to ophthalmology by Ehrilcher. It is used for various purposes in ophthalmology. It is coupled with slit-lamp examination for the assessment of:

- Epithelial defects, abrasions, or ulcers of the cornea
- *Tear film assessment*:
  - Test for dry eye—tear film break-up time (BUT)
  - To evaluate tear drainage—fluorescein disappearance test.
- Contact lens fitting
- Intraocular pressure measurement with applanation tonometer
- Seidel's test for wound leak.

The use of fluorescence is based on the fact that the fluorescein light can be spectrally separated from an exciting light. Structures absorbing the fluorescein dye are contrasted much better against the nonfluorescing environment. Observation of fluorescence requires a suitable excitation light source and a properly dosed concentration of fluorescein in the tear film.

The yellow-green fluorescence light is not monochromatic, with the emission maximum at 530–535 nm. Hence, for excitation, a radiation less than 530 nm is necessary. The efficiency of fluorescence is highest with blue light excitation in the wavelength range of 450–500 nm. The halogen lamp of the slit lamp serves as the excitation source. A cobalt blue filter is swung into the optical path of the slit lamp serving as an exciter filter. Stray light that would reduce contrast must be blocked by using a barrier filter. For this, a yellow filter >530 nm is used. This filter blocks the blue exciting light and transmits only the yellow-green fluorescence and longer wavelengths.

Concentration of Sodium Fluorescein

The optimum fluorescence effect is achieved with a sodium fluorescein concentration of 0.2–0.4% in the tear film.

This concentration is obtained by applying one drop of 2% sodium fluorescein or a fluorescein impregnated strip into the conjunctival sac of a patient with normal lacrimal secretion.

Assessment of Tear Film

The assessment of the tear film and the inspection of the lacrimal apparatus should be performed at the very beginning of the examination, particularly before contact lens fitting, as the quantity and composition of the lacrimal fluid may change during the course of examination, measurements as well as during the contact lens fitting process.

The daily tear secretion amounts to about 0.5–1.0 mL. Every contact lens needs a certain quantity of tear film so that it can float with minimal friction. Soft contact lenses additionally require a certain tear humidity to remain elastic.

The quality and quantity of the tear film can be examined simply and reliably with the slit lamp. The tear film BUT which shows the stability of the tear film is an important criterion for symptom-free wearing of contact lenses. To determine the BUT, 2% sodium fluorescein drops or an impregnated fluorescein strip moistened with nonpreserved saline is instilled into the lower fornix, without application of a local anesthetic. The patient is asked to blink several times. The tear film is then examined with a broad beam and a cobalt blue filter. The time interval between the last blink and the appearance of the first dry spot (breaking up of the tear film) gives the tear film BUT. During this examination, one must ensure that the patient is not dazzled (retinal irritation resulting in reflex secretion) as this would falsify the examination result. Tear film BUT greater than 10 seconds is normal.

Assessment of Nasolacrimal Duct Patency

Fluorescein disappearance test: Fluorescein is instilled into the conjunctival sac and observed for 2–3 minutes. On slit-lamp examination, prolonged retention of dye indicates inadequate tear drainage due to nasolacrimal duct (NLD) obstruction or atony of the sac.

Contact Lens Fitting

- Inspection of the anterior segment of the eye before inserting a contact lens
- Inspection of the contact lens fit on the eye with and without sodium fluorescein
- Inspection of the anterior eye segment, particularly the cornea on removal of the contact lens after it has been worn over a long period
- Thorough inspection of the contact lens.

Inspection of the Anterior Segment of the Eye before Inserting a Contact Lens

This inspection is carried out using diffuse or direct focal illumination with a wide, fully opened slit. The cornea, lids, sclera, conjunctiva, and tear film are examined.

Inspection of Contact Lens Fit

This requires diffuse illumination and a magnification of approximately 12×. The parameters assessed are:

- Fit of the lens and centration
- Lens movement (direction and speed)
- Presence of air bubbles or foreign bodies under the lens, and
- The state of the tear film.

Inspection of Contact Lens Fit with Sodium Fluorescein

This is applicable only for rigid contact lenses.

Flat Fitting (Fig. 17)

The fluorescence image of a flatly fitted contact lens on a spherical cornea shows a round, dark contact zone in the center (lens-cornea touch) surrounded by a wide fluorescing ring that becomes brighter toward the periphery (no lens-cornea touch). The fluorescence intensity increases continuously toward the edge (intense yellow-green).

Parallel Fitting

A contact lens fitted parallel to a spherical cornea shows a central, evenly round, and dark contact zone surrounded by a fluorescing ring that becomes brighter toward the periphery. The dark zone covers about 70–72%, the yellow-green ring about 28–30% of the area. The marginal area must jut out gently and continuously from the cornea with smooth transitions. If this is not so, the contact lens surface has a defect and should be removed immediately from the cornea.

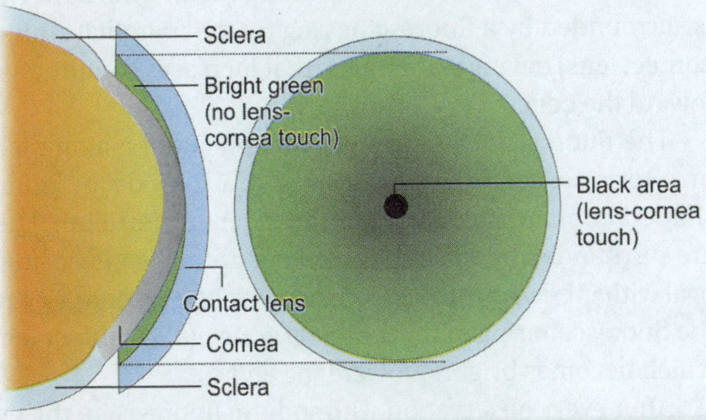

Fig. 17: Flat fit contact lens on spherical cornea.

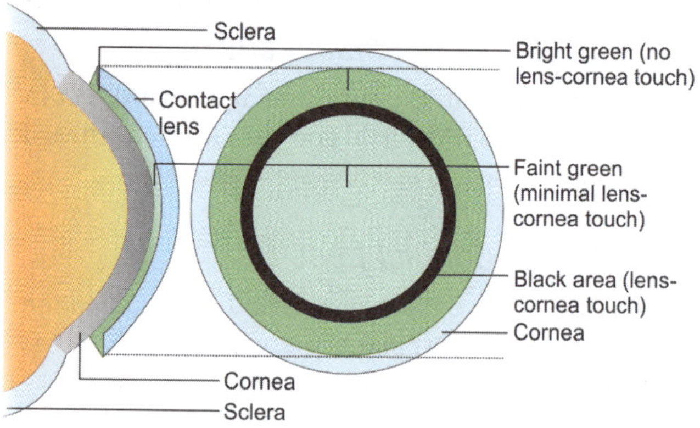

Fig. 18: Ideal fit contact lens on a spherical cornea.

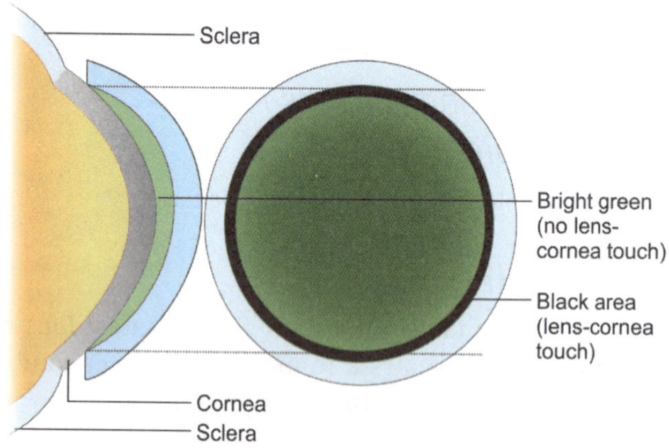

Fig. 19: Steep fit contact lens on a spherical cornea.

The fluorescence image of a parallel fitted contact lens on a toric cornea shows a central, dark contact zone with peripheral indentations in the steeper meridian. With increasing toricity of the cornea, a dark bone-shaped or butterfly-shaped contact zone is created. The contact lens rests on the flatter meridian, and juts out from the cornea in the steeper meridian. The marginal zone may project gently **(Fig. 18)**.

Steep Fitting (Fig. 19)

The fluorescence image of a steeply fitted contact lens on a spherical cornea shows a central fluorescing "lake" (no lens-cornea touch), surrounded by a paracentral, narrow, and dark fluorescence ring (lens-cornea touch). This dark ring is surrounded by a fluorescing ring (at the marginal zone of contact lens) having a brightness that increases continuously toward the edge.

The fluorescence image of a steeply fitted contact lens on a toric cornea shows paracentral, dark, sickle, or kidney shaped contact zones toward the steeper meridian. They are surrounded by a lacrimal lake that becomes increasingly oval with increasing toricity. At the periphery, it merges with the fluorescein ring of the marginal zone of the contact lens, which becomes brighter toward the edge.

After every observation with sodium fluorescein, the eye should be rinsed thoroughly with physiological saline to avoid infection.

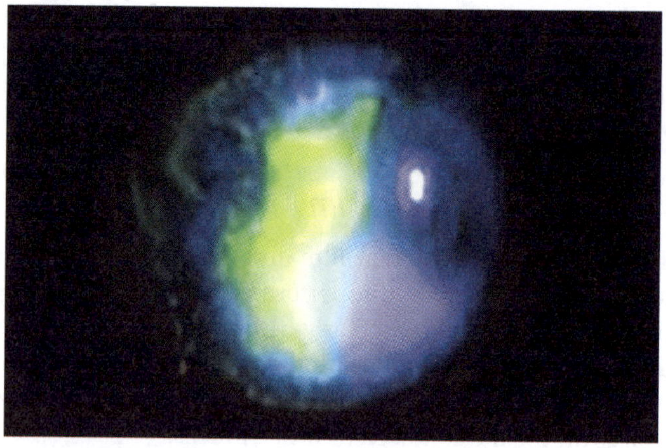

Fig. 20: Corneal abrasion following contact lens wear.

Inspection of the Cornea

The examination is performed with direct focal illumination (by optical section) and direct or scattering sclerocorneal illumination.

The cornea is checked for abrasions **(Fig. 20)**, erosions as well as possible deformation (air-bubble pits, edema). In addition, we can also examine the conjunctiva (pressure sores and allergic reactions) and the eyelids.

Inspection of Contact Lens

Contact lenses are inspected with diffuse and direct focal illumination. The lens should be supported during the inspection. The surfaces of the contact lens are checked for scratches, burr, and polishing marks. The edges of the contact lens are examined for cracks, chips, defects, and possible deposits.

Measurement of Intraocular Pressure

The most widely used accessory for the slit lamp is the Goldmann applanation tonometer. It is used for measuring the IOP. This method is characterized by high accuracy, reliability, and simplicity. In practical use, it is important that the tonometer is correctly mounted on the slit lamp so that it must be possible to move the applanation tonometer into the working position quickly and easily and at the same time, it should not hinder normal work with the slit lamp.

Procedure

The patient is positioned at the slit lamp with the forehead firmly against the headrest. Topical anesthetic drops and sodium fluorescein is instilled into the conjunctival sac of both eyes. The slit lamp must be adjusted as—maximum illuminated field, open slit, a blue filter, and the slit projector swung out laterally to about 50°, 8× or 12× microscope magnification. During measurement, the patient's eyes must be wide open. The examiner can assist in this by opening the patient's eyelids with thumb and forefinger. However,

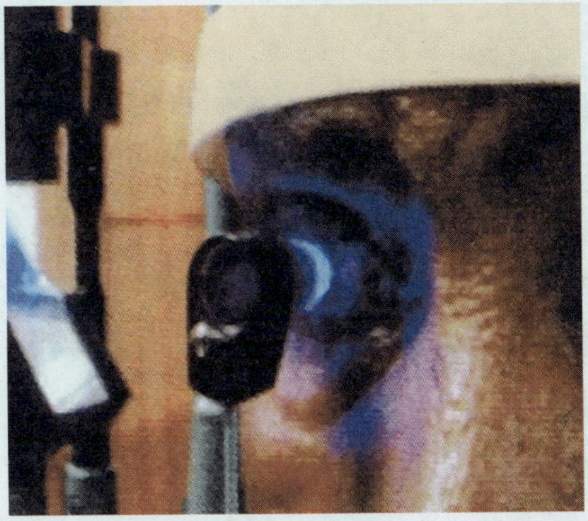

Fig. 21: Tonometry.

care should be taken not to exert inadvertent pressure on the globe. The fingers should rest only on the bony eye socket **(Fig. 21)**.

The measuring body of the applanation tonometer contains an image-doubling prism. When this prism is in contact with the cornea, the tear film ring between measuring body and cornea is divided into two green fluorescing semicircles. First, the prism is brought into contact with the cornea. Vertical adjustment is performed on the slit lamp so that both the semicircles are of equal size. The width of the rings should be about 0.2–0.3 mm and should oscillate with each pulse beat. For measurement of IOP, the dial on the tonometer is rotated, starting from scale division 1 on the measuring drum until the inner edges of the rings just touch each other. The corresponding value is read from the measuring drum and converted to mm Hg by multiplying by a factor of 10. If the measurement takes too long, the corneal epithelium will dry out and the measurements will not be reliable.

Seidel's Test for Wound Leak

Procedure: Fluorescein dye is instilled into the conjunctival sac; patient is asked to blink and observed under the slit-lamp. Leakage of aqueous directly into the tear film is seen by the Seidel's test as the dilution of fluorescein by the leaking aqueous at the site of leakage.

Marking the Axis on the Cornea for Toric Intraocular Lens

Slit-lamp can be used for the following procedures in toric intraocular lens (IOL) surgery:

- For marking of 0° and 180° reference axis
- For marking of the toric IOL placement axis
- Verifying the accuracy of the placement of toric IOL postoperatively.

Marking of 0° and 180° Reference Axis—Steps (Figs. 22A to D)

- Make a thin slit and position it at 0–180°.
- Align the illumination and observation column.
- Focus on the cornea and bisect the corneal Purkinje image.
- Mark with a fine marker pen or needle.

Marking of the Toric Intraocular Lens Placement Axis—Steps

- Make a thin slit and align it at the desired axis.
- Align the illumination and observation column.
- Focus on the cornea and bisect the corneal Purkinje image.
- Mark with a fine marker pen or needle **(Fig. 23)**.

Postoperative Verification of Toric Intraocular Lens Alignment

- Dilate the pupil well so that the toric IOL markings are seen **(Fig. 24)**.
- Align the slit on the markings present on the IOL **(Fig. 25)**.
- Read the axis from the scale.

GONIOSCOPY

The angle of the anterior chamber cannot be visualized directly through an intact cornea, because the light emitted from the angle undergoes total internal reflection at the anterior surface of the precorneal tear film. A goniolens eliminates total internal reflection by replacing the tear film-air interface with a new tear film-goniolens interface. There are two types of goniolenses, namely:

1. Indirect goniolenses provide an image of the opposite angle and can be used in conjunction with the slit lamp (e.g. Goldmann, Zeiss lenses).
2. Direct goniolenses provide a direct view of the angle. They are used with the patient in a supine position (e.g. Koeppe lenses).

The mirror contact lens is held either by hand (Goldmann) or with a special holder (Zeiss). The Goldmann is an indirect goniolens which has a contact diameter of approximately 12 mm. It has three mirrors. Modifications with one mirror and two mirrors are available. The Goldmann lens stabilizes the globe as well as provides an excellent view of the angle. It can be used for procedures like laser trabeculoplasty. The major disadvantage of Goldmann lens is that it cannot be used for indentation gonioscopy.

The Zeiss, Posner, and Sussman are indirect four-mirror goniolenses mounted on a handle. The contact surface of the lens has a diameter of 9 mm and a curvature that

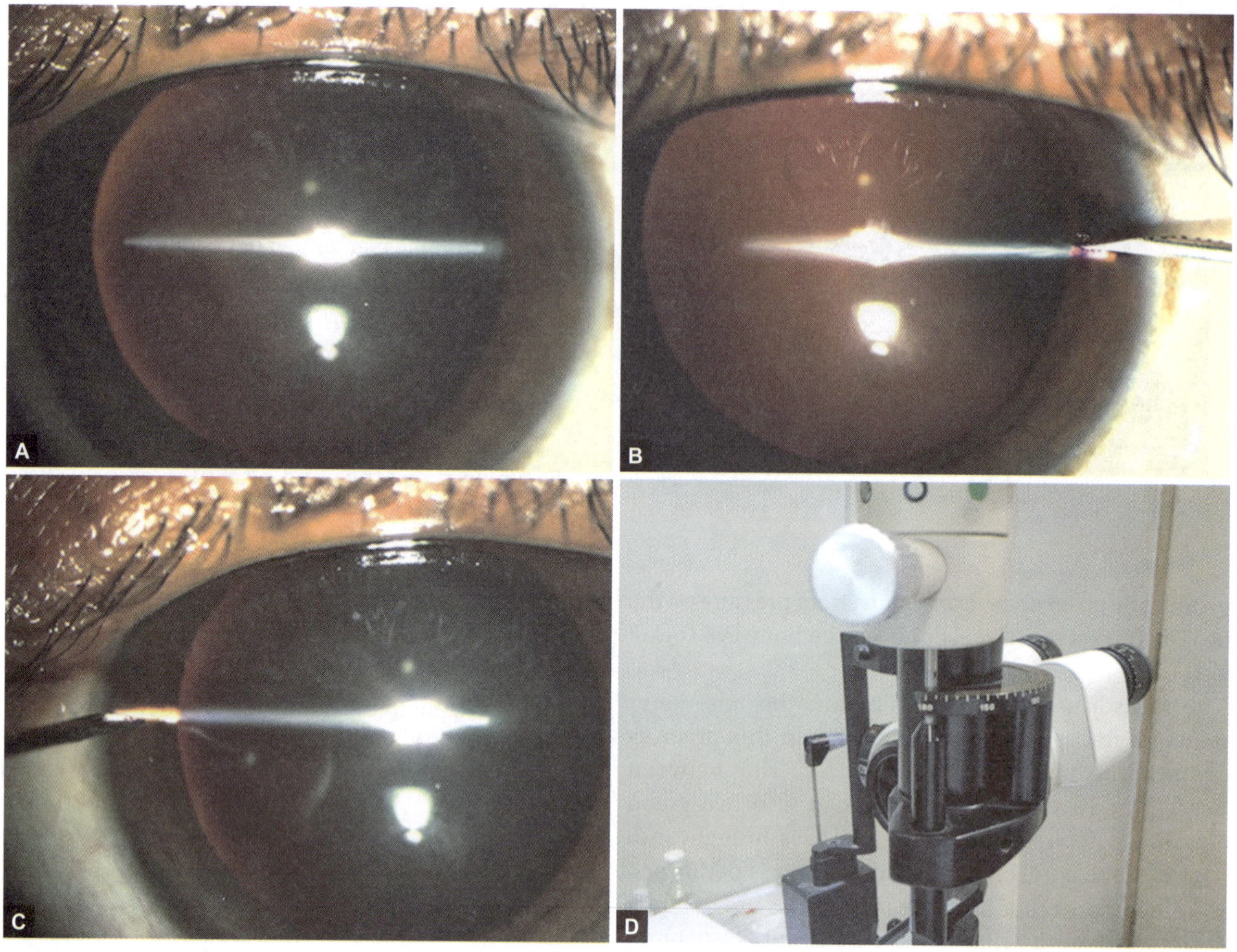

Figs. 22A to D: (A) Slit beam should be centered with reflex of illumination on the cornea; (B) Shift the slit beam peripherally (nasally) and mark the cornea beyond dilated pupil margin; (C) Shift the beam on other side and perform the same (Temporally); (D) The slit aligned at 180°.

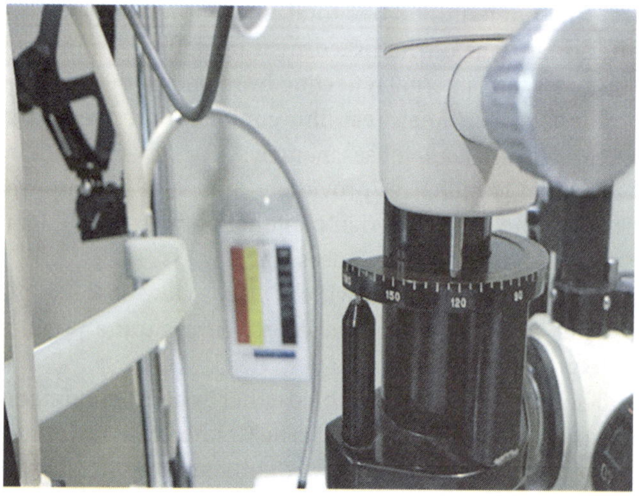

Fig. 23: The slit aligned at 120°.

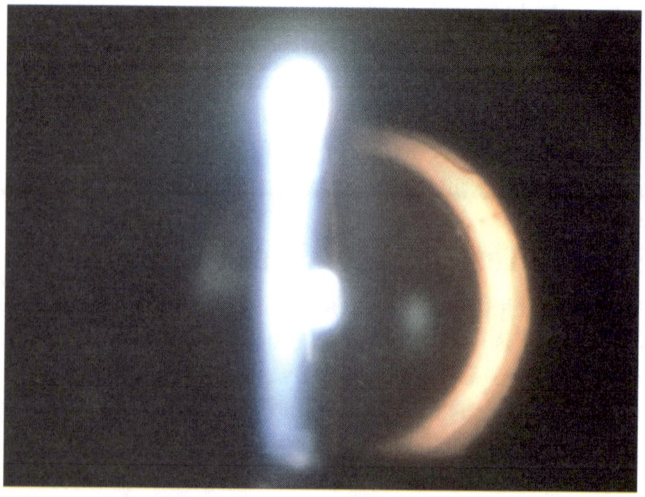

Fig. 24: Postoperative dilated pupil showing axis marking on the toric intraocular lens, with a vertical slit.

is flatter than that of the cornea, which negates the need for a coupling solution. The tear film provides adequate contact material and lubrication for the lens. The four-mirror permits quick and comfortable examination of the entire circumference of the angle with minimal or no rotation. The lens is useful for indentation gonioscopy, but since it does not stabilize the globe, it cannot be used for therapeutic procedures such as laser trabeculoplasty.

Procedure

The examination of the iridocorneal angle requires good stereoscopic observation through the slit-lamp

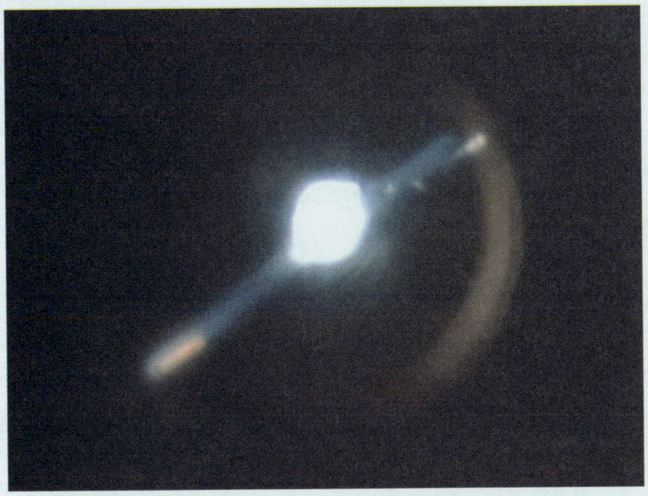

Fig. 25: The slit aligned on the toric intraocular lens marking.

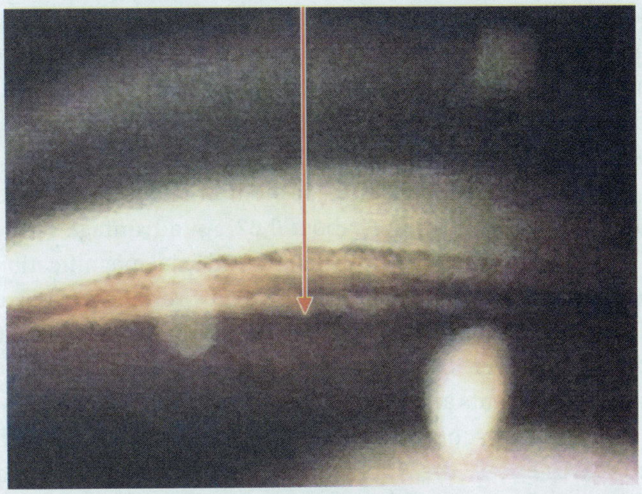

Fig. 26: An open angle on gonioscopy.

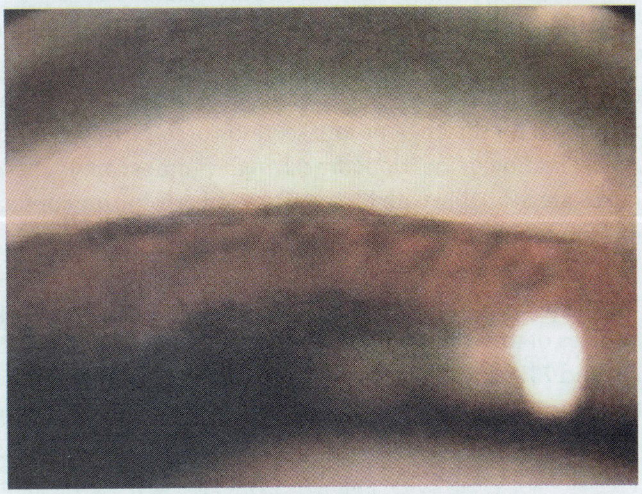

Fig. 27: A closed angle on gonioscopy.

biomicroscope. The patient should be informed about the procedure and the contact of the instrument with the eye. It is ideal to do gonioscopy in a dark room. After instillation of the topical anesthetic agent, coupling solution is filled into the cup of the contact lens. The patient is asked to look up and the inferior rim of the lens is inserted into the lower fornix and pressed gently against the cornea. Only gentle pressure should be exerted on the cornea because excessive pressure will inadvertently distort angle structures.

The slit beam should be as narrow as possible (2 mm) and care should be taken to avoid light falling on the pupil, because it may constrict the pupil and artifactually open the angle. For good reflex-free illumination, it is useful to rotate the slit so that it is perpendicular to the iridocorneal angle.

In case of single mirror lenses, the mirror is placed at 12 o'clock position and the inferior angle is identified first and then the mirror is rotated in the clockwise or anticlockwise direction. Each quadrant of the angle is visualized with the opposite mirror in a two-mirror or four-mirror gonioscope. The image that is seen is laterally reversed with the mirror in the horizontal and vertical meridian.

With a Goldmann gonioscope, it is possible to "see over the hill" by asking the patient to look in the direction of the mirror to get a view of angle obscured by the convex iris. With a four-mirror gonioscope, indentation gonioscopy can be performed by pressing the gonioscope posteriorly against the cornea. This forces the aqueous into the angle of the anterior chamber and pushes the peripheral iris posteriorly. Indentation gonioscopy helps to differentiate between appositional and synechial angle closure.

The angle of the anterior chamber may be open **(Fig. 26)** or closed **(Fig. 27)**.

Fundus Examination with Slit Lamp

It is not possible to visualize the fundus with a slit lamp alone due to the refractive power of the ocular media. In other words, the far point of the eye (punctum remotum) is so distant in front of (myopia) or behind (hyperopia) that the microscope cannot be focused. The use of auxiliary optics, generally a lens makes it possible to bring the far point within the focusing range of the microscope. Various auxiliary lenses are in use with a wide range of optical properties and practical application.

Based on the optics, the lenses are classified as:

- Concave optics
- Convex optics

Concave Optics

Concave lenses provide an upright, virtual, and intermediate image of the fundus. Due to this property, the normal working distance of the slit lamp to the patient is only changed slightly. As the pupil acts like a diaphragm, the stereoscopic field of view is limited with concave lenses.

There are two types of concave lenses widely in use:

1. Fundus contact lens
2. Gonioscope, namely the Goldmann 3-mirror or 4-mirror contact lens.

The Goldmann fundus contact lens is a negative contact lens. It has a refractive power of –64D thus compensating approximately for the refractive power of the cornea and permitting the examination of the posterior pole of the eye about 30° from the axis.

The lateral magnification for the normal eye is 0.91 and the axial magnification is about 0.62. An advantage of the Goldmann fundus lens is that lateral and axial magnification is virtually independent of the patient's refractive power. This is of particular importance while examining the vitreous body. However, contact lenses cannot be used on very sensitive patients and particularly patients just after surgery.

For fundus observation of a myopic patient with concave lenses, the microscope must be moved toward the patient. With myopia of –20D, the displacement is 18 mm, but only 7 mm for the Goldmann fundus lens.

With a fundus contact lens, only the central region of the fundus can be observed. Therefore, concave lenses are also available with built-in mirrors for observation of the different peripheral fundus regions and sections of the vitreous body or observation of the iridocorneal angle (gonioscopy). These lenses are available with three mirrors (three-mirror contact lens) and four mirrors (four-mirror contact lens).

The Goldmann lens consists of a central part and three mirrors set at different angles. The angles of the reflecting surfaces of the Goldmann three-mirror contact lens are 59°, 67°, and 73°. Since the curvature of the contact surface of the lens is steeper than that of the cornea, a viscous coupling solution with the same refractive index of the cornea is required to bridge the gap between the cornea and the Goldmann lens.

The axial region of the vitreous body and fundus can be observed by looking through the central part of these lenses (without a mirror). It provides a 30° upright view of the posterior pole. The equatorial mirror (which is the largest and oblong-shaped) enables observation of off-center areas of retina from 30° to the equator. The peripheral mirror (square-shaped and intermediate in size) enables visualization of the periphery of retina between the equator and the ora serrata. The gonioscopy mirror (smallest and dome-shaped) is used for observation of iridocorneal angle and also provides visualization of the extreme periphery and the pars plana. Therefore, the smaller the mirror, the more peripheral the view of the fundus obtained.

The mirror is positioned opposite to the area of the fundus to be examined. When viewing the vertical meridian, the image is upside down but not laterally reversed, as with indirect ophthalmoscopy, so that the lesions located to the left of the 12 o'clock meridian in the retina will also appear in the mirror on the left-hand side. When viewing in the horizontal meridian, the image is laterally reversed.

The four-mirror contact lens is a small pyramid, mainly of glass with the apex replaced with a ground-in recess with a radius of about 8 mm, which corresponds to the curvature of an average cornea. The angle of the reflecting surfaces is approximately 62°.

With these lenses, objects are seen as mirror images. Small peripheral holes in the retina that one may fail to see with an ophthalmoscope are easily discerned with a three-mirror contact lens.

Convex Optics

Convex lenses produce a reverse, real intermediate image of the fundus. For this reason, a longer distance is necessary between the slit lamp and patient's eye.

Convex lenses have very large monoscopic or stereoscopic field of view. This is because the convex lens images the entrance pupil of the microscope at reduced size in the patient's pupil which therefore does not act as a field stop.

Two types of convex lenses are available:

1. Contact lens after Schlegel; Panfundoscope
2. Aspheric plus lens such as auxiliary lens after Bayadi; +90D Volk lens, +78D, +60D, aspheric ophthalmoscopic lens AOL 90°

The latter is used in indirect ophthalmoscopy where the lens is held by hand about 9 mm in front of the patient's eye. Both slit projector and microscope should be set to a middle position, the slit fully opened, and a medium magnification (about 12×) set on the microscope. The distance between ophthalmoscopic lens and illuminating prism should be about 80 mm. The lens is illuminated in direct focal illumination.

It produces a reversed, real image of the fundus that is reduced in size. Without dilation of the pupil the retinal image is visible through the left-hand or right-hand eyepiece. Initially, this image will be obscured by reflections from the cornea. These reflections, however, are eliminated more easily with the Hruby lens by moving the joystick of the slit lamp laterally. Focusing is as with normal slit image observation. The small fundus image can be further magnified considerably using the magnification changer of the microscope. With a dilated pupil of more than 5 mm, the fundus of the eye can be viewed stereoscopically. The field angle is 60° at medium magnification and 40° at a magnification of 20×. With this method even for the inexperienced operator it is relatively easy to see the fundus.

Convex lenses are particularly well suited for the examination of strongly myopic eyes. When positioned correctly, lateral and axial magnifications become independent of the refractive power of the patient's eye. Simple convex lenses, however, exhibit abnormal field curvatures making them unsuitable for examination of the vitreous body.

So far, the conditions and methods of fundus observation with the slit lamp have been discussed. But without illumination, observation is impossible. Special requirements have to be met for illumination of the fundus through auxiliary lenses. For all types of auxiliary lens, the size of the pupil limits the maximum adjustable angle between observation and illumination though to a varying degree. This means it will not be possible in every case to bring both observation path and the illuminating beam together in the patient's pupil. The maximum adjustable illumination angle becomes smaller with increasing myopia. Convex lenses permit comparatively larger illumination angles with smaller pupils and higher myopia than concave lenses. For convex lenses with their real intermediate image plane, the homocentricity on the fundus between observation and illumination beams is better than with concave lenses. With all methods of examining the peripheral areas of the vitreous body and the fundus, the regions above and below are more easily examined than the lateral regions. This is a result of perspective distortion of the pupil. When observed from above or below, the pupil appears horizontally oval through which the two observation paths of the binocular microscope and the illumination path can easily pass but when viewing through the pupil from the side, it appears as vertically oval, and the three beams cannot pass through together. For this reason, the side regions are seen only monocularly.

To add, a conjunct laser delivery system is installed and mounted onto the slit lamp thereby facilitating laser procedures such as retinal photocoagulation, capsulotomy, iridotomy, trabeculoplasty, etc.

CONCLUSION

Slit-lamp is an instrument comprising of a biomicroscope with a high intensity light source to focus on different ocular structures. The types of illumination in a slit lamp are direct (diffuse and focal) illumination, retro illumination, sclerotic scatter, indirect illumination and specular reflection. The various procedures that the slit lamp aid are fundus examination, gonioscopy, applanation tonometry, contact lens fitting, etc.

CHAPTER 4

Corneal Topography

Francisco Arnalich Montiel, Jorge L Alió Del Barrio, Jorge L Alió y Sanz

BACKGROUND

The cornea is the most important refractive element of the human eye, providing approximately two-thirds of its optical power, accounting for about 43–44 diopters at the corneal apex. Because its surface is irregular and aspherical, it is not radially symmetric, and simple measurement techniques are inadequate.

The great upsurge in refractive surgery led to a need for improved methods to analyze corneal shape since refraction and keratometric data alone were insufficient to predict surgical outcomes. Understanding and quantifying corneal contour or shape has become essential in planning modern surgical intervention for refractive surgery, as well as in corneal transplantation, and it is also very valuable for assessing optical performance of the eye. The different methods for evaluating the anterior surface of the cornea, developed over several centuries, have, in the present era, led to the modern corneal topography.

First Steps in Corneal Measurement

In 1619, Scheiner analyzed corneal curvature by matching the image of a window frame reflected onto a subject's cornea with the image produced by one of his *calibrated spheres*.

Keratometer

In 1854, Helmholtz described the first true keratometer, which he called an *ophthalmometer*. With some minor improvements, it is still being used clinically for calculating refraction, intraocular lens power, and contact lens fitting normal corneas.

This apparatus is based on the tendency of the anterior corneal surface to behave like a convex mirror and reflect light. The projection of four point, mire, onto the cornea, creates a reflected image that can be converted into a corneal radius, "*r*", using a mathematical equation that considers distance from the mire to cornea (75 mm in the keratometer), image size and mire size (64 mm in keratometer). The corneal radius can be transformed into dioptric power using the formula:

$$DP = (\text{Index of refraction of the lens} - 1)/r$$

The *standard keratometric index* represents the combined refractive index of the anterior and posterior surfaces of the cornea, considers the cornea as a single refractive surface, and is 1.3375. Thus, the equation can be simplified to:

$$DP = 337.5/r$$

Although keratometers are still common in ophthalmology clinics, they do have specific limitations that need to be considered in order to avoid misleading conclusions.

- Most traditional keratometers measure the central 3 mm of the cornea, which only accounts for 6% of the entire surface.
- It assumes that the cornea is a perfectly spherocylindrical surface, which it is not. The cornea is aspheric in shape, flattening between the center and the periphery. Usually, the central corneal curvature is fairly uniform, and this is the reason why it can be used to calculate corneal power in normal patients. However, this is not true in some pathologies such as ectatic disorders or after refractive surgery.
- The keratometer provides no information as to the shape of the cornea either inside or outside the contour of the mire. Several corneal shapes can all give the same keratometric value, so this apparatus is of little use should it become necessary to reconstruct the whole corneal morphology.

Keratoscopy and Photokeratoscopy

Goode presented the first keratoscope in 1847. Placido was the first to photograph the corneal reflections of a series of illuminated concentric rings (known as Placido's rings) in 1880 **(Fig. 1)**. Finally, in 1896, Gullstrand was the first to develop a quantitative assessment of photokeratoscopy.

The keratoscope, like a keratometer, projects an illuminated series of mires onto the anterior corneal surface, usually consisting of concentric rings. The distance between the concentric rings or mires gives the observer an idea of the corneal shape. Areas where the *mires* appear closer together correspond to *steeper corneal* curvature, while flatter areas will spread the mires out. Surface irregularity is seen as mire distortion.

When a photographic camera is attached to the keratoscope, we have a photokeratoscope, which gives semiquantitative and qualitative information about the paracentral, midperipheral, and peripheral cornea.

Based on the mathematical equation, it is possible to calculate corneal power from object size. Still, photokeratoscopy gives limited information on the central area, which is not covered by the mires.

Videokeratoscopy

At the beginning of this century, modern corneal topographers were based on videokeratoscopy. A video camera is attached to the keratoscope, and the information is analyzed by a computer that displays a color-coded map of power distribution or corneal curvature of the anterior corneal surface **(Fig. 2)**. It overcomes some of the limitations of other methods, since it measures larger areas of the cornea, with a much larger number of points thus increasing resolutions. Computer technology makes it possible to create permanent records and do multiple data analyses.

FUNDAMENTALS AND TECHNOLOGICAL APPROACHES TO CORNEAL TOPOGRAPHY

Shape of the Normal Cornea

The anterior corneal surface is a refractive surface characterized by an almost spherical shape. The human cornea is not a perfect sphere and is usually assumed to have a conic section. This model could be represented in a simple way by means of the equation:

$$X^2 + Y^2 + (1 + Q)Z^2 - 2RZ = 0$$

where the Z-axis is the axis of revolution of the conic section, R is the radius at the corneal apex, and Q is asphericity, a parameter that is used to specify the type of conicoid.

For a *perfect sphere*, this parameter takes the value of zero ($Q = 0$), for an *ellipsoid* with the major axis in the X-Y plane (*oblate surface*) the asphericity is positive ($Q > 0$), for an *ellipsoid* with the major axis in the Z-axis (*prolate surface*) asphericity is negative ($-1 < Q < 0$), while for a paraboloid with its axis along the Z-axis the value is –1, and it is less than –1 for a hyperboloid.

Other parameters have been defined to classify the conicoid form of the cornea: "P", the shape factor ($P = Q + 1$), or the eccentricity value, "e", defined as $e = -\sqrt{Q}$.

Several studies have shown that the anterior corneal configuration tends to be prolate, i.e., the cornea progressively flattens out periphery by 2–4 diopters of flattening. The asphericity of the normal cornea depends on the study and ranges from –0.26 to –0.11.

This tendency can be detected in the topographic map. Toward the periphery, dioptric power appears to decline, and the nasal area flattens more than the temporal area **(Fig. 3)**. This could be helpful in distinguishing right eye topography from the left eye topography. The topographic patterns of the

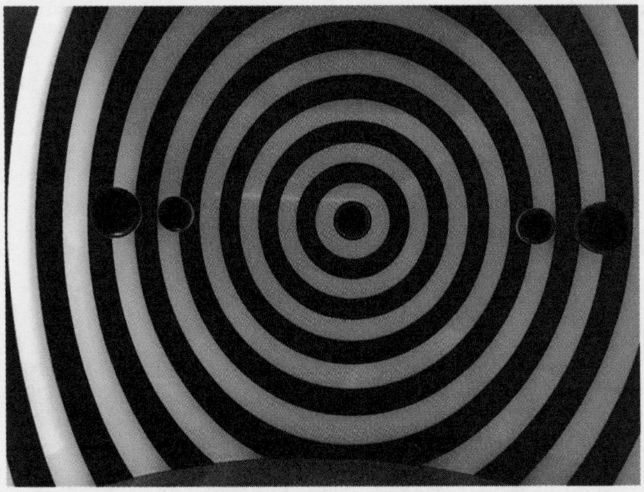

Fig. 1: Placido's rings.

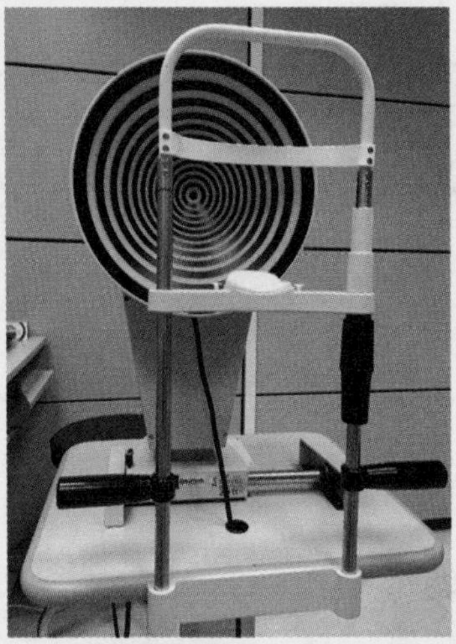

Fig. 2: Videokeratography system.

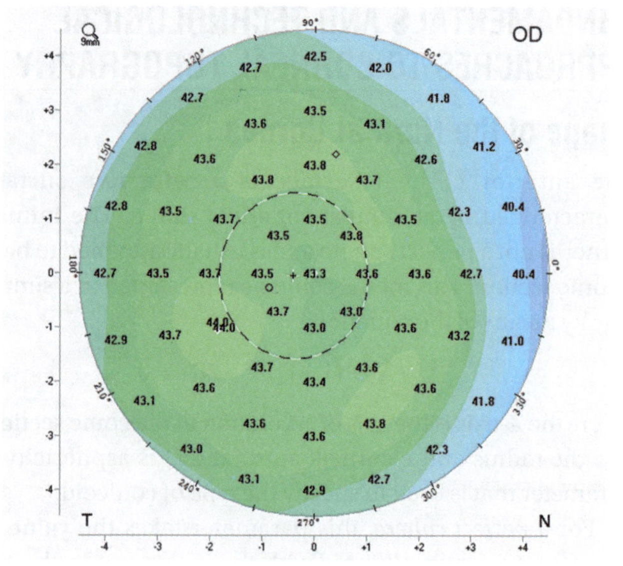

Fig. 3: Corneal topography in a normal right eye. There is a flattening toward the periphery, more pronounced at the nasal area.

two corneas of the same individual often show mirror-image symmetry.

Corneal topographic patterns **(Figs. 4A to D)** have been studied in normal eyes and the following shapes have been found—round (23%), oval (21%), symmetric bow-tie typical for regular astigmatism (18%), asymmetric bow-tie (32%), and irregular astigmatism (7%). In the round and oval shapes, there is an area of uniform dioptric power close to 43 diopters (D) in the center of the cornea. The bow-tie configuration reflects the existence of corneal astigmatism. Depending on the position of the axes, corneal astigmatism is defined as *against-the-rule* (the steepest axis is horizontal), *with-the-rule* (the steepest axis is vertical), or *oblique* (the steepest axis is near the meridian angles of 45° or 135°).

CORNEAL TOPOGRAPHY: CURRENT TECHNOLOGIES

Corneal topography is a noninvasive exploratory technique that graphically describes the geometric characterization

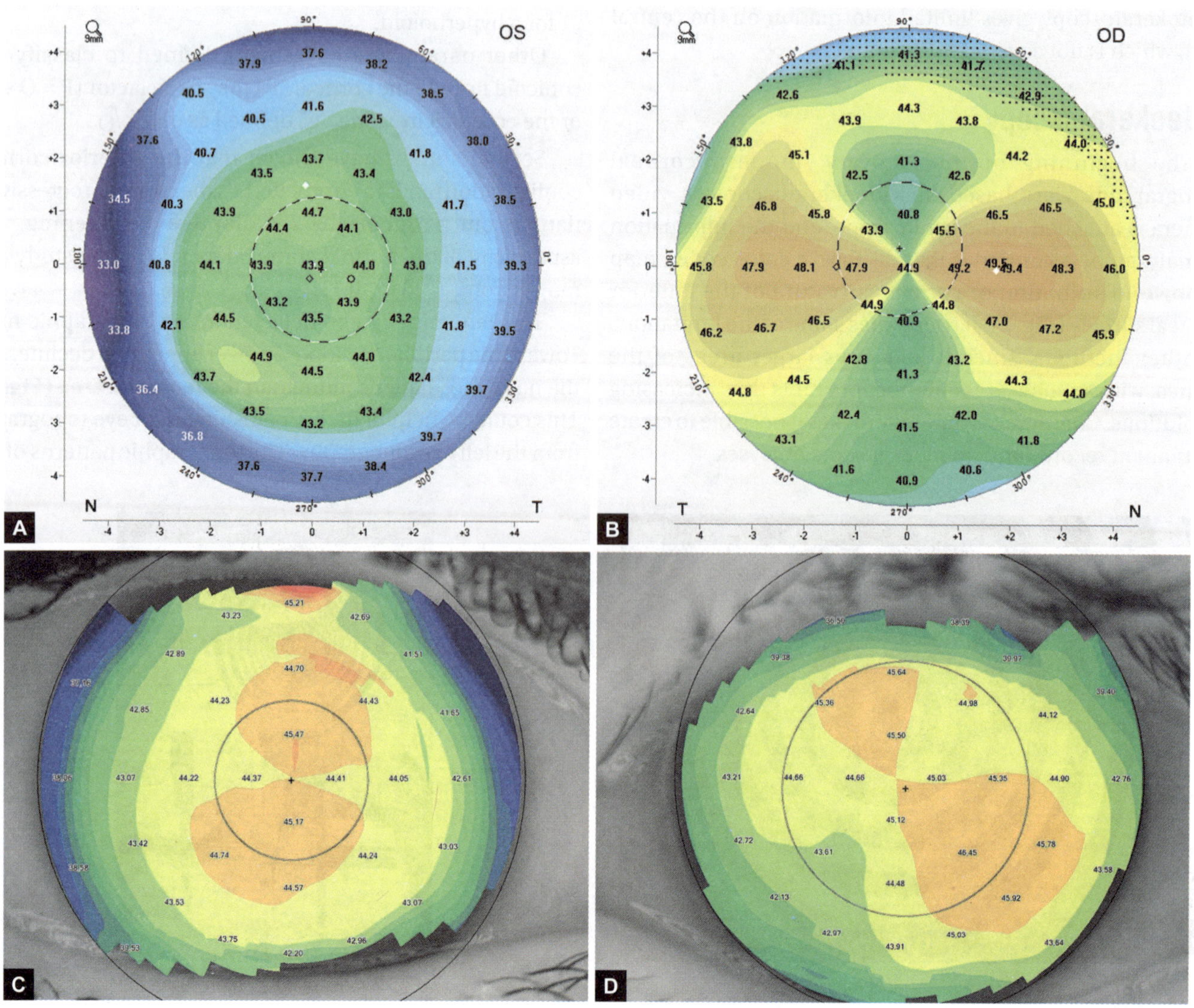

Figs. 4A to D: Normal corneal topographic patterns. (A) Oval topographic pattern; (B) Bow-tie pattern that shows an against-the-rule astigmatism; (C) With-the-rule astigmatism; (D) Oblique astigmatism.

of the morphology of the cornea, which permits us differentiating standard normal patterns from the pathological cornea. Current topographers are based on either systems based on the light reflection on the cornea, or systems based on the projection of a slit light into the cornea with different technology.

Systems Based on the Light Reflection on the Cornea: Curvature-based Topographers

Placido Disk System

A Placido disk system consists of a series of concentric illuminated rings or mires that are reflected off the cornea and recorded by video-computerized systems. The topographer uses an algorithm to translate these reflected images into radial curvature of the corneal surface. Height and slope data derived from the radial curvature of the anterior corneal surface are represented as a corneal keratometric map that follows a color scale developed by the University of Louisiana. Flat curves are represented with cool colors (blue or violet); while warm colors (red and orange) correspond to high curvature. Mild colors (green or yellow) correspond to medium curvature equal to the reference sphere.

Currently, several companies manufacture instruments called videokeratoscopes that picture corneal shape based on the Placido disk method, and, in fact, this approach has been the most clinically and commercially successful up to the last decade. Two types of Placido targets have been used:

1. *Large diameter target (disk-shaped)*: This is less sensitive to misalignment due to a long working distance, but there can be a loss of data due to interference by the patient's brow and nose.
2. *Small diameter target (cone-shaped)*: This is designed for a short working distance and can be influenced by automatic alignment and focusing or compensation of misalignment for accuracy. It does not present data loss due to shadows.

Limitations:

- Placido-based apparatus creates a 3D system by making geometric assumptions about the cornea since the apparatus does not measure corneal surface directly. These assumptions are not accurate for irregular and aspheric corneas.
- The reflection technique depends on the integrity and normality of the tear layer.

Interferometric Method-based Systems

In essence, a reference surface (or its hologram) is compared to the tested surface, the corneal surface, and interference fringes are produced as a result of differences between the two shapes, which can be interpreted as a contour map of surface elevations.

Interference techniques are used in the optical industry to detect lens and mirror aberrations of subwavelength dimensions. High accuracy is theoretically possible, but clinical use has not been very widespread as yet.

Moire Deflectometry-based Systems

The deflections of the rays reflected off the corneal surface are analyzed to build up a surface elevation map.

Systems Based on the Projection of a Slit Light onto the Cornea: Elevation-based Topographers

The common denominator of this technology is the projection of a slit light onto the cornea. Interestingly, many of these corneal topographies integrate a dual technology, and in a first stage, they use light reflection on the cornea by means of a Placido disk to obtain curvature and refractive power data, followed by capturing the image of the scattered light from the slit light to measure corneal elevations of the entire corneal segment. From these two-dimensional (2D) cross sections, it is possible to create a reliable 3D model.

Depending on the spatial arrangement of the photographic systems, we can distinguish two different systems.

Systems Based on the Principle of Normal Photography

Its main feature is that the plane of the camera lens is located parallel with the image. When the slit image is on the cornea, it splits into a specular reflection and a refracted beam that penetrates the corneal surface, and is scattered by the tissue of the cornea. An image of this scattered light within the corneal tissue is captured by an imaging system, which consists of a camera lens located in parallel with the image. It uses triangulation to measure the elevation of the anterior and posterior corneal surface with respect to a reference plane.

The most popular system using this principle is the Orbscan (Bausch & Lomb Incorporated, USA) **(Fig. 5)**, which was the first commercial device that was able to assess the posterior corneal surface. It has dual technology as it uses Placido disk and slit-based systems to obtain 40 slit images of the cornea. These images are captured over 1 second and are then recorded providing different maps of the anterior and posterior corneal surfaces, and also pachymetric data.

Systems Based on the Principle of Scheimpflug Photography

Its main feature is that the plane of the camera lens is placed sideways to the image. Scheimpflug imaging is based on the

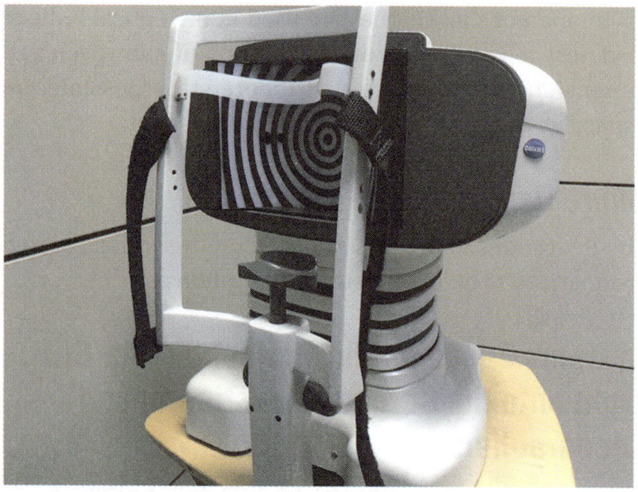

Fig. 5: Orbscan II system.

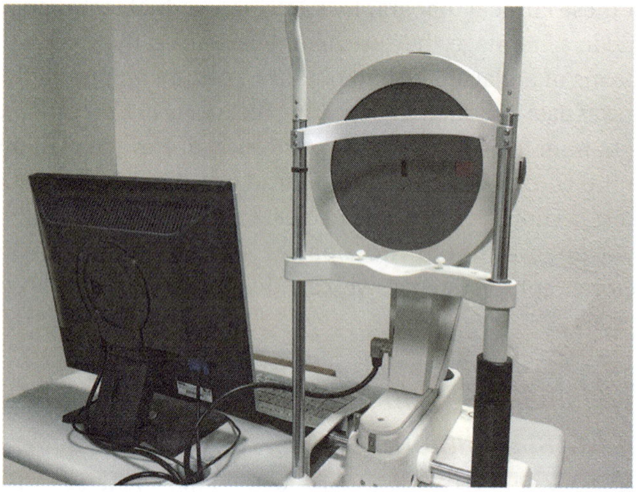

Fig. 6: Scheimpflug-based topographer—Pentacam.

Scheimpflug principle, which occurs when a planar subject is not parallel to the image plane. In this scenario, an oblique tangent can be drawn from the image, object and lens planes, and the point of intersection is the Scheimpflug intersection, where the image is in best focus. With a rotating Scheimpflug camera, the devices can obtain many Scheimpflug images in seconds. The main commercial systems based on this principle are Pentacam (Oculus, USA), Galilei (Ziemer, Switzerland), and Sirius (CSO, Italy), which offer repeatable measurements of the corneal curvature and other anatomical measurements of the anterior segment **(Fig. 6)**.

Although the instruments based on rotating Scheimpflug cameras are considered the most comprehensive and accurate, they also have some limitations. Lower imaging speed can increase the risk of motion artifacts, even though there is an inbuilt second camera to control for eye movements. For example, commercially available Pentacam uses a rotating Scheimpflug camera (180°) to provide a 3D scan of the anterior segment of the eye. It requires 2.0 seconds to complete 25 radial scans. Moreover, radial scanning may not provide sufficient scan density of the corneal periphery, needing interpolation. Another limitation is that the instruments using the Scheimpflug principle are less accurate in comparison to Placido-based ones in providing traditional curvature maps of the anterior surface, and only show moderate agreement in simulated keratometry values. The Sirius system has a dual technology and combines Scheimpflug camera and a small-angle Placido disk topographer with 22 rings. The data for the anterior surface are finally determined by merging the Placido image and the Scheimpflug images using a proprietary method.

Systems with a single Scheimpflug channel use a mathematical equation to estimate compensation for an off-center measurement; however, to properly compensate for an off-center measurement, a dual Scheimpflug technology is needed. Galilei uses a monochromatic slit-light source which combines dual Scheimpflug cameras and a Placido disk to measure both anterior and posterior corneal surfaces.

Systems Based on Optical Coherence Tomography

Optical coherence tomography (OCT) of the cornea and anterior segment is an optical method of cross-sectional scanning based on reflection and scattering of light from the structures within the cornea. Measuring different reflectivity from structures within the cornea by a method of optical interferometry produces the cross-sectional image of the cornea and other anterior segment structures.

In optical interferometry, the light source is split into the reference and measurement beams. The measurement beam is reflected from ocular structures and interacts with the reference light reflected from the reference mirror, a phenomenon called interference. The coherent or positive interference characterized by an increased resulting signal is measured by the interferometer, and, subsequently, the position of the reflecting structure of the eye can be determined.

In this way, the structures of the anterior segment can be visualized with a high degree of resolution (currently 18 microns axial and 60 microns transverse).

In 2005, a commercial 1,310 time-domain OCT system for anterior segment imaging was launched under the name Visante OCT (Carl Zeiss, Inc.). Currently, although it is widely used OCT device for dedicated in vivo anterior segment imaging and creates pachymetry maps, it cannot perform topographic analysis of the cornea, mostly because of limitations in acquisition time. The introduction of Fourier-domain OCT in 2002 with the primary advantage of increased sensitivity or speed and the possibility of 3D imaging promised to improve the ability of OCT to quantitatively assess the corneal topography. Nowadays, commercial high-speed 3D anterior-segment OCT, based on swept-source OCT, provides higher resolution cross-sectional images that can be used to obtain OCT-based corneal topography. The commercially available OCT-based topographer is SS-1000 CASIA (Tomey Corporation, Inc., Nagoya, Japan) **(Figs. 7 and 9)**.

PERFORMING A GOOD TOPOGRAPHY EXAMINATION

Corneal topography is a noninvasive imaging technique for mapping the surface curvature of the cornea. The specific method varies depending on the device used, but some aspects are common. The patient is seated facing a bowl containing an illuminated pattern which is focused on the anterior surface of his cornea. The reflected pattern is analyzed by a computer that calculates the shape of the cornea by means of different graphic formulae. Although computer programs are created to be very accurate, they cannot recognize, and account for, every problem. Critical points for precise measurement are accurate alignment, centering, and focusing. They depend on the ability of the examiner to take a good measurement. Another potential source of error is tear film irregularities, e.g. focal flattening over a dry patch. These may be most easily identified on the raw image.

Tear film breakup causes mistracking of the mires and artifacts in the topography pattern and will apparently look like significant irregularities **(Fig. 8)**. These corneal irregularities could suggest a corneal pathology, such as keratoconus, and result in wrong diagnosis **(Figs. 9A and B)**. To avoid disturbing the tear film, corneal topography should be performed before administering dilating drops and taking intraocular pressures.

In addition, one must avoid artifacts induced by the nose or the eyelids which can lead to a loss of information in certain areas **(Figs. 10A and B)**. These errors are transformed into black areas or areas without data on the topographic map. Correct positioning of the head, eyes and eyelid opening should be ensured to avoid these problems.

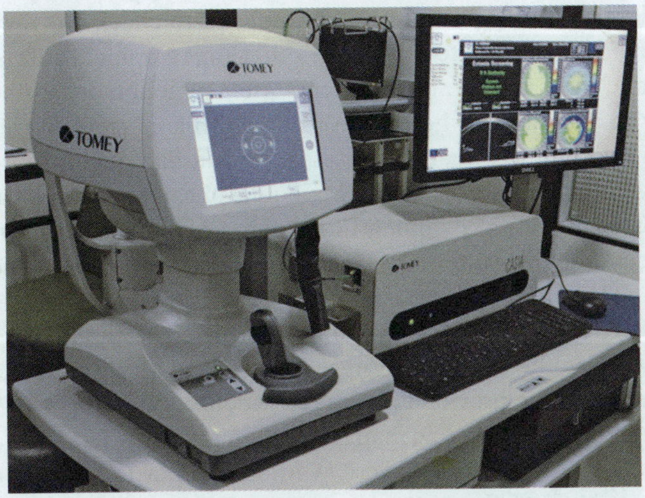

Fig. 7: OCT-based topographer—CASIA SS-1000. (OCT: optical coherence tomography)

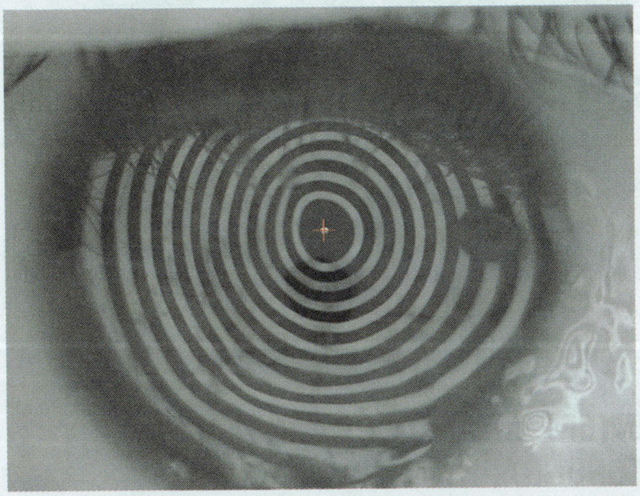

Fig. 8: Distortion of the Placido's rings because of tear film breakup.

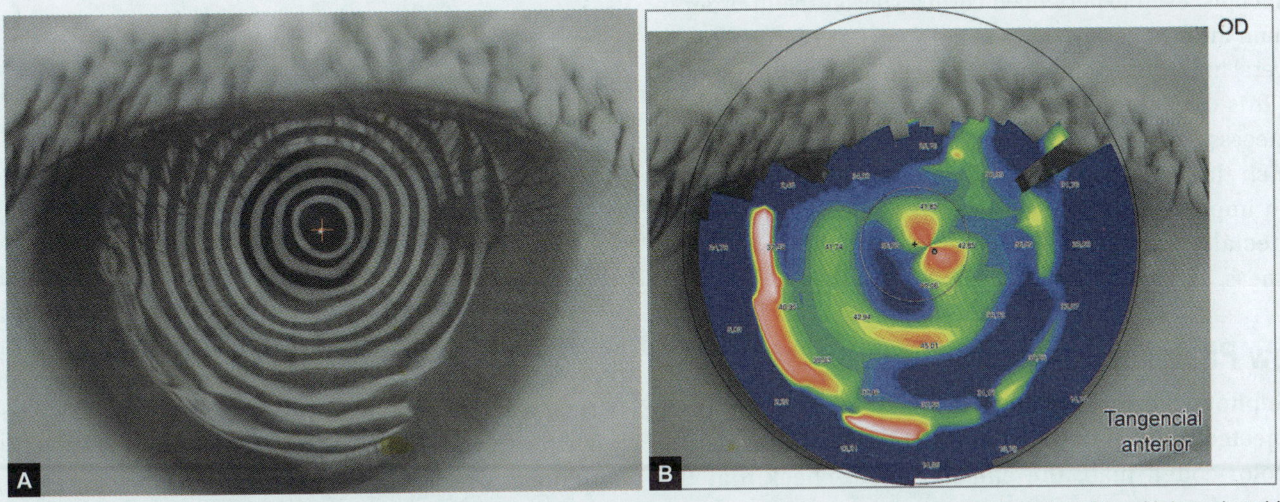

Figs. 9A and B: (A) Raw image; (B) Topographic irregularities and patches of the map in the same eye because of a tear film with large instability.

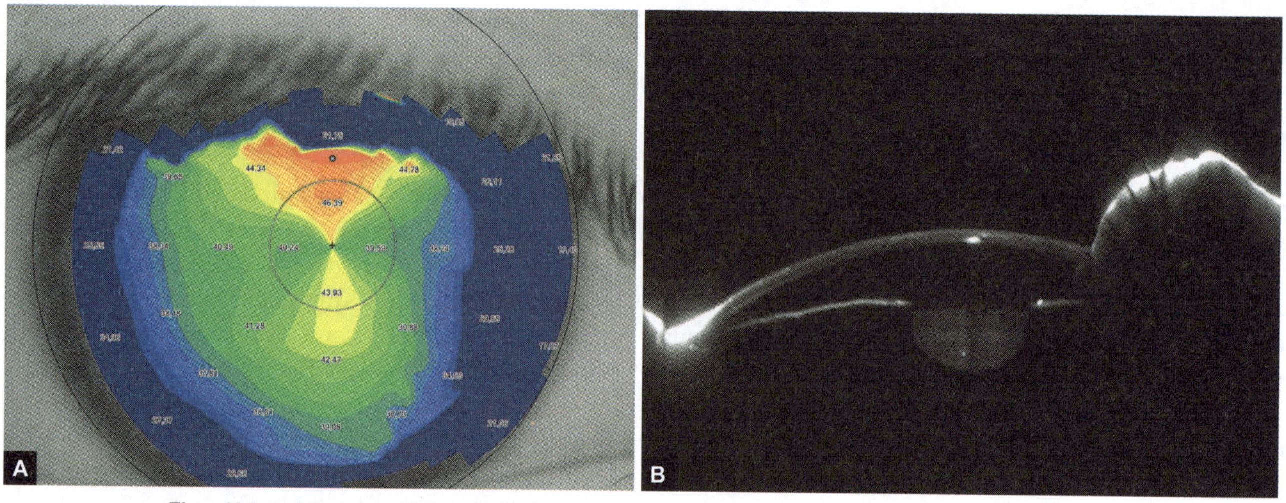

Figs. 10A and B: Loss of information of certain areas of the cornea due to eyelids not opened enough.

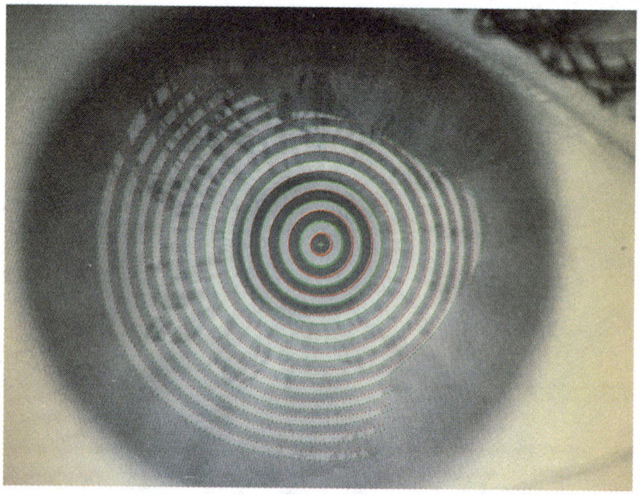

Fig. 11: Photokeratoscope raw image.

INTERPRETATION OF CORNEAL TOPOGRAPHY MAPS

Accurate interpretation of corneal shape using color-coded topographic maps is difficult and confusing for many clinicians, even experienced cornea specialists. In order to obtain the best performance in the analysis of corneal maps, several important points must be taken into consideration.

It is critical to check the raw image first. After that, it is necessary to focus on the scale and step intervals with which the color-coded topographic map is built up. It is also important to review different topographic displays, especially when evaluating irregular or postsurgery corneas.

Raw Photokeratoscope Image

The photokeratoscope image displays the Placido's rings projected onto the cornea **(Fig. 11)**. When considering a color-coded map, the clinician must check that the unprocessed data, upon which it is based, are reliable. If the videokeratoscope image is irregular, data cannot be processed by the instrument in a meaningful way.

Thus, for Placido disk-based computerized videokeratoscopes, the videokeratoscope image should not be ignored. In fact, it is recommended to check this map before referring to any of the other topographic displays, and to go back to it when there are any doubts regarding the accuracy of the displayed data. This image provides important information for assessing tear film quality, mire centering on the cornea, lid opening, or the causes of local irregularities, and other artifacts. If the device used displays computer tracking of the Placido mires it is important to rule out tracking errors.

Devices that rely only on scanning slit technology to analyze the anterior corneal surface lack of the valuable information provided by the raw videokeratoscope image. Whether the resulting map is based on reliable primary data or not is impossible to verify without the raw image. Some instruments identify regions of uncertainty, showing mire distortions that cannot be reliable, by leaving blank areas on the color-coded map. Other instruments merely extrapolate onto the uncertain regions information gathered from adjacent regions with reliable data.

For Scheimpflug technology, the Scheimpflug images should also be checked before looking at the resulting maps, and correct centration and focus should be assured.

Color-coded Scales

The shape of a cornea can be measured and represented by color-coded maps in which a given color indicates a different curvature or elevation. The usual color spectrum for corneal powers shows near-normal power as green, lower than normal power as cool colors (blues), and higher than normal powers as warm colors (reds). Most topographers offer absolute as well as normalized scales to allow the clinician to customize the information for maximal clinical value **(Figs. 12A and B)**:

- *Normalized scale (variable scale)* uses a given color for different curvatures or elevations on each cornea analyzed, depending on the range for that particular cornea, determined by its flattest and steepest values. These maps are difficult to interpret and can lead to an incorrect diagnosis since they may magnify subtle changes in corneal surface, if the scale is too narrow, or minimize large distortions, if the scale is too wide. In addition, color recognition, one of the primary clues used to interpret on corneal topography, is lost with a variable scale, since it uses different colors for different eyes.
- *Absolute scale (fixed scale)* uses the same color for the same curvature or elevation no matter which eye is examined. However, there are many different absolute scales since the examiner can choose different variables such as range or step size (intervals in color changes). For the specified scale, however, each display will use the same colors, steps and range. In order to facilitate comparisons over time and between patients, it is recommended to stick with a given fixed scale for routine examinations and to change the scale in the particular cases in which this becomes necessary. As an example, the popular Klyce/Wilson scale ranges from 28 D to 65 D in equal 1.5 D intervals. Currently, there is no consensus as to the best absolute scale, but in general, dioptric scales with intervals smaller than 0.5 D are not clinically useful and provide details that are not relevant and may complicate map interpretation. For corneas with large dioptric ranges, for instance in advanced keratoconus intervals greater than 0.5 D are recommended. Regarding scales for elevation maps, elevation steps of approximately 5 microns appear to be clinically useful.

As mentioned previously, color pattern recognition makes it possible to identify common topographic patterns such as the corneal cylinder **(Fig. 13)**, keratoconus (local area of inferonasal steepening) or pellucid marginal degeneration (butterfly-pattern or inferior arcuate steepening), as well as features associated with refractive surgery **(Fig. 14)**, such as optical zone size, centration, and central islands.

Topographic Displays: Corneal Maps

Maps can be obtained from the anterior and the posterior surface except in the case of pure Placido disk technology.

- *Axial map (sagittal map):* Although this is the original and most commonly used map, its values only provide a good approximation for the paracentral cornea **(Fig. 15A)**. The axial map measures the radius of curvature for a comparable sphere (with the same tangent as the point in question) with a center of rotation on the axis of the videokeratoscope. Localized changes in curvature and peripheral data are poorly represented because of the spherical bias of the reference optical axis. However, newer algorithms in some devices (e.g. arc-step method) have improved the accuracy of curvature measurements in the peripheral region.
- *Local tangential curvature map (instantaneous map):* The tangential map displays the tangential/instantaneous/local radius of curvature or tangential power, which is calculated by referring to the neighboring points and not to the axis of the videokeratoscope **(Fig. 15B)**. Tangential maps reflect local changes and peripheral data better than axial maps. They are very useful in detecting local irregularities, corneal ectatic diseases, or surgically induced changes. For example, in keratoconus corneas with a displaced apex, tangential maps are less influenced

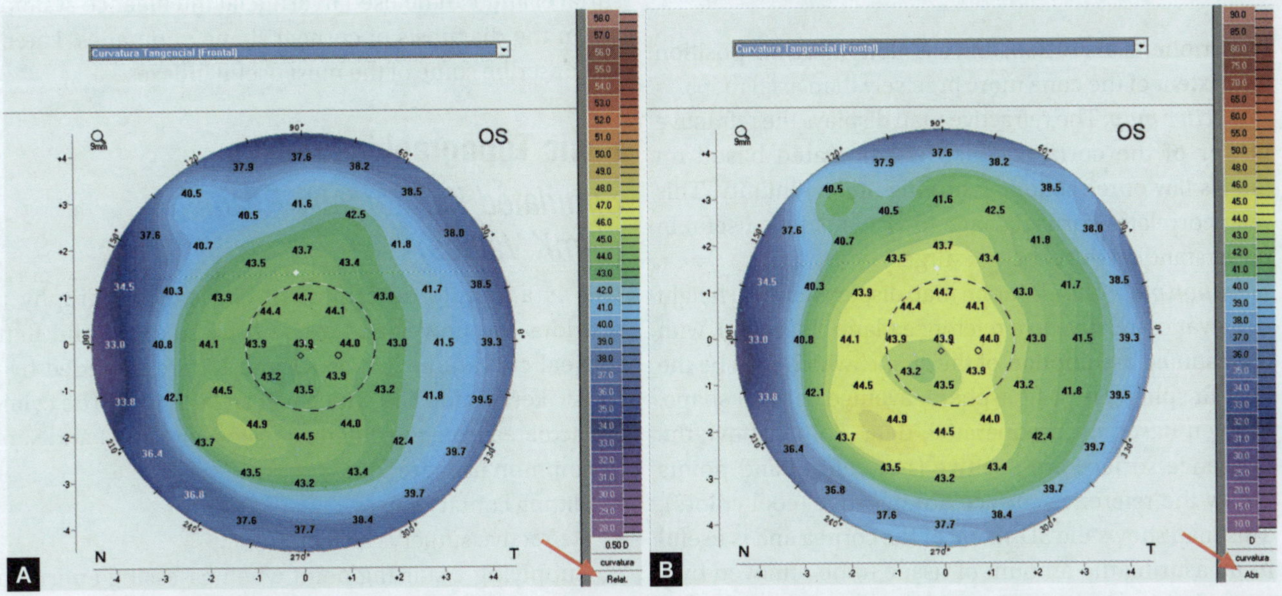

Figs. 12A and B: Corneal topography map represented using (A) a normalized relative scale, and (B) an absolute scale.

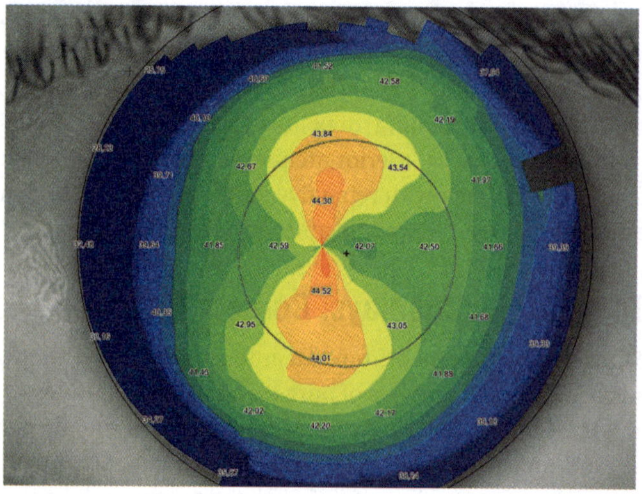

Fig. 13: Bow-tie pattern.

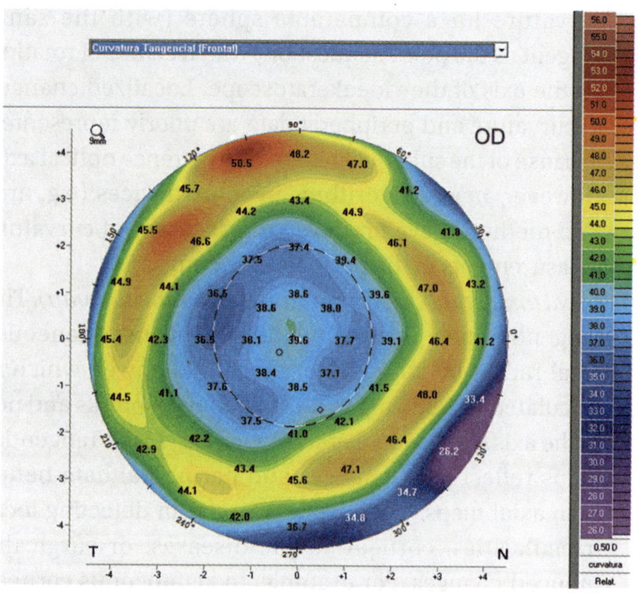

Fig. 14: Corneal topography after myopic LASIK.
(LASIK: Laser in situ keratomileusis)

by peripheral distortion, and can determine the position and extent of the cone more precisely than axial maps.

- *Refractive map:* The refractive map displays the refractive power of the cornea, which is calculated based on Snell's law of refraction, assuming optical infinity. This map correlates corneal shape to vision, and is useful in understanding the effects of surgery.
- *Elevation map:* The elevation map displays corneal height or elevation relative to a reference plane **(Fig. 15C)**, with a presumed assumption of the shape, which may be the best-fit sphere, best-fit asphere, average corneal shape, or even based on preoperative data. Points above the reference surface are positive (hot colors) and points below the reference surface are negative (cool colors). This map shows the 3D shape of the cornea and is useful in measuring the amount of tissue to be removed by a procedure, assessing postoperative visual problems, or planning and/or monitoring surgical procedures.
- *Difference map:* The difference map displays the changes in certain values between two maps **(Fig. 16)**. It is used to monitor any type of change, such as recovery from contact lens-induced warpage or surgery-induced changes.
- *Relative map:* The relative map displays some values by comparing them to an arbitrary standard (e.g. sphere, asphere, or normal cornea) and a specific mathematical model. This map enhances or magnifies unique features of the cornea being examined.
- *Corneal thickness maps* **(Fig. 15D)**: It is useful.
- *Irregularity map (surface quality maps):* The irregularity map uses the same technique as the elevation map, but takes as a reference surface the best-fit spherocylindrical toric surface. The difference between the actual surface and the theoretical surface represents that part of the cornea that cannot be optically corrected. Like refractive power maps, the irregularity map only has clinical meaning when considering the values over the pupillary area.

Numerous other displays, including 3D maps, astigmatic vector analysis, etc., are available but less used.

QUANTITATIVE DESCRIPTORS OF CORNEAL TOPOGRAPHY

Corneal Indexes

Color-coded maps provide a rapid visual method for clinical diagnosis, but do not supply numerical values that can be used for clinical management. Several corneal indexes describe different features of corneal topography quantitatively and are of great aid in contact lens fitting, for improved assessment of the optical quality of the corneal surface, and can be used in artificial intelligence systems to aid in the diagnosis of corneal shape anomalies. Later, we will describe some of the most useful indexes.

Basic Topographic Indexes

Simulated Keratometry Reading (SimK Values)

This is a simple descriptor of corneal topography that provides the power and axes of the steepest and flattest corneal curvatures just as K1 and K2 are provided by the classic keratometer, to which it correlates well. The cylinder is calculated from the difference between SimK1 and SimK2. Its common uses are:

- Fitting contact lenses
- Refractive surgery calculations
- Supplying a starting point when assessing an irregular corneal shape, since it gives the quantity and axis of astigmatism.

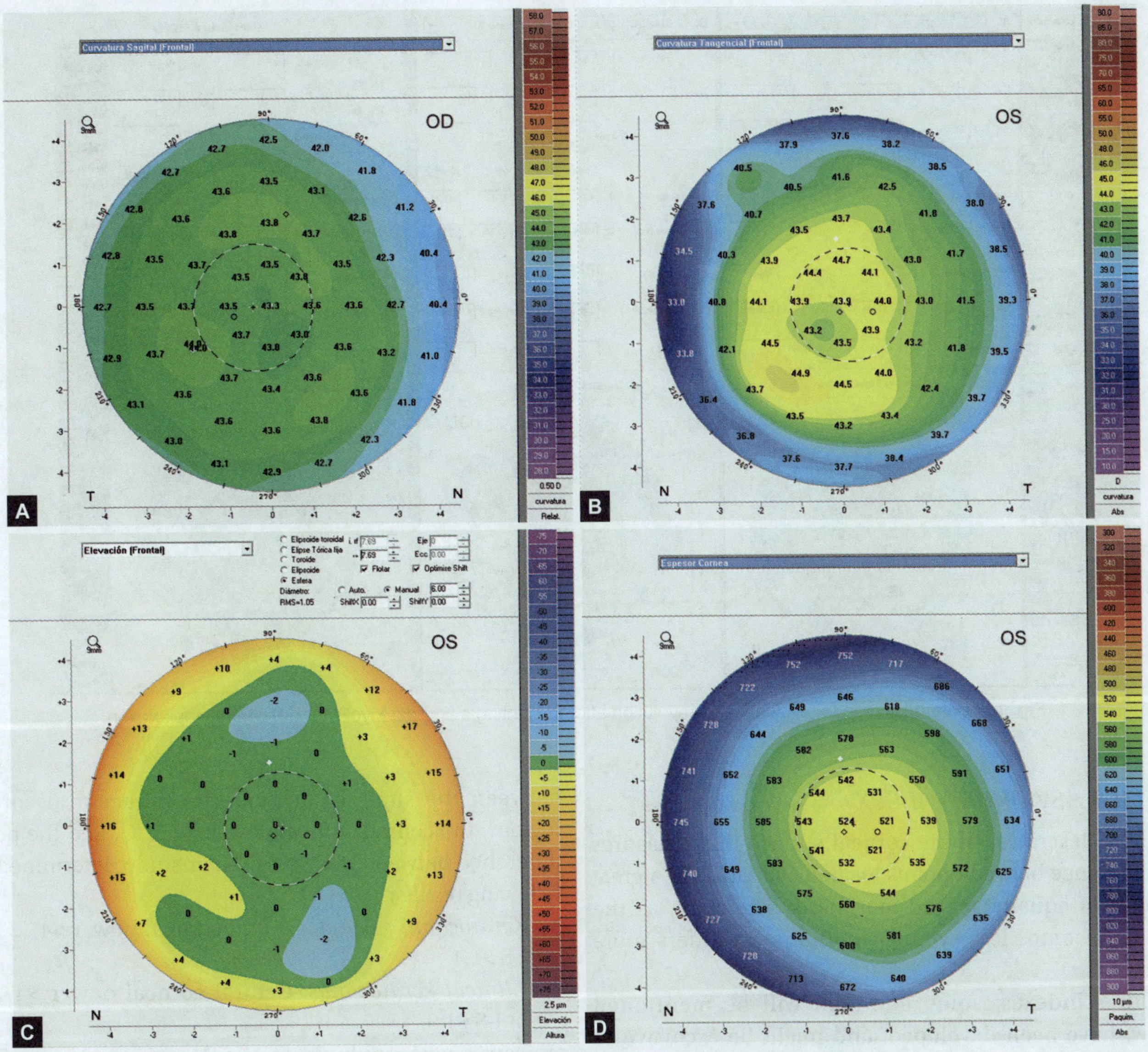

Figs. 15A to D: Different kinds of topography maps for the same cornea. (A) Sagittal axial map; (B) Instantaneous or tangential map; (C) Elevation map; (D) Pachymetry map.

Minimum Keratometry Reading (MinK)

This is the minimum meridional power from rings 7, 8, and 9. The average power as well as axis is displayed.

Corneal Eccentricity Index

This index estimates the eccentricity of the central cornea, and is calculated by fitting an ellipse to the corneal elevation data. A positive value is for a prolate surface, negative value for an oblate surface (e.g. flattened corneas after myopic refractive surgery), and zero value for a perfect sphere. Normal central corneas are prolate, meaning they are steeper in the center than in the periphery, and tend to be around 0.30. This value is used for fitting the contact lenses.

Average Corneal Power

This is the area-corrected average of corneal power in front of the pupil. It usually corresponds to the spherical equivalent of the classic keratometer, except after decentered refractive surgery. It may be helpful in determining central corneal curvature when calculating the appropriate intraocular lens.

Surface Regularity Index and Potential Visual Acuity

Surface regularity index (SRI) measures the regularity of the corneal surface that correlates with the best spectacle-corrected visual acuity assuming the cornea to be the only limiting factor. This index adds up the meridional mire-to-mire power changes over the apparent pupil entrance. The SRI value increases with increase in the irregularity of the corneal surface, and its normal value is less than 1.0. It measures optical quality.

Potential visual acuity (PVA) is a range of the expected visual acuity that is achievable based on the corneal topography and can be calculated based on SRI.

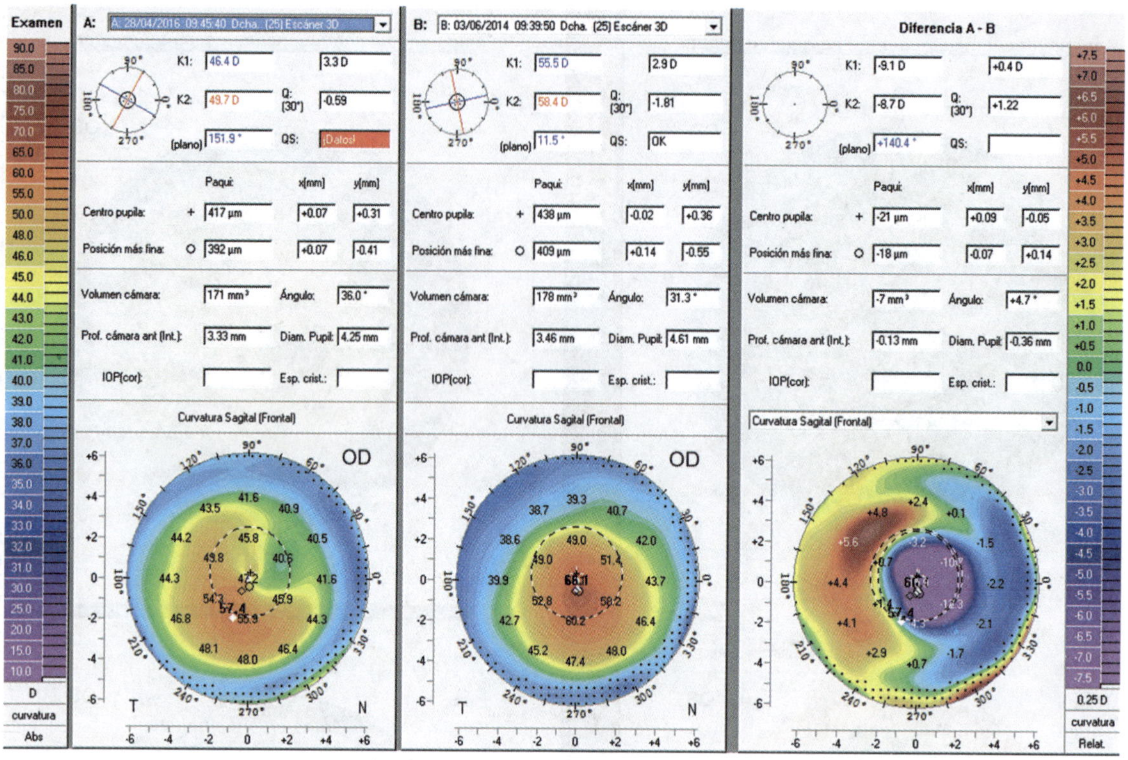

Fig. 16: Difference map for evaluating the evolution after implanting a corneal MyoRing with central applanation.

Surface Asymmetry Index

This is a descriptor of the corneal surface that measures the difference between points located 180° apart in a great number of equally spaced meridians. Therefore, as the cornea becomes less symmetric, the index differs more from 0.

Other indexes, some of which will be mentioned below, have been developed, and might be exclusive to one particular topographer. The clinician should evaluate the meaning, utility and validity of each index since some indexes have been tested in peer-reviewed literature while others have not.

Screening Tools and Artificial Intelligence Programs (Neural Networks) for Classification and Autodiagnosis

As mentioned previously, even for the experienced personnel, interpretation of topography can be difficult, particularly when trying to differentiate the early stages of a disease from a normal cornea (suspected keratoconus), or when trying to differentiate between two similar conditions (contact lens warpage vs. early keratoconus). Several mathematical algorithms have been developed to help solve this problem, with high sensitivity and specificity.

Rabinowitz and McDonnell developed the first numerical method for detecting keratoconus using only topographic data. They use the I-S value, which measures the differences between the superior and inferior paracentral corneal regions, the central corneal power (Max K), and the power difference between both eyes. Their study determined the following results:

- *Keratoconus suspect:* Central corneal power >47.2 D or I-S >1.4.
- *Clinical keratoconus:* Central corneal power >47.8 D or I-S >1.9.

However, using only these simple measurements for a diagnosis could create specificity problems. To solve the specificity problem, the new strategy must be able to detect and consider the unique characteristics of keratoconus maps, such as local abnormal elevations.

The Keratoconus Prediction Index

Keratoconus prediction index, developed by Maeda et al. is calculated from the differential sector index (DSI), the opposite sector index (OSI), the center/surround index (CSI), the surface asymmetry index (SAI), the irregular astigmatism index (IAI), and the percent analyzed area (AA). This method partially overcomes the specificity limitation.

Neural Network Model

Maeda et al. also developed the neural network model, based on artificial intelligence. It is a much more sophisticated method for classifying corneal topography and detecting different corneal topographic abnormalities; it employs indexes that were empirically found to capture specific characteristics of the different corneal pathologies, including keratoconus. Further modifications in neural network approach developed by Smolek and Klyce supposedly produce 100% accuracy, specificity, and sensitivity in diagnosing keratoconus.

The Pentacam system, for instance, has developed seven indexes of corneal irregularity within the central cornea for the grading and classification of keratoconus [tomographic keratoconus classification (TKC)], as well as the postoperative assessment **(Fig. 17)**. These indexes include index of surface variance (ISV), index of vertical asymmetry (IVA), keratoconus index (KI), central keratoconus index (CKI), index of height asymmetry (IHA), index of height decentration (IHD), and index of minimum radius of curvature (Rmin). This machine also provides with two diagrams that describe the change of corneal thickness in relation to location, and a progression index of this thickness/location relationship to suggest the presence or not of an ectatic disease. In addition to this, the Pentacam tomography includes a new software adaptation called the Belin/Ambrosio-enhanced ectasia display (BAD) that combines both the anterior and posterior elevation data and pachymetric data to orient in the diagnosis of corneal ectasia.

The Sirius system displays a keratoconus summary to aid in the diagnosis and the follow-up of keratoconus combining indices based on curvature, pachymetry and elevation such as the symmetry index of the front and back surface, or the Baiocchi Calossi Versaci front and back index (BCV f and BCV b) to evaluate coma and trefoil aberrations.

The Casia OCT system has a built-in software that estimates ectasia similarity of a scan, and this is calculated as the ectasia similarity score **(Fig. 18)**. This score is presented in percentage of similarity.

CORNEAL ABERROMETRY: FUNDAMENTALS AND CLINICAL APPLICATIONS

Whenever a point object does not form a point image on the retina, as it should be in an ideal optical system, one encounters an optical aberration. Although one may feel that he is measuring the total refractive error, when refracting a patient, one is actually only considering two components of a whole host of refractive components in the optics of the eye. However, these two components, sphere and cylinder do constitute the main optical aberrations of an eye. Even in a normal eye with no subjective need for refraction, optical aberrations can be detected.

Since the cornea has the highest refractive power, more than 70% of the eye's refraction, it is the principal site of aberrations, although the lens and the tear film may also contribute to aberrations.

MEASURING WAVEFRONT ABERRATION

Measuring Total Wavefront Aberration

It is possible to express ideal image formation by means of waves. An ideal optical system will provide a spherical converging wave centered at the ideal point image. However, in practice, the resulting wavefront differs from this ideal wavefront. The deviation from this ideal wavefront is called wavefront aberration, and the more it differs from zero, the more the real image differs from the ideal image and the

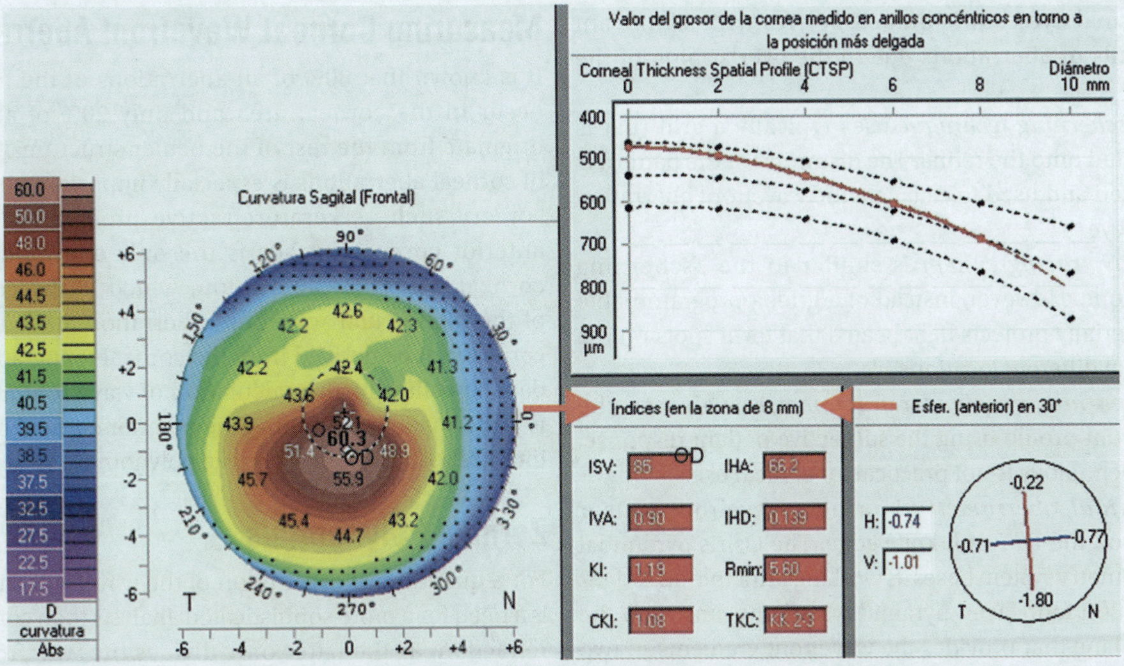

Fig. 17: Indices of cornea irregularity—Pentacam in a patient with keratoconus.

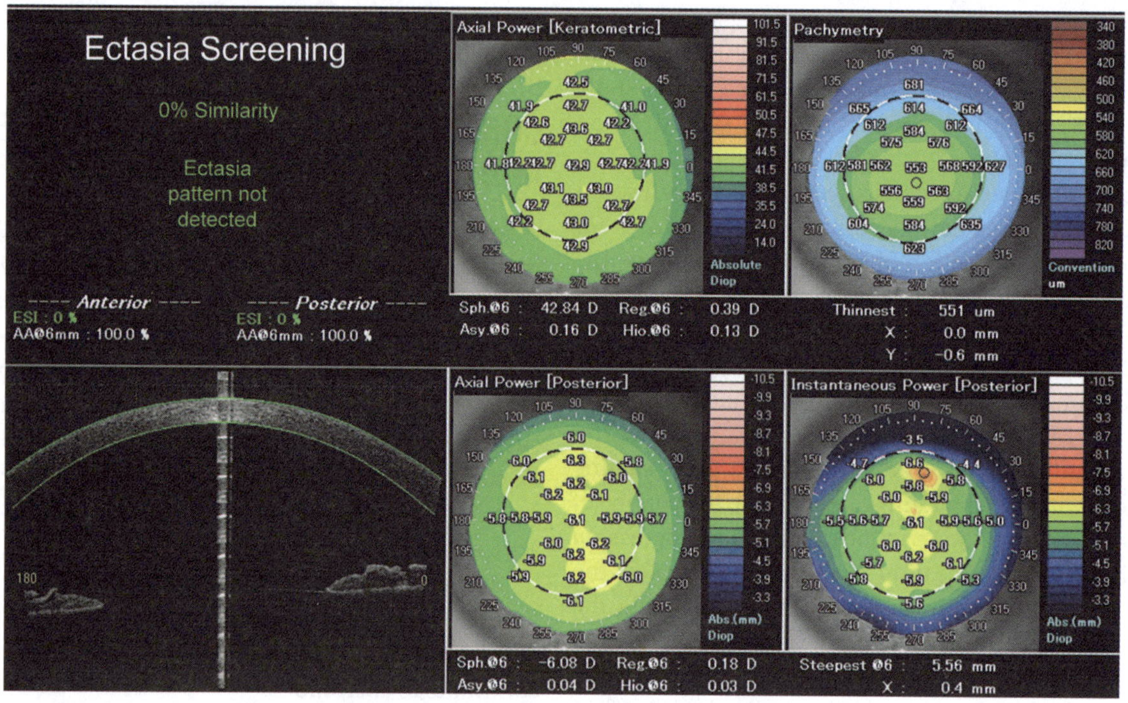

Fig. 18: Ectasia similarity score by CASIA S-100 of a normal cornea.

worse the image quality. Ocular wavefront sensing devices use five main technologies to determine the resulting or output wave:

1. *The Shack-Hartmann method* is the most widely used and is inspired by astronomy technology. It consists of analyzing the wave emerging from the eye after directing a small low energy laser beam. This reflected wave is divided by means of a series of small lenses (lenslet array), which generates focused spots. The position of spots is recorded and compared to the ideal one. This type of aberrometer provides reproducible measurements in normal eyes but is limited in eyes with significant amounts of aberrations due to the overlapping of the spots.
2. *The Tscherning technique* uses typically a grid that is projected onto the retina. The distortion of the pattern is analyzed and used to calculate the wavefront aberration of the eye.
3. *The ray tracing system* is similar to the Tscherning technique. However, instead of a grid, a programmable laser serially projects light beams that form spots on the retina at different locations.
4. *The spatially resolved refractometer* evaluates the wavefront profile using the subjective patient response. This technology is not practical for clinical use.
5. *Pyramidal aberrometry* is a new wavefront sensor based on the Foucault knife edge. The Osiris pyramidal aberrometry system bases its working principle on a high-resolution four-faced pyramid wavefront sensor on the focal plane that provides the wavefront gradients in two orthogonal directions and four pupil. Images (known as subpupil) distributed by their intensity—each subpupil performs a Foucault knife-edge test to derive slope and shape of the wavefront. Since wavefront is sampled in the very last stage of the optical path, the resolution of the device is extremely high compared to commercial sensors. Finally, the device seems to make possible the analysis of very irregular corneas probably due to his fuzzy dynamic range and to the absence of problems related to sample overlapping, so it might allow higher sensitivity than Hartmann-Shack wavefront sensor.

Measuring Corneal Wavefront Aberration

It is known that 80% of all aberrations of the human eye occur in the corneal area and only 20% of aberrations originate from the rest of the ocular structures. The effect of corneal aberrations is especially important after corneal surgery such as keratorefractive procedures since the anterior corneal surface is the only one modified. The corneal wavefront aberration, which is the component of the total ocular wavefront aberration attributed to the cornea, can be derived from the corneal topographic height data. Specifically, the calculation of wavefront aberrations is performed by expanding the anterior corneal height data into a set of orthogonal Zernike polynomials **(Fig. 19)**.

Zernike Polynomials

For a quantitative description of the wavefront shape, there is a need for a more sophisticated analysis than conventional refraction, as the latter only divides the wavefront in two basic terms—sphere and cylinder. One can obtain more

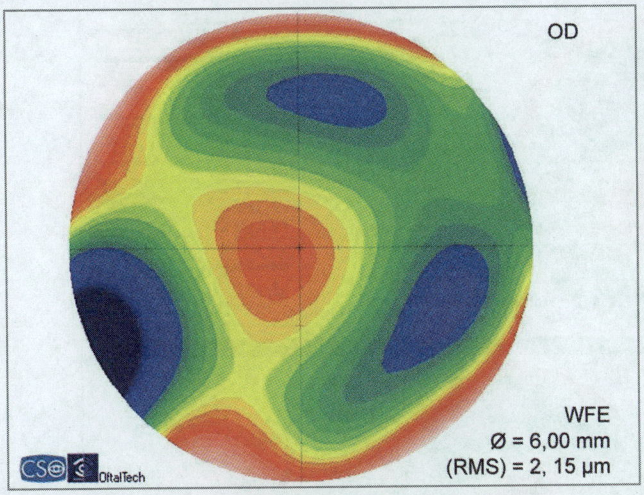

Fig. 19: Corneal wavefront analysis derived from height topography data.

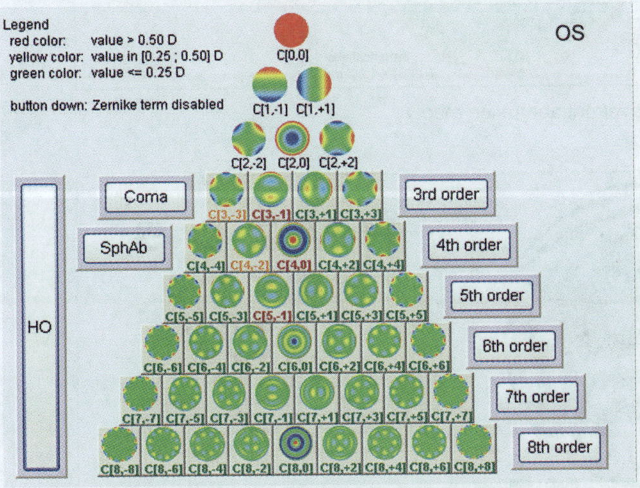

Fig. 20: Zernike polynomial expansion.

information by breaking down the wavefront into terms, which are clinically meaningful, besides the sphere and the cylinder. For this purpose, a standard equation has been universally accepted by refractive surgeons and vision scientists, known as Zernike polynomials.

Zernike polynomials are equations which are used to fit the wavefront data in a 3D way. The wavefront function is decomposed into terms that describe specific optical aberrations such as spherical aberration, coma, etc. **(Fig. 20)**. Each term in the polynomial has two variables, ρ (rho) and θ (theta), where ρ is the normalized distance of a specific point from the center of the pupil and θ is the angle formed between the imaginary line joining the pupillary center with the point of interest and the horizontal. According to that, we can imagine that aberrations are strongly influenced by pupil size, and, therefore, aberrometric measurements should be related to the diameter of the patient's pupil.

Zernike terms (Z_n^m) are defined using a double index notation—a radial order (n) and an angular frequency (m). When talking about first, second, third, etc. aberrations we point to indicate the radial order (n). Each radial order involves n + 1 terms. There are an infinite number of Zernike terms that can be used to fit an individual wavefront. However, for clinical practice, terms up to the fourth radial order are usually considered:

1. Zernike terms below third order can be measured and corrected by conventional optical means. *The first order term*, the prism, is not relevant to the wavefront as it represents tilt and is corrected using a prism. *The second order* terms represent *low order aberrations* that include defocus (spherical component of the wavefront) and astigmatism (cylinder component). Wavefront maps that measure only defocus and astigmatism can be perfectly corrected using spectacles and contact lenses.
2. After the second radial order comes the *high order aberration*. High order aberrations are not measured by conventional refraction or autorefraction. The aberrometer is the only method available that can quantify these complex kinds of distortions.
3. *Third order* terms describe coma and trefoil defects.
4. *Fourth order* terms represent tetrafoil, spherical aberration and secondary astigmatism components.

Because spherical and coma aberrations refer to symmetrical systems and the eye is not rotationally symmetrical, the terms spherical-like and coma-like aberrations are normally used **(Fig. 21)**.

Wavefront Maps

Wavefront map describes the optical path difference between the measured wavefront and the reference wavefront in microns at the pupil entrance. The wavefront error is derived mathematically from the reconstructed wavefront by one of the techniques described above. It is plotted as a 2D or 3D map for qualitative analysis in a similar fashion to corneal topography maps. In wavefront error maps, each color represents a specific degree of wavefront error in microns **(Fig. 21)**, and like in corneal topography maps, it is necessary to consider the range and the interval of the scale.

Optical and Image Quality

In order to evaluate the impact of aberrations on visual quality following quantitative parameters have been defined **(Fig. 22)**:

- *Peak to valley error (PV error):* This is a simple measure of the distance from the lowest point to the highest point on the wavefront and is not the best measurement of optical quality since it does not represent the extent of the defect.
- *Root mean square (RMS) error:* This measure is by far the most widely used. In a simple way, the RMS wavefront error is a statistical measure of the deviation of the ocular or corneal wavefront from the ideal **(Table 1)**. In other words, it describes the overall aberration and indicates how bad individual aberrations are.

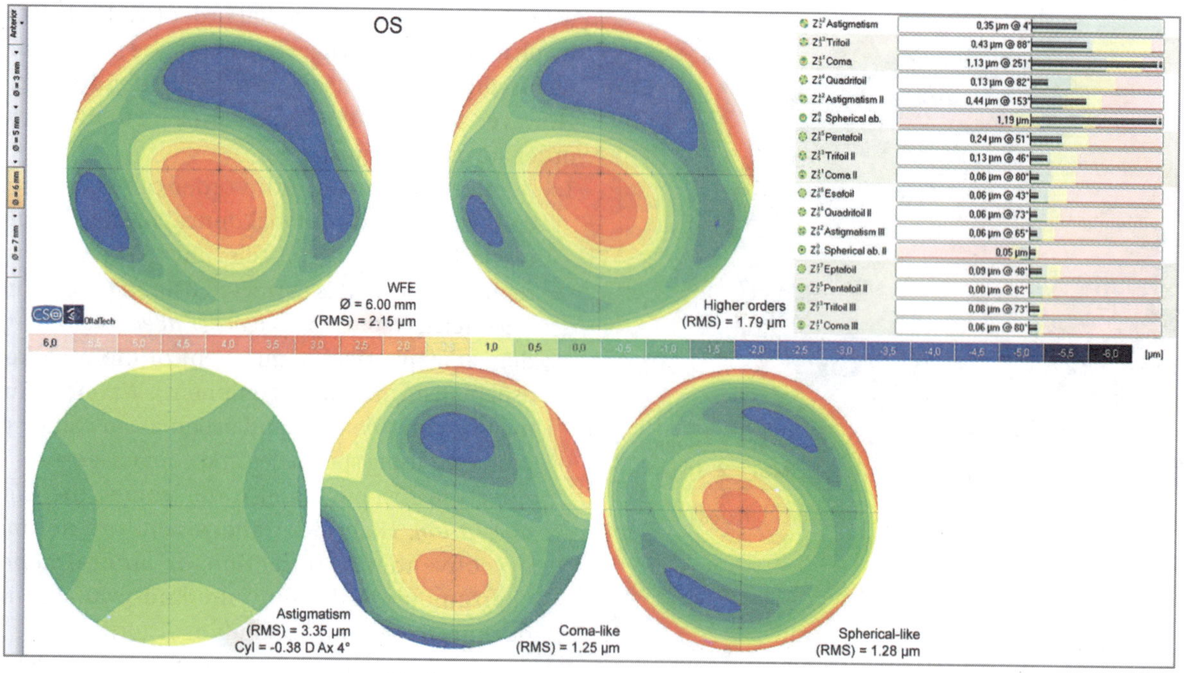

Fig. 21: Complete corneal wavefront aberration map.

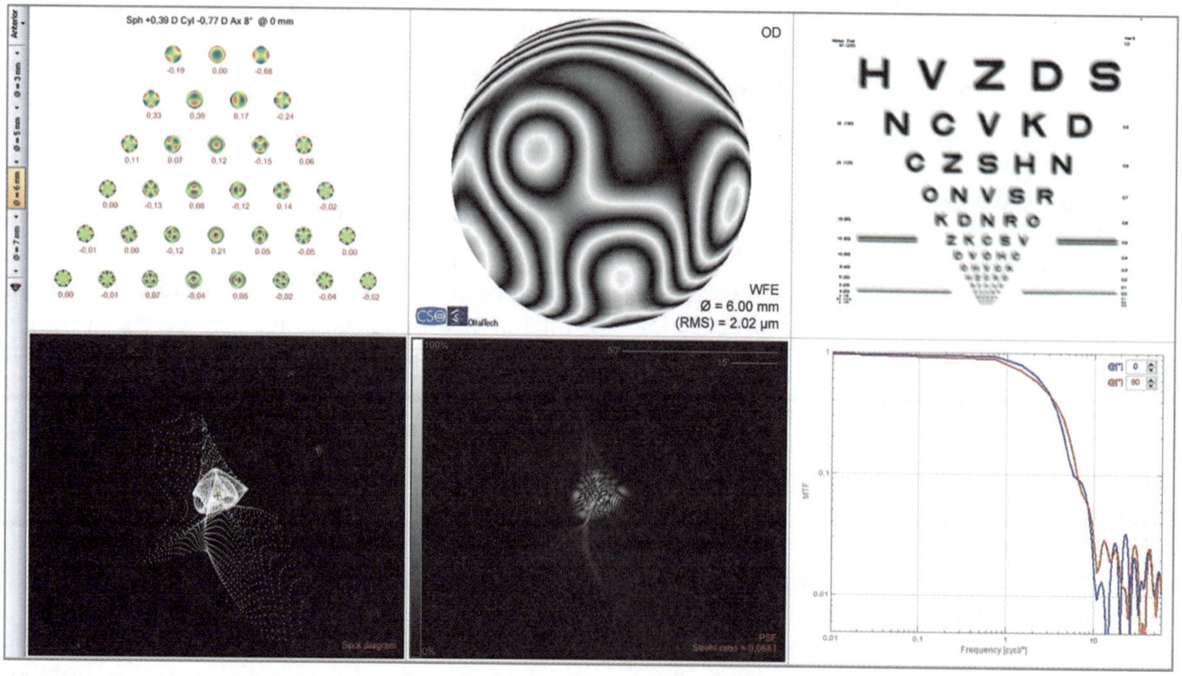

Fig. 22: Visual quality summary obtained with the Sirius CSO topographer. It is possible to visualize the wavefront map (gray scale), Strehl ratio, point spread function (PSF) and modulation transfer function (MTF) function.

Table 1: Reference values for corneal aberrations in the normal population.

Pupil (mm)	*Total RMS*	*Astigmatism RMS*	*Spherical aberration*	*Coma RMS*	*Spherical-like RMS*	*Coma-like RMS*
3	0.19 ± 0.07	0.14 ± 0.08	0.04 ± 0.03	0.05 ± 0.03	0.07 ± 0.02	0.09 ± 0.03
5	0.53 ± 0.21	0.43 ± 0.24	0.15 ± 0.05	0.14 ±0.08	0.18 ± 0.05	0.20 ± 0.08
7	1.26 ± 0.43	0.92 ± 0.53	0.52 ± 0.17	0.42 ± 0.23	0.57 ± 0.16	0.52 ± 0.22

(RMS: root mean square; Coma primary coma: terms Z_3; Spherical aberration primary spherical aberration: term Z_4; Spherical-like: terms fourth and sixth order; Coma-like: terms third and fifth order)

Source: Vinciguerra P, Camesasca FI, Cafossi A. Statistical analysis of physiological aberrations of the cornea. J Refract Surg. 2003;19(Suppl 2):S265-9.

- *Strehl ratio:* This represents the ratio of the maximum intensity of the actual image to the maximum intensity of the fully diffracted limited image, both being normalized to the same integrated flux. This ratio measures optical excellence in terms of theoretical performance results and it is linked to the RMS by the Maréchal intensity formula.
- *Point spread function (PSF):* This is the spread function observed on the retina when the object is a point in infinity. PSF measures how well one object point is imaged on the output plane (retina) through the optical system. In the eye, small pupils (approximately 1 mm) produce diffraction limited PSFs because of the pupil border. In larger pupils, aberrations tend to be the dominant source of degradation.
- *Modulation transfer function, phase transfer function and optical transfer function:* Sinusoidal gratings greatly simplify the study of optical systems because irrespective of the amount of eye aberrations, sinusoidal grating objects always produce sinusoidal grating images. Consequently, there are only two ways that an optical system can affect the image of a grating, by reducing contrast or by shifting the image at a specific resolution; are called respectively the *modulation transfer function* (MTF) and the *phase transfer function* (PTF). The eye's *optical transfer function* (OTF) is made up of the MTF and the PTF. A high-quality OTF is, therefore, represented by high MTF and low PTF.

CLINICAL APPLICATIONS

Aberrometers allow practitioners to gain a better understanding of vision by measurement of high order aberrations. These aberrations reflect a refractive error that is beyond conventional spheres and cylinders. There may be a large group of patients whose best-corrected visual acuity (BCVA) may improve significantly by removing the optical aberrations and this new refractive entity has been called *aberropia*. Reduced optical quality of the eye produced by light scatter and optical aberrations may actually be the root cause of blurred vision associated with dry eye syndrome and tear film disruption. Measurement of these aberrations are also helpful in keratoconus, post-graft fitting, irregular astigmatism or when refractive surgery has reduced the patient's optical quality.

Customized ablation patterns, currently in constant evolution, are the future step in laser technology that should address not only spherical and cylindrical refractive errors (low-order aberrations), but also high-order aberrations such as trefoil and coma **(Figs. 23A to C)**. Thus, vision can be optimized to the limits determined by pupil size (diffraction) and retinal structure and function.

CLINICAL USES OF CORNEAL TOPOGRAPHY

Pathological Cornea

Corneal topography is a very important tool in the detection of corneal pathologies, especially ectatic disorders. Screening

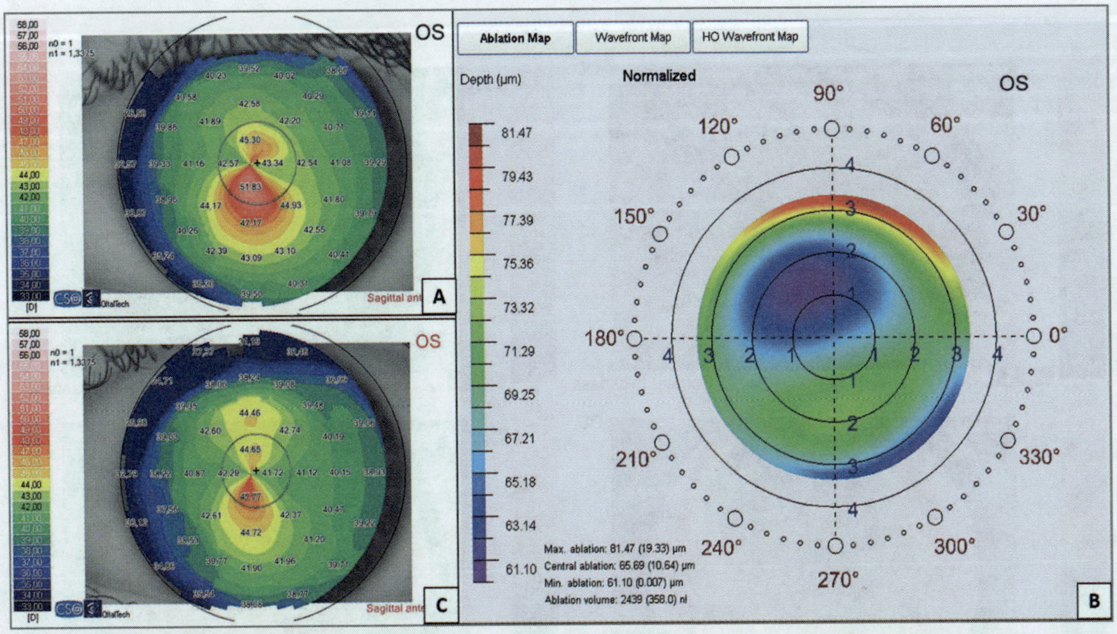

Figs. 23A to C: Customized ablation profile designed according to corneal aberrations: (A) Case of early keratoconus with an unaided and corrected distance visual acuity of 0.5; (B) Customized transepithelial PRK ablation profile in order to treat only the coma with the minimal possible ablation depth; (C) Topographic outcome 6 months after simultaneous transPRK and corneal collagen cross linking with an unaided vision of 0.8 and corrected distance vision of 1 due to the regularization of the astigmatism.

for these anomalies or their potential development is a critical point in preoperative evaluation for refractive surgery. Keratorefractive procedures are contraindicated in these abnormal corneas.

Keratoconus

Keratoconus is characterized by a localized conical protrusion of the cornea associated with an area of corneal stromal thinning, especially at the apex of the cone. The typical associated topographic pattern is the presence of an inferior area of steepening **(Fig. 24)**. In advanced cases, the dioptric power at the apex is at or above 55 D. In a small group of patients, the topographic alterations may be centered at the central cornea. In these cases, there may be an asymmetric bow-tie configuration, and usually the inferior loop is larger than the superior loop **(Fig. 23A)**. Keratoconic corneas have three common characteristics that are not present in normal corneas:

1. An area of increased corneal power surrounded by concentric areas of decreasing power
2. An inferior-superior power asymmetry
3. A skewing of the steepest radial axes above and below the horizontal meridian

Keratoconus suspects are problematic. They may signal impending development of a clinical keratoconus, but they may also represent a healthy cornea. The lack of ectasia in the fellow cornea does not indicate that the keratoconus suspect will not progress to true keratoconus. In these cases, the ideal management is close follow-up of the signs of keratoconus in order to check on their stability, and a thorough analysis of the videokeratographic indexes.

Pellucid Marginal Degeneration

Pellucid marginal degeneration is characterized by an inferior corneal thinning between 4 o'clock and 8 o'clock positions, a narrow band of clear thinned corneal stroma. The ectasia is extremely peripheral and it appears just over the thinned area, presenting a crescent-shaped morphology. This pattern has a classical "butterfly" appearance that results in a flattening of the vertical meridian and a marked against-the-rule irregular astigmatism **(Fig. 25)**.

Keratoglobus

Keratoglobus is a rare bilateral disorder in which the entire cornea is thinned out, most markedly near the corneal limbus, in contrast to the localized central or paracentral thinning of keratoconus. It is very difficult to obtain reliable and reproducible measurements in these cases due to the high level of irregularity and the poor quality of the associated tear film. Reliable topographic examinations show an arc of peripheral increase in corneal power (steepening) and a very asymmetrical bow-tie configuration.

Terrien's Marginal Degeneration

In Terrien's marginal degeneration, there is a flattening over the areas of peripheral thinning. When thinning is restricted to the superior and/or inferior areas of the

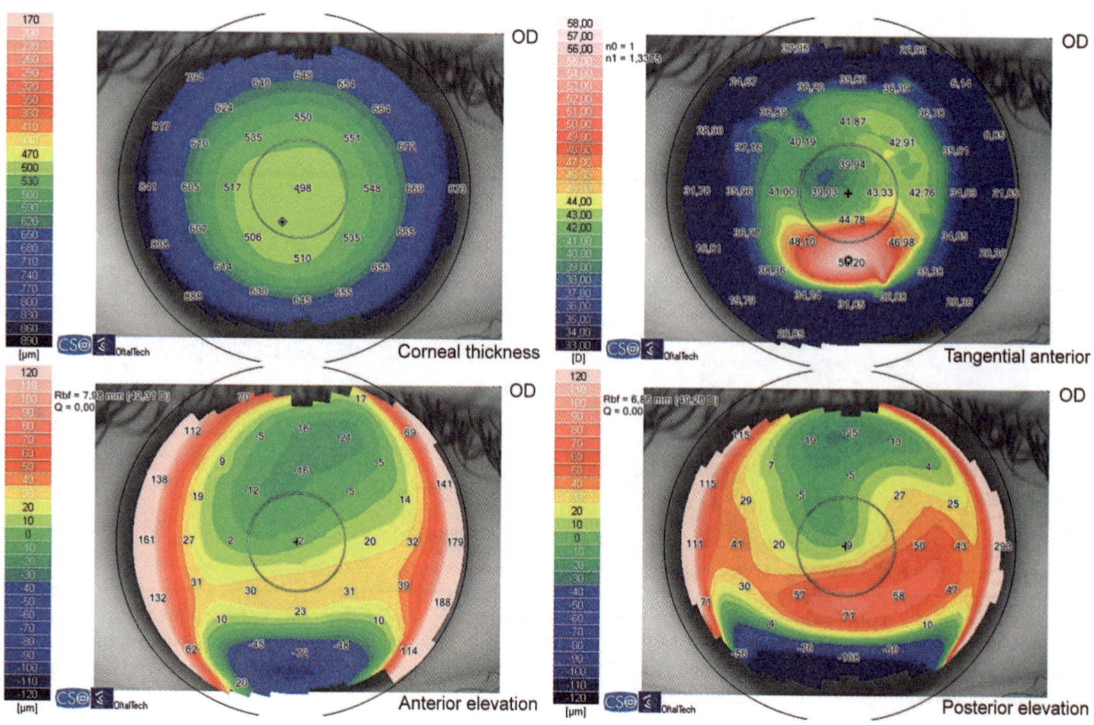

Fig. 24: Keratoconus topography pattern. Observe the inferior steepening with posterior elevation and corneal thinning.

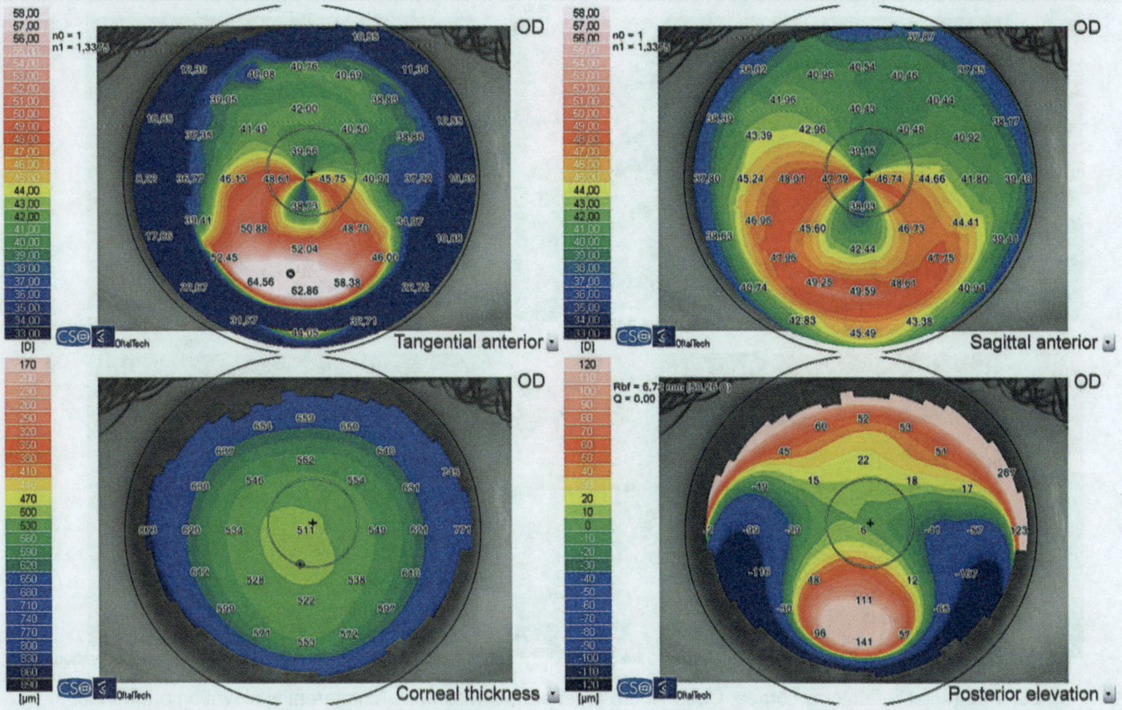

Fig. 25: Pellucid marginal degeneration topography pattern. Observe the crescent-shaped inferior ectasia with posterior elevation and inferior thinning.

peripheral cornea, there is a relative steepening of the corneal surface approximately 90° away from the midpoint of the thinned area. Therefore, high against-the-rule or oblique astigmatism is a common feature, as this disorder involves more frequently the superior and/or inferior peripheral cornea. If the area of thinning is small or if the disorder extends around the entire circumference of the cornea, central cornea may remain relatively spared with a spherical configuration.

Pterygium

Pterygium is a triangular encroachment of the conjunctiva onto the cornea usually near the medial canthus. When the lesion continues to grow out onto the cornea, it could lead to a high degree of astigmatism. When the growth of pterygium is about 2 mm or more, a flattening of the cornea at the axis of the lesion occurs. This produces marked with-the-rule astigmatism, even of more than 4 D. The evolution of the pathology and the surgical outcome could be monitored by changes in corneal topography.

POSTOPERATIVE CORNEA IN REFRACTIVE SURGERY

Keratorefractive procedures attempt to alter the curvature of the central and mid-peripheral cornea, and usually have a minimal effect on the corneal periphery. The area in which the curvature is modified is called the optical zone. This tends to be surrounded by a small zone of altered curvature before normal cornea is reached at the periphery. The corneal effect of surgery could be determined by analyzing the difference map between the preoperative and postoperative measurements.

Postradial Keratotomy

Radial keratotomy (RK) corrects myopia by placing a series of radial incisions (nearly full corneal thickness) leaving a central clear zone (optical zone). These incisions cause a flattening of the central cornea due to retraction of the most anterior collagen fibers and the outward pressure of the intraocular force. This area of flattening is surrounded at an approximately 7 mm zone by a bulging ring of steepening called the paracentral knee or inflection zone. This increases asphericity and corneal irregularity.

A very typical finding in these corneas is a topographic pattern with a polygonal shape. Depending on the number of incisions made, squares, hexagons or octagons can be seen. The angles of the polygons correspond closely to the central ends of the incisions **(Fig. 26)**.

Postastigmatic Keratotomy

Astigmatic keratotomy (AK) is a simple modification of the radial keratotomy that is used to correct astigmatism. Rather than placing incisions radially on the cornea, incisions are strategically placed circumferentially on the peripheral cornea at the steepest meridian. The incisions induce a flattening in that meridian, but provoke steepening in the perpendicular meridian, a process called coupling **(Figs. 27A and B)**. Coupling results from the presence of

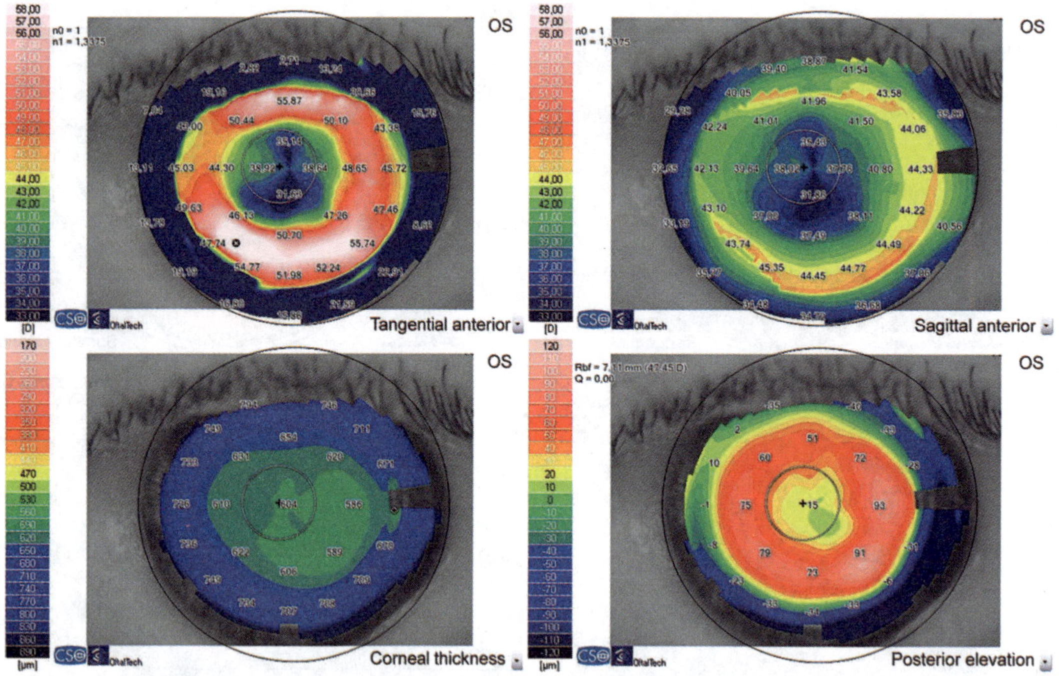

Fig. 26: Postradial keratotomy cornea. Observe the anterior and posterior circumferential elevation but without any alteration in the corneal pachymetry.

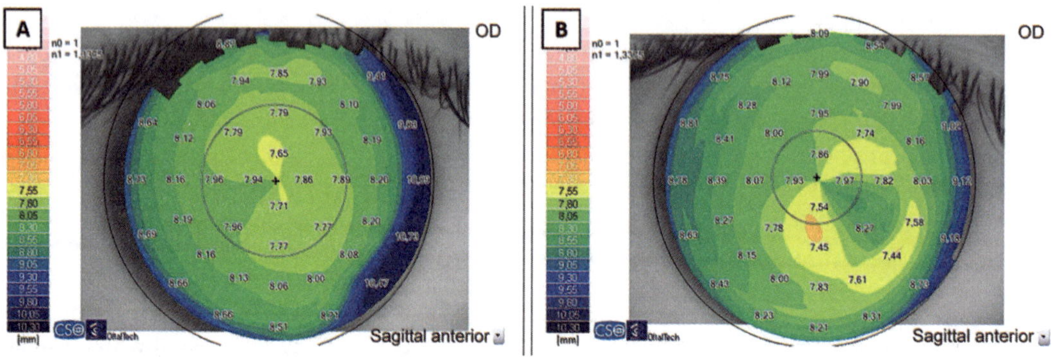

Figs. 27A and B: (A) Before and (B) after astigmatic keratotomy. Observe the considerable flattening induced by the keratotomy, in this case, excessive, generating a secondary significant astigmatism in the previously flat axis.

intact rings of collagen lamellae that run circumferentially around the base of the cornea. With the surgery, these rings become oval in the operated meridian and transmit forces to the untouched meridian. The astigmatic change achieved is the sum of the flattening in one meridian and the steepening on its perpendicular meridian.

Postphotorefractive Keratectomy

Photorefractive keratectomy (PRK) is a procedure which uses a kind of laser (excimer laser, a cool pulsing beam of ultraviolet light) to reshape the cornea. To correct myopia, the excimer laser flattens the central cornea by removing tissue in that area. However, the optical zone needs to be steepened to correct hyperopia. This is achieved by removing an annulus of tissue from the mid-periphery of the cornea.

The topographic pattern in myopic corrections shows a flattening of the central cornea, an oblate profile **(Fig. 28)**. Hyperopic corrections have a pattern of central steepening surrounded by a ring of relative flattening at the edge of the treatment zone, a prolate profile **(Fig. 29)**. In astigmatic corrections, the treatment zone is oval.

Inadequate ablations during surgery can be detected postoperatively by analyzing the resulting corneal topography. Decentrations can only be identified by a relatively asymmetric location of the treatment area **(Fig. 30)**. Other complicated patterns that may lead to severe visual disturbances are the presence of focal irregularities or central islands produced by an inhomogeneous laser beam or an irregular process of corneal healing.

Postlaser in situ Keratomileusis

Laser in situ keratomileusis (LASIK) is an excimer laser procedure-like PRK; but in this case, tissue is ablated under a superficial corneal flap in order to minimize the

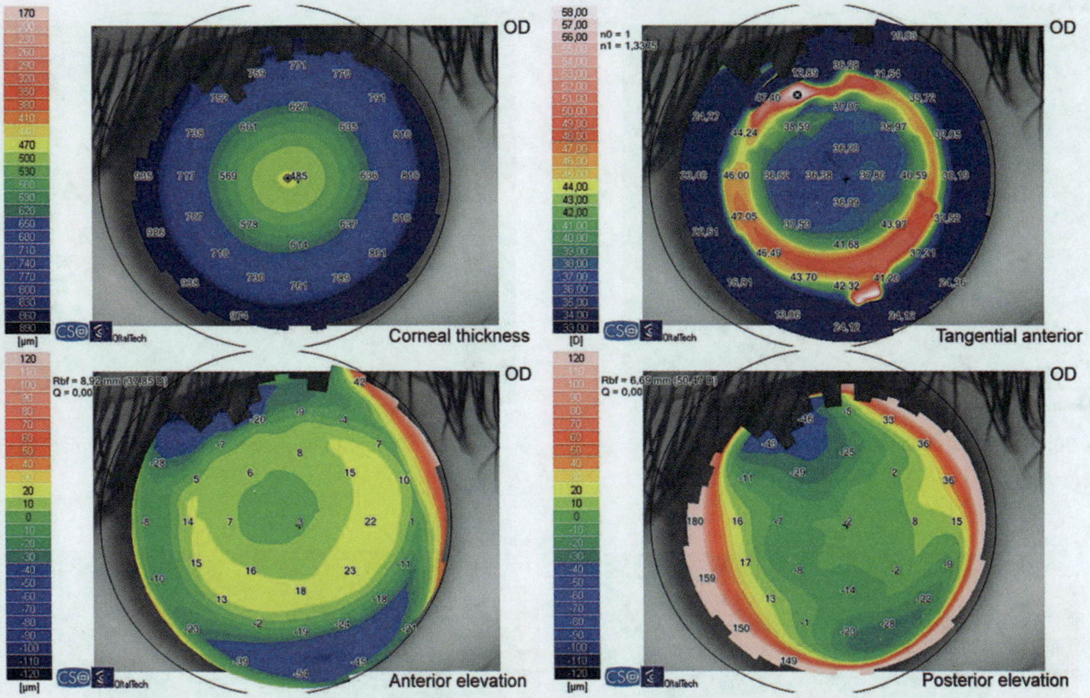

Fig. 28: Topographic pattern after myopic ablation.

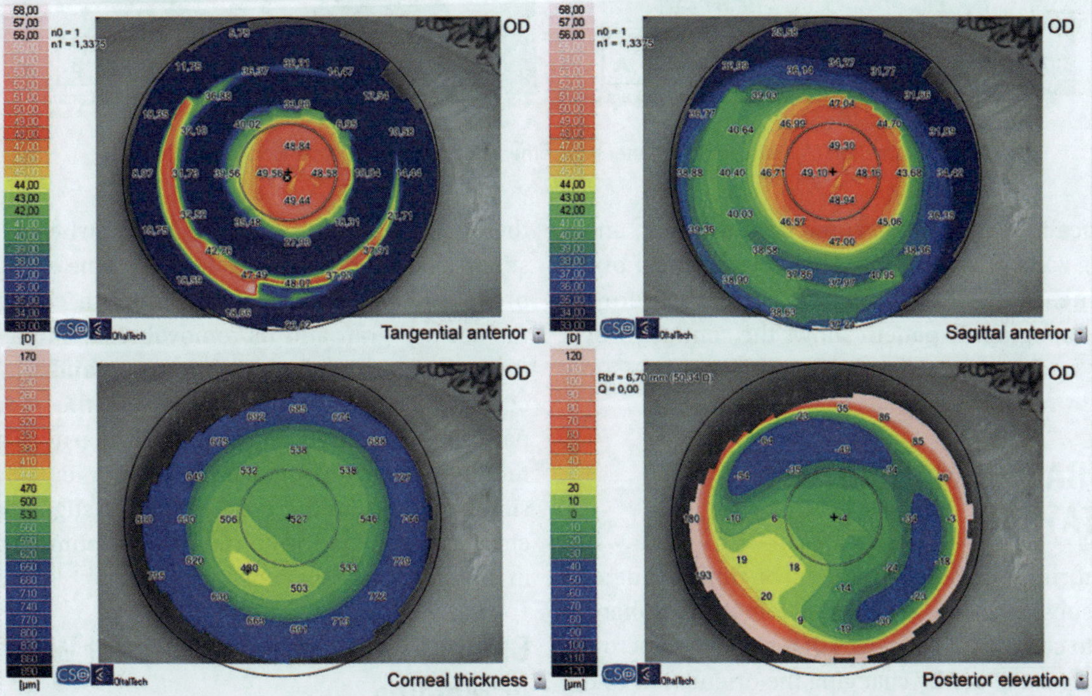

Fig. 29: Topographic pattern after a high hyperopic ablation. In contrast to a real corneal ectasia, after a hyperopic treatment the posterior corneal surface and the central corneal thickness are normal.

influence of the epithelium. The topographic patterns for myopic and hyperopic corrections are the same as in PRK **(Figs. 28 and 29)**. Although the ablation is covered by a flap of corneal tissue, surface irregularities and central islands may still occur. Decentrations may also occur in a LASIK ablation, depending on the patient's ability to maintain eye fixation during surgery **(Fig. 30)**. Epithelial in-growth at the periphery of the flap-stromal interface produces an area of steepening surrounded by an area of marked flattening making the corneal surface more irregular.

Postlaser Thermal Keratoplasty

In laser thermal keratoplasty (LTK), a Holmium laser is used to heat corneal stromal collagen in a ring around the outside of the pupil. The heat causes the tissue to shrink, producing

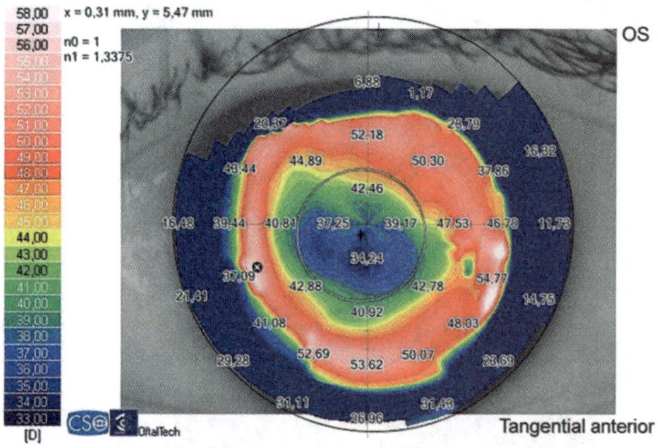

Fig. 30: Pattern of a decentered myopic ablation.

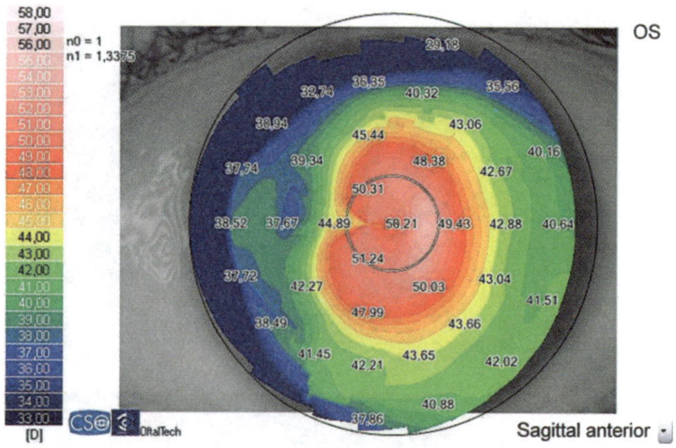

Fig. 31: Topographic pattern after laser thermal keratoplasty for hyperopia.

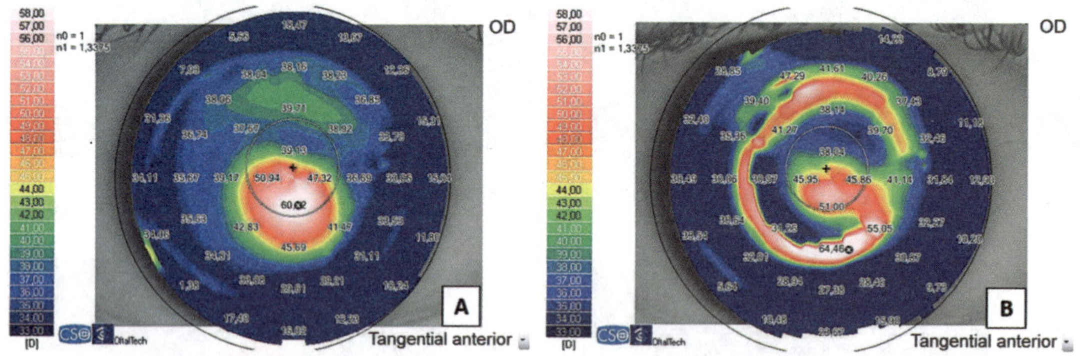

Figs. 32A and B: (A) Before and (B) after intracorneal ring segment implantation for keratoconus.

a zone of localized flattening centered on the spot, and a surrounding zone of steepening. This bulging effect of the central cornea makes it possible to correct hyperopia. The typical topographic pattern shows the central corneal steepening and a ring of flattening overlying the spots **(Fig. 31)**.

POSTINTRASTROMAL CORNEAL RINGS IMPLANTATION

Intrastromal rings are small segments or rings, made of a plastic-like substance, that are inserted into the periphery of the cornea to correct small degrees of myopia or hyperopia. They act as spacers and by changing the orientation of the collagen lamellae, depending on their shape and position, flatten or steepen the central cornea. Nowadays, intrastromal rings are mainly used to reduce the corneal steepening and irregular astigmatism associated with keratoconus **(Figs. 32A and B)**.

Postoperative Cornea in Keratoplasty Surgery

Keratoplasty topographies exhibit a wide variety of patterns, depending on the type of keratoplasty performed, the quality of the surgical procedure, whether sutures are still in place in the cornea, and the time elapsed after the procedure. Sutures usually induce a central bulge in the corneal graft and its removal results in a decrease of the astigmatic component **(Figs. 33A and B)**. The prolate configuration after keratoplasty is the most frequent pattern with a high degree of irregularity. There can be multiple regions of abnormally high or low power, or both simultaneously in the map. Irregular astigmatism over the entrance pupil may be detrimental to optimum visual acuity in the keratoplasty patient.

Contact Lens-induced Corneal Warpage or Molding

Corneal warpage is characterized by topographic changes in the cornea following contact lens wear [most frequently in wearers of hard or rigid gas permeable (RGP) lenses] as a result of the mechanical pressure exerted by the lens. There are at least four different forms of noticeable topography change that usually occur mixed with one another:

1. Peripheral steepening
2. Central flattening
3. Furrow depression
4. Central molding or central irregularity.

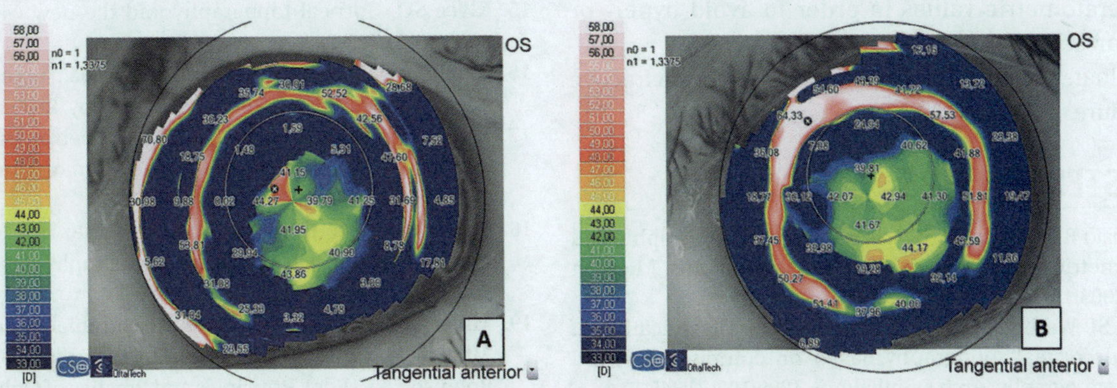

Figs. 33A and B: (A) Before and (B) after graft suture removal on a previous penetrating keratoplasty. Observe the significant reduction of the topographic cylinder.

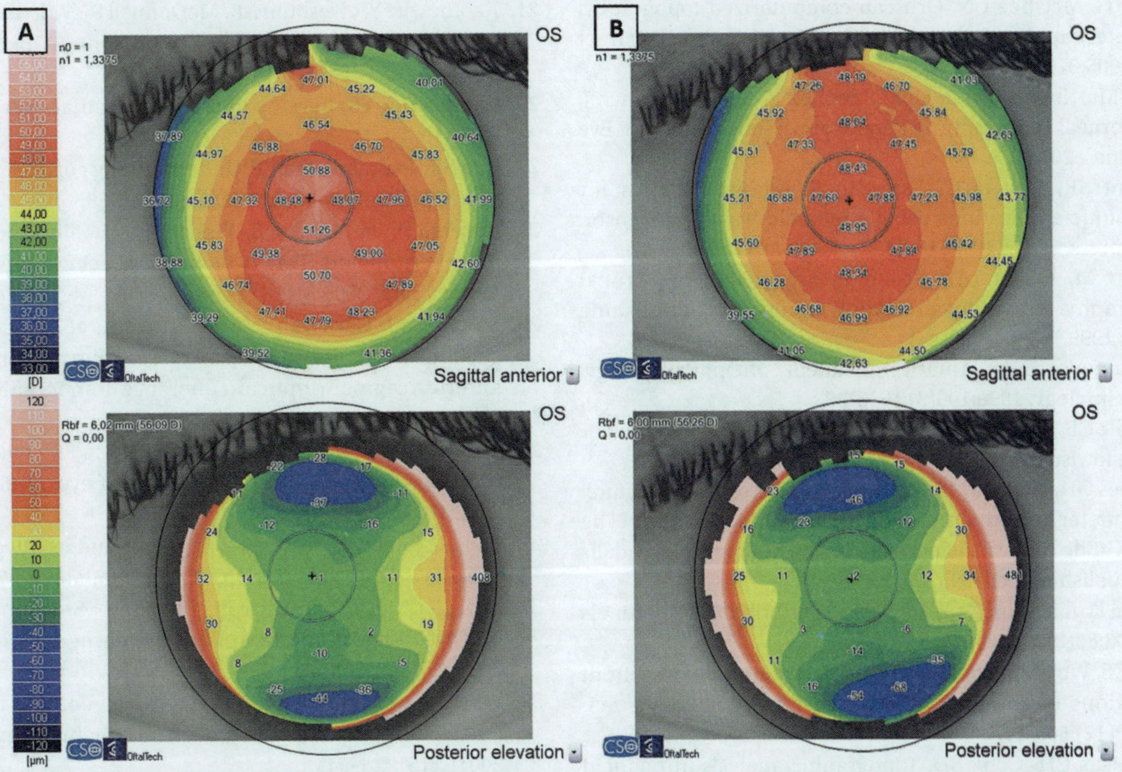

Figs. 34A and B: Corneal warpage. (A) Soft contact lens removed 1 day before the measurement; (B) Same patient 1 week later without using contact lenses. Observe the inferior asymmetry disappears on the topographic astigmatism.

Inferior corneal steepening (pseudokeratoconus) is caused by a superiorly riding contact lens that flattens above the visual axis with an apparent steepening below. The topographic image could appear similar to keratoconus, but both conditions are easily differentiated **(Figs. 34A and B)**. In corneal warpage, the shape indexes do not indicate any keratoconic condition, and the steep K is not as steep as it is in keratoconus.

OTHER USES OF CORNEAL TOPOGRAPHY

Corneal topography is a diagnostic tool, but it is also essential before all refractive procedures, to enable the surgeon to understand the refractive status of an individual eye, and plan the optimum refractive treatment. The corneal topography is also used for the following purposes:

- To guide removal of tight sutures after corneal surgery (keratoplasty, cataract surgery, etc.) that are causing steepening of the cornea **(Figs. 33A and B)**.
- To help in the AK surgical plan.
- To guide contact lens fitting—election of the probe lens and design of the lens.
- To calculate the keratometry values for the calculation of the required intraocular lens power before cataract surgery or refractive lens exchange. This is an important issue in corneas that have undergone previous refractive surgery because it is more difficult to estimate the

real keratometric values in order to avoid hyper- or hypocorrections.

- To evaluate the effect and evolution of a keratorefractive procedure.

SUGGESTED READING

1. Ambrósio R Jr, Klyce SD, Wilson SE. Corneal topographic and pachymetric screening of keratorefractive patients. J Refract Surg. 2003;19(1):24-9.
2. Bogan SJ, Waring GO 3rd, Ibrahim O, et al. Classification of normal corneal topography based on computer-assisted videokeratography. Arch Ophthalmol. 1990;108(7):945-9.
3. Boyd BF, Agarwal A, Alio JL, Krueger RR, Wilson SE (Eds). Wavefront Analysis Aberrometers and Corneal Topography. New Delhi: Jaypee Brothers Medical Publishers; 2003.
4. Cairns G, McGhee CN. Orbscan computerized topography: Attributes, applications, and limitations. J Cataract Refract Surg. 2005;31(1):205-20.
5. Cavas-Martínez F, De la Cruz Sánchez E, Nieto Martínez J, et al. Corneal Topography in Keratoconus: state-of-the-art. Eye Vis (Lond). 2016;3:5.
6. Chamot SR, Dainty C, Esposito S. Adaptive optics for ophthalmic applications using a pyramid wavefront sensor. Opt Express. 2006;14(2):518-26.
7. Corbett M, O'Brart D, Rosen E, Stevenson R. Corneal Topography: Principles and Applications. BMJ Publishing Group; 1999.
8. Corneal topography. American Academy of Ophthalmology. Ophthalmology. 1999;106(8):1628-38.
9. Courville CB, Smolek MK, Klyce SD. Contribution of the ocular surface to visual optics. Exp Eye Res. 2004;78(3):417-25.
10. Dabezies OH, Holladay JT. Measurement of corneal curvature: Keratometer (ophthalmorneter). In: Contact Lenses: The CLAO Guide to Basic Science and Clinical Practice. Kendall/ Hunt Publishing Co; 1995. pp. 253-89.
11. Hamam H. A new measure for optical performance. Optom Vis Sci. 2003;80(2):175-84.
12. Joslin CE, Wu SM, McMahon TT, et al. Higher-order wavefront aberrations in corneal refractive therapy. Optom Vis Sci. 2003;80(12):805-11.
13. Karabatsas CH, Cook SD. Topographic analysis in pellucid marginal corneal degeneration and keratoglobus. Eye (Lond). 1996;10(Pt 4):451-5.
14. Kaufman H, Barron B, McDonald M, Kaufman S. Companion Handbook to the Cornea. London: Butterworth Heinemann; 1999.
15. Klyce SD. Corneal topography and the new wave. Cornea. 2000;19(5):723-9.
16. Krachmer J, Mannis M, Holland E. Cornea. Surgery of Cornea and Conjunctiva. St. Louis; Elsevier-Mosby; 2005.
17. Maeda N, Klyce SD, Smolek MK. Neural network classification of corneal topography Preliminary demonstration. Invest Ophthalmol Vis Sci. 1995;36(7):1327-35.
18. Mejia-Barbosa Y, Malacara-Hernández D. A review of methods for measuring corneal topography. Optom Vis Sci. 2001;78(4):240-53.
19. Miller D, Greiner JV. Corneal measurements and tests. In: Albert DM, Jakobiec FA, Azar DT, Gragoudas ES, Power SM, Robinson NL (Eds). Principles and Practice of Ophthalmology. Philadelphia: WB Saunders; 1994.
20. Molebny VV, Panagopoulou SI, Molebny SV, et al. Principles of ray tracing aberrometry. J Refract Surg. 2000;16(5):S572-5.
21. Rabinowitz YS, Nesbum AB, McDonnell PJ. Videokeratography of the fellow eye in unilateral keratoconus. Ophthalmology. 1993;100(2):181-6.
22. Rabinowitz YS. Keratoconus. Surv Ophthahnol. 1998;42(4): 297-319.
23. Rao SK, Padmanabhan P. Understanding corneal topography. Curr Opin Ophthalmol. 2000;11(4):248-59.
24. Rozema JJ, Van Dyck DE, Tassignon MJ. Clinical comparison of 6 aberrometers. Part 1: Technical specifications. J Cataract Refract Surg. 2005;31(96):1114-27.
25. Steinberg J, Casagrande MK, Frings A, et al. Screening for subclinical keratoconus using swept-source Fourier domain anterior segment optical coherence tomography. Cornea. 2015;34(11):1413-9.
26. Thibos LN, Applegate RA, Schwiergerling JT, et al. Standards for reporting the optical aberrations of eyes. J Refract Surg. 2002;18(5):S652-60.
27. Vang L, Koch DD. Corneal topography and its integration into refractive surgery. Comp Ophthalmol Update. 2005;6:73-81.
28. Vincigerra P, Camesasca FI, Calossi A. Statistical Analysis of physiological aberrations of the cornea. J Refract Surg. 2003;19(Suppl 2):S265-9.
29. Wilson SE, Ambrosio R. Computerized corneal topography and its importance to wavefront technology. Cornea. 2001;20(5):441-54.
30. Wilson SE, Klyce SD. Advances in the analysis of corneal topography. Surv Ophthalmol. 1991;35(4):269-77.
31. Wilson SE, Lin DT, Klyce SD, et al. Terrien's marginal degeneration: corneal topography. Refract Corneal Surg. 1990;6(1):15-20.

CHAPTER

5 Corneal Confocal Microscopy

Manotosh Ray, George N Thomas

INTRODUCTION

Confocal microscopy is an advanced imaging technology that offers several advantages over conventional wide-field optical microscopy. The operator has the ability to control the depth of field, eliminate or reduce the background noise from the focal plane and the capability to obtain precise serial optical sections from thick specimens. The fundamental of confocal microscopy is its use of spatial filtering techniques to eliminate out-of-focus light or glare. The application of this technology permits the acquisition of images of high spatial resolution and contrast as compared to conventional microscopy. There has been tremendous interest in confocal microscopy in recent years, due in part to the relative ease of which extremely high quality images can be obtained from tissue samples, including the ability to image the cornea in vivo.

The major limiting factor of conventional light microscopy is that when a particular point of interest is viewed, the reflected light from the surrounding structures obscures the image produced. The fringing effect produced by this reflection reduces the image contrast. Therefore, the useful magnification in slit-lamp biomicroscopes and other similar ophthalmic instruments is limited to approximately 40 times. Further, magnification compromises the image quality and produces significant image blur. The confocal microscope, on the other hand, utilizes a principle in which both the illumination and observation system are focused on a single point. Thus, the spatial resolution is improved dramatically, and the system allows a usable magnification of up to 600 times.

Confocal microscopy employs an oscillating slit aperture in an ophthalmic microscope configuration, especially suitable for the analysis of cell layers of cornea. It can focus through the entire range of a normal cornea from epithelium to endothelium. A series of scans shows—(1) epithelium, (2) corneal nerves, (3) keratocytes, (4) endothelium, and (e) a computer-generated slice of cornea. There are distinct advantages of the confocal microscope over a regular light microscope. When a transparent tissue like the cornea is imaged with a regular microscope, the unfocused layers affect the visibility of the focused layer. A confocal microscope, on the other hand, can focus on a specific layer distinctly, without being affected by artifact from other layers.

OPTICS

A halogen light source passes through movable slits (Nipkow disk), which then is passed through a condenser lens (front lens) that projects the light to the cornea. Only a small area inside the cornea is illuminated to minimize light scatter. The reflected light passes through the front lens again and is directed to another slit of same size via a beam splitter. Finally, the image is projected onto a highly sensitive camera and displayed on a computer monitor **(Fig. 1)**.

The confocal microscope utilizes a transparent viscous sterile gel that is interposed between the front lens and cornea, to improve the optical interface between the two media. The front lens works on the "distance immersion principle". In this principle, the anteroposterior movement of the front lens enables scanning of the entire cornea starting from anterior chamber and corneal endothelium to most superficial corneal epithelium. The standard working distance (distance between front lens and the cornea) is 1.92 mm. Use of standard 40× immersion lens gives magnified cellular detail and an image field of 440 × 330 μm. Other lenses (e.g. 20×) can deliver a wide-field image, but with less distinct cell morphology. Newer confocal microscopes (such as the Confoscan 2.0) capture up to 350 images per examination at a rate of

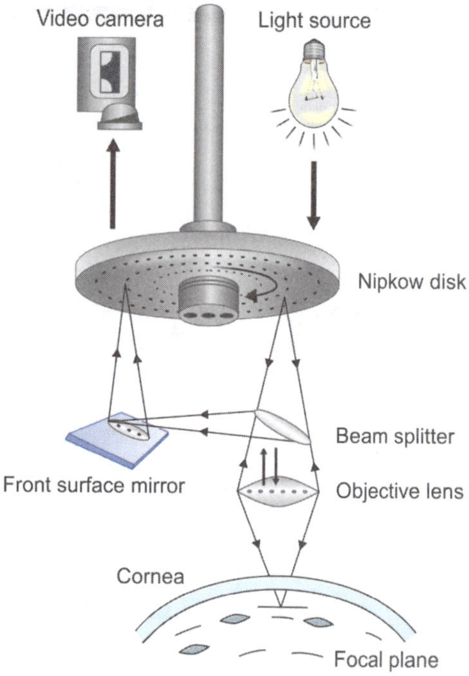

Fig. 1: Optics of confocal microscope.

25 frames per second. The thickness of the imaged layers can be varied from 3 microns to 5 microns depending on the scanning slit characteristics.

Every recorded image is characterized by its position on the "Z" axis of the cornea. Every time a confocal scan is performed, a displayed diagram shows the depth coordinate on the "Z" axis and the level of reflectivity on the "Y" axis. The diagram also displays the distance between two images along the anteroposterior line. This simultaneous graphic recording is called the "Z" scan graphic. The reflectivity on the "Z" scan is entirely dependent on the tissue being scanned. A transparent tissue displays low reflectivity, whereas a higher reflectivity is obtained from an opaque layer. Therefore, different corneal layers would display different reflectivities on the "Z" scan. The corneal endothelium displays the maximum reflectivity while that of the stroma is the lowest. An intermediate reflectivity is obtained from epithelial layers. A typical "Z" scan of entire normal cornea shows high endothelial reflection curves followed by low stromal reflection and then a late intermediate reflectivity from superficial corneal epithelium. Thus, confocal microscopy allows the user to perform corneal pachymetry or measure the distance between two specific corneal layers.

CONFOCAL MICROSCOPY OF THE NORMAL CORNEA

This is a noninvasive technique of imaging of corneal layers that provides excellent resolution and contrast. A well-executed scan can visualize the corneal endothelium, stroma, subepithelial nerve plexus, and epithelial layers distinctly. The limitations are the inability to image a normal Bowman's layer and Descemet's membrane, since these structures are not visible through this microscope. However, it is sometimes possible to view these structures when they are pathological. Eyes with corneal opacity or edema can also be successfully scanned.[1] The quality of an image depends on: (1) centration of the light beam, (2) stability of the eye, and (3) optimum brightness of the illumination.

Epithelium

The corneal epithelium has 5-6 layers. Three different types of cellular components are recognized in the epithelium.

1. Superficial (2-3 layers)—flat cells.
2. Intermediate (2-3 layers)—polygonal cells.
3. Basal cells (single layer)—cylindrical cells.

The superficial epithelial cells appear as flat polygonal cells with well-defined borders, prominent nuclei, and a uniform density of cytoplasm. The main identifying features of superficial epithelial cells are nuclei, which are brighter than surrounding cytoplasm and usually associated with perinuclear hypodense rings **(Fig. 2)**. The intermediate epithelial cells are similar polygonal cells as compared to the superficial layers, but their nuclei are not evident **(Fig. 3)**. Basal cell layers are smaller in size and appear denser than other two layers **(Fig. 4)**. The nucleus is also not evident in the basal layers. The corresponding Z-scans for the superficial and basal layers have been included, showing the depth of each scan.

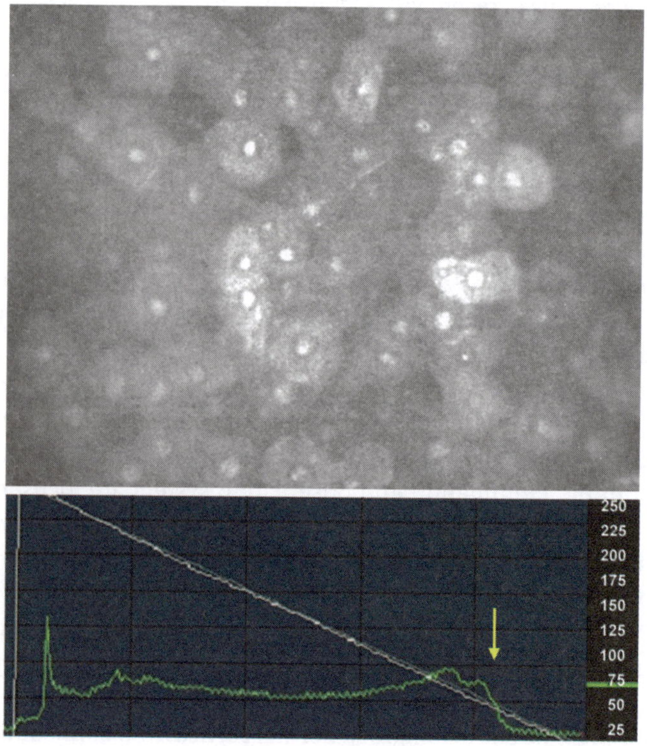

Fig. 2: Superficial epithelial cells with prominent nuclei with corresponding Z-scan.

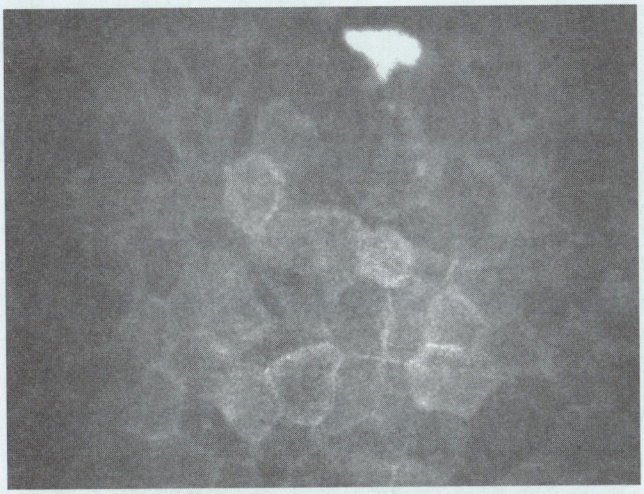

Fig. 3: Intermediate epithelial cells. High cell density with well-demarcated cell borders.

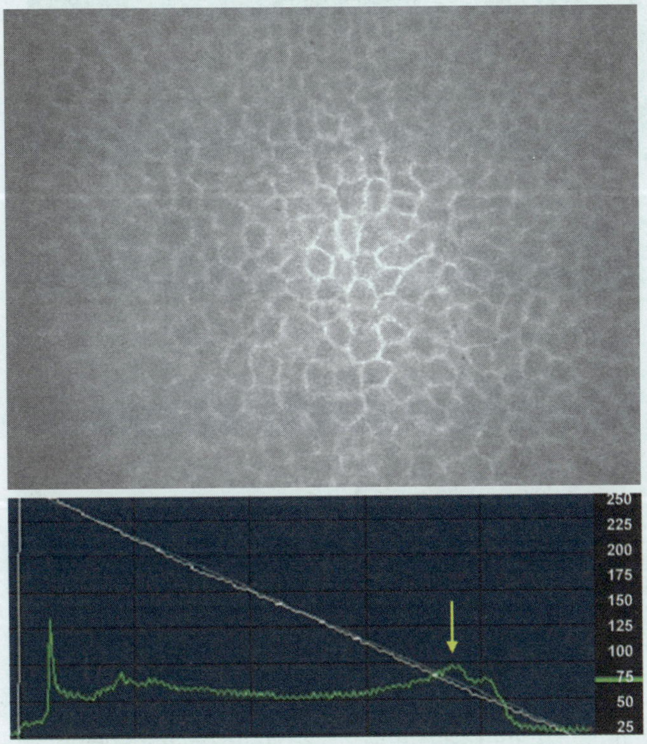

Fig. 4: Basal epithelial cells with corresponding Z-scan. A high cell density seen with well-demarcated cell borders.

Subepithelial Nerve Plexus

Corneal nerves originate from the long ciliary nerve, a branch of the ophthalmic division of the trigeminal nerve. Nerve fibers from the long ciliary nerve form a circular plexus at the limbus. Radial nerve fibers originate from this circular plexus and run deep into the stroma to form the deep corneal plexus. Deep vertical fibers that proceed from the deep corneal plexus run anteriorly to form the subbasal and subepithelial nerve plexuses. Small nerve fibers from the subbasal plexus terminate at the superficial epithelium.

This complex anatomy was not visualized in vivo until the advent of the corneal confocal microscope. Generally, the nerve fibers appear bright and are well contrasted against a dark background **(Fig. 5)**. Confocal microscopy can visualize the orientation, tortuosity, width, branching pattern, and other abnormalities of the corneal nerves.[2]

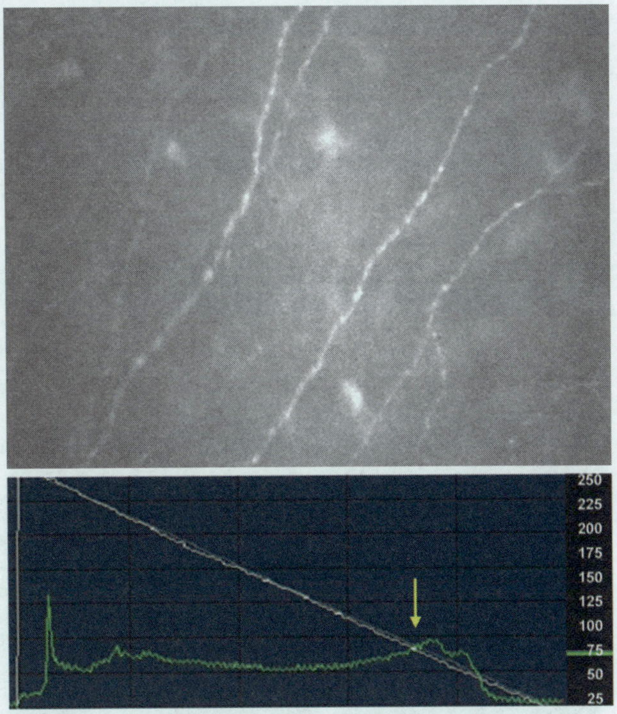

Fig. 5: Subepithelial nerve fibers with corresponding Z-scan.

Stroma

The corneal stroma represents 90% of the total corneal thickness. It has three components:

1. Cellular stroma—composed of keratocytes and constitutes 5% of the entire stroma.
2. Acellular stroma—represents the major component (90–95%) of the stroma, comprising regular collagen tissue (Type I, III, IV) and interstitial substances.
3. Neurosensory stroma—represented by stromal nerve plexus and nerve fibers originating from it.

The keratocyte concentration is much higher in the anterior stroma and progressively decreases toward the deep stroma. Generally, the keratocyte count is approximately 1,000 cells/mm^2 in the anterior stroma while the average value drops to 700 cells/mm^2 in the posterior stroma. The confocal image of stroma shows multiple irregularly oval, round, or bean-shaped bright structures that represent keratocyte nuclei. These nuclei are well contrasted against the dark areas which represent acellular matrix **(Figs. 6A to C)**. Anterior stromal keratocyte nuclei assume rounded bean-shaped morphology while the same in the rear stroma are more often irregularly oval. A bright highly reflective keratocyte represents a metabolically activated keratocyte of a healthy cornea. In a normal healthy cornea, collagen fibers and interstitial substances appear transparent to the confocal microscope and are impossible to visualize.

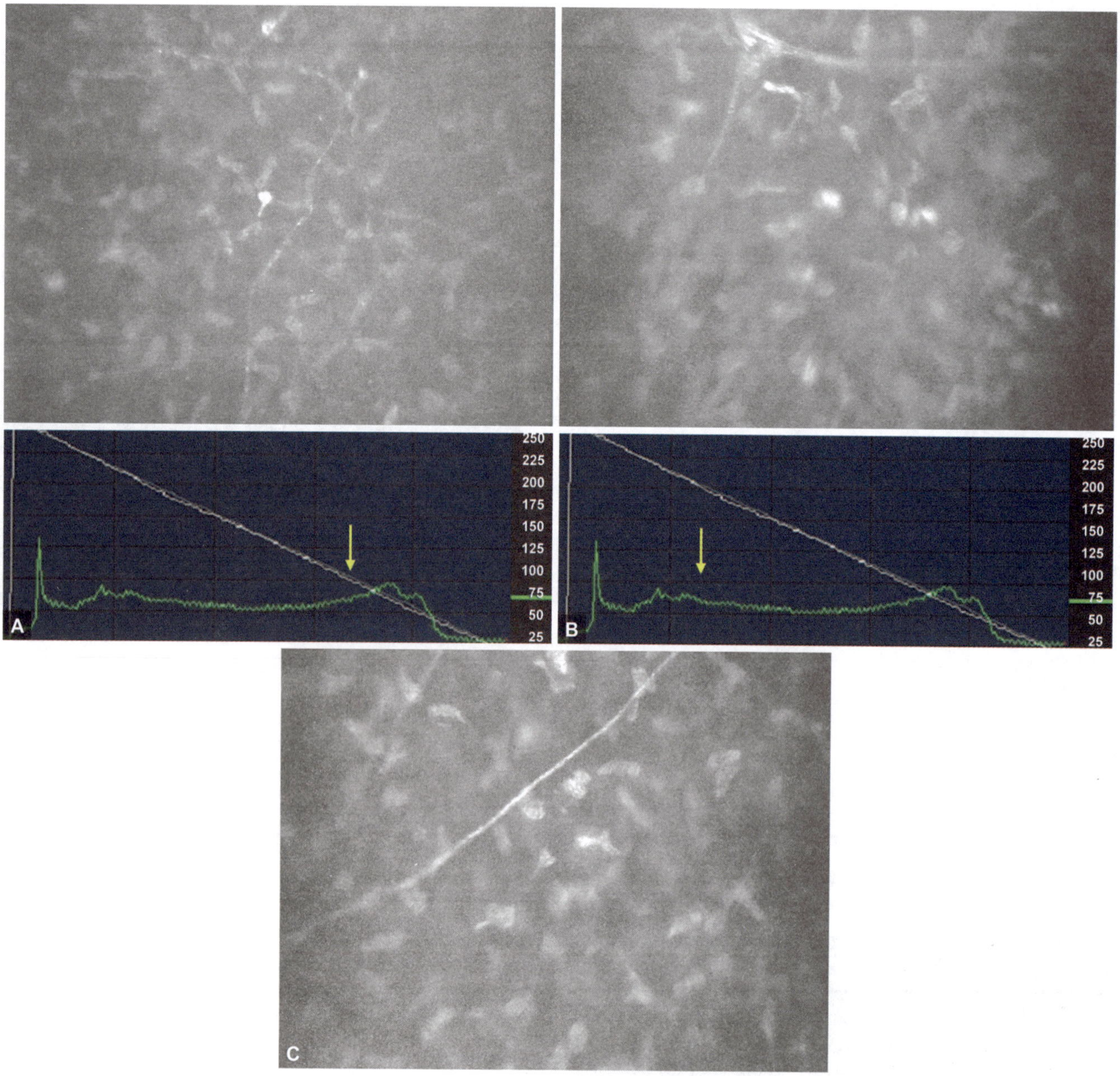

Figs. 6A to C: Anterior (A), intermediate (B), and deep (C) stromal keratocytes.

It is possible to identify stromal nerve fibers in the anterior and middle stroma. These nerve fibers belong to the deep corneal plexus and appear as linear bright thick lines. The stromal nerve fiber thickness is greater than epithelial nerves. Occasionally, nerve bifurcations are also clearly visible. Representative Z-scans have been included below for the anterior and intermediate stromal scans.

Endothelium

The endothelium is a noninnervated single layer of cells at the most posterior part of cornea. The endothelial cell density is maximal at birth and progressively declines with age. The normal endothelial cell count varies from 1,600 cells/mm^2 to 3,000 cells/mm^2 (average 2,700 cells/mm^2) in a healthy adult.[2-4] However, the cornea can still maintain its integrity until the cell count declines below 300–500 cells/mm^2.

Homogeneous hexagonal cells with uniform size and shape represent healthy endothelial cells. Increasing age and endothelial damage causes pleomorphism and polymegathism. Confocal microscopy easily identifies these endothelial cells. These cells appear as bright hexagonal and polygonal cells with no recognizable nucleus. The cell borders are represented by a thin, nonreflective dark line **(Figs. 7A and B)**. A 20× objective lens provides wide field with less magnification. It is possible to perform cell count and study the minute details of cellular morphology. **Figure 8** shows the corresponding Z-scan of the corneal endothelium. Newer confocal microscopes have the ability to perform reliable and accurate endothelial cell count measurements **(Fig. 9)**.

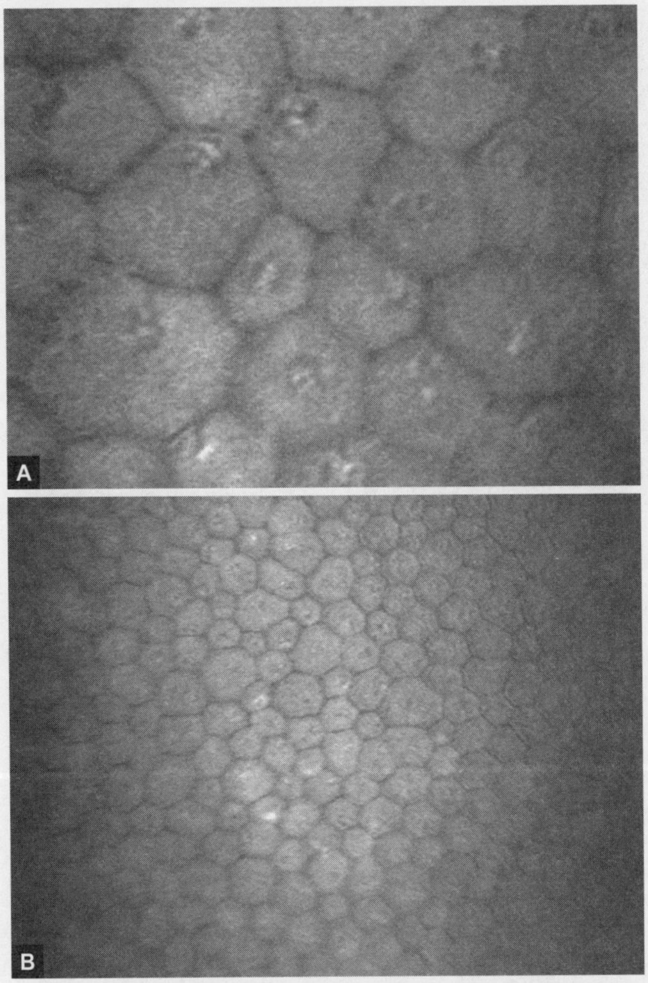

Figs. 7A and B: Hexagonal endothelial cells in a healthy cornea in high magnification (A) and low magnification (B).

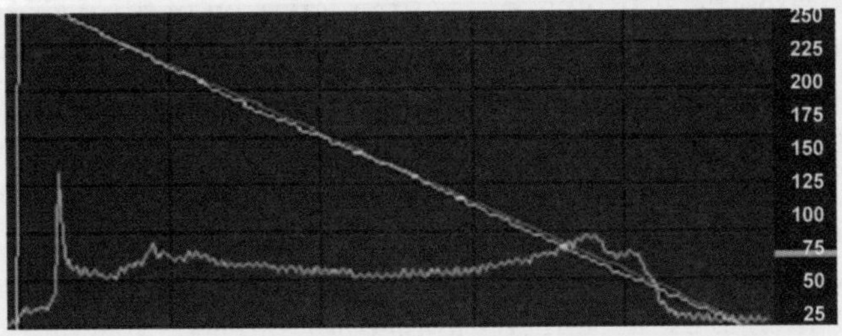

Fig. 8: Z-scan of the endothelium.

CONFOCAL MICROSCOPY IN CORNEAL PATHOLOGIES

Keratoconus

Keratoconus is a noninflammatory ectatic disorder of the cornea characterized by a localized conical protrusion associated with an area of stromal thinning. The thinning is most apparent at the apex of the cornea. The steep conical protrusion of the corneal apex causes high myopia with severe irregular astigmatism. Other features of keratoconus include an iron ring, known as Fleischer's ring, that partially or completely encircles the cone.[5] The cone appears as an "oil drop" reflex on distant direct ophthalmoscopy due to internal reflection of light. Deep vertical folds oriented parallel to the steeper axis of the cornea, at the level of deep stroma and Descemet's membrane are known as *Vogt's striae*. An acute corneal hydrops appears when there is a break in the Descemet's membrane. The corneal edema usually subsides after few months leaving behind a scar and flattening of the cornea. The corneal nerves become more readily visible due to thinning of the cornea. High irregular astigmatism precludes adequate spectacle correction. In the early stages, use of contact lenses may improve the visual acuity. However, contact lens fitting can be extremely difficult and in advanced cases it ceases to improve visual acuity optimally, necessitating corneal transplantation.

The most effective way to identify early cases of keratoconus is computerized corneal topography that has become a gold standard for diagnosis and follow-up of the disease in recent years.[6,7] Confocal microscopy is a relatively newer investigative modality to assess the keratoconic cornea. Morphological changes in keratoconus are mostly confined to the corneal apex and depend on the severity of the disease. The rest of the cornea may appear normal. The typical polygonal shape of superficial epithelial cells is lost. They appear distorted and elongated in an oblique direction with highly reflective nuclei **(Fig. 10)**. Cell borders are not distinguishable. There may be areas of basal epithelial loss as evident by a linear dark, nonreflective patch seen on confocal microscopy. The subepithelial nerve plexus generally appears normal. However, the subbasal nerve fibers are curved and take the course of stretched overlying epithelium. The corneal stroma is also affected by keratoconus. The confocal images of the stroma are highly specific to the disease. The characteristic stromal changes are multiple "striae" represented by thin hyporeflective lines oriented vertically, horizontally, or obliquely **(Fig. 11)**. These are confocal microscopic representation of Vogt's striae.[8] In advanced stages of keratoconus, the keratocyte concentration is reduced in the anterior stroma. The shape of the keratocytes is also altered. Occasionally, highly reflective bodies with tapering ends are visible in the anterior stroma near the apex. The nature of these abnormal bodies is not yet known, but it may represent altered keratocytes. The corneal endothelial changes vary from none to occasional pleomorphism and polymegathism.

Corneal Dystrophies

Corneal dystrophies are inherited abnormalities that affect one or more layers of cornea. Usually both eyes are affected but not necessarily symmetrically. They may present at birth but more frequently develop during adolescence and progress gradually throughout life. The effect on vision is highly variable, depending on the disorder.

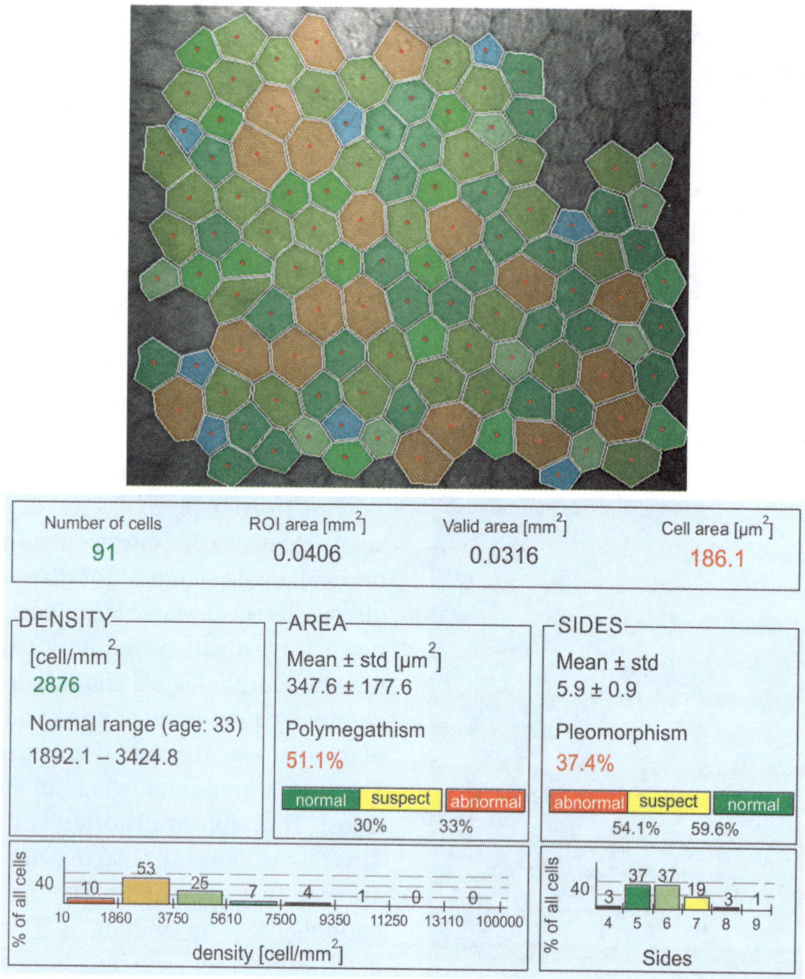

Fig. 9: Reliable automated endothelial cell counting by confocal microscopy.

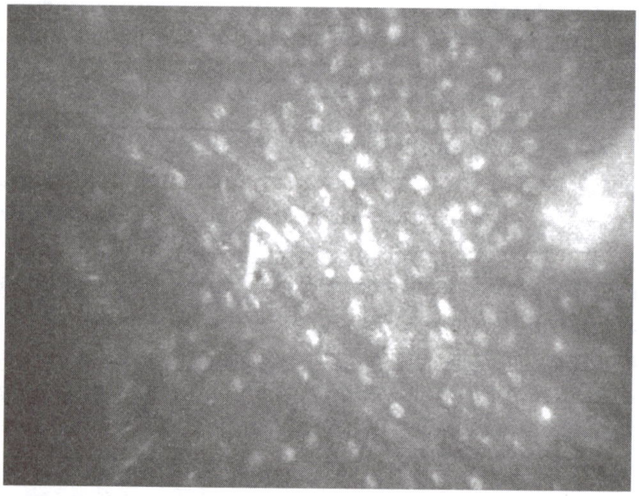

Fig. 10: Obliquely elongated superficial epithelium in keratoconus.

Granular Dystrophy

This is an autosomal dominant bilateral noninflammatory condition that results from deposition of eosinophilic hyaline deposits in the corneal stroma.[9] It specifically affects the central cornea and eventually can cause decreased vision and eye discomfort. Initially, the lesions are confined to superficial stroma, but with progression of the disease they can involve the posterior stroma as well.

Confocal microscopy reveals highly reflective, bright, and dense structures in the anterior and middle stroma. Keratocytes are not involved. Depth of stromal involvement may be ascertained by using the "Z" scan function. This is an added advantage over other contemporary investigations that enables the surgeon to plan for surgical procedures. Confocal microscopy is also useful in the differential diagnosis and follow-up of the disease.

Posterior Polymorphous Dystrophy

Posterior polymorphous dystrophy (PPMD) is a rare inherited disorder of the posterior layer of the cornea. It is a bilateral disorder with early onset, although early stage diagnosis is rare since most of the affected individuals remain asymptomatic. The characteristic endothelial changes are small vesicles or areas of geographic lesions. In fact, endothelial cells lining of the posterior surface of the cornea have epithelial-like features.[10,11] These cells can also cover the trabecular meshwork, leading to glaucoma in some patients. Most severe cases may develop

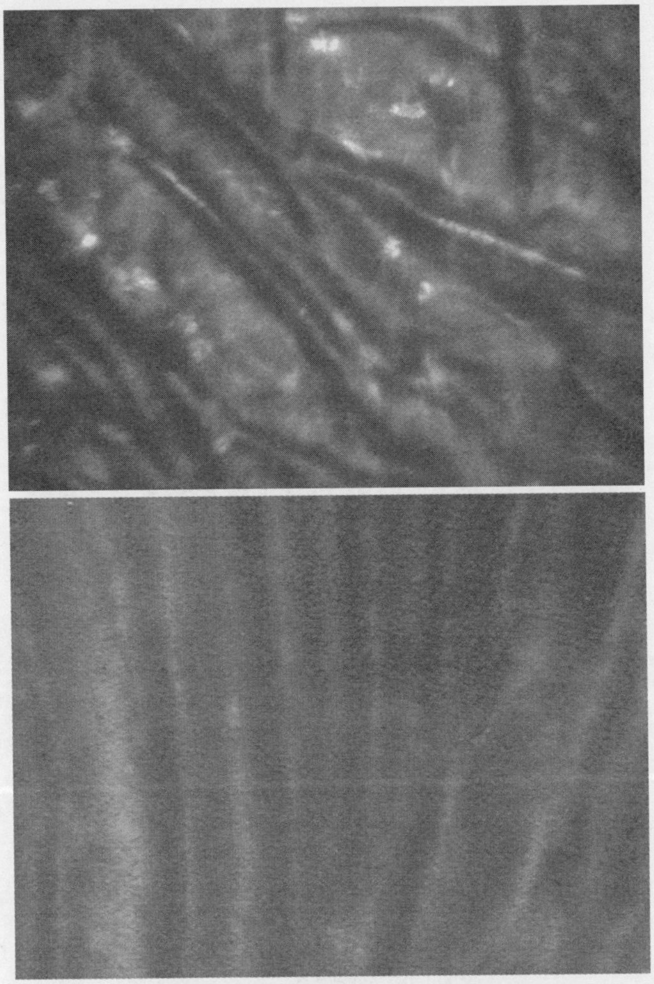

Fig. 11: *Advanced keratoconus*: Striae are seen in the stroma.

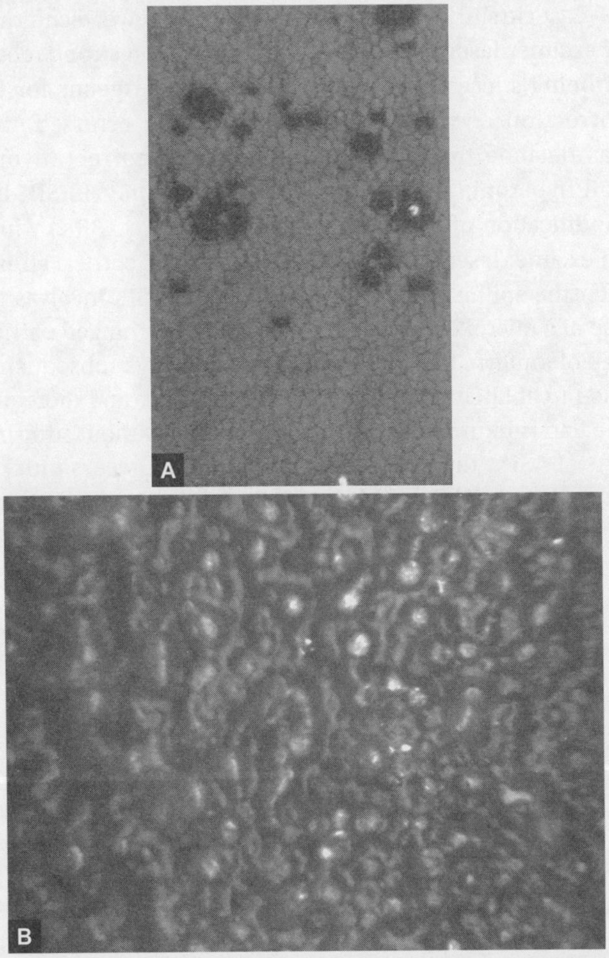

Figs. 12A and B: Guttata seen in the endothelium in mild Fuchs' endothelial dystrophy (A) and severe disease (B).

corneal edema due to compromised pump function of the endothelial cells.

Confocal microscopy shows multiple round vesicles at the level of Descemet's membrane and endothelium.[12] PPMD usually distorts the normal flat profile of the endothelial cells and present as large dark, cystic impressions on confocal scan. The endothelial cells surrounding the lesion appear large and distorted.

Fuchs Endothelial Dystrophy

Fuchs endothelial dystrophy is a chronic bilateral hereditary (variable autosomal dominant or sporadic) disorder of the corneal endothelium. It typically presents after the age of 50 years and is more common in females. There is a loss of endothelial cells that results in deposition of collagen materials in Descemet's membrane. These focal excrescences in Descemet's membrane are called corneal guttata, which is the hallmark of this disease. The integrity of the corneal endothelium is essential to maintain the metabolic and osmotic properties of the entire cornea. Corneal edema in Fuchs' dystrophy initially involves the posterior and middle stroma. As the disease advances, the edema progresses to involve the anterior cornea, resulting in bullous keratopathy.

Confocal microscopy is useful to visualize corneal guttata. This technique has a distinct advantage over conventional specular microscopy that fails to visualize the endothelium when there is significant corneal edema.[13] The corneal guttata appear dark with a bright central reflex **(Figs. 12A and B)**.[14] In advanced stages, the endothelial morphology is altered completely, but distorted cell borders can still be visualized.[14] In the early stages of bullous keratopathy, intraepithelial edema is seen as distorted cellular morphology with increased reflectivity. Confocal microscopy can also identify the bullae in the basal epithelial layer.

LASER IN SITU KERATOMILEUSIS

Traditionally, the cornea is evaluated with slit-lamp biomicroscopy and computerized corneal topography both pre- and postoperatively. Confocal microscopy adds a new perspective to the commonly employed investigations. The functional outcome of laser in situ keratomileusis (LASIK) depends on many factors including biomechanics, the healing process, and the inflammatory response of the flap interface that is created between the epithelial flap and stromal bed. A confocal scan is useful in the following scenarios.

Laser in situ keratomileusis is one of the newer techniques of excimer laser refractive surgery that has a strong record of being successfully used by refractive surgeons for the correction of various types of refractive errors. LASIK has become the technique of choice to correct myopia and hyperopia with or without astigmatism.[15] LASIK is a modification of photorefractive keratectomy (PRK) where an excimer laser is used to ablate superficial corneal stroma after the epithelium has been removed. LASIK involves the use of a microkeratome or laser to prepare a hinged corneal flap of uniform thickness. The excimer laser is subsequently used to ablate the mid-corneal stromal bed, and thereafter the flap is returned to its original position without suturing. After LASIK, the healing of corneal tissue occurs quickly, since there is minimal damage to the corneal epithelium and the Bowman's layer.

- Study of corneal flap thickness
- *Interface study*:
  - Healing process
  - Inflammatory response
  - Abnormal deposits
- Corneal nerve fiber regeneration
- Residual stromal thickness.

A well-designed flap is the key to a successful outcome in LASIK. Thinner flaps are at higher risk for developing flap complications. A few studies employing confocal microscopy had suggested that the actual flap thickness after LASIK is consistently lower than the predicted thickness.[16] The reasons are not yet understood. However, corneal edema that may be caused by microkeratome cut and suction may play an important role. Postoperative scarring and tissue remodeling could be other possible factors. Using a "Z" scan, it is possible to identify the interface that corresponds to a very low level of reflectivity. The flap thickness is obtained by measuring the distance between the highly reflective spike from the front surface of the cornea and the low reflective interface **(Fig. 13)**.

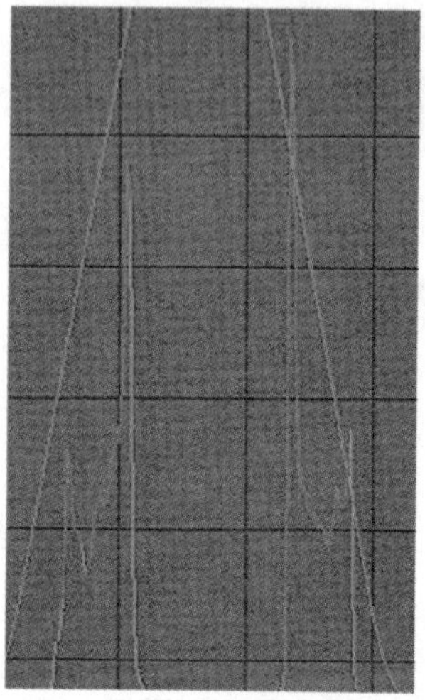

Fig. 13: Measurement of flap thickness in LASIK via Z-scan. (LASIK: laser in situ keratomileusis)

The interface usually appears as a hyporeflective space in between the relatively hyperreflective cellular stroma. This interface can be easily imaged by a confocal microscope. Typically, the keratocyte concentration is lower than normal in the interface. Bright particles and microstriae are consistently visible in the interface. These bright particles most probably originate from the microkeratome blade and are represented by highly reflective white bodies **(Fig. 14)**. Microstriae are present at the Bowman's layer. Excessive interface microstriae and bright particles may lead to astigmatism and eventually a poor outcome after LASIK. These microstriae can be imaged with a confocal microscope, even when the slit-lamp examination is unremarkable.

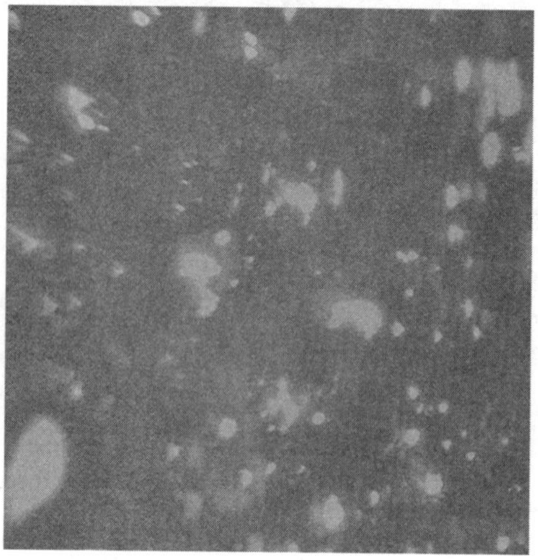

Fig. 14: Bright high reflective particles at the flap-stroma interface in LASIK. (LASIK: Laser in situ keratomileusis)

Diffuse lamellar keratitis (DLK) also known as the "Sands of Sahara syndrome", is a noninfectious inflammation of the interface. The etiology is not known, but it is assumed to be toxic or allergic in nature. In confocal scan, DLK appears as diffuse and multiple infiltrates in the interface with no anterior or posterior extension **(Fig. 15)**.

Subepithelial nerve fibers are also affected by LASIK. Nerves are not usually visible in immediate postoperative period. However, the regenerating nerve fibers appear as thin irregularly branching lines when a confocal scan is performed 5–7 days after surgery. The residual stromal thickness can also be measured using "Z" scan technique as described, while also evaluating the epithelial flap. A confocal scan image **(Fig. 16)** demonstrates a foreign body seen under the flap after LASIK.

INFECTIOUS KERATITIS

Acanthamoeba Keratitis

Accurate and prompt diagnosis of sight-threatening infectious keratitis is one of the major challenges in ophthalmic practice today. Delay in diagnosis and inappropriate treatment can adversely affect the visual

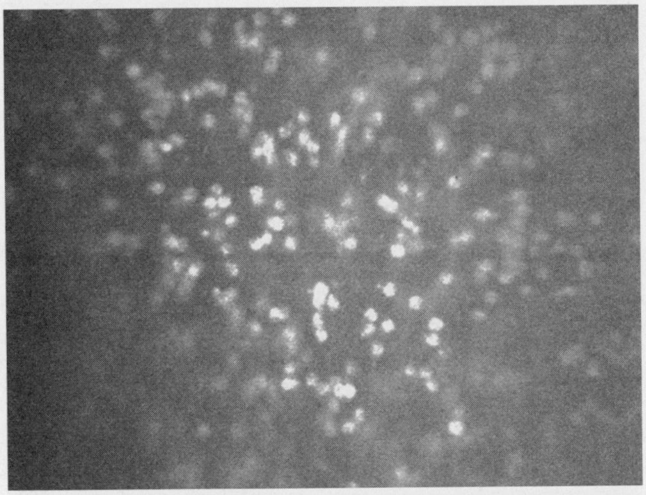

Fig. 15: Diffuse lamellar keratitis after LASIK. Multiple infiltrates are seen as bright spots.
(LASIK: laser in situ keratomileusis)

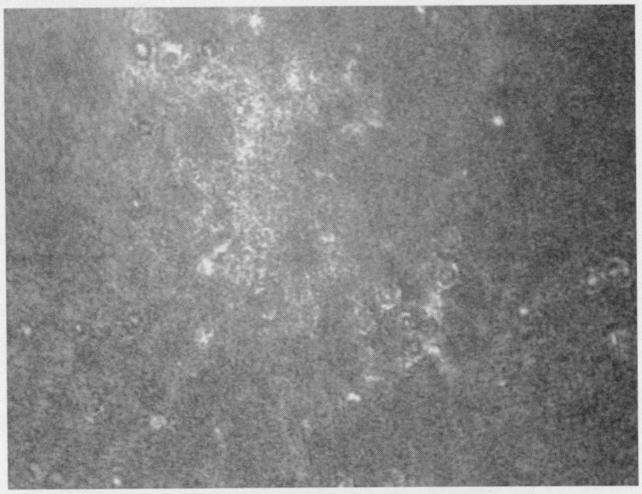

Fig. 17: In vivo confocal microscopy demonstrating active *Acanthamoeba* represented by bright refractile bodies. A few trophozoites are also visible.

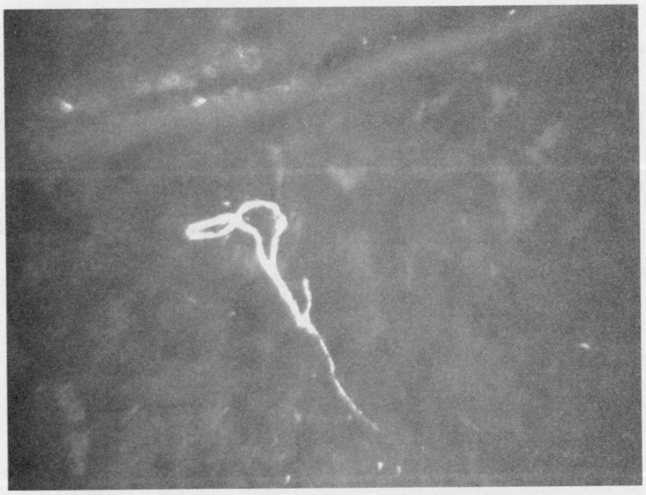

Fig. 16: A foreign body seen under the flap after LASIK.
(LASIK: laser in situ keratomileusis)

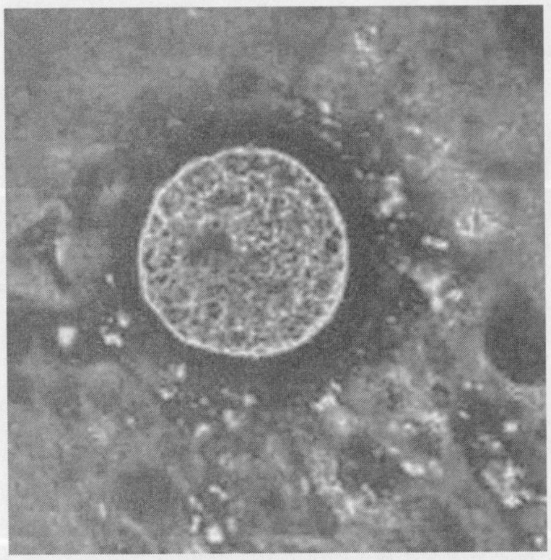

Fig. 18: In vivo confocal microscopy showing typical double-walled cystic form of *Acanthamoeba*.

outcome. Current microbiological diagnostic techniques can identify most of the offending organisms, if the tests are carried out meticulously. However, confocal microscopy can play a significant role in keratitis with prolonged course, polymicrobial keratitis, and in scenarios when conventional techniques are unable to identify any organism. The usefulness of confocal microscopy was demonstrated in eyes with *Acanthamoeba*[17] and fungal keratitis.[18,19]

It is frequently difficult to identify *Acanthamoeba* on the ocular surface, since its presentation can mimic herpetic keratitis and several forms of bacterial keratitis. This diagnostic dilemma has often led to delays in making the correct diagnosis and may affect the visual outcome significantly. Most cases of *Acanthamoeba* keratitis is diagnosed on tissue culture, corneal biopsy, and histological analysis.[20-22] Confocal microscopy offers a useful noninvasive technique to diagnose *Acanthamoeba* keratitis in vivo. Although confocal microscopy lacks sufficient resolution to be the only method of diagnosis, it can be used in screening patients suspected of having *Acanthamoeba* keratitis.[23,24] On confocal microscopy, *Acanthamoeba* are visualized typically as round or ovoid highly reflective structures ranging in size from 10 μm to 25 μm, which is larger than leukocytes **(Fig. 17)**. Sometimes the internal structure of *Acanthamoeba*, along with vacuoles is also visible. The double-walled cystic forms of the parasite are also often well visualized **(Fig. 18)**. *Acanthamoeba* are smaller and much more iridescent than corneal parenchymal cells such as epithelial cells and keratocyte nuclei.

Mycotic Keratitis

Mycotic keratitis is common in many countries, especially in tropical latitudes. Filamentous fungi are the most common cause of mycotic keratitis.[25] It is important to establish a specific diagnosis as early as possible, to ensure prompt institution of antifungal therapy. Although confocal microscopic examination may help in reaching a rapid

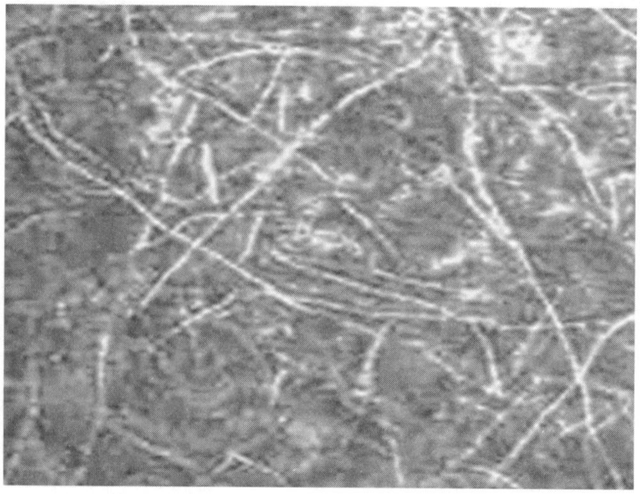

Fig. 19: In vivo confocal microscopy showing fungal hyphae.

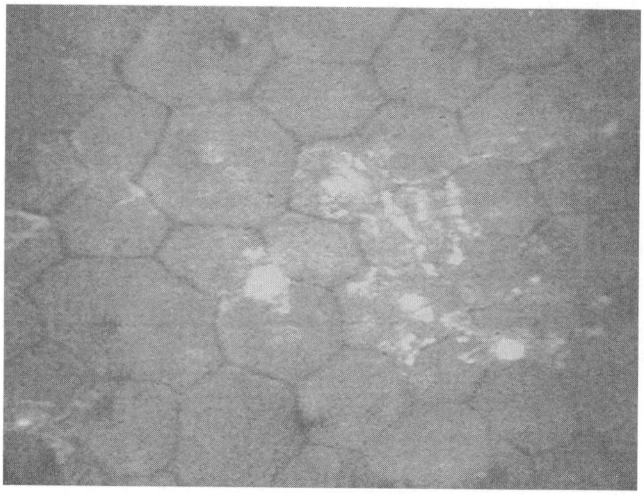

Fig. 20: Pleomorphism, polymegathism, and pre-endothelial deposits in a corneal graft.

presumptive diagnosis, the in vivo confocal microscopic characteristics of fungal keratitis continue to confuse ophthalmologists. A clear understanding of the confocal characteristics of fungal hyphae and spores may play an important role in establishing a rapid diagnosis. Identification of fungal organisms by confocal microscopy is important, not only for rapidly diagnosing fungal keratitis, but also for monitoring response to anti-fungal therapy. On confocal microscopy, the mycotic organisms appear as thin, extensively branching, and beaded filaments. Sometimes round to oval spores also can be found **(Fig. 19)**. In vivo confocal microscopy reveals four types of morphologies of mycotic keratitis, such as: (1) branching hyperreflective structures, (2) long linear hyperreflective structures, (3) short rod hyperreflective structures, and (4) round to oval structures (spores). The hyphae must not be confused with corneal nerves, which appear regular, elongated and uniform with sharp margins.

CORNEAL GRAFTS

The confocal microscope is a useful tool to follow up corneal grafts and to detect abnormalities that may occur postoperatively. It provides images at the cellular level to identify pathological changes even before they become clinically evident. It can also be used to assess the donor cornea.

Corneal graft survival is heavily dependent on the number of healthy endothelial cells present. Endothelial cell loss occurs rapidly after corneal transplantation.[26] Majority of cell loss takes place during the first two postoperative years.[27] Several studies have suggested that endothelial cell loss is much higher after corneal grafting when the primary indications are bullous keratopathy or hereditary stromal dystrophy in comparison to keratoconus and corneal leukomas.[28,29] Another interesting fact is that endothelial cell loss is greater when corneal transplantation is performed on phakic eyes than on aphakics.[30]

Confocal microscopy supersedes conventional specular microscopy while evaluating endothelial cell characteristics, especially in eyes with stromal edema. During the immediate postoperative period, endothelium looks normal and healthy. However, as time progresses, endothelial cell density decreases as evidenced by pleomorphism and polymegathism. Occasionally, bright pre-endothelial deposits appear, the significance of which is not yet known **(Fig. 20)**.

Reinnervation after grafting is another clinical phenomenon that is imaged well by confocal microscopy. The first sign of innervation that starts a few months after keratoplasty is new nerve growth at the periphery of the graft stroma. However, complete innervation may take many years to develop. Regenerated nerve fibers look similar to those found in the normal cornea. Occasionally, they may take a tortuous and convoluted course depending on age (e.g. older patients) and primary indications of keratoplasty (e.g. bullous keratopathy and corneal dystrophies).

It is well known that allograft rejection is one of the most common causes of graft failure. Graft rejection can be classified as epithelial, subepithelial, and endothelial rejection, of which the endothelial subtype has the worst prognosis. The confocal microscopic features of epithelial rejection are distorted basal epithelial cells with altered subepithelial reflectivity. Subepithelial rejection is identified by discrete opacities underneath the epithelial layer.[31] Endothelial rejection, on the other hand, is characterized by coexistence of normal looking and degenerated endothelial cells, focal endothelial cell lesions, and bright highly reflective microprecipitates **(Fig. 21)**.[32]

INTRACORNEAL DEPOSITS

Sources of intracorneal deposits can be exogenous or endogenous. They can involve various layers of cornea individually or in combination.

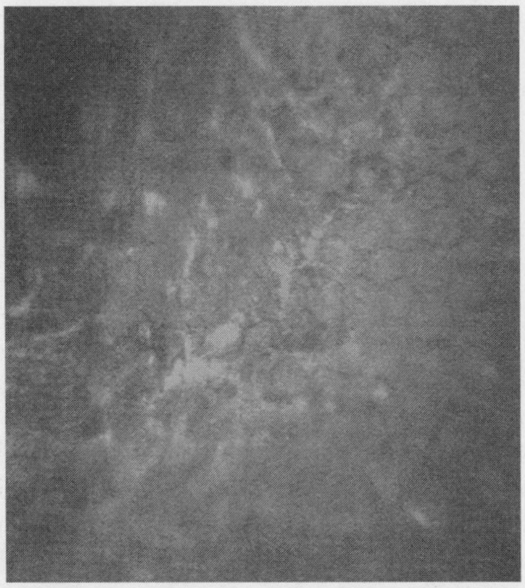

Fig. 21: Coexistence of degenerated and normal endothelial cells in early endothelial allograft rejection.

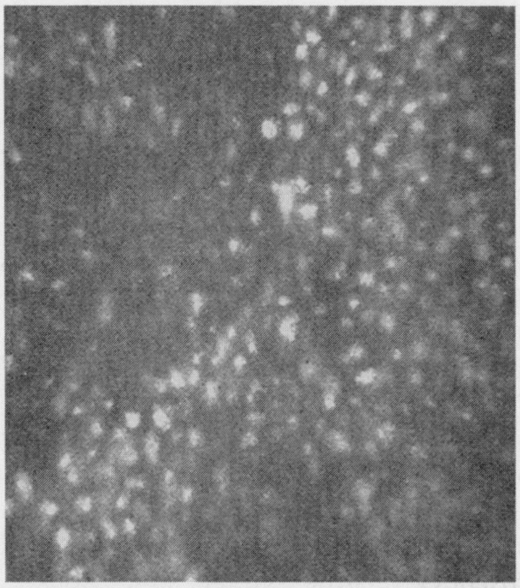

Fig. 22: Intracellular deposits at basal epithelial layer in amiodarone toxicity.

Exogenous sources:
- Long-term use of contact lenses
- Refractive surgery
- Vitreoretinal surgery using silicone oil
- Drugs including amiodarone and chloroquine.

Endogenous sources:
- Wilson's disease
- Hyperlipidemia
- Fabry's disease
- Hemosiderosis.

The clinical diagnosis of these conditions is based on slit-lamp biomicroscopy and systemic features. The knowledge of confocal microscopic features in these disorders is limited, except in drug-induced keratopathies.

VORTEX KERATOPATHY

Vortex keratopathy, also known as *cornea verticillata,* is characterized by whorl-like corneal epithelial deposits. It can be induced by various drugs, e.g. amiodarone (used for cardiac arrhythmias) and antimalarials (chloroquine and hydroxychloroquine). Clinically, vortex keratopathy is manifested as golden-brown opacities at the level of the inferior corneal epithelium. On electron microscopy, they appear as intracytoplasmic lysosome-like lamellar inclusion bodies located at the basal epithelial layer.[33] Confocal microscopy adds a new perspective to the imaging of this condition. It demonstrates involvement of the entire cornea, although vortex keratopathy is primarily a corneal epithelial pathology. The characteristic features are presence of highly reflective, bright intracellular deposits at the basal epithelial layer **(Fig. 22)**. The overlying epithelium is usually normal. In advanced cases, these microdeposits may extend to the stroma and eventually to the endothelium.[34] Stromal keratocyte density is often reduced.

CONCLUSION

Ophthalmic investigations and imaging modalities have advanced tremendously over the past few decades. The confocal microscope is one of these wonderful innovations that has shed much light on the anatomy and pathology of the human cornea. It is becoming increasingly useful in clinical practice and its indications are continually expanding. Confocal microscopy is truly an exciting tool that can be useful for the clinical diagnosis, follow-up, and analysis of many corneal lesions.

ACKNOWLEDGMENTS

We would like to acknowledge Nidek Technologies for their contribution of clinical photographs, as well as Aria Mangunkusumo and Vanathi Ganesh for their help.

REFERENCES

1. Weigand W, Thaer AA, Kroll P, et al. Optical sectioning of the cornea with a new confocal in vivo slit-scanning videomicroscope. Ophthalmology. 1995;102(4):485-92.
2. Oliveira-Soto L, Efron N. Morphology of corneal nerves using confocal microscopy. Cornea. 2001;20(4):374-84.
3. Tuft SJ, Coster DJ. The corneal endothelium. Eye (Lond). 1990;4(Pt 3):389-424.
4. Nucci P, Brancato R, Mets MB, et al. Normal endothelial cell density range in childhood. Arch Ophthalmol. 1990;108(2): 247-8.
5. Gass JD. The iron lines of the superficial cornea. Arch Ophthalmol. 1964;71:348-58.
6. Maguire LJ, Bourne WM. Corneal topography in early keratoconus. Am J Ophthalmol. 1989;108(2):107-12.
7. Maguire LJ, Lowry JC. Identifying progression of subclinical keratoconus by serial topography analysis. Am J Ophthalmol. 1991;112(1):41-5.

8. Somodi S, Hahnel C, Slowik C, et al. Confocal in vivo microscopy and confoal laser-scanning fluorescence microscopy in keratoconus. Ger J Ophthalmol. 1996;5(6):518-25.
9. Werner LP, Werner L, Dighiero P, et al. Confocal microscopy in Bowman's and stromal corneal dystrophies. Ophthalmology. 1999;106(9):1697-704.
10. Hirst LW, Waring GO 3rd. Clinical specular microscopy of posterior polymorphous endothelial dystrophy. Am J Ophthalmol. 1983;95(2):143-55.
11. Mashima Y, Hida T, Akiya S, et al. Specular microscopy of posterior polymorphous endothelial dystrophy. Ophthalmic Paediatr Genet. 1986;7(2):101-7.
12. Chiou AG, Kaufman SC, Beuerman RW, et al. Confocal microscopy of posterior polymorphous endothelial dystrophy. Ophthalmologica. 1999;213(4):211-3.
13. Chiou AG, Kaufman SC, Beuerman RW, et al. Confocal microscopy in cornea guttata and Fuchs' endothelial dystrophy. Br J Ophthalmol. 1999;83(2):185-9.
14. Rosenblum P, Stark WJ, Maumenee IH, et al. Hereditary Fuchs' dystrophy. Am J Ophthalmol. 1980;90(4):455-62.
15. Reviglio VE, Bossana EL, Luna JD, et al. Laser in situ keratomileusis for myopia and hyperopia using the Lasersight 200 laser in 300 consecutive eyes. J Refract Surg. 2000;16(6): 716-23.
16. Durairaj VD, Balentine J, Kouyoumdjian G, et al. The predictability of corneal flap thickness and tissue laser ablation in laser in situ keratomileusis. Ophthalmology. 2000;107(12):2140-3.
17. Cavanagh HD, Petrol WM, Alizadeh H, et al. Clinical and diagnostic use of in vivo confocal microscopy in patients with corneal disease. Ophthalmology. 1993;100(10):1444-54.
18. Winchester K, Mathers WD, Sutphin JE. Diagnosis of aspergillus keratitis in vivo with confocal microscopy. Cornea. 1997;16(1):27-31.
19. Florakis GJ, Moazami G, Schubert H, et al. Scanning slit confocal microscopy of fungal keratitis. Arch Ophthalmol. 1997;115(11):1461-3.
20. Mathers WD, Sutphin JE, Folberg R, et al. Outbreak of keratitis presumed to be caused by Acanthamoeba. Am J Ophthalmol. 1996;121(2):129-42.
21. Auran JD, Starr MB, Jakobiec FA. Acanthamoeba keratitis: a review of the literature. Cornea. 1987;6(1):2-26.
22. D'Aversa G, Stern GA, Driebe WT Jr. Diagnosis and successful medical treatment of Acanthamoeba keratitis. Arch Ophthalmol. 1995;113(9):1120-3.
23. Winchester K, Mathers WD, Sutphin JE, et al. Diagnosis of Acanthamoeba keratitis in vivo with confocal microscopy. Cornea. 1995;14(1):10-7.
24. Chew SJ, Beuerman RW, Assouline M, et al. Early diagnosis of infectious keratitis with in vivo real time confocal microscopy. CLAO J. 1992;18(3):197-201.
25. Wang L, Zhang J, Sun S, et al. In vivo confocal microscopic characteristics of fungal keratitis. Life Sci J. 2008;5(1):51-4.
26. Harper CL, Boulton ML, Marcyniuk B, et al. Endothelial viability of organ cultured corneas following penetrating Keratoplasty. Eye (Lond). 1998;12(Pt 5):834-8.
27. Vasara K, Setälä K, Ruusuvaara P. Follow-up study of human corneal endothelial cells, photographed in vivo before eneucleation and 20 years later in graft. Acta Ophthalmol Scand. 1999;77(3):273-6.
28. Obata H, Ishida K, Murao M, et al. Corneal endothelial cell damage in penetrating keratoplasty. Jpn J Ophthalmol. 1991;35(4):411-6.
29. Abott RL, Fine M, Guillet E. Long-term changes in corneal endothelium following penetrating keratoplasty: a specular microscopic study. Ophthalmology. 1983;90(6):676-85.
30. Ing JJ, Ing HH, Nelson LR, et al. Ten-year postoperative results of penetrating keratoplasty. Ophthalmology. 1998;105(10): 1855-65.
31. Cohen RA, Chew SJ, Gebhardt BM, et al. Confocal microscopy of corneal graft rejection. Cornea. 1995;14(5):467-72.
32. Cho BJ, Gross SJ, Pfister DR, et al. In vivo confocal microscopic analysis of corneal allograft rejection in rabbits. Cornea. 1998;17(4):417-22.
33. Ghose M, McCulloch C. Amiodarone-induced ultrastructural changes in human eyes. Can J Ophthalmol. 1984;19(4):178-86.
34. Ciancaglini M, Carpineto P, Zuppardi E, et al. In vivo confocal microscopy of patients with amiodarone-induced keratopathy. Cornea. 2001;20(4):368-73.

CHAPTER

6 Tonometry

Shefali Parikh, Rajul Parikh

INTRODUCTION

Role of intraocular pressure (IOP) in the definition, diagnosis, and management of glaucoma has been on a roller coaster. Till few years back, glaucoma was synonymous with an increased IOP. If the IOP was more than 22 mm Hg, IOP lowering agents were started; this is still practiced by quite a few ophthalmologists. IOP was one of the most important components in the definition of glaucoma. However, with the knowledge gathered from various population-based studies, it is realized that a high number of patients with glaucoma (at least 50%) in various population-based studies shows IOP less than 21 mm Hg. Also, the information about the natural history of glaucoma helps us to know that despite lowering IOP, glaucomatous optic neuropathy continues to progress in a few patients. These observations exposed the limitation of IOP as a main criterion for diagnosis of glaucoma. In 1996, the American Academy of Ophthalmology has preferred practice pattern for primary open-angle glaucoma and recognized that IOP is neither a component of definition of glaucoma nor a clinical characteristic of it. Presently, IOP is considered as one of the causal risk factors for glaucoma and its progression. However, the fact remains that, at present, in the armamentarium of glaucoma management, lowering of IOP is the only available treatable option that reduces retinal ganglion cell (RGC) loss.

WHAT IS INTRAOCULAR PRESSURE?

The IOP is the pressure inside the eye to maintain the integrity of the globe. Maintenance of IOP is a faculty of aqueous humor which is continuously secreted from the ciliary epithelium of ciliary processes. It is dependent on two factors: (1) rate of aqueous humor formation, and (2) facility of aqueous outflow. If the former is more or the latter is less, IOP may rise.

The IOP in an individual, like blood pressure, is a dynamic variable. It shows temporal variation (fluctuation over days) and diurnal variation (fluctuation over 24 hours) in every individual. "Normal IOP" in an individual is not a fixed number but a range. In a large population-based survey conducted on Caucasians, it was observed that 95% of individuals had an average IOP of 15.7 ± 2 SD (standard deviation) which if translated in integers, falls between 10 mm Hg and 21 mm Hg. If we take 3 SD, then 99% of population would lie between 6 mm Hg and 24 mm Hg. Studies conducted in south Indian population (Vellore and Andhra Pradesh Eye Disease studies) also reported mean IOP of 15.5 mm Hg (2 SD: 9–22.6 mm Hg). Normal distribution of IOP in a population is not Gaussian **(Fig. 1)**, but is skewed toward right. This skew indicates that in a population, individuals with IOP > 21 mm Hg should be more than 2.5%. One can draw inference from this that there is no upper cutoff for normal IOP and that 5% of the normal individuals would have IOP above or below this range.

Intraocular Pressure Measurements

There are various ways to measure IOP. Different techniques of measurement of IOP are given below and types of tonometer are shown in **Box 1**.

Direct Method

A catheter is inserted into the anterior chamber of the eye, and the other end is connected to a manometric device from which the pressure is calculated. Though this is the most accurate method available, it is not feasible in human being because of its invasive nature.

Indirect Method

It is based on eyes' response to an applied force.

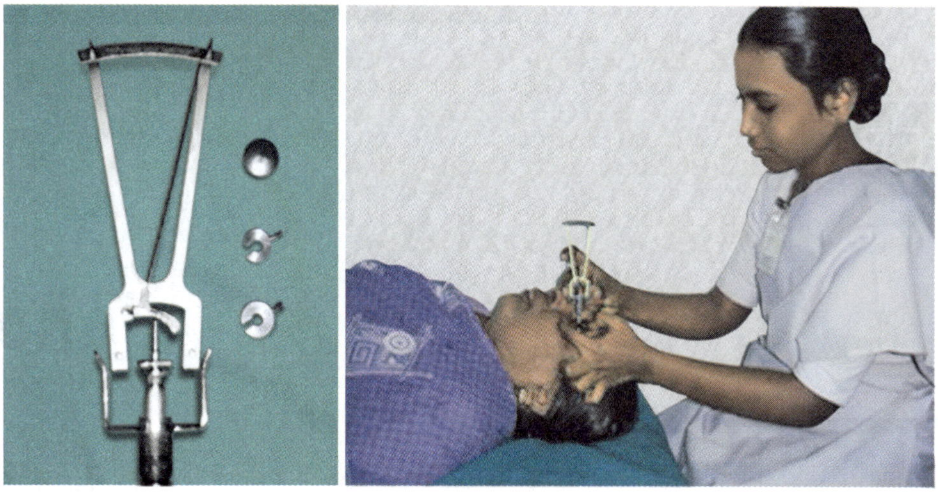

Fig. 1: Schiötz tonometer.
(*Source*: Professor R Ramakrishnan, Aravind Eye Hospital, Tirunelveli)

Box 1: Classification of tonometers.

I. *Invasive instruments*:
    A. Needles and cannulas (manometry)
    B. Transensors
II. *Noninvasive instruments (tonometers)*:
    A. *Instruments that touch the eye*:
        1. *Static instruments*:
            a. *Applanation tonometers*:
                (i) Constant area (Goldmann, Mackay-Marg)
                (ii) Constant force (Maklakoff)
            b. *Indentation tonometers*:
                (i) Constant indentation
                (ii) Constant force (Schiötz)
        2. *Dynamic instruments*:
            a. *Ballistic tonometers*:
                (i) Impact acceleration
                (ii) Impact duration
                (iii) Rebound velocity
            b. Vibration tonometers (Krakau)
    B. Instruments that do not touch the eye (noncontact tonometers) (Grolman)

Palpation Method

Intraocular pressure is estimated by response of eye to pressure applied by finger pulp (indents easily/firm to touch). This method cannot give accurate IOP reading and is not used as an IOP measurement technique.

The indirect methods can be broadly divided into contact and noncontact methods. Basic types of contact tonometer differ according to shape and magnitude of deformation.

Contact Tonometers

Intraocular pressure measurement is performed by deforming the globe and correlating the force responsible for deformation to the pressure within the eye. Both indentation and applanation tonometers effect a deformation of globe, but the magnitude varies.

Indentation Tonometers

Indentation tonometer is used to measure the amount of deformation or indentation of the globe in response to a standard weight applied to the cornea or the area flattened by a standard force. The shape of corneal deformation is truncated cone. It displaces large intraocular volume so conversion tables based on empirical data is used to estimate IOP. The prototype is Schiötz tonometer.

Applanation Tonometers

Applanation tonometers are used to measure force necessary to flatten a small, standard area of cornea. The shape of corneal deformation is simple flattening. The shape is constant, so IOP is derived from mathematical calculation. There are two types of tonometers on the basis of variable that is measured.

1. *Variable force:* Area of cornea on applanation held constant, force varies. Prototype is Goldmann tonometer.
2. *Variable area:* Force applied to cornea held constant, area varies. Prototype is Maklakoff tonometer. The volume displacement is sufficiently large to require a conversion table.

Noncontact Tonometer

Noncontact tonometer (NCT) measures time required to deform a standard area of corneal surface in response to a jet of air.

Schiötz Tonometer (Indentation Tonometer)

Schiötz tonometer consists of metal plunger that slides through a hole in a concave metal plate. The plunger supports a hammer device connected to needle that crosses a scale. The extent to which cornea is indented by plunger is measured as the distance from the foot plate curve to the plunger base, and a lever system moves a needle on calibrated scale. The indicated scale reading and the plunger weight are converted to an IOP measurement. More the plunger indents the cornea, higher the scale reading and lower the IOP.

Basic Concept

The weight of tonometer on the eye increases the actual IOP (Po) to a higher level (Pt). The change in pressure from Po to Pt is an expression of the resistance of the eye (scleral rigidity) to the displacement of fluid. Determination of Po from a scale reading Pt requires conversion which is done according to Friedenwald conversion tables. Friedenwald generated an empirical formula for linear relationship between the log function of IOP and the ocular distension. This formula has "C" a numerical constant, the coefficient of ocular rigidity which is an expression of distensibility of eye. Its average value is 0.025.

Procedure

Patient should be in supine position, looking up at a fixation target, while examiner separates lids and lowers the tonometer plate to rest on the anesthetized cornea so that plunger is free to move vertically **(Fig. 1)**. A fine movement of needle on scale is in response to ocular pulsations. Scale reading is an average of the extremes of these excursions. The 5.5 g weight is initially used. If scale reading is 4 or less, additional weight is added to plunger. Conversion table is used to derive IOP in millimeter of mercury (mm Hg) from scale reading and plunger weight. The instrument is calibrated before each use to check scale reading is zero.

Sources of Error

Accuracy is limited as ocular rigidity varies from eye to eye. As conversion tables are based on an average coefficient of ocular rigidity, eye that varies significantly from this value gives erroneous IOP. High ocular rigidity is seen in high hyperopia, long-standing glaucoma, age-related macular degeneration, and vasoconstrictor therapy. Low ocular rigidity is found in high myopia, advanced age, miotics, use of vasodilators, after retinal detachment (RD) surgery (vitrectomy, cryopexy, scleral band), and intravitreal injection of compressible gas. The variable expulsion of intraocular blood during Schiötz tonometry may influence IOP measurement. Repeated measurements lower IOP. Either a steeper or a thicker cornea causes greater displacement of fluid during tonometry and gives a falsely high IOP measurement.

Goldmann Applanation Tonometry

Tonometer Principle

The Goldmann applanation tonometer (GAT) was introduced in 1957 by Hans Goldmann and Theo Schmidt. The optimum design for the tonometer tip was derived from empirical experimentation.

The Imbert-Fick principle states that the pressure *(P)* of a body of fluid encapsulated within a sphere is directly proportional to the force *(W)* required to applanate an area *(A)* of the sphere:

$$W = PA \qquad \text{(equation 1)}$$

The principle assumes that the surface encapsulating the sphere under examination is infinitely thin, perfectly elastic, perfectly dry, and perfectly flexible and that the only force being exerted upon it is the force from the applanating surface. In reality, none of these is true when applied to the cornea. Goldmann recognized that having a finite corneal thickness, a measurable corneal rigidity and the capillary attraction forces of the pre-corneal tear film would affect the accuracy of the tonometer. It was also acknowledged that a variation in central corneal thickness (CCT) would affect the accuracy of IOP readings, but it was felt that in the absence of corneal pathology, the CCT did not vary much around 500 μm. Based on these assumptions, a modification of the Imbert-Fick principle was devised that included factors to consider the resistance of the cornea to applanation and the surface tension of the tear meniscus surrounding the tonometer prism during measurement:

$$W + s = PA + b \qquad \text{(equation 2)}$$

Where W = tonometer force, s = surface tension of precorneal tear film, P = intraocular pressure, A = area of applanation, b = corneal rigidity/resistance to bending **(Fig. 1)**.

With this formula it was determined that on applanating an external corneal area of approximately 7.35 mm^2, the effects of corneal rigidity and tear film surface tension forces would cancel **(Fig. 2)**. In addition, a force of 0.1 g would correspond to an IOP of 1 mm Hg.

Procedure

The GAT is available as a slit lamp mounted or handheld device **(Fig. 3)**. Corneal anesthesia is required. The use of

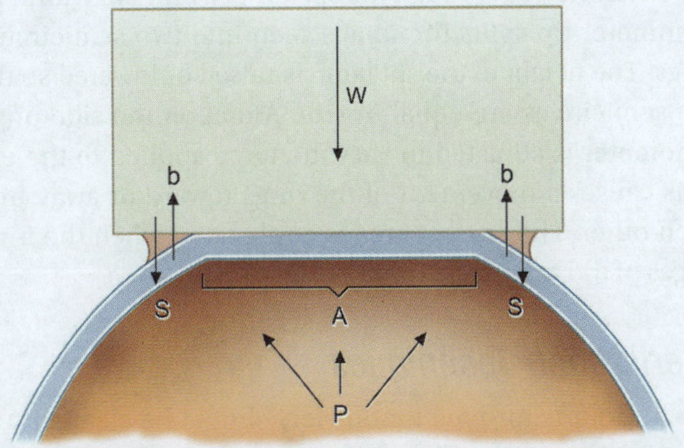

Fig. 2: Representation of force involved during applanation tonometry. (W = tonometer force; s = surface tension of precorneal tear film; P = intraocular pressure; A = area of applanation; b = corneal rigidity/resistance to bending).

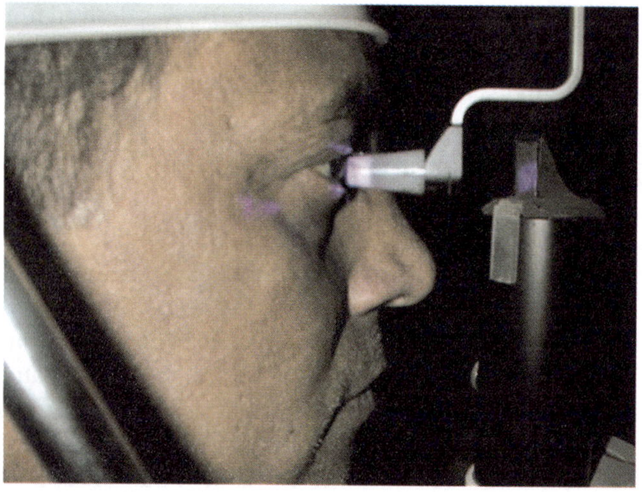

Fig. 3: Goldmann applanation.

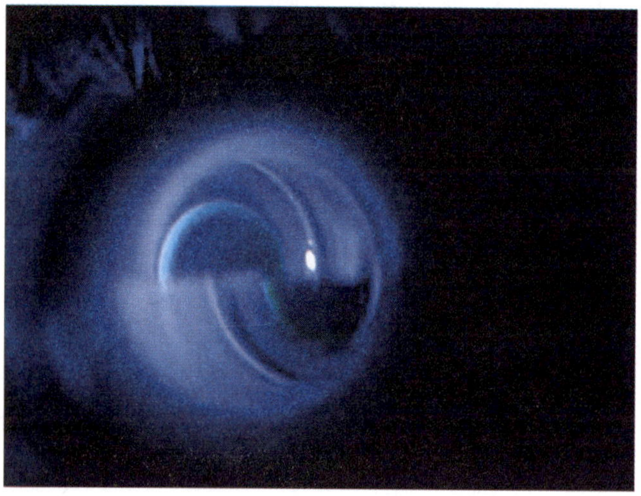

Fig. 4: Ideal mire with applanation tonometer.

fluorescein sodium facilitates the IOP reading—the tears fluorescein a cobalt blue light, making it easier to determine the area applanated. The slit-lamp illumination arm is positioned at an angle to the observation arm to maximize illumination of the tonometer head. The instrument is brought closer to the eye until corneal contact is made.

When viewed through the slit lamp, a biprism within the tonometer tip splits the image seen into two semicircular rings. The height of the slit lamp is raised or lowered so that the semicircles are equal in size. A dial on the side of the tonometer is adjusted to vary the force applied to the eye. This causes a movement of the rings toward or away from each other. The correct area is applanated when the inner edges of the semicircles touch **(Fig. 4)**.

Sterilization Techniques

Tip of Goldmann-type tonometers should be cleaned with an alcohol soaked sponge followed by drying for at least 1–2 minutes before using again.

Sources of Error

Goldmann applanation tonometer measurements are potentially affected by corneal curvature, corneal astigmatism, magnitude of capillary attraction, and tear film fluorescence.

- *Corneal curvature:* In patients with with-the-rule astigmatism, regular *corneal astigmatism* over 4D will result in an underestimate of IOP, and against-the-rule astigmatism, an overestimate of IOP by 1 mm Hg. Clinically, GAT IOP measurement error of 1 mm Hg is insignificant. A practical way to overcome this problem is to take two successive measurements, one with the prism oriented horizontally and the other vertically, and then simply take the average of the two. In irregular corneal astigmatism GAT mires will be distorted and reproducible results may not be obtained. The use of Tono-Pen could be suggested in such irregular corneas.
- *Magnitude of capillary attraction:* The radius of contact is greater with wide mires, which leads to overestimation and is lesser with thin mires leading to underestimation. To get consistent readings, optimal mire widths should be between 0.4 mm and 0.6 mm that corresponds approximately to one-fourth to one-third of the radius of the applanated area.
- *Adequate tear film fluorescence:* It is needed for the clear visualization of the contact point between the GAT tip and the cornea. Hypofluorescence leads underestimation of IOP and hyperfluorescence leads overestimation of IOP.
- *Posture*: IOP is higher in the supine position when compared with the sitting position. Total inversion of the body, like in "sirsasana", results in a significant and rapid rise in IOP.
- *Obesity:* Measuring the IOP with the Goldmann tonometer in obese patients may give high readings. This is due to thorax compression and breath holding, which causes transitory rises of IOP. In overweight patients, Perkins handheld applanation tonometer is recommended to obtain accurate IOP.
- *Valsalva maneuver/Necktie use:* This leads to an increase in IOP.
- *Eyelid squeezing*: An attempt to eyelid closure increases IOP measured both with Tono-Pen and with Goldmann applanation tonometry by at least 2–4 mm Hg.
- *Central corneal thickness*: All forms of tonometry currently available are affected by CCT. GAT tonometer is affected most. The effect of CCT on dynamic contour tonometer (DCT) IOP measurement is about half that of the CCT effect on GAT IOP measurement. NCT and rebound tonometry are also significantly affected by CCT. Although it is known that CCT does significantly affect GAT IOP measurement, its contribution to the measurement error in individual patients is unknown.

Most population studies find that the relation between CCT and GAT measurement error is about 2.5 mm Hg per 100 microns CCT. IOP "correction" nomograms in individual patients have not been validated and have the potential to lead ophthalmologists off target in their clinical decision-making.

Noncontact Tonometry

Principle

The NCT was developed by Grolman in the early 1970s and uses a jet of air to applanate the anterior corneal surface. The system consists of a central air plenum flanked either side by a light emitter and detector. When the cornea is in the resting state, light emitted is scattered by the convex corneal surface. As the pressure of the air pulse directed to the cornea increases to deform the cornea, the corneal surface behaves like a plane mirror reflecting light to the detector. At the point of maximal light detection when the cornea is completely applanated, the instrument switches off the air pressure pulse **(Figs. 5A and B)**. The newer machines have pressure transducer, so that the IOP is determined from the actual air jet pressure required to applanate the cornea. The NCT is simple to use and requires minimal training to master. The NCT usually measures IOP higher than GAT and also limited by all errors which GAT is prone for. It is as best as a screening tool, and all high IOP needs to be reconfirmed by GAT.

Pneumotonometry

Principle

The principle of using a pneumatic device to measure IOP was first described by Durham and was modified by Langham in 1969. The pneumotonometer is a contact applanation tonometer that consists of four main components:

1. A sensor that responds to IOP when applied to the cornea.
2. A transducer that converts the pneumatic signal to an electrical signal.
3. A combined amplifier and recorder that amplifies the signal and provides a readout of the signal recorded.
4. An air supply unit that supplies compressed air to the tonometer probe.

The probe has a hollow central tube flanked circumferentially by side exhausts. The probe tip is covered by a flexible inert silicone elastomer diaphragm (Silastic membrane), which comes into contact with the cornea. A constant flow of air is passed through the central tube, forcing a small gap between the diaphragm and probe edge forcing air out through the side exhausts. When placed against cornea, the force of air eventually results in the cornea being applanated to the edge of the probe, forcing the membrane gap to close. Air pressure within tube rises until it balances the IOP and membrane mechanics of the cornea, at which point air can escape. At this point, the air pressure within the tube is proportional to the IOP.

The pneumotonometer is also able to measure the fluctuations in IOP caused by the cardiac cycle. These variations are manifestations of ocular blood flow and are recorded as the ocular pulse amplitude (OPA).

Procedure

The tonometer is a slit-lamp mounted device and requires corneal anesthesia prior to IOP measurement. A disposable tip is placed over the pneumatic probe. When the probe tip is in contact with the cornea, a whistling sound indicates good contact. The pitch varies with the ocular pulse. A minimum of seven cycles is required for an adequate ocular blood flow (OBF) reading.

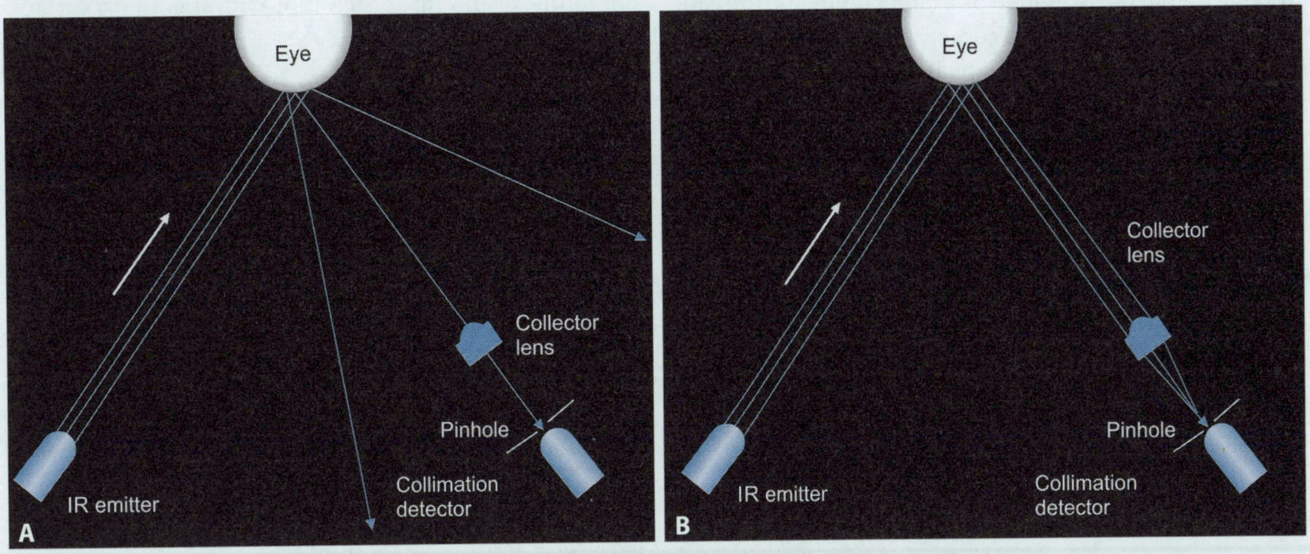

Figs. 5A and B: Noncontact tonometer principle.

The Reichert Ocular Response Analyzer

The ocular response analyzer (ORA; Reichert Corporation; New York, USA) measures the corneal response to indentation by a rapid air pulse. The principles of the ORA are based on those of NCT. A metered air pulse is directed at the cornea until an applanation event is reached. This first "force-in" applanation acts as a trigger to switch off the air pulse, after a small further increase in air pressure, which causes a degree of corneal indentation. The air pressure steadily reduces until it is completely removed. The instrument makes two measurements—the force required to flatten the cornea as the air pressure rises ("force-in" applanation, P1) and the force at which the cornea becomes flat again as the air pressure falls ("force-out" applanation, P2). The second applanation occurs at a lower pressure than the first, and this has been attributed to the dampening effects of the cornea. The difference between the two pressures is termed *corneal hysteresis (CH)* **(Fig. 6)**. CH is a direct measure of the biomechanical properties of the cornea and can completely describe the contribution of corneal resistance to IOP measurements than CCT alone.

The ORA produces two measurements of corneal biomechanical properties, CH and the corneal response factor (CRF). While CH represents the absolute difference between the applanation pressures P1 and P2, the CRF is derived from the formula (P1- *k*P2), where *k* is a constant. It has been suggested that CH predominantly reflects the viscous properties of the cornea, whilst CRF better reflects the elastic properties.

The Tono-Pen

Principle

The Tono-Pen is based on the principle of the MacKay-Marg tonometer. The device consists of a central 1.02 mm diameter moveable plunger surrounded by a larger footplate. Pressing the instrument tip against the cornea activates a strain gauge that senses the force generated by the plunger to applanate the central cornea. As the rest of the tonometer comes into contact with the cornea, the force exerted on the plunger reduces until the plunger is flush with the footplate. The effect of corneal rigidity is transferred to the surrounding footplate and, at that point, the force exerted on the plunger is considered to be only the IOP. This change in force generates a waveform tracing which is analyzed by a microprocessor.

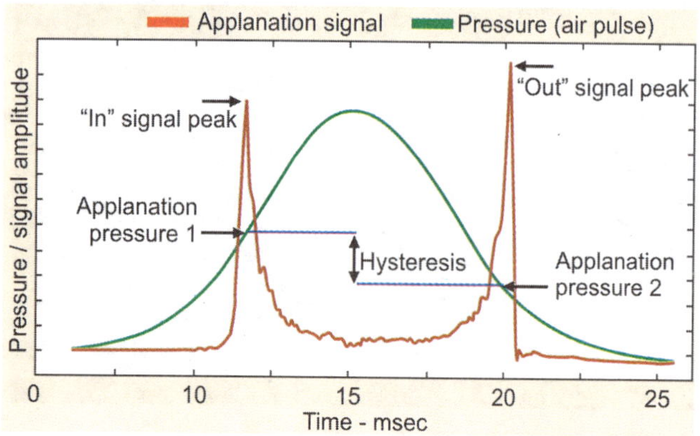

Fig. 6: Ocular response analyzer.

Procedure

The device requires corneal anesthesia for measurements. Disposable tips are changed between patients. The Tono-Pen is handheld and positioned upon the central cornea. When the instrument has generated a satisfactory waveform, an audible click is sound, and the operator repeats small pecking movements onto the cornea until 6–10 readings are accepted. These are automatically averaged and a digital display provides the final reading along with the percentage variability between the highest and lowest value.

The Pascal® Dynamic Contour Tonometer

The Pascal® Dynamic Contour Tonometer (DCT; Swiss Microtechnology® AG, Port, Switzerland) was first introduced in 2002. The design purposed was to develop a noninvasive and direct method for IOP measurement that would be relatively unaffected by the interindividual variations of corneal biomechanics. The tonometer is a nonapplanating, slit-lamp mounted, contact tonometer **(Fig. 7)**.

Principle

The principle is based on contour matching, which assumes that if the eyes were enclosed by a contoured, tight fitting shell, the forces generated by IOP would act on the shell wall. Replacing part of the shell-wall with a pressure sensor would enable measurement of these forces and therefore the IOP.

The DCT has a contoured tonometer tip surface that aims to match the contour of the cornea. The radius of curvature of the tip is 10.5 mm with a contact surface of

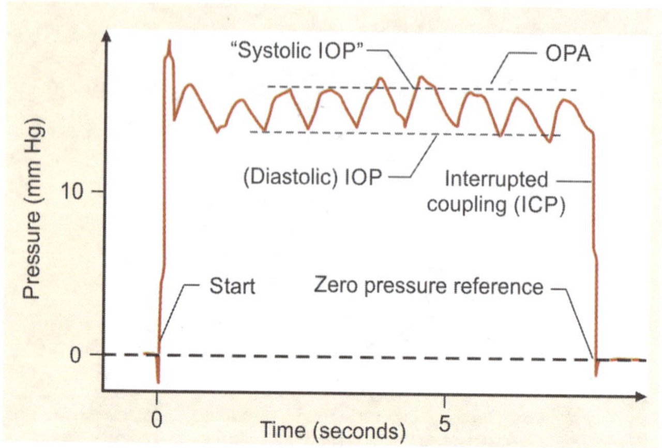

Fig. 7: Pressure curve from DCT recording. The instrument displays the diastolic IOP and ocular pulse amplitude.
(DCT: dynamic contour tonometer; IOP: intraocular pressure; OPA: ocular pulse amplitude)

approximately 7 mm diameter. A piezoresistive pressure sensor of diameter ~1.2 mm is integrated flush within the contour surface, enabling transcorneal measurements of the anterior chamber fluid pressure. The tip is mounted into housing, similar to that used for GAT, which provides a constant appositional force of 1 g. IOP readings are sampled at 100 Hz and data are computed with a resolution of 0.1 mm Hg. Diastolic IOP is displayed on an LCD screen within the housing. The dynamic sampling of IOP also yields pressure curves from which the OPA is determined **(Fig. 7)**. The OPA value displayed on the LCD screen is a peak-to-peak difference of the average systolic IOP and average diastolic IOP, in units of mm Hg. The DCT provides an audible signal, the pitch of which modulates regularly, indicating pulse oscillations.

Procedure

Corneal anesthesia is required. A disposable silicone tip is placed on the tonometer head, and is changed between patients. A minimum of 5 cardiac cycles need to be recorded for an adequate reading, although between 5 cycles and 8 cycles is recommended. Once adequate measurements are obtained, the LCD display will generate an IOP and OPA value (in mm Hg), and a "quality score". Readings of value "1" and "2" only should be accepted, although the manufacturer reports that readings up to quality "3" are acceptable. Readings of "4" or "5" should be discarded.

Rebound Tonometry

Principle

Rebound tonometry **(Fig. 8)** uses a dynamic electromechanical method for measuring IOP. The device consists of two coils, a solenoid propelling coil and a sensing coil positioned around a central shaft containing a lightweight magnetized probe. The application of a transient electrical current to the solenoid coil propels the probe to the cornea. This movement of the magnetized probe induces a voltage within the system which is monitored by the sensor, allowing the speed and direction of probe movement to be determined. As the probe impacts cornea, it decelerates and rebounds from surface; deceleration is less at low compared with high IOPs.

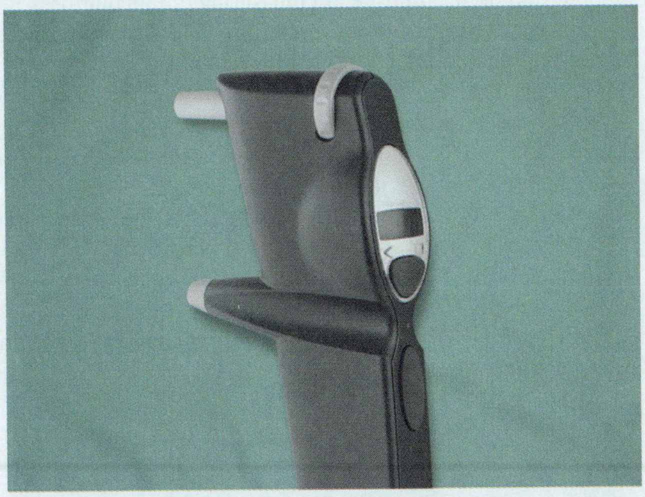

Fig. 8: Rebound tonometry.

Procedure

No corneal anesthesia is required. The instrument is a handheld device and on activation of the measurement button automatically takes six readings of IOP, automatically discarding the highest and lowest reading before presenting a digital readout of the average IOP.

Draeger Tonometer

Draeger tonometer is similar to Perkins but uses different set of prisms and operates with a motor adjusting the force on these prisms.

MacKay-Marg Tonometer

Principle

Force is required to keep the flat plate of a plunger flush with a surrounding sleeve against the pressure of corneal deformation. Tonometer incorporates a 1.5 mm diameter plunger affixed to a rigid spring that extends 10 μ beyond the plane of surrounding rubber sleeve. Movement of plunger is electronically monitored by a transducer and recorded on a moving paper strip. When the tonometer is placed against cornea, the tracing that represents the force applied to the plunger begins to rise. At 1.5 mm of corneal area applanation, tracing reaches a peak and the force applied = IOP + Force required to deform the cornea. At 3 mm flattening, force required to deform cornea is transferred from plunger to surrounding sleeve, creating a dip in tracing corresponding to IOP. Flattening of >3 mm of area gives artificial elevation of IOP. It is accurate in eyes with scarred, edematous, and irregular corneas.

Other MacKay-Marg-type Tonometers: CAT 100 Applanation and Biotronics Tonometers

They have an internal logic program which automatically selects the acceptable measurement and three or more good IOP readings are averaged and displayed on screen.

SPECIAL CONSIDERATIONS

Contact Lenses

Contact lenses can make changes in corneal shape and/or corneal thickness, and there is evidence that many soft contact lens wearers may develop corneal edema throughout the day as a result of lens wear. Silicone hydrogel contact lenses should provide sufficient oxygen to the cornea to prevent corneal edema during the day.

Corneal Edema

Large amounts of corneal edema produce a lower IOP when the IOP is measured with applanation tonometry.

Refractive Surgery

Following many forms of keratorefractive surgery, including laser in situ keratomileusis (LASIK), laser-assisted subepithelial keratectomy (LASEK), and photorefractive keratectomy (PRK), there is a mean decline in measured IOP using static tonometry. This may be due to the changes in corneal biomechanics and elasticity, which can have an overriding effect on static IOP measurement, in addition to changes in corneal curvature.

SUGGESTED READING

1. Armaly MF. On the distribution of applanation pressure. I. Statistical features and the effect of age, sex, and family history of glaucoma. Arch Ophthalmol. 1965;73:11-8.
2. Bengtsson B. Comparison of Schiotz and Goldmann tonometry and tonography in a population. Acta Ophthalmol. (Copenh) 1972;50:455.
3. Craven ER, Butler SL, McCulley JP, et al. Applanation tonometer tip sterilization for adenovirus type 8. Ophthalmology. 1987;94(12):1538-40.
4. Drance SM. The coefficient of scleral rigidity in normal and glaucomatous eyes. Arch Ophthalmol. 1960;63:668-74.
5. Dunn JS, Brubaker RF. Perkins applanation tonometer: clinical and laboratory evaluation. Arch Ophthalmol. 1973;89(2): 149-51.
6. Durhan DG, Bigliano RP, Masino JA. Pneumatic applanation tonometer. Trans Am Acad Ophthalmol Otolaryngol. 1965;69(6):1029-47.
7. Finlay RD. Experience with the Draeger applanation tonometer. Trans Ophthalmol Soc UK. 1970;90:887-92.
8. Forbes M, Pico G Jr, Goldman B. A noncontact applanation tonometer: description and clinical evaluation. Arch Ophthalmol. 1974;91(2)134-40.
9. Friedenwald JS. Contribution to the theory and practice of tonometry. Am J Ophthalmol. 1937;20(10):985-1024.
10. Friedenwald JS. Standardization of tonometers decennial report. Trans Am Acad Ophthalmol Otolarymgol. 1954;58.
11. Friedman E, Ivry M, Ebert E, et al. Increased scleral rigidity and age-related macular degeneration. Ophthalmology. 1989;96(1):104-8.
12. Glouster J, Perkins ES. The validity of the Imbert-Fick law as applied to applanation tonometry. Exp Eye Res. 1963;2:274.
13. Grolman B. Non-contact applanation tonometry. Optician. 1973;166:4.
14. Hollows FC, Graham PA. Intra-ocular pressure, glaucoma, and glaucoma suspects in a defined population. Br J Ophthalmol. 1966;50(10):570-86.
15. Imbert A. Theories ophthalmotonometers. Arch Ophthalmol. 1885;5:358.
16. Kaufman HE, Wind CA, Waltman SR. Validity of MacKay-Marg electronic applanation tonometer in patients with scarred irregular corneas. Am J Ophthalmol. 1970;69(6):1003-7.
17. Khan JA, Davis M, Graham CE, et al. Comparison of Oculab Tono-Pen readings obtained from various corneal and scleral locations. Arch Ophthalmol. 1991;109(10):1444-6.
18. Krieglstein GK, Waller WK. Goldmann applanation versus hand-applanation and schiötz indentation tonometry. Albrecht Von Graefes Arch Clin Exp Ophthalmol. 1975; 194(1):11-6.
19. Kronfeld PC. Tonometer calibration: empirical validation. Trans Am Acad Ophthalmol Otolaryngol. 1957;61(1):123-6.
20. Langham ME, McCarthy E. A rapid pneumatic applanation tonometer: comparative findings and evaluation. Arch Ophthalmol. 1968;79(4):389-99.
21. Macro FJ, Brubakar RF. Methodology of eye pressure measurement. Biorheology. 1969;6(1):37-45.
22. Markiewitz HH. The so-called Imbert-Fick law. Arch Ophthalmol. 1960;64:159.
23. McMillan F, Forster RK. Comparison of MacKay-Marg, Goldmann, and Perkins tonometers in abnormal corneas. Arch Ophthalmol. 1975;93(6):420-4.
24. Moses RA. Fluorescein in applanation tonometry. Am J Ophthalmol. 1960;49:1149-55.
25. Moses RA. The Goldmann applanation tonometer. Am J Ophthalmol. 1958;46(6):865-9.
26. Pepose JS, Linette G, Lee SF, et al. Disinfection of Goldmann tonometers against human immunodeficiency virus type I. Arch Ophthalmol. 1989;107(7):983-5.
27. Perkins ES. Hand-held applanation tonometer. Br J Ophthalmol. 1965;49(11):591-3.
28. Petersen WC, Schlegel WA. Mackay-Marg tonometry by technicians. Am J Ophthalmol. 1973;76(6):933-6.
29. Posner A. An evaluation of the Maklakov applanation tonometer. Eye Ear Nose Throat Mon. 1962;41:377-8.
30. Posner A. Practical problems in the use of the Maklakov tonometer. Eye Ear Nose Throat Mon. 1963;42:82-3.
31. Rootman DS, Insler MS, Thompson HW, et al. Accuracy and precision of the Tono-Pen in measuring intraocular pressure after keratoplasty and epikeratophakia in scarred corneas. Arch Ophthalmol. 1988;106(12):1697-100.
32. Schields MB. The non-contact tonometer: its value and limitations. Surv Ophthalmol. 1980;24(4):211-9.
33. Schmidt TA. The clinical application of the Goldmann applanation tonometer. Am J Ophthalmol. 1960;49:967-78.
34. Schwartz NJ, Mackay RS, Sackman JL. A theoretical and experimental study of the mechanical behavior of the cornea with application to the measurement of intraocular pressure. Bull Math Biol. 1966;28(4):585-643.
35. Starrels ME. The measurement of intraocular pressure. Int Ophthalmol Clin. 1979;19:9.

CHAPTER

7 Gonioscopy

Ronnie Jacob George, A Parivadhini, A Narayanaswamy, L Vijaya

INTRODUCTION

Gonioscopy, the visualization and assessment of the anterior chamber angle, is an essential procedure in the diagnosis and management of glaucoma. Gonioscopy serves two purposes:

1. To identify the eyes at risk for angle-closure
2. To detect any abnormalities in the angle.

Both of which can help in differentiating one type of glaucoma from another and provide guidance for appropriate therapy. The term gonioscopy was coined by Trantas in 1907. Subsequently, Goldmann introduced the gonioprism, and Barkan mastered the art of gonioscopy and highlighted its role in the management of glaucoma. All cases of glaucoma should undergo a routine and periodic gonioscopic evaluation for complete ophthalmic examination. The procedure is fairly easy to perform, but experience is needed in accurate assessment and interpretation.

OPTICAL PRINCIPLES

The anatomy of the eye is such that the angle recess is not visualized by routine instrumentation due to total internal reflection of rays emerging from the angle recess. The gonioscope was evolved to overcome this optical problem of critical angle at the air-cornea interface (46*) **(Figs. 1A to C)**.

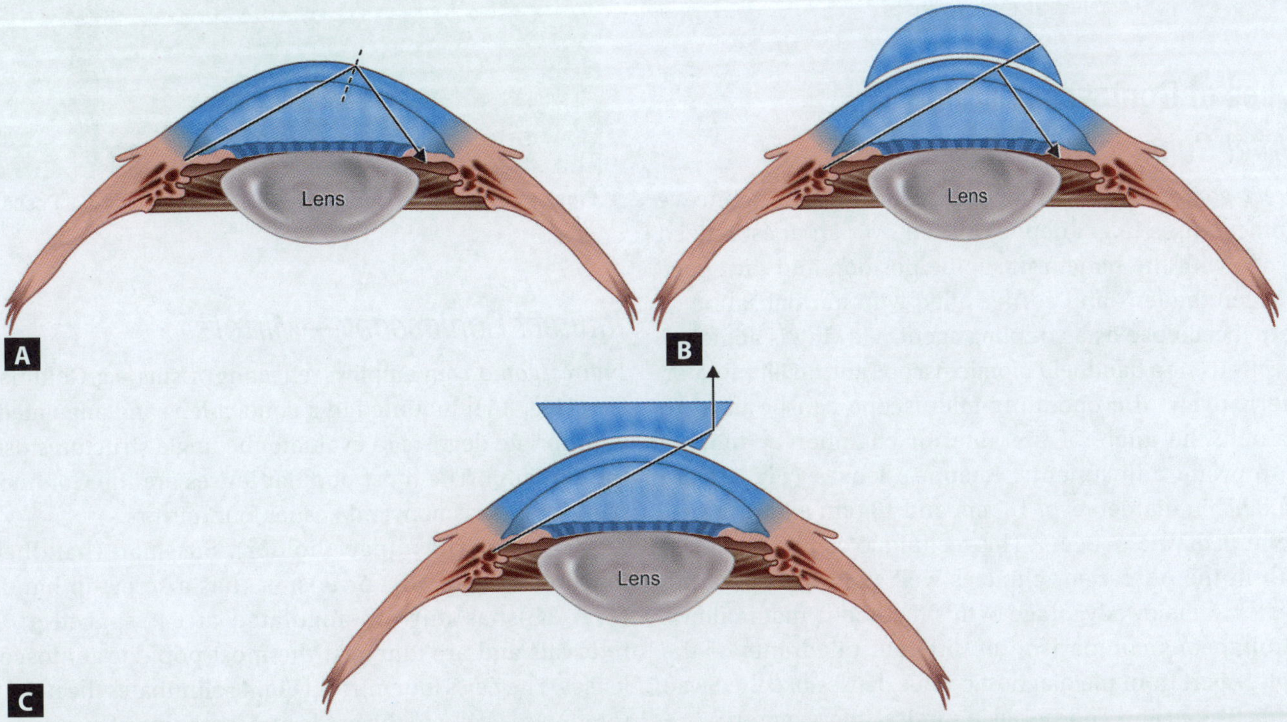

Figs. 1A to C: *Optical principles of gonioscopy*: (A) Incident light from the angle exceeds critical angle resulting in total internal reflection and preventing visibility of the recess; (B and C) The goniolens optically eliminates the cornea as shown in the schematic diagrams and allows visibility of the angle.

Table 1: Contact lenses used for gonioscopy.

Type	Lenses	Features
Direct		
	• Koeppe • Barkan • Thorpe • Swan-Jacob • Layden	• Diagnostic lens-50 diopter concave lens available in two sizes, for infants (16 mm) and adults (18 mm) • Surgical lens—available in various sizes and has blunted edges allowing access for goniotomy • Surgical and diagnostic lens • Surgical lens for goniotomy • Diagnostic lens for evaluating neonatal angle
Indirect		
	• Goldmann single mirror and three mirrors • Zeiss and Posner four mirrors • Sussman four mirrors • Ritch trabeculoplasty lens	• Diagnostic and therapeutic lenses provide excellent images with good magnification and globe stability • Ideal diagnostic lenses, patient friendly and very valuable in evaluating narrow angles and to perform indentation gonioscopy • Handheld four mirrors—similar advantages as the Zeiss lenses • Four-mirror lens with pairs inclined at 59°and 62°. One of each set has a convex lens over it providing magnification—both diagnostic and therapeutic

Goldmann lenses **(Fig. 3A)** are of two types: (1) Single-mirrored lens has a mirror angulated at 62° and (2) three-mirrored lens has mirrors at 59° (tongue-shaped, used to evaluate the angle), 67° (midsized, used to view midperipheral fundus) and 73° (long, used to view peripheral fundus and ciliary body) (59 + 8 = 67 + 6 = 73). The central well has a diameter of 12 mm and radius of curvature of 7.38 mm. A newer modified version with 8.4 mm radius of curvature eliminates the need of using a coupling solution. The three mirrors also aid in retinal evaluation and laser therapy.

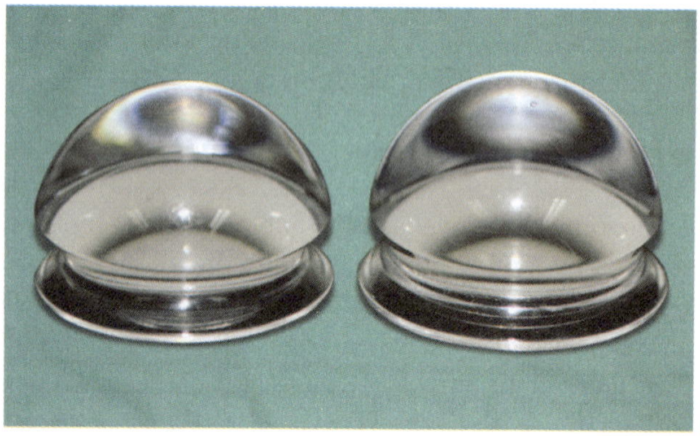

Fig. 2: Koeppe lenses.

Types of Gonioscopy (Table 1)

Direct Gonioscopy—Lenses

Direct gonioscopy is performed with the aid of concave contact lenses (e.g. Koeppe) placed over an anesthetized cornea with the patient in supine position and the space between the lens and cornea filled with normal saline or methyl cellulose as a coupling agent. Viewing is achieved directly using a handheld biomicroscope and an illuminator. Alternatively, the operating microscope can be used to evaluate the angle of the anterior chamber by making appropriate adjustments. Koeppe's lenses **(Fig. 2)** are available in diameters of 16 mm and 18 mm allowing easy use in pediatric patients. This technique can be practiced both in the outpatient clinic as well as in the operation theater. A major advantage of this method is that it allows simultaneous comparison of different quadrants of the angle. Apart from the diagnostic value, lenses like the Swan Jacob, Barkan and Thorpe aid in surgical intervention.

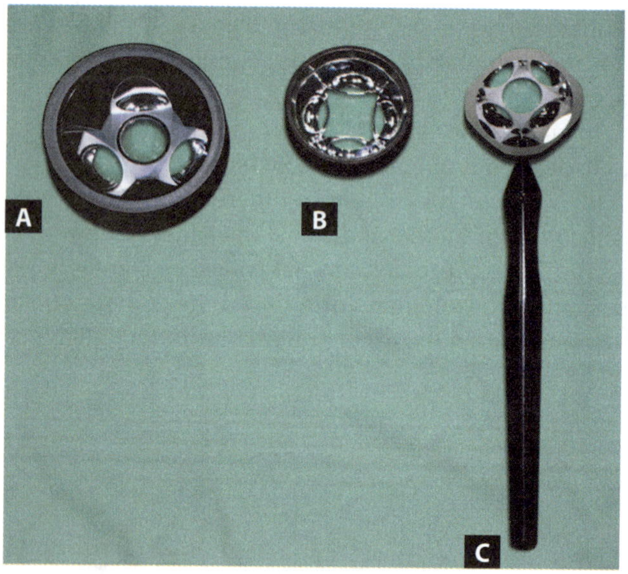

Figs. 3A to C: (A) Goldmann lens; (B) Sussman lens; (C) Posner four-mirror lens.

Indirect Gonioscopy—Mirrors

Indirect gonioscopy employs reflecting prisms [e.g. Goldmann lens **(Fig. 3A)**] mounted in a contact lens and angulated at appropriate degrees to evaluate the angle structures using the slit lamp. The most popular lenses are the Goldmann type, Zeiss, Sussman, and Posner four mirrors.

Zeiss lens (has unger holder), Sussman (handheld) four mirror **(Fig. 3B)** or Posner (has a screw-in handle) **(Fig. 3C)** has mirrors angulated at 64° spaced at 90° intervals and are amongst the most popular gonioscopy lenses. The Zeiss four mirror **(Fig. 4)** eliminates the need for rotation to evaluate the angle and its radius of curvature is

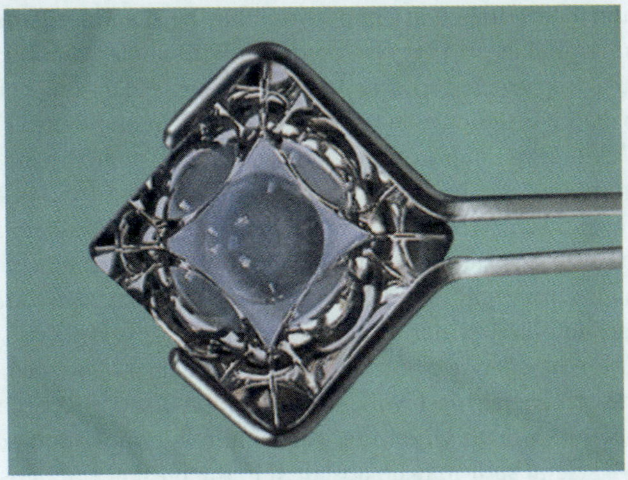

Fig. 4: Zeiss four-mirror lens.

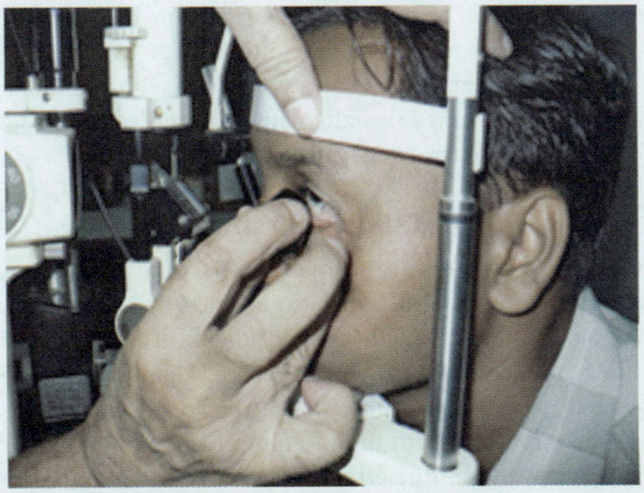

Fig. 5: The inferior rim of three-mirror gonioscope is inserted in the lower fornix with patient in upgaze as shown and swiftly tilted on to the cornea preventing loss of any coupling fluid.

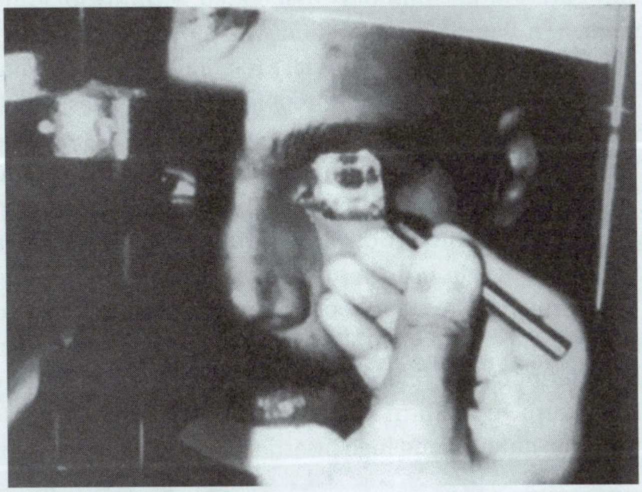

Fig. 6: The four-mirror gonioscope is applied gently and directly on to the cornea. Fingers rested over cheek to ensure adequate support and prevent inadvertent pressure over the globe.

7.8 mm, closer to the corneal curvature, thereby eliminating the need for a viscous coupling agent. The diameter of the lens is 9.0 mm which aids in dynamic or compression gonioscopy, an important technique in evaluating narrow angles and angle-closure glaucomas.

Manipulative gonioscopy can be performed by Goldmann two-mirror lenses in which the patient is asked to look in the direction of angle to be visualized with pressure on the cornea. Indentation gonioscopy can be performed with Zeiss, Posner, and Sussman lenses wherein indentation of the central cornea displaces the aqueous into peripheral AC, pushes the iris backward and widens the chamber angle.

Protocol for a Routine Gonioscopy

- Explain the procedure to the patient.
- Reassure the patient and ensure cooperation.
- Corneal surface is examined to rule out any contraindication for gonioscopy (abrasion, infection, significant corneal edema, or opacity).
- Adequate anesthesia is ensured using either 0.5% topical proparacaine or 4.0% lignocaine.
- The patient and examiner should be in a comfortable posture with adequate support to examiner's forearm and elbow to make sure of good control and minimal pressure over the eye throughout the procedure.
- The lens is held in the examiner's left hand for evaluating the right eye and vice versa.
- The three-mirror gonioscope is filled with viscous solutions and inserted as shown in **Figure 5**. The four-mirror Zeiss lens is applied directly **(Fig. 6)**.
- The patient is asked to maintain a straight gaze once the lens is in situ.
- Low, but adequate illumination (dark room) and small beams (1 mm) are focused on the mirror, with viewing and illumination maintained in the same axis. The illumination arm is moved paraxial when needed to evaluate the nasal and temporal recesses. Magnification and illumination can be increased when needed to evaluate finer details like new vessels and foreign bodies.

One quadrant can be evaluated at a time with the three-mirror by sequential rotation while with the four-mirror all four quadrants can be evaluated without rotation and with minimum adjustments of the slit lamp. Always remember the opposite quadrant (e.g. with mirror at 7 o'clock, the 1 o'clock angle) is being evaluated and the image is reversed but not crossed.

Other dynamic maneuvers like compression and over-the-hill evaluation are subsequently done. Over-the-hill maneuver involves asking the patient to look in the direction of the mirror; which in turn gives access to viewing angle recess over the convex iris. Compression techniques will be dealt with subsequently.

- Disinfection of lenses is necessary prior and after every use because of the potential of transmitting infection. Lenses can be swiped dry with bacillocid (2% glutaraldehyde) or alternatively lenses can be rinsed with soap solution and water, and allowed to dry.

Gonioscopic Anatomy and Interpretation

Repeated and routine normal gonioscopic studies are essential in adding to one's experience in evaluating a pathological angle. A methodical evaluation of each structure either from iris plane to Schwalbe's line **(Fig. 7)** or from iris plane to Schwalbe's should curtail errors in interpretation.

To start with, from the peripheral iris plane one can follow upward to the insertion of iris root. The contour of iris has several variations. The normal adult eye has a slightly convex contour. The same may be exaggerated in hyperopic eyes, wherein the anterior segment it is crowded. A flat iris configuration is commonly associated with myopia and aphakia. A flat iris configuration with a peripheral convex roll or hump of iris that lies in close relation to the trabecular meshwork and can be seen in phakic normal eyes which often mimics a narrow angle and is referred to as *plateau iris configuration*. Contours could also be concave and are associated with high myopes and pigment dispersion syndrome. The insertion of iris root may vary from a posterior, anterior or high insertions, thereby determining the visibility of the ciliary body band and the contour and depth of angle recess. The ciliary body band is composed of the anterior end of ciliary muscle and is seen as a slate gray or dark brown uniform band when insertion of iris root is posterior, anterior and high insertions preclude its view. An unusually wide ciliary body band may be seen in myopes and aphakes and may be confused with angle recession, but comparative gonioscopy and other signs of trauma help to distinguish between the normal and the pathological.

The next anterior transition is the scleral spur, the most prominent and most important landmark, identification of which is vital in terms of orientation of the angle. The scleral spur is the posterior lip of the scleral sulcus and is attached to the ciliary body band posteriorly and to the corneoscleral portion of trabecular meshwork anteriorly. It is visible as a glistening opaque white line between the ciliary body band and trabecular meshwork, however, identification at times may be difficult when the trabeculum is nonpigmented. The scleral spur may be obscured in the presence of dense pigmentation of angle structures like in post-traumatic or postsurgical situations. Iris processes, which are fine uveal strands arising from anterior iris surface and running up to the corneoscleral meshwork may also prevent a good view especially when they are prominent, as seen in congenital glaucomas. The spur is not visible in the presence of peripheral anterior synechiae (PAS) or appositional angle-closure on routine gonioscopy.

The trabecular meshwork has a posterior functional, more pigmented portion and a less functional nonpigmented anterior portion. The corneoscleral part of the meshwork extends from the scleral spur to the Schwalbe's line. The pigmentation of the meshwork varies with the kind of eyes, age and other pathological conditions. Brown eyes and adult eyes tend to have a deeper pigmentation compared to blue eyes and younger individuals. A nonpigmented trabecular meshwork may often present a tricky situation

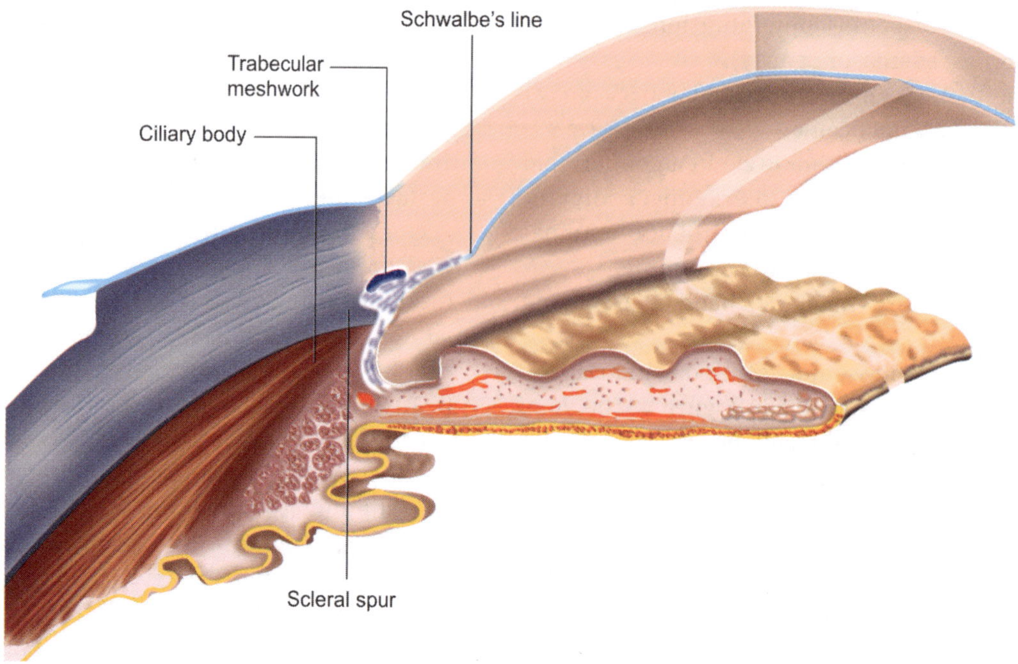

Fig. 7: Gonioscopic landmarks of a normal angle of the anterior chamber.

as far as accurate assessment is concerned, since its color and texture seems to merge with the scleral spur. However, a careful evaluation reveals it to be a more translucent and less white structure. The *parallelepiped effect* is a useful adjunct that can be used in situations wherein the landmarks are indistinguishable. This effect causes a narrow-slit-beam of light that is reflected from the anterior and posterior corneal surfaces to collapse at the Schwalbe's line. Once this point is identified the other landmarks can be assessed based on the distance from the line.

The Schlemm's canal is usually not visible, but can be seen through a less pigmented posterior trabeculum when reflux blood fills up either due to raised episcleral venous pressure, or rarely as a normal phenomenon. Excess pressure over the globe especially with a three-mirror gonioscope can also cause artifactual filling up of the Schlemm's canal with blood.

Schwalbe's line as described before represents the peripheral termination of the Descemet's membrane. Usually optically identified by the parallelepiped method, it also at times appears as a prominent white ridge known as *posterior embryotoxon*, a misnomer. This ridge is better appreciated when the patient looks in the direction of the mirror and is more prominent in the temporal quadrants. The line may occasionally be pigmented and is referred to as *Sampaolesi line* as seen in pseudoexfoliation and pigment dispersion syndrome.

Pediatric Eye

The pediatric eye has definite but subtle variations in its anatomy. The iris contour in a newborn is usually flat and its insertion is posterior to scleral spur with the anterior extension of ciliary body band visible. This contour does eventually become convex as the angle recess develops in 6–12 months. The trabecular meshwork is nonpigmented and appears thick and translucent. Congenital glaucomas present with anterior insertions of the iris directly on to the trabeculum and at times the anterior iris stroma sweeps upward in a concave fashion to insert onto the trabecular meshwork.

Grading and Recording of Gonioscopic Findings

Though multiple individual variations in assessment and grading gonioscopic details are being followed, it is important to follow a certain protocol of documentation, which aids in follow-up of the disease process. Among the systems described **(Table 2)**, the Spaeth's system is thought to be complete as it covers details with regard to angle width, iris insertion, and configuration. Any gonioscopic data should contain (1) width of angle recess, (2) iris contour and insertion of iris root, (3) degree of pigmentation, and (4) presence of abnormal structures in each quadrant. **Figure 8** shows a wide-open angle (Shaffer's grade IV or Spaeth's D40r) with regular iris contour and deep recess. All the landmarks—iris root, ciliary body band, scleral spur, and trabecular meshwork are visible. When insertion of iris occurs at scleral spur, the peripheral iris appears slightly convex, the angle of the anterior chamber still remains open (Shaffer's grade III or Spaeth's C30r, **Fig. 9**).

Classification of Primary Angle-closure

- *Primary angle-closure suspect (PACS):* An eye in which appositional contact between the peripheral iris and posterior trabecular meshwork is possible (if posterior trabecular meshwork is not visualized for >270), is considered PACS.
- *Primary angle-closure (PAC):* An eye with an occludable drainage angle and features indicating that trabecular

Table 2: Classification systems for gonioscopy.

System	*System basis*	*Angle structures and classification*	
Scheie (1957)	Extent of angle structures visualized	• All structures visible • Angle recess not seen • Ciliary body band not seen • Posterior trabeculum obscured • Only Schwalbe's line visible	• Wide open • Grade I narrow • Grade II narrow • Grade III narrow • Grade IV narrow
Shaffer (1960)	Angular width of recess	• Wide open (30°–45°) • Moderately narrow (20°) • Extremely narrow (10°) • Partly or totally closed	• Grade 3–4, closure impossible • Grade 2, closure possible • Grade 1, closure probable • Grade 0, closure present
Spaeth (1971)	• Insertion of iris root • Angular approach to the recess configuration of peripheral iris	• Anterior to Schwalbe's line • Behind (posterior) to Schwalbe's line • At scleral spur • Deep into ciliary body band • Extremely deep • 0–40° • Regular (slightly convex) • Queer (posterior bowing) steep	A B C D E r q s

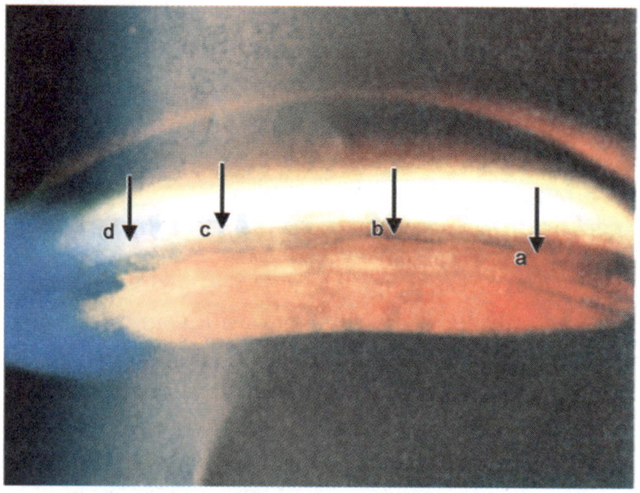

Fig. 8: *Goniophotograph of a grade IV Shaffer's angle (corresponds to Spaeth-D40r)*: (a) Iris root; (b) Ciliary body band; (c) Scleral spur; (d) Trabecular meshwork. Iris contour is regular with a deep recess.

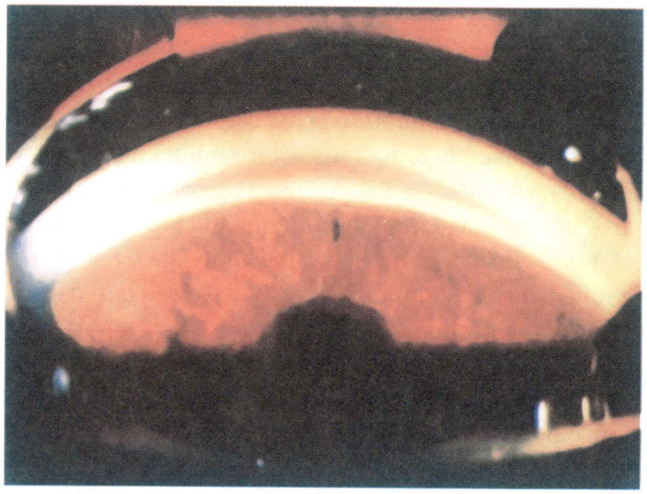

Fig. 10: A narrow angle visible up to the Schwalbe's line.

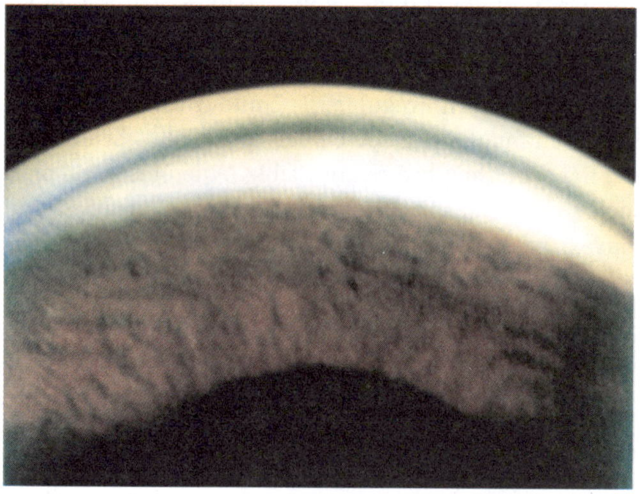

Fig. 9: Goniophotograph of a grade III Shaffer's angle (corresponds to Spaeth-C30r). Landmarks are visible up to scleral spur with a mild iris convexity.

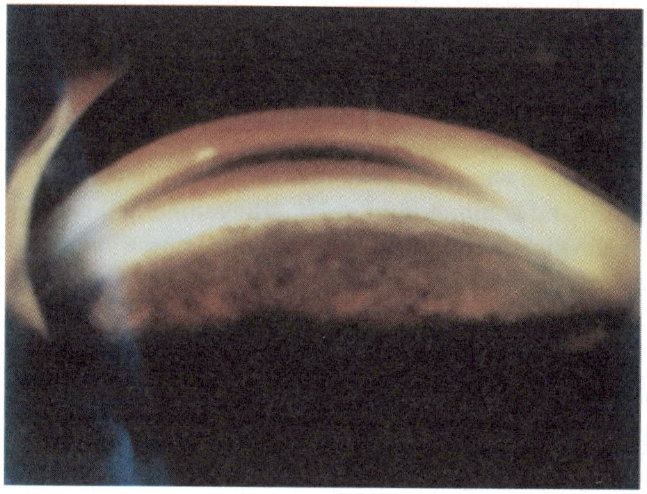

Fig. 11: The same angle on compression widens to reveal landmarks up to scleral spur.

obstruction by the peripheral iris has occurred, such as PAS, elevated intraocular pressure, iris whorling (distortion of the radially orientated iris fibers), "glaucomflecken" lens opacities, or excessive pigment deposition on the trabecular surface. The optic disk does not have glaucomatous damage.

- *Primary angle-closure glaucoma (PACG):* Primary angle-closure glaucoma is defined when primary glaucoma is present with the evidence of angle-closure.

Compression Gonioscopy

Compression or indentation gonioscopy is a simple and invaluable technique that one needs to know to assess narrow angles **(Fig. 10)** and chronic angle-closure situations. It helps distinguish appositional angle-closure from synechial angle-closure. The technique employs exerting external pressure over the cornea using the Zeiss, Posner or Sussman four-mirror lenses, thereby forcing the lens iris diaphragm posteriorly and allowing visualizing the hidden angle recess **(Fig. 11)**.

The technique involves a routine assessment of all quadrants, following which, if one subsequently decides the angle is narrow, each quadrant is reevaluated using a narrow slit-beam (to prevent miosis causing artifactual opening of the angle recess), pressure is applied directed toward the center of the eye. It results in deepening of the anterior chamber in the area of recess caused by bowing back of peripheral iris along with stretching of the limbal scleral ring and straightening of the angle recess; following this one can see structures that were not visible earlier, or confirm the presence of PAS. Corneal folds often distort the view but this can be minimized with appropriate technique in application of pressure. The physiological principles involved in compression gonioscopy have been depicted in **Figures 12A to C**. Compression may not be effective when intraocular pressures are beyond

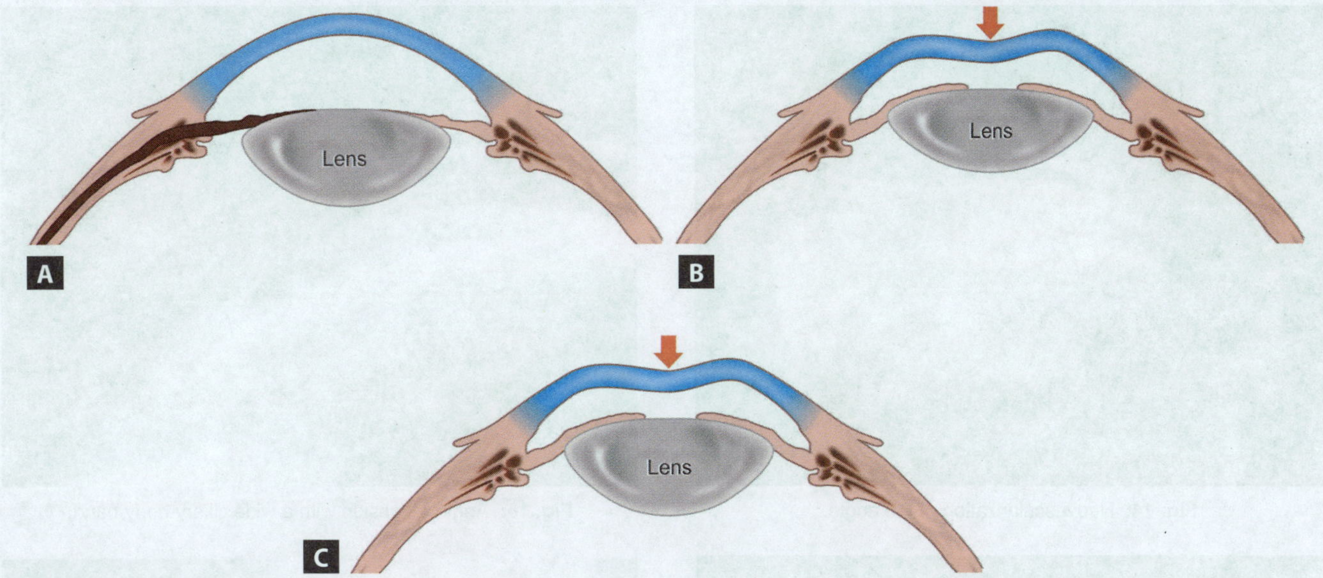

Figs. 12A to C: *Compression gonioscopy*: (A) The narrow angle appears closed on a routine gonioscopy; (B) Compression fails to allow visibility of angle structures due to PAS; (C) Compression widens the recess and allows a view of all structures in the absence of PAS.
(PAS: peripheral anterior synechiae)

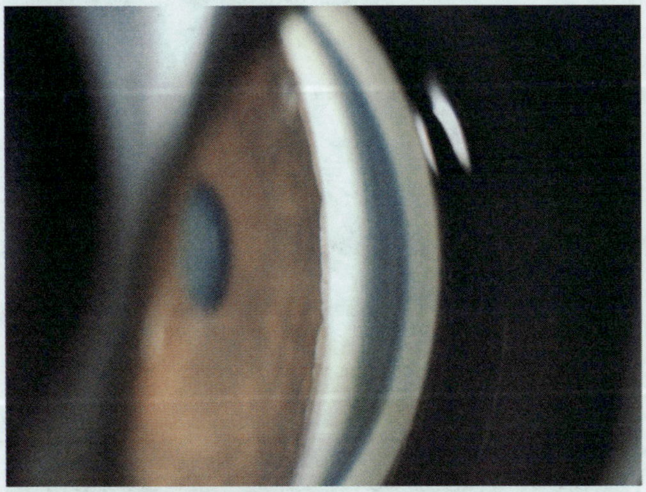

Fig. 13: Peripheral anterior synechiae.

Table 3: Differences between iris processes and peripheral anterior synechiae.

Iris processes	*PAS*
Delicate and lacy	Broad and irregular
Follows concavity of angle recess	Bridges the angle recess
Does not obscure underlying structures	Obscures underlying structures
Does not inhibit posterior movement of the iris on indentation	Inhibits posterior movement
	Drag normal iris vessels with them
	Pigmentation of the cornea anterior to the synechiae may be present

(PAS: peripheral anterior synechiae)

40 mm Hg as this limits the expansion of the limbal scleral ring.

Common Gonioscopic Findings and their Variations

Peripheral Anterior Synechiae

The PAS **(Fig. 13)** is a pathological term referring to the adhesions of peripheral iris to the anterior angle structures, most often the functional trabecular meshwork, or rarely, extending to the Schwalbe's line. Typically seen associated with PACG, uveitic and other secondary angle-closure glaucomas, PAS may often be confused with iris processes, which are normal fine lacy cords of uveal tissue extending from the peripheral iris to the trabecular meshwork. The PAS on the other hand are broad adhesions commonly localized to quadrants with areas in between widening with indentation technique of gonioscopy **(Table 3)**. An angle that is closed 360° may often present a dilemma but one can follow the slit-beam from the posterior surface of the cornea which normally does not meet the beam on the iris directly in an angle that is open but instead lies alongside the other. A direct continuation of the beam without a break is suggestive of a closed-angle. Clinical correlation and experience will often help overcome this hurdle.

Blood Vessels

Normally all vessels in the angle are restricted to the ciliary body band and iris root, and do not extend to the scleral spur or trabecular meshwork. Anomalous vessels are not rare; they, however, can readily be distinguished from neovascularization **(Fig. 14)**, which are vessels usually arising from the peripheral iris surface and branching out in an arborizing and lacy pattern onto the corneoscleral portion

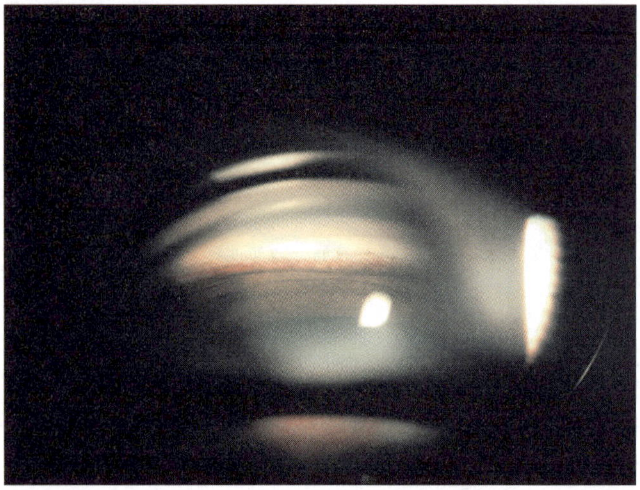

Fig. 14: Neovascularization of the angle.

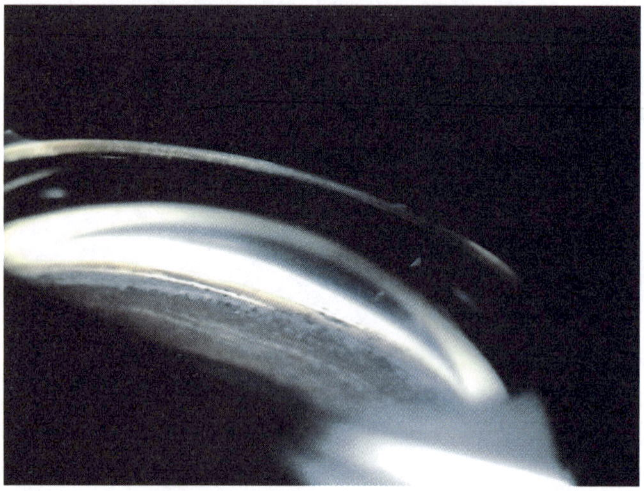

Fig. 16: Angle recession with a wide ciliary body band.

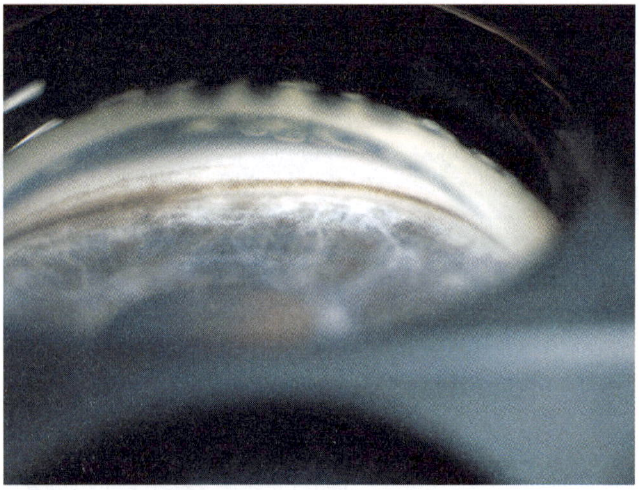

Fig. 15: Patchy pigmentation of the angle.

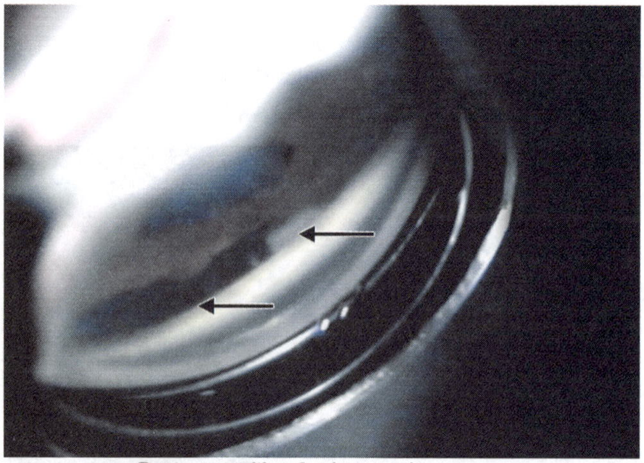

Best seen with a 3 mirror gonioscope

Fig. 17: Iridodialysis with a ciliary body cleft.

of trabecular meshwork. Varying amounts of PAS may also be associated depending on the stage of disease process.

Pigmentation

The trabecular meshwork has a varying amount of pigmentation varying from 0 to 4, which is a subjective grading that correlates to none (0), faint (1), average (2), heavy (3), and very heavy (4). Pigmentation increases with age under normal physiological conditions. Excessive pigmentation is usually pathological and is associated with pseudoexfoliation syndrome, pigment dispersion syndrome, and traumatic and uveitic glaucomas. Patchy trabecular meshwork pigmentation can be seen corresponding to areas of gonioscopically identifiable previous closure **(Fig. 15)**.

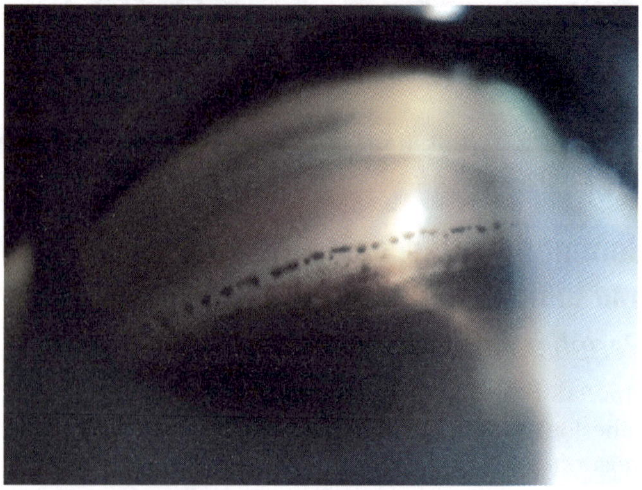

Fig. 18: Keratic precipitate in angle.

Other Abnormal Findings

A variety of surprises may be hidden in the angle recess. Angle recession may be seen as irregular widening of ciliary body band **(Fig. 16)**, iridodialysis, CD cleft **(Fig. 17)**, KPs **(Fig. 18)**, trabeculectomy stoma **(Fig. 19)** can also be observed. Blood in Schlemm's canal appears as a uniform linear reddish hue just anterior to pigmented trabecular meshwork and is associated with raised episcleral venous pressure. It can also be observed under normal conditions and as an artifact when excess external pressure is exerted during gonioscopy.

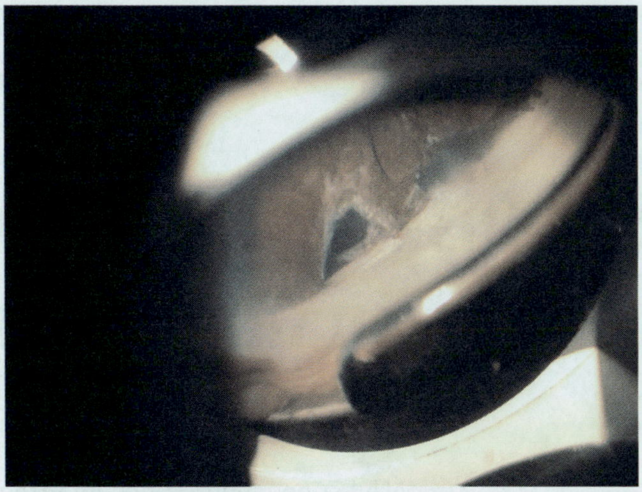

Fig. 19: Trabeculectomy stoma.

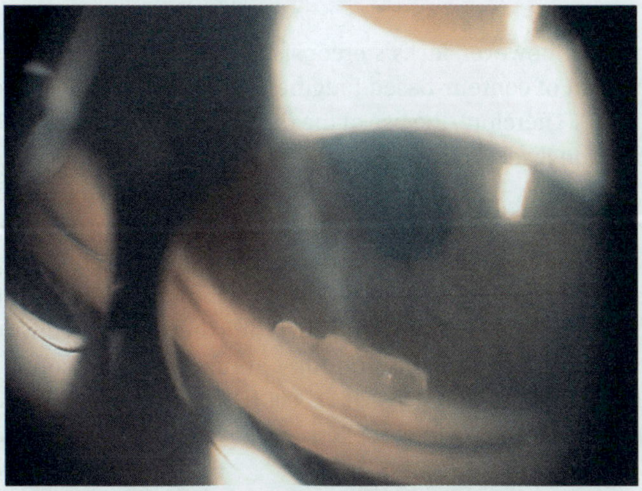

Fig. 20: Foreign body in the angle.

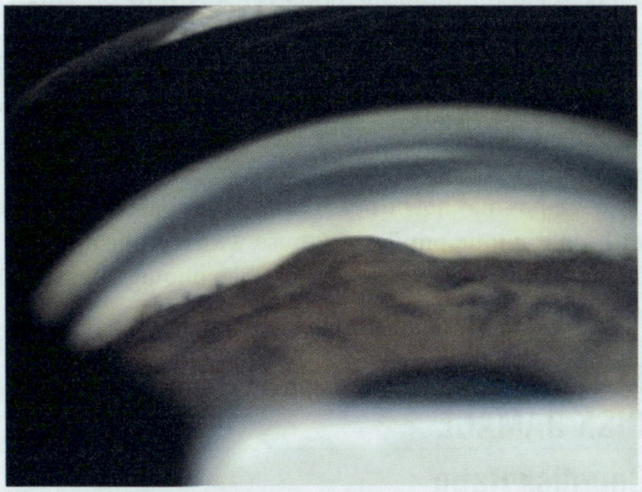

Fig. 21: Iris cyst.

Pseudoexfoliative material, microscopic hyphema, and hypopyon can be visualized. Foreign bodies **(Fig. 20)**, iris cyst **(Fig. 21)**, and emulsified silicone oil globules **(Fig. 22)** are among the other things that can be picked up by a careful gonioscopy.

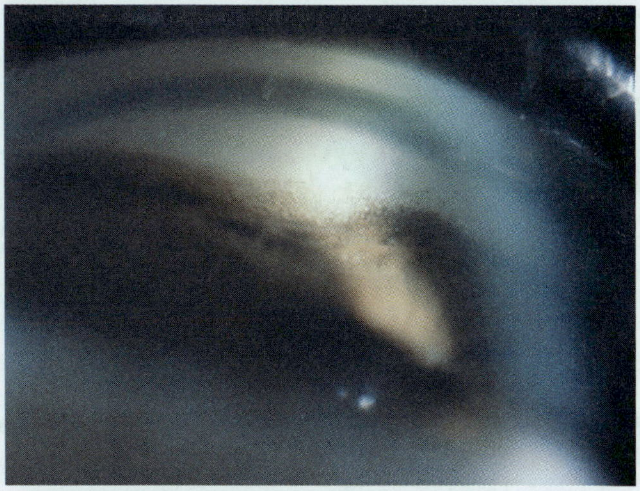

Fig. 22: Silicone oil globules in the angle.

CONCLUSION

The diagnostic basis of any glaucoma should be in correlation to the gonioscopic findings whenever possible. The management and prognosis of the disease depends on a complete diagnosis that includes a routine and periodic gonioscopic evaluation. Gonioscopy widens our scientific understanding of the disease process and guides us to manage the disease more effectively.

SUGGESTED READING

1. Alward WL. A history of gonioscopy. Optom Vis Sci. 2011;88(1):29-35.
2. Foster PJ, Buhrmann R, Quigley HA, et al. The definition and classification of glaucoma in prevalence surveys. Br J Ophthalmol. 2002;86(2):238-42.
3. Foster PJ, Gazzard GA, Garway-Heath T, et al. Pattern of trabecular surface pigment deposition in primary angle closure. Arch Ophthalmol. 2006;124(7):1062.
4. Friedman DS, He M. Anterior chamber angle assessment techniques. Surv Ophthalmol. 2008;53(3):250-73.
5. Grant WM, Schumen JS. The angle of the anterior chamber. In: Epstein DL, Allingham RR, Schuman JS (Eds). Chandler and Grant's Glaucoma, 4th edition. Baltimore: Williams & Wilkins; 1996.
6. Kanski JJ, James AM, John FS. Glaucoma: A Colour Manual of Diagnosis and Treatment, 2nd edition. London: Butterworth-Heinemann; 1996.
7. Neil TC, Diane CL. Atlas of Glaucoma. London: Martin Dunitz; 1998. p. 39.
8. Savage JA. Gonioscopy in the management of glaucoma. In: Focal Points: Clinical Modules for Ophthalmologists. San Francisco: American Academy of Ophthalmology (AAO); 2006.
9. Stamper R, Liebermann M, Drake M. Becker-Shaffer's Diagnosis and Therapy of the Glaucomas, 8th edition. Mosby; 2009.
10. Thomas R, Thomas S, Chandrashekar G. Gonioscopy. Indian J Ophthalmol. 1998;46(4):255-61.

CHAPTER

8

Optic Disk Assessment in Glaucoma

Nikhil S Choudhari, G Chandra Sekhar

INTRODUCTION

Glaucoma is the second leading cause of blindness worldwide. The estimated number of people with open-angle and angle-closure glaucoma for 2020 using prevalence models is 79.6 million.[1] At least 50% of patients do not know that they have glaucoma since the disease is usually asymptomatic.[2] Recent time has seen rapid advances in imaging technologies such as confocal scanning laser ophthalmoscopy, scanning laser polarimetry, and optical coherence topography for detection of glaucomatous damage. However, these technologies have only moderate ability to pick up glaucoma at an early stage.[3-5] New psychophysical tests such as short wavelength automated perimetry, frequency doubling perimetry, and motion automated perimetry are targeted at specific visual functions and have been shown to be more sensitive and specific than standard automated perimetry for identifying early glaucomatous damage.[6-8] However, these techniques may not be available to all clinicians and have the limitations of any subjective test. Several studies have shown that abnormalities in the appearance of the optic disk may precede visual field defects.[9,10] Conventional stereoscopic clinical evaluation and imaging of the optic disk with fundus photographs is still the most frequently used and sensitive means of diagnosing glaucoma.[11] With some training, it is possible to clinically evaluate optic nerve head and retinal nerve fiber layer stereoscopically and detect early glaucomatous damage. The aim of this chapter is to highlight the techniques of clinical evaluation of the optic disk, describe the morphological changes of the optic nerve in glaucoma, and discuss the differential diagnosis.

METHODS OF OPTIC DISK EXAMINATION

Traditionally, the direct ophthalmoscope has been used for the evaluation of the optic nerve head. Though it has the advantage of providing a magnified view of the optic nerve head, it however, lacks stereopsis and permits color-based instead of contour-based judgment of the neuroretinal rim (NRR). Therefore, the use of the direct ophthalmoscope is to be strongly discouraged.

A variety of contact and noncontact lenses are available, which allow stereoscopic view of the fundus on the slit-lamp. Contact lenses such as Goldmann lenses are relatively uncomfortable for the patient, take longer time and the coupling fluid can cause transient blurring and difficulty in obtaining good quality fundus photographs. Noncontact lenses include +60 D, +78 D, +90 D, and Volk superfield lenses. These provide excellent stereoscopic and magnified view of the optic disk.

It is important to draw the appearance of the optic nerve head based on these methods **(Figs. 1 and 2)**. Though drawing of the optic disk suffers from the disadvantage of being subjective in nature, this does offer a quick and inexpensive method of monitoring the optic nerve head in patients with glaucoma over time. It also serves as a check against incomplete examination of the optic disk. Moreover, photographs may not be possible in all cases such as patients with rigid miotic pupils and those with significant media opacities. However, wherever possible, photographs are an indispensable adjunct to clinical evaluation.

FEATURES OF GLAUCOMATOUS DISK DAMAGE

Cup-disk Ratio

Early studies by Armaly et al. have reported that the vertical and horizontal cup-disk diameters ratio are useful for the quantification of glaucomatous optic neuropathy and for early detection of glaucoma.[12] The ratio has limited value in the identification of glaucomatous damage because of the wide variability in the size of the optic cup in the normal population.

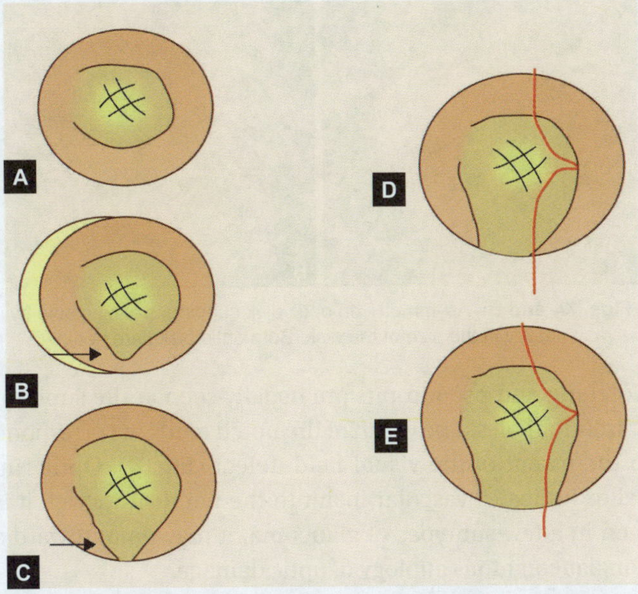

Figs. 1A to E: Optic disk drawing. Conventionally, the outline of the cup is not drawn on the temporal side. Therefore, all these drawings are of right disk. The arrow indicates inferior excavation in (B) and inferior notch in (C). Note relation of vessel to the notch in (D) and (E).

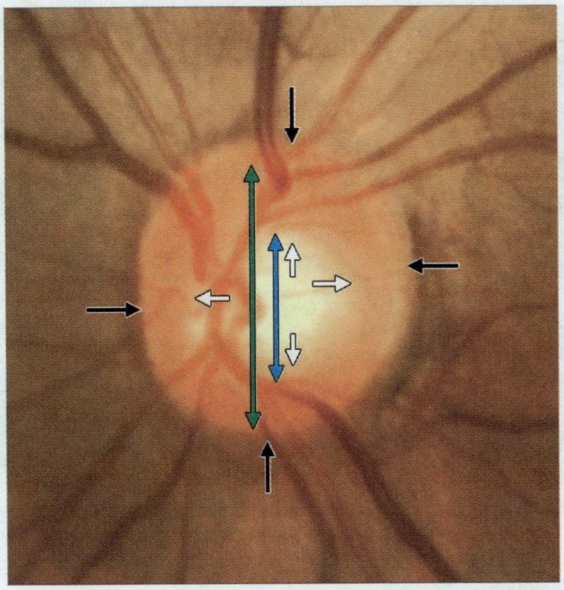

Fig. 3: Disk margin (black arrow) and cup margin (white arrow). Maximum vertical diameter of the cup (blue arrow) and the disk (green arrow).

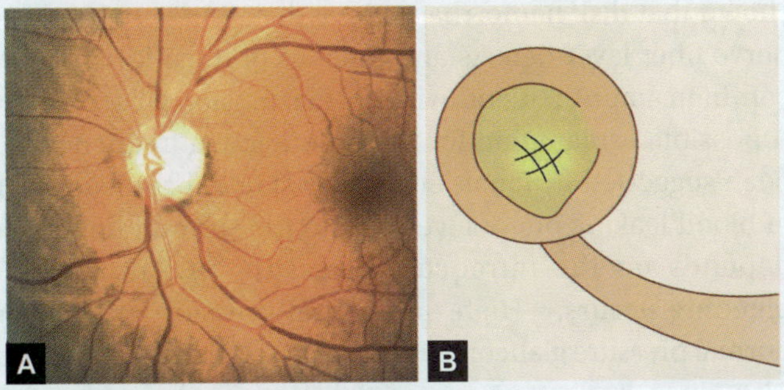

Figs. 2A and B: Optic disk documentation. Note the inferior excavation and the inferior nerve fiber layer defect outlined by the two lines in the optic disk drawing.

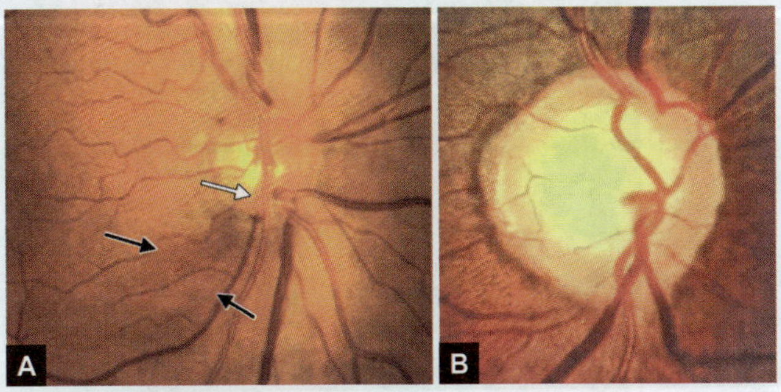

Figs. 4A and B: Cup-disk ratio in relation to optic disk size. The optic disk on left is small with small cup and still has inferior excavation (white arrow) with nerve fiber layer defect (black arrow). In contrast, the optic disk right has a large physiological cup.

Disk margin is defined by inner edge of white scleral ring (outer arrows), and the optic cup is the level at which NRR steeps (inner arrows) **(Fig. 3)**. A large cup-disk ratio can be normal if the optic disk is large,[13] and a small cup-disk ratio may be glaucomatous if the optic disk is small **(Figs. 4A and B)**.[14] The problem with estimating cup-disk ratio as a measure of glaucomatous damage is that it is difficult to decide if the cup is physiological in a large disk or pathological in a small or normal sized disk. In a study by Garway-Heath et al. vertical cup-disk diameter ratio *corrected for the optic disk size* was the best parameter to separate between normal subjects and patients of ocular hypertension with retinal nerve fiber layer defect.[15] Therefore, in the clinical description of the optic nerve head, it is important to state the vertical cup-disk diameter ratio in combination with the estimated disk size. The disk diameter can be measured by adjusting the slit-lamp beam height to the edges of the disk while viewing the disk with a 60 D lens **(Fig. 5)**.[16] The measurement by this method is roughly equal to the measurement obtained by the planimetry of disk photographs by Litmann's correction. Measurements can also be made with other lenses by multiplying the measured value with the appropriate magnification factor, Goldmann contact lens X1.26 and Volk superfield lens X1.5.[16]

It is important to differentiate contour cupping from color cupping. The margin of the cup should be determined by the bend of the small vessels across the disk rim and not by the central area of disk pallor **(Fig. 6)**.

Asymmetry of Optic Disk Cupping

Asymmetry of cupping is seldom seen in normal eyes and until proven otherwise, must be taken as an indication of early glaucomatous damage. However, while assessing asymmetry, it is important to rule out asymmetry of the disk size, which can be physiological or be the result of

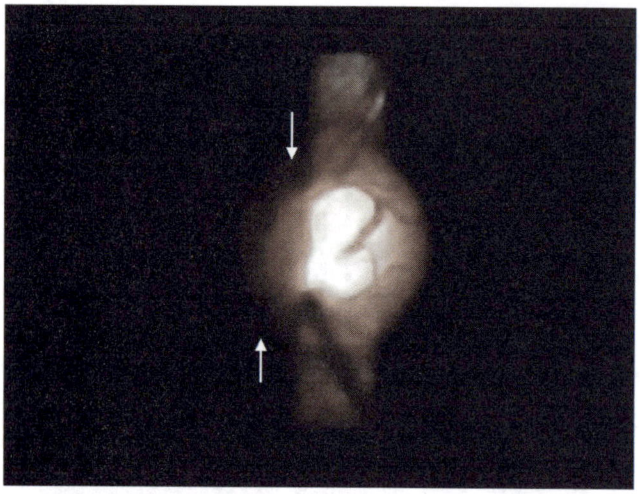

Fig. 5: During slit-lamp biomicroscopy, adjust the height of the slit-lamp beam to the vertical disk diameter, read the height of the beam and then multiply it by the correction factor of handheld lens to obtain vertical optic disk diameter.

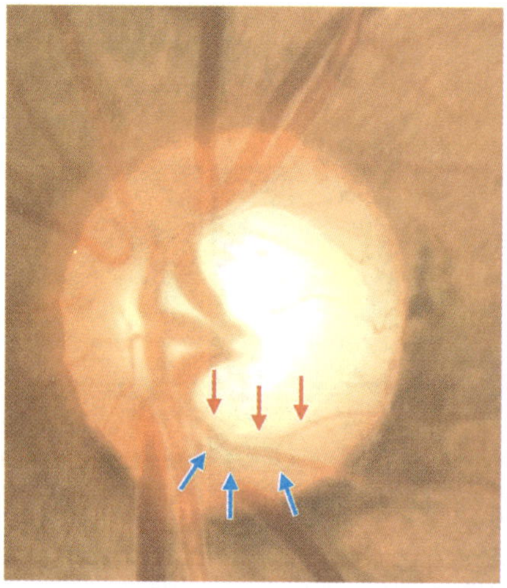

Fig. 6: Margin of color cup (red arrows) versus contour cup (blue arrows). The former may miss the inferior excavation.

anisometropia. Inter-eye asymmetry in the size of the optic disk may result in difference in the cup-disk ratio between two eyes in the absence of glaucoma **(Figs. 7A and B)**.

Neuroretinal Rim Evaluation

A focal or diffuse loss of the NRR is typical in glaucoma. Focal damage usually involves a particular area of the rim. If the rim is completely lost in a focal area, it is called complete notch **(Fig. 8)**, whereas localized thinning of the rim is called incomplete notch or excavation **(Figs. 2 and 9)**. Diffuse damage results in symmetrical enlargement of the cup. The inferior > superior > nasal > temporal (ISNT) rule states that normally the inferior rim is the thickest followed by the superior, the nasal and then the temporal **(Fig. 10)**.[17] During optic nerve head evaluation, one must look carefully for any areas of thinning of the NRR or for notching. If the cup is especially deep in the notch, it is known as a pseudo-pit.

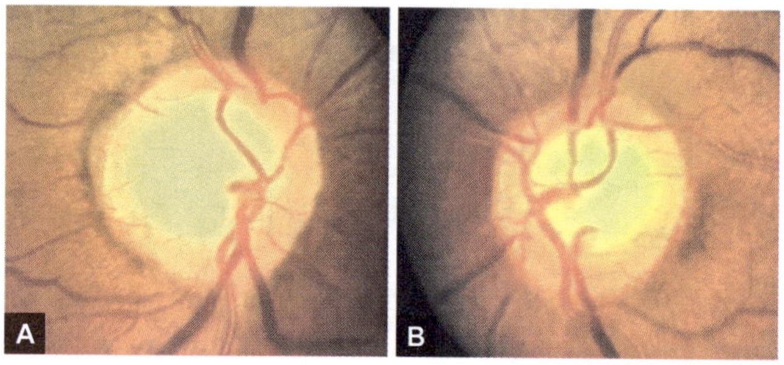

Figs. 7A and B: Asymmetry on optic disk cupping is explainable by asymmetry in the size of the disk. Both optic disks are healthy.

Notching and pseudo-pits are usually seen at the superior or inferior poles. The width of the notch tends to correspond to the extent of the visual field defect **(Fig. 8)**. Optic rim pallor indicates vascular insult to the nerve. Although it is seen in a few subtypes of glaucoma, it may point toward a nonglaucomatous etiology of optic damage.

Vascular Changes

Splinter hemorrhages on the optic disk are a common finding in glaucoma patients **(Figs. 9 and 11)**. Various studies have shown that disk hemorrhages in association with localized nerve fiber layer defects and notches of the NRR are more common among patients with normal tension glaucoma.[18,19] A possible explanation for the difference in frequency has been suggested by Jonas, et al. They stated that the amount of blood leaking out of a vessel into the surrounding tissue depends on the intraocular pressure (IOP) when the bleeding occurs.[19] High transmural pressure gradient in normal pressure glaucoma leads to larger disk hemorrhages. Also, since the absorption rate of disk hemorrhages depends on the size of the disk bleed, the hemorrhages in patients of normal pressure glaucoma may take a longer time to disappear and thus have a higher chance to be detected than the disk hemorrhages in patients of high pressure glaucoma.[20]

Hemorrhages in glaucoma usually appear as splinter-shaped or flame-shaped hemorrhages on the disk surface **(Fig. 9)**.[21] They usually precede NRR changes and visual field defects. The visual field defects corresponding to the location of the hemorrhage may be expected to appear weeks to year later.[22] The presence of disk hemorrhage(s) is considered an indication for further IOP lowering in the management of glaucoma.

Configuration of Vessels

The retinal vessels on the optic nerve head can provide clues about the topography of the disk. Nasalization of the vessels and baring of circumlinear vessels can be seen in glaucoma as well as in other diseases of the optic nerve. Bayoneting of the vessels can be seen if the rim is absent or very thin.

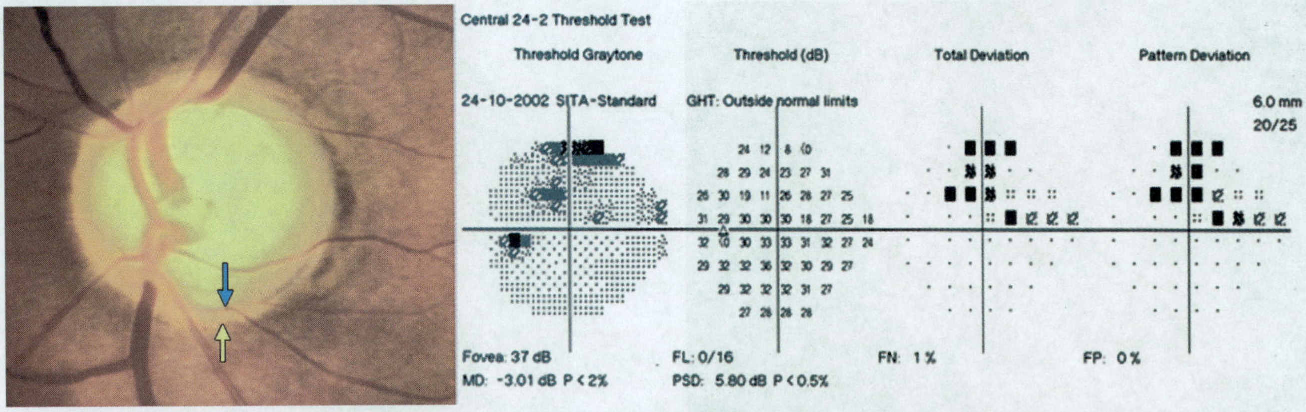

Fig. 8: Inferior optic disk notch (yellow arrow) and the visual field defect. The visual field defect corresponds with the glaucomatous changes in the optic disk. Blue arrow indicates bayoneting sign.

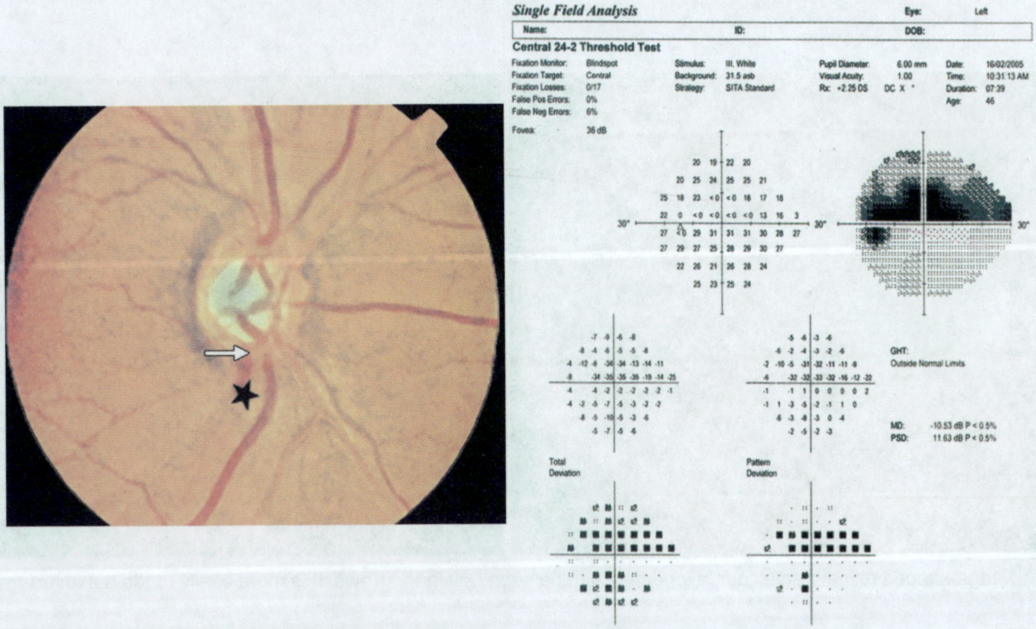

Fig. 9: The optic disk photograph shows early inferior excavation (arrow) with corresponding superior arcuate field defect. Note optic disk hemorrhage (star).

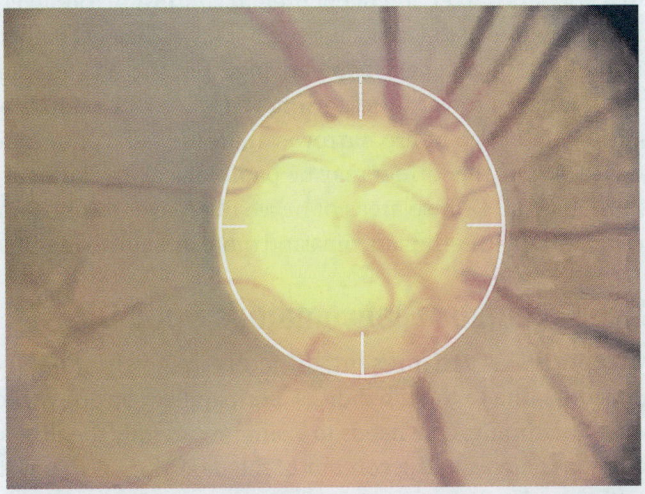

Fig. 10: *ISNT (inferior > superior > nasal > temporal) rule*: The inferior rim is the thickest followed by the superior, the nasal and then the temporal.

This causes the vessels to pass under the overhanging edge of the cup and then make a sharp bend as they cross the disk surface. This convoluted appearance of the vessels is called "bayoneting" **(Fig. 8)**.

Peripapillary Atrophy

The zone closer to the optic nerve head with retinal pigment epithelium (RPE) and choroidal atrophy and baring of sclera is known as *zone*-β. The more peripheral zone with only RPE atrophy is called *zone*-α **(Fig. 12)**. A highly significant correlation has been reported between the location of peripapillary atrophy and visual field defects.[23] Changes may represent congenital anomalies, especially in myopic eyes. However, appearance of these changes *de novo* or their presence in small, nonmyopic disks should be viewed

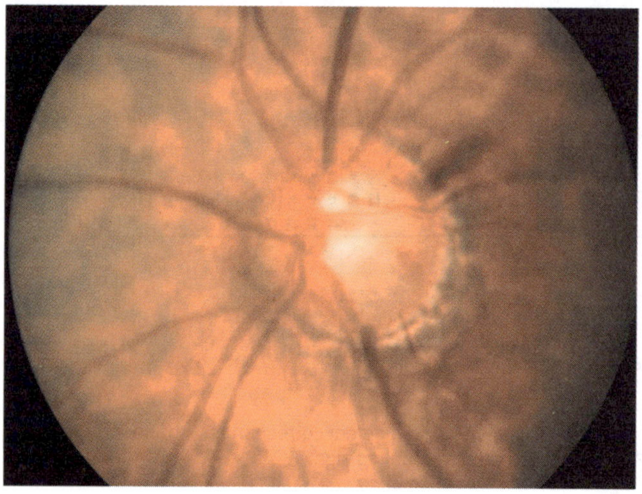

Fig. 11: Disk hemorrhage.

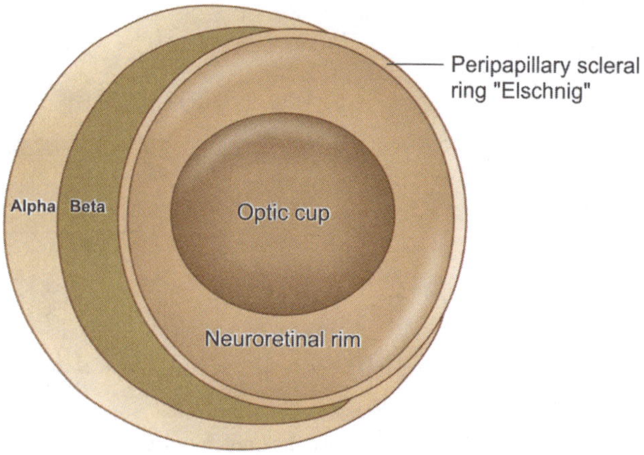

Fig. 12: Peripapillary atrophy. The diagram shows atrophic zone closer to the optic nerve head called zone-β and the more peripheral zone called zone-α.

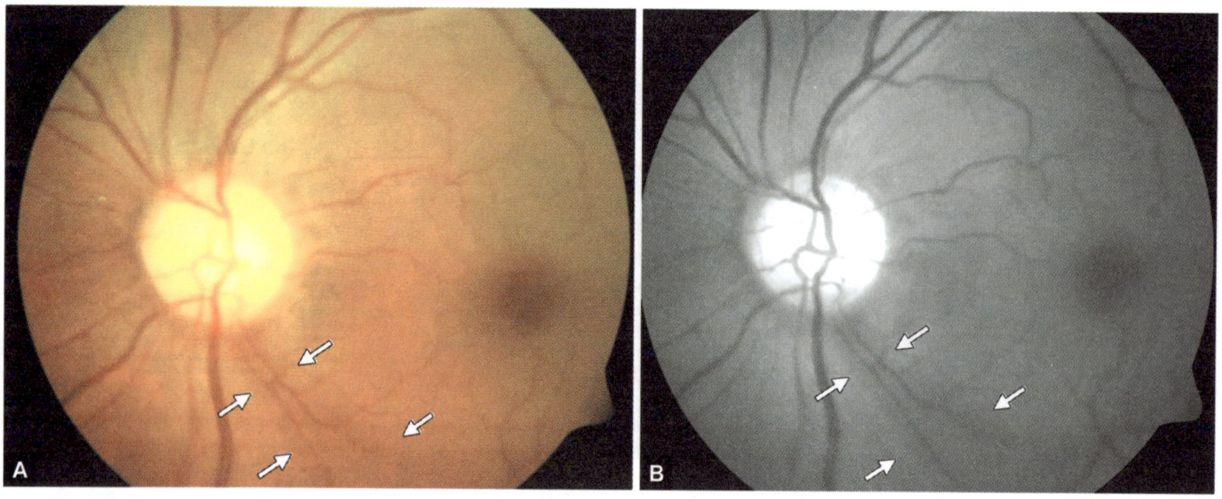

Figs. 13A and B: A wedge-shaped retinal nerve fiber layer defect can be seen between arrows. It is more easily made out in red-free photograph.

with suspicion. Peripapillary atrophy may be a focal or circumferential **(Figs. 6, 8, and 11)**.

Retinal Nerve Fiber Layer Abnormalities

Examination of the nerve fiber layer is often useful in detecting early glaucomatous damage with normal disk appearance and normal visual fields. The NRR is formed by axons converging from the retina to the scleral canal. Since the axons are spread out in a thin layer in the retina, even minor losses of the axons can be observed in the retinal nerve fiber layer. In healthy eyes, the nerve fiber layer in the arcuate region appears slightly opaque with radially oriented striations. The small retinal blood vessels have a blurred and crosshatched appearance, as they lie buried in the nerve fiber layer. The best way to assess the nerve fiber layer is by doing slit-lamp biomicroscopy through a dilated pupil using red free light, a wide-slit beam and high magnification. In the presence of nerve fiber layer atrophy, the small retinal blood vessels become more clearly visible and appear unusually sharp, clear, and well-focused. The fundus in the affected area appears darker and deeper red in contrast to the silvery or opaque hue of the intact nerve fiber layer. Defects may be in the form of a wedge shape arising from the disk margin and widening toward the periphery **(Figs. 13A and B)** or slit-like defects that are narrower than the adjacent blood vessels. While the former may be pathological, the latter are physiological. Diffuse areas of nerve fiber layer atrophy are less common in early glaucoma and more difficult to identify.

Myopic Versus Glaucomatous Optic Disk

Myopic disks can present difficulty in evaluation for glaucoma due to the tilted disks, peripapillary atrophy, and shallow cupping. One needs to examine carefully the disk to look for changes in the contour of the blood vessels, as well delineate the disk margin from the peripapillary changes **(Fig. 14)**.

Differential Diagnosis

In addition to glaucoma, other abnormalities can cause excavation and/or pallor of the optic disk and it is, therefore, important to rule out these possibilities before making the diagnosis of glaucoma.

- *Physiological cupping:* Assessment of the size of the optic disk, careful examination of the NRR and the retinal nerve fiber layer can help distinguish physiological cupping from glaucomatous damage in most cases **(Figs. 15A and B)**.
- *Optic nerve coloboma:* Optic nerve colobomas typically demonstrate enlargement of the papillary region, partial or complete excavation, blood vessels entering and exiting from the border of the defect and a glistening white surface. The visual field defects can be in the form of generalized constriction, centrocecal scotomas, altitudinal defects, arcuate scotomas, enlargement of the blind spot and ring scotomas that can mimic those found in glaucomatous eyes.

Morning glory syndrome is a variant of optic disk coloboma and is characterized by a large excavated disk, central core of white or gray glial tissue surrounded by an elevated annulus of variably pigmented subretinal tissue **(Fig. 16)**. The retinal vessels appear to enter and exit from the margins of the disk, are straightened and often sheathed.

- *Congenital optic disk pit:* Congenital optic disk pits appear gray or yellowish white, round or oval, localized depression within the optic nerve **(Fig. 17)**. They are located within the temporal aspect of the disk in over half of the cases and centrally in about one-third. Involvement is usually unilateral in about 80% cases and the optic disk is larger on the involved side. Approximately 55–60% of the eyes have a field defect in the form of arcuate scotomas, paracentral scotoma, altitudinal defect, generalized constriction, and nasal or temporal steps.[24]

In the absence of other indicators of congenital anomaly like associated fundus coloboma, the differential

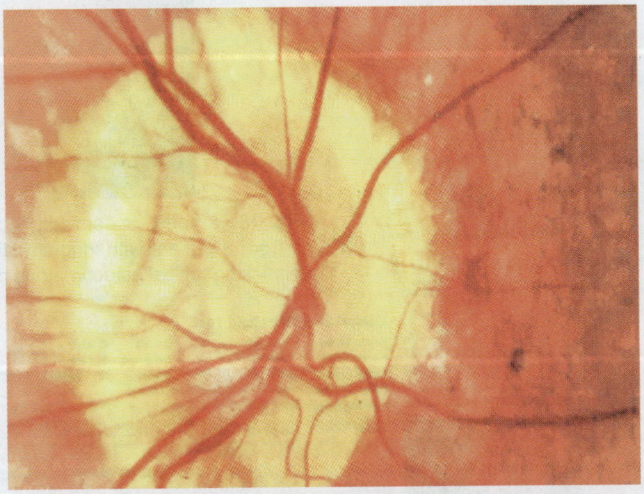

Fig. 14: Myopic disk with primary open-angle glaucoma.

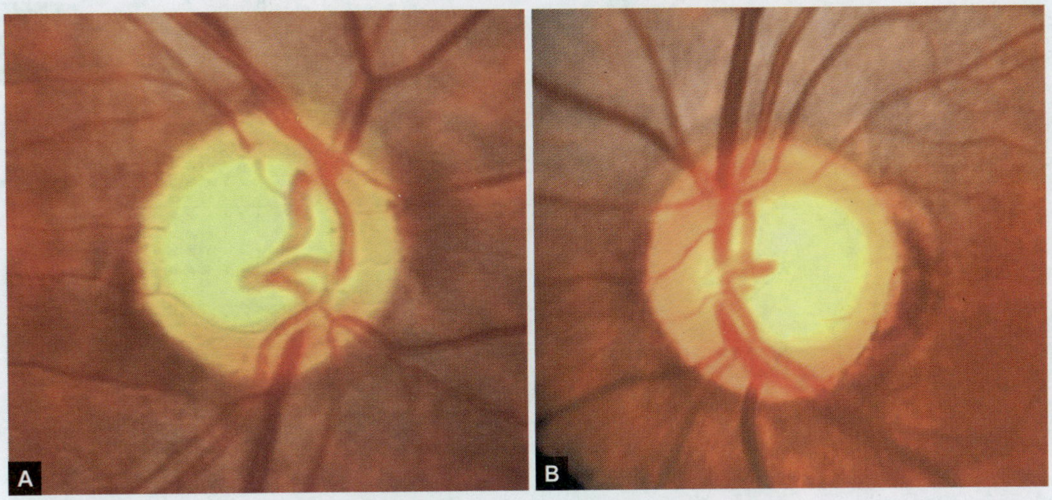

Figs. 15A and B: Physiological optic disk cupping.

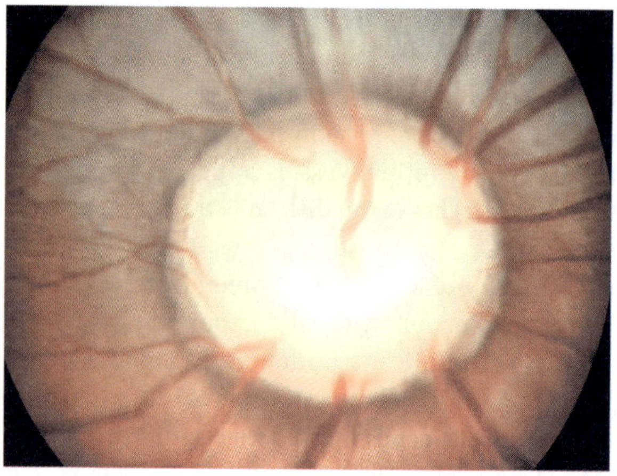

Fig. 16: Morning glory optic disk.

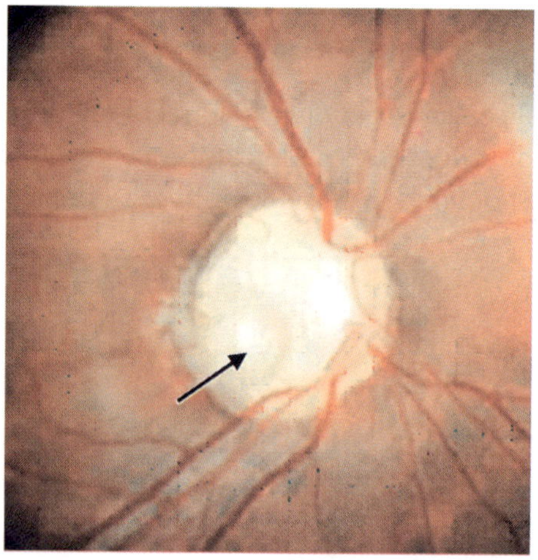

Fig. 17: Congenital optic disk pit (arrow).

diagnosis may be difficult and the absence of progression on follow-up may be the only indicator that the patient has a congenital anomaly and not glaucoma.

- *Anterior ischemic optic neuropathy:* A history of acute visual loss, initial swelling of the optic disk, absence of marked cupping, presence of centrocecal scotoma or altitudinal defects, rise in erythrocyte sedimentation rate (ESR) can help differentiate it from glaucoma. In the late stages the cupping in some cases may be exactly the same as is seen in glaucoma **(Fig. 18)**.
- *Neurological causes:* Younger age, unusual history of onset and progression, normal IOP, and pallor of the NRR

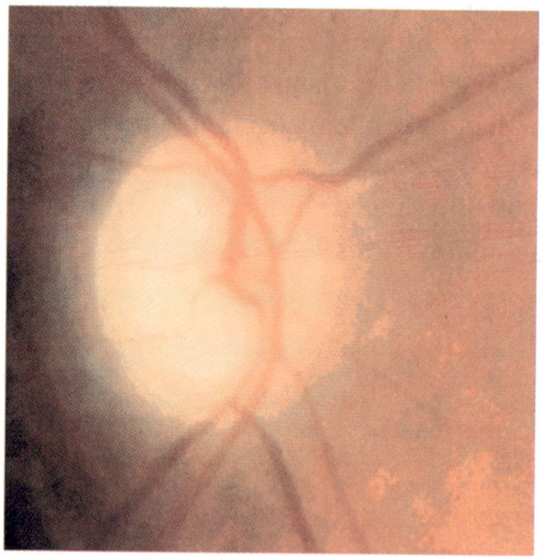

Fig. 18: Anterior ischemic optic neuropathy. The optic disk photograph is from a patient with long-standing anterior ischemic optic neuropathy mimicking typical glaucomatous cupping.

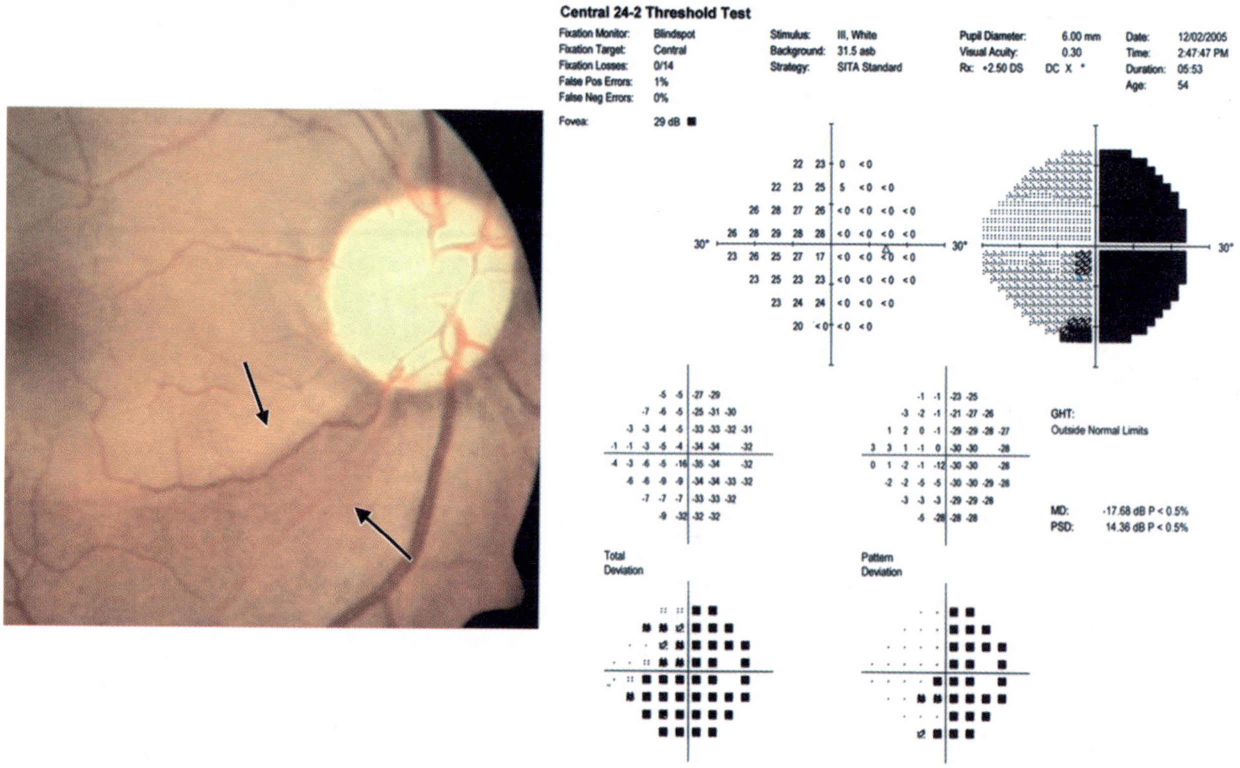

Fig. 19: Optic disk photograph showing significant cupping, but with disproportionate pallor, with visual field defect showing a temporal hemifield defect suggestive of chiasmal compression.

disproportionate to cupping should arouse suspicion of a neurological disorder causing optic disk damage **(Fig. 19)**. Presence of visual field defects that respect vertical midline and the pattern of the field defects should be able to suggest the possible site of the intracranial lesion.[25]

SUMMARY

In summary, the optic disk evaluation in glaucoma is best done stereoscopically at the slit lamp with a dilated pupil using one of the 60D, 78D, or 90D lenses. Changes in the NRR, optic disk hemorrhage(s), peripapillary atrophy and nerve fiber layer defect(s) are more important features than the cup-disk ratio. The cup-disk ratio is to be documented and interpreted along with the disk size and not in isolation. One should avoid the urge to instantaneously diagnose glaucoma based on the cup to disk ratio alone. The diagnosis of glaucoma depends on multiple factors including the presence of a visual field defect that correlates with the anatomic changes on the optic nerve head and the peripapillary retina.

REFERENCES

1. Quigley HA, Broman AT. The number of people with glaucoma worldwide in 2010 and 2020. Br J Ophthalmol. 2006;90(3): 262-7.
2. Dandona L, Dandona R, Srinivas M, et al. Open-angle glaucoma in an urban population in southern India: the Andhra Pradesh eye disease study. Ophthalmology. 2000;107(9):1702-9.
3. Zangwill LM, Bowd C, Berry CC, et al. Discriminating between normal and glaucomatous eyes using the Heidelberg Retina Tomograph, GDx Nerve Fiber Analyzer and Optical Coherence Tomograph. Arch Ophthalmol. 2001;119(7):985-93.
4. Bowd C, Zangwill LM, Berry CC, et al. Detecting early glaucoma by assessment of retinal nerve fiber layer thickness and visual functions. Invest Ophthalmol Vis Sci. 2001;42(9):1993-2003.
5. Medeiros FA, Zangwill LM, Bowd C, et al. Comparison of the GDx VCC scanning laser polarimeter, HRT II confocal scanning laser ophthalmoscope, and stratus OCT optical coherence tomograph for the detection of glaucoma. Arch Ophthalmol. 2004:122(6):827-37.
6. Johnson CA, Adams AJ, Casson EJ, et al. Blue-on-yellow perimetry can predict the development of glaucomatous field loss. Arch Ophthalmol. 1993;111(5):645-50.
7. Bayer AU, Maag KP, Erb C. Detection of optic neuropathy in glaucomatous eyes with normal standard visual fields using a battery of short-wavelength automated perimetry and pattern electroretinography. Ophthalmology. 2002;109(7):1350-61.
8. Sample PA, Bosworth CF, Blumenthal EZ, et al. Visual function-specific perimetry for indirect comparison of different ganglion cell populations in glaucoma. Invest Ophthalmol Vis Sci. 2000;41(7):1783-90.
9. Quigley HA, Dunkelberger GR, Green WR. Chronic human glaucoma causing selectively greater loss of larger optic nerve fibers. Ophthalmology. 1988;95(3):357-63.
10. Sommer A, Pollack I, Maumenee AE. Optic disc parameters and onset of glaucomatous field loss. I. Methods and progressive changes in disc morphology. Arch Ophthalmol. 1979;97: 1444-8.
11. Greaney MJ, Hoffman DC, Garway-Heath DF, et al. Comparison of optic nerve imaging methods to distinguish normal eyes from those with glaucoma. Invest Ophthalmol Vis Sci. 2002; 43(1):140-5.
12. Armaly MF, Saydegh RE. The cup-disc ratio. The findings of tonometry and tonography in the normal eye. Arch Ophthalmol. 1969;82(2):191-6.
13. Jonas JB, Zäch FM, Gusek GC, et al. Pseudoglaucomatous physiologic large cups. Am J Ophthalmol. 1989;107(2): 137-44.
14. Jonas JB, Fernandez MC, Naumann GO. Glaucomatous optic nerve atrophy in small disks with low cup-to-disc ratios. Ophthalmology. 1990;97(9):1211-5.
15. Garway-Heath DF, Ruben ST, Viswanathan A, et al. Vertical cup/disc ratio in relation to optic disc size: its value in the assessment of the glaucoma suspect. Br J Ophthalmol. 1998; 82(10):1118-24.
16. Jonas JB, Dichtl A. Advances in the assessment of the optic disk changes in early glaucoma. Cur Opin Ophthalmol. 1995;6(2):61-6.
17. Jonas JB, Gusek GC, Naumann GO. Optic disc, cup and neuroretinal rim size, configuration and correlations in normal eyes. Invest Ophthalmol Vis Sci. 1988;29(7):1151-8.
18. Kitazawa Y, Shirato S, Yamamoto T. Optic disc hemorrhage in low-tension glaucoma. Ophthalmology. 1986;93(6):853-7.
19. Jonas JB, Budde WM. Optic nerve head appearance in juvenile-onset chronic high-pressure glaucoma and normal-pressure glaucoma. Ophthalmology. 2000;107(4):704-11.
20. Jonas JB, Xu L. Optic disk hemorrhages in glaucoma. Am J Ophthalmol. 1994;118(1):1-8.
21. Drance SM, Fairclough M, Butler DM, et al. The importance of disc hemorrhage in the prognosis of chronic open angle glaucoma. Arch Ophthalmol. 1977:95(2):226-8.
22. Heijl A. Frequent disc photography and computerized perimetry in eyes with optic disc haemorrhage: a pilot study. Acta Ophthalmol (Copenh). 1986:64(3):274-81.
23. Jonas JB, Naumann GO. Parapapillary chorioretinal atrophy in normal and glaucoma eyes. II. Correlations. Invest Ophthalmol Vis Sci. 1989:30(5):919-26.
24. Brown GC. Congenital fundus abnormalities. In: Duane TD (Ed). Clinical Ophthalmology. Philadelphia: JB Lippincott; 1991.
25. Choudhari NS, Neog A, Fudnawala V, et al. Cupped disc with normal intraocular pressure: the long road to avoid misdiagnosis. Indian J Ophthalmol. 2011;59(6):491-7.

CHAPTER

9

Perimetry

Devendra Sood, NR Rangaraj

INTRODUCTION

The central 30° visual field examination is the current gold standard in evaluation, management, and follow-up of glaucoma. Characteristic visual field changes are typically diagnostic of glaucoma and other parameters like intraocular pressure (IOP), structural changes in the optic nerve head, and central corneal thickness help in the evaluation of glaucoma **(Fig. 1)**. The Octopus series and the Humphrey visual field analysis machines are popular and clinically evaluated, hence this chapter would focus on these two perimetry systems.

EVOLUTION OF OCTOPUS PERIMETER

Visual field as a tool for diagnosis has been used since Mariotte discovered the blind spot. The first standardized visual field mapping was the introduction of the Goldmann perimeter **(Fig. 2)** in 1945. This perimeter offered a standard background illumination with fixed target sizes. A highly trained operator was needed to administer the visual field test. Goldmann perimeter was the gold standard despite the limitations.

Automated computer assisted perimetry was developed in 1972 by Fankhauser et al. **(Fig. 3)**. Sphar investigated the basic concept of threshold determination. Bebie, Fankhauser, and Hirsbrunner contributed the concepts, which formed the mathematical and statistical model into a workable software for the automated static perimetry which included behavior pathology of the tested locations over time. The advantage of a computerized automated perimeter is the ability to collect the visual field data of the test done on an individual and compare the values statistically with normal values of the visual field data for the particular age match in a given location in the visual field. The normal data is derived

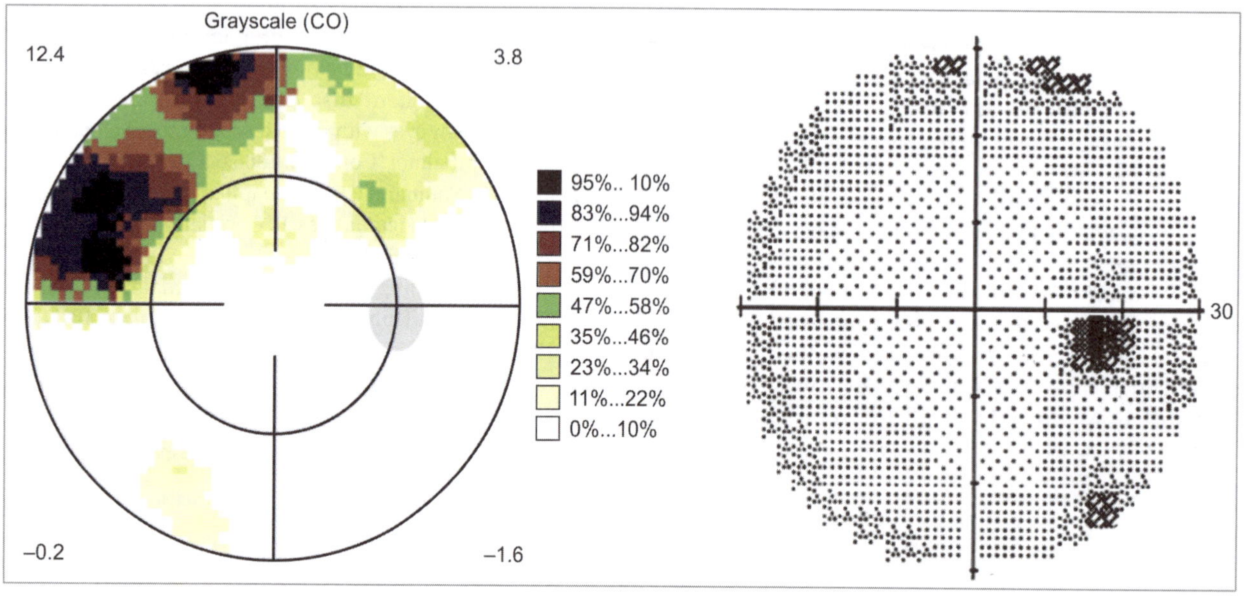

Fig. 1: Gray color scale: Octopus and Humphrey fields.

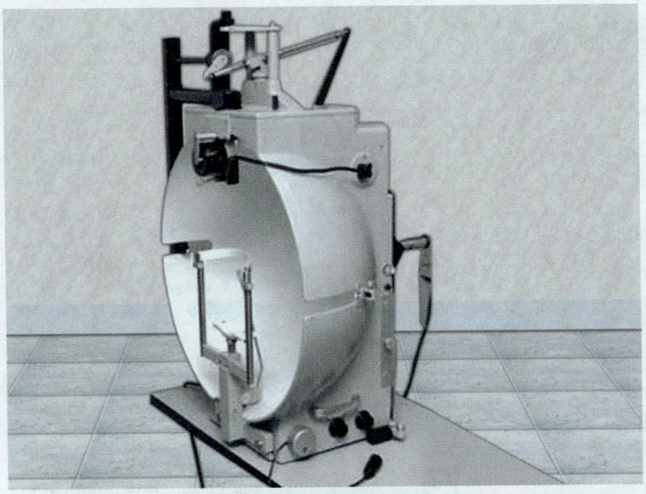

Fig. 2: Goldmann perimeter.

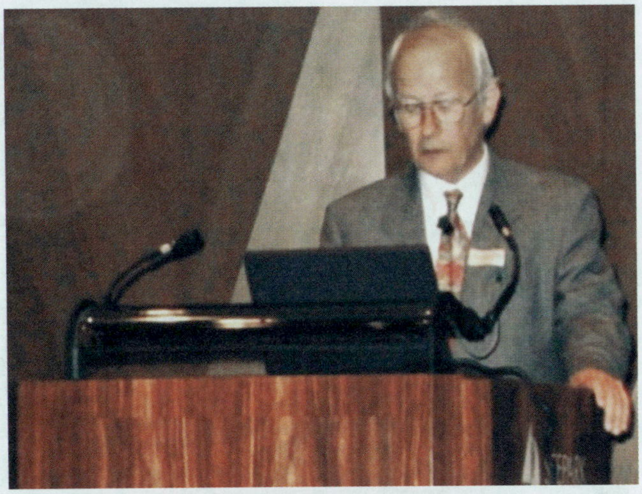

Fig. 4: Professor Hans Bebie.

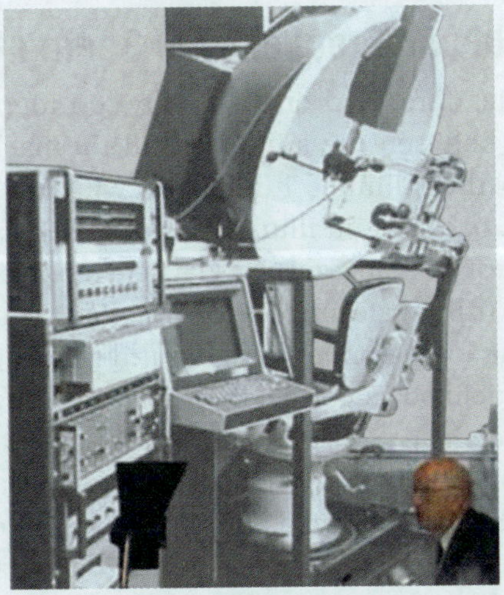

Fig. 3: Fankhauser with original perimeter (note the dental chair).

as follows. For example, data collected from 100 normals of a particular age match for a given location in the visual field are tested and the higher 95% values are labeled as "normal" and the 5% whose values fall below "normal" are termed abnormal. Hence, this statistical concept assumes that the values that fall below the "normal" are abnormal. Even though the software detects the value as abnormal, clinical correlation is necessary for diagnosis to label the visual field defect as glaucoma.

The automated perimeter was in continuous evolution, and in 1985, the G1 program was introduced by Flammer which was based on the topography of the retinal nerve fiber. The G1 program had 59 test point locations and tested the visual field specifically for pathology related to glaucoma. Bebie **(Fig. 4)** provided additional information from the basic data and it was reorganized based on the measured test point sensitivity from the highest sensitivity to the lowest in the form of defect curve called Bebie curve. The strategy of visual field testing also underwent refinements to divide the test into stages and phases where the area of likely pathology was first tested to improve the diagnostic yield. Humphrey automated field analyzer (HFA) developed the full threshold strategies and the Statpac program which performed an in-depth analysis of test results which was out of reach for most doctors. The Swedish interactive threshold algorithm (SITA) was a smart testing strategy to improve the diagnostic value as well as save the time taken to perform the test by the patient. Heijl, Greve, and others contributed to the present concepts in the Humphrey visual field analyzer over the years.

Octopus introduced faster strategies to determine the differential light sensitivity like the "TOP" by Professor González de la Rosa in the 90s. The tendency oriented perimetry (TOP) strategy was based on the algorithm of repetitive extrapolation of local visual field information at the tested location and in neighborhood groups of the tested locations. This strategy allowed 59 tested points as in G1 to be extrapolated with 294 adjustments to give the final results in the visual field results. The TOP strategy can give a completed visual field result in 3 minutes comparable to the full threshold visual field testing which takes 10–15 minutes each eye. The dynamic strategy on the Octopus perimeters was introduced by Dr Webber. This strategy was based on the original threshold strategy but steers the staircase test according to the steepness of the frequency of seeing curve (FOSC) at every point tested to give good quality of visual field report in a much shorter time, about 5–6 minutes.

The Octopus and the HFA perimeter have undergone major design evolution since the first clinical models were introduced. The Octopus perimeters have two models, the latest 900 series cupola perimeter and the infinity projection perimeter of the 300 series **(Figs. 5A to C)**. All computing is done on the external desktop computer. The perimeters have flash memory cards, which do all relevant computing functions on the visual filed machine. The advantage being new strategies and programs may be upgraded by switching to new memory cards in the older machine without

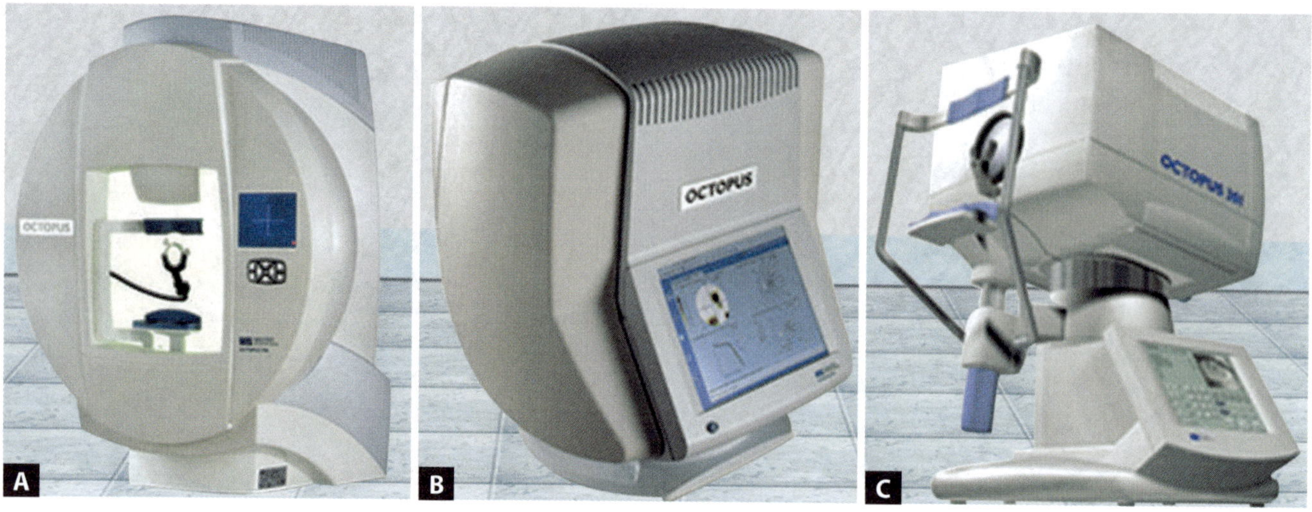

Figs. 5A to C: Octopus perimeter.

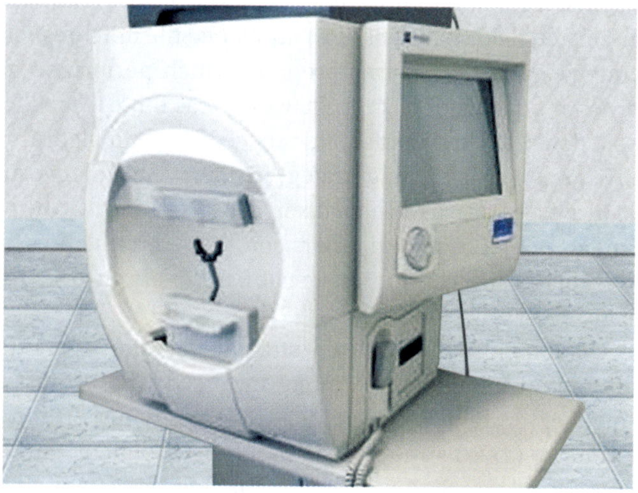

Fig. 6: Humphrey automated field perimeters.

having to replace the machine. New version upgrades may also be downloaded and upgraded on the visual field machine itself. The Humphrey perimeters have been traditionally designed around the cupola, and the computing is done on a self-contained computer in the machine itself. The storage of data is on an internal hard disk **(Fig. 6)**, the printer being the only external peripheral device connected to the machine.

BASIC TERMINOLOGIES IN PERIMETRY

Visual Field

Visual field is area measured by a steadily fixating eye under standard conditions of color, stimulus size, and background for a particular machine. The machine seeks to measure the least difference between the stimuli against the background illumination. This is known as the differential light sensitivity and plotted as decibels on the visual field report as raw data or graphically as the color or grayscale. All visual field analyzers have the same basic concepts.

Threshold and Frequency of Seeing Curve

The patient's threshold or the ability to differentiate the difference between the stimulus and the background is defined as the stimulus luminance which is perceived for a given background illumination. The threshold for a particular test point in a given visual field report is expressed in decibel (dB) scale in clinical practice. The ability to perceive the least amount of light for a given age and test location is defined as normal threshold. The brightest light stimulus is defined as 0 dB and the least bright as 40 dB. This means a 34 dB response is more sensitive than a threshold of 25 dB. The computerized automated perimeter analyzes normal threshold values from the normal data against which the patient data is compared for a given age and test location. These normal values are incorporated into the statistical calculations and result before the final results are displayed and printed out.

The probability of 50% chance of seeing or not seeing this difference between the background and stimulus is graphically described by the FOSC as function of stimulus luminance. In reality the threshold is not a fixed point, it fluctuates during the test when it is being conducted and long over periods of time at the same test points. Normally, the FOSC is very steep; this is due to the very consistent response to the projected light stimulus during visual field examination. This ability to perceive the 50% threshold illumination is very accurate in normal individual at all test points in the visual field, about 4 dB of the expected value for the test point location **(Fig. 7)**. The test points which are abnormal due to disease show inconsistency of response and the bandwidth of response becomes more than 4 dB which makes the FOSC flat **(Fig. 8)**. Generalized depression of the field causes the FOSC shift to the right but remains steep when the visual field is affected by cataracts and other opacities in the media. The FOSC is for a theoretic understanding of how each test point is tested and the result

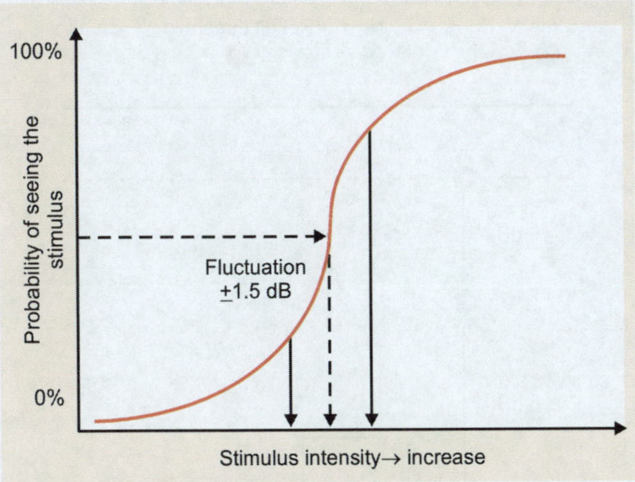

Fig. 7: Normal frequency of seeing curve.

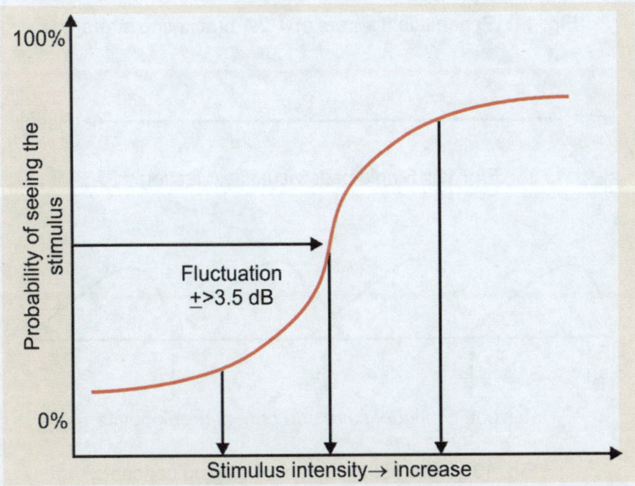

Fig. 8: Frequency of seeing curve is flat in pathology due to fluctuations.

thus obtained. The FOSC is not graphically represented on the visual field report and only the test result in decibels is represented.

Hill of Vision

Background illumination plays an important part in the shape of the hill of vision. The hill of vision is again a theoretic understanding of how the overall shape of the visual field looks like, more akin to a geographic map of a country. Lower background illumination in static perimetry increases the dynamic range and highlights areas of depressed sensitivity better because of the flatter slope of the hill of vision **(Fig. 9)**. The drawback of lower background illumination is longer period of adaptation before the test is started. The Goldmann kinetic perimetry and the HFA use a 31.5 asb as the background illumination for detection of threshold. The direct projection perimeters like the Octopus 123 and 300 use a background illumination of 31.5 asb, hence can be used in normal clinic lighting conditions with a shortened adaptation time.

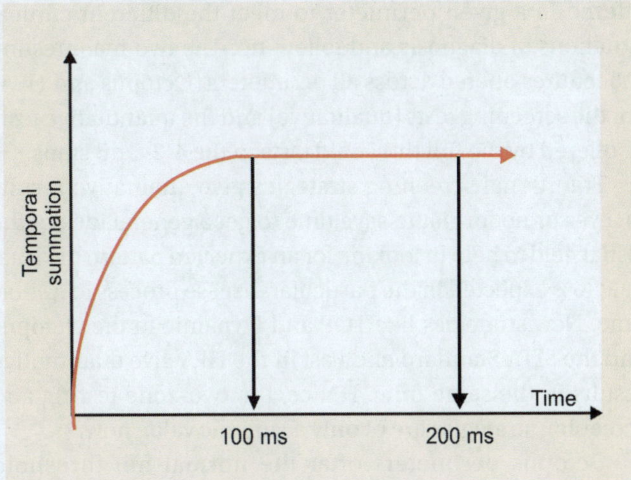

Fig. 9: Hill of vision.

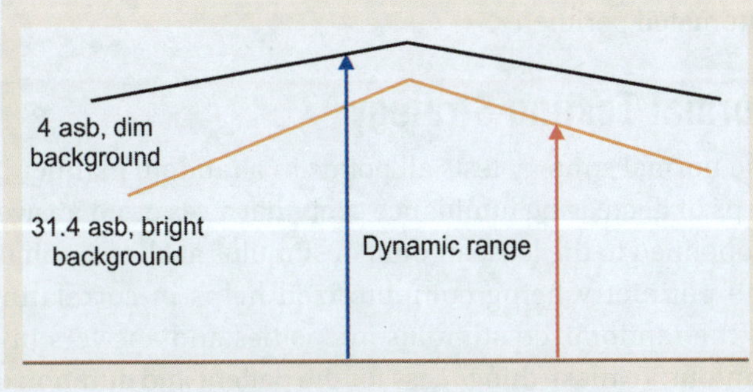

Fig. 10: Stimulus duration in milliseconds.

Stimulus Exposure Time

The stimulus exposure time is fixed for a particular machine and cannot be changed. The stimulus time is an important factor in minimizing patient errors and obtaining correct result for the tested point. The stimulus exposure time is 100 ms in the Octopus perimeter and the HFA uses 200 ms, since this time is enough to reach temporal summation of the stimulus luminance. Any exposure longer than 200 ms will provoke fixation reflex and give erroneous results **(Fig. 10)**. Setting the stimulus interval takes into consideration the NO answer and the next stimulus. The adaptive stimulus presentation keeps track of the average time of response and proceeds with the completion of the test either faster or slower to adapt to the patient's speed of answering a test stimulus. The normal interval is set between 1.5 seconds and 4 seconds. The SITA strategy uses this stimulus interval to do away with false positive catch trials and save time.

MEASUREMENT STRATEGIES

The evaluation of visual field takes into consideration the program or "where" of the visual field or the test point locations are. The strategy is the "how" the test points are evaluated. A choice of test strategies and programs are offered in a given perimeter to meet the different clinical situations of diagnosis and follow-up. The two main testing procedures offered across all perimeters (Octopus and HFA) are the screening tests (qualitative) and the quantitative tests as offered by the full threshold tests in the 4-2-1 dB steps.

Traditional screening strategies give qualitative results in a yes or no format to save time to get a general idea of the visual field to help in looking for an expected pattern of visual field loss expected in the particular disease process in a short time. New strategies like TOP and Dynamic in the Octopus and the SITA Standard and Fast in the HFA give quantitative results in the same time. Hence, the two-zone testing and screening strategies are of only academic value now.

Octopus perimeters offer the normal full threshold testing strategy, the Dynamic strategy (Weber), and TOP. It is important to understand the classical normal strategy introduced by Flammer in 1972 since it forms the basis of all automated perimetry.

Normal Testing Strategy

The normal strategy tests all points in a random manner in steps of decreasing luminance such that a yes or no answer is obtained to the least amount of stimulus at all test points. The perimetry being computerized helps in correlating all the randomized stimulus intensities and answers in a printout. To make things easy for the patient and duration of test shorter, testing starts at one point in each of four visual field quadrants called anchor points. The anchor points test the general slope of the hill of vision to the age corrected normal values. The visual field determination starts at all test points from the expected age corrected minus 4 dB. A "no" answer drops the stimulus luminance by 6 dB if the first response to a minus 4 dB start is negative. A brighter light stimulus is projected which is 8 dB less to quickly approach the depressed sensitivity of the test point. Once the anchor points are determined, further testing in a 4-2-1 dB step approach at each of the predetermined test points is determined from the data obtained from the estimated hill of vision rather than starting from normal hill of vision values which would make the testing tedious. This is approximately five questions per test point hence sensitive enough to detect shallow pathology. Normal strategy takes about 15–18 minutes per eye to complete a visual field examination **(Fig. 11)**. These strategies are similar in principle into both Octopus and HFA.

Octopus and the HFA introduced new strategies to minimize the effects of physical and retinal fatigue, which are implemented in all models of the perimeters as below:

- Staging and phases
- Dynamic strategy
- Tendency oriented perimetry
- SITA fast and SITA standard for the HFA perimeters.

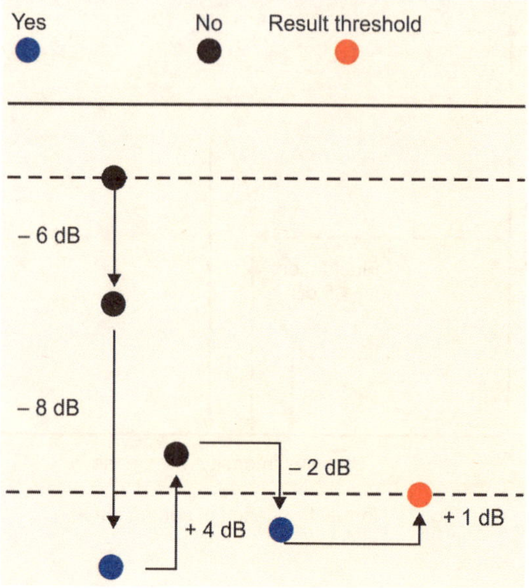

Fig. 11: Schematic diagram of 4-2-1 bracketing strategy.

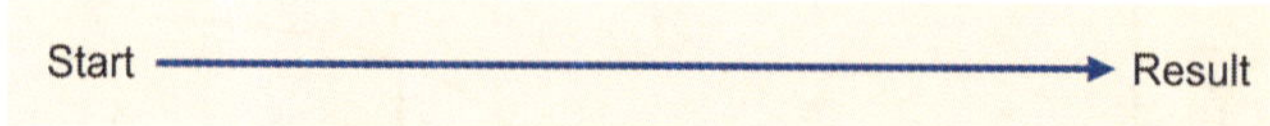

Fig. 12: Single pass visual field testing.

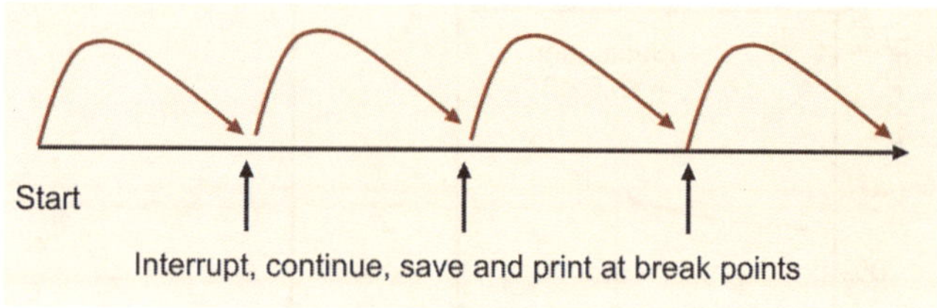

Fig. 13: Schematic diagram of staging concept.

Octopus Staging and Phases

Staging of visual field: Visual field analysis testing was traditionally done in a single pass, i.e. the first to last test result is needed before a test result is printed out **(Fig. 12)**. Normal strategy typically takes 18–20 minutes to complete for final results of the test. The single pass visual field test was modified by Octopus into staged modules to run in a sequence of diagnostically relevant stages and test points so that the first tested points give the best results without the influence of fatigue, physical, or retinal. Each of the four stages behaving as independent test with result outcome accumulated thus far. The need to continuation into the next stage may depend on more diagnostic information. This visual field result can now be saved, printed or restarted from the last tested point. The results obtained in the first two stages account for almost 80% of the result **(Fig. 13)**. The Octopus perimeters have a "defect level" indicator in the screen which statistically facilitates if the current visual field examination is "normal", "borderline" or "depressed". In cases of borderline, the test could be continued in the next two stages of the visual field test to get a complete analysis.

Test phases in Octopus perimeter: After one or two stages of visual field testing in the first phase, one of four options now exists in second phase of visual field testing. (1) The test may be saved, printed, or stopped; (2) The test points may be retested to ascertain the short-term fluctuations (SFs); (3) Quantify relative defects; (4) When data already indicates deviation from normal then additional peripheral test points may be tested to confirm clinical findings. This concept of phasing allows standardized data to be obtained by selectively testing for a specific pathology at the expected test points with very little loss of information and economizing the time duration taken for the test **(Fig. 14)**.

Dynamic Test Strategy

Webber introduced the Dynamic strategy of visual field testing. The stimulus luminance step size (bracketing) adapts to the slope of the FOSC. When the depth of the defect is deep, the step size increases from increments steps of 2–10 dB to achieve final calculated value from the last two tested values. The accuracy obtained with this test is comparable to the regular full threshold test with a 4-2-1 dB strategy. This strategy provides quantitative data, which may be represented as the grayscale, Bebie curve, and global indices. Quantitative values are useful for follow-up and to track changes over time. The test duration is about 40–50% in severely depressed fields and 30–40% in marginally depressed fields when compared to normal threshold. SF values may also be calculated by retesting all locations in the second phase if additional information is needed. Dynamic strategy provides data of the visual field comparable to the regular full threshold determination done in four stages **(Figs. 15A and B)**.

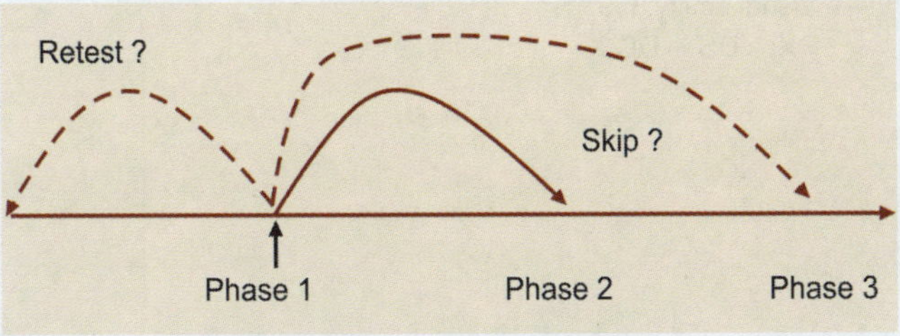

Fig. 14: Test phases after 1st stage.

Tendency Oriented Perimetry

Tendency oriented perimetry strategy introduced by Professor González de la Rosa reduces the time taken to complete the visual field analysis by 80% to the time taken by normal threshold. TOP takes into consideration the neighboring test locations into account when the results are interpreted. TOP strategy can be applied to all test methods like blue on yellow and flicker or programs like macular-M2. The neighboring zones exhibit a topographical interdependence, which establishes a tendency between adjacent points under examination.

The TOP evaluates every "yes" and "no" in two ways, the test location under test is evaluated for the differential sensitivity, which is called the vertical bracketing and the neighboring points are also adjusted by interpolation. A "yes" answer at the test location will influence the neighboring point positively and a "no" answer will influence the neighboring point negatively on the decibel scale. Regular full threshold perimetry every test location is tested at least 4–6 times before arrival at the final value of differential sensitivity. A single answer in TOP is adjusted five times from the results of the neighboring test locations in the grid for final results.

The TOP divides the test location in the visual field into evenly intermingling grids. The four grids are examined one after another and the locations of the other three matrices are adjusted to get new values by interpolation. The examination starts at half the value of the expected age corrected value, which in decibel is 8/16 of the expected normal value. Then the testing begins with steps in relation to the patient's age corrected value, i.e. 4/16, 3/16, 2/16 and finally a 1/16. These steps may be in either direction to determine the final threshold of di-sensitivity **(Fig. 16)**. Grayscales show a rounded effect in TOP compared to regular threshold grayscale values because of the adjustments of the neighboring points. Hence, the average sensitivity values obtained may be a little "shallow" compared with regular threshold testing **(Fig. 16)**. This difference is not of any significance when the parameter in follow-up is only changes over time, since the pathology is already established and the patient compliance is improved for follow-up testing. Note the difference in mean deviation (MD) values of only 0.1 between the two strategies **(Fig. 16)**. The gray/color scale shows some spread and shallowness of the color scale in the TOP strategy.

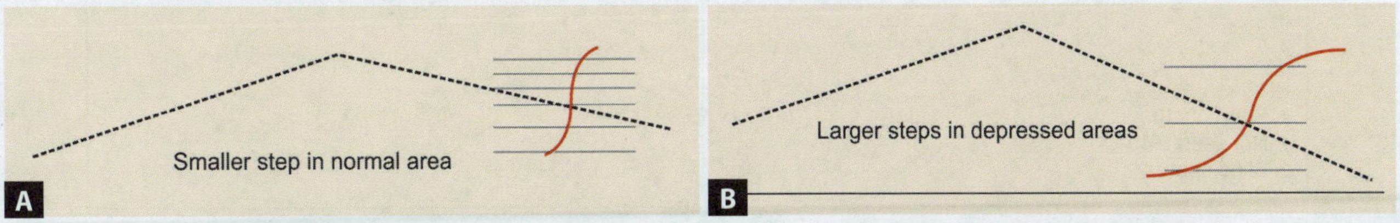

Figs. 15A and B: (A) Smaller steps in normal test locations; (B) Larger steps in depressed areas.

HUMPHREY VISUAL FIELD ANALYZER

Swedish Interactive Threshold Algorithm Strategy

The Swedish interactive threshold algorithm was developed for the Humphrey visual field analyzer to save time up to 50% while maintaining better sensitivity, accuracy, and reproducibility. SITA works by continuous estimation of the measurement and the staircase estimation is interrupted when the mathematical and statistical evaluation reach the predetermined error levels. The visual field model is continuously evaluated from a predefined one and retesting of tested points avoided and results in saving time. The false positive catch trials are not done in SITA, since this is continuously evaluated by the software depending on the time taken by the patient to react to the presented stimulus. The SITA standard combined with a 24-2 testing program saves time and has acceptable accuracy and reproducibility in the detection of glaucomatous abnormalities.

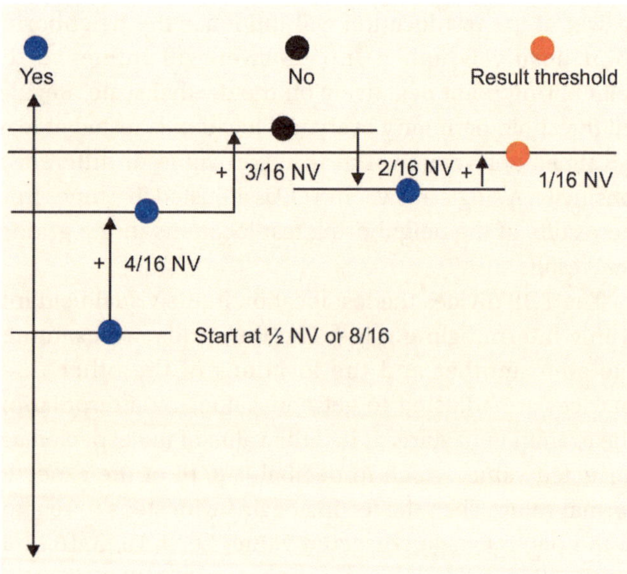

Fig. 16: Schematic representation of the bracketing in tendency oriented perimetry.

Qualitative Two Level Testing

With the introduction of faster full threshold testing, these screening tests are almost obsolete. Two-level testing uses a maximum of two questions per location and provides a simple quantification of the tested location. The test starts with a stimulus -4 dB, less than the age corrected value. A "yes" answer sums up the test result of that location. A "no" answer provides the same location the brightest stimuli and a "yes" tags the test location as relative defect. A "no" to the brightest stimulus is classified as an absolute defect. The Octopus perimeter allows these relatively tested points to be quantified in the second phase and thus converts a qualitative test result into a quantified test result. Example of a 40 point two zone testing which gives a yes or no answer is given in **Figure 17**.

Octopus Examination Programs

A white on white visual field testing procedure needs two questions to be answered, "which" locations need to be tested—program and "how" should it be tested—strategy. A third additional question could be—"what method"—flicker, kinetic or blue on yellow perimetry should be used?

A combination of test program, test strategy, and perimetry method may be appropriately chosen for a given pathology under investigation. Octopus perimeter offers test locations or programs for specific pathology, e.g. glaucoma, macular degeneration, or neurological examination.

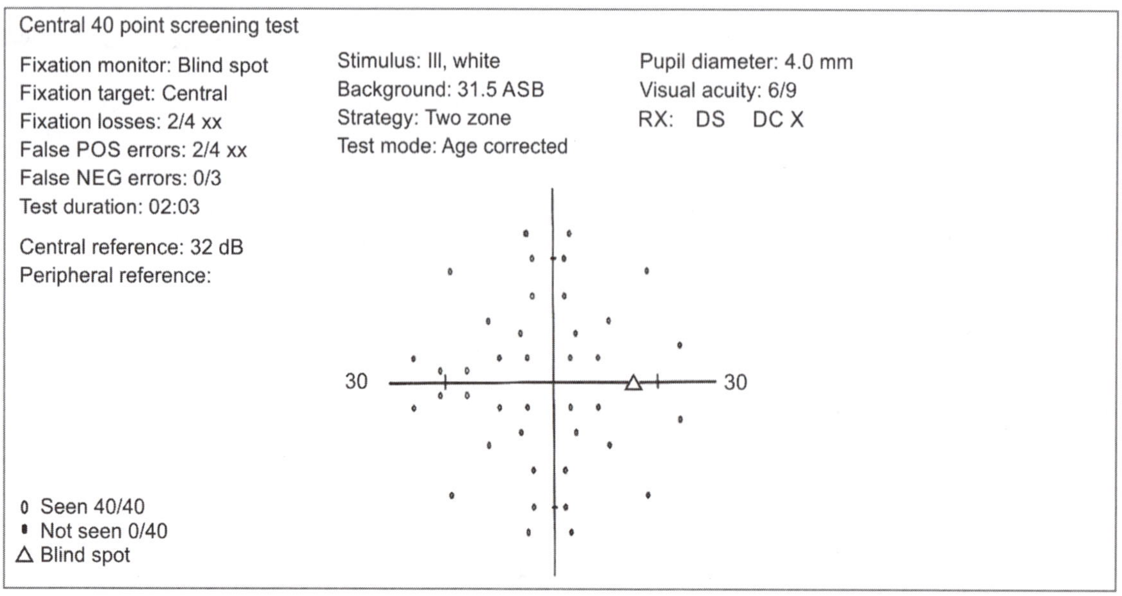

Fig. 17: Two-zone testing in Humphrey field analyzer.

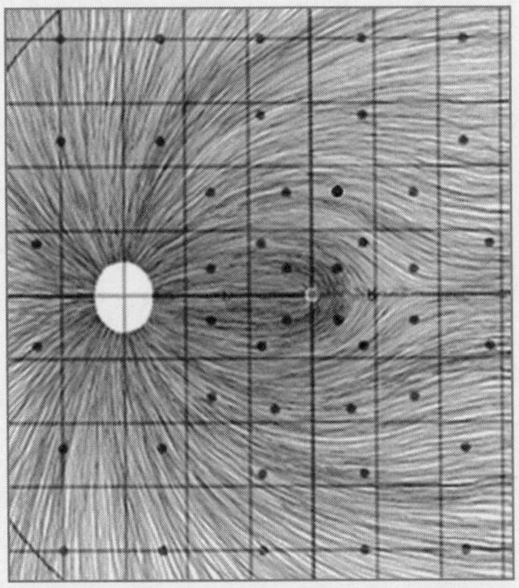

Fig. 18: G1 test points superimposed on the nerve fiber layer.

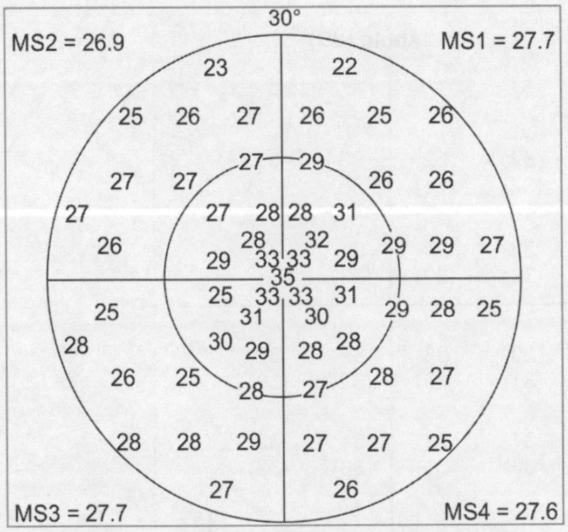

Fig. 19: Typical G1 locations of test points.

The test programs that are offered on the Octopus perimeters, which are commonly used, are as follows:

Program G1/G2

The two programs are identical in the central 30° consisting of 59 test point locations and differ only in the peripheral 15 additional points tested between the 30° and 60° in G2. The G2 is a program optimized for Octopus 101/900 series perimeter. The G1 program test locations respect the topography of the nerve fiber layer and are weighted to detect the nasal step in glaucoma **(Fig. 18)**. The foveal and paracentral areas have resolution of 2.8° in the G1/G2 programs compared to 4.2° resolution in a classical program 32 test location. The increased resolution in the foveal area gives a good follow-up when there is a fixation threat, without the need of an additional visual field test for the fovea. Depressed areas have a high false negative behavior because of a flatter FOSC and extend the test duration.

All strategies can run on the G1 and G2 program **(Fig. 19)**. The 300 Octopus perimeters allow the phase 2 retesting of all the test locations in the Dynamic and Normal strategy. The phase 3 (screening the periphery) and phase 4 (quantifying the periphery) run in the 101 and 900 series these perimeters are used in research and teaching settings. The 4 dB background illumination increases the dynamic range of the tested locations. Most clinical needs are satisfied with the 300 series Octopus perimeter. Having an additional test point between the 30° and 60° of testing does not give additional information but only confirms what is seen in the central 30° field.

Program 32 (Octopus) and the 30-2 Humphrey Field Analyzer

This is the classic "off axis" program introduced by Octopus and later by other perimeters as the 30-2 program. There are 76 test locations in a grid pattern with a resolution of 6°. This program is not related to the topography of the nerve fiber layer or pathology with both eyes having identical pattern of test locations. The area where the blind spot appears marks the right and left eye. The program 32 is still an option since old follow-up was done with this program. It may also be used in neurological cases where this program defines the vertical and horizontal meridians well. Phase 2 testing may be done to assess the short-term fluctuations (SF) in Normal and Dynamic strategy **(Fig. 20)**. HFA also introduced the 24-2 program, which does not include the edges and reduces time taken to complete the examination.

Program M2

The macular program was designed for detection and follow-up of central and paracentral visual field defects in patients with neurological diseases, macular or perimacular diseases. The M2 program has 45 test locations which are tested in two stages consisting of the central 4° and the area between 4° and 9°. The 45 test locations in the central 4° gives a 0.7° resolution with a Goldmann Size III which is 0.43° in diameter **(Fig. 21)**. The additional 36 test locations situated in the outer 4°–9° give this program the highest resolution in the central 10° of the visual field. Additional test locations may also be tested between 9.5° and 26° if need be. The M2 program can be run using the TOP, Dynamic or Normal strategy to define the visual field pathology in question.

Systematic Interpretation of Octopus Seven-in-One Single Field Report, "The Ten Step Approach"

The new Octopus Seven-in-One printout from the EyeSuite contains both the raw results from the visual field examination and easy-to-read data interpreting the results of the visual field test. The single field printout also presents the statistical calculations, images, graphs, plots,

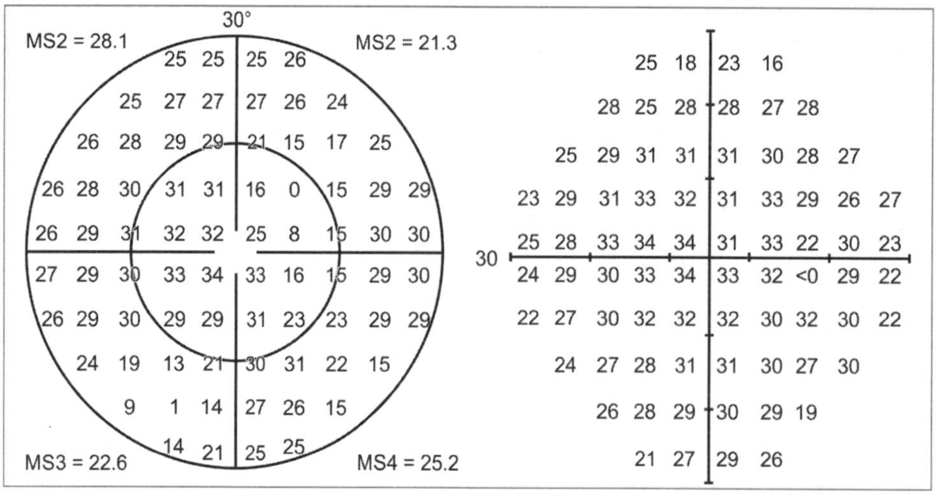

Fig. 20: Test point locations in the P32 (Octopus) and the 30-2 in Humphrey field analyzer program.

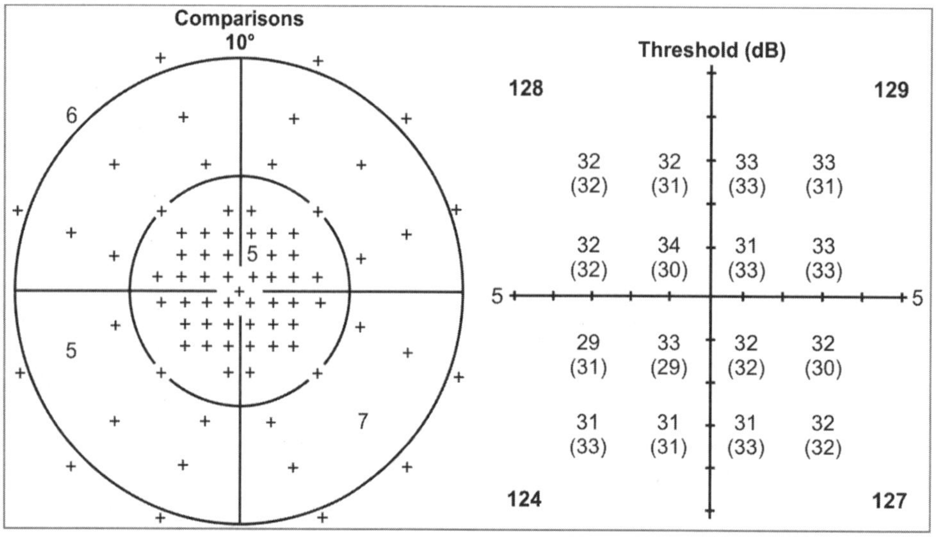

Fig. 21: Test point locations in the M2 program and the Humphrey field analyzer macular program.

and indices. The "Ten Step Approach" to the single field printout makes the interpretation of visual fields in a clinic setting easy to read and correlate the clinical findings **(Fig. 22)**. The new format of the Seven-in-One single field-printout from the EyeSuite software presents changes in the Bebie curve in the way the diffuse loss of sensitivity is calculated. In the Ten Step Approach, the Seven-in-One visual field is divided into 10 areas which are specific to a particular aspect of interpretation.

The Seven-in-One Single Field Report is interpreted in the following order:

1. *Patient data:* Information about the patient.
2. *Examination particulars:* The eye examined, date, and type of printout.
3. *Examination details:* The program and strategy used, reliability factors, pupil size, and examination parameters.
4. *Value table:* This table shows the actual measured values. The statistical and graphical details of the Seven-in-One printouts are derived from this set of raw data.
5. *Comparison table:* Represents the local difference between the measured values and the normal values corrected for the patient's age.
6. *Grayscale (in color or in B/W):* This graphic display is now derived from the comparison table, hence clutter-free and brings to attention to the defect in question.
7. *Cumulative defect Bebie curve:* An arrangement of all test data from the highest value to the least from left to right which is overlaid on a statistically age corrected normal for comparison.
8. *Corrected comparison table:* Uncovers any defect from any uniform depression caused by a cataract or other diffuse loss, e.g. uncorrected refractive errors, cataract, etc. These values are derived from the Bebie curve.
9. *Probability plots:* The data presented in the probability and corrected probabilities are symbolic representation of the defect, from the comparisons and corrected comparisons tables, respectively.
10. *Visual field indices:* Condenses the visual field results in a few numbers.

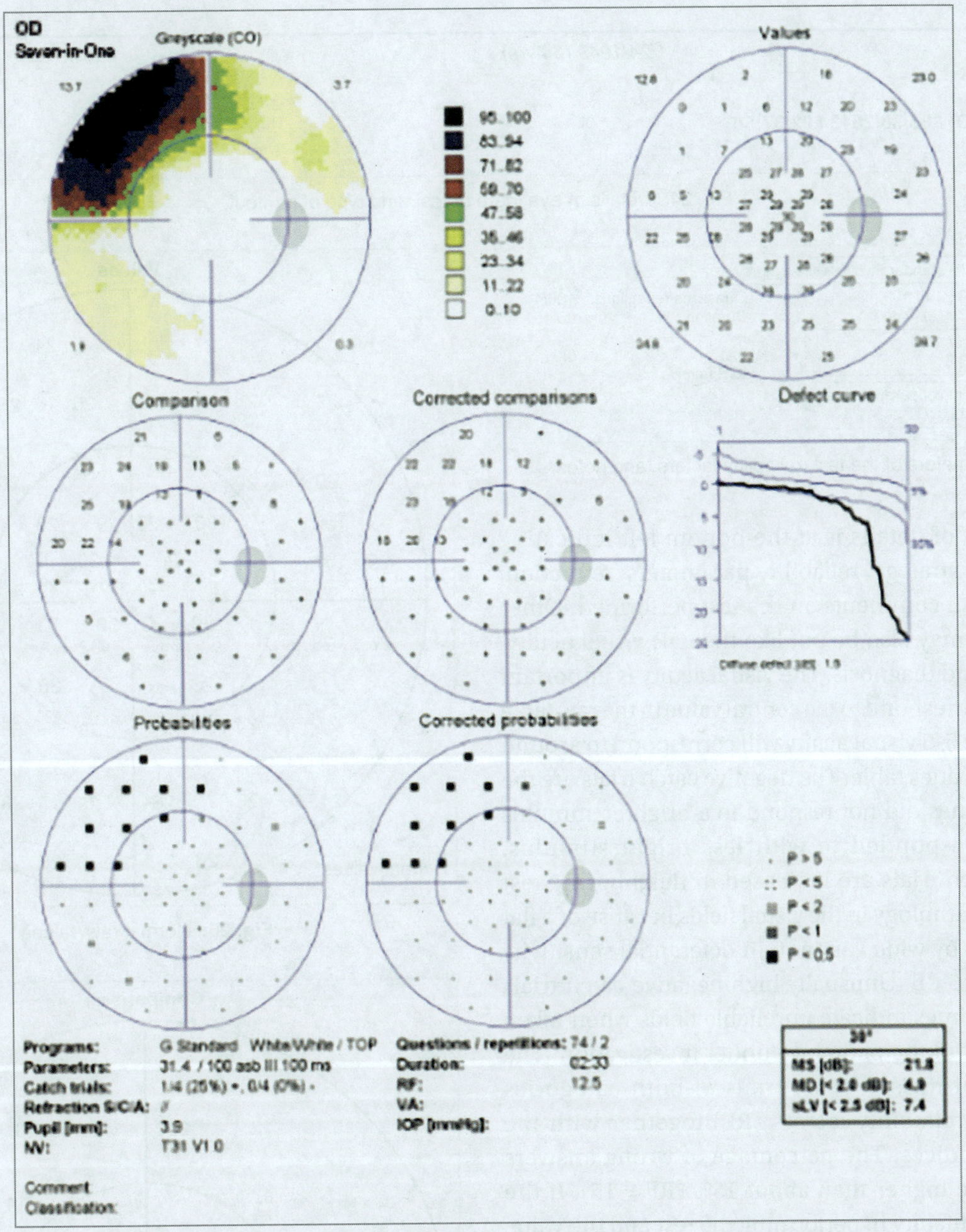

Fig. 22: Seven-in-One printout.

Premier Eye Care and Surgical Center
15, Luz Avenue, Mylapore, Chennai 600004, Ph +91 44 24992722
24x7 +91 9841582722

S	*P*	*, 1/24/1949 (64 yrs)*
ID 1	*1*	

Fig. 23: Date of birth and ID of patient.

The Ten Step method of interpreting the Seven-in-One printout takes all the presented data in a systematic approach to give a meaningful evaluation of the visual field **(Fig. 22)**.

1. *Patient data:* Demographic information about the patient. The name and date of birth should be entered correctly since these parameters assign a unique entry in the database. The date of birth is used for age the corrected values and comparison. A wrong date of birth (older) will show unusually high sensitivity expected for the given age **(Fig. 23)**.
2. The eye that was examined, examination date and the printout format details are marked out clearly for follow-up. It is important to remember that the same program and strategy are to be used for follow-up when analysis is done with the EyeSuite Software **(Fig. 24)**.

S P , 1/24/1949 (64 yrs)
ID 1 1
Right eye (OD) / 03/30/2013 / 02:37:50
Seven-in-One

Fig. 24: Details of eye, date of test, and type of printout.

Programs:	G standard/white/white dynamic		
Parameters:	31.4 III 100 ms	Questions/repetitions:	160/4
Catch trials:	3/8(+), 0/8(-)	Duration:	06:15
Refraction S/C/A:	-5/-1/85	RF:	18.7
Pupil (mm):	3.6	VA:	6/9
		IOP (mmHg):	
Comment:	Patient cooperation good		
Classification	POAG, CCT 543		

Fig. 25: Parameters of the test, reliability factors, and notes.

3. The third set of details is at the bottom left indicating the program, strategy, reliability parameters, refraction, pupil size, and comments on the test performed. Other entered data may also be put like the IOP, visual acuity, comments, and diagnosis. The visual acuity is important since it will correspond to the central value in the raw table **(Fig. 25)**. The 6/6 visual acuity will correspond to around 30 dB in the values table. The negative catch trials are the number of times did not respond to a brighter stimulus which was responded to with less bright stimulus. Negative catch trials are increased in neighboring test locations of pathology in the visual fields because of a flat FOSC caused by wide variation in deferential sensitivity of more than 5 dB. Unusually high negative catch trials do not sometimes indicate unreliable fields when taken in the context of the pathology under investigation. The percentage of missed catch trials of both categories defines the "reliability factor" (RF) together with the visual field indices. The percentage of wrong answers should not be higher than about 15% (RF = 15). If the patient has difficulty in performing the test and the value is higher than 20%, this is noted so as to use this data in subsequent follow-up.
4. The values table represents the raw data in numerical values and shows high central values with lower peripheral values and gives an understanding of the general height and shape of hill of vision **(Fig. 26)**.
5. The comparisons table adjusts for the age of the patient and represents data in a simple easy-to-understand format. A "+" symbol represents a normal value corrected for the age match. A number in this table represents a deviation from the normal expected value greater than 4 dB from normal values expected for the given test location. A black square represents absolute defects indicating the brightest light did not evoke any response **(Fig. 27)**. Note the + symbol, black squares and numerals indicating the extent of deviation from normal age match.

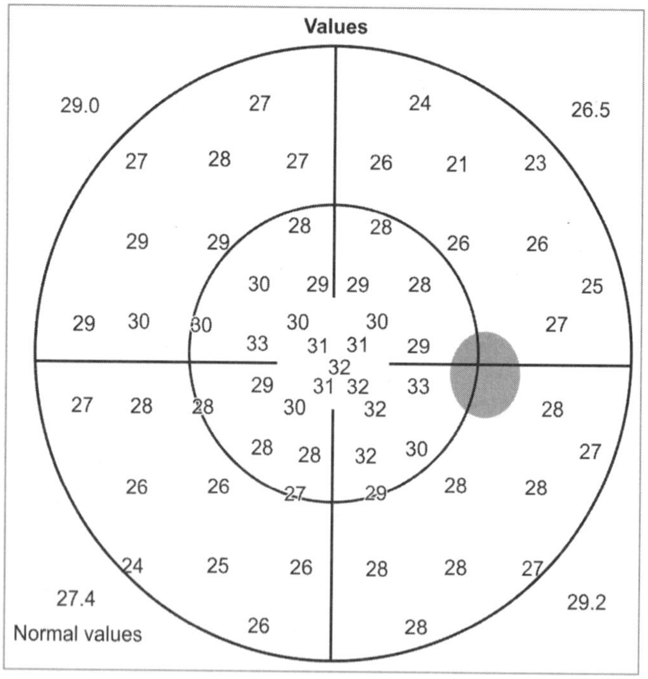

Fig. 26: Normal raw values.

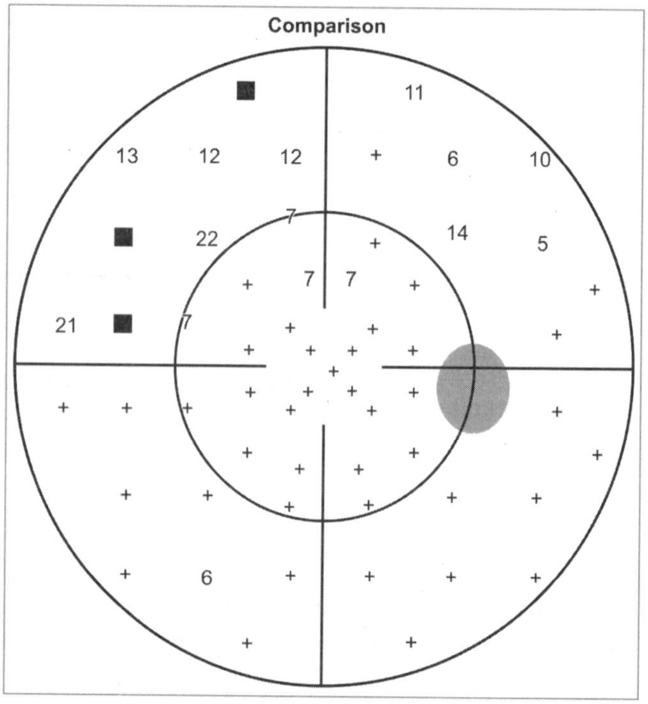

Fig. 27: Comparison.

6. The gray/color scales are derived from the numerical values of the comparisons table in the new Seven-in-One single visual field format and provide more information

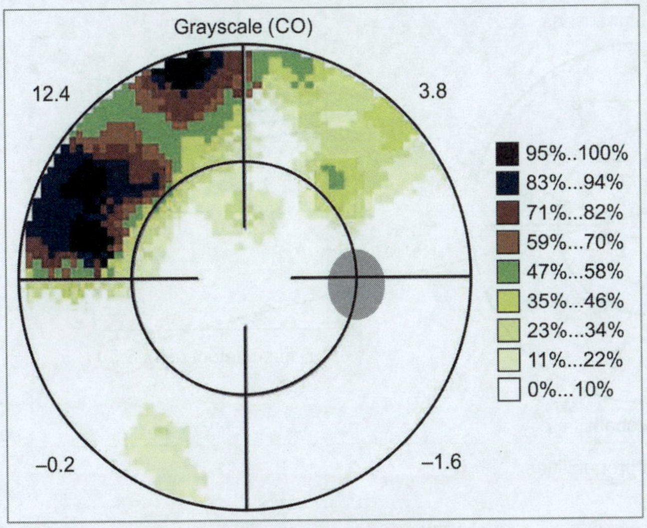

Fig. 28: Gray/color scale.

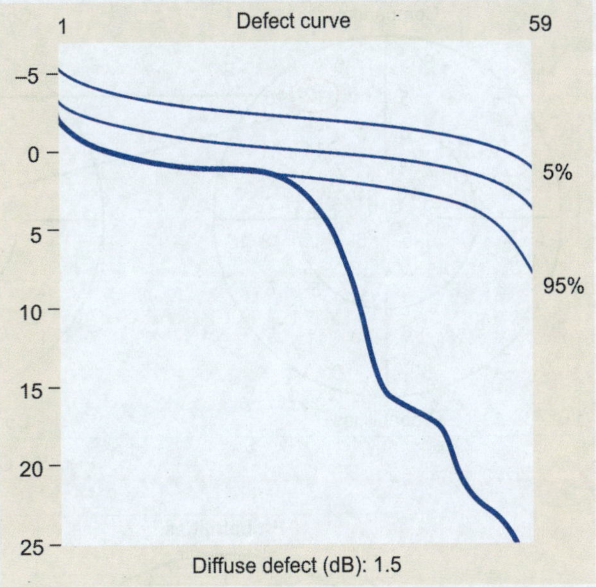

Fig. 29: Cumulative defect/Bebie curve.

since it is age corrected match, at a glance to the topography and depth of the defect. This makes it easy to explain to the patient the darker color representing abnormality and the white being normal **(Fig. 28)**.

7. *Cumulative defect Bebie curve:* This graphical display is an arrangement of all test data from the highest value to the least from left to right which is overlaid on a statistically age corrected normal for comparison. The values are a rank list and do not give the topography of the defect. The Bebie curve contains information on the MD and loss variance (LV). The normal age corrected range is displayed and the current patient examination is displayed for comparison. The Bebie curve is used to calculate the diffuse defect from the averages of the 12th–16th reading from the left. Diffuse defect separates the local defect from the diffuse loss. Diffuse defect is stable even when 20% of test locations are affected. Value of the diffuse defect is displayed at the bottom of the table **(Fig. 29)**.
8. *Corrected comparison table:* It shows the defects discounting any uniform depression caused by a cataract or other diffuse loss, e.g. cataract, corneal opacities, miosis, and uncorrected refraction. The values of this table are derived from the value of the diffuse defect from the Bebie curve when subtracted from the comparisons. The corrected comparisons uncover focal loss hidden behind a diffuse loss as in a case of an eye with cataract with glaucomatous visual field defects **(Fig. 30)**.
9. Probability plots are the last two tables which use probabilities symbol at the test points to display the normal and deviation. The probabilities plot displays the comparison table and the corrected probabilities plot displays the corrected comparisons. These tables bring to attention of the clinician the statistical probability of the points under consideration, the probability of being normal. The symbols range from $P < 0.5$ to $P > 5$. The significance of $P < 0.5$ is understood as the tested point is normal in 0.5% of the population and hence the probability of the test point being abnormal is very high. A structure to function correlation helps to detect the abnormal test point **(Fig. 31)**. The example below when corrected for diffuse defect reveals a normal visual field, and corrected defective field is shown in **Figure 32**.
10. Global indices in the new format is summary display of the visual field tested, i.e. 30° or 10°. The indices displayed are mean sensitivity (MS), MD and the square root of loss variance (sLV). Visual field indices summarize the characteristics of the visual field into few key numeric values. These indices provide a global perspective of the visual field and indicate at a glance the diffuse and focal loss and are useful in comparing visual fields over time. Flammer is credited with the introduction of these indices in 1985. The global indices are more precise since the effect of scatter and inaccuracies of test points are reduced by averaging the results over all tested locations. The fluctuations are also reduced by the square root of the number of test locations by a factor of 8 in a typical G1 program. Hence, deviation from the normal values indicates pathology.

Mean sensitivity is the first index to be displayed **(Fig. 33)**. MS is the average of all test locations which are measured in decibel. MS is the arithmetic mean of all test locations and is a raw value, hence cannot be compared. MS gives a general picture of the sensitivity or the shape of the hill of vision in a visual field for a given patient responses.

Mean defect is the age corrected mean sensitivity **(Fig. 33)**. This age correction makes MD independent of age. The normal value of MD is zero. Ninety percent of fields have a normal value between –2.0 and +2.0. Borderline MD values of more than +2.4 or more need a retest to confirm damage.

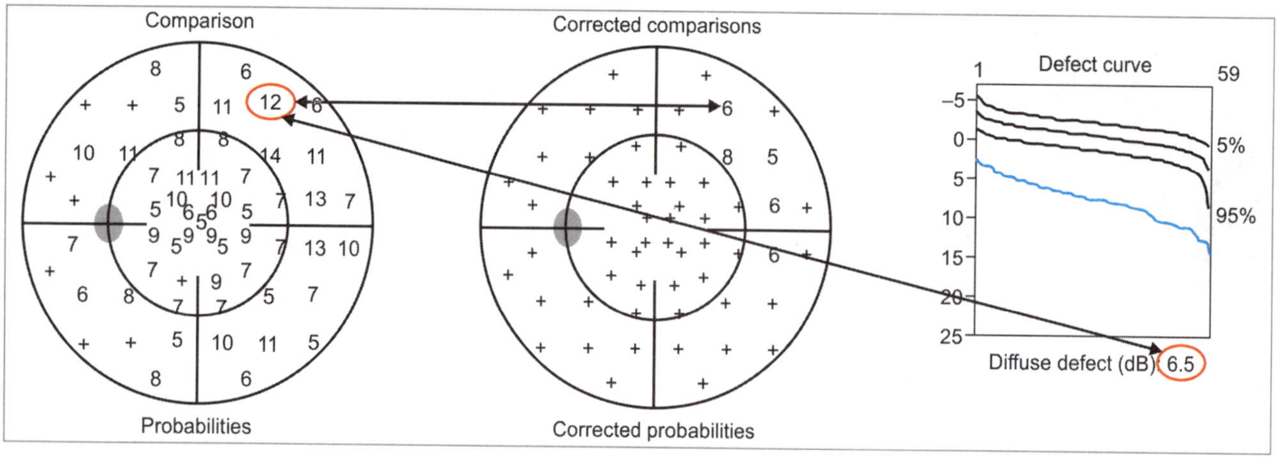

Fig. 30: Corrected probabilities.

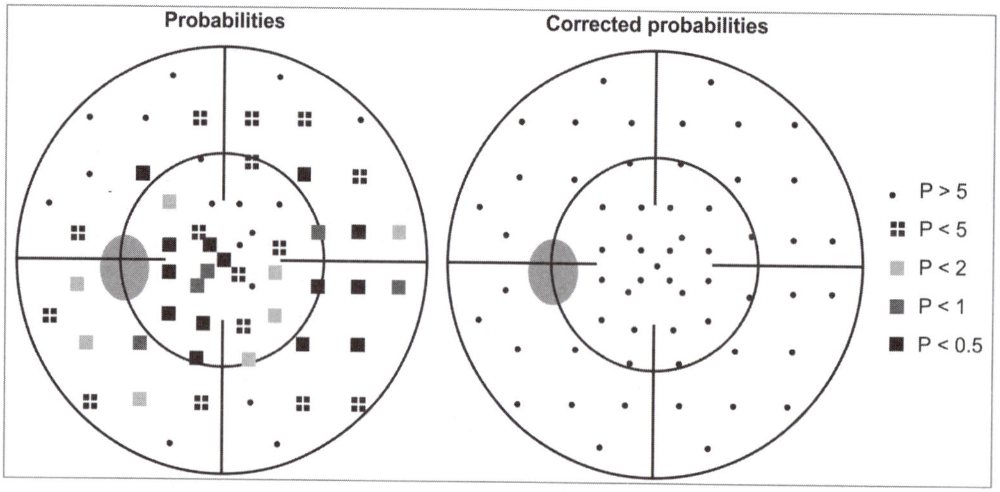

Fig. 31: Corrected probabilities showing visual field defect in a symbolic representation.

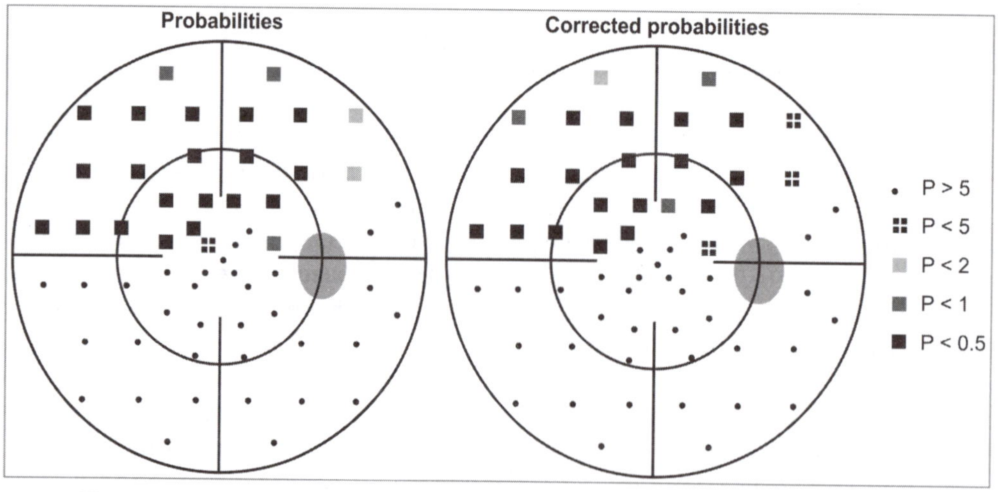

Fig. 32: Corrected probabilities showing normal fields after correcting for the diffuse defect.

The trend of MD over time is a good indicator of global damage. This value may be affected by cataract, opacities of cornea, miosis, and uncorrected refractive errors.

sLV is the square root of loss variance **(Fig. 33)**. LV is the square value of the standard deviation of the local defects in the comparisons tables. LV is a very sensitive index to

	30°
MS (dB):	19.7
MD (<2.0 dB) :	7.6
sLV (<2.5 dB):	9.3

Fig. 33: Global indices with the area of visual field tested.
(MS: mean sensitivity; MD: mean deviation; sLV: square root of loss variance)

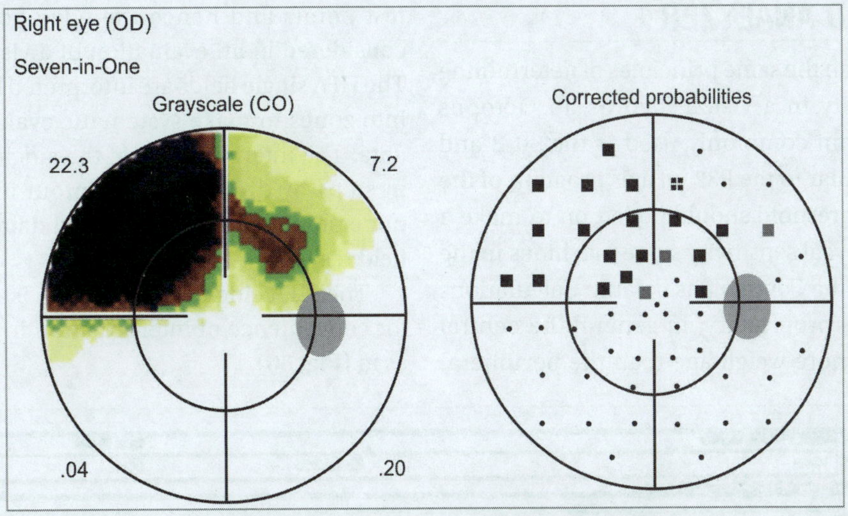

Fig. 34: Field report showing superior arcuate defect.

early localized damage; its use in follow-up is limited since it increases exponentially and difficult to chart progression against other global indices. sLV as a number being the square root is more smooth on a follow-up trend analysis graph. sLV as an index is now featured in a single field analysis report. sLV gives an idea of the extent of focal defect and provides an index for progression analysis follow-up over time. sLV is derived from corrected values of the comparisons table and hence have a bandwidth of normal values of less than 2.5 dB.

Summary of Interpretation

The Seven-in-One printout in **Figure 22** may be summarized as follows:

- Step 3 provides the details of the catch trials 0/4, hence the patient was attentive with the RF value showing 0. The refraction values have been noted in the visual field.
- Step 8 shows the corrected comparisons which are corrected for age and factors that affect the height of hill of vision. The table shows black squares indicative of area of absolute scotoma; the numerals show the extent of deviation from normal in areas of pathology; and the "+" symbol indicates the areas of normal values. The topography of the defect is also displayed on the probability plots with the statistical significance of the tested points which display values that may be normal in only <0.5% of population.
- Step 10 summarizes the global indices, the MD 8.9B (<2 dB) and the sLV 9.0 dB (<2 dB). The visual field which is reliable shows test points that are depressed to a level of significance that would be found in population of <0.5%, hence abnormal. The test points respect the horizontal meridian and the points across the meridian have a difference of more than 14 dB. The defective test point location exhibits an arcuate shape typical of glaucomatous visual field loss. The global indices MD and sLV are well above the range of normality. Clinical interpretation requires that these visual field defects should correlate with the damage in the optic disk before being labeled as "Glaucoma".

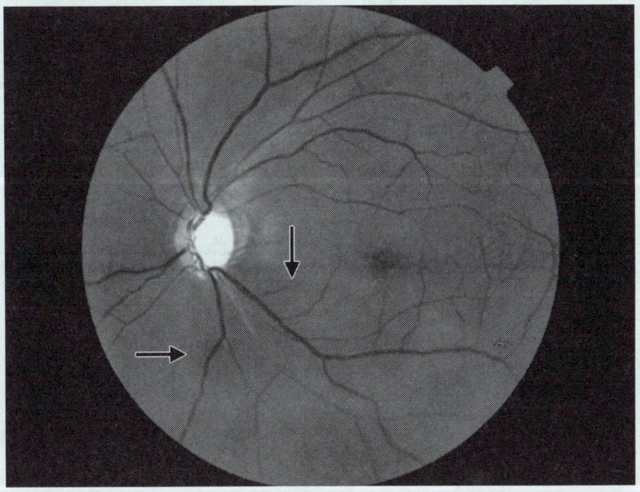

Fig. 35: Red-free fundus picture showing corresponding nerve fiber layer defect.

Structure-function Correlation

The visual field printout report **(Fig. 34)** should be always correlated with the clinical fundus **(Fig. 35)** findings and should be consistent for a proper analysis of the patient's eye condition. Pitfalls in interpretation are very common, hence clinical decisions on therapy and surgery should always have a structure-function correlation. A fundus picture is a good additional tool for follow-up, though a good disk diagram should be enough when cost considerations are constraints. The automated perimeter, sophisticated software, and statistical analysis performed on a computer do not replace clinical judgment.

HUMPHREY FIELD ANALYZER

The HFA is also based on the same principles of determining threshold of sensitivity in a visual field as an Octopus perimeter. The program commonly used is the 30-2 and the 24-2 which are similar to the P32 off axis program of the Octopus. The foveal threshold should be left on to make a measurement of the foveal sensitivity some machines in the HFA series come with the Fovea off as default. Calculations of the final results are proprietary, in general the central test points are given more weightage than the peripheral test points and hence the edge points in a 30-2 are not considered in an evaluation of a visual field for glaucoma. The HFA single fields are interpreted by dividing the printout into zones to make systematic evaluation of the statistical data. The interpretation of the single field printout is done in steps by dividing the printout into five zones for easy understanding of the statistical data of the patient's visual field result.

The HFA single field printout is divided into five zones for convenience of interpretation in a systematic approach as in **(Fig. 36)**.

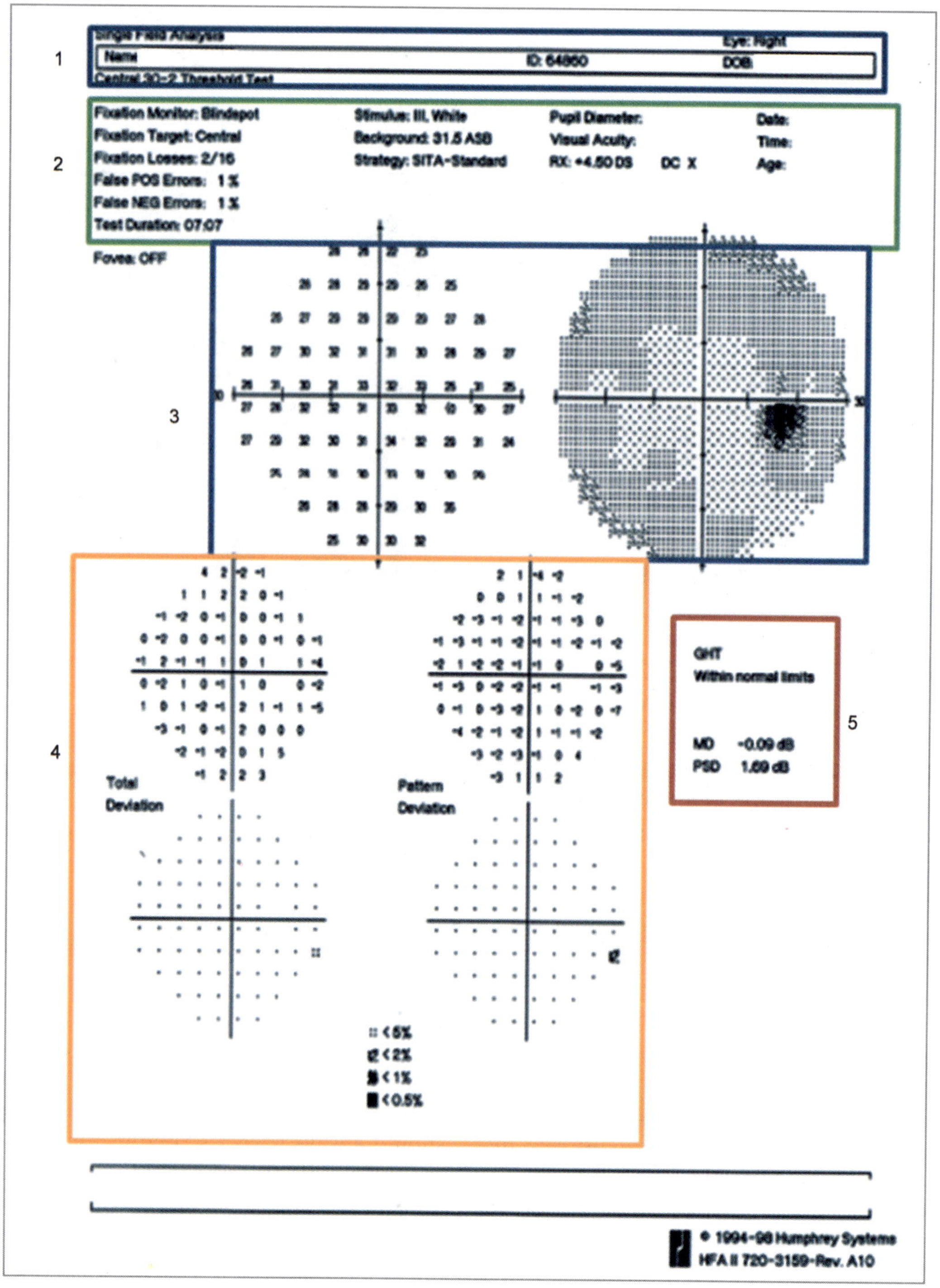

Fig. 36: Humphrey field analyzer single field printout divided into five zones.

Single field analysis | Eye: Right

Name	ID: 64860	DOB

Central 30-2 Threshold test

Fig. 37: Zone 1.

Fixation monitor: Blind spot
Fixation target: Central
Fixation losses: 2/16
False POS errors: 1.%
False NEG errors: 1.%
Test duration: 07:07

Stimulus: III, white
Background: 31.5 ASB
Strategy: SITA-standard

Pupil diameter:
Visual acuity:
RX: +4.50 DS DC X

Date:
Time:
Age:

Fig. 38: Zone 2.

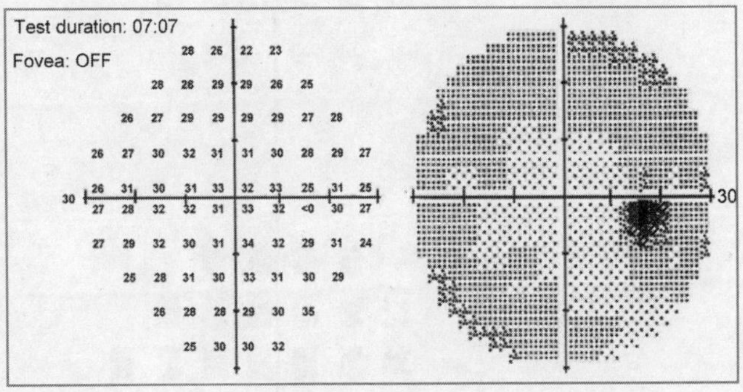

Fig. 39: Zone 3.

Zone 1

The zone 1 **(Fig. 37)** is the demographics of the patient, type of test that was conducted, the tested eye, patient details with the name, ID number, date of birth, and the program used for testing the eye. This example was a single field analysis in which the right eye was tested with the name, ID number, and date of birth. The program used was central 30-2 threshold test. The name and date of birth should be entered carefully each time for the particular patient since variation in spelling would be recognized as different patients by the machine. Wrong date of birth entry would result in comparison of normative data of the age match that was entered wrong. A lower age entered for an older patient would result in increased sensitivity.

Zone 2

The zone 2 **(Fig. 38)** contains the monitoring data such as the fixation losses, false positive errors, false negative errors, and the reliability of the particular field test on the left-hand side. The data in the middle two columns of zone 2 gives the color of the stimulus used, the strategy used, e.g. SITA-standard along with the pupil size, visual acuity which is entered by the operator, and the corrective glasses used. The visual acuity entered provides a ready reference to tally with the foveal sensitivity. A 6/6 visual acuity would have sensitivity of around 32–34 dB. The last column in the zone 2 is the date and time on which date is done along with the current age derived from the date of birth entered.

Zone 3

The zone 3 **(Fig. 39)** is the graphical representation of the raw values of the test performed with the grayscale representation of the raw values. The raw test values are useful to glance how the test has been performed, and a general look at the numbers should indicate higher values toward the center and lower values in the periphery. For example, values such as 33 dB and 32 dB are more central and values such as 24 dB is toward the periphery in normal fields. These numbers provide a general height of the hill of vision. Areas of depressed sensitivity would be abnormal and appear as darkened areas in the grayscale representation. The grayscale also gives a general idea of the topography of the defect. The grayscale is useful to show patients the extent of the visual field defect and the need for management and follow-up.

Zone 4

The zone 4 displays the total deviation and the pattern deviation. The two grayscale plots below the respective numerical tables display the same information in a statistically evaluated grayscale plot from p values that are significant from <5% in the form of dots to >0.5% represented as black squares. The total deviation is the point-to-point difference in the threshold values of the patient with the age match normal. **Figure 40** shows numerical values of the difference from the expected age corrected values. This example shows a general overall reduction in the height of the hill of vision with higher values of deviation across the horizontal meridian on the upper nasal quadrant. The pattern deviation plot below also shows areas of statistically significant deviation p values to the extent of <0.5%, but does not uncover the hidden loss due to pathology. The pattern deviation is not only corrected for age match, the overall lower height of the hill of vision is also corrected and the hidden loss is uncovered. The pattern deviation plot in the example below displays the statistically significant loss (0.5%) on the upper nasal quadrant. The clinician need not be an expert statistician to infer the clinical significance since the machine does all the statistical evaluation with

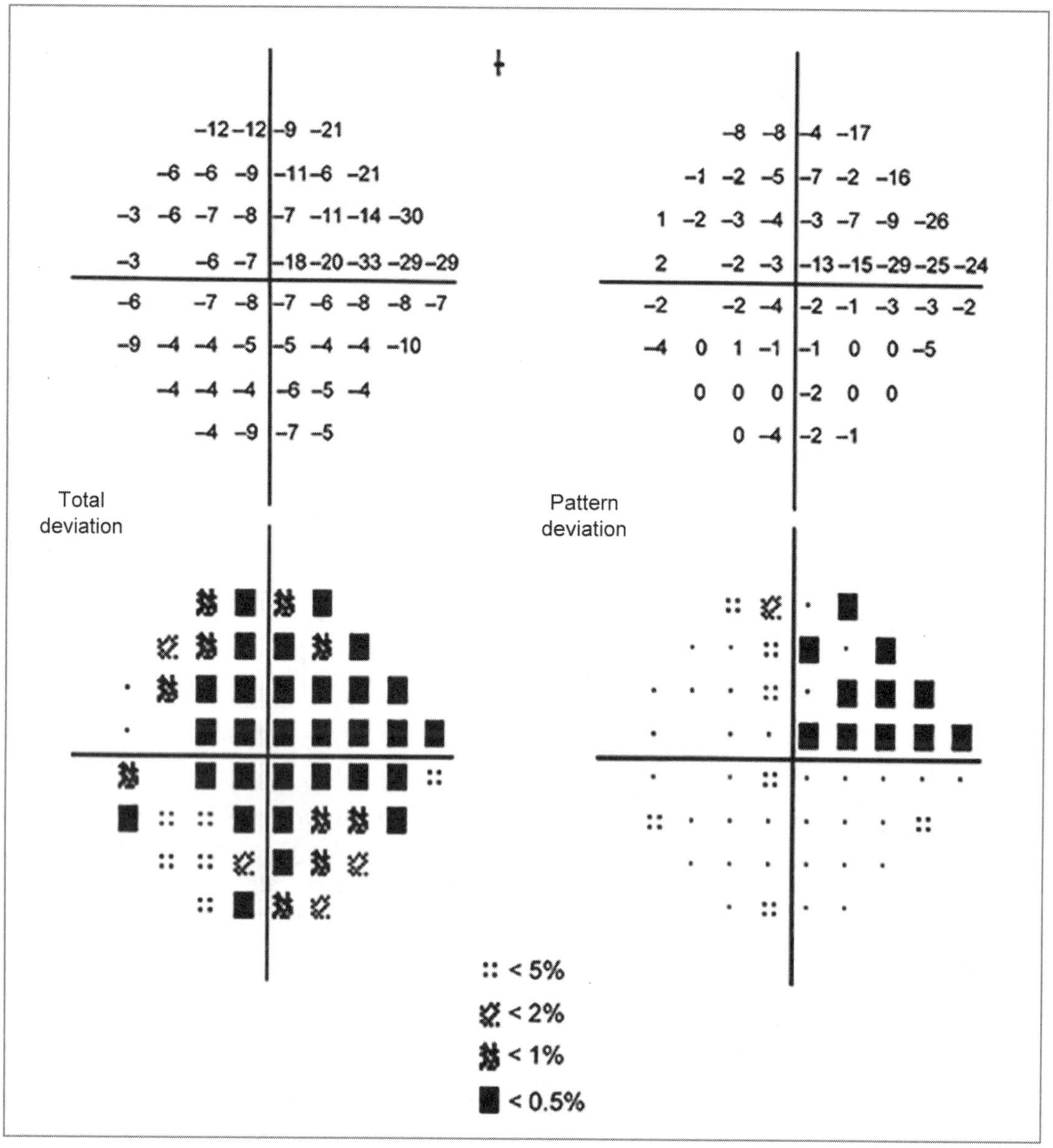

Fig. 40: Zone 4.

onboard computing to provide a printout result. The grayscale values showing the statistical significance of the plotted symbols are also provided for ready reference. This example illustrates the uncovering of the hidden loss due to depressed areas of threshold sensitivities despite an overall loss in the sensitivities due to diffuse loss as in cataract, corneal opacities, or miosis.

Zone 5

The zone 5 contains the glaucoma hemifield test (GHT) and the global indices giving additional important information of the given visual field test **(Fig. 41)**. The GHT provides simple remarks on the visual field test result and the global indices MD and pattern standard deviation (PSD) are values which summarize the visual field into result with the statistical significance of the deviation from normal values, if any **(Fig. 41)**.

The glaucoma hemifield compares the five sectors in the upper field with the five mirror images in the lower field. All areas are covered except the temporal area where a wedge-shaped defect may be missed.

The GHT gives the following messages that appear above the GHT symbol on the printout; within normal limits, outside normal limits, borderline, general reduction in sensitivity, abnormally high sensitivity, and low patient reliability. These messages should be correlated with the clinical findings to make meaningful clinical decisions. These results are based on the shaded sectors tested as seen in **Figure 42**.

The visual field index (VFI) is a value similar to the MD; was added to the printout several years ago. The VFI

GHT
Borderline

VFI	98%
MD	–0.48 dB
PSD	1,87 dB p < 10%

Fig. 41: Global indices in HFA single field analysis.
(GHT: glaucoma hemifield test; HFA: Humphrey field analyzer; MD: mean defect; PSD: pattern standard deviation; VFI: visual field index)

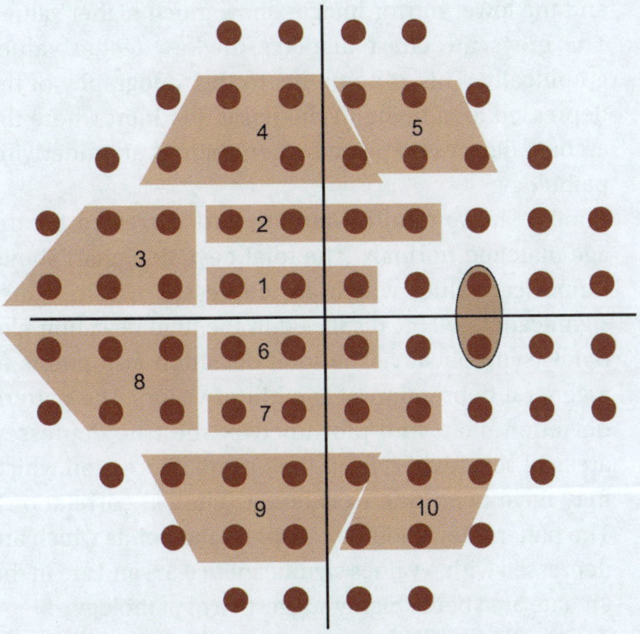

Fig. 42: Glaucoma hemifield test sectors compared across the horizontal meridian.

is a staging index for the total amount of field loss. It is reported to be less sensitive to cataracts. Values range from 100% (normal) to 0% (perimetrically blind) **(Fig. 41)**. The percentage value can be tracked over series of tests and used as one indicator for progression.

Global Indices

There global indices in HFA printout appear as set of numbers on the right-hand side along with the GHT message. The global indices make calculations which help the clinician to assess the field result as a whole rather than a point-by-point basis. The global indices are calculated from age corrected normals data, hence the p values for the indices are again not corrected for age. The four indices used in HFA are the MD, the PSD, the SF, and the corrected pattern standard deviation (CPSD) **(Fig. 43)**. The older full threshold test printout carries all the four indices and the newer strategy like the SITA carries only the MD and PSD **(Fig. 44)**, since newer algorithms do away with test and retest a point and economize on the catch trials to give an idea of the overall height of the hill of vision and the depth of the local defect in a shorter time period.

MD	–5.32 dB	p < 2%
PSD	5.85 dB	p < 2%
SF	2.55 dB	p < 5%
CPSD	5.09 dB	p < 1%

Fig. 43: Global indices in a full threshold Seven-in-One printout.
(CPSD: corrected pattern standard deviation; MD: mean defect; PSD: pattern standard deviation; SF: short-term fluctuation)

MD	–0.09 dB
PSD	1.69 dB

Fig. 44: Global indices in SITA strategy Seven-in-One printout.
(MD: mean defect; PSD: pattern standard deviation; SITA: Swedish interactive threshold algorithm)

Mean Deviation

Mean deviation is the elevation or depression of the patient's overall field compared to the normal reference field. A significant MD may indicate an overall depression or that there is loss in one sector and not in the other sectors. In the above example **(Fig. 43)**, the MD is –5.32 dB with a p value that is <2%; this means that less than 2% of normal population show an MD value larger than the value found in this test. The categories for the p values are p < 10%, p < 5%, p < 2%, p < 1% and p < 0.5%. MD is best interpreted in relation to the total and PSD charts.

Pattern Standard Deviation

Pattern standard deviation is a measure of the degree to which the shape of the patient's measured field departs from the age corrected reference field. A low PSD indicates a smooth hill of vision and a high PSD indicates an actual visual field irregularities or variability in patient response. The same categories of p values are used to indicate the statistical significance. The example in **Figure 43**, the PSD is 5.85 dB with a p value of <2%. This means that less than 2% of the normal population shows a PSD larger than the value found in this example.

Short-term Fluctuation

Short-term fluctuation is an index of consistency of the patient's answers during the test and is obtained by testing twice at 10 preselected points. For example, in **Figure 43**, the SF value is 2.55 dB with a p < 5%; this means that less than 5% population will show an SF value larger than that found in this example. The same categories of p values are used to indicate the statistical significance. The SF is used to calculate the CSPD. SF is a global index in full threshold printouts.

Corrected Pattern Standard Deviation

Corrected PSD is a measure of how much the total shape of the patient's hill of vision deviates from the shape of the hill of vision of normals for the patient's age, after correcting for intra-test variability. For example, in **Figure 43**, the CPSD is 5.09 dB with a p < 1%. CPSD attempts to remove the effects of patient variability during the test and highlight only irregularity caused by actual field loss. The categories of p values are the same as for MD values. CPSD is a global index in full threshold printouts.

Reading Humphrey Field Analyzer Seven-in-One Printout

The HFA printout gives the clinician a well-documented statistical visual field result which has been compared for the age matched normals. Now the problem is how the clinician assesses if a visual field defect is indeed due to pathology or significant. There are three well-known criteria by which the test result may be assessed. These criteria help to establish if the depressed area is due to glaucoma. All three criteria or even any one of them is sufficient to make a diagnosis depending on the clinical findings.

Criterion-1: There should be three or more non-edge points that are depressed to an extent that would be found in less than 5% of the population and one of those points should be depressed to an extent found expected in 1% of the population. These points should be clustered in the arcuate area. The arcuate area is important because these test points are on the nerve fiber layer which corresponds to the damage on the neuroretinal rim. The non-edge points are disregarded only in the 30-2 and not in the 24-2 program.

Criterion-2: The PSD should be depressed to an extent found in less than 5% of the population. The PSD is more commonly regarded since it is used most frequently by the clinician. The CSPD is more appropriate when a full threshold strategy is performed to iron out the intra-test variability.

Criterion-3: The GHT message reads "outside normal limits". This message is taken into account depending on the overall clinical assessment of the patient to determine if the pathology is due to glaucoma.

Interpretation of visual field based on the above noted criteria would be a useful exercise to reinforce the way a visual field analysis read and used for clinical decision **(Fig. 45)**.

The systematic approach to reading the printout is to look at the zones in a stepwise manner and apply the criteria to gauge the clinical relevance of the charts and values in the printout. The stepwise approach is described as follows:

- Zone 1 identifies the patient name, ID number, the date of birth, left eye, and this test was a 24-2 threshold test.
- Zone 2 shows that the visual field test had 1 fixation loss, 1% false positive error, no false negative error and the strategy used to test the visual field was SITA Standard, and the date of examination. The test duration was 7.45 minutes. The reliability parameters, the strategy used and the refractive correction and visual acuity are displayed. The operator entered parameters like the visual acuity and refractive correction. The operator needs to enter every time the test is performed and improves the quality of visual field test result yield.
- Zone 3 shows values of 0 along the horizontal meridian and the lower mirror images show much higher values. The grayscale chart displays the raw tested values graphically. This zone points to the topography of the depressed area being in the nasal quadrant where the arcuate defect is expected when there is an underlying pathology.
- Zone 4 shows total deviation chart corrected for the age matched normals. The total deviation chart shows numerical values which are depressed with p values significant to <0.5% displayed in the total deviation plot below symbolically. The total deviation also points to a general depression of the hill of vision. The pattern deviation chart and plot uncover the true depressed areas of sensitivities from the overall depression which may have been due to cataract (clinical correlation). The pattern deviation plot displays the points which are depressed with p values significant to 0.5% and are in the arcuate area being highly suggestive of pathology.
- Zone 5 shows GHT message which reads as "outside normal limits" which means that it is normal only in 0.5% of the population, indicating the significance of the depressed areas of sensitivity. The global indices MD and PSD also show p values that are significant to <0.5%. Applying the three criteria one can find:

1. There are three non-edge points depressed to <0.5%,
2. Pattern standard deviation is significant to p <0.5%, and
3. The GHT message is "outside normal limits".

In conclusion, the above interpretation when combined with clinical examination of the optic disk (ISNT rule) points to the diagnosis of the defect uncovered by the automated perimeter (HFA 720).

PROGRESSION ANALYSIS IN GLAUCOMA

Progression is present even in well controlled glaucoma patients. The average rate of progression in well controlled glaucoma is around 0.1 dB per year and in the worst case it is around 2 dB. The Octopus EyeSuite software is now used in conjunction with all models of Octopus perimeters. The software can be used to import, store, manage, display, and print. The software can be used in a PC network and all stations on the network may view the visual field test files. The graphic display of the results of the follow-up makes it easy to understand the changes and progression.

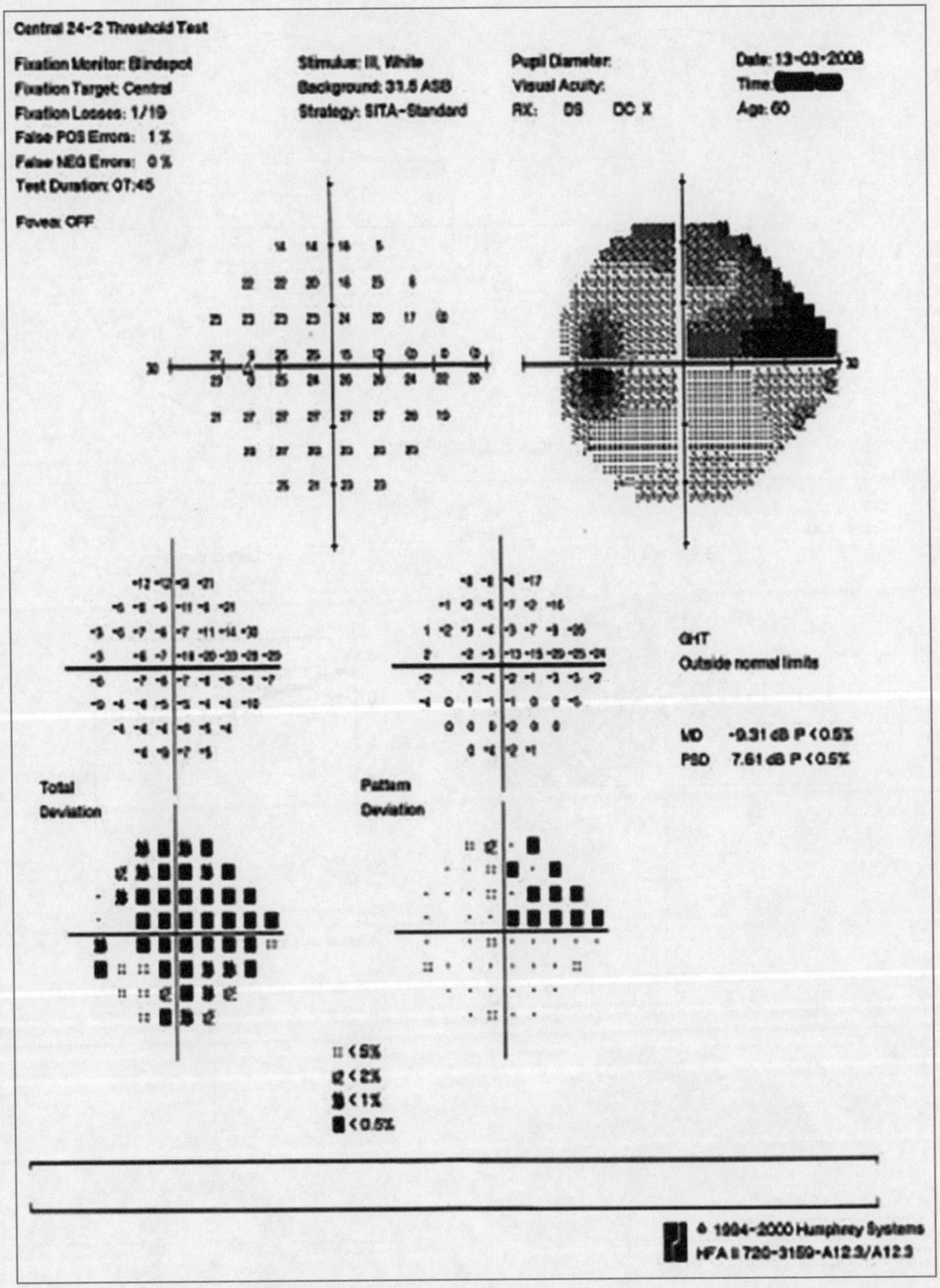

Fig. 45: Example of a Seven-in-One printout.

On screen "mouse over" display ensures that the level of significance of a particular value on display symbolically is highlighted. Follow-up requires same strategy and program each time the patient comes back this is marked and selected automatically in EyeSuite software. Hence, a TOP strategy will not be compared with Dynamic strategy or a P32 program be compared with G1. The EyeSuite software automatically groups the tests from the same patient together classified into right and left eye. The last six tests as a default are selected for display. The tests can further be manually selected or deselected using the Ctrl and select feature as in any windows-based operating system personal computer.

Visual function changes and progression are characteristic in glaucoma by definition. Major trials have also demonstrated progression as inevitable in well managed and untreated glaucoma. In the light of this knowledge, management and follow-up of glaucoma is based on tracking visual field progression which may be global or

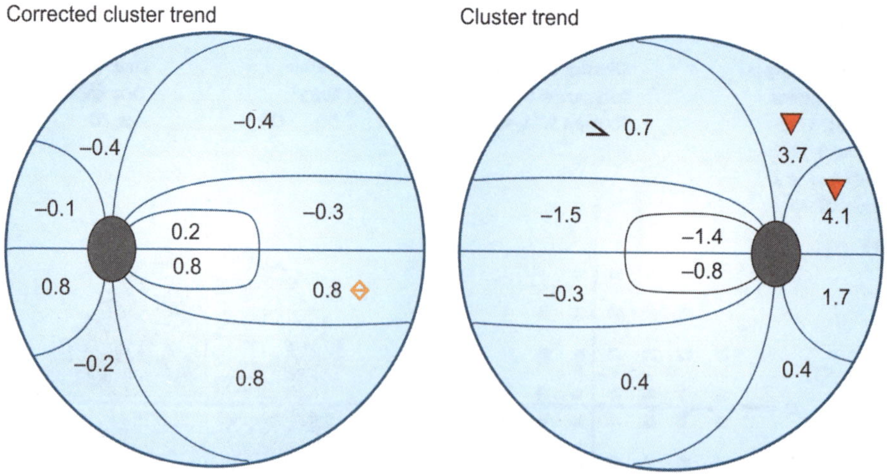

Fig. 46: Cluster trend.

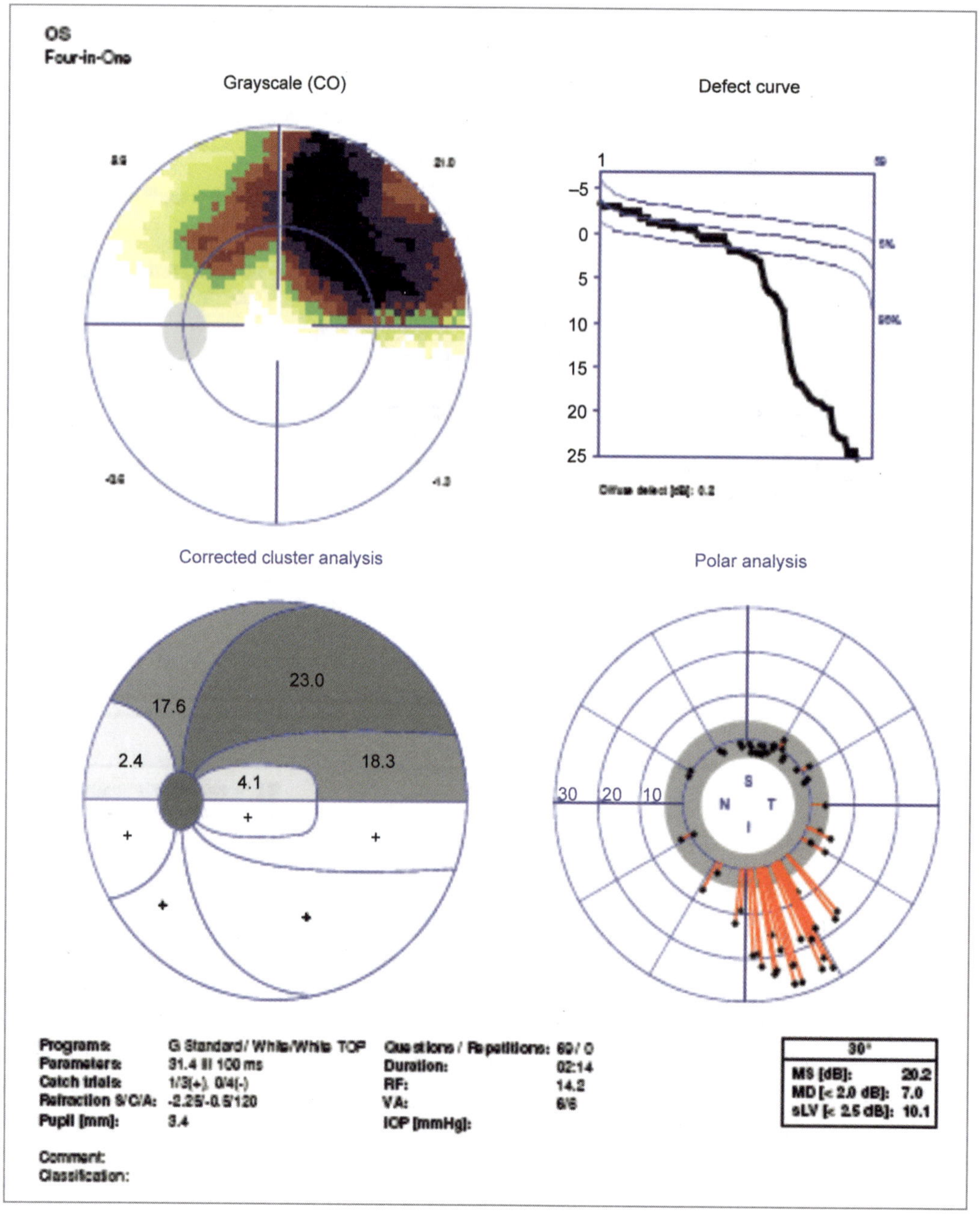

Fig. 47: Four-in-One printout in EyeSuite.

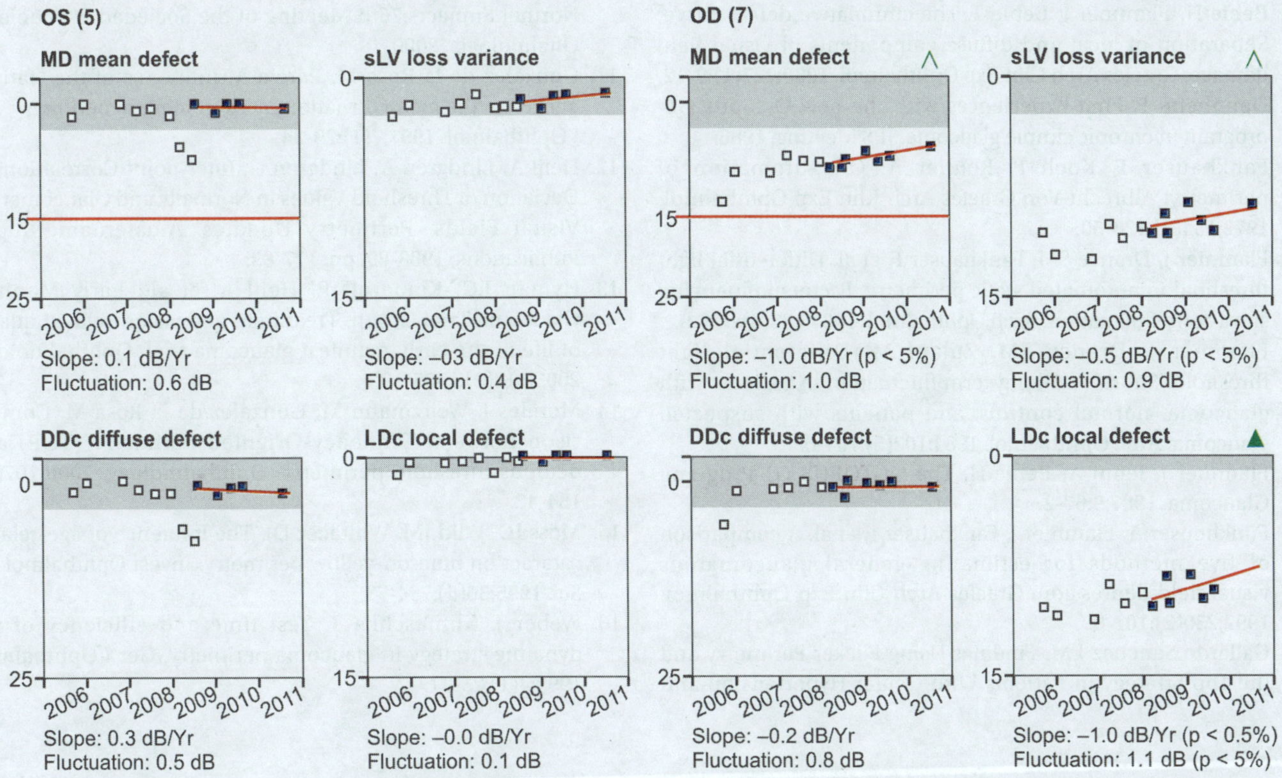

Fig. 48: Mean defects, loss variance, diffuse defects, and local defects.

focal in nature. The rate of progression of the glaucoma in turn influences the therapeutic decision to alter treatment to suite the changing needs and the quality of vision for the patient.

The Octopus EyeSuite uses both global indices along with sectors of visual field clusters to analyze and detect the rate of progression and change in visual fields over time. There is evidence that normal as well as pathological visual fields have test locations which are relative to one another and can fluctuate up to 8 dB. Analysis of cluster of points in a sector minimizes the test to retest variability rather than the point-to-point analysis as in other progression analysis software **(Fig. 46)**. The symbolic representation over the sectors makes interpretation easy and correlate with the damage on the optic disk at a glance. Below is an example of the combination of printout (Four-in-One) of gray/color scale corrected comparison, defect curve, cluster analysis, and polar analysis. The printout makes interpretation of change obvious and points to subtle changes in the structure and function correlation with the polar analysis which can be correlated with the optic disk directly in its orientation as well **(Fig. 47)**.

The trend analysis of global indices MD and sLV along with the new indices introduced in the EyeSuite like the local defects and diffuse defects takes into consideration **(Fig. 48)** the loss in sensitivity due to cataract in follow-up analysis. The gray band in the graphical plot indicates the area of normal values. The red line in the MD plot indicates the 15 dB mark to highlight worsening of quality of vision.

EyeSuite perimetry software displays global changes along with regional changes, when functional changes correlate with structural defects even subtle changes are correctly interpreted and detected. The trend-based analysis detects the rate of progression and the event-based analysis detects that change has indeed progressed. The EyeSuite perimetry software is able to display the global trends and cluster trends to detect the rate of progression globally and in sectorwise changes.

The EyeSuite software is a software program used for analysis of single fields as well as progression in glaucoma and storage of data. The software allows selection of various printouts required by the clinician for follow-up and therapeutic or surgical decisions for a given patient.

ACKNOWLEDGMENT

All diagrams, pictures, and visual fields are reprinted with the kind permission of HAAG-STREIT AG.

SUGGESTED READING

1. Anderson DR, Patella VM. Automated Perimetry, 2nd edition. St. Louis: Mosby and Co; 1999.
2. Bebie H, Fankhauser F, Spahr J. Static perimetry: strategies. Acta Ophthalmol (Copenh). 1976;54(3):325-38.

3. Bebie H, Flammer J, Bebie T. The cumulative defect curve: Separation of local and diffuse components of visual field damage. Graefes Arch Clin Exp Ophthalmol. 1989;227(1):9-12.
4. Dannheim F. First experiences with the new Octopus G1-program in chronic simple glaucoma. IPS Meeting. 1986.
5. Fankhauser F, Koch P, Roulier A. On automation of perimetry. Albrecht Von Graefes Arch Klin Exp Ophthalmol. 1972;184(2):126-50.
6. Flammer J, Drance SM, Fankhauser F, et al. Differential light threshold in automated static perimetry. Factors influencing short-term fluctuation. Arch Ophthalmol. 1984;102(6):876-9.
7. Flammer J, Drance SM, Zulauf M. Differential light threshold. Short- and long-term fluctuation in patients with glaucoma, normal controls, and patients with suspected glaucoma. Arch Ophthalmol. 1984;102(5):704-6.
8. Flammer J, Jenni A, Bebie H. The OCTOPUS G1 Program. Glaucoma. 1987;9:67-2.
9. Funkhouser A, Flammer J, Fankhauser F, et al. A comparison of five methods for estimating general glaucomatous visual field depression. Graefes Arch Clin Exp Ophthalmol. 1992;230(2):101-6.
10. Gallardo Sánchez LM. Findings Using Flicker Perimetry and the Top Strategy in Patients With Ocular Hypertension and Normal Subjects.76th Meeting of the Sociedad Española de Oftalmología. 2000.
11. González de la Rosa M, Pareja A. Influence of the "fatigue effect" on the mean deviation measurement in perimetry. Eur J Ophthalmol. 1997;7(1):29-34.
12. Heijl A, Lindgren A, Lindgren G. Inter-point Correlations of Deviation of Threshold Values in Normally and Glaucomatous Visual Fields. Perimetry Updates. Amsterdam: Kugler Publications; 1988-89. pp. 177-83.
13. Hyman LG, Komaroff E, Heijl A, et al.; Early Manifest Glaucoma Trial Group. Treatment and vision-related quality of life in the early manifest glaucoma trial. Ophthalmology. 2005;112(9):1505-13.
14. Morales J, Weitzmann M, González de la Rosa M. Comparison between Tendency-Oriented Perimetry (TOP) and octopus threshold perimetry. Ophthalmology. 2000;107(1): 134-42.
15. Moss ID, Wild JM, Whitaker DJ. The influence of age-related cataract on blue-on-yellow perimetry. Invest Ophthalmol Vis Sci. 1995;36(5):764-73.
16. Weber J, Klimaschka T. Test time and efficiency of the dynamic strategy in glaucoma perimetry. Ger J Ophthalmol. 1995;4(1):25-31.

CHAPTER

10 Imaging in Glaucoma

Rajul Parikh, Shefali Parikh

INTRODUCTION

Glaucoma is a chronic, progressive neurodegenerative disease. It is defined as chronic progressive optic neuropathy with typical optic disk and retinal nerve fiber layer (RNFL) changes with corresponding visual field defect. Intraocular pressure (IOP) is considered only a major risk factor and not a diagnostic criterion.

At present, clinically visible RNFL defects are considered as the sensitive indicator for early diagnosis of glaucoma. Experimental studies have shown that localized RNFL defects can ophthalmoscopically be detected if more than 50% of the thickness of the RNFL is lost.[1] The gold standard for detection of the functional damage in glaucoma is automated perimetry. It has been reported that locations with a 5 dB decrease in sensitivity on white on white perimetry (WWP) already had a 20% loss of retinal ganglion cells; this was 40% at locations with a 10 dB decrease in sensitivity. As the optic nerve and RNFL damage is irreversible, the early diagnosis of glaucoma is important.[2]

Retinal ganglion cell loss is detected as:

- Thinning of the RNFL (RNFL defect)
- Changes in the shape of the optic nerve head (ONH) (neuroretinal rim loss).

Currently, optic disk photography is considered a gold standard to detect changes to the ONH. Photographs should be taken at baseline and at follow-ups. However, for routine clinical use optic disk photography has several limitations. With the advent of high-resolution new imaging technologies like Heidelberg retina tomogram (HRT), scanning laser polarimetry, and optical coherence tomography (OCT), it has become possible to objectively quantify RNFL thinning, which may appear before manifest field defects on WWP.[3,4] The objective quantification with photography is possible but it is tedious, time consuming and requires training.

Currently, following techniques are available for structural assessment of optic disk and RNFL:

- Optic disk photography,
- Retinal nerve fiber layer photography,
- Confocal scanning laser ophthalmoscopy (HRT—**Fig. 1A**),
- Scanning laser polarimetry (GDx VCC—**Fig. 1B**), and
- Optical coherence tomography (OCT—**Fig. 1C**).

In this chapter, we will discuss only basic of imaging for the diagnosis of glaucoma, and limit our discussion to newer imaging technologies, namely HRT, GDx VCC, and OCT.

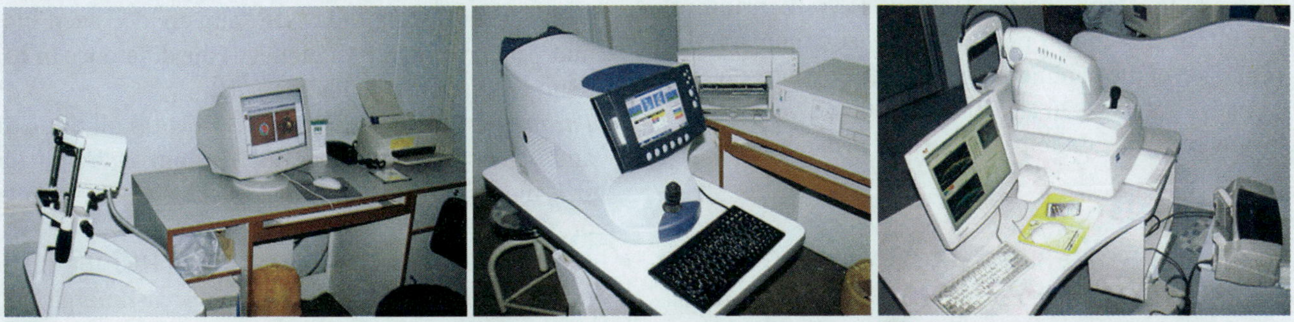

A Confocal scanning laser ophthalmoscope B Scanning laser polarimeter C Optical coherence tomogram

Figs. 1A to C: Different optic nerve head and RNFL imaging modalities. (RNFL: retinal nerve fiber layer)

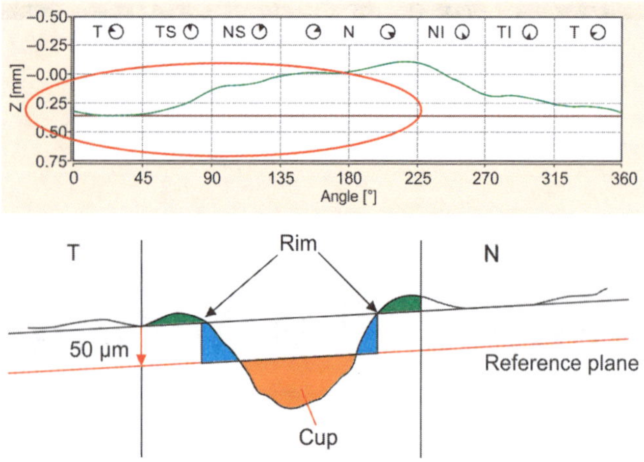

Fig. 2: Relationship between the ONH, the contour line, and the reference plane.
(ONH: optic nerve head)

HEIDELBERG RETINAL TOMOGRAM (HRT II/HRT III)

Heidelberg retinal tomogram is based on confocal scanning laser ophthalmoscopy principle. This technique allows the acquisition of 3-D images of the ONH. In brief, the fundus is scanned by a low-power laser beam (670 nm). The light that reflects back from the scanned points is detected by a photodetector. The images formed from this detection are digitized and stored on computer.

In HRT, sequential confocal scans are acquired in depth at the level of the ONH, and then merged by the in-built software into a 3-D image. Measurements are made from this image. The current models are HRT II and HRT III, which acquire a series of up to 64 optical sections in depth at intervals of 1/16 mm.

For analysis, a contour line should be manually placed by the operator to demarcate the limits of the ONH. The in-built software then places an inferior limit which is parallel, and in-depth, to the retinal surface. This limit is termed *Reference Plane* and is placed 50 microns below the contour line. Measurements are made based on this imaginary plane. **Figure 2** shows the relationship between the ONH, the contour line, and the reference plane. **Figure 3** shows HRT II printout and **Figure 4** shows HRT III printout. The printout provides topographic measurements and a classification of the parameters based on a comparison with a normative database. In HRT III, the optic disk parameters are compared with ethnic-based normative database.

Parameters Table

Parameter table shows the parameters measured from an acquired scan. A normal range is also provided. This normal range is calculated from a normative database, which is different from that used for Moorfields regression analysis. The HRT III has an ethnic specific database, which includes Indian data also. It also provides statistical value comparing patient result to normative database ($p < 0.05$ = borderline, $p < 0.001$ = outside normal limits).

- *Patient and examination data:* This data include given name, date of birth, ID number, gender, and scan date. Scan data are also provided—focus, depth, and operators' initials. We can also include IOP.
- *Quality score:* It is a "topography standard deviation" and indicates quality of an image. (A value <40 usually indicates good quality images).
- *Mean height contour graph:* It is available in HRT II printout. The green line in **Figure 2** (upper image) represents the retinal surface height profile along the contour line. The red line (**Fig. 2**, lower image) represents the reference plane. The dark black line parallel to the reference plane (**Fig. 2**, lower image) represents the mean peripapillary retinal surface height.
- *Horizontal height profile:* It is available in HRT II printout. Horizontal profile represents the height profile along the white horizontal lines across the ONH in the topography image. The parallel red line on the graph represents the reference plane and the two perpendicular black lines represent the borders of the disk as defined by the contour line previously drawn.
- *Vertical height profile:* It is available in HRT II printout. "Vertical profile" has the same characteristics as "horizontal profile" but the height profile represented is along the vertical lines across the ONH in the topography image.
- *Reflection image:* It is a "false" color picture representing changes in reflectivity for each region of the ONH. It is divided into six sectors, which are compared with a normative database using the Moorfields regression analysis software. This comparison takes into account the relationship between ONH size and rim area, and classifies each sector as "within normal limits" (green tick), "borderline" (yellow exclamation mark), or "outside normal limits" (red cross).
- *Topography image:* Topography image is a "false" color image representing the height of the scanned area (the brighter the color, the more depressed the region, and vice versa). On the ONH, "cup area" is seen in red and "rim area" in blue and green (the difference in color denotes difference in height levels).
- *Parameters:* In HRT II, printout provides all optic disk and RNFL parameters. In HRT III, along with optic disk size, the software also identifies disk as "small", "average", or "large".
- *RNFL profile graph:* This is available in HRT III printout. It displays the height values at the optic disk margin going around the optic disk from the temporal side, to superior, nasal, inferior, and back to temporal (TSNIT). The green shaded area is the normal range, yellow is borderline, and

Scan: Focus: 1.00 dpt Depth: 2.75 mm Operator: IOP: ---

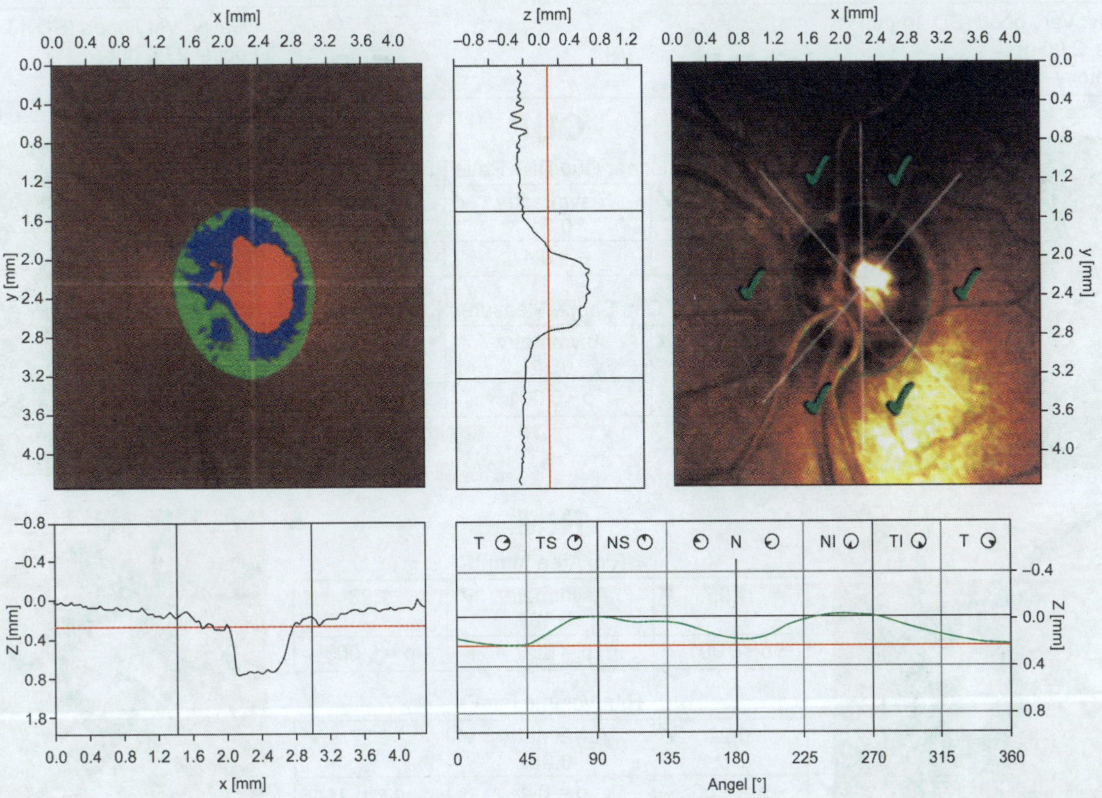

Stereometric Analysis ONH		Normal Range
Disk Area	2.133 mm^2	1.69 - 2.82
Cup Area	0.598 mm^2	0.26 - 1.27
Rim Area	1.535 mm^2	1.20 - 1.78
Cup Volume	0.158 cmm	-0.01 - 0.49
Rim Volume	0.234 cmm	0.24 - 0.49
Cup/Disk Area Ratio	0.280	0.16 - 0.47
Linear Cup/Disk Ratio	0.529	0.36 - 0.80
Mean Cup Depth	0.211 mm	0.14 - 0.38
Maximum Cup Depth	0.634 mm	0.46 - 0.90
Cup Shape Measure	-0.226	-0.27 - -0.09
Height Variation Contour	0.295 mm	0.30 - 0.47
Mean RNFL Thickness	0.155 mm	0.18 - 0.31
RNFL Cross Sectional Area	0.801 mm^2	0.95 - 1.61
Reference Height	0.263 mm	
Topography Std Dev.	12 μm	

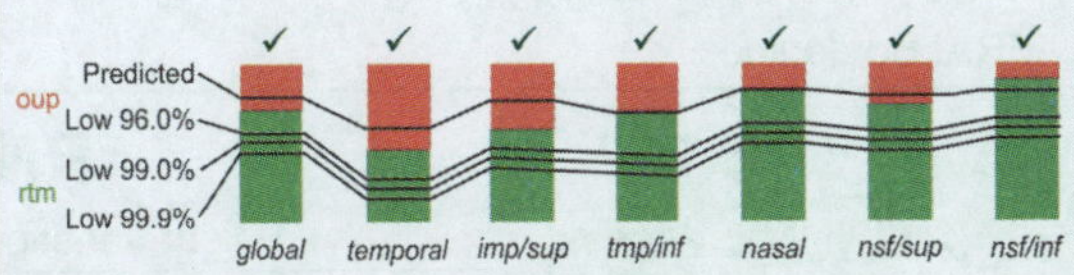

Moorfields Classification Within normal limits (*)

(*) Moorfields regression classification (Ophthalmology 1998; 105; 1557–1563 Classification based on statistics. Diagnosis is physician's responsibility.

Comments:

Date: **Signature:**

Fig. 3: Heidelberg retinal tomography II printout.
(IOP: intraocular pressure; ONH: optic nerve head; RNFL: retinal nerve fiber layer)

the red zone indicates outside normal limits compared to the selected ethnic-specific normative database.

- *Inter-eye asymmetry:* It evaluates the symmetry of the RNFL profile between eyes. If the correlation between eyes is good, the value will be near 0%.

Important Diagnostic Criteria for Heidelberg Retina Tomograph

- *Moorfields regression analysis*[5] ***(Fig. 5)***: The column height represents the ONH (or sector) area. It is divided into the percentage of rim area (green) and percentage of cup area (red). This is compared with age-matched data.

If the percentage of the rim is larger than or equal to the 95% limit, the respective sector is classified as "within normal limits". This would be marked as a green tick.

If the percentage of the rim is between the 95% and the 99.9% limits, the respective sector is classified as "borderline". This would be marked as a yellow exclamation mark.

If the percentage of the rim is lower than the 99.9% limit, the respective sector is classified as "outside normal limits". This would be marked as a red cross.

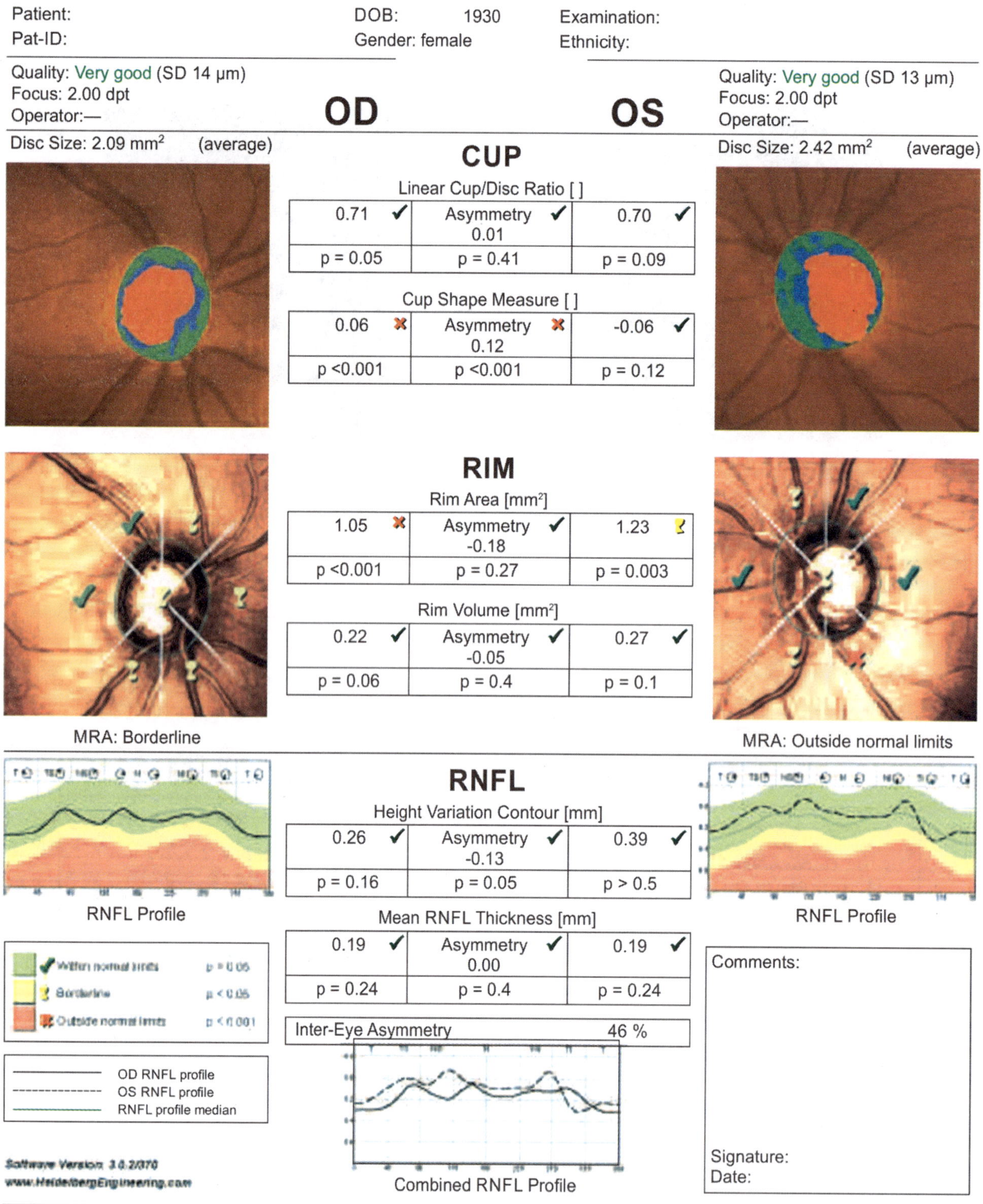

Fig. 4: Heidelberg retinal tomography III printout.

In the HRT printout, there is a classification for the whole disk (1st column) and a classification for each single sector (2nd–7th column).

- *FSM discriminant function:*[6] It was developed by Swindale and coworkers.[7] The discriminant function is a linear combination of the three parameters—cup shape measure, rim volume, and contour line height variation **(Fig. 6)**. An eye is classified as being normal if the discriminant function value F is positive; it is classified as glaucomatous if F is negative. Mikelberg et al. reported a sensitivity of 87% and a specificity of 84%.[6]
- *RB discriminant function:* This discriminant function has high specificity but poor sensitivity for the diagnosis of early glaucoma.

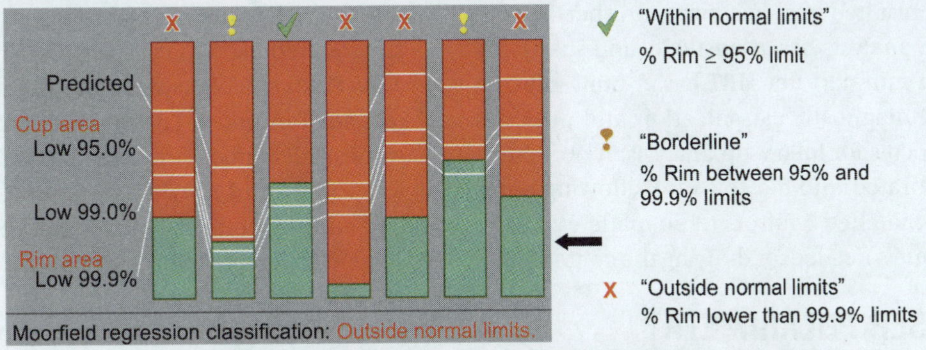

Fig. 5: Classification and confidence limit for Moorfield regression analysis.

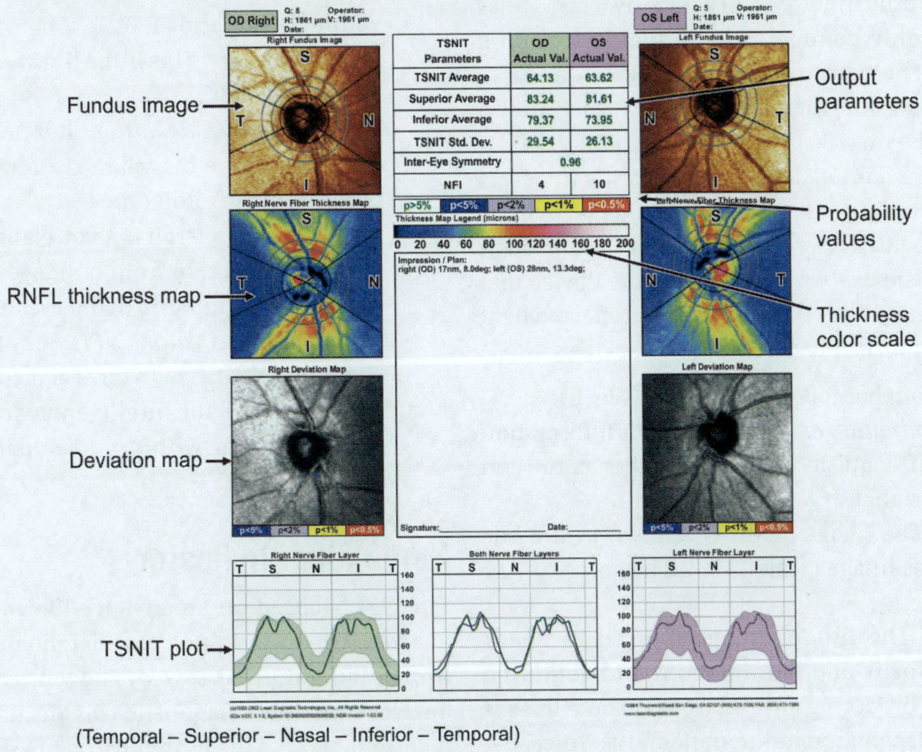

Fig. 6: GDx VCC printout.

- *Ranked sector distribution curves:* Here, the ONH is divided into 36 sectors, each 10° wide, to compute the stereometric parameter values in each segment, and to sort these 36 values in descending order. The result is a graphical representation of the ONH configuration similar to the Bebie curves used in the Octopus perimetry. From a normal population data, normal ranked sector distribution (RSD) curves; the 5th and 95th percentile curves have been calculated. To test a specific eye, its RSD curve is simply plotted together with the normal RSD curves. This is not widely used for diagnosis.
- *Glaucoma probability score:*[8] Glaucoma probability score (GPS) utilizes large, ethnic-selectable databases and artificial intelligence (relevance vector machine), which derives the probability of damage consistent with glaucoma. The GPS provides immediate results without drawing contour lines or relying on reference planes. It has similar sensitivity and specificity to the Moorfields regression analysis. This 3-D model combines the optic disk topographic information with the peripapillary RNFL information. The model uses five parameters—three characterize the shape of the optic disk (capturing information from the cup size, depth and slope of the rim); two characterize the RNFL (capturing information from the RNFL curvature both horizontally and vertically across the image). A normal result is displayed using a green tick, a borderline result using a yellow exclamation point, and an abnormal result using a red X.

Diagnostic Accuracy

Heidelberg retinal tomography measurements have been shown to have high diagnostic accuracy for detecting glaucoma.[5,7,8] The Moorfields regression analysis had a sensitivity and specificity of 84% and 96%, respectively.[5] An analysis based on the shape of the optic disk and surrounding RNFL resulted in a sensitivity and specificity of 89% and 89%.[7] GPS analysis has a sensitivity and specificity of 91% and 90%.[8] In summary, the HRT has in-built software that allows overall diagnostic classification and provides measurement protocols for follow-up analysis. A normative database is incorporated into the software, allowing comparisons with age-matched controls to be made. With the HRT, observer's input is needed for drawing the contour line.

SCANNING LASER POLARIMETRY

The scanning laser polarimetry (GDx VCC) is done with a scanning laser polarimeter marketed by Carl Zeiss Meditec. It is the only commercially available scanning laser polarimeter. The device is a confocal scanning laser ophthalmoscope with integrated polarimeter, which uses a near-infrared laser beam (780 nm) to scan the retina.

The principle of scanning laser polarimetry is to assess RNFL thickness according to light retardation. This involves scanning the retina with a laser beam, which passes through it and reflects from the deeper layers toward the device that releases the laser beam. The retardation of the reflected light is then measured for an estimation of RNFL thickness.

The GDx VCC printout has following features **(Fig. 6)**:

- *Patient and examination data:* This contains information about the patient, acquisition site, ID number, name and surname, gender, ancestry, and date of birth.
- *Image quality:* The image quality is shown in the box above the fundus image (scale 1–10). The score of 7 or more is desirable.
- *Fundus image:* The fundus image is used to check image quality, focus and illumination, and centering of the "ellipse" (black ring around ONH). The ellipse is automatically placed around the optic nerve. In case it is misplaced, its size and position can be easily modified to allow a correct placement. A correctly centered ellipse allows the "calculation circle" (area between the gray rings) to be placed at the peripapillary area.
- *Thickness map:* The thickness map is a color coded representation of RNFL thickness. Thick RNFLs are colored in yellow, orange and red (the warmer the color, the thicker the RNFL), while thin RNFL values are colored dark and light blue (the deeper the blue, the thinner the RNFL). Generalized RNFL loss results in a more uniform blue appearance, and a focal ("wedge") defect appears as a dark blue band originating at the ONH, extending through the bundle.
- *Deviation map:* The deviation map reveals the location and severity of RNFL defects over the entire thickness map. It analyzes a 20 × 20 degree region centered on the optic disk using a gray scale and fundus image of the eye as a background. The map is averaged into a grid of 32 × 32 squares, where each square (super pixel) is compared with the age-matched normative database. Super pixels that fall below the normal range are flagged by colored squares, representing varying probabilities of normality.
- *TSNIT curve:* TSNIT stands for Temporal-Superior-Nasal-Inferior-Temporal. The graph displays RNFL thickness values calculated within the calculation circle, starting temporally and moving superiorly, nasally, inferiorly, and ending temporally for both eyes (darker line). The shaded area represents the normal range for that age.
- *Parameters table* **(Fig. 7)**:
  - *TSNIT average:* It is the average of the RNFL thickness within the calculation circle.
  - *Superior average:* This is the thickness measured within the superior 120°.
  - *Inferior average:* This is the thickness measured within the inferior 120°.
  - *TSNIT standard deviation:* It represents the standard deviation of the overall measurement; the bigger the number, the healthier the eye.
  - *Inter-eye symmetry:* It is a correlation coefficient of the total measurement from both eyes. A value close to 1 means high symmetry of the eyes.
  - *Nerve fiber indicator (NFI):* It is an indicator of the likelihood of an eye to have glaucoma. It is calculated with an artificial intelligence software using data obtained from within and outside the calculation circle.

Nerve Fiber Indicator

The NFI is based on an advanced form of neural network analysis, which is trained to differentiate optimally normal from glaucomatous eyes. The entire RNFL profile is analyzed, and the diagnostic classification of the output is determined using the normative database (data from normal eyes). The 95th percentile is used as the cutoff for classifying the RNFL as "normal" (between 0 and 30) or "borderline" (between 31 and 50). The 99th percentile is used as the cutoff for classifying the RNFL as glaucomatous (between 51 and 100).[9]

Diagnostic Accuracy

The reported sensitivity and specificity of GDx in the early diagnosis of glaucoma ranges from 72% to 78% and 56% to 92%, respectively.[10-14] In literature, most of researchers have not found any single parameter with high diagnostic accuracy. The use of combination of more than one parameter can be used to improve the diagnostic accuracy of GDx VCC. For example, NFI >50 has maximum specificity positive, likelihood ratio at both the 5% and 30% prevalence level. If positive, it can be used to virtually "rule in" the disease. NFI >20 has maximum sensitivity, negative likelihood ratio at both 5% and 30% prevalence. If negative, it can be used to "rule out" the disease.

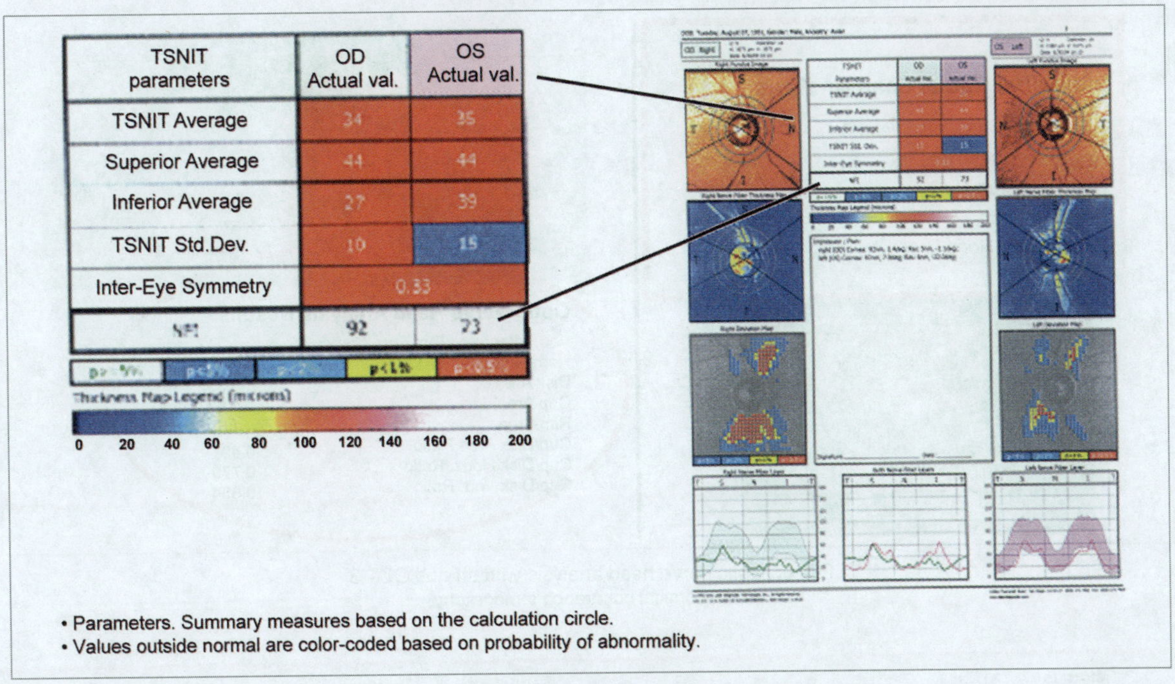

Fig. 7: Global parameters.

Future Potential

The enhanced corneal compensation (ECC) is a software solution to reduce the atypical pattern that can be found in some scans. The ECC will allow the reduction of noise in scans. In summary, the GDx VCC is a new technology, which has in-built software which allows overall diagnostic classification. A normative database is incorporated into the software, allowing comparisons with age-matched controls to be made.

OPTICAL COHERENCE TOMOGRAPHY

Optical coherence tomography can be used to scan the ONH, peripapillary retina, and macular region. An 820-nanometer near-infrared light beam is used, and the reported depth resolution is less than or equal to 10 microns. It is a noncontact, noninvasive imaging technique that provides high-resolution cross-sectional images of the retina. The principle is similar to ultrasound but here light is used to scan the retina. The intensity of light signal reflecting from retinal structures is used to create a tomographic image. The combined use of low-coherence light and an interferometer provides high depth resolution, which yields near-histological differentiation of the structures studied. This is based on Michelson interferometer principle.

Optical coherence tomography has ONH analysis, RNFL analysis, and macular parameter analysis.

Printout—Optic Nerve Head

The useful parameters for an OCT printout of the ONH **(Fig. 8)** are:

- The raw and composite ONH scans. The composite scan is obtained from 6 to 24 scans.
- The individual and global stereometric parameters.

Printout—Retinal Nerve Fiber Layer

The useful parameters for an OCT printout of the RNFL **(Fig. 9)** are:

- Total, quadrant and clock-hour sectors of RNFL thickness. Clock-hour sectors consist of 12 equal 30° sectors.
- An in-built normative database allows the comparison between acquired measurements and data and normal, age-matched data. Comparison is made if one of the sector-type is selected.
- The differences between the two eyes (inter-eye differences), as both eyes are measured.

As RNFL analysis is widely reported and used, it is discussed briefly.

Printout—Retinal Nerve Fiber Layer

- *Patient and examination data:* It includes name, date of birth, gender, and ID number. It also includes scan protocol used, date of the scan, and analysis protocol selected.
- *Fundus photography:* It is obtained immediately after scanning, and is used to evaluate the correct position of the circular scan around the ONH.
- *Signal strength:* The signal strength is shown in the box on the right (scale 1–10). The signal strength of 7 or more is desirable.
- *Retinal nerve fiber layer thickness analysis of both eyes:* It is a graphic representation of the RNFL thickness

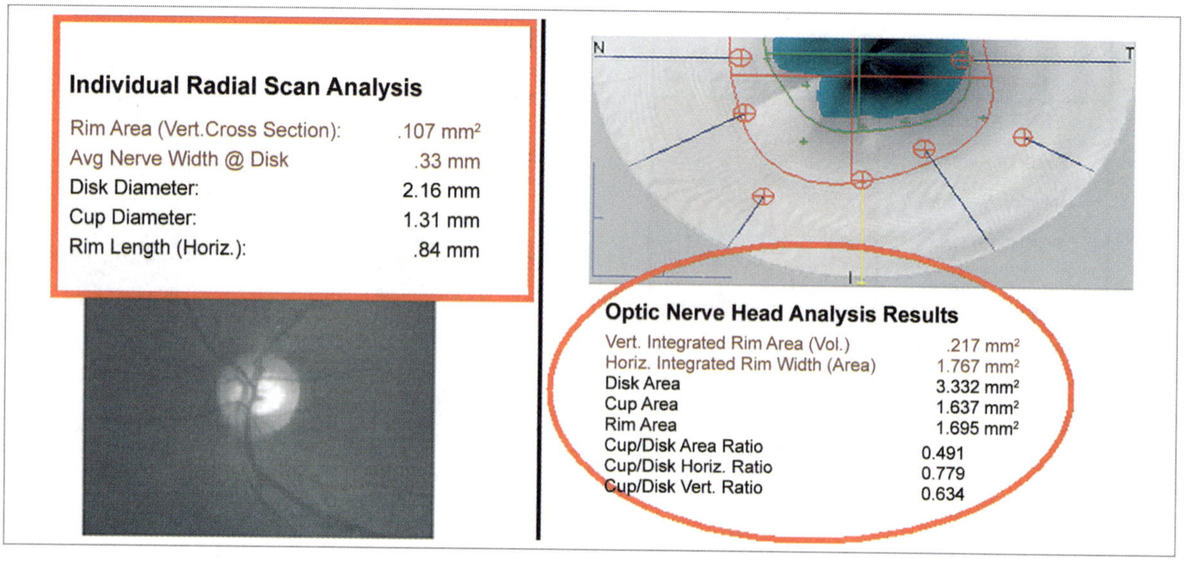

Fig. 8: Optic nerve head analysis with stratus OCT 3.
(OCT: optical coherence tomography)

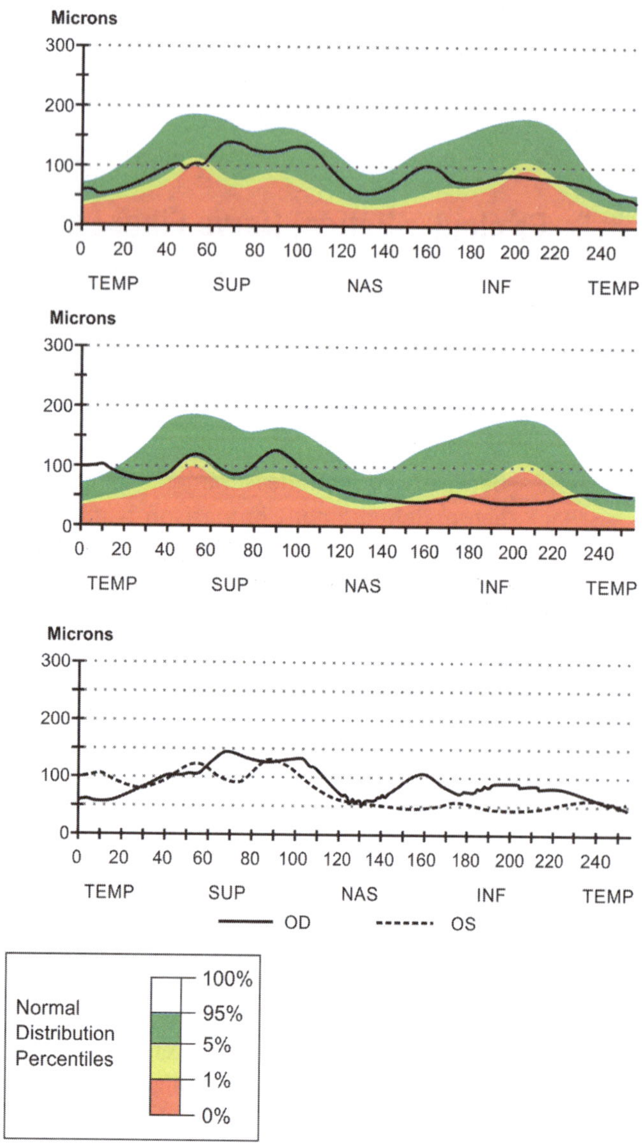

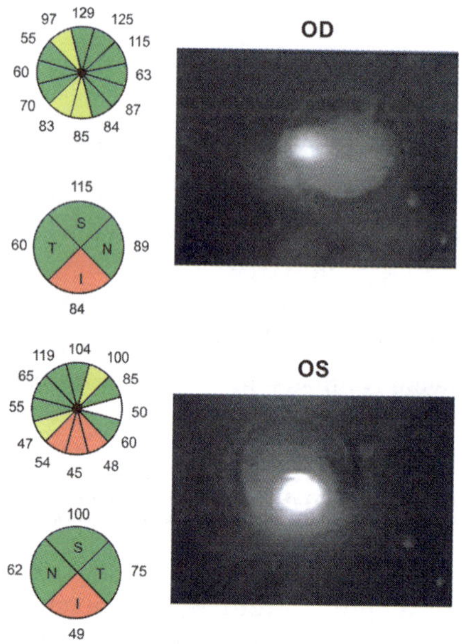

	OD (N = 3)	OS (N = 3)	OD–OS
Imax/Smax	0.73	0.44	0.29
Smax/Imax	1.37	2.28	-0.91
Smax/Tavg	2.23	1.75	0.48
Imax/Tavg	1.62	0.77	0.86
Smax/Navg	1.59	2.11	-0.52
Max-Min	91.00	90.00	1.00
Smax	140.00	131.00	9.00
Imax	102.00	58.00	44.00
Savg	118.00	107.00	11.00
Iavg	84.00	49.00	35.00
Avg.Thick	88.46	73.14	15.32

Fig. 9: Optical coherence tomography printout (RNFL analysis).

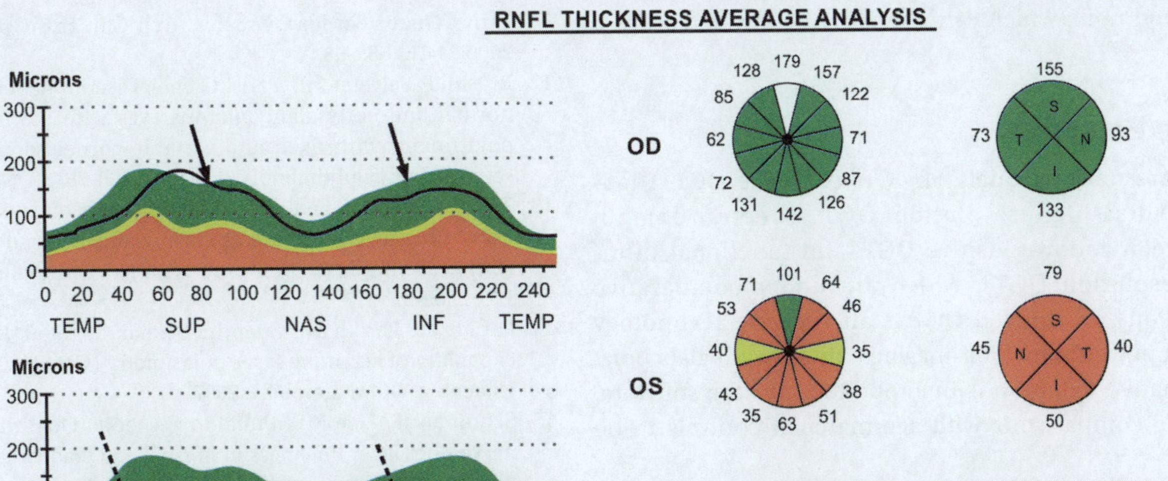

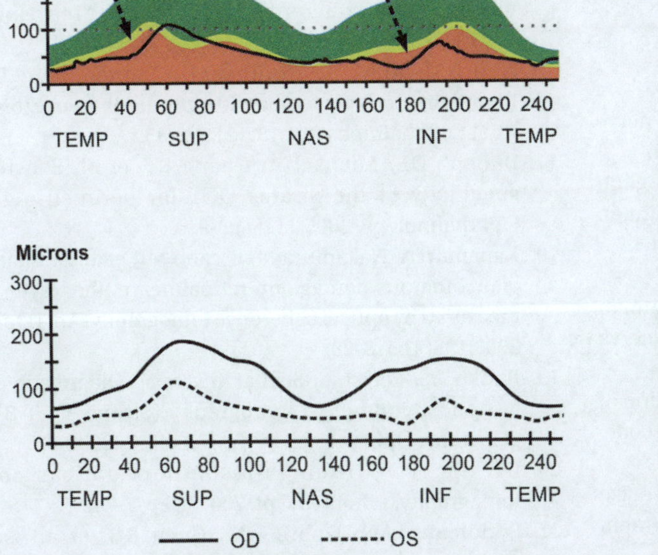

Patient/Scan Information	
PD - OD Normal OS Early Glaucoma DOB: 06/23/1979, ID: NA, Male	
Scan Type	Fast RNFL Thickness (3.4)
ScanDate	01/29/2002
ScanLength	10.87

	OD (N = 3)	OS (N = 3)	OD–OS
Imax/Smax	0.80	0.67	0.13
Smax/Imax	1.25	1.50	–0.24
Smax/Tavg	2.49	2.78	–0.29
Imax/Tavg	1.99	1.86	0.13
Smax/Navg	1.96	2.43	–0.47
Max–Min	126.00	82.00	44.00
Smax	183.00	110.00	73.00
Imax	146.00	74.00	72.00
Savg	155.00	79.00	76.00
Iavg	133.00	50.00	83.00
Avg.Thickness	113.60	53.57	60.03

In RNFL graph, the black line represents patient's RNFL thickness with normative database.
The right eye RNFL is within normal limit (black arrow). The left eye RNFL is abnormal (dotted arrow)

Fig. 10: Retinal nerve fiber layer analysis.
(RNFL: retinal nerve fiber layer)

around the ONH. On the X-axis, the sector of the RNFL is represented according to the TSNIT sequence—the circular scan is linearly represented, starting from the temporal region, continuing toward the superior, nasal, inferior regions, and terminating in the temporal region. On the Y-axis, thickness is expressed in microns **(Fig. 10)**. The patient's RNFL graph is compared with age-matched normative database.

- Retinal nerve fiber layer thickness measurements made around the ONH for each eye are presented as two circles—the top one is divided into 12 clock-hour sectors and the bottom one into four equal 90° sectors. Each sector is represented with a number and color code. The number represents the thickness expressed in microns, and the color code indicates the possibility of that value being found in the normal population:
  - Green and white values found in up to 95% of the normal population.
  - Yellow values found in less than 5% of the normal population.
  - Red values found in less than 1% of the normal population.
- *Parameters table:* The parameters table presents data from both eyes plus inter-eye differences. Color indicates the probability of finding similar values in a normal population. The color coding and its statistical significance are same as discussed above in RNFL profile.

Diagnostic Accuracy

Several studies have evaluated the diagnostic significance of OCT parameters. RNFL thickness in the inferior region often had the best ability to discriminate healthy eyes from those with glaucoma, with sensitivities ranging between 67% and 84% for specificities of more than 90%. We have observed 6-clock, RNFL thickness parameter with very high positive likelihood ratio, which can virtually rule in the disease if positive.[10,15-19]

Future Potentials

There are newer models of OCTs (En-Face OCT, High-speed ultra-high resolution OCT, Spectral-domain OCT, Polarization-sensitive OCT, and functional ultra-high resolution OCT), which are under comparative evaluations.[20-25] Indeed OCT is an evolving technology and is a powerful tool for imaging patients with glaucoma. A normative database is incorporated into the software, allowing comparisons with age-matched controls to be made.

REFERENCES

1. Quigley HA, Addicks EM. Quantitative studies of retinal nerve fiber layer defects. Arch Ophthalmol. 1982;100(5):807-14.
2. Quigley HA, Dunkelberger GR, Green WR. Retinal ganglion cell atrophy correlated with automated perimetry in human eyes with glaucoma. Am J Ophthalmol. 1989;107(5):453-64.
3. OCT Manual. Dublin, CA: Carl Zeiss Meditac; 2004.
4. Quigley HA, Dunkelberger GR, Green WR. Chronic human glaucoma causing selectively greater loss of larger optic nerve fibers. Ophthalmology. 1988;95(3):357-63.
5. Wollstein G, Garway-Heath DF, Hitchings RA. Identification of early glaucoma cases with the scanning laser ophthalmoscope. Ophthalmology. 1998;105(8):1557-63.
6. Iester M, Mikelberg FS, Drance SM. The effect of optic disc size on diagnostic precision with the Heidelberg retina tomograph. Ophthalmology. 1997;104(3):545-8.
7. Swindale NV, Stjepanovic G, Chin A, et al. Automated analysis of normal and glaucomatous optic nerve head topography images. Invest Ophthalmol Vis Sci. 2000;41(7):1730-42.
8. Bowd C, Chan K, Zangwill LM, et al. Comparing neural networks and linear discriminant functions for glaucoma detection using confocal scanning laser ophthalmoscopy of the optic disc. Invest Ophthalmol Vis Sci. 2002;43(11):3444-54.
9. Reus NJ, Lemij HG. Diagnostic accuracy of the GDx VCC for glaucoma. Ophthalmology. 2004;111(10):1860-5.
10. Bowd C, Zangwill LM, Berry CC, et al. Detecting early glaucoma by assessment of retinal nerve fiber layer thickness and visual function. Invest Ophthalmol Vis Sci. 2001;42(9):1993-2003.
11. Da Pozzo S, Fuser M, Vattovani O, et al. GDx-VCC performance in discriminating normal from glaucomatous eyes with early visual field loss. Graefes Arch Clin Exp Ophthalmol. 2006;244(6):689-95.
12. Brusini P, Salvetat ML, Parisi L, et al. Discrimination between normal and early glaucomatous eyes with scanning laser polarimeter with fixed and variable corneal compensator settings. Eur J Ophthalmol. 2005;15(4):468-76.
13. Tjon-Fo-Sang MJ, Lemij HG. The sensitivity and specificity of nerve fiber layer measurements in glaucoma as determined with scanning laser polarimetry. Am J Ophthalmol. 1997;123(1):62-9.
14. Parikh RS, Parikh SR, Chandra Sekhar GS, et al. Diagnostic capability of scanning laser polarimetry (GDx VCC) in early glaucoma. Ophthalmology. 2007.
15. Schuman JS, Hee MR, Puliafito CA, et al. Quantification of nerve fiber layer thickness in normal and glaucomatous eyes using optical coherence tomography. Arch Ophthalmol. 1995;113(5):586-96.
16. Nouri-Mahdavi K, Hoffman D, Tannenbaum DP, et al. Identifying early glaucoma with optical coherence tomography. Am J Ophthalmol. 2004;137(2):228-35.
17. Budenz DL, Michael A, Chang RT, et al. Sensitivity and specificity of the Stratus OCT for perimetric glaucoma. Ophthalmology. 2005;112(1):3-9.
18. Kanamori A, Nakamura M, Escano MF, et al. Evaluation of the glaucomatous damage on retinal nerve fiber layer thickness measured by optical coherence tomography. Am J Ophthalmol. 2003;135(4):513-20.
19. Parikh RS, Parikh S, Sekhar GS, et al. Diagnostic capability of optical coherence tomography (Stratus OCT 3) in early glaucoma. Ophthalmology. 2007;114(12):2238-43.
20. Drexler W. Ultrahigh-resolution optical coherence tomography. J Biomed Opt. 2004;9(1):47-74.
21. Podoleanu AG, Dobre GM, Cucu RG, et al. Combined multiplanar optical coherence tomography and confocal scanning ophthalmoscopy. J Biomed Opt. 2004;9(1):86-93.
22. Nassif N, Cense B, Park BH, et al. In vivo human retinal imaging by ultrahigh-speed spectral domain optical coherence tomography. Opt Lett. 2004;29(5):480-2.
23. de Boer JF, Cense B, Park BH, et al. Improved signal-to-noise ratio in spectral-domain compared with time-domain optical coherence tomography. Opt Lett. 2003;28(21):2067-9.
24. Cense B, Chen TC, Park BH, et al. Thickness and birefringence of healthy retinal nerve fiber layer tissue measured with polarization-sensitive optical coherence tomography. Invest Ophthalmol Vis Sci. 2004;45(8):2606-12.
25. Bizheva K, Pflug R, Hermann B, et al. Optophysiology: Depth-resolved probing of retinal physiology with functional ultrahigh-resolution optical coherence tomography. Proc Natl Acad Sci USA. 2006;103(13):5066-71.

CHAPTER

11

Ophthalmoscopy

Pukhraj Rishi, Tarun Sharma

INTRODUCTION

A comprehensive eye examination is a must for a complete assessment of the anterior and posterior segments of the eye—be it a diagnostic or preoperative evaluation. Although there are several methods of eye examination viz. slit-lamp biomicroscopy, gonioscopy, perimetry, tonometry, ultrasonography, ophthalmoscopy remains an important tool for a complete evaluation of the posterior segment of the eye. In December 1850, Helmholtz announced the invention of an "eye-mirror", which was the original ophthalmoscope. It was mounted with a holder for one lens, and lenses had to be changed constantly for eyes of different refraction. Rekoss introduced a revolving disk carrying a series of lenses.

PRINCIPLES OF OPHTHALMOSCOPY

The basic principle of ophthalmoscopy is shown in **Figure 1**. If the patient's eye is emmetropic, light rays emanating from a point in the fundus emerge as a parallel beam. If this beam enters the pupil of an emmetropic observer, the rays are focused on the retina and an image is formed. This is called direct ophthalmoscopy.

The fundus can be seen only when the observed and the illuminated areas of the fundus overlap. In the emmetropic eye this can happen only if the light source and the observer's pupil are optically aligned. Under normal conditions this does not happen, hence the pupil normally appears dark **(Fig. 2)**.

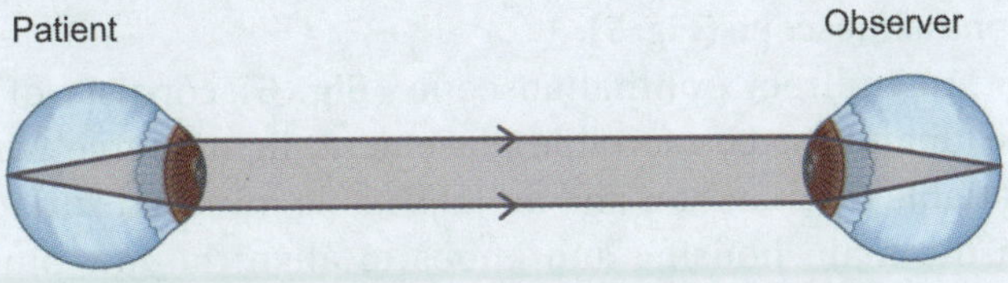

Fig. 1: Optics of image formation in an emmetropic eye.

The illuminating and the observing beams are aligned using a semireflecting mirror or a prism allowing fundal view **(Fig. 3)**.

INDIRECT OPHTHALMOSCOPY

Ruete introduced indirect ophthalmoscopy in 1852. Several types of indirect ophthalmolscopes are available. One must understand the optical principles of indirect ophthalmoscopy to carry out an ocular examination (including fundus angioscopy) **(Fig. 4)**. The indirect ophthalmoscope can be used in the treatment of disorders of the posterior segment.

There are five indirect ophthalmoscopy techniques. These are slit-lamp indirect, head mounted indirect, monocular indirect, modified monocular indirect, and penlight ophthalmoscopy. Indirect ophthalmoscopy is carried out in a dark room with fully dilated pupils.

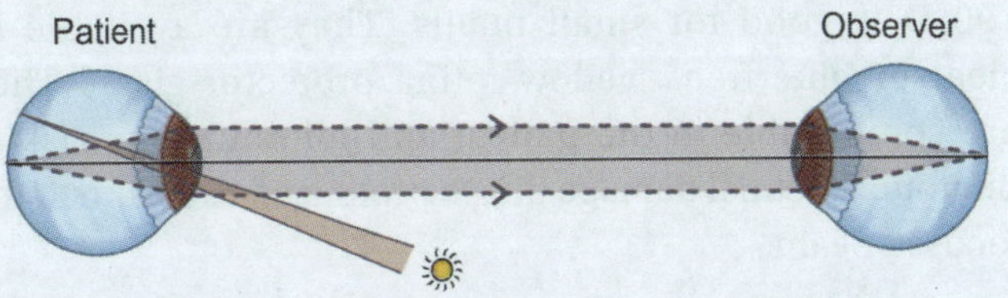

Fig. 2: The light source and the observer's pupil are not optically aligned.

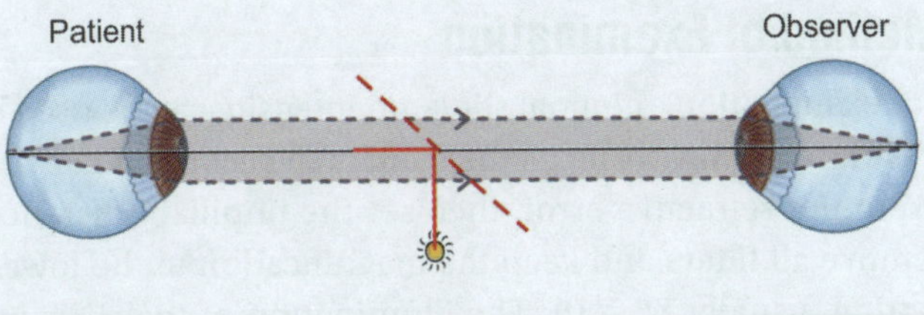

Fig. 3: The light source and the observer's pupil are optically aligned.

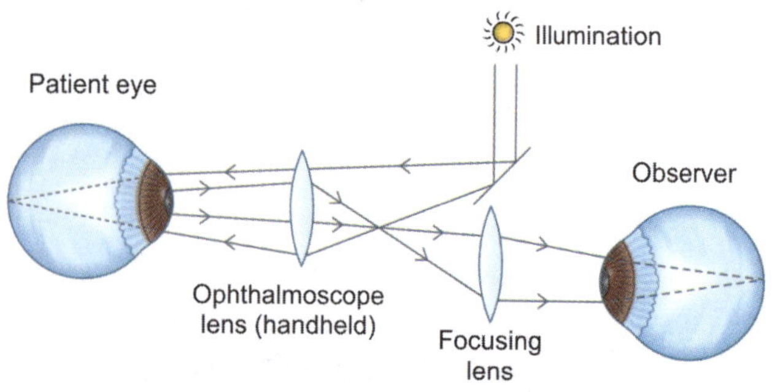

Fig. 4: Optics of indirect ophthalmoscope.

Table 1: Field of view and image magnification obtained by different contact lenses.

Lens	*Field of view*	*Image magnification*	*Laser spot*	*Working distance*
SuperQuad 160®	160°/165°	.5x	2.0x	Contact
Staurenghi Lens	150°	0.23x	4.34x	Contact
Equator Plus®	114°/137°	.44x	2.27x	Contact
Quad Pediatric	100°/120°	.55x	1.82x	Contact
QuadrAspheric®	120°/144°	.51x	1.97x	Contact
PDT Laser	115°/137°	.67x	1.5x	Contact
TransEquator®	110°/132°	.7x	1.44x	Contact
Area Centralis®	70°/84°	1.06x	.94x	Contact
Super Macula® 2.2	60°/78°	1.49x	.67x	Contact

The equipments required for slit-lamp indirect ophthalmoscopy includes slit lamp and condensing lens. The condensing lens may be either noncontact or contact lens.

Noncontact lenses: They are plus-powered with two convex aspheric surfaces. The +60 D version has the greatest magnification and is best used for the disk and macula. The +78 D version is a commonly used diagnostic lens and the +90 D is good for small pupils. They are available in clear or blue-free, "yellow retina protector glass". They are comfortable to the patient and minimize the risk of phototoxic retinal damage due to prolonged exposure to the focused beam.

Contact lenses: Goldmann, Mainster, SuperQuad, Equator Plus, Area centralis, and Super Macula lenses are often used. Field of view and image magnification obtained by these lenses are listed in **Table 1**.

Method of Examination

For examination, minimal slit-lamp intensity can be used in a darkroom. Always focus the oculars to accommodate any examiner refractive error, then set the pupillary distance, remove all filters and keep the magnification to the lowest setting, usually X6–X10. The illumination of the slit lamp should be adjusted for an intermediate slit height and a 2 mm width, and then placed in the straight ahead position between the oculars (zero degrees or coaxial). Before examination, ensure that the condensing lens surfaces are clean. Hold the lens vertically between the thumb and index finger of the left hand to examine the patient's right eye and vice versa.

Examination Procedure

Instruct the patient to fixate straight ahead, to stare wide and to blink normally. Center the beam in the patient's pupil and focus on the cornea. Now the lens is placed in front of the patient's eye, directly in front of the cornea so the back surface just clears the lashes. Examiner's fingers may be placed on either the brow bar or the patient's forehead. Using the joystick, focus on the fundus image by slowly moving away from the cornea, keeping the beam centerd in the pupil. Once the retinal image is focused, the magnification may be increased. Scan across the entire lens keeping it steady. In order to view the peripheral retina, ask the patient to change fixation into the nine cardinal positions of gaze. The lens is realigned and refocused the slit lamp as necessary. To reduce interfering reflections, tilt the lens or move the illumination arm up to 10° on either side, once the fundus has been focused. For fine-tuning the fundus view, lateral and longitudinal adjustments of the lens may be made to optimize the field of view. When viewing finer fundus details, intensity and magnification of slit lamp should be increased.

HEAD MOUNTED BINOCULAR INDIRECT OPHTHALMOSCOPY

Binocular indirect ophthalmoscopy (BIO) is a technique used to evaluate the entire ocular fundus. It provides for stereoscopic, wide-angled, and high-resolution views of the entire fundus and overlying vitreous. Its optical principles and illumination options allow for visualization of the fundus regardless of high ametropia or hazy ocular media.

Light beams directed into the patient's eye produce reflected observation beams from the retina. These beams are focused to a viewable, aerial image following placement of a high plus-powered condensing lens at its focal distance in front of the patient's eye. The resultant image is real, inverted, magnified, laterally reversed, and located between the examiner and the condensing lens. The observer views this image through the oculars of the headborne indirect ophthalmoscope **(Fig. 5)**.

An indirect ophthalmoscope **(Fig. 6)** consists of a headband for comfortable placement, light source with variable illumination and an adjustable mirrored surface in the main housing and knobs to align the low plus-powered eyepieces (+2.00 D to +2.50 D) with the examiner's

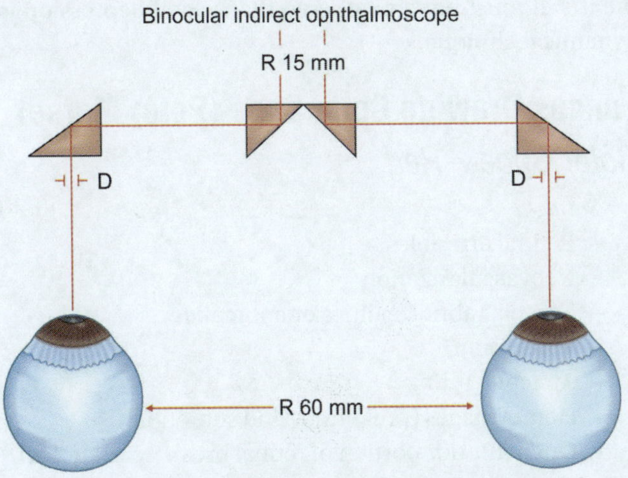

Fig. 5: Optics of binocular indirect ophthalmoscopy.

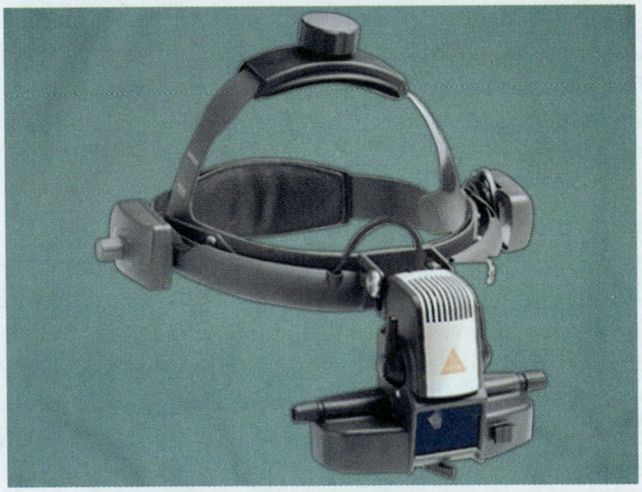

Fig. 6: Indirect ophthalmoscope.

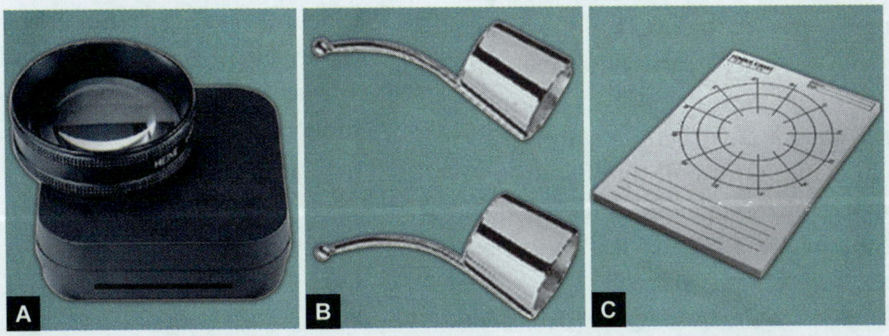

Figs. 7A to C: (A) 20 D condensing lens; (B) A pair of scleral depressors; (C) Fundus drawing sheet.

interpupillary distance. A 20 D condensing lens **(Fig. 7A)**, a pair of scleral depressors **(Fig. 7B)**, and fundus drawing sheet **(Fig. 7C)** are needed for proper indirect ophthalmoscopy and documentation.

Examination Procedure

Proper placement and adjustment of the BIO is an important step in the examination. Place the loose BIO onto the head and position the bottom of the front headband one index finger width above the eyebrows. Tighten the crown strap until this headband position begins to stabilize, then position the back head strap on or below the occipital notch and tighten until secured. Now the knobs that control the instruments main housing (oculars and light tower) should be loosened and fixate straight ahead and level in vertical position the oculars and aligned tangential to or slightly angled downward from the ocular surface; this should maximize observer's visual field and minimize horizontal diplopia. Horizontally align each ocular by closing one eye and fixating a centrally positioned thumb of an outstretched hand. Turn on the light source and fixate straight ahead on a wall at 40–50 cm looking at the projected light source. Use the mirror knob to vertically place the light source at the upper one-half to one-third of the field.

The headset is adjusted and the voltage set to midrange (occasionally the sneeze reflex may start from the periphery first). The choice of condensing lens depends upon the need for a panoramic view or detail; a 30 D provides panoramic view while fundus details can be obtained with 14 D. Stereopsis is important and depends on the choice of lens. A full stereopsis is obtained with 14 D, three-quarter with 20 D, and one-half stereopsis with 30 D. A 30 D lens can be used to get a view of fundus in patients with small pupil. The condensing lens should be held between the tip of the flexed index finger and the ball of the extended thumb of the nondominant hand and the scleral depressor with the dominant hand. The extended third finger acts as the pivot. The more convex surface should be toward the observer and the white-ringed edge closest to the patient so as to avoid bothersome light reflexes. These reflexes can be made to move in opposite direction from each other by slightly tilting the lens. Condensing lenses have their surfaces coated to reduce such flexes. The lens must be smudge-free.

The patient should have at least some idea of what to expect in the examination. Although the patient may be examined in either sitting or supine position, it is best to recline the patient on a couch with the face directed toward the ceiling to avoid stooping. The couch or table should be just high enough to reach the examiner's hips. The examiner stands opposite to the clock hour position to be examined. The patient is instructed to keep both the eyes open and fixate toward his outstretched hand which points to the meridian of interest.

From a working distance of 18–20 inches, direct the light beam into the pupil, producing a complete red pupillary reflex. Pull backward on the lens, maintaining the central position of the pupil reflex, until the entire lens fills with the fundus image. Fine adjustments are made in the lens tilt and vertex distance to produce a distortion-free full lens view. The patient must be repeatedly urged to open the fellow eye. Good cycloplegia is the most important single factor in getting cooperation in this regard. The eye with inadequate cycloplegia is very photophobic.

All the vital elements involved in the visualization of the fundus, namely observer's macula, the eyepiece of the scope, center of the condensing lens, patient's pupil and the object observed in the fundus must be kept on an axis to maintain the fundal view. In order to develop and achieve a continuous sweeping picture of the fundus, a major retinal blood vessel must be picked out from the posterior pole and followed as anteriorly as possible by the observer's movements alone. This vessel should be then followed back to the optic disk. This maneuver needs constant practice to master it.

The problem of orientation in the fundus may be solved by learning to accurately draw the image exactly as we see in the condensing lens. The drawing chart may be placed inverted over the patient's chest. Positioning 180° away from the area of interest, the observer must think in terms of anterior in the fundus or posterior in the fundus (or central and peripheral). Draw the image seen in the lens on that part of the fundus chart that is closest to the observer.

Since 30% of the retina lies anterior to the equator, failure to study this region will result in overlooking serious pathology in many cases. Scleral depression not only allows for an easy and complete view of the ora serrata and the pars plana but also allows a better evaluation of the retinal topography making lesions such as horseshoe tears or vitreoretinal traction more visible. It is of particular value in differentiating a retinal hemorrhage from a retinal break, in recognizing a raised from a depressed lesion and in detecting whether a foreign body lies on or anterior to the retina. The absence of an overhanging orbital margin superonasally makes initial attempts at scleral depression easier. The depressor is applied to the superior lid, without pressure, at the tarsal margin. The patient looks up and the depressor slides posteriorly parallel to the surface of the globe, as the lid retracts. The depressor is gently pressed against the globe at the equatorial region, and a grayish mound is seen to come up in view from the inferior part of the fundus. In viewing the ora, it is sometimes necessary to tilt the condensing lens somewhat forward, into a plane more nearly parallel to the iris. It must be remembered that scleral depression is a dynamic technique.

Fundus Drawing Color Code (Peter Morse)

Color Code—Red

- *Solid*:
  - Retinal arterioles
  - Neovascularization
  - Vascular abnormalities or anomalies
  - Vortex vein
  - Attached retina
  - Hemorrhages (pre-, intra- and subretinal)
  - Open interior portion of retinal break (tears, holes)
  - Normal foveola (drawn as red dot).
- *Cross lined*:
  - Open portion of giant tears or large dialysis
  - Inner portion of chorioretinal atrophy
  - Open portion of retinal holes in inner layer of retinoschisis
  - Inner portion of the areas of retina.

Color Code—Blue

- *Solid*:
  - Detached retina **(Fig. 8)**
  - Retinal veins
  - Outlines of retinal breaks (tears, holes)
  - Outline of ora serrata (dentate processes, ora bays)
  - Meridional, radial, fixed star-shaped and circumferential folds

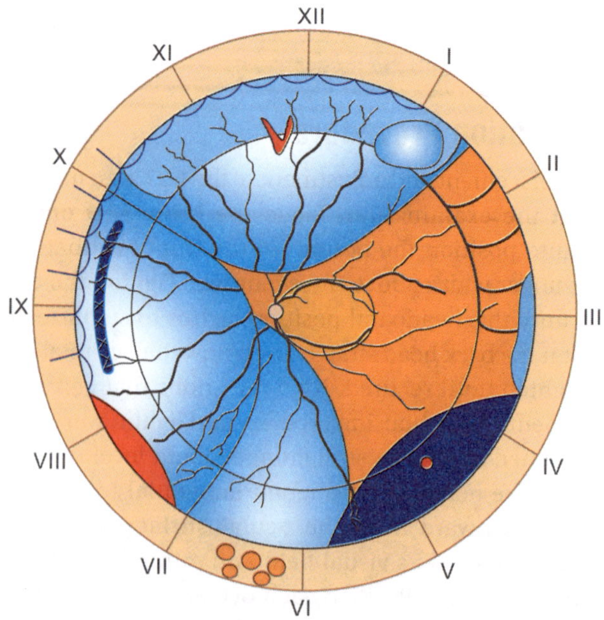

Fig. 8: A long-standing, partial, rhegmatogenous retinal detachment with demarcation lines and intraretinal macrocyst. A horseshoe tear, lattice degeneration, and a retinal dialysis are also seen. An improperly placed scleral buckle effect is made out. Pars plana is detached, nasally. Retinoschisis with inner layer hole is seen in inferotemporal periphery. Pars plana cysts are seen inferiorly.

- Vitreoretinal traction tufts
- Retinal granular tags and tufts (cystic, noncystic)
- Outline of flat neovascularization
- Outline of lattice degeneration (inner chevrons or Xs)
- Outline of thin areas of retina
- Intraretinal cysts (with overlying curvilinear stripes to show configuration).

• *Cross lines*:
  - Inner layer of retinoschisis
  - White with or without pressure
  - Detached pars plana epithelium anterior to separation of ora
  - Outer surface of retina seen in rolled edge of retinal tears, inverted flap of giant retinal tear.
• *Stippled or circles*: Cystoid degeneration.
• *Interrupted lines*: Outline of change in area or folds of detached retina because of shifting fluid.

Color Code—Green

• *Solid*:
  - Opacities in the media (cornea, anterior chamber, lens, and vitreous)
  - Vitreous hemorrhage
  - Vitreous membranes
  - Hyaloid ring
  - Intraocular foreign bodies
  - Retinal opercula
  - Cotton wool patches
  - Ora serrata pearls
  - Outline of elevated neovascularization.
• *Stippled or dotted*:
  - Asteroid hyalosis
  - Frosting or snowflakes on cystoid, retinoschisis, and lattice degeneration.

Color Code—Brown

• *Solid*:
  - Uveal tissues
  - Pars plana cysts
  - Ciliary processes (pars plicata)
  - Striae ciliaris
  - Pigment beneath detached retina
  - Subretinal fibrosis demarcation lines
  - Choroidal nevi
  - Malignant choroidal melanomas
  - Metastatic and other choroidal tumors
  - Choroidal detachment.
• *Outline*:
  - Chorioretinal atrophy beneath detached retina
  - Posterior staphyloma
  - Edge of buckle beneath detached retina.

Color Code—Yellow

• *Solid*:
  - Intraretinal edema
  - Intraretinal or subretinal hard yellow exudates
  - Deposits in retinal pigment epithelium
  - Detached maculae in some retinal separations
  - Retinal edema as a result of photocoagulation, cryotherapy, or diathermy
  - Long and short posterior ciliary nerves
  - Retinoblastoma.
• *Stippled or dotted*: Drusen.

Color Code—Black

• *Solid*:
  - Pigment within the detached retina (lattice, flap of horseshoe tear, and paravascular pigmentation)
  - Pigment in choroid or pigmented epithelial hyperpigmentation in areas of attached retina
  - Pigmented demarcation lines at the attached margin of detached retina or within detached retina
  - Hyperpigmentation as a result of previous treatment with cryotherapy, photocoagulation, or diathermy
  - Completely sheathed retinal vessels.
• *Outline*:
  - Partially sheathed vessels (lattices and retinoschisis)
  - Edge of buckle beneath attached retina
  - Long posterior ciliary nerves and vessels (pigmented)
  - Short posterior ciliary nerves and vessels
  - Chorioretinal atrophy.

Indirect Ophthalmoscopy in Operating Room

Many problems may be encountered whilst operating and performing an indirect ophthalmoscopy. The fundus to be examined is usually a difficult one, with a retinal detachment and/or proliferative vitreoretinopathy (PVR). The cornea may become edematous or abraded during the course of surgery. Particular care must be taken in patients having undergone laser in situ keratomileusis (LASIK) surgery to prevent dislocation of corneal flap. The fundus picture may change with each step in surgery. The advantages of indirect ophthalmoscopy in the operation room stem from its safe working distance from the sterile operating field, in accurate localization of all retinal breaks and other fundus landmarks by scleral depression. It helps in obtaining a fine needle aspiration biopsy and treatment of choroidal or retinal tumors.

Indirect ophthalmoscopy is a valuable tool in the examination of children and uncooperative adults. Since the field of view is much larger with an indirect ophthalmoscope, fundus examination is possible even in moving eye. A quick comparison with the other eye is also possible. Children

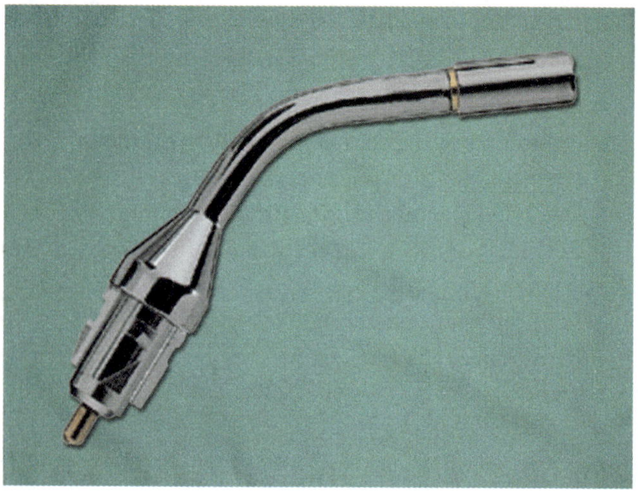

Fig. 9: Transillumination probe.

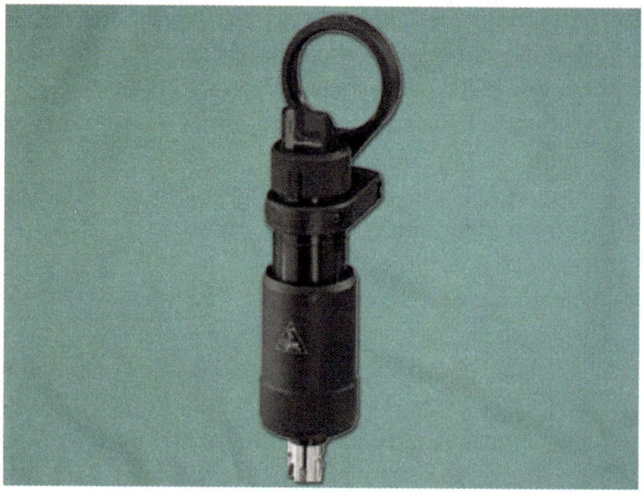

Fig. 10: Monocular indirect ophthalmoscope.

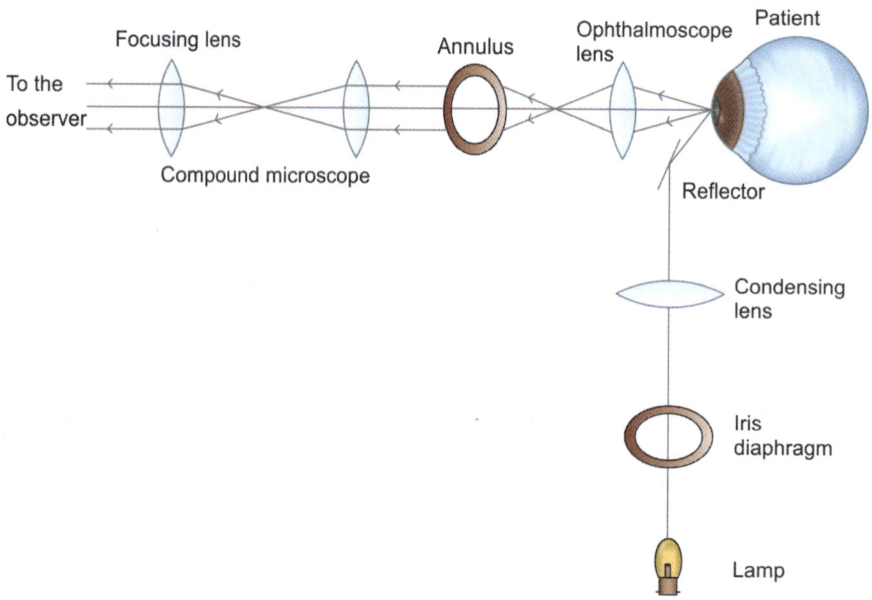

Fig. 11: Optics of monocular indirect ophthalmoscopy.

would generally react more favorably to the more impersonal distance of indirect examination. It is also useful equipment in examining the anterior segment for rubeosis and tumor seedings in children with advanced retinoblastoma.

Fundus angioscopy and transillumination **(Fig. 9)** can be performed using indirect ophthalmoscopy, which helps in differentiating various types of fundus mass lesions. Nystagmus, aniridia, albinotic fundus, partial vitreous hemorrhage, fundus coloboma, microphthalmos, and persistent hyperplastic primary vitreous can be diagnosed with the help of indirect ophthalmoscope.

MONOCULAR INDIRECT OPHTHALMOSCOPY

Monocular indirect ophthalmoscopy combines the advantages of increased field of view (indirect ophthalmoscopy) with erect real imaging (direct ophthalmoscopy). By collecting and redirecting peripheral fundus-reflected illumination rays, which cannot be accomplished with the direct ophthalmoscope. The indirect ophthalmoscope **(Fig. 10)** extends the observer's field of view approximately four to five times. An internal lens system then reinverts the initially inverted image to a real erect one **(Fig. 11)**, which is then magnified. This image is focusable using the focusing lever/eyepiece lever. It gives a field of view of approximately 30°, yet it is important that the patient looks in 6–8 different directions to see as much of the fundus as possible. The optical system of the monocular indirect ophthalmoscope (MIO) has a lens which erects the image and allows seeing things as they actually appear anatomically. It also gives a greater working distance from the patient of 5–6 inches. The MIO has a yellow filter that allows one to see deeper details of the retina at about the level of the choroid. The cost of the MIO is nearly equal to that of a good BIO and of course it does not allow a stereoscopic view of the retina.

Examination Procedure

To examine the right eye, remove the patient's spectacle correction, stand to the patient's right side, and ask him to fixate straight ahead and level with the left eye. The observer should wear his refractive correction. The iris diaphragm lever is pushed fully to the left to maximally increase the aperture size. Center the red dot on the filter dial to open the aperture for normal viewing. The observers head should be against the forehead rest and align the eye through the instrument with the patient's right eye. Then position several inches in front of the patient and focus through the pupil onto the fundus using the thumb and focusing lever. Adjust the focus and iris diaphragm to produce a clear maximally illuminated fundus view. Continue to approach the patient until the observer's knuckle lightly touches the patient's cheek, as the working distance decreases, fundus magnification increases. Angle the light slightly nasally to illuminate and visualize the optic disk.

MODIFIED MONOCULAR INDIRECT OPHTHALMOSCOPY

A thorough fundus examination is important and required in all young patients with strabismus or amblyopia in order to rule out organic causes of amblyopia prior to the initiation of treatment. The patient cooperation obtained with head mounted BIO (using a 20 D lens) and slit-lamp biomicroscope (using a 90 D) is usually difficult or impossible on younger children. Also the magnification of the fundus may be inadequate to allow accurate evaluation of posterior pole details. The direct ophthalmoscope is often the best available instrument for detailed retinal examination in young patients.

However, children often become frightened as the examiner approaches closely, as is necessary with the direct ophthalmoscope and cooperation is lost. Additionally, children often fix the ophthalmoscope light and track it as the examiner moves it, allowing examination of the macula but not of the disk. The field of view is small and the magnification is more than is usually necessary. This will prevent the examiner from seeing the large area of fundus. To avoid these difficulties the direct ophthalmoscope can be used in conjunction with a 20 D condensing lens. This combination provides a moderately magnified and wider angle view of the posterior pole. This avoids the close proximity between the patient and examiner required when using a direct ophthalmoscope alone. The technique is called modified monocular indirect ophthalmoscopy and has been noted for its ability to provide a good view of the retina through a small pupil.

Examination Procedure

To begin the examination a red reflex is visualized through the direct ophthalmoscope held approximately 18 cm from the patient's eye. A 20 D lens is then placed 3–5 cm in front of the patient's eye in the path of the ophthalmoscope light beam, the examiner then needs to move slightly toward or away from the patient until a clear image of the retina is observed.

An inverted, aerial image of the retina is produced, located between the observer and the lens. The apparent magnification will gradually increase as the examiner moves closer to this image (i.e. closer to the patient), allowing more detailed examination. Moving closer to the image obtains a magnification of ×4 to ×5. As the examiner moves closer, additional lenses in the ophthalmoscope are needed to keep the image clear depending on the accommodative needs of the examiner. A viewing distance of approximately 18 cm from the patient is optimal, providing suitable magnification and a wide field of view.

A disadvantage of the technique, as with conventional direct ophthalmoscopy is the lack of a true stereoscopic view, however, lateral movement and rotation of the direct ophthalmoscope during the examination gives good parallax clues to depth.

PENLIGHT OPHTHALMOSCOPY

This is a very old, basically a bedside technique that originally utilized a penlight and a high plus lens. The patient must be dilated to get as much binocularity as possible and large field of view. The ophthalmoscope is held just below the eyes and its light directed into the patient's eye. The patient's eye is viewed from over the top of the ophthalmoscope while a 20 D lens is placed approximately 3–4 cm from the patient's eye. The light leaving the condensing lens must come to focus within the pupil allowing the fullest field of view of the retina, approximately 30°. The image is inverted and laterally reversed and located between the ophthalmoscope and the condensing lens. The degree of stereopsis depends on how fully the pupil is dilated and one's ability to converge and accommodate on the image. It still gives a larger field of view than an MIO though less magnification. This is an alternative method to examine small infants. Should the bulb burn out in a BIO one has an alternative means to get a good view of the peripheral fundus? Do not put hands on the patient's shoulder or head. Instead, use the back of the chair to steady yourself.

DIRECT OPHTHALMOSCOPY

Direct ophthalmoscope **(Fig. 12)** is most commonly used instrument in ophthalmic practice. The ophthalmologist must familiarize oneself with the use of the direct ophthalmoscope in an appropriate manner.

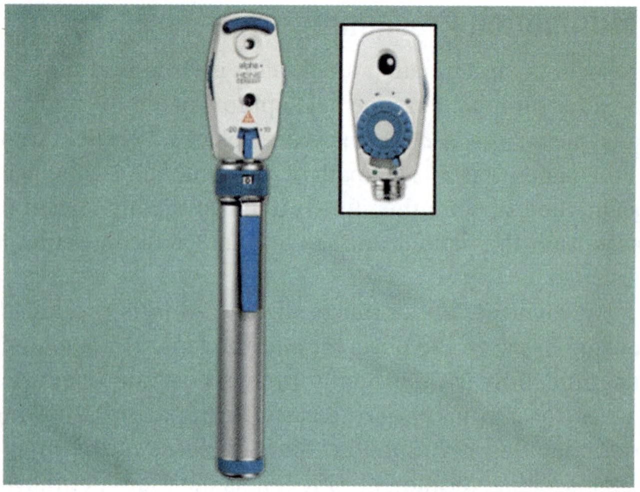

Fig. 12: Direct ophthalmoscope.

Before being able to recognize the abnormalities in fundus, one must know what normal looks like. It is advisable to examine as many of your colleagues as possible both inside and outside clinic hours. Good observational and recording skills can be developed with practice.

Examination Procedure

Direct ophthalmoscopy is best carried out in a darkroom with fully dilated pupils. One must be familiar with the color coding of the lens wheel and the various apertures and filters. Instruct the patient to look at a distant target (the white spotlight on the vision chart) and to "pretend" to still see it even if obscured with your head. The patient may blink as required. Your left eye and left hand should be used to examine the patient's left eye. The field of view of the fundus is increased when examiner goes closer to the patient's eye. When patients with low myopes or low hyperopes are to be examined, it is better to remove their glasses. However, for myopes and hyperopes above ±3.00 DSph and for astigmats above 2.50 DCyl, it is advisable to keep the glasses on in order to overcome problems associated with magnification, minification, and distortion. The extra reflexes produced by the spectacle lenses will at first prove distracting but can be overcome with practice.

Using a large diameter aperture, examine the external features of the eye including pupils. With a +1 D or +2 D lens in the ophthalmoscope, view the pupils at a distance of 40–66 cm from the patient. Look for media opacities. To find the location of the opacity, note movement of the opacity with relation to the movement of the ophthalmoscope, using the pupillary plane as a reference point. If the opacity moves in the same direction as the ophthalmoscope, the opacity is located behind the iris. If the opacity moves in the opposite direction to the ophthalmoscope, the opacity is located in front of the iris.

Using the ophthalmoscope as a light source, which is held tangential to the iris one looks for any shadow that appears on the nasal side. If the nasal irido-corneal angle has no shadow, it denotes a wide-open angle. However, as this shadow increases in width relative to the overall cornea size, the angle seems narrow.

Dial up +10 DSph lens in the lens wheel and observe the eye from a distance of 10 cm. Study the red reflex to detect any media opacity. The position of opacity can be inferred from its parallax with respect to the pupil. When the patient looks up and the opacity appears to move in the same direction within the red-reflex then it is located anterior to the pupil plane (i.e. in the cornea or in the anterior chamber). Opacity that remains stationary lies in the plane of the pupil, but when it moves in the opposite direction to that of the patient's gaze, it lies posterior to the pupil plane (i.e. the posterior lens or vitreous). It may be easier to move yourself slightly from side to side rather than ask the patient to move his eye to achieve the same effect. During ophthalmoscopy it is advisable to keep both eyes open and suppress the image from the other eye. It may take some practice to accomplish this.

It is better to move closer to the patient and gradually reduce the power of the lens in the wheel and focus on the crystalline lens, the vitreous and finally the fundus. The power of lens necessary to focus on the fundus will depend on patient's and observer's uncompensated refractive error and accommodation. Once a blood vessel on the fundus is located, move along it and locate the point at which it branches. Then move your field of view in the direction in which the apex of the branch is pointing till you reach the optic disk.

If one controls his accommodation, it allows for an estimation of the patient's refractive error by focusing the optic disk. Retinal blood vessels should be examined in each quadrant after locating the disk. Artery to vein ratio (A/V), arteriolar light reflex (ALR), branching of vessels to all four quadrants, and crossing phenomenon must be assessed.

Once again focus the disk and move nasally to view the macula. In this position you may obscure the fixation target, cause the pupil to constrict, dazzle the patient, and notice some troublesome corneal reflections. These factors make the macula a difficult area to visualize. It may be useful to use a smaller aperture beam. The patient should not be asked to look into the light when viewing the macula through an undilated pupil. The patient will accommodate and this together with the bright light from the ophthalmoscope will make the pupil even smaller reducing the ability to view the whole macular area.

Finally ask the patient to look in the eight cardinal directions to view the peripheral fundus. You will need to adjust the lens in the wheel slightly as the periphery is closer to you than the optic disk requiring more focusing power (plus lens). The red-free filter makes small macroaneurysms and small hemorrhages stand out more clearly. It can also be helpful in estimating the C/D ratio.

It is also used to differentiate between retinal nevus and choroidal nevus. The retinal blood supply and its retinal pigment epithelium (RPE) act like a red filter. Therefore, a nevus that lies behind the retina and located in the choroid will not be seen when viewed with the red-free filter. On the other hand a nevus located on or in the retina will still be seen with the red-free filter in place. A cobalt-blue filter is useful in detection of nerve fiber drop out.

The direct ophthalmoscope gives a magnification of approximately ×15 and a field of view of 6.5–10°. The formula M = 60 D/4 holds well for up to ±10 Ds of refractive error.

HRUBY LENS DIRECT OPHTHALMOSCOPY

The use of the slit-lamp biomicroscope allows a stereoscopic view of the retina. The auxiliary lenses provide high magnification with excellent resolution. The Hruby lens (–55 D) produces an upright virtual image that is not laterally reversed.

Examination Procedure

Patient cooperation can be enhanced by attention to comfort and with the use of a fixation device. Once the illuminated slit is imaged in the patient's pupil, the Hruby lens is introduced in front of the patient's eye as close as possible without contacting the cornea or lashes.

This mode of direct ophthalmoscopy can provide a very high level of magnification, even greater than that of the monocular handheld direct ophthalmoscope. The actual level of magnification depends on that available through the slit lamp. Stereopsis is provided to a greater degree than all other examination techniques.

The main disadvantage of this technique is the field of view. It is smaller than all other examination methods with the exception of direct monocular ophthalmoscopy (less than two disk diameters for an emmetropic patient). More dilation is required than in other binocular techniques. The quality of the image is easily degraded by media opacities; however, increasing the slit-lamp illumination can reduce this problem. As the magnification is so high, small movements of the observer, lens, or patient have an immediately noticeable effect on image quality.

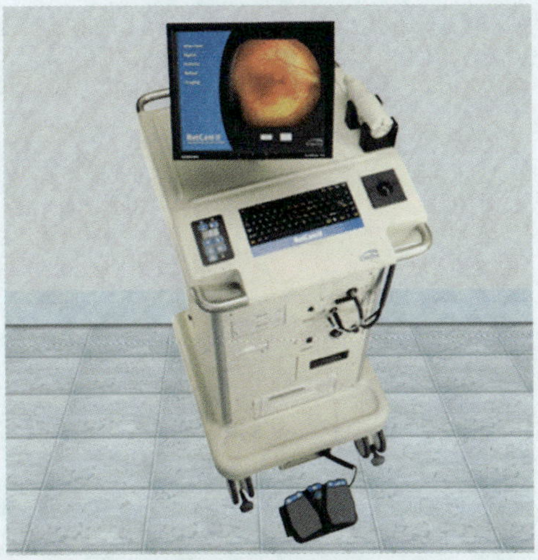

Fig. 13: RetCam viewing system.

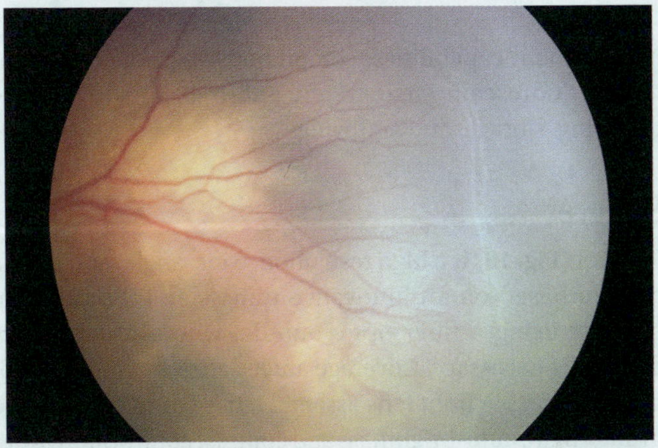

Fig. 14: Wide-angle fundus photograph (RetCam) of a premature infant showing retinopathy of prematurity with a demarcation ridge clearly made out.

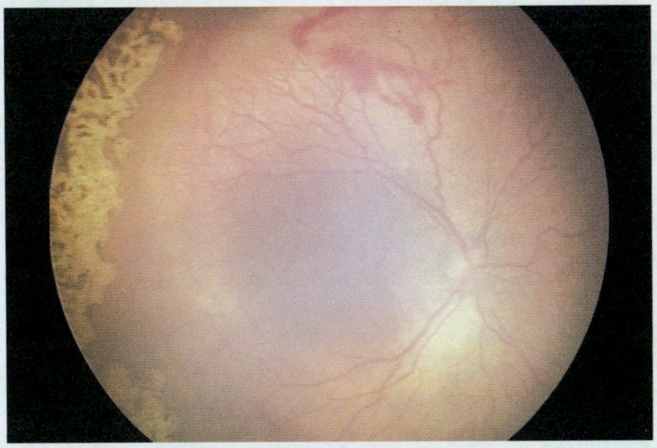

Fig. 15: Fundus photograph (RetCam) of a premature infant showing retinopathy of prematurity with laser photocoagulation marks. Preretinal hemorrhage is seen beyond the superotemporal vascular arcade.

WIDE-ANGLE VIEWING SYSTEM

RetCam

The RetCam **(Fig. 13)** has a 3-CCD (charge-coupled device) chip video camera. It is lightweight, easy to position, and has a long cable for easy patient access. It has five changeable lenses: 130°, 120°, 80°, 30°, and Portrait. It has a large LCD display with 20 seconds of real time video per clip and a frame-by-frame or real-time video review. It has a lighted control panel, a dual DVD-RAM for easy backup, multi-image data recall and display, side-by-side image comparison, high resolution 24 bit color image, instant-digital image capture and is US Food and Drugs Administration (FDA) approved. It provides a 130° view for easy screening for retinopathy of prematurity **(Figs. 14 and 15)**, integrated image and patient

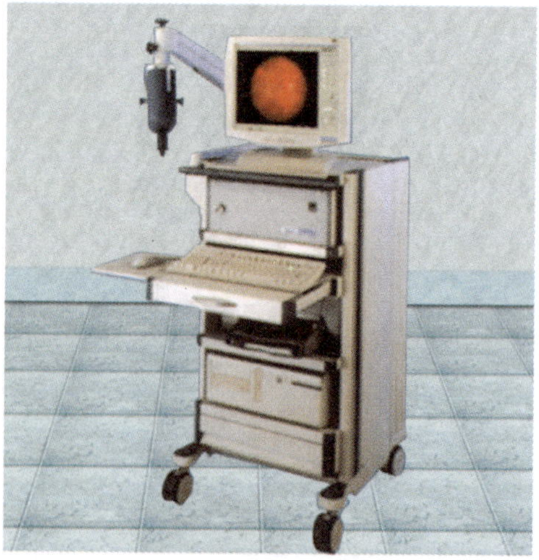

Fig. 16: Panoret.

management capabilities, comprehensive photodocumentation, fluorescein angiography and built-in software for reporting, storage, and archiving.

Panoret

Panoret **(Fig. 16)** is a high resolution, wide-angle, and retinal camera based on an innovative transscleral illumination concept using a fiber optic bundle, where no pupillary dilation is necessary. Coverage angles are 50° and 100° with interchangeable front lens assembly. It is computer assisted in auto-light, auto-brightness and contrast control along with auto-disk storage. Fundus illumination may, however, be limited in heavily pigmented eyes. DVD recording is possible. DICOM 3.0 connectivity is available for telemedicine.

Optos Ultra-wide Camera

The Optos camera employs scanning laser ophthalmoscopy technology and is capable of producing wide-field images with 200° field of view, which equates roughly to 82.5% of the retinal surface area. The technology utilizes an ellipsoid mirror to obtain images of the retinal periphery without the need for bright illumination or a contact lens, and in some patients, pupillary dilation. The current model uses a red (633 nm) and green laser (523 nm) to scan the retina and obtain the images. The images created by each of these laser wavelengths may be separated into their individual components, providing more detailed information. The Optos camera is also capable of producing high-resolution fluorescein angiogram images of the retinal periphery.

SUGGESTED READING

1. Benson WE, Regillo CD. Retinal Detachment: Diagnosis and Management, 3rd edition. Philadelphia: Lippincott-Raven; 1998. pp. 75-99.
2. Havener WH, Gloekner S. Atlas of Diagnostic Tecniques and Treatment of Retinal Detachment. St. Louis: Mosby; 1967. pp. 1-51.
3. Michels RG, Rice TA, Wilkinson CP. Retinal Detachment, 2nd edition. St. Louis: Mosby; 1997. pp. 347-70.
4. Regillo CD, Brown GC, Flynn Jr HW. Vitreoretinal Disease: The Essentials. New York: Thieme; 1999. pp. 41-9.
5. Rosenthal ML, Fradin S. The technique of binocular indirect ophthalmoscopy. Highlights Ophthalmol. 1967;9:179-257.
6. Schepens CL, Hartnett ME, Hirose T. Schepens' Retinal Detachment and Allied Diseases, 2nd edition. Boston: Butterworth-Heinemann; 2000. pp. 99-129.
7. Yanoff M, Duker JS, Augsburger JJ, et al. Ophthalmology, 2nd edition. St. Louis: Mosby; 2004.

CHAPTER

12 Ophthalmic Photography

Sadao Kanagami

INTRODUCTION

Among all types of medical photography, the specialty of ophthalmic photography is perhaps the most difficult to master as it requires in-depth knowledge of not only the ocular structures, and the disease process of the eye, but it also requires special photographic skills in regard to the equipment needed to record ocular pathology on silver base media or electronic medium. Captured ophthalmic images often have a direct influence on not only the diagnosis but also the treatment choice as in the case of fundus fluorescein angiography (FFA) or indocyanine green (ICG) angiography. The responsibility of accurately capturing this information needed by the treating ophthalmologist becomes critical and weighs heavily on the shoulder of the ophthalmic photographer—especially with the advent of teleophthalmology where images may be captured hundreds of miles away from the treating ophthalmologist.

The ophthalmic photography differs greatly from biological photography in general as the images captured by the ophthalmic photographer are part of the treatment decision process or utilized in the management of ophthalmic patients. Recent trends in ophthalmic photographic equipment include computerized equipment that further adds to the long list of specialized technique and changes in ophthalmic imaging.

Some of the ophthalmic photography and imaging equipment include the following in the long list of tools used in our field.

35-mm CAMERA

A 35-mm camera with a motorized drive to automatically advance the film should be fitted with a long macro lens in the order of 135–150 mm (or a medical lens such as the Nikon Medikor lens) in order to keep facial distortion to a minimum. This is very important especially when taking photographs in the specialty area of *plastics*. A macro lens should be selected to include fields of one eye to full face; a second macro lens could include head/shoulder to full body. The selected 35-mm camera should also be fitted with either a double-sided macro flash or a built-in ring flash. These macro flashes are typically meant for short range (<1 m) photography for optimum illumination. When photographing patients for *plastics* or for full body photography, a studio flash setup is still the recommended approach **(Fig. 1)**.

FUNDUS CAMERA

Mydriatic Fundus Camera

Conventional noncorneal contact mydriatic fundus camera **(Fig. 2)** can range between 20° and 60° view of the ocular fundus. The ophthalmic photographer can choose the angle of view that will best reflect the needs of the photo documentation as, e.g. in imaging the optic nerve for glaucoma one would use a view of 20°, while in the case of a large melanotic choroidal tumor one would select

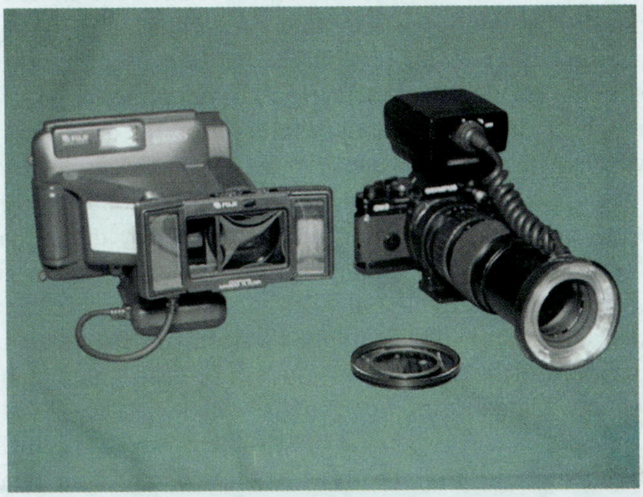

Fig. 1: Macro lens for close-up photography.

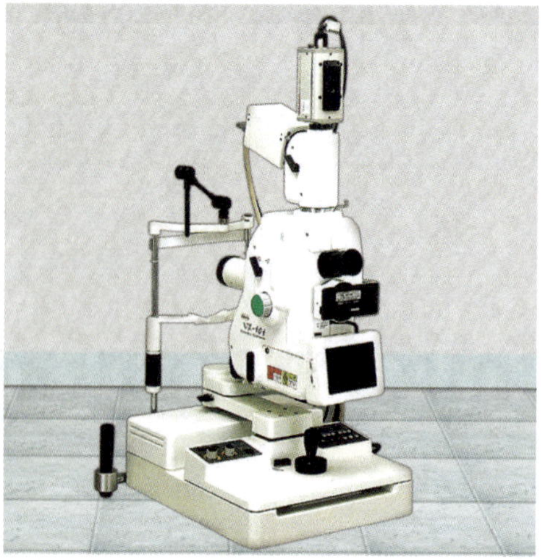

Fig. 2: Fundus camera.

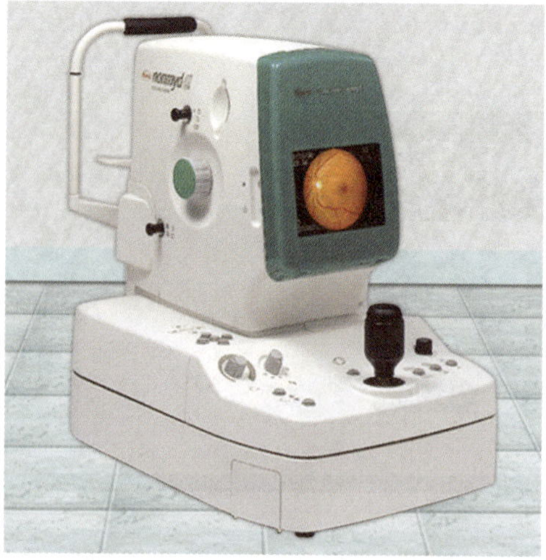

Fig. 3: Nonmydriatic fundus camera.

a wider 60° field of view. Mostly, these retinal cameras capture full color images of the retina as well as having capabilities of capturing monochromatic and angiographic images (fluorescein and ICG). Determining the exposure level of electronic flash is completely different from the regular 35-mm camera used in external photography. Usually, these values are predetermined (factory setting) by the angle of view selected on the retinal camera as well as the film sensitivity used. Other determining factors for flash intensity can be the use of a plus diopter setting and angiographic or monochromatic selections (such as cobalt blue and red-free). Typically, retinal cameras have two or more camera backs; a 35-mm camera for color or monochromatic black and white film, a polaroid camera and in some cases certain retinal camera manufacturers offer optional video camera (analog or digital) to show the images on the monitor and store them in imaging software program on the computer system.

Nonmydriatic Fundus Camera

As the name suggests, the nonmydriatic fundus camera does not require the use of mydriatic agents to dilate the patient's pupil. The nonmydriatic fundus camera usually requires a natural dilation of 4 mm; this can be a limiting factor on patients over the age of 60 years old that typically do not naturally dilate well. These fundus cameras are usually very easy to operate as they have no viewfinder but instead they use a large 4-inch monochromatic TV monitor [or in some more modern nonmydriatic cameras, a liquid crystal display (LCD) screen] where the patient's fundus can be seen by way of an infrared video alignment camera. Since the viewing lamp utilizes infrared wavelength, the patient is not aware of the examination process. The flash illumination when using a low lux video charge-coupled device (CCD) camera is usually very low as these cameras have a very high sensitivity. The lower the lux level of the color CCD camera, the faster the pupillary recovery time and thus, the faster the

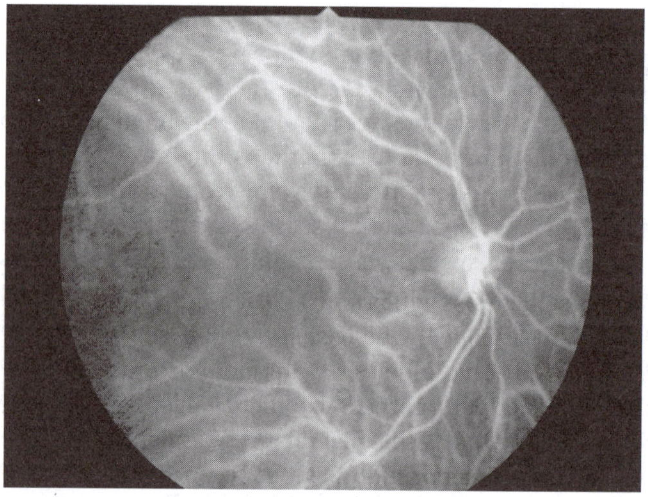

Fig. 4: Indocyanine green angiogram.

photographic procedure. There are many manufacturers of nonmydriatic fundus cameras some have the ability to capture angiographic images. When one uses mydriatic cameras in the mode of nonmydriatic, these cameras are usually confined for mid-phase only as a waiting period of at least 1 minute must be allowed to permit full pupillary recovery time. Nonmydriatic cameras can download their captured images to a computerized filing system. Often, nonmydriatic cameras **(Fig. 3)** are used to photograph diseases of the posterior segment of the eye.

The camera is very small and light weighted, it can be easily taken outside of the clinic. Fundus images have been stored on a personal computer directly from the camera using USB cable and an exclusive software.

Indocyanine Green Angiography

Indocyanine green angiography can be performed with near-infrared illumination using a retinal camera. ICG angiography examines the dynamic flow circulation of the choroidal vessels and adjunct structures **(Fig. 4)**. Typically, a retinal camera that has been designed with

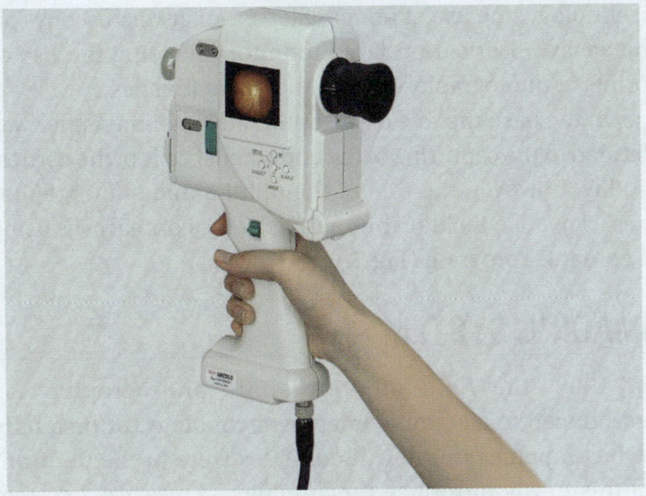

Fig. 5: Digital handheld fundus camera.

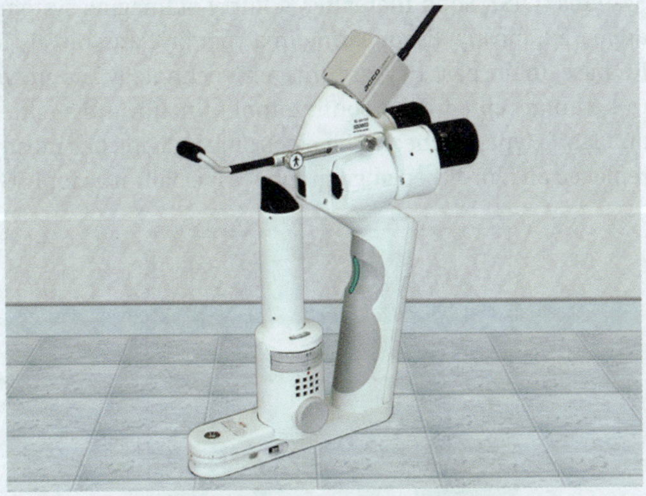

Fig. 6: Kowa Genesis with slit-lamp attachment.

special filters uses a black and white near-infrared CCD video camera (analog or digital) and records static megapixel images stored in a computer bank or dynamic images on videotapes as in the case of the scanning laser ophthalmoscope (SLO).

Digital Handheld Fundus Camera

Digital handheld fundus camera is recently introduced. This camera is designed for digital images; therefore, it becomes light and easy to operate compared to the previous model. The fundus images are displayed on a small LCD monitor and can be checked. These images can be stored on a memory card.

There is an adapter for indirect images. The adapter is very useful while taking the fundus photographs of the premature babies **(Fig. 5)**.

PHOTO SLIT LAMP (KOWA ATTACHMENT)

The handheld Kowa Genesis camera has a special attachment **(Fig. 6)** that allows for anterior segment photo

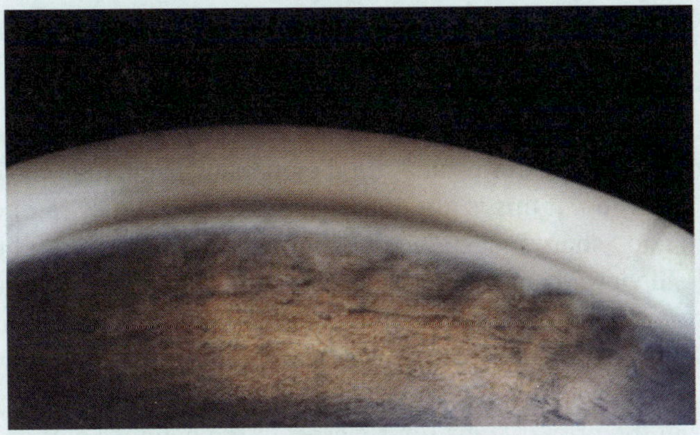

Fig. 7: Gonio photography.

documentation using a slit adapter. It allows the user to take images on either 35-mm film, video or fully digital backs. Once the adapter is connected, it is possible to capture conventional anterior segment images including of gonioscopy **(Fig. 7)**. For gonioscopy, topical anesthetic agent and a transparent gel such as Goniosol should be used. A lens that has antireflection coating should be preferred.

Use of gonioscopic lenses needs special techniques; however, combined with the use of a video camera it makes it easier to preview the captured field as opposed to capturing on conventional 35-mm film and waiting for the film to be processed to evaluate the photographic technique. However, using video-captured image does not equal the quality of 35-mm film (resolution, hue, color, contrast) but most surgeons agree that the trade-off of immediacy in seeing the images is well worth the quality of the 35-mm film. For publication a conventional 35-mm film can also be used in conjunction with the video images.

Portable Slit Lamp with Video Camera

Portable slit lamp is very useful when taking pictures of bed-ridden patients and/or small children. This slit lamp can adapt a very small video camera and can take patients' anterior segment photographs or video images.

PHOTOGRAPHY IN OPERATING THEATER

There are two main ways of capturing images in the operating theater, the first consists of positioning the camera next to the operator using a bedside approach, while the other technique is to attach a camera directly to the operating microscope and have the operator take all images using one of the optical pathways of the microscope (right or left). Using this technique means that the photography port will be taken through a 70/30 (%) type of prism and that the operator will have to look through only the optical pathway that is occupied by the camera. Using this technique will ensure the operator that what he/she sees is what is actually captured. Additionally, using this technique will give a good preview of the nonstereo image that is captured by the recording device since only one optical pathway is equipped with a recording device (usually the right optical pathway is best). It is critical that the microscope should be set for focusing for the recording device and not the operator's actual dioptric correction. If this is not done, captured images may not be in good sharp focus. The operator will also notice that the field viewed and the field photographed is not exactly the same area (usually the photographed field is smaller) but with practice and years of experience, very good results may be achieved. It is critical as in any other type of photography that the primary lens (lens closest to the patient's cornea) be free of artifacts such as dust, fingerprints, water stains, fluorescein stains. Attentive care should be given to the lens cleaning techniques to avoid possible damage to the costly lens. If this is not done, the quality and color of the captured images will be very low with color shift and low contrast images as well as poor optical resolution.

SPECULAR MICROSCOPY

Photography of the corneal endothelial cells can be easily performed using a slit-lamp photomicroscope and resulting images can be analyzed using a computer program. Typically, these images can show the borders of the cells that reflect the light toward the high magnification microscope lens when used in conjunction with specular illumination methods. This illumination can be achieved by using the illumination tower set at 45° (incident light) from the apex of the cornea while observing the return light (reflected light) through the objective when the observation tower is set at 45° from the opposite side of the illumination tower. Recent trends in specular microscopy are the use of noncontact specular microscope that causes little trauma to the patient and risk of cross contamination is minimal as no corneal contact is required with the system.

In **Figure 8**, one can easily compare the size and/or the arrangement of the corneal cells. With innovative imaging technology, the use of noncontact specular microscopy can be easily observed on large monitor obviating the use of prints or photography on silver highlight film base.

In the past, the role of the ophthalmic photographer was limited to the capturing of the endothelial cells of the cornea. Today, however, the role of the ophthalmic photographer has evolved to include the analysis of the corneal cells using a computer program **(Fig. 9)**.

IMAGING SYSTEM

In 1990, the field of ophthalmic photography was introduced to electronic imaging technology. At first, only two companies in the United States were in the forefront of this newly introduced technology—Kowa VK-2 system **(Fig. 10)**, Topcon ImageNet and Ophthalmic Imaging Systems (OIS). Soon thereafter, a flurry of imaging systems appeared, mostly disappearing in a year or 2 and mostly in PC base. In the past 10 years, this new technology has grown to be an accepted daily routine tool of major universities and HMO type practices. The electronic imaging has mostly replaced all film-based angiography (especially true for ICG)

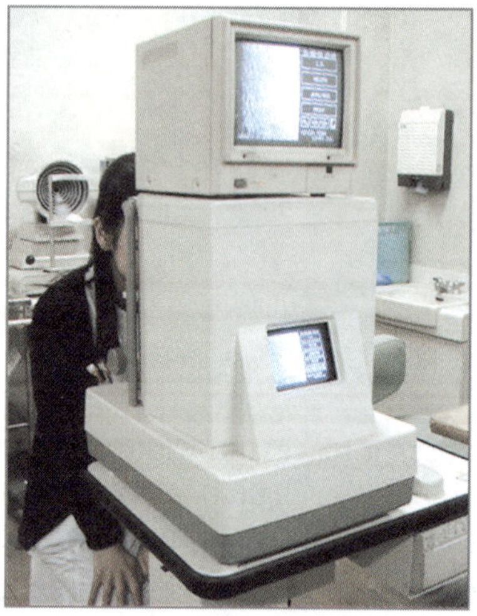

Fig. 9: Noncontact Robo.

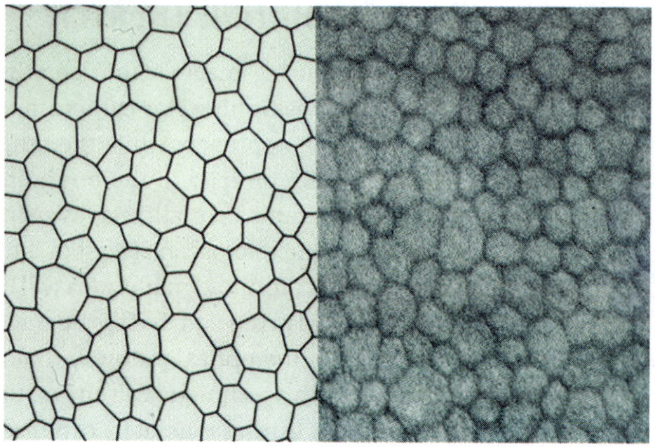

Fig. 8: *Specular photography*: Endothelial cells.

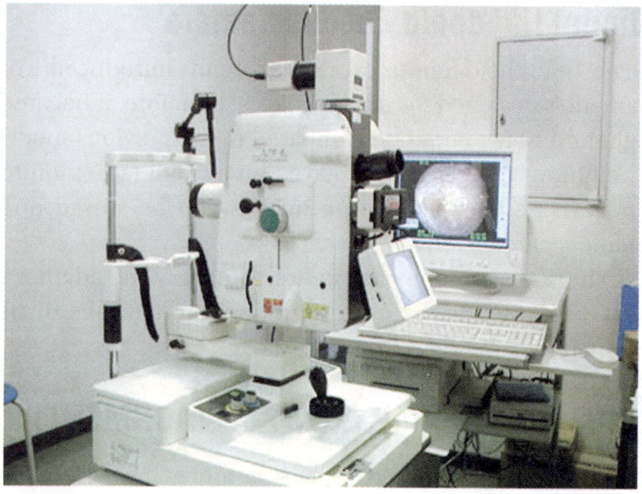

Fig. 10: *Digital imaging system*: Kowa VK-2 system.

avoiding the long darkroom delays. Although this technology is not comparable to film-based technology, yet as far as resolution and gray scale, it does offer certain advantages, such as, instant results viewable on large cathode-ray tube (CRT) screens, image processing or enhancement, transfer of images through the internet for teaching, screening or second opinion (teleophthalmology).

Imaging system has following advantages:

- Captured images are displayed on a monitor immediately.
- Displayed images are large, so the patients who are dilated or have low vision can appreciate them.
- Images may be reviewed by the treating ophthalmologist as they are being captured.
- Prints can be produced immediately on thin paper so it is easy to put on a patient's chart.
- Images may be stored in the computer data base system for easy review and follow-up.

Imaging system has following disadvantages:

- The computer systems are quite expensive and technology changes rapidly making systems obsolete in 1 year.
- Computer, large CRT screen and printer require additional space.
- Operation of the computer and system software requires training and maintenance.
- Quality of image is not yet comparable with 35-mm film.

Imaging systems in ophthalmology typically means that the conventional ophthalmic camera recording device such as the 35-mm or polaroid type back is replaced with a CCD that may be either analog (video signal) or digital (higher resolution than video signal). These CCDs usually can add significantly to the cost of the fundus or slit-lamp camera especially if they are digital in nature. Digital CCD can be either a single chipped red, green and blue chipped or could be three chipped, one for each of the RGB wave lengths. The latter is far more expensive than the single chip but the color separation with the three-chip-CCD is superior. The area of sensitization of the CCD chip (usually varying from inch-to-inch) being much smaller than of the 35-mm surface (24 mm × 36 mm) or of the polaroid sheet, the light (flash intensity) required to expose the light sensitive CCD is significantly less than that of traditional film base emulsion to expose the same area of the eye. Much like the film base emulsion, CCD comes in a variety of sensitivity calculated in lux values. The lower the value in front of the lux, the more sensitive (and usually more expensive) the CCD is. However, it can also be said that the more sensitive the CCD is, the more electronic "noise" (comparable to large grain when referring to film) can be produced (comparable to higher sensitivity film such as 1,600 or 3,200 ISO). More recently, ophthalmic manufacturers have introduced nonmydriatic retinal cameras with purely digital recording devices. Nonmydriatic cameras are usually equipped with two CCD, one is a black and white infrared low resolution used for alignment of the patient's retina (image is viewable on a small CRT screen located on the base of the nonmydriatic retinal camera), while the second is used to actually capture the color image of the retina through the naturally dilated pupil in a dimly lit room. One of the main advantages of the low light CCD chip used in the nonmydriatic camera is that retinal images can be captured sequentially without having to wait 4–5 minutes as with instant type photography (polaroid). The captured retinal images typically do not affect seriously the natural dilation of the pupil. Pupillary recovery is usually very fast as opposed to when using instant type film. Additionally, some nonmydriatic retinal cameras can capture ICG angiography since in some cases the infrared cameras used higher resolution.

Photography of Both Eyes

To take the photographs of ocular movements especially in case of strabismus, amblyopia, and ocular muscle disorder, 9 directions eye gaze position should be captured **(Fig. 11)**. To achieve this type of photography, simply place the patient's head in a straight forward position referred to as primary gaze. Having selected a long lens such as 135-mm macro or 150-mm macro combined with a ring flash, is asked to fixate at a gaze of 30° in each o'clock position such as 12 o'clock, 1:30, 3, 4:30, 6, 7:30, 9 and 10:30 and take photographs in each of these positions. Make certain that the patient maintains his or her head in the primary straight forward position and avoid side-to-side head shifts or frontal and backward tilts. When taking photographs in downward gazes (4:30, 6, 7:30 o'clock), an assistant should help in lifting the eyelids in order to expose those gaze positions. For an overall even illumination, the use of a ring flash should be used, as the ring flash will create a ring pattern on the patient's corneas, will be equidistant and could be considered as a Heirshberg ring. The long macro lens (135- to 150-mm macro) will avoid facial distortion and give accurate facial renderings.

Photography of Face and Skin

For full face photography of patients, the practice of using a long 135- to 150-mm macro lens still applies in order to maintain correct facial proportions and avoid the distortion created by wider-angle non-macro lenses. It is important that the patient wipes the facial sweat or heavy makeup used by some women as well as any ocular ointment used onto the eyes prior to taking photographs. This practice will avoid getting any unwanted or irregular flash reflexes. Typically, it is a good idea to use an electronic set of flashes mounted as in a photo studio. This type of illumination helps to accentuate areas of interest by creating shadows. If no flash is available, it is possible to use natural outdoor

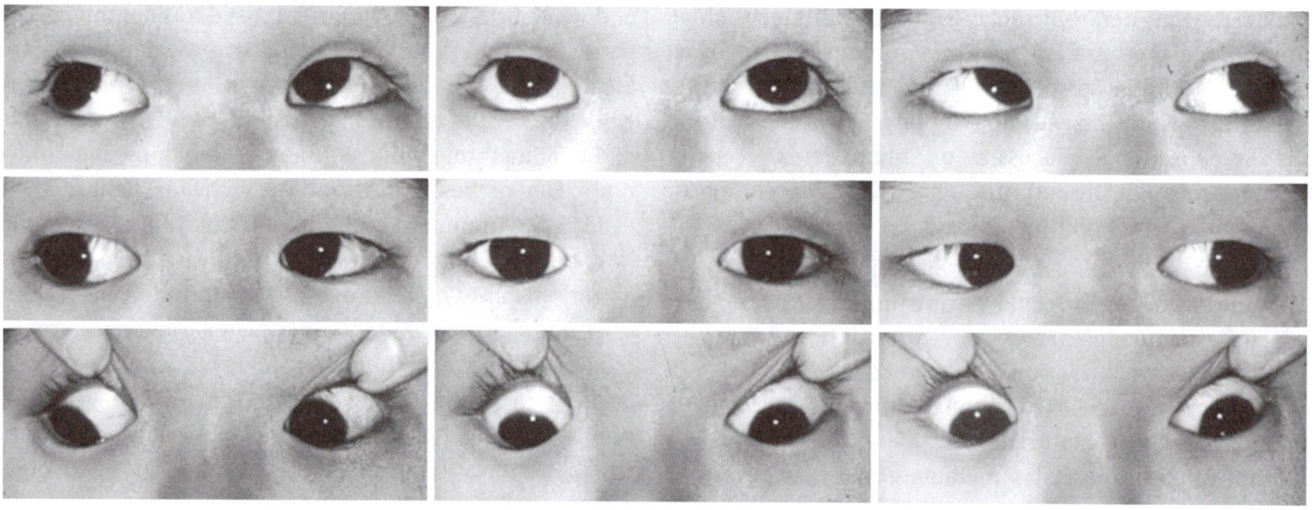

Fig. 11: Eye gaze position in nine directions.

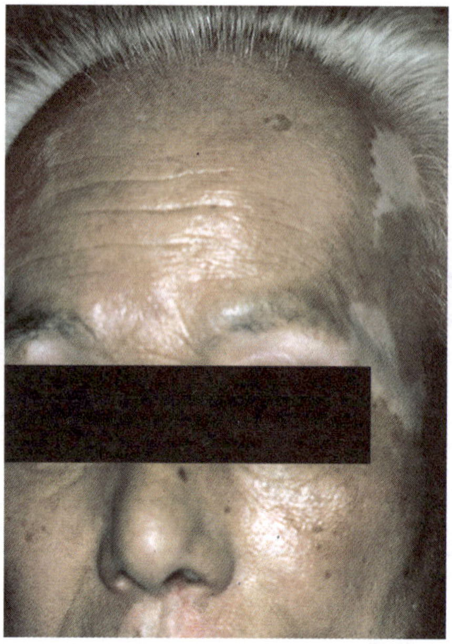

Fig. 12: Face and skin photograph.

sunlight illumination but caution should be used not to overexpose the area of interest and use a standard blue or gray background. To document proptosis, the best position is to capture the image from above the patient's head using two macro-type electronic flashes set at 90° from the patient. This technique will create the appropriate shadows that will help define areas of interest to the plastic ophthalmic surgeon **(Fig. 12)**.

Photography of Pupil

In some cases of neuro-ophthalmology, it is important to document the pupillary changes of patients and to differences between the right and the left pupil (as both may dilate differently from each other under similar lux conditions). The best way to record these differences is to use a black and white camera that is mounted on a tripod (for added steadiness) and have the patient place his chin in a chin rest (also for added steadiness). The room is then darkened and about 5 minutes is needed to allow for each pupil to either dilate or constrict depending on the particular condition of the patient (at times a flash light, white light, may be used to provoke a specific pupillary reaction that is recorded on video). Analog iris recorders are available that use infrared CCD cameras in combination with an infrared illumination system that is not perceivable to the patient and where the patient's pupil does not react. Images are then recorded as either a series of still images or as a string of segments (continuous video images) that are then transferred to a computer for numeric processing. Typically when performing these studies, no mydriatic agents are used unless otherwise indicated by the examiner.

EXTERNAL PHOTOGRAPHY

When taking photographs of the cornea and the lens, the choice instrument is a photo slit lamp since it has the correct optical magnification and the appropriate flash to accomplish the task at hand. However, when a photo slit lamp is not available, a 35-mm SLR camera with macro lens and electronic flash or even a fundus camera (using a plus diopter) may be used. External close-up photography of one eye for the purpose of documentation of ocular trauma or tumors can be taken with a macro type lens (usually a long lens) and a side macro flash (usually mounted on either side of the front of the macro lens) to avoid disturbing flash reflexes often found when using a ring flash type systems. Careful evaluation of where the flash reflex will fall is critical in obtaining useful photo documentation. Many macro type electronic flashes have what is called a *modeling light* that is mounted directly next to the flash tube. These modeling lights will illuminate the field of interest and give a good idea of where the flash reflexes will show-up when the photograph is captured. Since the cornea and sclera are highly reflective surfaces, special attention needs to be given to the illumination technique. It is possible to limit these reflections by using polarizing filters on the flash and lens; however, the reflexes will only partially disappear and the iris detail is made very dark.

Conventional 35-mm SLR Camera

When using a 35-mm macro lens for ophthalmic photo documentation, it is critical to select a lens that will keep the true perspective of the area of interest. Nikon Corporation introduced in the market a special macro lens with intergraded ring type macro flash tube. This special macro lens called *Nikon Medikor lens*, it comes in two focal lengths. This lens works somewhat differently in that the photographer selects the required magnification on the lens and then simply focuses by physically moving toward or away from the patient. Other possible choices for macro lenses are:

- One eye—135-mm macro to 150-mm macro lens
- Two eyes—105-mm macro lens to 135-mm macro lens
- Full face—105-mm macro lens to 135-mm macro lens
- Torso—50-mm macro lens to 105-mm macro lens
- Full body—50-mm macro lens to 105-mm macro lens.

Use of Fundus Camera in External Photography

The handheld fundus camera (Kowa Genesis) may be especially useful in close-up external photography as the system uses a powerful distortion-free macro lens along with a coaxial illumination in the fundus camera that produces a small reflex on the cornea or sclera. This camera is particularly well suited in the pediatric population **(Fig. 13)**.

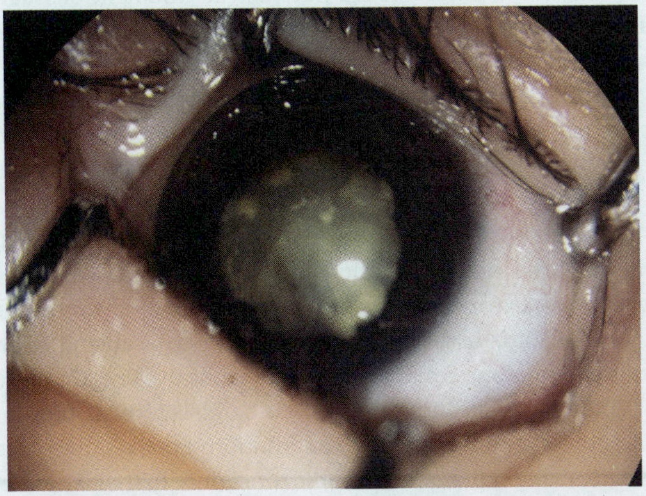

Fig. 13: External eye with handheld fundus camera.

Some table-top retinal cameras are also well suited for external (single eye) photo documentation of the eye; these retinal cameras are usually fitted with a frontal concave lens. To capture the images, simply position the patient in the chin rest as you would for conventional retinal photography and select a plus diopter setting (as well as in some cases selecting a higher magnification lens) by focusing the retinal camera until the images become clear. Film type and flash exposure is the same as for regular fundus photography **(Fig. 14)**. For taking fluorescein stain photography of the cornea or sclera, the retinal camera may be the most useful instrument since it already has both the exciter and barrier filters in place **(Fig. 15)**. When performing iris angiography, again the retinal camera is best suited for this purpose not only due to the filters but also because these cameras are equipped with an internal timer that is critical for fluorescein studies requiring dynamic flow analysis **(Fig. 16)**. Black and white films ISO 400 or instant type (polaroid or Fuji) film can be used and processed in a similar way as for retinal angiography.

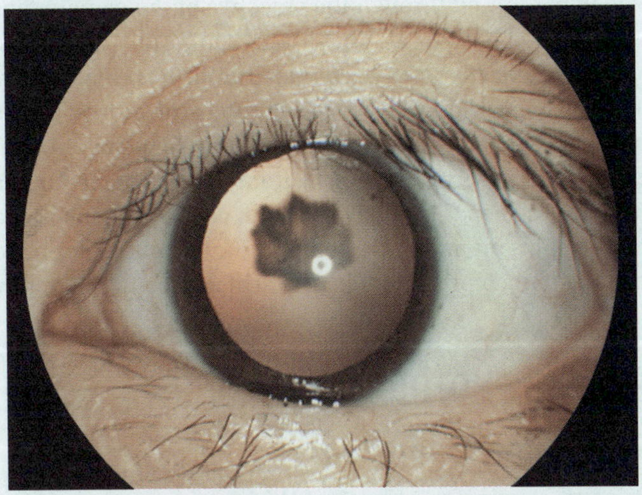

Fig. 14: External eye with table-top fundus camera.

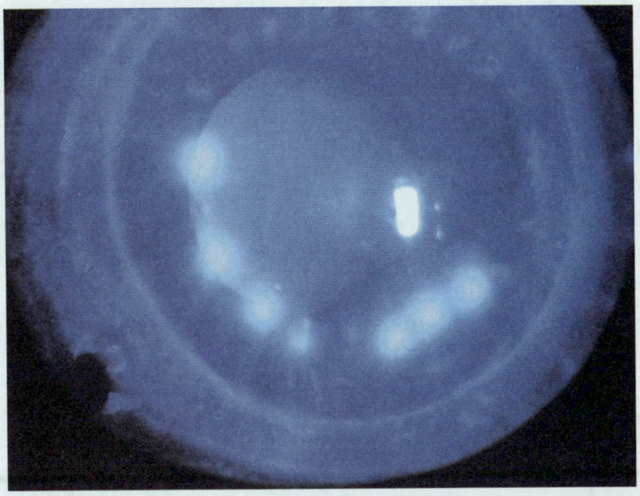

Fig. 15: Fluorescein stain photography.

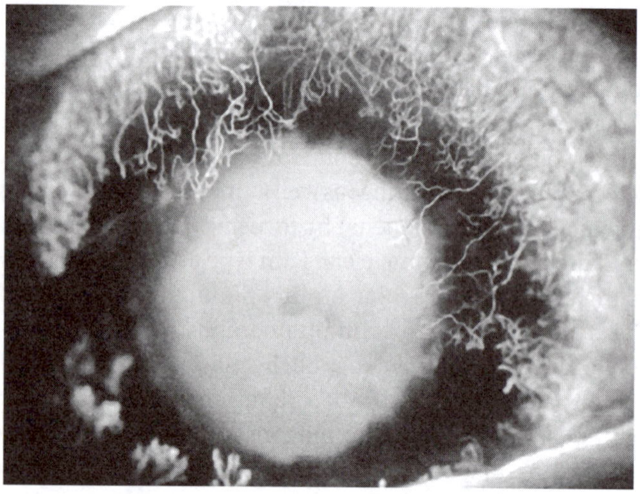

Fig. 16: Anterior segment fluorescein angiogram.

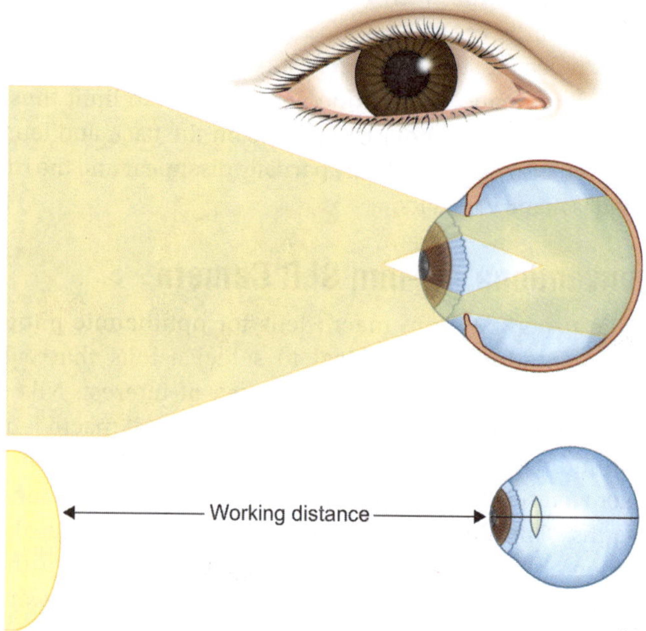

Fig. 17: Working distance.

OPTICAL SYSTEM OF FUNDUS CAMERA

Fundus camera's optical system can be compared to the Galilean type telescope and is characteristic by incorporating an internal coaxial type illumination and electronic flash. The light emitted through the objective of the camera lens is a ring-shaped image. The distance from this ring to the surface of objective lens is referred to as the *working distance* and is of great importance in taking good artifact-free fundus photographs. The actual position of this ring-shaped light can be best observed by looking from the side of the fundus camera. To keep this relative position constant is one of the most important and basic points in fundus photography to insure good color saturation and artifact-free photography **(Fig. 17)**.

FUNDUS PHOTOGRAPHY

Preparatory Operations

Prior to starting the photographic session, the patient's eye must be dilated with a mydriatic agent to achieve best possible pupillary dilation (optimally a pupillary dilation of over 8 mm is desirable). The objective lens should be clean and free from dust and smear. Any dust particles must be carefully removed with a manual blower while smear should be removed with lens cleaning paper. Check that the film is correctly loaded and flash intensity control is properly set according to the film sensitivity as well as the retinal pigmentation. Also adjust the eyepiece diopter scale to match the operator's dioptric correction **(Fig. 18)**. Adjust the height of the motorized camera table as well as the operator's and patient's stool so both may be as comfortable as possible in front of the fundus camera **(Fig. 19)**.

Operational Procedures

The patient rests his/her chin on the chin rest and presses his/her forehead lightly against the forehead bar. Adjust the patient's lateral canthus with the head rest of the fundus camera and align the patient's eye with the illumination beam and optical pathway of the fundus camera. If necessary, adjust the optical table for optimal patient comfort.

Looking through the viewfinder of the fundus camera, focus the camera until you obtain a sharp image of the posterior segment of the eye. Slightly adjust the joystick (left-right-forward and backward) to set the camera to a position in which the subject's eye is evenly illuminated. It should be free from flares and reflections. One should try to achieve maximum color saturation. Ask the patient to gaze at the fixation target until you have the desired area of the fundus in your viewfinder. It is important for operator to ask the patient to keep both eyes open throughout the entire photographic session. Also, make certain that the eyelids as well as eyelashes should not obstruct the light passage. The light beam should be projected entirely into the pupil to avoid artifacts to be recorded on the film **(Fig. 20)**.

If pictures are taken before the above conditions are fully satisfied, reflections and/or artifacts will be produced and it will result in a lower picture quality and poor contrast. Once all these conditions have been fully satisfied, capture the image with a minimum delay, otherwise the patient may be tired and lose fixation and concentration. When the patient is asked to keep his eye open for over 30 seconds, the tear film starts breaking and cornea gets dry causing a low contrast photograph. It is important to always keep in mind that the patient's comfort and well-being is critical in order to achieve good photo documentation. Speak slowly and clearly explain the photographic procedure to the patient in order to lessen his or her anxiety.

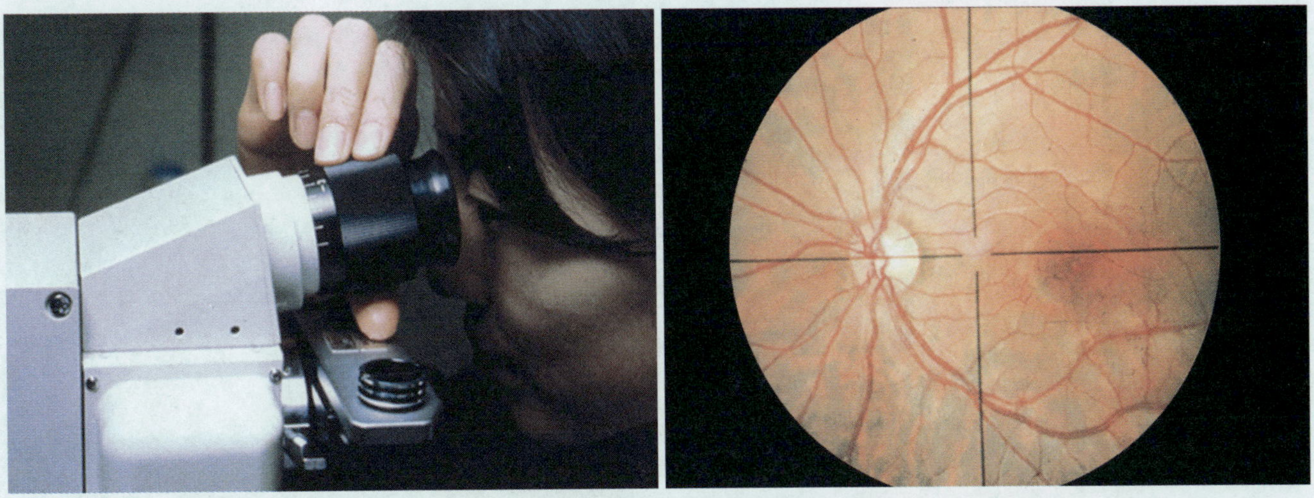

Fig. 18: Dioptric correction.

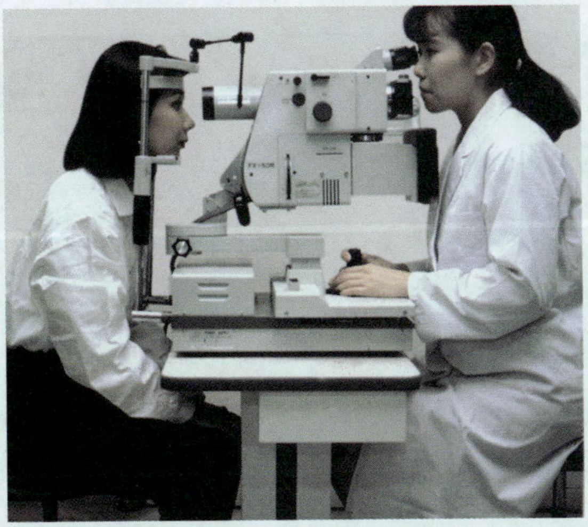

Fig. 19: Comfortable position.

FLUORESCEIN ANGIOGRAPHY

Ophthalmic photography is unique because the medical photographers also perform dynamic flow studies of the iris, retina or choroid using dyes such as sodium fluorescein or ICG. These studies provide a vital piece of information needed by the treating ophthalmologist in order to understand the vision problems of a patient. Fluorescein angiography is often more complex than conventional color retinal photography. This, however, is not the case, the main differences between color retinal photography and angiography are a set of filters (usually a set of exciter and barrier filter) and remembering the correct sequence of the flow study (area to be photographed in the early, mid or late phase that are usually recorded with a timer).

Principle of Sodium Fluorescein Angiography

Sodium fluorescein is mainly used to perform dynamic flow studies of the integrity of retinal vessels (in some cases,

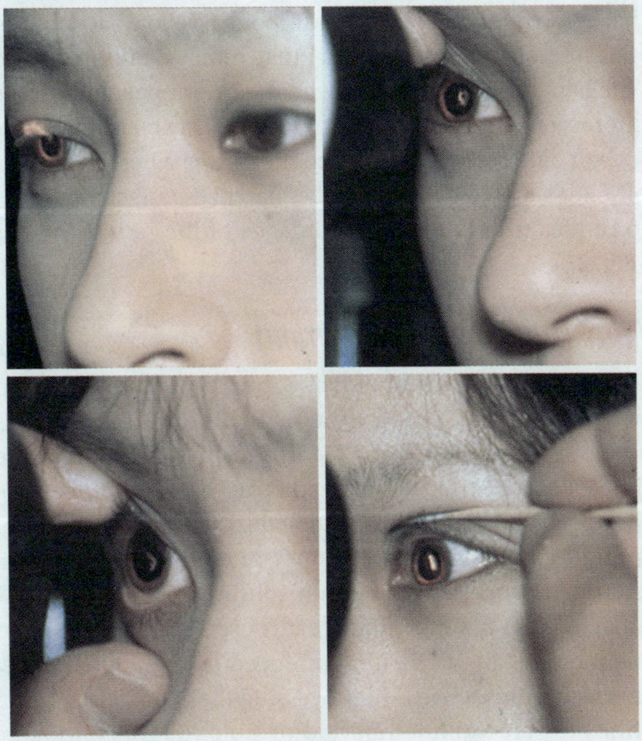

Fig. 20: Beam pathway.

sodium fluorescein may also be used in the study of the vascular integrity of the anterior segment). Once the pupils are sufficiently dilated, a solution with a concentration of 10% (2.5 cc of volume) or 25% (1 cc of volume) of sodium fluorescein is injected in the patient's vein. Injection volume should be carefully controlled in children or patients weighing less than 100 pounds. When using a concentration of 10% of sodium fluorescein, a recommended dose of 0.066 cc/kg should be used. It not only avoids adverse reactions but gives a good fluorescence standard in the dynamic flow study. The dye travels throughout the body's circulatory system (first throughout the veins) including the retinal vessels. When observing the retina with a cobalt blue light (referred to as the exciter light set at about 490 nm), sodium

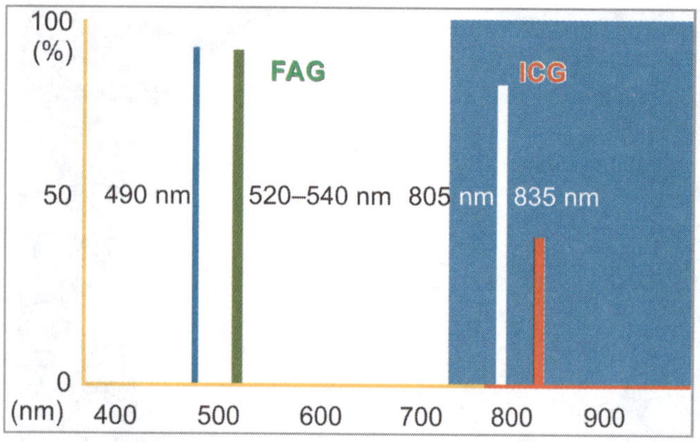

Fig. 21: Fluorescein absorption and emission. (FAG: fluorescein angiography; ICG: indocyanine green)

fluorescein reflects a green fluorescence toward the film plane of the retinal camera. Before arriving to the film plane, that green fluorescence passes through a yellow barrier filter (referred as the barrier filter) that removes all unwanted blue light that may interfere with the true appearance of the fluorescence found at about 520 nm. These exciter filters (cobalt blue set at 490 nm) and the barrier filter (sharp cut-off filter set at 520 nm) must be matched perfectly in order to render true fluorescence images of the retinal vessels **(Fig. 21)**.

Film Type and Development

The amount of fluorescence perceived by the film when properly excited by cobalt blue illumination is somewhat low; therefore, a highly sensitive black and white film such as ISO 400 film should be used. When processing this black and white film (in total darkness), use a medium to high-contrast fresh developer in conjunction with an extended processing time in a solution set at 20°C/68°F. Push process is a technique that is used in angiography to see more detail on the film produced by the fluorescence; this technique consists of processing the exposed sensitive (film) for an extended period of time (50–100% longer) or to process the film in a warmer solution say 2–4°C higher.

Photographic Procedures

Fluorescein angiographic study consists of several phases based on time sequence. Depending on the particular ocular disease, dynamic flow studies vary between 3 minutes and 15 minutes. Fluorescein angiography has following phases:

- *Preinjection or control photograph*: It is a photograph in which both the *exciter* and *barrier* filters are in place and a photograph is taken without the presence of sodium fluorescein. This is usually done to determine the presence of pseudofluorescence or autofluorescence such as in the case of *drusen*.

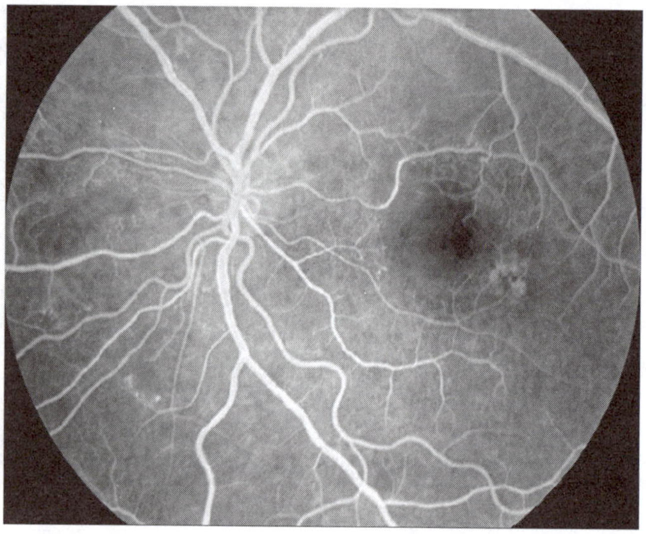

Fig. 22: Arterial/venous phase of fundus angiography.

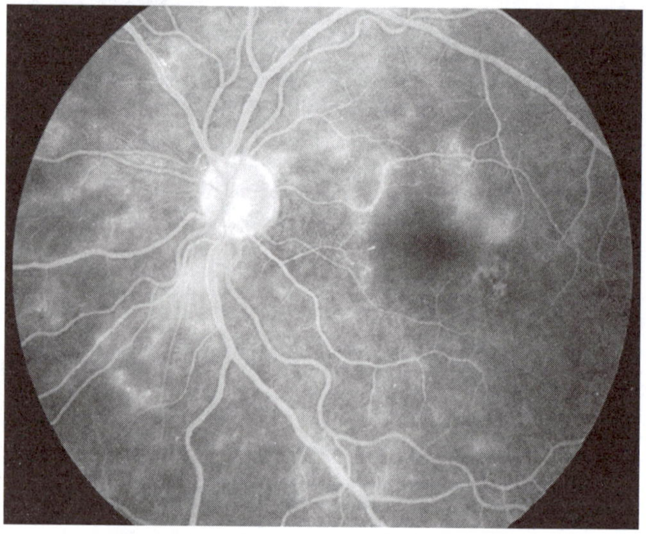

Fig. 23: Late phase of FA fundus angiography.

- *Arterial and venous phase*: This is the early phase of the angiogram study usually within 14–30 seconds after injection of sodium fluorescein **(Fig. 22)**.
- *Mid-phase*: When all retinal vessels have been filled (stained) with sodium fluorescein (from 30 seconds to 120 seconds).
- *Late phase:* This is the last phase and varies in duration depending on the disease of the patient. In diabetic retinopathy, this phase may vary from 3 minutes to 5 minutes, whereas in some ocular tumors, it may last as long as 15–20 minutes **(Fig. 23)**.

The fluorescein angiography helps in understanding various retinal diseases and abnormalities. One needs to study carefully the retinal drawing of the patient's chart and look for notes or direction from the retina specialist to understand the areas of interest and the main phase of the study (early, mid or late). It is critical to follow precisely the retina specialist's notes to understand the diseased eye to be first studied (right or left eye). How soon the retina

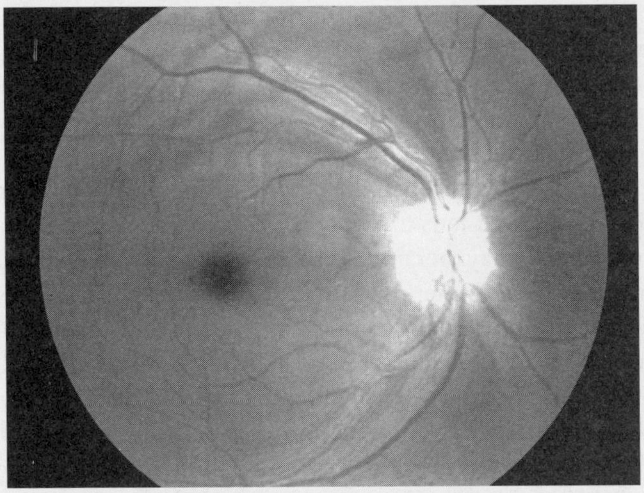

Fig. 24: Nerve fiber layer with blue filter.

specialist needs to evaluate the results of the angiogram? Does the retina specialist need to treat the patient with laser immediately after the angiographic study. This is referred to as a STAT angiogram. A good practice is to carefully study the diseased retinal areas when performing color photography, usually done prior to an angiography. Once you understand the ocular disease, you can start the angiographic procedure with a good plan. Number of images in each phase, early, mid and late phases as well as area of interest are dependent on a particular study. It is, however, important to get different results from what were initially anticipated. In fact, at times, angiographic pattern may be completely different from what was anticipated, a retinal vessel that was thought to be leaking may be intact and a normal one may be found leaking. Anticipating the unexpected findings comes with years of angiographic experience and a good set of standardized angiographic protocol.

MONOCHROMATIC FUNDUS PHOTOGRAPHY

Various monochromatic wavelengths penetrate at different layers of the eye revealing specific structures as well as foreign bodies in those layers. With the appropriate monochromatic wavelength filter (cobalt blue filter), it is possible to isolate the first layer of the retina where you can find the nerve fiber layers **(Fig. 24)**. This may be very useful while documenting a patient with glaucoma to demonstrate nerve fiber dropout. A green filter (referred to as red-free) will cut out all red-light making those areas black (red is seen as black) creating a nice high-contrast image of the posterior pole. Red filters will allow the longer wavelengths of the visible spectrum to penetrate deep into the ocular structures to reveal the choroidal vascular pattern (choroidal vessels appear as white while retinal vessels will appear as black as shown in **Figure 25**) and a choroidal nevus or melanoma **(Fig. 26)**. These photographs, in particular those taken with red-free light, are very suitable for printing use. Take one shot before starting fluorescein angiography.

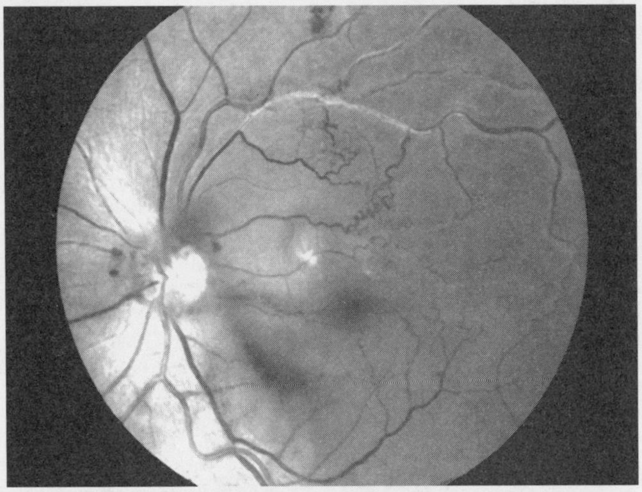

Fig. 25: Red-free photography.

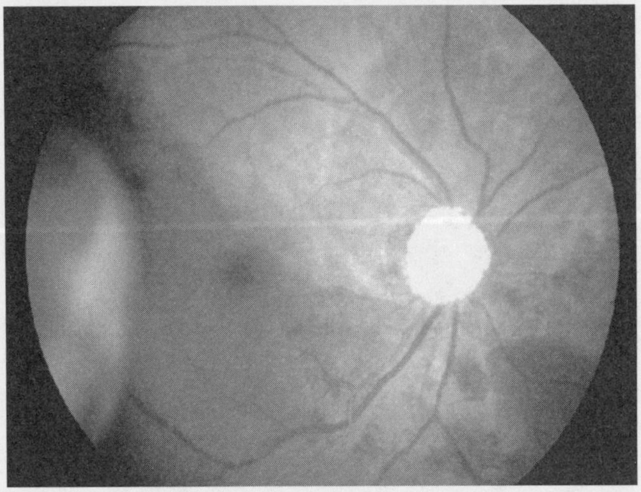

Fig. 26: Choroidal pigment with red filter.

PHOTO SLIT-LAMP BIOMICROGRAPHY OF ANTERIOR SEGMENT

The anterior segment is usually photographed with a photo slit-lamp biomicroscope. It is similar to the clinical slit-lamp biomicroscope that is used in our daily work; with the exception that it incorporates a camera (static or motion such as video) and an electronic flash light **(Fig. 27)**. Needless to say, photographers need a good understanding of the clinical instrument before they can become skillful in capturing clinically useful images of the anterior segment **(Fig. 28)**. Different from fundus photography, photo slit-lamp biomicroscopy is perhaps the most challenging type of photography in the field of ophthalmology. It requires a good understanding of the ocular structures; disease process as well as illumination techniques to illustrate the area of interest to the clinician. The illumination is of key importance.

Since pathology varies greatly and may appear differently for each case, simple changes of slit-width, height angle of the illumination tower or even the use of diffuser, the same

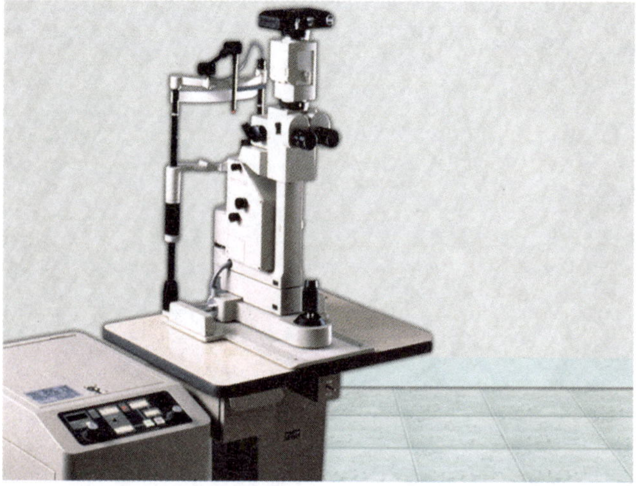

Fig. 27: Photograph of slit lamp.

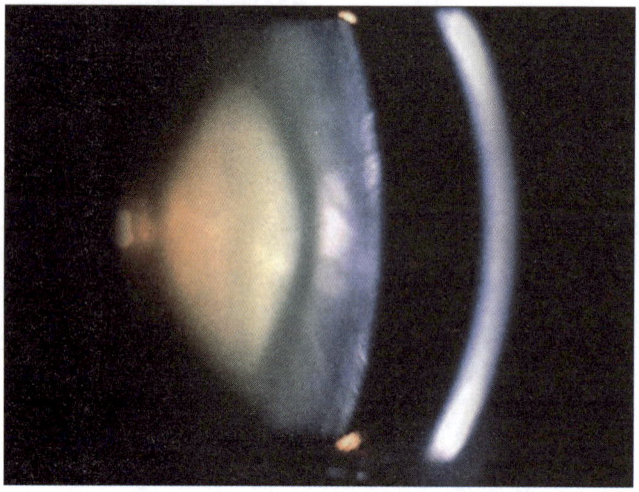

Fig. 28: Slit-lamp photograph of lens with various nuclei.

pathology may show itself quite differently in the final picture. It becomes essential to select most suitable lighting technique for each situation. This challenge is perhaps what gives the photographer greatest pleasure in taking pictures: to be able to illustrate best an area of interest.

In observing through the slit-lamp, the reflections from the cornea and lens are not so offensive. However, same reflections may become disturbing and even harmful in hiding areas of interest when taking photographs. Carefully adjust the illumination tower angle to avoid unwanted reflections. When using auxiliary light (often referred to as fill light), it is necessary to pay attention to avoid the reflection that light may produce on the cornea. Carefully place the area of interest in the field to be photographed while making certain that you are using the best possible form of illumination. Use appropriate magnification to ensure that not only the area of interest is captured but you leave enough room to have a point of reference for follow-up photographic sessions, e.g. in photographing an iris melanoma; use of medium magnification would allow for a portion of the iris to be seen for identification that the mass is located at 12, 3, 6 or 9 o'clock and provides an idea about the size of the mass.

SUGGESTED READING

1. Fogla R, Rao SK. Ophthalmic photography using a digital camera. Indian J Ophthalmol. 2003;51:69-72.
2. Kwan A. A simple slit lamp digital photographic system. Eye News. 2000;6:18-21.
3. Prasad S. Digital video in a surgical setting. J Cataract Refract Surg. 2004;30:2302-3.

CHAPTER

13

Fundus Autofluorescence Applications in Retinal Practice

Anand Rajendran, Vinay PG, Vishal MY

INTRODUCTION

Autofluorescence (AF), originating from the lipofuscin-laden retinal pigment epithelium (RPE) cells, has been recognized and evaluated for a few decades now. In the RPE, lipofuscin is largely located in phagocytosed photoreceptor outer segments (OS) whereas in various other cell types, it is generated internally by autodigestion.[1,2] Phagocytosis of the apices of the photoreceptor OS, and their consequent digestion by lysosomes, is one of the cardinal functions of the RPE.[1-3] Although the digestion of these OS is nearly complete, a fractional portion stays undigested—the lipofuscin. The accumulation of fluorescent material in the RPE reflects the level of metabolic activity, which is largely determined by the quanta of photoreceptor OS renewal. Over the age of 70, approximately 20–33% of the cytoplasmic volume may be comprised of lipofuscin and melanofuscin granules.

Hence, AF imaging is, quintessentially, a topographic "metabolic mapping" of the lipofuscin in the RPE and other fluorophores in the outer retina and subretinal space. This retinal AF is understood to reflect a balance between accumulation and removal of lipofuscin in the RPE. The lipofuscin in the RPE cells is extraordinary, as this is largely formed as a result of the light energy trapping function of the retina. The lipofuscin is primarily concentrated in the RPE of the central retina, the region possessing the highest concentration of visual pigment as well as receiving the greatest amount of light. These retinoid-derived fluorophores abound in conjugated double bonds which explains the long wavelength fluorescence emission from the lipofuscin.[4]

DEMONSTRATION OF FUNDUS AUTOFLUORESCENCE

Vitreous fluorophotometry gave us the first in-vivo evidence of fundus autofluorescence (FAF). A distinct "retinal" peak was noted in the preinjection scans, whose magnitude increased with age in keeping with the known properties of lipofuscin fluorescence.[5,6] These studies led to the development of a fundus spectrofluorometer[7,8] created to evaluate, specifically, the excitation and emission spectra of the AF from small retinal foci (2° diameter) of the fundus and to permit absolute measurements of the emanated fluorescence.

Fundus Autofluorescence Imaging Modalities

Confocal Scanning Laser Ophthalmoscope

Although originally developed by Webb and coworkers, it was in 1995 that von Ruckmann et al. first described FAF imaging with the confocal scanning laser ophthalmoscope (cSLO).[9,10]

The FAF signal has, compared to fundus reflectance or fluorescence angiography, a very low intensity. In order to enhance image contrast and reduce background noise, several single FAF images are recorded in series.[9,11-14] The mean image (of 4–16 frames) is then calculated, and the pixel values are normalized. The high rate of up to 16 frames per second and the high sensitivity of the cSLO allow FAF imaging to be recorded in rapidly and at minimal excitation energies.[15]

Three different cSLO systems have thus far been developed for creating FAF images—Heidelberg retina angiograph [HRA classic, HRA 2 and Spectralis HRA, Heidelberg Engineering, Heidelberg, Germany; Rodenstock cSLO (RcSLO; Rodenstock, Weco, Dusseldorf, Germany), and Zeiss prototype SM 30 4024 (ZcSLO; Zeiss, Oberkochen, Germany)]. Only the former is commercially available. These instruments use an excitation wavelength of 488 nm generated by an argon or solid-state laser for FAF imaging.

An additional development of the cSLO (Spectralis HRA + OCT, Heidelberg Engineering, Heidelberg, Germany) is combination with spectral-domain optical coherence tomography (OCT) in the same instrument. This permits simultaneous cSLO and OCT recordings. With the cSLO system, any lateral eye movement can be detected in real time and input into the scanning system of the OCT modality, facilitating a very accurate registration of the OCT A-scans.

Another key feature is that, with the use of any of the cSLO imaging modes (reflectance, FAF, or angiography) as the reference image, retinal locations on the fundus image can be mapped to cross-sectional OCT findings with precision. The extremely high resolution of these images has likened them to "optical biopsies" of the retina.

Fundus Camera

The lipofuscin can be stimulated, by direct illumination, to fluoresce and has a wide emission band ranging from about 500 nm to 750 nm.[16] However, other structures in the eye in front of the retina also fluoresce—the crystalline lens, being one of the foremost. In order to obtain clear and good quality AF images, the instrument has to be able to either reject or circumvent the fluorescence from the lens.

Scanning laser ophthalmoscopes has a confocal capability in which only conjugate points on the fundus are imaged. Points not lying on the conjugate planes are rejected. This allows cSLOs to use excitation and barrier wavelengths similar to those used in fluorescein angiography to obtain AF photographs.

While the initial camera-based systems were restricted by lower contrast and narrower fields of view, the next generations involved shifting the excitation and emission wavelengths toward the red end of the spectrum to preclude AF from lens.[17,18] Image quality was enhanced using a new set of filters. A band-pass filter centered at about 580 nm for excitation and another centered at about 695 nm as a barrier filter were used. The nuclear sclerosis of the lens does not attenuate these. Additionally, as the lens fluorescence occurs with wavelengths shorter than the upper cutoff of the barrier filter, lens AF rarely is a problem with moderate degrees of nuclear sclerosis. The limitations of this system for AF include all those associated with a typical fundus camera especially, for patients with small pupils.

Differences between the Autofluorescence Images Taken with a Confocal Scanning Laser Ophthalmoscope and a Fundus Camera

The wavelengths used with the commercially available cSLO are absorbed more by blood as compared with the wavelengths in the modified fundus camera. This makes the contrast between the vessels and background more in cSLO images than in the images from the fundus camera. This possibly, is the reason why the optic nerve often shows more fluorescence with a fundus camera system than with the cSLO. Light scattering affects fundus camera systems more than cSLO systems. All these factors may lead to a lesser ability of the fundus camera system to discern smaller retinal vessels as compared to the cSLO. Macular pigments or fluorescein does not absorb the wavelengths used in the fundus camera. Fundus cameras utilize a cone of light entering the eye, hence, small pupillary apertures reduce the intensity of AF. Fundus camera images need manual removal of the excess lens AF from patients with advanced degrees of nuclear sclerosis.

ASSESSING THE FUNDUS AUTOFLUORESCENCE IMAGE

When a FAF image is being evaluated, any abnormal recording should be discerned, and a plausible cause should be investigated for. The characteristics of a normal FAF image which need to be understood are as follows:

The *optic nerve head* is devoid of the RPE and the autofluorescent lipofuscin and is hence, characteristically dark. The *retinal vessels* are also dark because of absorption from blood constituents. The *macular area* has the FAF signal most markedly reduced at the fovea. Beginning from the foveal center, a faint yet discernible increase in the signal can be observed at about the margin of the fovea, with a further steady increment toward the outer macula.

Beyond these areas with decrements in FAF intensity, the FAF signal appears evenly distributed **(Figs. 1A and B)**.

The quality of the recorded image determines the accuracy with which abnormalities in the FAF image are depicted. Any opacities in the cornea, vitreous, the lens, or the anterior chamber may affect the detection of pathologies at the level of the RPE and the neurosensory retina.

CAUSES FOR A REDUCED FUNDUS AUTOFLUORESCENCE SIGNAL

Reduction in Retinal Pigment Epithelium Lipofuscin Density

- Retinal pigment epithelium atrophy [such as geographic atrophy (GA)]
- Hereditary retinal dystrophies (such as RPE65 mutations).

Increased Retinal Pigment Epithelium Melanin Content

For example, RPE hypertrophy.

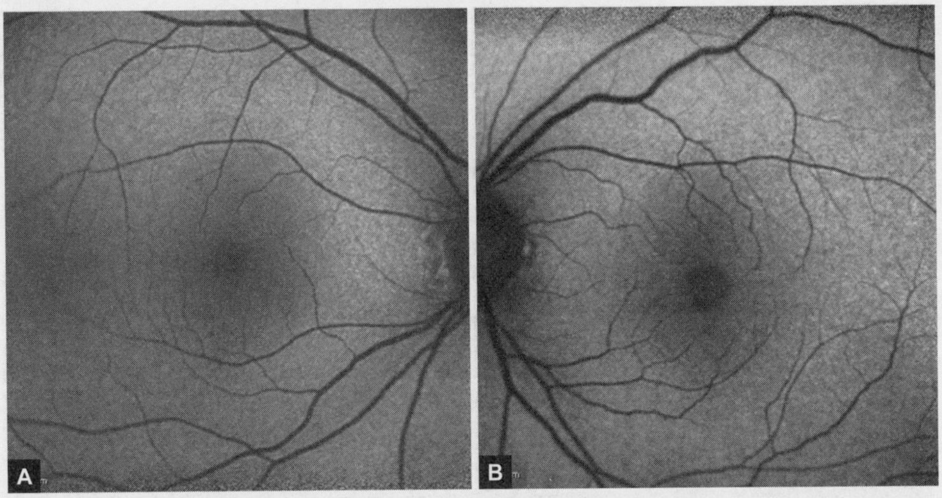

Figs. 1A and B: The normal fundus autofluorescence patterns seen in the (A) right and (B) left eye of a patient.

Absorption from Extracellular Material/ Cells/Fluid Anterior to the Retinal Pigment Epithelium

- Intraretinal fluid (such as macular edema)
- Migrated melanin-containing cells
- Crystalline drusen or other crystal-like deposits
- Fresh intraretinal and subretinal hemorrhages
- Fibrosis, scar tissue, borders of laser scars
- Retinal vessels
- Luteal pigment (lutein and zeaxanthin)
- Media opacities (vitreous, lens, anterior chamber, and cornea).

CAUSES FOR AN INCREASED FUNDUS AUTOFLUORESCENCE SIGNAL

Excessive Retinal Pigment Epithelium Lipofuscin Accumulation

- Lipofuscinopathies, including Stargardt disease, Best disease, pattern dystrophy, and adult vitelliform macular dystrophy
- Age-related macular degeneration (AMD), such as RPE in the junctional zone preceding enlargement of occurrence of GA.

Occurrence of Fluorophores Anterior or Posterior to the Retinal Pigment Epithelium Cell Monolayer

- Intraretinal fluid (such as macular edema)
- Subpigment epithelial fluid in pigment epithelial detachments
- Drusen in the subpigment epithelial space
- Migrated RPE cells or macrophages containing lipofuscin or melanolipofuscin (seen as pigment clumping or hyperpigmentation on funduscopy)
- Older intraretinal and subretinal hemorrhages
- Choroidal vessel in the presence of RPE and choriocapillaris atrophy, such as in the center of laser scars or within patches of RPE atrophy
- Choroidal nevi and melanoma.

Lack of absorbing material:

- Depletion of luteal pigment, such as in idiopathic macular telangiectasia (IMT) type 2
- Displacement of luteal pigment, such as in cystoid macular edema.

CLINICAL APPLICATIONS

Macular and Retinal Dystrophies

In several macular and retinal dystrophies, autofluorescent material does aggregate in the RPE and the extracellular deposits in the neurosensory space may also be fluorescent. FAF imaging enables detection of the abnormal phenotype in some disorders when it is not otherwise evident **(Figs. 2A to D)**.

Clinically discernible pale yellowish deposits at the level of the RPE/Bruch's membrane in Best's disease **(Figs. 3A to D)**, adult vitelliform macular dystrophy, fundus albipunctatus **(Figs. 4A to D)**, and Stargardt's macular dystrophy or fundus flavimaculatus are associated with markedly increased FAF intensities.[16,19] The focal flecks in Stargardt's disease are much more clearly highlighted on FAF images in comparison to fundus photographs **(Figs. 5A and B)**. They show a bright FAF signal that may weaken as atrophy develops. Cone dystrophies also have a typical circular ring of hyper-AF as seen in **Figure 6**.

Age-related Macular Degeneration I: Early Manifestation

Age-related macular degeneration, a complex disease with both genetic and environmental factors, has become the

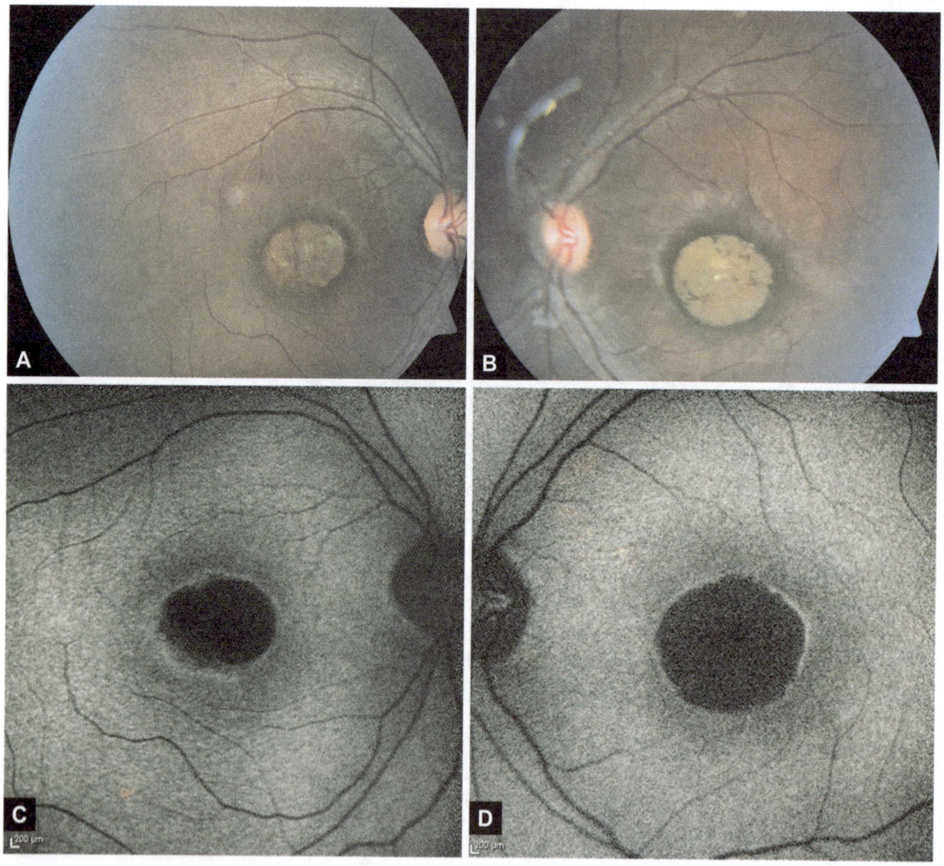

Figs. 2A to D: A patient diagnosed as advanced atrophic Stargardt's disease with the fundus photographs (A and B) and the fundus autofluorescence images (C and D) revealing central hypoautofluorescence reflecting the RPE atrophic pathology surrounded by the hyperautofluorescent ring.

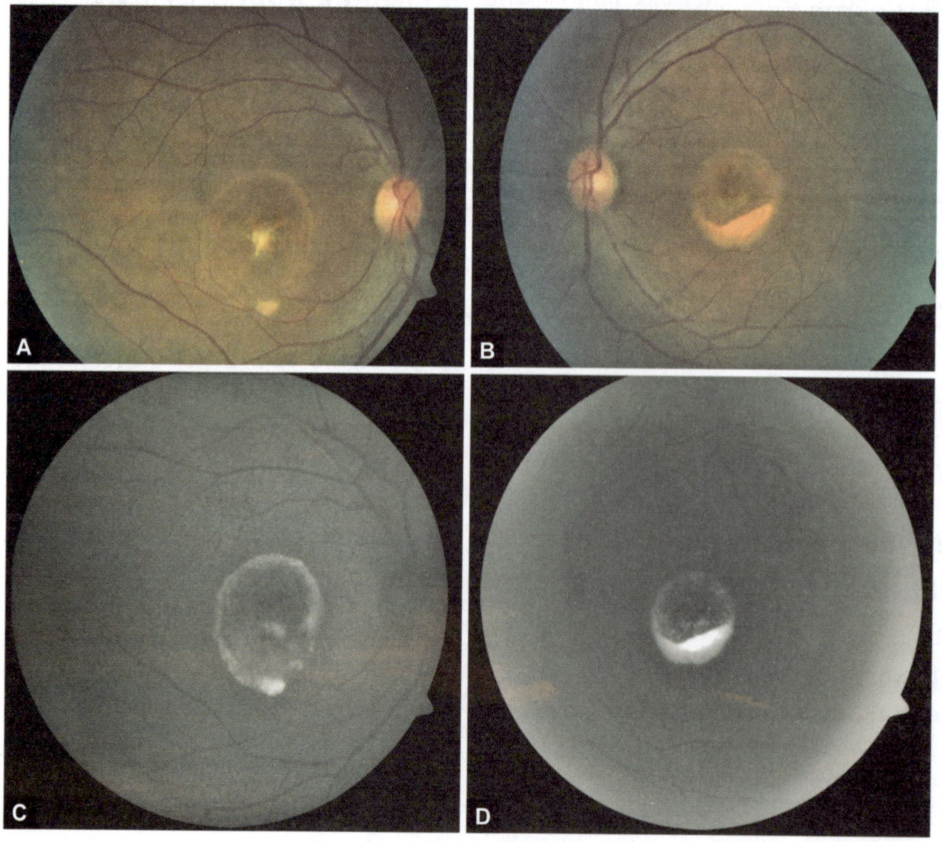

Figs. 3A to D: The fundus pictures (A and B) and the corresponding fundus autofluorescence pictures of a patents with Best's disease; (C and D) demonstrating the hyperautofluorescence emanating from the accumulated lipofuscin-laden deposit in the neurosensory space.

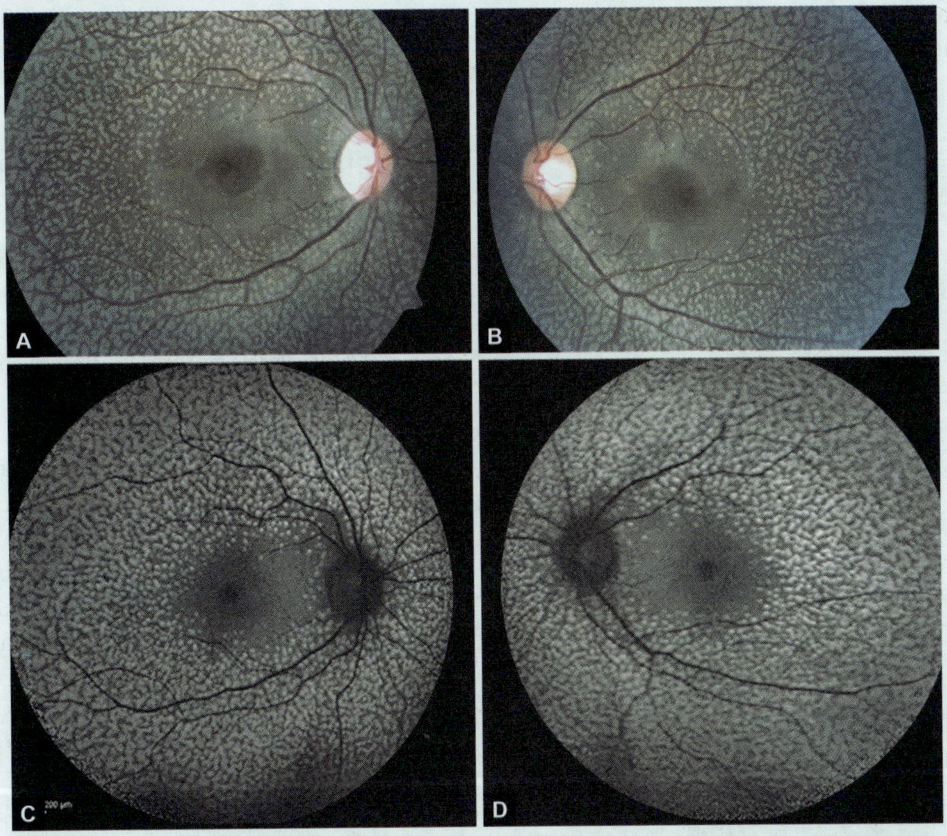

Figs. 4A to D: A patient with fundus albipunctatus with fundus pictures (A and B) and corresponding autofluorescence images (C and D) showing the hyperautofluorescent specks.

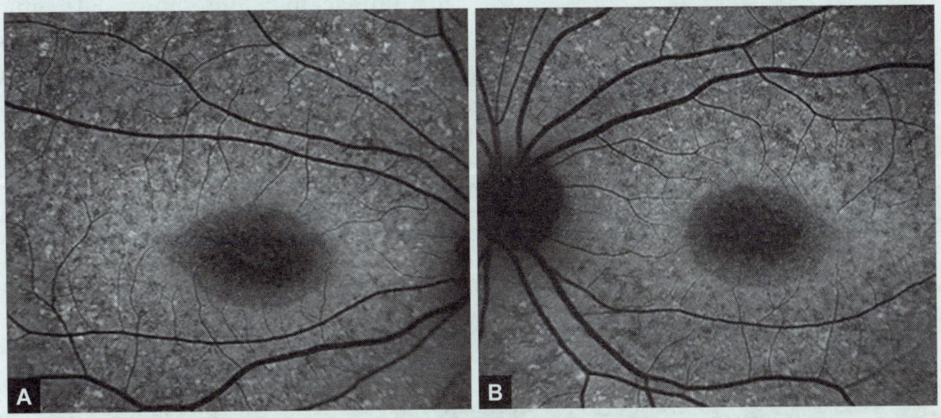

Figs. 5A and B: A patient with the classical Stargardt's fundus autofluorescence patterns—with a central mottled hypoautofluorescence surrounded by hyperautofluorescent flecks radiating from the macula with hypoautofluorescent speckles around in the right (A) and left (B) eyes.

most common cause of legal blindness in industrialized countries.[20-23] A hallmark of ageing is the accumulation of lipofuscin granules in the cytoplasm of RPE cells **(Figs. 7A and B)**.

Fundus autofluorescence as an imaging modality has been studied recently in patients with AMD. These help us to know the spatial correlation of FAF findings with established early AMD changes such as focal hypo- and hyperpigmentation and drusen.

One important observation in patients with early AMD is that alterations in the FAF signal are not necessarily associated with corresponding funduscopically or angiographically visible changes such as drusen and irregular hyper- or hypopigmentations.[18,23,24]

This indicates that FAF findings may represent an independent measure of disease stage and activity.

CLASSIFICATION OF FUNDUS AUTOFLUORESCENCE PATTERNS IN EARLY AGE-RELATED MACULAR DEGENERATION

Fundus autofluorescence findings in patients with early AMD were recently published by an international workshop on FAF phenotyping in early AMD.[3] Pooling data from several retinal centers, researchers developed a classification system with eight different FAF patterns.

It demonstrates the relatively poor correlation between visible alterations on fundus photography and notable FAF changes. Based on these results, it was speculated that FAF findings in early AMD may indicate more widespread abnormalities and diseased areas.

These changes on FAF imaging at the RPE cell level may precede the occurrence of visible lesions as the disease progresses.

RETICULAR DRUSEN

Reticular drusen can be identified as a peculiar pattern on FAF images, with multiple relatively uniform roundish or elongated spots with decreased intensities and surrounded by an interlacing network of normal-appearing FAF signals.[23]

These are readily identified on FAF images and easily detected than on funduscopy or fundus photographs. The exact anatomic location (i.e. sub-RPE, Bruch's membrane, and choriocapillaris) and morphological pattern is not clearly understood.

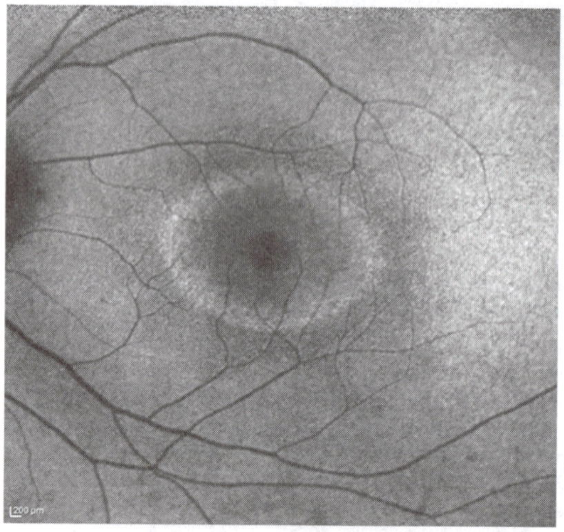

Fig. 6: Autofluorescence pattern of a patient with cone dystrophy with the central hypoautofluorescent nidus along with the typical hyperautofluorescent perimacular halo.

Age-related Macular Degeneration II: Geographic Atrophy

Geographic atrophy represents the atrophic late-stage manifestation of "dry" AMD, characterized by development of atrophic patches that may initially occur in the parafoveal area.[25-27] During the natural course of the disease, atrophy slowly enlarges over time, and there is foveal sparing until later.

Due to the distinct changes of the topographic distribution of RPE lipofuscin, which is the dominant fluorophore for FAF imaging the signal is markedly reduced over atrophic areas, while high-intensity FAF levels can be observed in the junctional zone surrounding the atrophic patches. FFA and fundus photography do not show any morphological changes at this stage.

DETECTION AND QUANTIFICATION OF ATROPHY

As FAF signal intensity is markedly reduced, areas of atrophy can be readily visualized on FAF images. In contrast to fluorescein angiography, FAF imaging represents a noninvasive imaging method and is less time consuming.

The advantages of FAF imaging in GA have been used to detect and precisely quantify atrophic areas on FAF images using customized image analysis software.[28,29] This software allows the automated segmentation of atrophic areas by a region algorithm. Interfering retinal blood vessels that have a similar FAF intensity compared with atrophic areas are recognized by the software and can be excluded from the measurements.

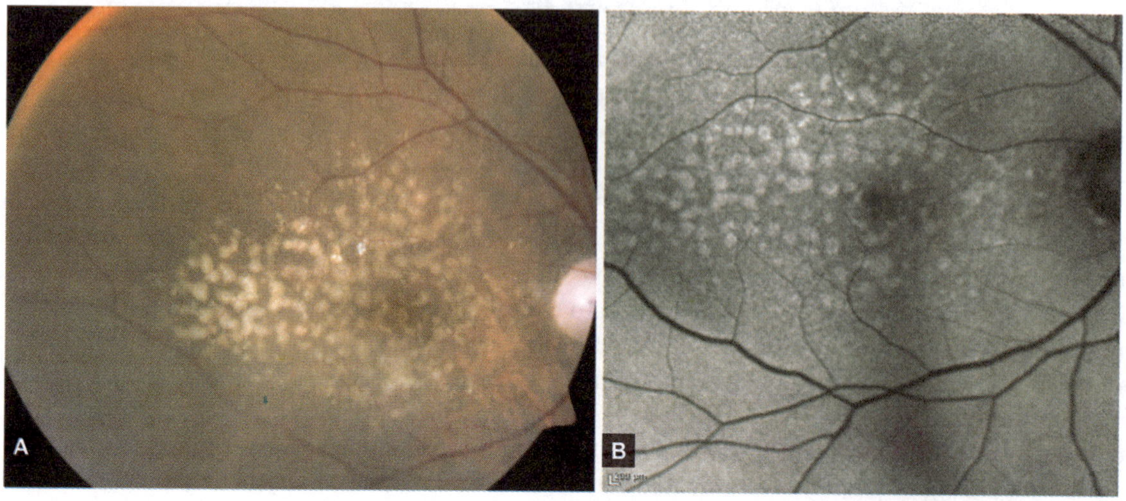

Figs. 7A and B: The fundus picture (A) and autofluorescence image (B) highlighting the copious autofluorescence from the drusenoid material.

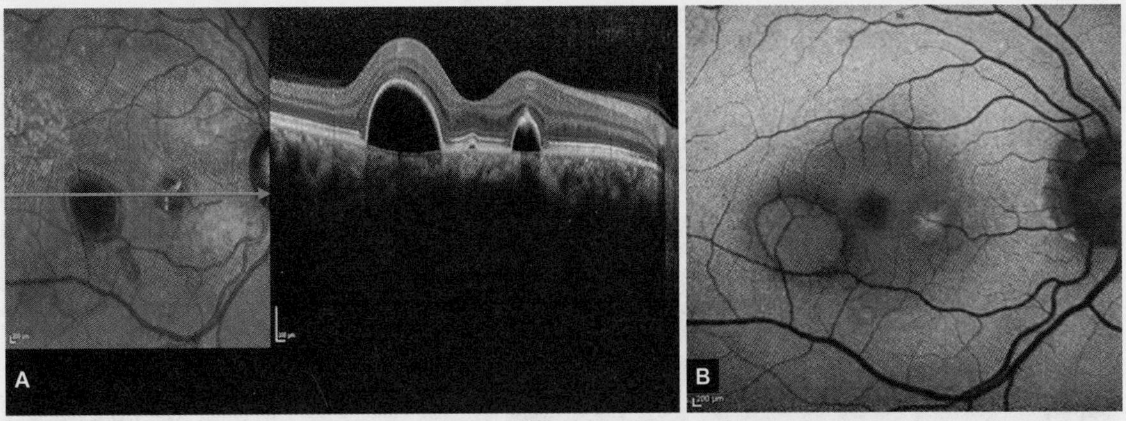

Figs. 8A and B: The optical coherence tomography picture (A) and corresponding fundus autofluorescence image (B) showing a large detachment of the retinal pigment epithelium with intermediate fundus autofluorescence signal with surrounding well-defined less autofluorescent halo-delineating the entire border of the lesion.

Further developments include the alignment of FAF images at different examinations using retinal landmarks in order to correct for different scan angles and magnifications. This allows accurate assessment of atrophy progression overtime and can be used in longitudinal observations, including interventional trials.

Age-related Macular Degeneration III: Pigment Epithelium Detachment

Retinal pigment epithelial detachments (PEDs) are a common feature of advanced AMD. Conventional imaging techniques such as fundus photography, fluorescein, or indocyanine green angiography cannot detect the variations in the area of PED which can be seen by FAF signal in that area.

Changes in FAF intensities in patients with PED secondary to AMD can be classified into four groups. Other dominant fluorophores with similar excitation and emission spectra inside the PED, such as extracellular fluid or degraded photoreceptors, may be present and contribute to typical patterns with abnormal FAF intensity **(Figs. 8A and B)**. FAF phenotypes may reflect not only different stages in the evolution of a PED but also heterogeneity on a cellular and molecular level in the disease process, and may thus be relevant for future molecular genetic analyses.

Age-related Macular Degeneration IV: Choroidal Neovascularization

Choroidal neovascularization (CNV) is a common cause of visual loss in patients with AMD and represents the growth of subretinal new vessels in the macular region.

FUNDUS AUTOFLUORESCENCE FINDINGS IN EARLY CHOROIDAL NEOVASCULARIZATION

Eyes with "recent-onset" CNV were found to have patches of "continuous" or "normal" AF corresponding to areas of hyperfluorescence on the comparative fluorescein angiograms. This implied that RPE viability was preserved at least initially in CNV development.

Fundus autofluorescence imaging was able to delineate the edge of CNV lesions better than FFA and it was statistically larger.[30]

FUNDUS AUTOFLUORESCENCE FINDINGS IN LATE STAGE CHOROIDAL NEOVASCULARIZATION

In eyes with long-standing CN, decreased areas of AF were seen, implying nonviable RPE, and lack of photoreceptor outer segment renewal. These represent areas of RPE atrophy beneath the CNV scars in the late stages of disease,[30] whereas areas of increased FAF seen inferior to lesions were thought to be due to a gravitational effect of fluid tracking under the retina, similar to that seen in central serous retinopathy.[31,32] Increased FAF signal has also been described around the edge of lesions that are thought to represent proliferation of RPE cells around the CNV.[30,31]

FUNDUS AUTOFLUORESCENCE FINDINGS IN RELATION TO CHOROIDAL NEOVASCULARIZATION CLASSIFICATION

Classic Choroidal Neovascularization

Purely classic lesions showed low or decreased FAF signal at the site of the CNV, with a ring of increased FAF around some lesions **(Figs. 9A and B)**.

Occult Choroidal Neovascularization

According to McBain et al., foci of decreased FAF were seen scattered within the lesion. These were felt to be due to small areas of RPE loss or damage caused by the chronic, more indolent lesions growing underneath the RPE. Areas

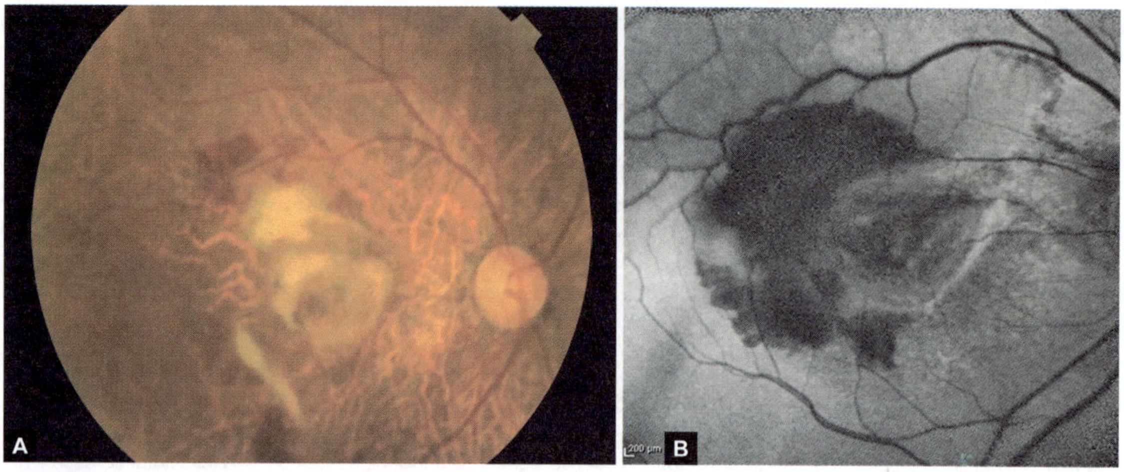

Figs. 9A and B: The fundus picture (A) and autofluorescence image (B) showing the choroidal neovascular membrane.

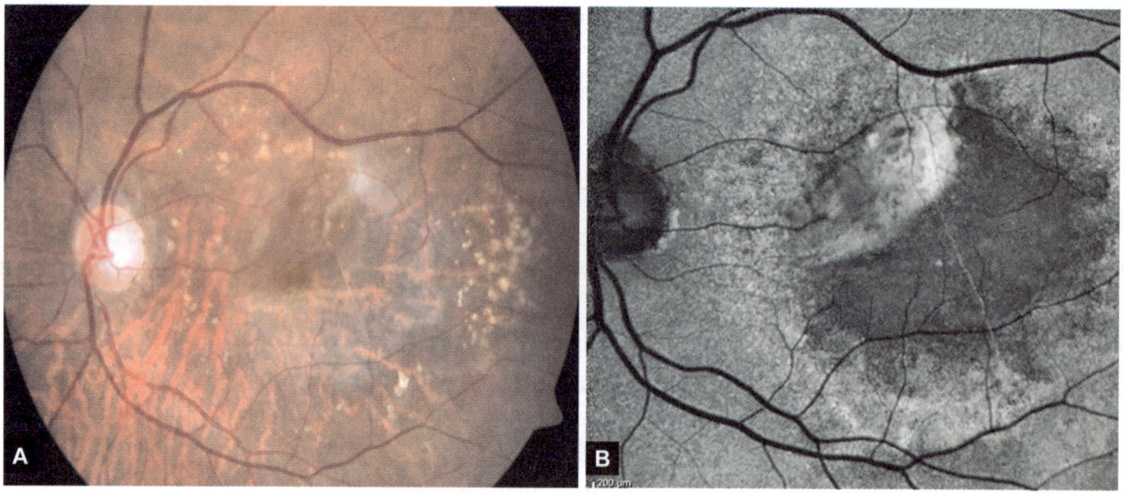

Figs. 10A and B: The fundus picture (A) and autofluorescence image (B) showing retinal pigment epithelium tear following development of choroidal neovascularization secondary to age-related macular degeneration.

of increased FAF were less frequently associated with the edge of occult lesions compared with predominantly classic lesions.

Retinal Pigment Epithelium Tears

Areas with RPE loss are characterized by a very low signal and intense hypo-AF because of a complete lack of RPE and loss of lipofuscin. They are sharply demarcated. The adjacent area with rolled-up RPE is characterized by heterogeneous signal of distinct increased FAF. Thus, the exact location of the tear can be delineated in most cases **(Figs. 10A and B)**.

IDIOPATHIC MACULAR TELANGIECTASIA

Idiopathic macular telangiectasia (also known as idiopathic parafoveal telangiectasis) is a descriptive term for different disease entities presenting with telangiectatic alterations of the juxtafoveolar capillary network with a predominant location temporal to the fovea **(Figs. 11A and B)**.[31,33]

Fundus Autofluorescence in Type 1 Idiopathic Macular Telangiectasia

Fundus autofluorescence imaging may show an increased signal that may be explained by a reduced macular pigment optical density (MPOD) due to retinal tissue defects in the area with cystoid changes. However, overall the distribution is normal, with the highest MPOD in the fovea and attenuation toward the periphery.

Fundus Autofluorescence in Type 2 Idiopathic Macular Telangiectasia

Macular pigment optical density is typically reduced in the macular area, and the area of depletion largely corresponds to angiographic late-phase hyperfluorescence and increased confocal blue reflectance. In early stages, FAF shows minimal alteration, whereas in late stages, it may be grossly abnormal. When intraretinal pigment clumping has occurred, FAF may show a reduced signal due to a blockade phenomenon.

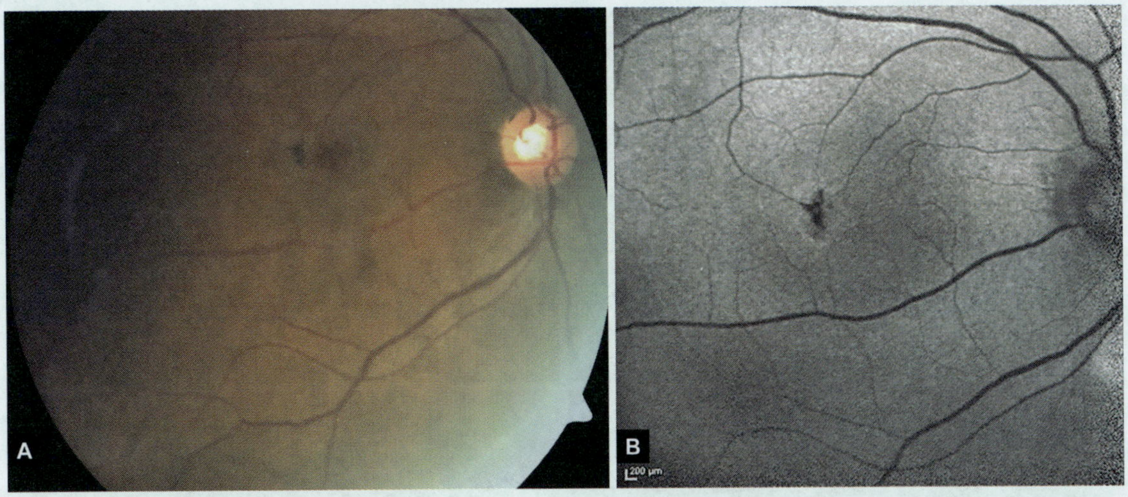

Figs. 11A and B: A patient with MacTel or IJT—the clinical picture (A) and the fundus autofluorescence; (B) showing the intense hypoautofluorescence of the pigment deposits.
(MacTel: macular telangiectasia; IJT: idiopathic juxtafoveolar retinal telangiectasis)

Table 1: Ocular diseases with their autofluorescence patterns and corresponding clinical features.

Ocular disease	*FAF pattern*	*Correlation with fundus finding*
Choroidal neovascularization	• Hypofluorescence—hemorrhage, exudates, and atrophy • Hyperfluorescence—active LF and RPE proliferation	FAF signal typically extends beyond the edge defined by color fundus image and fluorescein angiography
Stargardt's and Best's disease	• Hyperfluorescence ranging from intense to moderate on LF concentration • Hypofluorescence areas in end stage and with RPE atrophy	RPE atrophy is not initially visible on fundus examination
Central serous chorioretinopathy	*Acute*: Hyperfluorescent areas in the active stages *Chronic*: Hypofluorescent areas	*Acute*: FAF highlights edge of the detachment that may or may not be visible on fundus examination *Chronic*: RPE cell death not visible on fundus examination
Pan retinal photocoagulation	Hypofluorescent signal followed by weak hyperfluorscence due to RPE proliferation/scar formation	Laser scar correlate with hypofluorescence

(FAF: Fundus autofluorescence; LF: lipofuscin; RPE: retinal pigment epithelium)

Autofluorescence patterns and clinical morphology of diseases are shown in **Table 1**.

Chorioretinal Inflammatory Disorders

Autofluorescence photography complements other methods of imaging the ocular fundus. The amount of AF is governed by the amount of fluorophores in any given area in the fundus.

Choroidal neovascularization associated with intraocular inflammation is a common complication, and this secondary CNV produces characteristic AF findings. By observing AF characteristics, we can estimate the extent of damage, diagnose sequelae such as secondary CNV, learn more about the inflammatory process in question, and possibly anticipate future problems caused by disease **(Figs. 12A to D)**.

ACUTE POSTERIOR MULTIFOCAL PLACOID PIGMENT EPITHELIOPATHY

In the acute phases of acute posterior multifocal placoid pigment epitheliopathy (APMPPE), more lesions are visible by either fluorescein angiography or ophthalmoscopy than are visible by AF photography.[34]

The areas of decreased pigmentation with increased fluorescence and decreased AF suggest atrophy or absence of functional RPE cells. Given the finding of increased pigmentation and AF centrally with a depigmented hypoautofluorescent surround, it is possible that with healing of the lesions there was a centripetal contraction of each placoid lesion with retraction of the edges inward.

The implication of these findings is that the RPE is affected secondarily to the choroidal changes, and the RPE undergoes alterations well after the choroid is affected.

ACUTE SYPHILITIC POSTERIOR PLACOID CHORIORETINITIS

Acute syphilitic posterior placoid chorioretinitis (ASPPC) shares similarities to APMPPE in that both conditions can cause yellowish plaque-like changes in the posterior pole.[35] There are important differences in appearance, and probably in pathophysiology. ASPPC usually causes a solitary yellow placoid lesion that has a more prominent color and

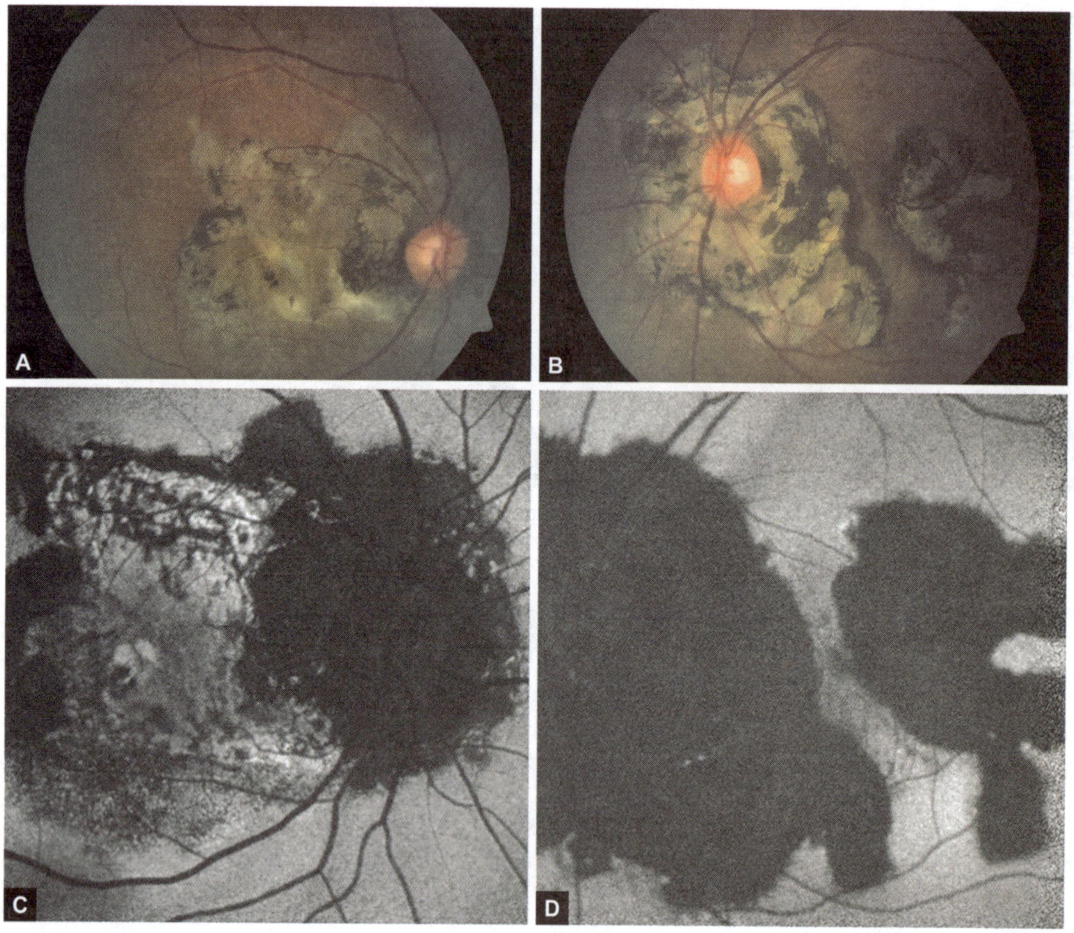

Figs. 12A to D: The clinical picture (A and B) of a case of healed geographic helicoid peripapillary choroidopathy with the fundus autofluorescence images (C and D) demonstrating the deep hypoautofluorescence of the scarred area and the neighboring mottled hyperautofluorescence.

opacification at its outer borders. The AF abnormalities are confined only to the placoid region.

MULTIFOCAL CHOROIDITIS AND PANUVEITIS

Autofluorescence photography of multifocal choroiditis and panuveitis (MCP) demonstrates clinically visible chorioretinal scars as hypoautofluorescent.[36] However, AF photography often shows many more times the number of hypoautofluorescent spots than the number of chorioretinal scars. Subsequent development of visible chorioretinal spots has occurred in areas occupied by the hypoautofluorescent spots seen by AF imaging. Thus AF appears to show areas of RPE damage from MCP that are more numerous and extensive than what the choroidal scars would indicate.

Secondary CNV is visible as a butterfly-shaped area of hyper-AF. The borders of the AF show prominent attachments to hypoautofluorescent MCP scars. The hyper-AF of past CNV persists despite subsequent treatment. Of interest is the finding of small hyperautofluorescent spots or rings in the vicinity of MCP scars.

ACUTE ZONAL OCCULT OUTER RETINOPATHY

The autofluorescent findings in acute zonal occult outer retinopathy (AZOOR) are limited largely because AZOOR is a rare disease. AF photography showed that the outer border was intensely autofluorescent, consistent with the presence of lipofuscin, and that the central area of the lesion was hypoautofluorescent, consistent with atrophy of the RPE. The patient had visual field abnormalities in the eye consistent with the location and size of the AF abnormality.

BIRDSHOT CHORIORETINOPATHY

Autofluorescent abnormalities are usually associated with the depigmented lesions, while the early lesions do not necessarily cause autofluorescent abnormalities.

FUTURE DIRECTIONS AND LIMITATIONS

It may be used in patients with retinal dystrophies to access the potential functional preservation of the outer retina,

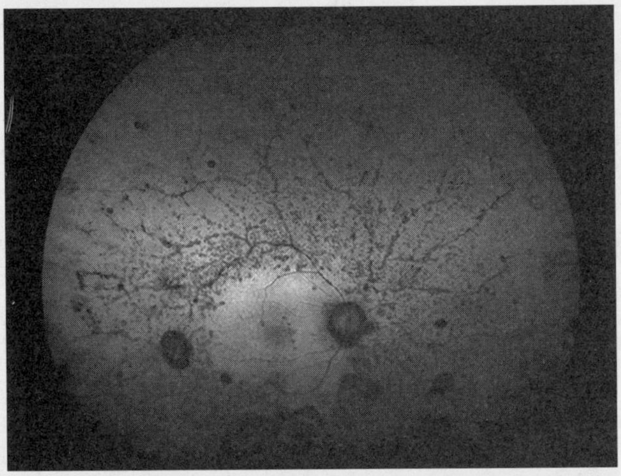

Fig. 13: A ultra-widefield fundus autofluorescence image with over 100° in a single capture using scanning laser ophthalmoscopy.

which would therefore have implications in monitoring or evaluation of treatments for this in the future.

At present, most limitations are due to the resolution of the image. The optical media and the lens which may present confounding background noise, can influence the intensity of fluorescence coming from the retina with increasing age, fluorescent properties also change, which makes the uses of FAF in older patients more difficult to interpret.

Ultra-widefield Autofluorescence

A typical fundus camera delivers a 50° field of view, but now ultra-widefield imaging can deliver 100° or more. Optos 200Tx using scanning laser ophthalmoscopy can image the peripheral retina to 200° with a single capture **(Fig. 13)**.

Perspectives in Imaging Technologies

Today, over a decade after the first visualization of the topographic distribution of lipofuscin accumulation over larger retinal areas in vivo using cSLO, FAF imaging is increasingly been used in research and in the clinical setting.[9] FAF findings now also serve to identify high-risk features and rapid progressors in an ongoing large interventional trial of patients with GA secondary to AMD. There are limitations to currently used FAF imaging devices, these include resolution and quantification issues as well as distinction of different underlying fluorophores according to spectral characteristics. Novel emerging imaging techniques offer new perspectives.

REFERENCES

1. Cuervo AM, Dice JR. When lysosomes get old? Exp Gerontol. 2000;35:119-31.
2. Sparrow JR, Boulton M. RPE lipofuscin and its role in retinal photobiology. Exp Eye Res. 2005;80:595-606.
3. Yin D. Biochemical basis of lipofuscin, ceroid, and age pigment-like fluorophores. Free Rad Biol Med. 1996;21:871-88.
4. Feeney-Burns L, Hilderbrand ES, Eldridge S. Aging human RPE: morphometric analysis of macular, equatorial, and peripheral cells. Invest Ophthalmol Vis Sci. 1984;25: 195-200.
5. Delori FC, Bursell SE, Yoshida A, et al. Vitreous fluorophotometry in diabetics: study of artifactual contributions. Graefe's Arch Clin Exp Ophthalmol. 1985;222:215-8.
6. Kitagawa K, Nishida S, Ogura Y. In vivo quantification of autofluorescence in human retinal pigment epithelium. Ophthalmologica. 1989;199:116-21.
7. Delori FC. Fluorophotometer for noninvasive measurement of RPE lipofuscin. Noninvasive assessment of the visual system. OSA Technical Digest. 1992;1:164-7.
8. Delori FC. Spectrophotometer for noninvasive measurement of intrinsic fluorescence and reflectance of the ocular fundus. Applied Optics. 1994;33:7439-52.
9. von Ruckmann A, Fitzke FW, Bird AC. Distribution of fundus autofluorescence with a scanning laser ophthalmoscope. Br J Ophthalmol. 1995;79:407-12.
10. Webb RH, Hughes GW, Delori FC. Confocal scanning laser ophthalmoscope. Appl Optics. 1987;26:1492-9.
11. Bellmann C, Holz FG, Schapp O, et al. Topography of fundus autofluorescence with a new confocal scanning laser ophthalmoscope. Ophthalmologe. 1997;94:385-91.
12. Bindewald A, Jorzik JJ, Roth F, et al. cSLO digital fundus autofluorescence imaging. Ophthalmologe. 2005;102:259-64.
13. Jorzik JJ, Bindewald A, Dithmar S, et al. Digital simultaneous fluorescein and indocyanine green angiography, autofluorescence, and red-free imaging with a solid-state laser-based confocal scanning laser ophthalmoscope. Retina. 2005;25:405-16.
14. Solbach U, Keilhauer C, Knabben H, et al. Imaging of retinal autofluorescence in patients with age-related macular degeneration. Retina. 1997;17:385-9.
15. American National Standards Institute (2000). American national standard for the safe use of lasers: ANSI Z136.1. Laser Institute of America, Orlando, FL. [online] Available from: https://www.lia.org/resources/laser-safety-information/laser-safety-standards/ansi-z136-standards [Last accessed on November, 2019].
16. Delori FC, Dorey CK, Staurenghi G, et al. In vivo fluorescence of the ocular fundus exhibits retinal pigment epithelium lipofuscin characteristics. Invest Ophthalmol Vis Sci. 1995;36:718-29.
17. Delori FC, Fleckner MR, Goger DG, et al. Autofluorescence distribution associated with drusen in age-related macular degeneration. Invest Ophthalmol Vis Sci. 2000;41:496-504.
18. Spaide RF. Fundus autofluorescence and age-related macular degeneration. Ophthalmology. 2003;110:392-9.
19. von Rückmann A, Fitzke FW, Bird AC. In vivo fundus autofluorescence in macular dystrophies. Arch Ophthalmol. 1997;115:609-15.
20. Holz FG, Pauleikhoff D, Spaide RF, et al. Age-related macular degeneration. Berlin: Springer; 2004.
21. Holz FG, Pauleikhoff D, Klein R, et al. Pathogenesis of lesions in late age-related macular disease. Am J Ophthalmol. 2004;137:504-10.

22. Klein R, Klein BE, Tomany SC, et al. Ten-year incidence and progression of age-related maculopathy: the Beaver Dam eye study. Ophthalmology. 2002;109:1767-79.
23. Lois N, Owens SL, Coco R, et al. Fundus autofluorescence in patients with age-related macular degeneration and high risk of visual loss. Am J Ophthalmol. 2002;133:341-9.
24. Bindewald A, Bird AC, Dandekar SS, et al. Classification of fundus autofluorescence patterns in early age-related macular disease. Invest Ophthalmol Vis Sci. 2005;46:3309-14.
25. Blair CJ. Geographic atrophy of the retinal pigment epithelium. A manifestation of senile macular degeneration. Arch Ophthalmol. 1975;93:19-25.
26. Maguire P, Vine AK. Geographic atrophy of the retinal pigment epithelium. Am J Ophthalmol. 1986;102:621-5.
27. Schatz H, McDonald HR. Atrophic macular degeneration. Rate of spread of geographic atrophy and visual loss. Ophthalmology. 1989;96:154151.
28. Deckert A, Schmitz-Valckenberg S, Jorzik J, et al. Automated analysis of digital fundus autofluorescence images of geographic atrophy in advanced age-related macular degeneration using confocal scanning laser ophthalmoscopy (cSLO). BMC Ophthalmol. 2005;5:8.
29. Schmitz-Valckenberg S, Jorzik J, Unnebrink K, et al. Analysis of digital scanning laser ophthalmoscopy fundus autofluorescence images of geographic atrophy in advanced age-related macular degeneration. Graefes Arch Clin Exp Ophthalmol. 2002;240:73-8.
30. Dandekar SS, Jenkins SA, Peto T, et al. Autofluorescence imaging of choroidal neovascularization due to age-related macular degeneration. Arch Ophthalmol. 2005;123:1507-13.
31. Lafaut BA, Bartz-Schmidt KU, Vanden Broecke C, et al. Clinicopathological correlation in exudative age related macular degeneration: histological differentiation between classic and occult choroidal neovascularization. Br J Ophthalmol. 2000;84:239-43.
32. Charbel Issa P, Scholl HP, Helb HM, et al. Macular telangiectasia. In: Holz FG, Spaide RF (Eds). Medical Retina. Heidelberg: Springer; 2007. pp. 183-97.
33. Helb HM, Charbel Issa P, Pauleikhoff D, et al. Macular pigment density and distribution in patients with macular telangiectasia. Invest Ophthalmol Vis Sci. 2006;5701/B795.
34. Spaide RF. Autofluorescence imaging of acute posterior multifocal placoid pigment epitheliopathy. Retina. 2006;26:479-842.
35. Matsumoto Y, Spaide RF. Autofluorescence imaging of acute syphilitic posterior placoid chorioretinitis. Retina. 2007;1(3):123-7.
36. Haen SP, Spaide RF. Fundus autofluorescence in multifocal choroiditis and panuveitis. Am J Ophthalmol. 2008;145(5): 847-53.

CHAPTER 14

Fundus Fluorescein Angiography

Pradeep Venkatesh

INTRODUCTION

Fluorescein angiography is a dynamic study of the retinochoroidal status following the administration of the dye sodium fluorescein. Despite the advent of several other technologies, fluorescein angiography continues to be the mainstay diagnostic modality to determine the health of the inner and outer blood retinal barriers. Although fluorescein angiography provides valuable additional information, it is not a substitute for meticulous clinical evaluation. The investigation has to be undertaken with specific objectives in mind and never as a test to reveal the cause of an unexplained loss of vision. In almost all cases wherein fluorescein angiography is necessary, the fundus already has changes discernible on ophthalmoscopy.

The retina depends for its survival on two circulations—the choroidal circulation and the central retinal arterial circulation. Fluorescein angiography helps us evaluate the retinal circulation but is unable to reveal the status of the choroidal circulation. Indocyanine green (ICG) angiography is necessary to study the choroidal vasculature.

The outer third of the retina is supplied by choroidal blood flow and the inner two-thirds by retinal blood flow. These two circulations complement each other. The retinal arteriolar vasculature is an end-arterial system, and so lacks anastomoses (exception being the cilioretinal artery which is seen in about 20% of the population). The retinal arteriolar rami do not penetrate deeper than the inner nuclear layer and the capillaries have nonfenestrated endothelial cells. The endothelial cell-to-pericyte ratio is 1–2:1. Capillary density is maximum at the macula and absent at the extreme periphery, adjacent to the retinal vessels themselves and within the foveal avascular zone. The inner blood retinal barrier is constituted by the retinal capillary endothelium, and the outer blood retinal barrier is constituted by the retinal pigment epithelium (RPE)–Bruch's membrane complex. The inner barrier is highly impermeable to passage of solutes and keeps the intravascular component from merging with the extravascular space (however minimal) within the retina. The Bruch's membrane is permeable to the passage of fluorescein dye. The impermeability of the outer blood retinal barrier is due to the tight intercellular junctions, the zonulae occludens, along the apical ends of the retinal pigment epithelial cells. The outer barrier keeps the choroidal compartment separate from the retinal layers.

Another feature of the ocular tissue that has a bearing on the appearance of the fluorescein angiogram is the presence of three important pigments: melanin (absorbs the entire visible wavelength), xanthophyll (absorbs blue wavelength), and hemoglobin (absorbs predominantly green wavelength). Melanin absorbs light rays over the entire visible spectrum. Owing to this absorption characteristic, melanin within the RPE prevents visualization of fluorescein dye that passes out easily through the choriocapillaris. As infrared light is not absorbed, ICG angiography enables visualization of the choroidal vasculature. Xanthophyll is a pigment that is unique to the macular region. Here, it is present within its deeper layers, particularly in the inner fiber of the cones (Henle's layer). Xanthophyll has the property of absorbing blue light and so acts like a blue minus filter. The exciter light used during fluorescein angiography is also blue. Hence, xanthophyll, by absorbing this blue light, contributes to the dark color of the macular region on a normal angiogram. Hemoglobin is the pigment that transports oxygen in the blood and so is usually confined to the intravascular compartment. Abnormally; however, it may reach the extravascular space whenever the vessels rupture from any cause. Hemoglobin has the property of absorbing light maximally at the green end of the visible spectrum. The emitted light by fluorescein sodium is also green. As a result, the concentration of hemoglobin within the bloodstream also has a bearing on the contrast of the angiogram. In fact, it may be near impossible to derive any useful information by undertaking angiography in a patient with severe polycythemia. In addition, blood that is present in the extravascular spaces prevents angiographic visualization of the underlying structures by acting as a physical, opaque barrier to the passage of light.

The permeability of a solute across different membrane barriers in the body is determined by the physiochemical properties of the solute (herein sodium fluorescein), such as molecular weight, protein binding affinity, etc. and the nature of the junctional complexes (zonulae occludens, macula occludens, and zonulae occludens) across the cellular and acellular barriers. Fluorescein sodium is a xanthene derivative with a molecular weight that is "large" enough (376 kD) to prevent its passage across the tight barriers of the outer and inner blood retinal barriers. It has a high affinity for binding to the plasma proteins, mainly albumin (70–80% is normally protein bound). In addition, it also binds to the erythrocytes. Sodium fluorescein, bound or unbound does not normally pass across both the outer and inner blood retinal barriers. Although binding of fluorescein molecules reduces the amount of free fluorescein available for excitation, it facilitates the separation of the absorption (465 nm) and emission wavelengths (530 nm) by the filters more efficiently. Though mild-to-severe adverse events have been reported during fluorescein angiography, sodium fluorescein is a relatively inert dye. It is highly water soluble and is removed out of the body within 24–48 hours, mainly by the renal route.

PROCEDURE OF FUNDUS FLUORESCEIN ANGIOGRAPHY

As fluorescein angiography is an invasive procedure, written informed consent is mandatory before undertaking the test. Also, ensure that the emergency equipment is readily available in case of need. Inform the patient about why the test is being performed and the need for his cooperation to ensure quality images and information is gathered. The pupil must be well dilated and the patient must be seated comfortably at the fundus camera. At our center we inject 3 mL of sodium fluorescein 20% dye into the antecubital vein (preferred site for intravenous injection) using a 23 G needle (one may also inject the dye through a preplaced venflon or scalp vein). The timer is started as soon as injection of the dye commences; another click (which creates a blank image) is made at the end of the dye injection. This time interval indicates the injection time (ideally between 6 seconds and 8 seconds). To slow an injection creates poor image contrast while too rapid an injection may increase the risk of adverse events like nausea and vomiting. Then take sequential pictures so as to capture adequate frames during each of the four phases of the angiogram (read later). Capturing images every 1–2 seconds during the early phase was recommended during the era of analog fundus imaging (using film roll). In the current era of digital imaging, taking images so frequently is no longer a necessity because one gets real-time feedback about the quality of the image captured. Once the procedure is complete, the patient must be asked to be seated at the waiting area for about half an hour and inform the angiography team in case any rashes or itching develops. This and other adverse events must be managed adequately before releasing the patient from your observation. In case the patient develops significant side effects during the procedure, this must be written clearly in bold letters on the patient records and he/she must be advised to avoid getting the test again.

Fluorescein angiography can be performed using the blue filter on a direct or indirect ophthalmoscope, but this method is not efficient and does not allow for documentation of the findings. Hence, the standard method for performing fluorescein angiography is through use of a fundus camera. The fundus camera, other than being able to capture color, red free images, etc. has the ability to capture fluorescein angiographic images because of special filters incorporated into the machine. These filters (a pair of barrier and exciter filters) become introduced into the optical pathway when angiography mode is activated. The exciter filter allows the passage of only blue light (465 nm) corresponding to the maximum absorption characteristics of fluorescein sodium. The barrier filter allows the passage of only green light (525 nm) corresponding to the maximum emission characteristic of the dye **(Fig. 1)**. The quality of filters also shows a tendency to deteriorate over a period of time. Whenever there is a mismatch or overlap between the exciter and barrier filters, the quality of the angiogram suffers. In fact, the phenomenon of pseudofluorescence results from the camera having a significant overlap of exciter and barrier filters wavelengths. In the nondigital era, analog cameras were used to capture the images and the results were read from film negatives or contact prints. The quality of images captured using analog cameras has superior

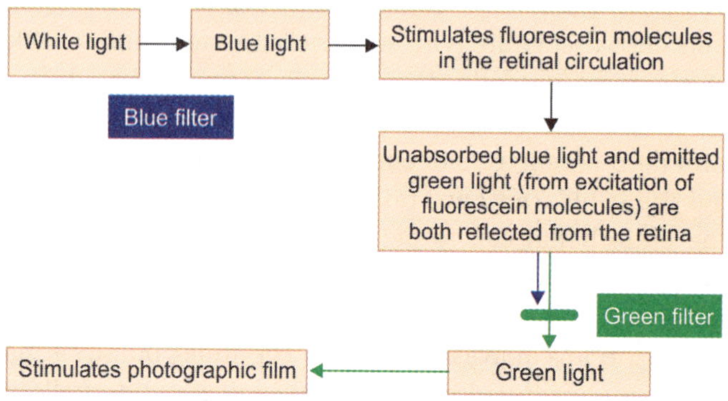

Fig. 1: Role of exciter and barrier filter in the optical pathway during fluorescein angiography.

resolution compared to most digital cameras. Despite this, they are no longer manufactured due to ergonomic reasons. Therefore, all fundus cameras currently in use are digital in nature and capture images using confocal or nonconfocal pathways. Most digital cameras allow image capture up to 60°, unless special wide-field lenses are used. Optos is a fundus camera that allows 200° ultrawide-field fluorescein angiography without any need for using special lenses.

INDICATIONS

Fluorescein angiography is normally undertaken if it is likely to change the diagnosis, likely to alter the treatment or to assess the progress and response to treatment, and also as a baseline in diseases that may change over a period of time. It is impossible to interpret the progress of a disease or to assess response to treatment by looking a single angiogram. The availability of a color photograph is also very useful for the proper interpretation of a fluorescein angiogram. Before making an attempt at interpretation, it would be prudent to note if the eye and the area on the angiographic pictures matches those of intended study, and whether all the phases of the angiographic study are present.

PHASES OF FUNDUS FLUORESCEIN ANGIOGRAPHY

Although there is a considerable overlap, four phases are recognized during fluorescein angiographic study. These phases are the prefilling, transit, recirculation, and late phases. Each phase appears after an approximate interval following dye injection into the antecubital vein, and each phase has a certain importance as shown in **Figure 2**. In the prefilling phase (interval between A and B) one can recognize autofluorescence and early pseudofluorescence. Transit phase (interval between B and C) encompasses the arterial, arteriovenous (AV) (capillary), venous, peak, and late venous phase. The foveal avascular zone is best recognized in the peak phase when fluorescence in the choroidal and retinal vasculature (arteries and veins) is uniform. The staining of tissues is best appreciated in the recirculation phase (C and D) while the late phase (D and E) is important to diagnose angiographic cystoid macular edema and occult choroidal neovascular membranes. Late pseudofluorescence is also detected when present in the last phase of the angiogram.

INTERPRETATION OF FUNDUS FLUORESCEIN ANGIOGRAPHY

On interpretation, the functional integrity of the retinochoroidal layers may be classified into the following categories: Normal, variant of normal, and abnormal. An abnormal angiogram may reveal areas of hyperfluorescence, hypofluorescence or a combination of the two **(Flowchart 1)**. One must be careful not to interpret artifacts as abnormalities in the retina. For the accurate classification of an angiogram, the early, mid, and late phases must be viewed in sequence. Any attempt at making a diagnosis based on a single frame of the angiographic study may

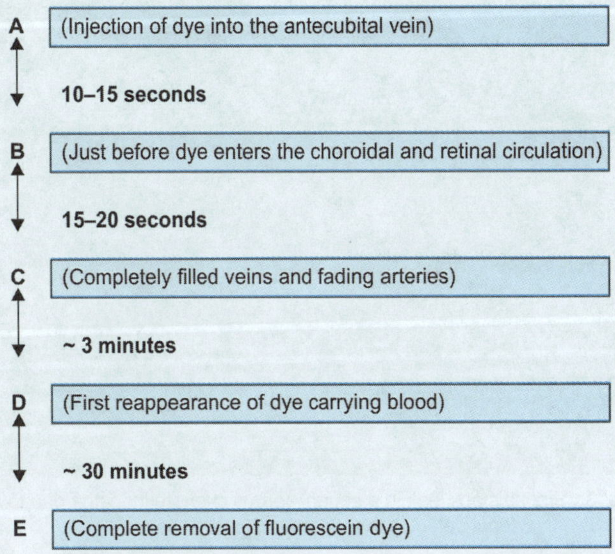

Fig. 2: Various phases of fluorescein angiography.

Flowchart 1: Interpretation of fundus fluorescein angiography.

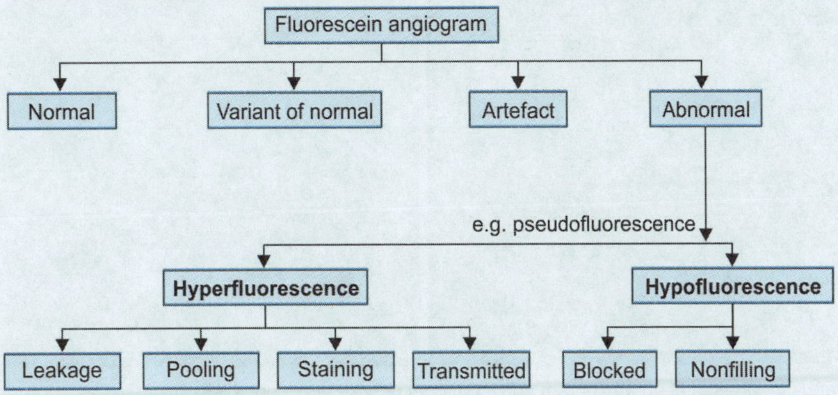

prove to be erroneous. As a generalization, it may be said that on an angiographic picture any "white" lesion is indicative of hyperfluorescence, and any "dark" lesion, of hypofluorescence. The cause of hyperfluorescence is the leakage of fluorescein dye by a breach in the outer [e.g. central serous retinopathy (CSR); **Fig. 3**] and/or inner [e.g. neovascularization on the disk (NVD), neovascularization elsewhere (NVE), and vasculitis; **Fig. 4**] blood-retinal barrier. When the hyperfluorescence is frank and increases from the early to the late phase in both size and intensity, it is known as a leakage as in cases of CSR and neovascularization. When the hyperfluorescence increases in intensity and the size remains constant on looking at the various phases, then it is called pooling (e.g. pigment epithelial detachment; **Figs. 5A and B**). Hyperfluorescence that is minimal in the early and mid phases, but which becomes marked in the late phases is likely to be due to staining. In some cases [e.g. acute posterior multifocal placoid pigment epitheliopathy (APMPPE) and active choroiditis], a black lesion (hypofluorescent) in the early phases may become a whiter lesion (hyperfluorescent) in the late phases. A mottled hyperfluorescence that appears very early and remains unchanged in the later phases is most likely to be due to a "window defect" which is otherwise called transmitted hyperfluorescence.

A dark lesion (hypofluorescence) that remains constant through all the phases is indicative of a blocked hypofluorescence. A hypofluorescence that is most prominent in the AV phase of the angiogram, and which is associated with the nonfilling of the dye due to a functional or anatomical closure of the retinal vessels is indicative of capillary nonperfusion **(Fig. 6)**. It is necessary to note that blocked fluorescence can imply a blocked choroidal background fluorescence or a blocked retinal and choroidal fluorescence. The former is indicative of a subretinal pathology while the latter of a preretinal/subhyaloid hemorrhage. The most common cause of blocked fluorescence is a preretinal/subretinal hemorrhage. Rarely, it is caused by pigment epithelial hyperplasia and hypertrophy. Peripheral lesions are best studied using wide-field angiography **(Fig. 7)**.

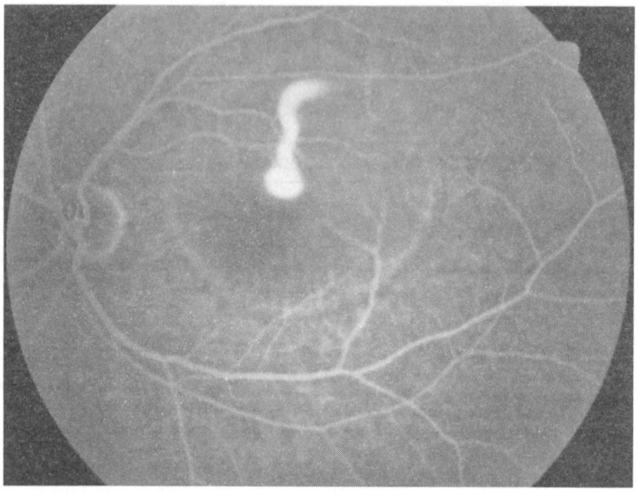

Fig. 3: Smoke stack leak in a central serous chorioretinopathy due to a focal defect in the outer blood-retinal barrier.

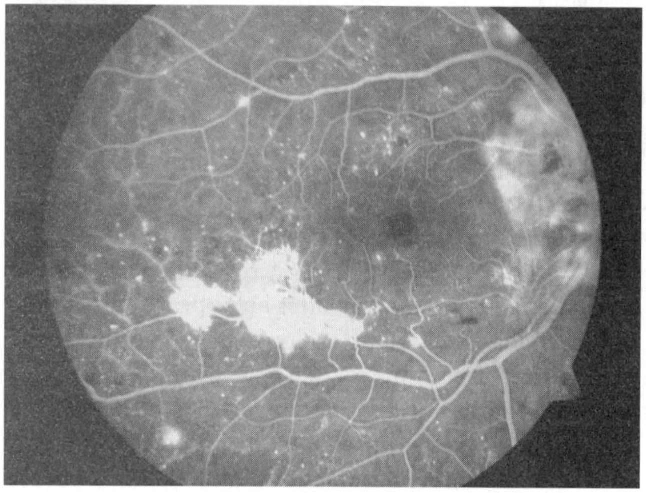

Fig. 4: Leakage from neovascularization on the disk (NVD) and neovascularization elsewhere (NVE) on the retina; this is indicative of an immature inner blood-retinal barrier within these abnormal vessels.

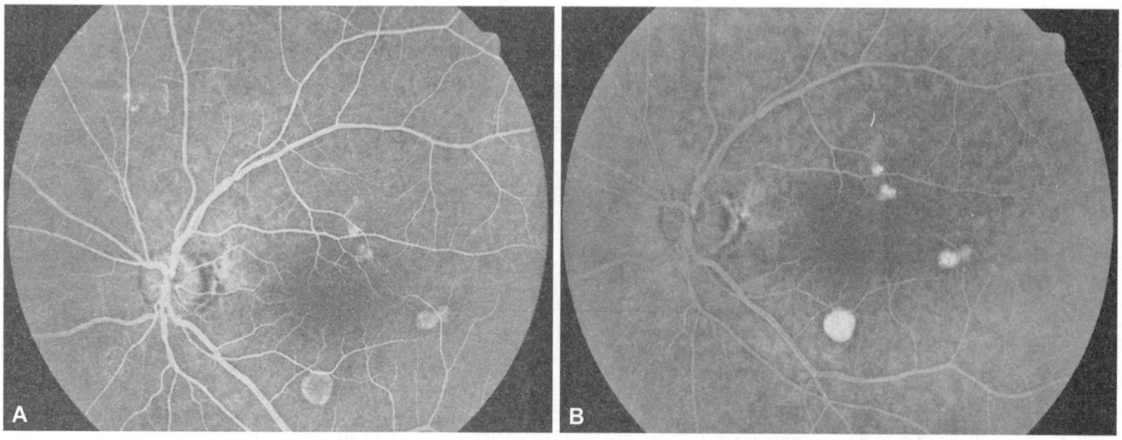

Figs. 5A and B: The early and late phases of an angiogram showing focal hyperfluorescence which increases in intensity but not in size; it results from the pooling of dye within the retinal pigment epithelial detachment.

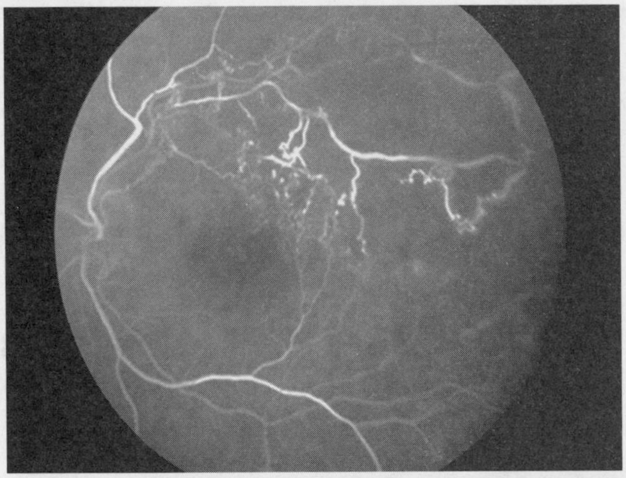

Fig. 6: Extensive capillary nonperfusion in the superotemporal retina of a patient with branch-retinal vein occlusion.

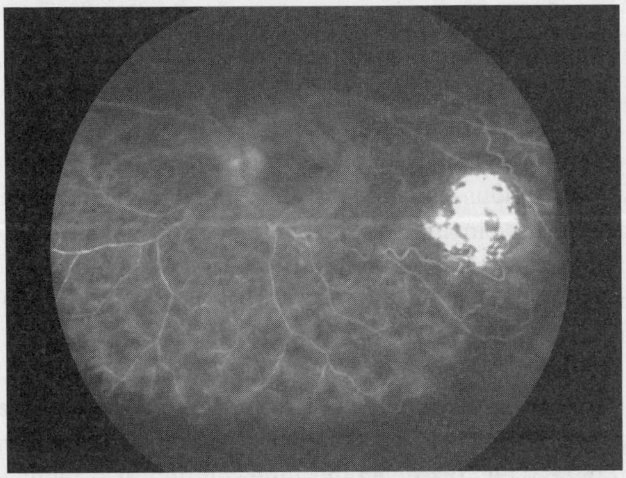

Fig. 7: Wide-field fluorescein angiographic image of a patient with a vasoproliferative tumor of the retina.

CONCLUSION

In conclusion, it may be said that the interpretation of an angiogram is likely to be more accurate and fruitful if we seek answers to each of the following questions:

- Is it normal or abnormal? If abnormal,
- Is the abnormality black or white or mixed?
- What are the time characteristics of the abnormality?
- Are all the retinal vessels filling normally?
- What happens to the size of the abnormality in the various phases of the angiogram (constant/increases/decreases)?
- What happens to the intensity of the color in the late phases compared to the mid and early phases (becomes more white/no change)?
- How is the distribution of the abnormal fluorescence (patchy/homogenous)?
- How are the margins of the abnormality, poor or clearly defined?
- How do answers to the above correlate with the fundus picture?

SUGGESTED READING

1. Rabb MF, Burton TC, Schatz H, et al. Fluorescein angiography of the fundus—a systematic approach to interpretation. Surv Ophthalmol. 1978;28:387-403.
2. Venkatesh P, Garg S, Azad RV. Retinal Imaging. New Delhi: Jaypee Brothers Medical Publishers (P) Ltd; 2008.
3. Venkatesh P, Garg S, Verma L, et al. Step by step fundus fluorescein and Indocyanine green angiography. New Delhi: Jaypee Brothers Medical Publishers (P) Ltd.; 2007.

CHAPTER 15

Indocyanine Green Angiography

Rajesh Ramanjulu, P Mahesh Shanmugam, Pradeep Sagar

INTRODUCTION

Indocyanine green angiography (ICGA) allows the study of choroidal circulation and hence is specifically suited for studying sub-retinal pigment epithelial (RPE) diseases, such as occult choroidal neovascularization (CNV), polypoidal choroidal vasculopathy (PCV), and central serous chorioretinopathy (CSC).

HISTORY

The entry of indocyanine green (ICG) into medicine was in the mid-1950s. Irwin Fox, who was in search of a biocompatible dye that could be detected in blood, was the first to recognize the dye at Eastman Kodak laboratories. ICG exhibited peak absorption of near-infrared light at 805 nm; this is the same wavelength at which the optical densities of oxygenated and reduced hemoglobin in blood are approximately equal. This relationship made it possible to measure ICG concentration in blood in terms of its optical density at 805 nm, regardless of oxygen saturation.

As the dye was unstable in aqueous solution, it was referred to Hynson Westcott and Dunning, a small Baltimore pharmaceutical company, for development into the stable lyophilized form that remains in use today.

The first medical use of ICG was in 1956 in cardiology for measuring the time-varying dilution of ICG in whole blood. From this, cardiac output could be determined and valvular septal defects could be characterized. The dye is excreted exclusively by the liver and this subsequently led to its application for measuring hepatic function and blood flow.

The first attempt at using ICG for angiography was made by Kogure et al. when they demonstrated the infrared absorption angiography of the canine brain vasculature. In 1971, Bernie Hochheimer demonstrated in cats that the infrared absorption angiography method could be simplified. He illuminated the fundus with a narrow band of near-infrared wavelengths and used Kodak high-speed infrared black and white films. Importantly, the ICG dye in the vessels could be imaged after filtering light from a standard fundus camera. This suggested that the technique might be used in human subjects. It took considerable effort to produce the first intravenously injected ICG fluorescence angiogram image in 1972. This was the first ever published human ICG fluorescence angiogram.

Indocyanine green is a tricarbocyanine dye with both hydrophilic and lipophilic properties.[1] The empirical formula of ICG is $C_{43}H_{47}N_2NaO_6S_2$. The molecular weight is 775 D. When dissolved in saline solution, ICG tends to form polymers if the solution concentration is high; and, monomers, if the concentration is low. For this reason, the dye is dissolved in water for intravenous injections. ICG is stimulated with near-infrared wavelength light at 810 nm, and the emission spectrum is at 830 nm. The ICG molecule can be considered active at a wavelength between 790 nm and 830 nm.

Following intravenous administration, ICG binds to blood lipoproteins (fundamentally phospholipids) in a proportion that can reach 98%.[2-4] The emitted fluorescence intensity increases as a result of such binding. ICG is weakly fluorescent and exhibits only 4% of the fluorescence exhibited by sodium fluorescein. Elimination takes place in the liver, with secretion in the bile.

The ICG molecule has biophysical properties that make it useful for visualizing the choroidal circulation. The dye is excited by light close to infrared (longer operating wavelength), thereby increasing its ability to fluoresce better through pigment, lipid, and hemorrhage than fluorescein dye. ICG circulates almost entirely bound to plasma proteins, and gradually diffuses across the choriocapillaris; this retention of ICG in the choroidal circulation, coupled with low permeability, allows better visualization of the choroidal circulation. These properties make it possible to visualize CNV beneath blood exudates or retinal pigment epithelial detachments (PEDs)[5,6] by differentiating (in the latter case) between the hypofluorescent serous component and the hyperfluorescent vascular component.

Indocyanine green is also useful in delineating the abnormal aneurysmal outpouchings of the inner choroidal vascular network seen in PCV and the focal areas of choroidal hyperpermeability in CSC. It is an additional aid in differentiating abnormal vasculature in intraocular tumors, and in distinguishing the abnormal fluorescence patterns seen in choroidal inflammatory conditions such as serpiginous choroidopathy, acute multifocal placoid pigment epitheliopathy (AMPPE), to mention a few.

PHASES OF INDOCYANINE GREEN ANGIOGRAPHY

Indocyanine green angiography is typically divided into three phases—the arterial (initial dye filling pattern), venous phase, and late stage:

1. *Arterial phase*: Choroidal hyperfluorescence usually begins in the subfoveal region and progresses in a radial fashion towards the periphery. A vertical watershed passing through the disk is well defined in this phase.
2. *Venous phase*: Choroidal veins become delineated in ICGA by 15–20 seconds after the injection of the dye. Approximately 25% of the individuals demonstrate a classic horizontal watershed area passing through the disk and fovea. The draining veins are arranged in a symmetrical fashion and divided into upper and lower beds, thus defining the watershed level (**Fig. 1**). An interesting fact is that 75% of the venous drainage is preferential for ST area and the remaining 25% in the IT and SN areas.

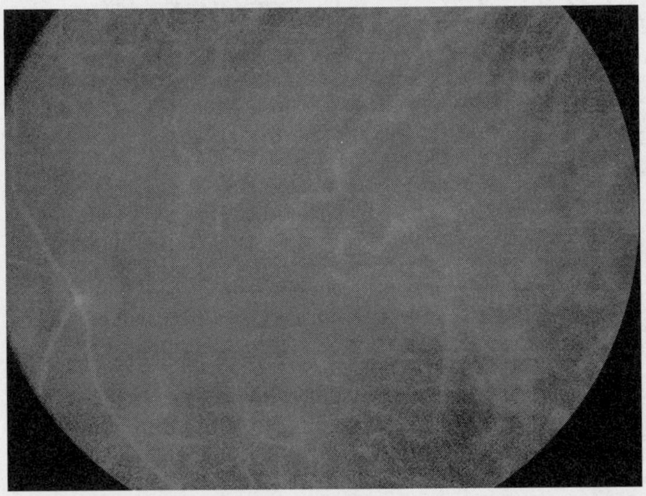

Fig. 1: One of early phases in indocyanine green angiography showing horizontal watershed demarcation, bisecting the disk, and running along the macular area.

3. *Late phase*: ICG images several minutes into the late phases do not change much. The ability to discern choroidal vessels decreases with extravasation of dye, dye dilution, and its clearance.

The ICG dye disappears from the circulation quickly and its retention rate at 15 minutes is less than 10%. Late phase ICGA pictures are obtained 15–20 minutes later, the persistence of the dye shows anomalous vasculature.

ADVERSE REACTIONS

Adverse reactions are similar to those observed with fluorescein, but are less frequent.[1] The dye should not be used in patients with shellfish or iodine allergies, liver disease, and end-stage renal disease. No studies in animal models have been made regarding the use of the dye in pregnancy. However, current practice patterns regarding the use of ICG angiography in pregnant patients may be unnecessarily restrictive.[7]

APPLICATIONS IN OPHTHALMOLOGY

Let us consider the advantages of ICGA over FA before discussing its clinical application:

- *Hazy media*: ICGA can be performed in conditions where the media preclude fundus fluorescein angiography (FFA). This is due to the Rayleigh scatter (a phenomenon seen when the scattering particles are smaller than the incident wavelength, scatter intensity being larger for shorter wavelengths).
- Indocyanine green angiography can be performed even in the presence of vitreous hemorrhage, due to the phenomenon of Mie or forward scatter.
- Infrared light used is barely visible and so photophobic patients tolerate it.
- It measures the occult choroidal neovascular membrane (CNVM) more precisely as compared to FFA, which might under/overestimate.

DIAGNOSTIC APPLICATIONS

Nonexudative (Dry) Age-related Macular Degeneration

Indocyanine green angiography has been used to facilitate the diagnosis of basal laminar drusen and to differentiate them from reticular pseudodrusen. However, ICGA is not routinely used to study dry age-related macular degeneration (AMD) except in cases of drusenoid PED to confirm the absence of CNV.

Recently, ICGA has been reported to be useful for evaluating the atrophic areas present in Stargardt disease, in comparison with the atrophy of dry AMD.[8] The hypofluorescence evidenced by ICGA in the atrophic areas ("dark atrophy") has been shown to be more frequent in Stargardt disease than in atrophic AMD, suggesting a possible selective damage of the choriocapillaris in Stargardt disease.

Exudative (Wet) Age-related Macular Degeneration

Classic Choroidal Neovascularization

Classic CNV or type II CNVM is clearly defined by FA.[9,10] ICGA does not offer relevant supplementary information unless associated large PED/occult CNV is present. A classic CNVM may be seen much less distinctly in ICGA as compared with FFA **(Figs. 2A to D)**.

Occult CNVMs (type 1—beneath the RPE) demonstrate one of the following features on ICGA:

- Hot spot (<1 disk diameter area)—a well-defined leakage increasing in its size and intensity into the later phases.
- Plaque (>1 disk diameter area)—a leakage with borders partly obscured and/or ill defined.
- Mixture—of the above two patterns in a single or contiguous lesion.

Plaque was found to be the most common type (61% of the cases) and had a poor visual prognosis, whereas the focal spots or "hotspots" (29%) had a better prognosis, and they were considered to be potentially treatable by ICG-guided laser photocoagulation.[11,12]

The term "occult" refers to a type of CNV that is difficult to visualize, analyze, and localize on FA.[13] The fundamental advantage of ICGA is that it allows early detection and localization of occult CNV.

Occult CNV can be grouped into two main types:

1. *Occult CNV without serous PED*: Fibrovascular PED (fibrovascular pigment epithelium detachment with irregular and poorly demarcated hyperfluorescence on FFA) **(Figs. 3A to D)**. FA shows irregular and poorly delimited hyperfluorescence with late phase ill-defined leakage. This complemented with the optical coherence tomography (OCT) is sufficient in confirming the diagnosis and evaluating its activity.
2. *Occult CNV associated with serous PED*: Serous PED may be avascular or vascular, and FA fails to delineate the area of the underlying neovascular complex. This is primarily due to the hyperfluorescence of the PED, which masks the underlying CNV complex **(Figs. 4A to D)**. When ICGA is used, the PED appears as a hypofluorescent lesion in all phases of the angiogram. In rare situations, it may appear isofluorescent or at minimum hyperfluorescent in comparison to its

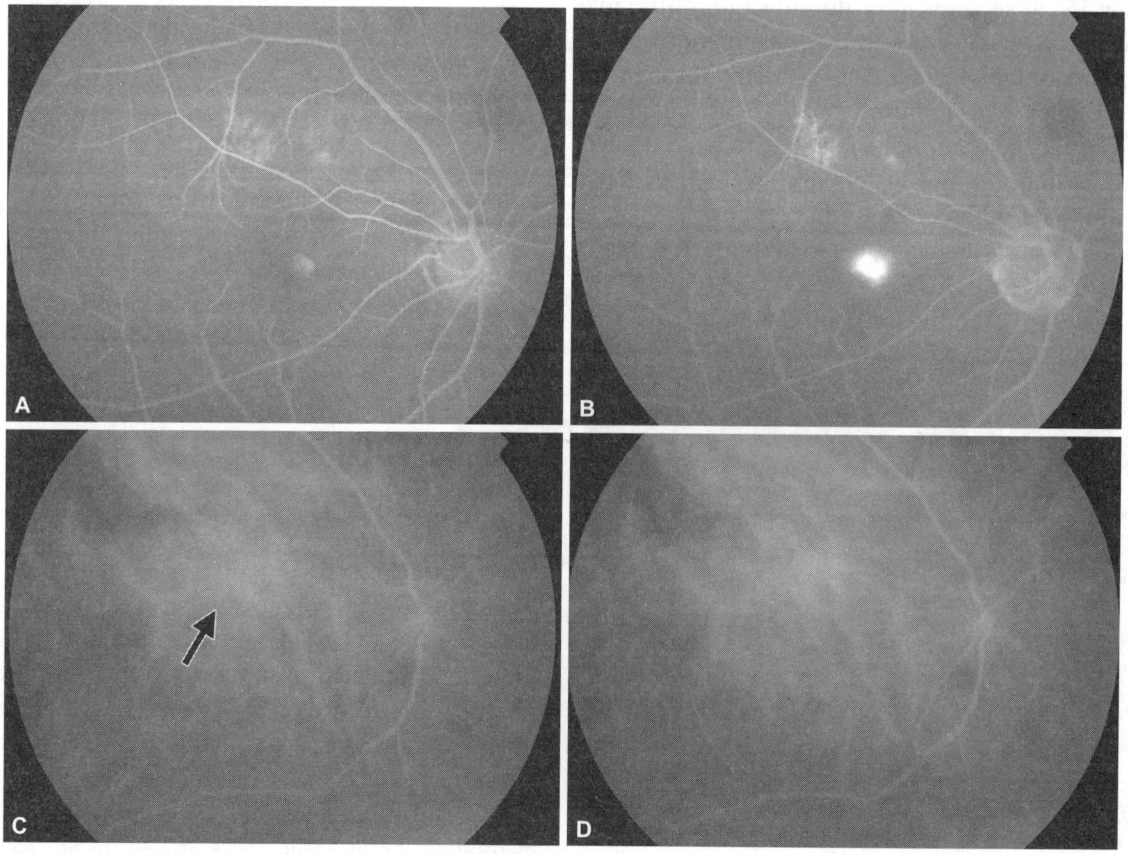

Figs. 2A to D: (A and B) Fundus fluorescein angiography shows defined hyperfluorescent lesion increasing in intensity and size in the later phases stage of classic choroidal neovascular membrane; (C and D) Indocyanine green angiography in this condition shows the same leakage area and so does not add much to our knowledge (arrow).

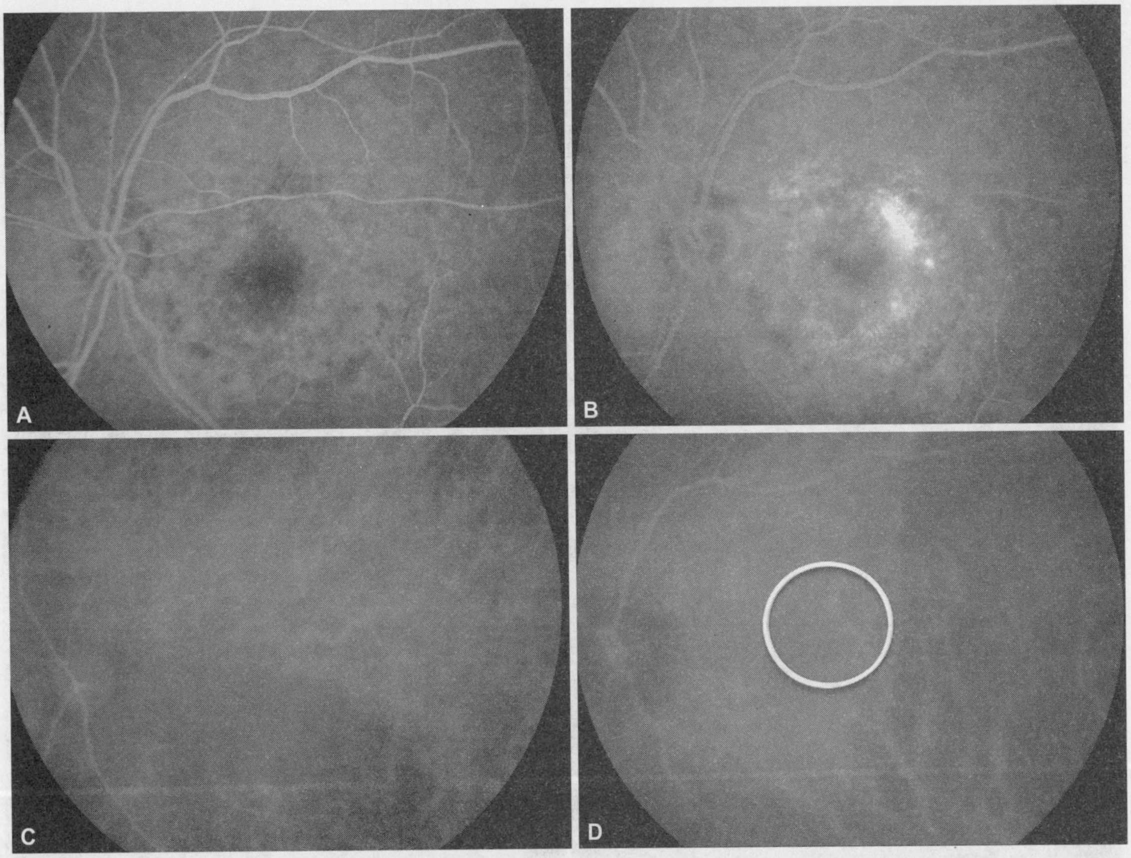

Figs. 3A to D: (A and B) Fundus fluorescein angiography (FFA) shows late leakage of undetermined source with a pigment epithelium detachment (fibrovascular); (C and D) Indocyanine green angiography shows a plaque leakage at the site of stippled leakage (on FFA).

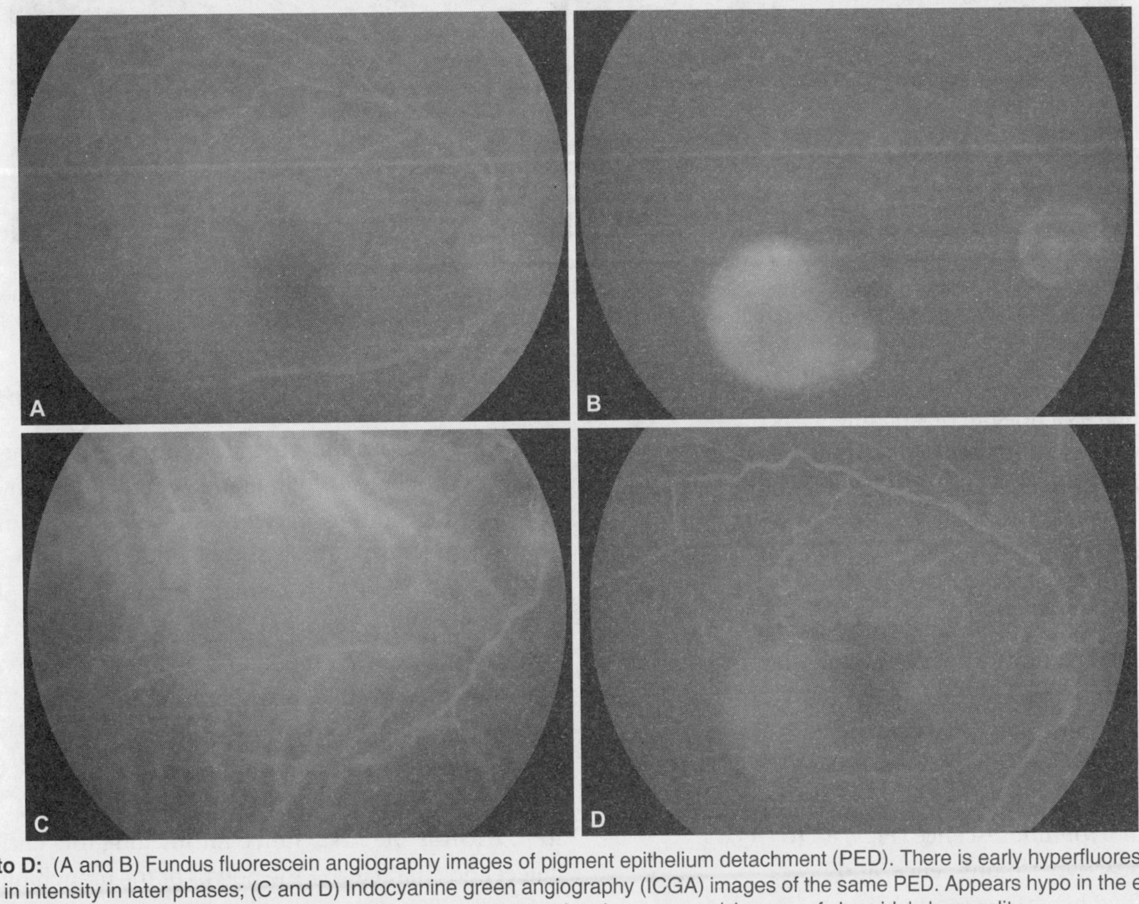

Figs. 4A to D: (A and B) Fundus fluorescein angiography images of pigment epithelium detachment (PED). There is early hyperfluorescence which increases in intensity in later phases; (C and D) Indocyanine green angiography (ICGA) images of the same PED. Appears hypo in the early and late phases without any activity in the choroid. Thus, ICGA helps us in showing the presence/absence of choroidal abnormality.

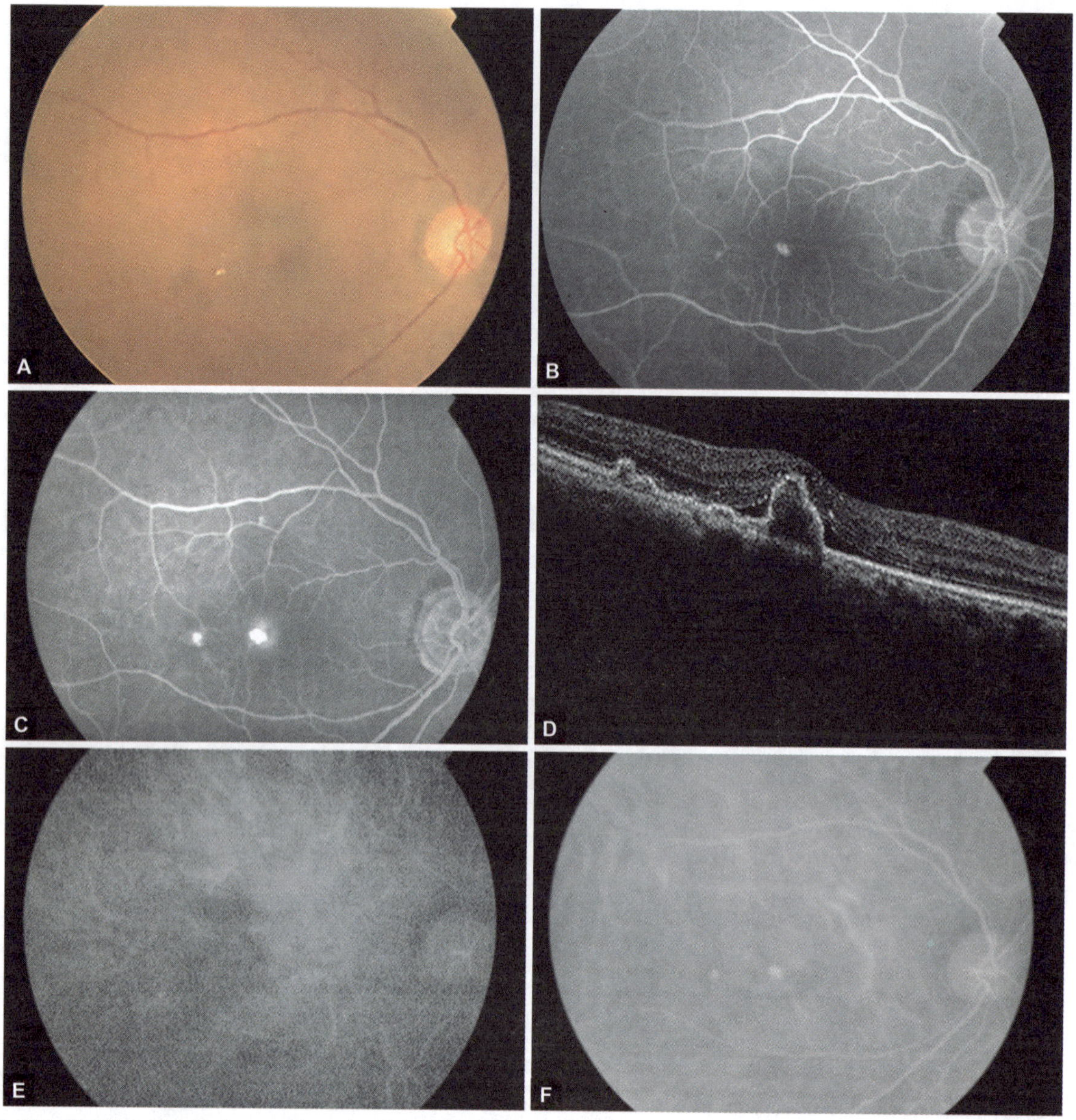

Figs. 5A to F: (A to C) CP and fundus fluorescein angiography (FFA) of a patient with retinal angiomatous proliferation (RAP); Early hyperfluorescence, as early as the beginning of the arterial phase with leakage in later phases stage of RAP; (D) Optical coherence tomography shows pigment epithelial detachment, intraretinal fluid, and exudates; (E and F) Indocyanine green angiography corresponds to the finding of RAP and further confirming the diagnosis.

surrounding and the underlying CNVM complex can be discerned as a hotspot or a plaque.

A type III variant, more popularly termed as retinal angiomatous proliferation (RAP) was identified by Yannuzzi et al. (2001).[14,15]

On the basis of the FA, RAP mimics the angiographic signature of the occult or minimally classic CNV and not typically of a vascularized PED.[16]

Some groups have described five different patterns of ICG angiograms in RAP, during the transit phase of high-speed ICG.[17] These are:

- Focal hyperfluorescence **(Figs. 5A to F)**
- Irregular hyperfluorescence
- Circular hyperfluorescence **(Figs. 6A to E)**
- Multifocal hyperfluorescence, and
- Combined hyperfluorescence.

POLYPOIDAL CHOROIDAL VASCULOPATHY

Polypoidal choroidal vasculopathy is a primary abnormality of the choroidal circulation characterized by an inner choroidal vascular network of vessels ending in an aneurysmal bulge or outward projection. Clinically, it is visible as a reddish-orange, spheroid, and polyp-like structure.[18] The disorder is associated with multiple, recurrent, serosanguineous detachments of the RPE and neurosensory retina, secondary to leakage and bleeding from the peculiar choroidal vascular abnormality.[19] Although FA, sometimes, can establish the diagnosis of PCV when the vascular elements are large and located beneath atrophic RPE, ICGA is the first choice for imaging this entity. It can detect and characterize the polyps or the branching vascular network with enhanced sensitivity and specificity.[19,20]

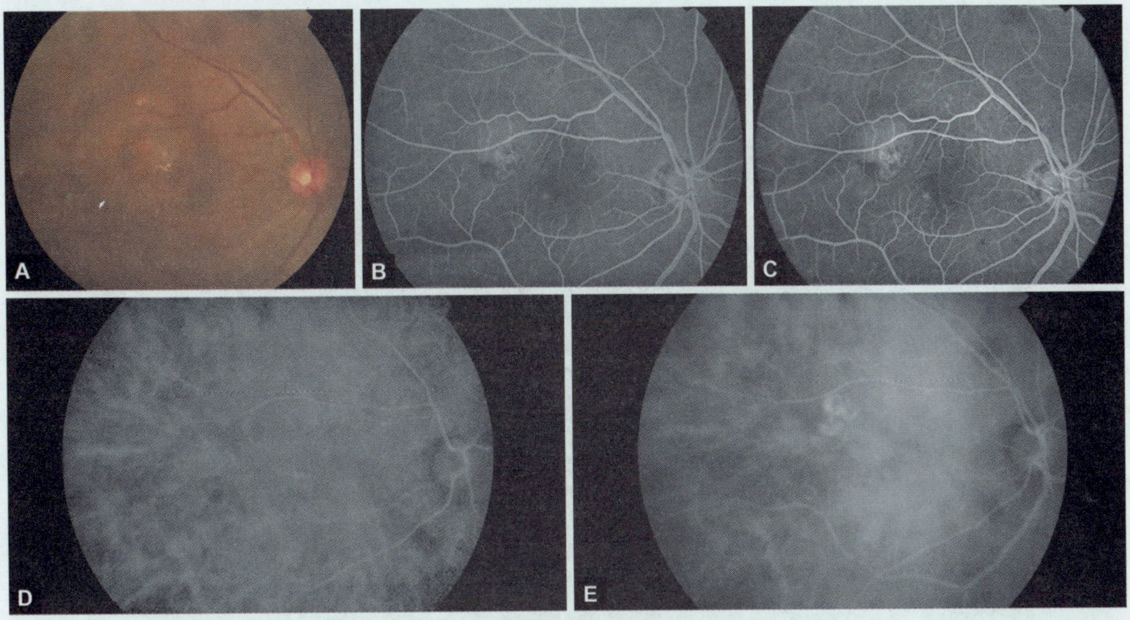

Figs. 6A to E: (A to C) A retinoretinal anastomosis well demonstrated on the indocyanine green angiography; (D and E) Thereby diagnosing the condition as retinal angiomatous proliferation.

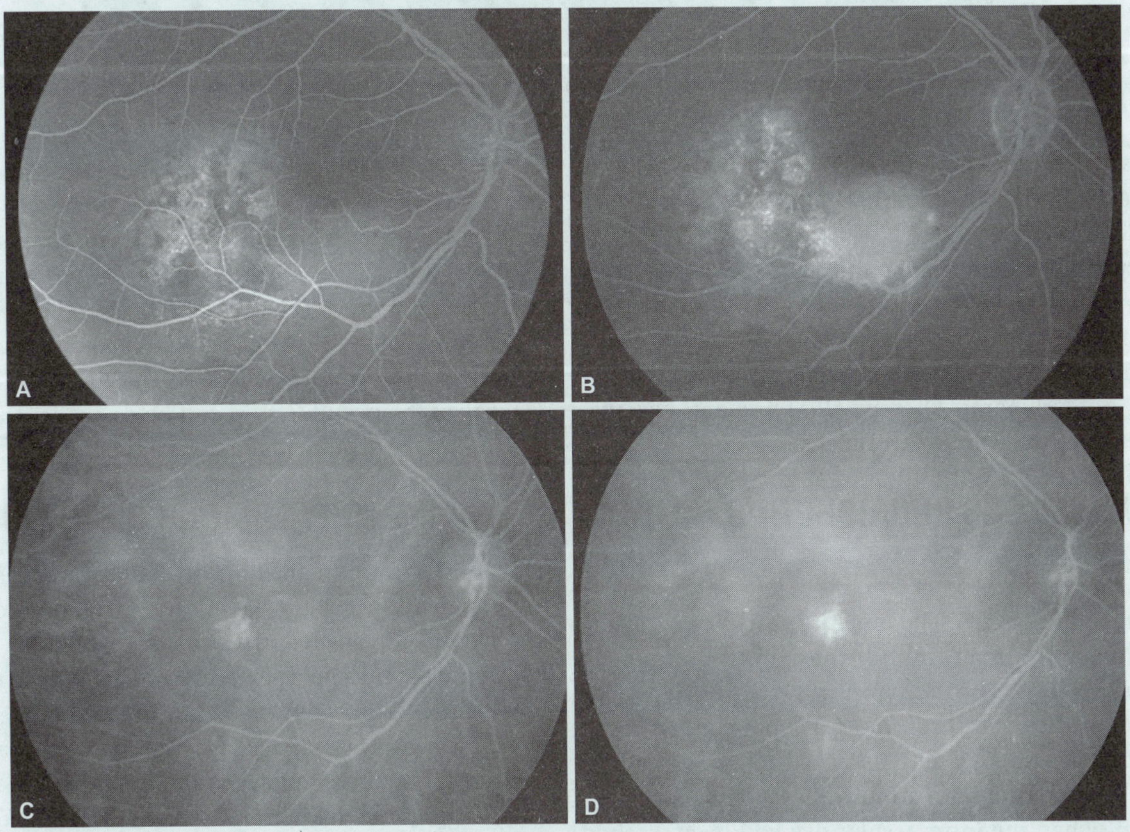

Figs. 7A to D: (A and B) Fundus fluorescein angiography (FFA) images demonstrating mottled hyperfluorescence with a large subfoveal pigment epithelium detachment. FFA fails to recognize the etiology of the underlying leakage; (C and D) Indocyanine green angiography, on the other hand, easily demonstrates a bunch of polyps confirming the diagnosis of polypoidal choroidal vasculopathy.

The early phase of ICG angiogram shows a distinct network of vessels within the choroid, which are usually prominent in their size in comparison to the surrounding choroidal vessels. Shortly after the network is identified, small hyperfluorescent polyps become visible within the choroid **(Figs. 7A to D)**. These polypoidal structures may correspond to the reddish-orange choroidal excrescence seen clinically, but the clinical examination typically does not show all the polyps, whereas the ICGA does. In the later phase of the angiogram, there is a uniform disappearance

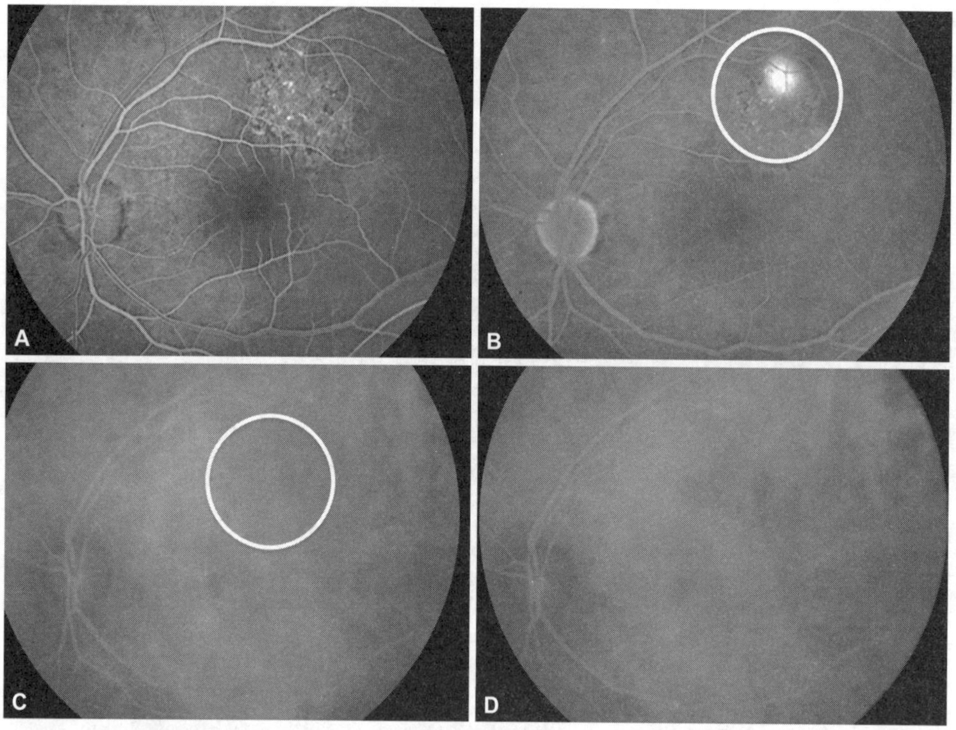

Figs. 8A to D: (A and B) Acute on chronic central serous chorioretinopathy (CSC). Fundus fluorescein angiography (FFA) images in the early phase shows window defects corresponding to the retinal pigment epithelial (RPE) changes in the chronic CSC. A hyperfluorescent spot shows up a bit late and increases in size and intensity showing leakage; (C and D) Viewed on indocyanine green angiography shows epicentral hypo- and surrounding hyper- and much larger areas of RPE alteration missed out on FFA.

of the dye ("washout") from the bulging polypoidal lesions. The particular late ICG staining of occult CNV is not seen in the PCV.[19]

Indocyanine green angiography has led to the early discovery of polyps in the peripapillary, the macular and the extramacular areas.[21] Identification of the polyps would allow treatment with laser photocoagulation if extrafoveal, and with photodynamic therapy (PDT) or anti-vascular endothelial growth factor (VEGF) agents.

CENTRAL SEROUS CHORIORETINOPATHY

Acute Phase

The leaking point of CSC seen on FA appears as a localized hypofluorescent area around the point of leakage **(Figs. 8A to D)**. These hypofluorescent areas are continuously observed throughout dye passage. In these regions, biomicroscopy and FA showed no abnormalities such as RPE detachment or atrophy. In the late phase ICG angiogram (when the intravascular dye had been washed out), abnormal choroidal hyperfluorescence may be seen. The sizes of the hyperfluorescent areas can range from 0.5 to 3.0 disk diameters and they were observed surrounding the leakage point seen in FA.[22]

Chronic Phase

In patients with a long-standing disease, when choroidal hyperfluorescence fades, hypofluorescent spots became increasingly evident, revealing pigment epithelial alterations not shown by FA. RPE atrophic tracts can be well-visualized and appear hyperfluorescent in cases with minimal amount of RPE atrophy and more hypofluorescent in cases with marked RPE atrophy **(Figs. 9A to D)**.

Another great advantage of ICGA is the detection of concomitant/complicated secondary CNVM. A distinct leakage of the occult CNVM can be easily detected among the focal leakage point of the CSC or the PED.

INFLAMMATORY LESIONS OF THE CHOROID

The most common finding on FA that corresponds to areas of active choroiditis is of early hypofluorescence with late hyperfluorescence; whereas in ICGA, they appear as hypofluorescent spots showing more extensive areas of involvement than seen on FA. In inflammatory disorders less information is obtained from the analysis of early phases as against the altered pattern of filling in intermediate and late phases of the ICGA. ICGA per se provides very limited information about the activity of the disease and to interpret the ICGA images, clinical and FA correlation is very essential.

To mention a few lesions and their ICGA findings:

- *Serpiginous choroiditis*: Hypofluorescent dots in all phases.
- *Multifocal choroiditis*: Large irregular spots of hypofluorescence and many more in number as compared to those seen in FFA. Late homogeneous background fluorescence.

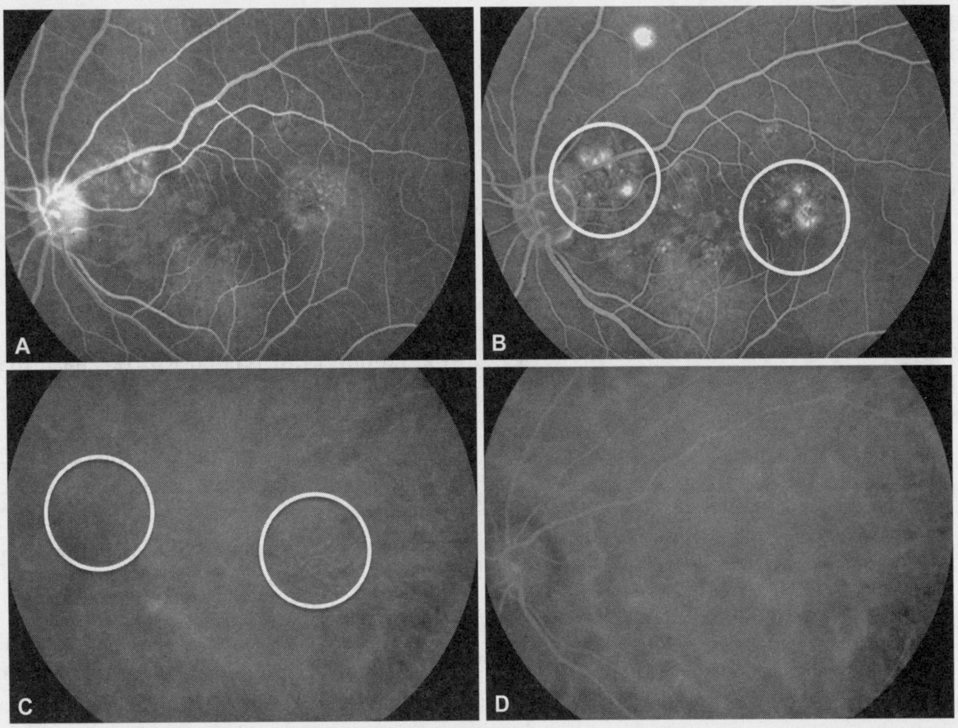

Figs. 9A to D: (A and B) Fundus fluorescein angiography images of the left eye (LE), in the early and late phases in a patient with multifocal chronic central serous chorioretinopathy; (C and D) The circled areas show epicenters of leakage. Indocyanine green angiography reveals interesting points as enumerated in the text. Early phases show hypofluorescence in the epicenter of the leakage (marked with the circles) with mild hyperfluorescence in the surrounding area. In the later phases, it achieves a ground-glass appearance.

- *Acute posterior multifocal placoid pigment epitheliopathy (APMPPE)*: Well-demarcated, hypofluorescent lesions in all phases.

TUMORS

Indocyanine green angiography has been described in four basic lesions of the choroid.

MELANOMA AND NEVUS

The patterns of ICG videoangiography are varied, depending on the degree of tumor pigmentation, thickness, and vascularity. Pigmented melanoma shows hypofluorescence in the early phases, while the less pigmented ones may demonstrate the intrinsic choroidal vasculature. Late phase angiograms usually show mild hyperfluorescence due to the leakage from underlying vessels. Rarely, a three-ring pattern can be appreciated in some melanomas during the later phases: (1) a central region of dense hypofluorescence, (2) a ring of mild hyperfluorescence, and (3) a peripheral ring of hypofluorescence.[23]

Choroidal Metastasis

Indocyanine green angiography shows a pattern of subtle diffuse homogeneous fluorescence of the tumor. In the late frames metastatic lesions showed ill-defined isofluorescence without hyperfluorescence, and in the late frames they were hypofluorescent overall.[24]

Choroidal Hemangioma

A lacy diffuse hyperintense pattern with a filling of the peripheral portion of the hemangioma first, and then the central portion as imaged with rapid sequence photography is observed in ICGA. The normal choroidal pattern is obscured by the vascular channels of the tumor. The fluorescence clears at variable rates leaving traces of fluorescence in the vascular channels giving the silhouettes of the vascular channels.[24]

Choroidal Osteoma

As one can anticipate, it shows an overall hypofluorescence as compared to the surrounding choroid.[24]

THERAPEUTIC APPLICATIONS

- Indocyanine green angiography with the confocal scanning laser ophthalmoscope (SLO), capturing at the rate of 10 frames per second can identify choroidal feeder vessels supplying CNVM. A laser treatment to such extrafoveal feeder vessels, particularly in membranes that are large or subfoveal, may be effective in closing the feeder vessel and CNVM with the preservation of the fovea and central vision.[25]
- Indocyanine green enhances the efficacy of transpupillary thermotherapy (TTT), as the peak absorption spectrum of ICG is the same as the peak emission of the diode laser. This allows selective ablation of the chorioretinal

lesions using ICG-augmented TTT. ICG-enhanced TTT to effectively treat retinoblastoma refractory to conventional focal treatments without deleterious ocular side effects has been reported.[26]

CONCLUSION

Indocyanine green angiography allows visualization of choroidal vascular pathology, being particularly useful in the diagnosis of PCV and occult CNVMs. It has helped in expanding the knowledge of certain disease such as CSC, wherein ICGA shows more extensive choroidal vascular pathology than what can be seen on FA. It also aids in selectively identifying and treating the feeder vessels of resistant CNVM.

REFERENCES

1. Hope-Ross M, Yannuzzi LA, Gragoudas ES, et al. Adverse reactions due to indocyanine green. Ophthalmology. 1994;101:529-33.
2. Cherrick GR, Stein SW, Leevy CM, et al. Indocyanine green: observations on its physical properties, plasma decay, and hepatic extraction. J Clin Invest. 1960;39:592-600.
3. Baker KJ. Binding of sulfobromophthalein (BSP) sodium and indocyanine green (ICG) by plasma alpha-1 lipoproteins. Proc Soc Exp Biol Med. 1966;122(4):957-63.
4. Brown N, Strong R. Infrared fundus angiography. Br J Ophthalmol. 1973;57(10):797-802.
5. Guyer DR, Yannuzzi LA. Occult choroidal neovascularization. In: Yannuzzi LA, Flower RW, Slakter JS (Eds). Indocyanine Green Angiography. St. Louis, Missouri: Mosby; 1997. pp. 157-80.
6. Guyer DR, Puliafito CA, Mones JM, et al. Digital indocyanine-green angiography in chorioretinal disorders. Ophthalmology. 1992;99(2):287-91.
7. Fineman MS, Maguire JI, Fineman SW, et al. Safety of indocyanine green angiography during pregnancy. Arch Ophthalmol. 2001;119:353-5.
8. Giani A, Pellegrini M, Carini E, et al. The dark atrophy with indocyanine green angiography in Stargardt disease. Invest Ophthalmol Vis Sci. 2012;53(7):3999-4004.
9. Hoang QV, Gallego-Pinazo R, Yannuzzi LA. Long-term follow-up of acute zonal occult outer retinopathy. Retina. 2013;33(7):1325-7.
10. Sorenson JA, Yannuzzi LA, Slakter JS, et al. A pilot study of digital indocyanine green videoangiography for recurrent occult choroidal neovascularization in age-related macular degeneration. Arch Ophthalmol. 1994;112(4):473-9.
11. Guyer DR, Yannuzzi LA, Slakter JS, et al. Classification of choroidal neovascularizaton by digital indocyanine green videoangiography. Ophthalmology. 1996;103:2054-60.
12. Guyer DR, Yannuzzi LA, Ladas I, et al. Indocyanine green-guided laser photocoagulation of focal spots at the edge of plaques of choroidal neovascularization. Arch Ophthalmol. 1996;114:693-7.
13. Coscas G. Age-related Macular Degeneration. In: Coscas G (Ed). Atlas of Indocyanine Green Angiography Fluorescein Angiography, ICG Angiography and OCT Correlations. Philadelphia: Elsevier; 2005. p. 118.
14. Yannuzzi LA, Freund KB, Takahashi BS. Review of retinal angiomatous proliferation or type 3 neovascularization. Retina. 2008;28(3):375-84.
15. Gass JD. Serous retinal pigment epithelial detachment with a notch: a sign of occult choroidal neovascularization. Retina. 1984;4:205-20.
16. Rouvas AA, Papakostas TD, Ntouraki A, et al. Angiographic and OCT features of retinal angiomatous proliferation. Eye (Lond). 2010;24(11):1633-42.
17. Yannuzzi LA, Sorenson JS, Spaide RF, et al. Idiopathic polypoidal choroidal vasculopathy. Retina. 1990;10:1-8.
18. Spaide RF, Yannuzzi LA, Slakter JS, et al. Indocyanine green videoangiography of idiopathic polypoidal choroidal vasculopathy. Retina. 1995;15:100-10.
19. Yannuzzi LA, Ciardella AP, Spaide RF, et al. The expanding clinical spectrum of idiopathic polypoidal choroidal vasculopathy. Arch Ophthalmol. 1999;115:478-85.
20. Yannuzzi LA, Wong DW, Sforzolini BS, et al. Polypoidal choroidal vasculopathy and neovascularized age-related macular degeneration. Arch Ophthalmol. 1999;117:1503-10.
21. Yannuzzi LA, Nogueira FB, Spaide RF, et al. Idiopathic polypoidal choroidal vasculopathy: a peripheral lesion. Arch Ophthalmol. 1998;116:382-3.
22. Kitaya N, Nagaoka T, Hikichi T, et al. Features of abnormal choroidal circulation in central serous chorioretinopathy. Br J Ophthalmol. 2003;87(6):709-12.
23. Atmaca LS, Lu FB, Atmaca P. Fluorescein and indocyanine green videoangiography of choroidal melanomas. Jpn J Ophthalmol. 1999;43:25-30.
24. Shields CL, Shields JA, De Potter P. Patterns of indocyanine green videoangiography of choroidal tumours. Br J Ophthalmol. 1995;79:237-45.
25. Lee WK, Kim HK. Feeder vessel laser photocoagulation of subfoveal choroidal neovascularization. Korean J Ophthalmol. 2000;14(2):60-8.
26. Francis JH, Abramson DH, Brodie SE, et al. Indocyanine green enhanced transpupillary thermotherapy in combination with ophthalmic artery chemosurgery for retinoblastoma. Br J Ophthalmol. 2013;97(2):164-8.

CHAPTER

16

Optical Coherence Tomography Angiography in Retinal Diseases

Chaitra Jayadev, Rohit Agrawal, Santosh Gopikrishna Gadde

INTRODUCTION

Abnormalities in the retinal and choroidal vasculature have been implicated in the pathogenesis of various retinal disorders. Fundus fluorescein angiography (FA) and indocyanine green angiography (ICGA) have been traditionally used to study retinal and choroidal vasculature, respectively. However, it has a major drawback of being an invasive test.

Optical coherence tomography angiography (OCTA) is a new, noninvasive imaging technique that generates volumetric angiography images in a matter of seconds thus producing high-resolution, 3-D angiograms of the retinal and choroidal vascular networks.

PRINCIPLE

The OCTA makes use of moving red blood cells (RBCs) as an intrinsic contrast agent. OCTA acquires repeated OCT B-scans at the same location to detect motion of the RBCs and thus creates an en face view of the retinal circulation. Various approaches have been described for quantifying this change through assessment of the phase, intensity, or both parameters of the OCT signal and are accordingly classified as phase-signal-based OCTA techniques, intensity-signal-based OCTA techniques, and complex-signal-based OCTA techniques **(Table 1)**.[1]

The images acquired and tools available for analysis depend on the machine platform as well as the algorithm used to acquire the image. In this chapter we will restrict our discussion to AngioVue software of the RTVue XR Avanti spectral-domain OCT (SD-OCT) (Optovue, Inc, Fremont, CA), which uses a split-spectrum amplitude decorrelation angiography (SSADA) algorithm **(Fig. 1)**.

The device obtains volumetric scans of 304 × 304 A-scans at 70,000 scans per second in approximately 3 seconds.

Table 1: Commercially available OCTA machines.

OCTA	*OCT platform*	*Algorithm*
AngioVue	OptoVue	SSADA
AngioPlex	Zeiss CIRRUS™ OCT	OMAG
SS-OCT Angio™	Swept Source OCT DRI OCT Triton series system (TOPCON)	OCTARA™
Spectralis® OCT angiography	Heidelberg	Amplitude decorrelation
AngioScan	Nidek RS-3000	Modified OMAG

(OCTA: optical coherence tomography angiography; OCTARA: optical coherence tomography angiography ratio analysis; OMAG: optical microangiography; SSADA: split-spectrum amplitude-decorrelation)

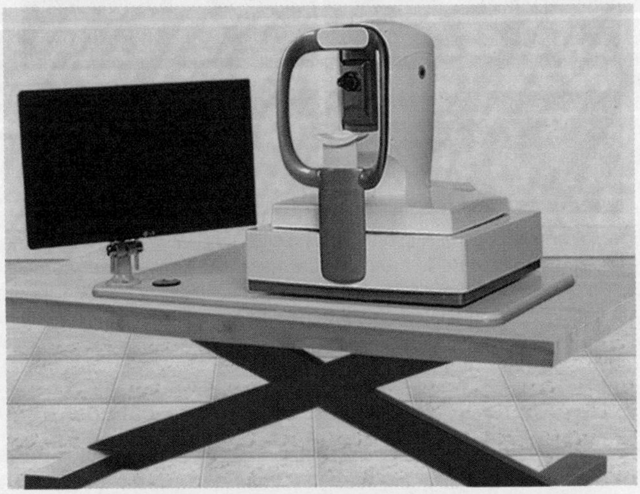

Fig. 1: RTVue XR Avanti spectral-domain optical coherence tomography (SD-OCT) (Optovue, Inc., Fremont, CA).

Angiograms can be captured in the following dimensions—8 × 8 mm, 6 × 6 mm, 3 × 3 mm, and 2 × 2 mm. The software automatically segments the full-thickness retinal scans into the "superficial" and "deep" inner retinal vascular plexuses, outer retina, and choriocapillaris (CC) **(Figs. 2A to E)**.[2]

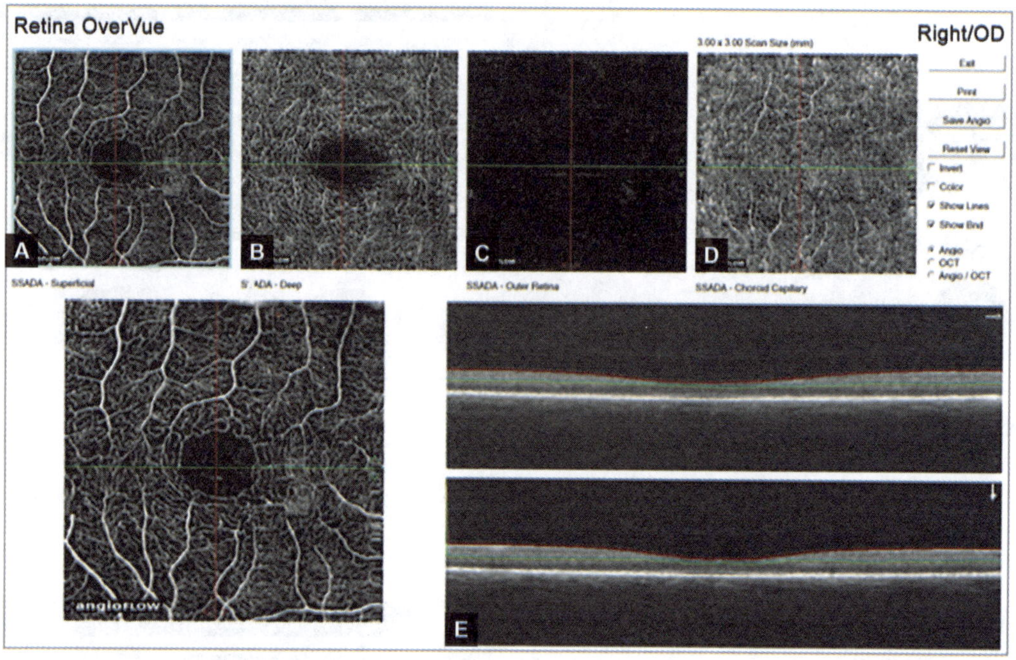

Figs. 2A to E: The OCT angiogram fields of view and segmentation layers on AngioVue. The normal right eye of a 30-year-old Indian man using the AngioVue optical coherence tomography angiography (OCTA) software of the RTVue XR Avanti (Optovue, Inc., Fremont, CA). (A) 3 × 3 mm OCT angiogram of the "superficial" inner retina; (B) 3 × 3 mm OCT angiogram of the "deep" inner retina; (C) 3 × 3 mm OCT angiogram of the outer retina shows absence of vasculature. The white represents noise; (D) 3 × 3 mm OCT angiogram of the choriocapillaris is generally homogeneous. There is back shadowing from retinal vessels; (E) OCT B-scan image.

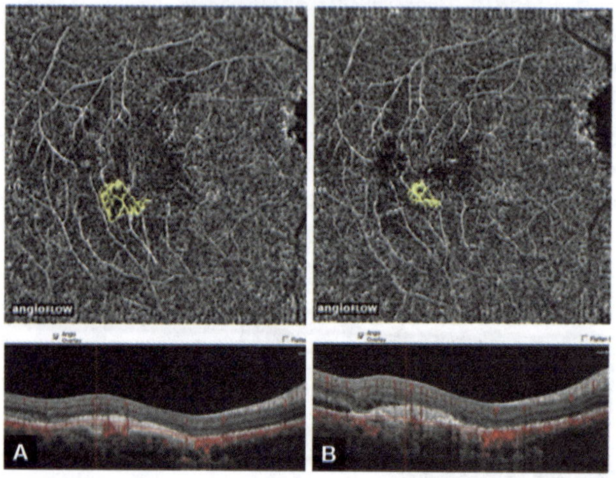

Figs. 3A and B: Use of AngioAnalytics (OptoVue RTVue XR AVANTI, Inc. Fremont, CA) software to measure flow area. (A) Neovascular complex (yellow network) at first presentation; (B) Neovascular complex 1 month post anti-VEGF demonstrating decreased flow area.

The AngioVue has a built-in software called AngioAnalytics which can perform basic function like calculating flow/non-flow area as well as vessel density **(Figs. 3A and B)**.

OPTICAL COHERENCE TOMOGRAPHY ANGIOGRAPHY OF RETINAL DISORDERS

Diabetic Retinopathy

Microaneurysms can be detected as focally dilated and abnormaliy shaped capillaries in superficial vascular plexus (SVP) and/or deep vascular plexus (DVP) in OCTA images. In addition, microaneurysms are found to be more abundant in DVP than SVP.[3,4] The detection rate of microaneurysms by OCTA is significantly lower than by FA.[4] The velocity of blood flow through the microaneurysms determines its detection on OCTA **(Figs. 4A and B)**.

Many studies have demonstrated a widening of the foveal avascular zone (FAZ) before the clinical detection of diabetic retinopathy. Thus, OCTA could serve as a predictor of diabetic retinopathy. In patient with diabetic retinopathy, FAZ enlargement has been noted in both SVP and DVP; the findings being more pronounced in DVP **(Figs. 5A and B)**.[4]

Optical coherence tomography angiography has been used to study vessel tortuosity, an indicator of the severity of nonproliferative diabetic retinopathy (NPDR).[5,6] In NPDR, an increase in the vessel tortuosity with the progression of the retinopathy either in superficial retinal layers or in deep retinal layers has been detected. It can also detect venous beading as contiguous focal dilations of retinal vessels.[7] Cotton-wool spots and intraretinal hemorrhages, on both FA and OCTA, correspond to areas of decreased or no perfusion.[8]

Optical coherence tomography angiography has allowed us to visualize the morphology of intraretinal microvascular abnormality (IRMA) using en face images. They are seen as dilated or looping vessels adjacent to areas of capillary nonperfusion. The caliber of these loops are noticeably larger on the OCTA than that of surrounding normal capillaries, thereby allowing easier distinction from normal vasculature.[9]

Optical coherence tomography angiography is not able to assess vascular leakage. This can be advantageous when

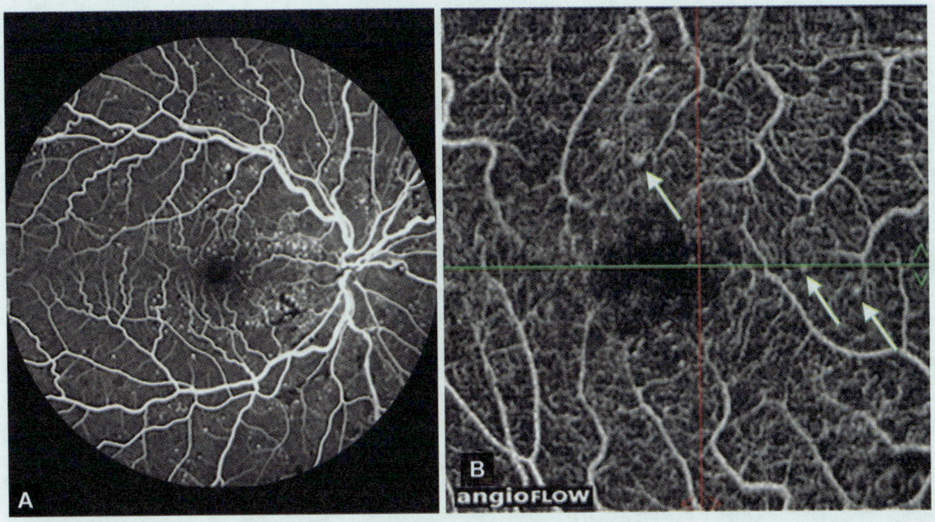

Figs. 4A and B: (A) The FA of a 65-year-old female patient with moderate NPDR showing multiple pin point hyperfluorescent areas indicating microaneurysms and vascular beading; (B) OCTA (OptoVue RTVue XR AVANTI, Inc., Fremont, CA) image of SCP of the same eye showing microaneurysms (white arrows), lesser in number compared to FA.
(FA: fluorescein angiography; NPDR: nonproliferative diabetic retinopathy; OCTA: optical coherence tomography angiography; SCP: superficial capillary plexus)

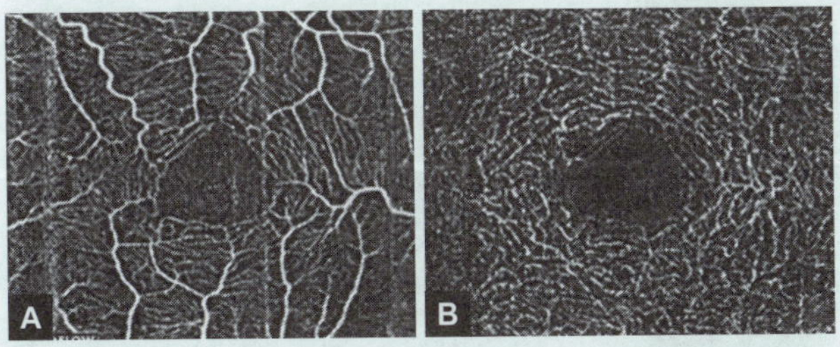

Figs. 5A and B: 3 × 3 mm OCTA (OptoVue RTVue XR AVANTI, Inc., Fremont, CA) scan of a 50-year-old male, diabetic patient with moderate NPDR demonstrating FAZ enlargement. The findings are less marked in SVP (A) compared to DCP (B).
(DCP: deep capillary plexus; FAZ: foveal avascular zone; OCTA: optical coherence tomography angiography; NPDR: nonproliferative diabetic retinopathy; SVP: superficial vascular plexus)

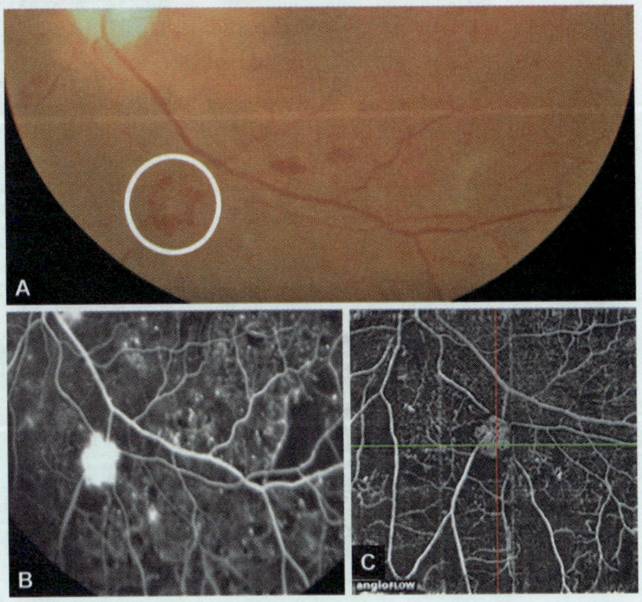

Figs. 6A to C: (A) Color fundus photograph of the left eye of a 52-year-old male affected by proliferative diabetic retinopathy showing neovascular tuft (white circle); (C) Optical coherence tomography angiography (OCTA) (6 × 6 mm) of the superficial capillary plexus (SCP) allows a better delineation of new vessels when compared to (B) fluorescein angiography.

trying to delineate boundaries of the new vessel complex. It can help the clinician to better differentiate between microaneurysms from small neovascular tufts, which are seen on FA as smaller areas of focal leakage **(Figs. 6A to C)**.[7]

Optical coherence tomography angiograms of patients affected by proliferative diabetic retinopathy (PDR) show lower retinal capillary density, higher capillary tortuosity, dilated capillary segments, capillary dropouts, capillary loops, and enlarged FAZ with asymmetric contour **(Figs. 7A and B)**.[10] OCTA can also be used to assess response to treatment. Shrinkage of new vessels post anti-vascular endothelial growth factor (VEGF) or pan-retinal photocoagulation has been seen.

Thus, OCTA is a useful tool when it comes to detecting vascular changes in diabetic retinopathy; it can be used as an adjunct with OCT and FA to better study the retinal changes caused by diabetes mellitus.

Retinal Artery Occlusion

A few studies and case reports have detailed the utility of OCTA in retinal artery occlusions. A good agreement between FA and OCTA has been noted. OCTA shows reduced flow in the area adjacent to the arterial embolus. Additionally the capillary ischemia seems to be more marked in the SVP than the adjacent DVP.[11] This area of ischemia correlates well with the areas of delayed filling on FA **(Figs. 8A to I)**.

It has been seen that in the acute phase both central retinal artery occlusion (CRAO) and branch retinal artery occlusion (BRAO) show decreased perfusion in the SVP and the DVP. However, the DVP shows improvement in vascularity in chronic cases probably due to the reorganization of the vascular network.[11,12]

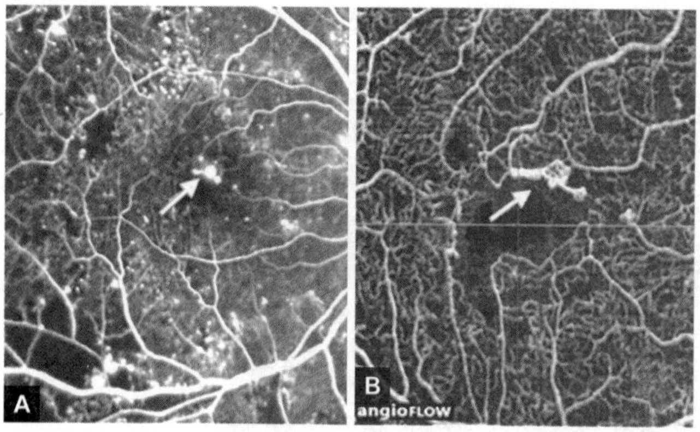

Figs. 7A and B: (A) The FA showing venous looping (white arrow) and distorted FAZ; (B) OCTA (OptoVue RTVue XR AVANTI, Inc., Fremont, CA) image of same eye showing well-delineated venous looping (white arrow) and distorted FAZ.
(FA: fluorescein angiography; FAZ: foveal avascular zone; OCTA: optical coherence tomography angiography)

Retinal Vein Occlusion

Both central retinal vein occlusion (CRVO) as well as branch retinal vein occlusion (BRVO) has been studied with OCTA. The features include FAZ enlargement in both SVP and DVP, capillary nonperfusion corresponding to the area involved, microvascular abnormalities, vascular congestion, telangiectasia, collateral formation, and neovascularization.[13,14]

The 3 mm × 3 mm scans demonstrate good agreement with FA; however, because of its limited field of view peripheral vascular changes may be missed out.[15,16]

Compared to FA, OCTA shows superior capability of delineating and measuring FAZ diameter. The FAZ diameter is increased in the SVP and DVP, with the DVP showing a larger FAZ when compared to SVP.[14,17] While imaging

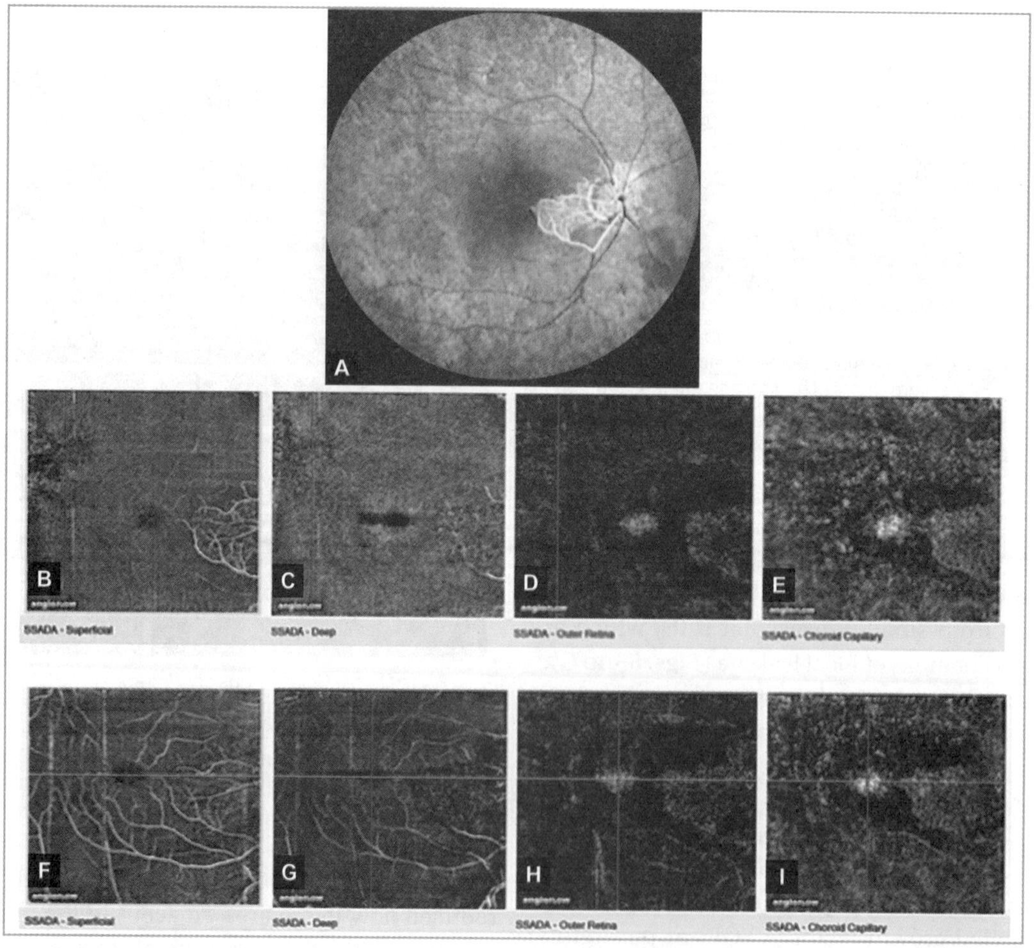

Figs. 8A to I: (A) The FA at 20 seconds showing filling of the cilioretinal artery with retrograde flow into the veins. The area perfused by the cilioretinal artery does not involve the fovea. Optical coherence tomography angiography OptoVue RTVue XR AVANTI, Inc., Fremont, CA (SSADA algorithm) done pre- and immediately post-paracentesis. OCTA done before paracentesis (B to E) showing no perfusion in the superficial plexus (B) except a localized area supplied by the cilioretinal artery that is perfused; deep plexus (C) shows disruption in the vascular areas with coarse texture and the choriocapillaris are not affected. An altered area on choroidal level (E) can be noticed which may be reduced back signals due to the retinal edema due to CRAO. The OCTA changes correspond very precisely to the early frames of FFA. The brighter areas on choroid capillary layer correspond to the better contrast of the fovea and perfused cilioretinal artery in comparison with the dark arc-like area seen in outer retina and choroid as this dark area is the representation of the retinal edema due to CRAO itself. OCTA done post-paracentesis (F to I) reveals increased perfusion of the retinal vasculature in both superficial and deep layers. The superficial layer (F) shows reperfusion quite clearly with an established centripetal pattern. The deep layer (G and H) shows artifacts of the vessels of superficial plexus. The choroidal layer (I) shows no alteration.
(CRAO: central retinal artery occlusion; FA: fluorescein angiography; FFA: fundus fluorescein angiography; SSADA: split-spectrum amplitude-de-correlation; OCTA: optical coherence tomography angiography)

of peripheral vasculature is a limiting feature, certain OCTA parameters such as disruption of the perifoveal capillary arcade in SVP, capillary network disruption in DVP, and deep capillary bed nonperfusion correlate with peripheral ischemia **(Figs. 9A to C)**.[18]

The retina's deep capillary plexus (DCP) appears to be the most affected vascular network in retinal vein occlusion (RVO). OCTA, with its ability to study each vascular bed separately, offers an opportunity to detect changes in each bed individually.

Dry Age-related Macular Degeneration

Optical coherence tomography angiography of eyes with dry age-related macular degeneration (AMD) shows a reduced vascular density in both the retinal vascular plexuses. An altered blood flow in SVP, DVP and CC is seen in early as well as later stages of AMD. In addition, the CC flow is severely compromised in areas of geographic atrophy **(Fig. 10)**.[19,20]

Wet Age-related Macular Degeneration

Type I Choroidal Neovascularization

Type I choroidal neovascularization (CNV) has a distinctive appearance within the CC slab on OCTA. It is seen as a highly organized complex of pruned vascular tree or tangled network or vascular loop. Often a central feeder vessel is seen with neovascular tree radiating centrifugally in a medusa pattern or branching in a sea-fan pattern. A hyporeflective halo surrounding the CNV has been also noted.[21,22] This halo might just be a shadow artifact from the retinal pigment epithelium (RPE), or compression of CC or flow void area or a combination of all the above **(Figs. 11A and B)**. Additionally, type I CNV lesion tends to appear smaller on OCTA

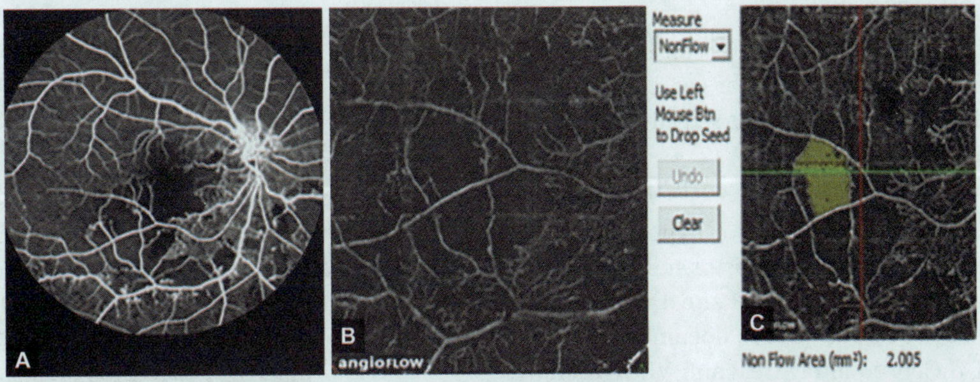

Figs. 9A to C: (A) The FA in a case of inferotemporal BRVO demonstrating capillary nonperfusion areas; (B) OCTA demonstaring capillary nonperfusion areas that correlate well with FA; (C) Use of angio-analytics to quantify nonperfusion areas.
(BRVO: branch retinal vein occlusion; FA: fluorescein angiography; OCTA: optical coherence tomography angiography)

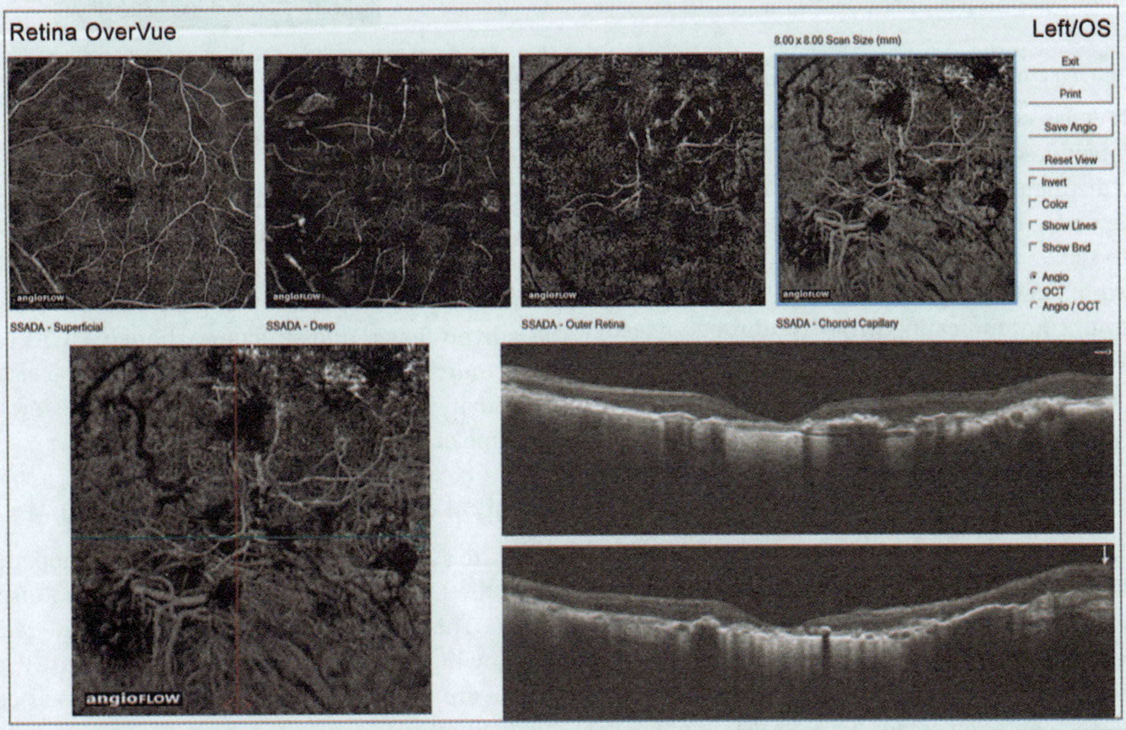

Fig. 10: Optical coherence tomography angiography (OCTA) of a 70-year-old man with geographic atrophy showing altered vasculature in choriocapillaris (CC) level.

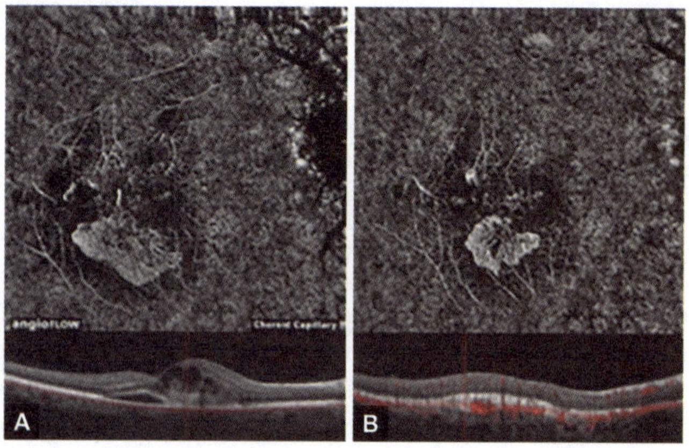

Figs. 11A and B: (A) The OCTA images of the CC layer showing a well-defined network of fine vessels suggestive of CNVM complex. A hyporeflective halo surrounding the CNVM can also be made out; (B) OCTA image of the same eye 2 weeks post-intravitreal anti-VEGF treatment showing decrease in the size of the CVVM complex.
(CNVM: choroidal neovascular membrane; OCTA: optical coherence tomography angiography; VEGF: vascular endothelial growth factor)

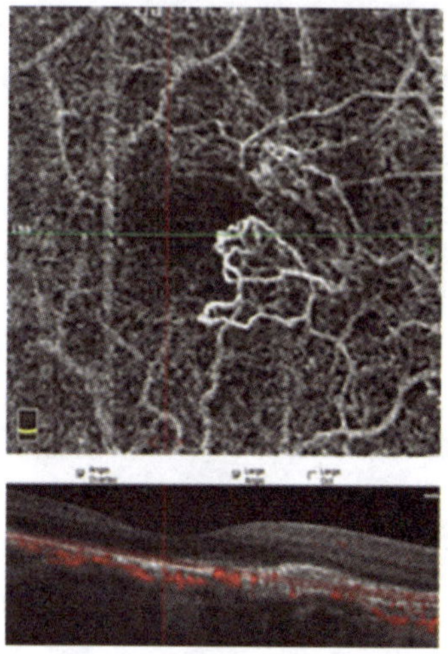

Fig. 12: Optical coherence tomography angiography demonstrating branched vascular network (BVN) as a hyperflow lesion in choriocapillaris segmentation.

when compared to ICG.[22] While OCTA can detect type I CNV with similar sensitivity as ICG or OCT, multimodal imaging is shown to further improve the sensitivity.[23]

Type II Choroidal Neovascularization

Type II lesions on OCTA present as a hyperflow lesion in the outer retina, with a glomerulus or medusa shape, surrounded by a dark halo. The SVP and DVP show no abnormal flow.[24] OCTA can be used to document response of a mixed type I-II CNV to intravitreal anti-VEGF therapy. Being noninvasive, it helps to monitor the retinal and choriocapillaris microvasculature in patients with CNV, thus, aiding in diagnosis and treatment decisions.

Type III Choroidal Neovascularization

Type III CNV, also known as retinal angiomatosis proliferans (RAP) is considered as an AMD variant that is sometimes difficult to distinguish from classic CNV. The sensitivity of OCTA in detecting type III CNV has been reported to range from 34% to 100%.[25] On OCTA, type III CNV appears as a tuft of bright, small, and curvilinear vessel in the outer retinal segmentation, communicating with DCP through a feeder vessel. Often, a small clew-like lesion is seen on the CC segmentation.[26]

POLYPOIDAL CHOROIDAL VASCULOPATHY

Polypoidal choroidal vasculopathy (PCV) is a disease entity characterized by multiple, bilateral, recurrent, serous, and serosanguinous RPE detachments in association with multiple polypoidal vascular abnormalities and branching vascular network (BVN) in the choroidal vasculature.

Branching vascular network is seen as a hyperflow lesion in CC segmentation of the OCTA. Its details are better seen when compared to ICG **(Fig. 12)**. It usually takes the appearance of a medusa or sea fan of tangled vascular pattern. The appearance of polyps on OCTA varies depending on the blood flow. They can be seen as either hyperflow round lesions with surrounding dark halo in some cases or as a hypo-flow round structure. Though, OCTA can display BVN more clearly, it cannot detect polypoidal lesions with a sensitivity comparable to ICG possibly due to low blood flow in some of the polyps.[27]

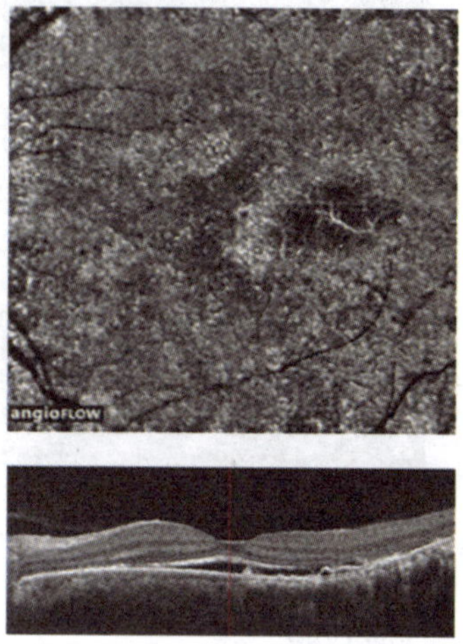

Fig. 13: A case of central serous chorioretinopathy showing a characteristic altered texture in the area involved. The pigment epithelial detachment seen as a dark well-circumscribed area on the choroidal level of the optical coherence tomography angiography.

Central Serous Chorioretinopathy

In acute stages of central serous chorioretinopathy (CSCR), only the CC slab shows altered texture and displays dark areas. This could correspond to either flow reduction or shadowing from SRF or both.[28] The SVP, DCP, and outer retina are normal. Abnormal choroidal vessels correspond to distinct, well-delineated, high-flow, and tangled pattern areas in the CC layer **(Fig. 13)**.

In chronic central serous retinopathy (CSR), the picture is further complicated by the development of CNV, persistent SRF and RPE alterations. No abnormalities are noted in the SVP and DVP. On the other hand, abnormal flow signals in outer retinal slab, altered CC texture and higher flow signals may be seen in the chronic disease.[28-30] Signs consistent with CNV include altered CC texture, abnormal flow in the avascular outer retinal slab, and abnormal vasculature in CC. OCTA, has been shown to be more effective in picking up CNV when compared to fundus fluorescein angiography (FFA)/ICG.[29]

MACULAR TELANGIECTASIA TYPE 2

Several authors have described OCTA findings of macular telangiectasia type 2 (MacTel2), showing a great concordance between FA and OCTA in the detection of associated vascular changes.

Superficial Layer

Stages 1–3 show enlargement of the FAZ, beginning temporally with a progressive horizontal increase in the FAZ diameter in the later stages. An increase in the intervascular space with progressive capillary rarefaction has been shown. These changes are accompanied by abnormal anastomoses between the capillary networks of the superficial and deeper layers. The finer vascular anastomoses could be appreciated as discrete bunches at multiple areas, more in the temporal aspect of the macula. The changes in larger blood vessels are more pronounced in the later stages with an abrupt ending and posterior dipping which can be traced into the deeper layers with adjustment of segmentation. Stages 4 and 5 demonstrate a gross decrease in retinal thickness and extensive empty spaces showing prominent larger blood vessels with radiating branches and widespread dark gray empty areas **(Figs. 14A to C)**.

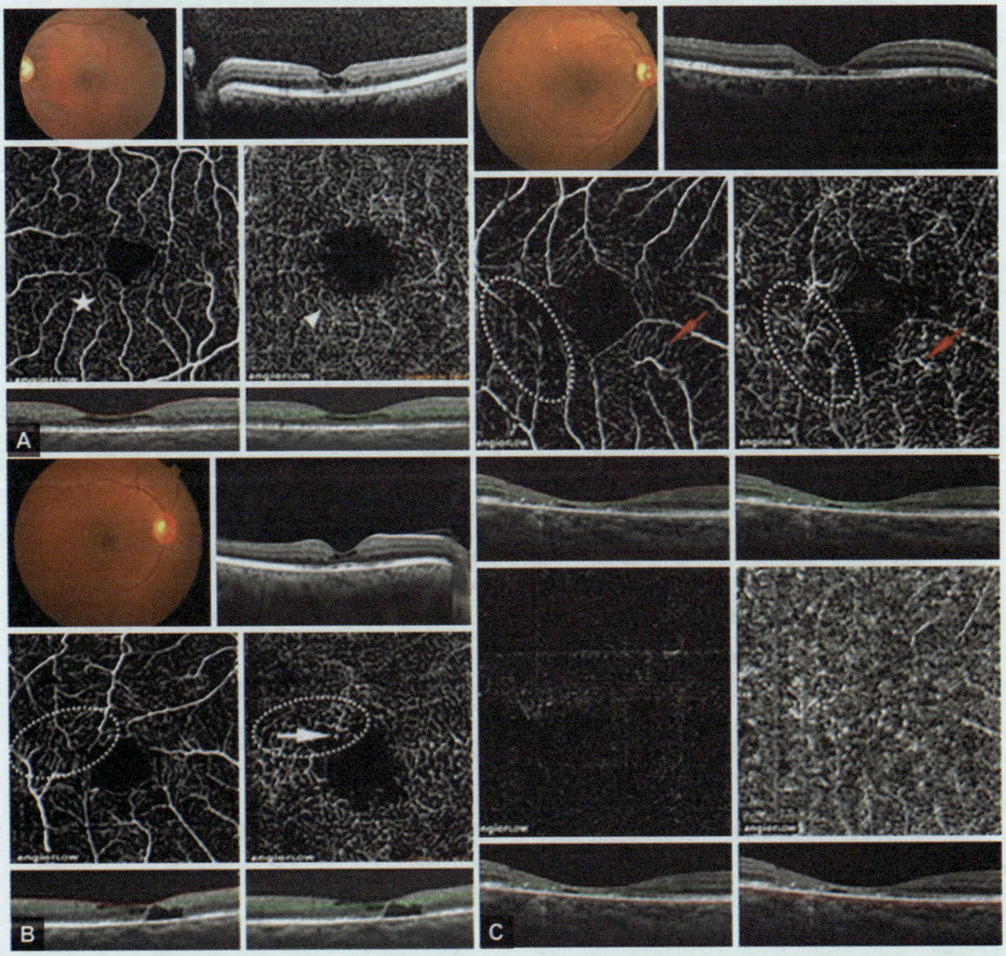

Figs. 14A to C: (A) *Stage 1*: Color fundus photograph showing dull foveal reflex and optical coherence tomography (OCT) reveals intraretinal hyporeflective spaces with changes in photoreceptor layer. OCTA-macular telangiectasia type 2 (MacTel2) showing mild irregularity of the foveal avascular zone (FAZ) and minimally increased intervascular spaces more in the superficial plexus (*) and broken regular network of FAZ with broken twig-like capillaries at deep plexus (arrowhead); (B) *Stage 2*: Color fundus photograph showing altered fovea with slight graying of perifoveal area with OCT showing intraretinal hypo-reflective spaces and internal limiting membrane drape at the fovea. On OCTA, besides stage 1 changes, there is progressive temporal enlargement and capillary rarefaction of FAZ in superficial layers (dotted circled area). Deep layer shows decrease in perifoveal capillary density but more pronounced and brighter capillary twigs, lost FAZ ring (dotted circle) and few aneurysmal dilatations (arrow). Outer retina and choroid are uninvolved; (C) *Stage 3*: Color fundus image showing vascular telangiectasia with graying of perifoveal retina. OCT shows decreased central foveal thickness, intraretinal hyporeflective spaces and photoreceptor loss. OCTA shows gross segmental loss of perifoveal capillary network, more temporally in both superficial and deep layers with increase in the FAZ and also noticeable distortion, more in the deeper plexus (dotted circled area). The right-angled vessel dipping can be appreciated and traced from superficial to deep plexus (red arrows). Outer retina and choroid are uninvolved.

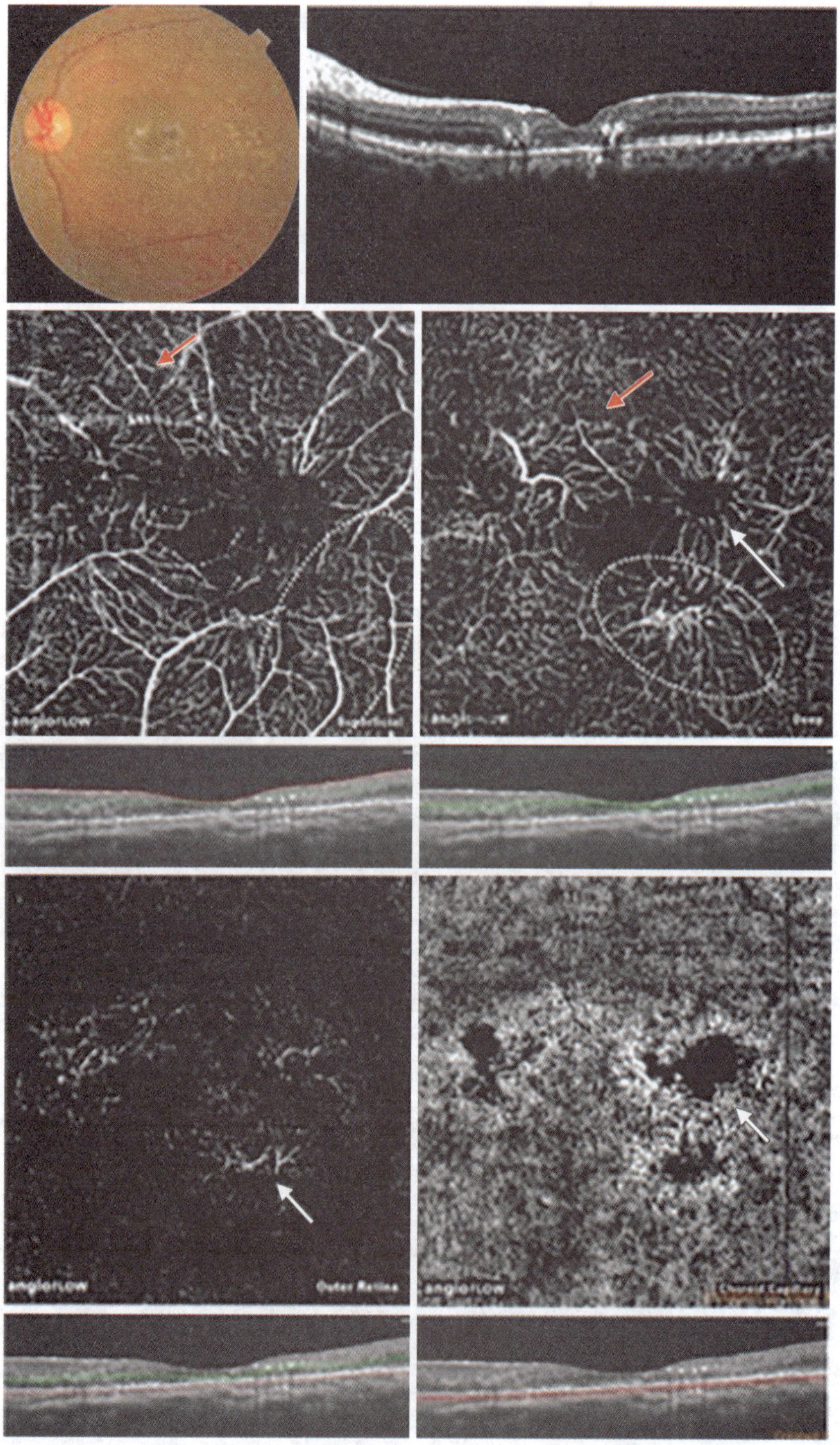

Fig. 15: *MacTel Stage 4*: Color fundus photograph showing pigment clumps and retinal pigment epithelium (RPE) alteration at macula. Optical coherence tomography (OCT) shows intraretinal hyper-reflectivity with backscattering and disruption of photoreceptor layer with variable retinal thinning. OCTA shows increased foveal avascular zone diameter and intervascular spaces, more horizontally with complete loss of perifoveal regular capillary meshwork in the superficial and deep layers with prominent larger vessels. A brush-like localized branching of vessels (dotted circles) with right-angled dipping can be seen around darker areas (arrows) suggestive of RPE hyperplasia. Outer retina reveals blood vessels corresponding to areas around RPE hyperplasia (arrows). Choroid reveals dark areas surrounded by gross alteration of texture surrounding it. Red arrows depict the anastomosis between the superficial and deep layers.

Deep Vascular Plexus

This layer demonstrates changes earlier than the superficial layer in the initial stages. The close-knit ring of perifoveal capillaries appears more pronounced and brighter with a decrease in vessel density. As the disease progresses, there is an increase in the FAZ diameter. Brush-like branching pattern of smaller vessels is noted. Prominent larger vessel segments with blunt ends suggestive of vessel dipping and gross capillary rarefaction can be appreciated **(Fig. 15)**.

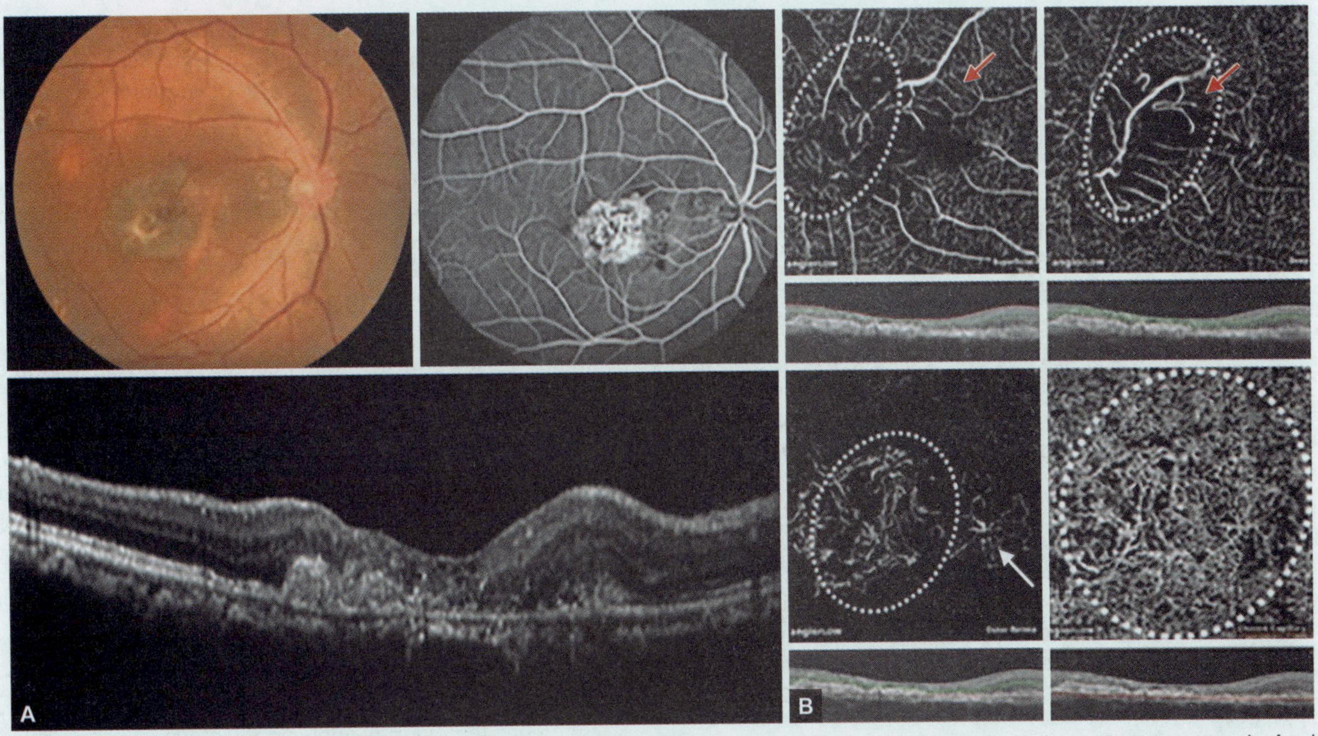

Figs. 16A and B: (A) *MacTel Stage 5*: A predominantly scarred neovascular membrane due to macular telangiectasia type 2 as seen on color fundus photograph, mid-phase frame of fluorescein angiography and optical coherence tomography scan; (B) Superficial and deep layers show complete distortion of foveal avascular zone, gross capillary rarefaction and dilated vessels that can be traced through different layers with abnormal anastomosis (dotted circles). Outer retina shows dense vascular network corresponding to the area of the scar (dotted circles) with an additional area of network of vessels (arrow) not corresponding to other layers suggestive of extensive areas of involvement. Choroid shows gross alterations in the texture with porous/spongy appearance, larger blood vessels with interspersed finer vessels in the area of the scar (larger dotted circle). Red arrows depict the anastomotic vessels between the superficial and deep network.

Outer Retina

It remains featureless in early disease. When present, the vascular network of the choroidal neovascular membrane (CNVM) with its blood vessels of varying caliber can be noted.

Choroid Layer

The later stages with RPE hyperplasia and CNVM scarring show bright areas with altered choroidal architecture that are porous with a sponge-like or coral-like appearance with prominent larger vessels that seem embedded in the substance of choroid with a network of interspersed finer vessels corresponding to the area of the scar and the changes seen in the other layers **(Figs. 16A and B)**.

CONCLUSION

Optical coherence tomography angiography has been shown to be a useful imaging modality for the evaluation of several retinal diseases. In the future as newer algorithms are developed and as scanning speeds become faster, larger fields of view with higher resolution is bound to become available to the clinician. Thus, OCTA is poised to become an invaluable tool in imaging the retina.

REFERENCES

1. Gao SS, Jia Y, Zhang M, et al. Optical coherence tomography angiography. Investig Opthalmol Vis Sci. 2016;57(9):OCT27-36.
2. de Carlo TE, Romano A, Waheed NK, et al. A review of optical coherence tomography angiography (OCTA). Int J Retina Vitreous. 2015;1:5. eCollection 2015.
3. Couturier A, Mané V, Bonnin S, et al. Capillary plexus anomalies in diabetic retinopathy on optical coherence tomography angiography. Retina. 2015;35(11):2384-91.
4. Ishibazawa A, Nagaoka T, Takahashi A, et al. Optical coherence tomography angiography in diabetic retinopathy: a prospective pilot study. Am J Ophthalmol. 2015;160(1):35-44.e1.
5. de Carlo TE, Chin AT, Bonini Filho MA, et al. Detection of microvascular changes in eyes of patients with diabetes but not clinical diabetic retinopathy using optical coherence tomography angiography. Retina. 2015;35(11):2364-70.
6. Lee H, Lee M, Chung H, et al. Quantification of retinal vessel tortuosity in diabetic retinopathy using optical coherence tomography angiography. Retina. 2018;38(5):976-85.
7. Hwang TS, Jia Y, Gao SS, et al. Optical coherence tomography angiography features of diabetic retinopathy. Retina. 2015;35(11):2371-6.
8. Matsunaga DR, Yi JJ, De Koo LO, et al. Optical coherence tomography angiography of diabetic retinopathy in human subjects. Ophthalmic Surg Lasers Imaging Retina. 2015;46(8):796-805.

9. Schaal KB, Munk MR, Wyssmueller I, et al. Vascular abnormalities in diabetic retinopathy assessed with swept-source optical coherence tomography angiography wide field imaging. Retina. 2019;39(1):79-87.
10. Choi W, Waheed NK, Moult EM, et al. Ultrahigh speed swept source optical coherence tomography angiography of retinal and choriocapillaris alterations in diabetic patients with and without retinopathy. Retina. 2017;37(1):11-21.
11. de Castro-Abeger AH, de Carlo TE, Duker JS, et al. Optical coherence tomography angiography compared to fluorescein angiography in branch retinal artery occlusion. Ophthalmic Surg Lasers Imaging Retin. 2015;46(10):1052-4.
12. Lee AY, Zhang Q, Baughman DM, et al. Evaluation of bilateral central retinal artery occlusions with optical coherence tomography-based microangiography: a case report. J Med Case Rep. 2016;10(1):307.
13. Rispoli M, Savastano MC, Lumbroso B. Capillary network anomalies in branch retinal vein occlusion on optical coherence tomography angiography. Retina. 2015;35(11):2332-8.
14. Adhi M, Bonini Filho MA, Louzada RN, et al. Retinal capillary network and foveal avascular zone in eyes with vein occlusion and fellow eyes analyzed with optical coherence tomography angiography. Investig Ophthalmol Vis Sci. 2016;57(9):486-94.
15. Suzuki N, Hirano Y, Yoshida M, et al. Microvascular abnormalities on optical coherence tomography angiography in macular edema associated with branch retinal vein occlusion. Am J Ophthalmol. 2016;161:126-32.e1.
16. Nobre Cardoso J, Keane PA, Sim DA, et al. Systematic evaluation of optical coherence tomography angiography in retinal vein occlusion. Am J Ophthalmol. 2016;163:93-107.e6.
17. Casselholmde Salles M, Kvanta A, Amrén U, et al. Optical coherence tomography angiography in central retinal vein occlusion: correlation between the foveal avascular zone and visual acuity. Investig Ophthalmol Vis Sci. 2016;57(9):OCT242-6.
18. Coscas F, Glacet-Bernard A, Miere A, et al. Optical coherence tomography angiography in retinal vein occlusion: evaluation of superficial and deep capillary plexa. Am J Ophthalmol. 2016;161:160-71.e1-2.
19. Toto L, Borrelli E, Di Antonio L, et al. Retinal vascular plexuses' changes in dry age-related macular degeneration, evaluated by means of optical coherence tomography angiography. Retina. 2016;36(8):1566-72.
20. Moult EM, Waheed NK, Novais EA, et al. Swept-source optical coherence tomography angiography reveals choriocapillaris alterations in eyes with nascent geographic atrophy and drusen-associated geographic atrophy. Retina. 2016;36 (Suppl 1):S2-11.
21. Jia Y, Bailey ST, Wilson DJ, et al. Quantitative optical coherence tomography angiography of choroidal neovascularization in age-related macular degeneration. Ophthalmology. 2014;121(7):1435-44.
22. Costanzo E, Miere A, Querques G, et al. Type 1 choroidal neovascularization lesion size: indocyanine green angiography versus optical coherence tomography angiography. Investig Opthalmol Vis Sci. 2016;57(9):OCT307.
23. Inoue M, Jung JJ, Balaratnasingam C, et al.; COFT-1 Study Group. A comparison between optical coherence tomography angiography and fluorescein angiography for the imaging of type 1 neovascularization. Invest Ophthalmol Vis Sci. 2016;57(9):OCT314-23.
24. El Ameen A, Cohen SY, Semoun O, et al. Type 2 neovascularization secondary to age-related macular degeneration imaged by optical coherence tomography angiography. Retina. 2015; 35(11):2212-8.
25. Kuehlewein L, Dansingani KK, de Carlo TE, et al. Optical coherence tomography angiography of type 3 neovascularization secondary to age-related macular degeneration. Retina. 2015;35(11):2229-35.
26. Miere A, Querques G, Semoun O, et al. Optical coherence tomography angiography in early type 3 neovascularization. Retina. 2015;35(11):2236-41.
27. Kim JY, Kwon OW, Oh HS, et al. Optical coherence tomography angiography in patients with polypoidal choroidal vasculopathy. Graefe's Arch Clin Exp Ophthalmol. 2016;254(8):1505-10.
28. Costanzo E, Cohen SY, Miere A, et al. Optical coherence tomography angiography in central serous chorioretinopathy. J Ophthalmol. 2015;2015:134783.
29. Quaranta-El Maftouhi M, El Maftouhi A, Eandi CM. Chronic central serous chorioretinopathy imaged by optical coherence tomographic angiography. Am J Ophthalmol. 2015;160(3):581-7.e1.
30. de Carlo TE, Rosenblatt A, Goldstein M, et al. Vascularization of irregular retinal pigment epithelial detachments in chronic central serous chorioretinopathy evaluated with OCT angiography. Ophthalmic Surg Lasers Imaging Retina. 2016;47(2):128-33.

CHAPTER

17 A-scan Ultrasonography

Nazneen Nazm, Arup Chakrabarti, Meena Chakrabarti

INTRODUCTION

A-scan ultrasonography (USG) is one of the most common performed noninvasive diagnostic modality in ophthalmology. It is an indispensable tool which helps in accurate measurement of the axial length (AL) of the eye—an essential prerequisition for intraocular lens (IOL) power calculation. It is also a very useful tool in determining the reflectivity of intraocular and intraorbital lesions when used in conjunction with the B-mode. This article aims to provide a comprehensive coverage of the various uses of A-mode ultrasound scan.

HISTORY

Since the time Sir Harold Ridley experienced a postoperative refractive surprise of 21 diopters (21 D) in IOL power calculation in the first two patients in 1949–50, biometry and IOL power calculation has come a long way. In 1956, Mundt and Hughes first reported the use of diagnostic ultrasound for ocular use. They reported the use of industrial flaw detection equipment for A-mode examination of in vitro enucleated eyes and patients with intraocular tumors. Oksala and Lehtinen from Finland described the use of handheld A-mode transducer for clinical use. Around the same time, Baum and Greenwood developed the technique of B-scan USG using the immersion method.

There were a number of teething problems initially in the development of and use of ultrasound for ophthalmic purpose. Initial transducers were unfocused and had poor resolution. Displays were generated on oscilloscopes and photography was used for recording. Rulers were used to measure echo time intervals on these photographs to compute biometry results, making the technique quite inaccurate.

Increasing transducer frequencies and more advanced time measurement techniques (rather than the previous method of ruler measurements of photographed A-mode displays) paved the way for advances in biometry precision. In 1967, Giglio and Ludlam developed a system which used a 20-MHz focused transducer with multitrace oscilloscope display. This provided improved measurement precision. Later, Coleman and Carlin developed a system which used high-frequency focused transducer. Start and stop gates were available and could be adjusted to bracket echoes of interest, and the interval between them could be electronically measured, averaged, and displayed as an alphanumeric value. The use of digital technique improved the measurement precision to about 20 mm.

PHYSICS OF ULTRASOUND

Principle of USG is based on the use of high-frequency sound waves (2–15 MHz) to generate an image. Sound is defined as a vibration which propagates in a wave pattern through a transmission medium such as solid, liquid, or gas. Sound waves are audible when they have a frequency between 20 Hz and 20 KHz. Ultrasound waves possess a frequency greater than 20,000 Hz (20 KHz) and are not audible by human beings. Most A- and B-scans used for ophthalmic purpose have a probe frequency of approximately 10 million Hz or 10 MHz. Such high sound frequency has a dual advantage: (1) it allows restricted depth of penetration into ocular tissue, and (2) it allows for excellent resolution of minute structures.

The velocity of sound depends on the density of medium through which it travels. Sound travels faster through solids than liquids. Therefore, sound doesn't travel at a uniform velocity as it passes through eye since human eye is made up of both solid and liquid structures. Sound therefore, continuously changes velocity as it passes through the different structures in the eye: through solid cornea, the liquid aqueous, the solid lens, the liquid vitreous, the solid retina, choroid, sclera, and finally the orbital tissue. The velocity of

Table 1: The velocity of sound as it passes through different ocular structures.

Ocular structure	*Velocity of sound*
Cornea	1,641 m/s
Lens (average lens velocity in cataract group)	1,641 m/s
Aqueous	1,532 m/s
Vitreous	1,532 m/s

sound as it passes through these media is summarized in the **Table 1**.

The average sound velocity (Vc) through a phakic eye is 1,550 m/s, through an aphakic eye is 1,532 m/s and through a pseudophakic eye is 1,532 m/s plus the correction factor (CF) for the IOL material (discussed later).

A-scan biometry uses reflected sound waves to measure intraocular lengths. "A" stands for "amplitude" and is a measure of strength of echo. In A-scan biometry technique, a thin sound beam of approximately 10 MHz is emitted from the probe tip. As the sound beam strikes each interface (i.e. junction between two media of different densities such as the aqueous/anterior lens surface and posterior lens capsule and anterior vitreous), an echo bounces back into the probe tip. These echoes received by the probe tip as a result of sound waves hitting different interfaces, are converted by the instrument to spikes arising from baseline. If the difference of Vc at interface is small, the echo produces is weak and the resultant spikes produced are short. On the contrary, if the difference between the two media at an interface is high, the resultant echo is strong and the spike high. Therefore, if the difference in the Vc in the two media across an interface is not high, the echo produced is weak and the resultant spike short and vice versa. There are certain other factors which affect the height of resultant spike such as:

- *Shape and smoothness of surface*: The more irregular the surface, the weaker the echoes. This is because some of the sound waves returning from the surface undergo reflection and refraction.
- The angle of incidence of sound beam to the surface (i.e. the orientation of probe to the corneal surface).
- *Reflection and refraction of sound waves (similar to light waves) and also the absorption of sound waves*: This is the reason for reduced retinal spike in case of very dense cataract since the cataractous lens absorbs a significant portion of the sound waves.

B-scan USG is the other type of ophthalmic USG. "B" in B-scan refers to "brightness". Here, an oscillating sound beam is emitted and passed through the eye. As it passes through the eye, it strikes the intraocular structures. An echo is reflected back to the probe and this is converted into an electric signal. The echoes are seen as a series of dots that together form a two-dimensional image. Stronger the echo, brighter the dot. The process is repeated 1,000 times per second to produce a real-time display. B-scan USG is used to image intraocular structures especially when direct visualization of structures is difficult or impossible such as in case of dense cataract, corneal opacities, or vitreous hemorrhage. It is a valuable tool for diagnostic purpose even when the pathology is clinically invisible. The B-scan is complimentary to the A-scan in diagnostic utility because it displays topographic features such as shape and anatomic relationship to different structures.

ULTRASOUND BIOMETRY INSTRUMENTATION

A variety of A-scan equipment are available today. An A-scan biometry machine consists of four basic parts—(1) pulser, (2) probe, (3) receiver, and (4) display screen. These are all housed within a single unit. The transducer is located at the tip of the probe. Pulsing electricity is delivered to the probe tip which contains the piezoelectric crystal. The crystal vibrates and emits the sound beam. After a few microseconds the returning echoes are received by the probe tip and transformed into electric signals and converted to spikes on display; also called echograms. Here, in this context three terms are important—(1) gain, (2) resolution, and (3) gates.

1. *Gain:* Gain is defined as the degree of echo amplification. It is measured in decibel (dB). When the gain setting in the instrument is set at the highest, the spike height and the sensitivity of display screen are set at the maximum. This enables visualization of weaker signals. However, one must remember that increasing gain decreases resolution (discussed below). Conversely, when the gain setting is reduced, the amplitude of spike and display sensitivity is decreased but resolution is increased. At the beginning of examination, the gain should be set at a relatively high level. A high gain setting helps to grossly align the sound beam with structures along the visual axis to assess the overall appearance of the echogram. Once aligned, the gain setting should be reduced during examination to medium in order to improve resolution of spikes. Gain settings need to be increased in dense cataract because dense cataract absorbs sound.
2. *Resolution:* Resolution is defined as the ability of the biometry machine to display two interfaces which lie in close proximity, one directly behind the other, as separate spikes or echoes. Resolution is inversely proportional to gain.
3. *Gates:* Gates are electronic markers or cursors or calipers on the screen display that provides the measurement of distance between two (or more) anatomic points/interfaces. For more accurate scans, gates must be visible on the display. Also, the operator should be able to change the gate position in case they are not correctly aligned on

the correct anatomical structure because misalignment of gate will cause the entire ocular length calculation to be wrong. In the manual mode, the gate position is selected by the examiner while in the automatic mode the gate position is determined by the instrument. Usually, the biometer automatically places a gate on (1) corneal spike, (2) anterior lens spike, (3) posterior lens spike, and (4) the retinal spike. The biometer then measures the distance between each pair of gates at given Vc.

Ultrasound uses the formula "distance = velocity × time", to calculate the distance (and thereby the length) between each pair of gates. This distance is the total distance from probe to ocular structures and back to the probe. Therefore this distance is divided by 2 after proper selection of measurement mode (aphakic, phakic, or pseudophakic) to account for the difference in Vc in different situations.

Probe orientation for B scan: The B-scan can be oriented in three ways—(1) transverse, (2) longitudinal, and (3) axial. In a transverse scan the probe is directed tangential to the limbus while it is positioned perpendicular to the limbus with the probe marker pointing to the center of cornea in longitudinal scan. An axial scan is procured by placing the probe on the center of cornea with the patient looking straight ahead.

EXAMINATION PROCEDURE

Meticulous attention to technique during examination is important. The procedure is described below:

- *History:* A detailed history must be elicited prior to the procedure. This includes history of trauma and any previous ocular surgery. It is important to know, if the eye is aphakic or pseudophakic or if the patient underwent retinal detachment (RD) surgery (such as sclera buckling) or if there is silicon oil injected in the eye. A history of diabetes, age-related macular degeneration (ARMD) is important because macular pathology such as gross edema/macular thickening or macular detachment can lead to erroneous measurement of axial length (shorter AL). A previous history of RD surgery with sclera buckle is important as it can induce a change in the AL measured (erroneously long AL).
- *Patient preparation:* The procedure should be explained to the patient. Topical anesthesia, i.e. proparacaine eyedrops is instilled in the eye if patient is not allergic to it. The patient is then asked to wipe off excess anesthetic eyedrops/tears before the procedure since the presence of even small amounts of tears or fluids on cornea can lead to erroneous AL measurements (false high reading). The patient is positioned comfortably. Check the instrument for settings—measurement mode (phakic/pseudophakia/aphakia), gate position, and gain settings prior to examination is important. The probe tip must be cleaned before each use (discussed later). Always ensure that the tip is dry. Reassure the patient again and ask him/her to fixate in primary gaze, preferably at the light within the probe. However, remember to position the fixation light far enough from the patient's eyes to not stimulate convergence. Stimulating convergence would lead to erroneous readings since the sound beam will not be perpendicular to the eye and will not pass through the fovea. Always perform the examination in both eyes to compare measurements of the two eyes. Any unusual measurements can thus be detected and this can help to minimize errors.
- *Keratometry:* The keratometer is an instrument to measure the radius of curvature of anterior corneal surface. Keratometry readings are essential for and used in conjunction with A-scan biometry for IOL power calculation. Keratometry readings must always be obtained prior to AL readings because placement of probe of biometry can produce distortion of mires on cornea and can lead to inaccurate keratometry readings. Therefore, always perform keratometry before A-scan biometry.

TECHNIQUE FOR MEASUREMENT OF AXIAL LENGTH FOR INTRAOCULAR LENS POWER CALCULATION

There are two main techniques of A-scan biometry: (1) The contact technique; and (2) The immersion technique.

Contact Technique

In this technique, the probe is in contact with the cornea and hence the name. The probe is gently placed on the center of cornea and the sound beam directed from corneal vertex toward macula. The contact technique includes the "hand-held method" and the "applanation" method. The procedure is as follows:

- Select the correct mode (aphakic/phakic/pseudophakic) depending on the type of eye to be scanned.
- Ask the patient to fixate on the red light.
- Excess drops or tears must be wiped off lightly from the eye as presence of tears on cornea can lead to wrong AL calculation (false high AL readings).
- Place the probe lightly on the center of cornea. Avoid corneal compression with the probe as this can lead to false low AL calculation.
- Remove the probe and ask patient to blink to keep cornea moist.
- The procedure is repeated several times till three or requisite numbers of high quality readings are obtained.
- Avoid excessive manipulation of probe on cornea as this can produce an epithelial defect.

Hand-held Method

In this technique, a hand-held probe is used for AL measurement. The patient is seated comfortably either upright or reclining with the patient's head positioned in front of the display screen of biometer. The examiner is seated on an adjustable stool facing the patient with his/her arm resting on patient's shoulder and the side of the hand (holding the probe) on patient's cheek. It is important for the examiner to rest his hand comfortably on patient's shoulder in order to avoid exerting undue pressure (and thereby compression) on the cornea. Being seated in this way allows the examiner to both view the instrument display and patient's fixation. Because of the possibility of corneal compression, the contact method has been replaced by other more accurate techniques of biometry.

Applanation Method

In this method, a chin rest is used. The patient is seated comfortably with the chin on chin-rest and the forehead pressed against the headrest. The probe is fixed in a sleeve or probe holder. A pressure-sensitive probe holder helps to minimize corneal compression. The patient is asked to fixate in primary gaze at the fixation light within the center of probe tip. Initially, the joystick is retracted away from the patient and then gradually advanced toward the cornea till the probe gently applanates the cornea and A-scan readings are obtained.

Potential Sources of Errors with Contact Method

There are several potential sources of errors with this method. The sources of error are:

- *Corneal compression:* This is the most common source of error and occurs due to inadvertent pressure on cornea. This leads to falsely low AL calculation. This can be minimized by placing the probe gently on cornea and removing the probe in-between measurements (the "on-and-off technique"). One can also view the cornea from the side and place the probe lightly on corneal apex. One must also keep an eye on the anterior chamber depth (ACD) measurements because undue compression on cornea causes ACD to decrease.
- Presence of fluid either on probe tip or in the eye in the form of excess tears or presence of eyedrop/ointment can lead to formation of a "fluid meniscus" between the eye and the probe tip leading to falsely high AL readings. This can be avoided by checking that the probe tip is dry prior to placing it on the cornea and also by asking the patient to wipe off excess tears or fluid from the eye prior to the procedure.
- Error may also be produced due to incorrect settings in the eye, e.g. failing to choose "aphakia mode" when the eye is aphakic. Errors may also occur due to improper gate placement (discussed above). Therefore one must always keep an eye on the machine display during the procedure.

Immersion Technique

The immersion technique became popular because it avoids the inherent disadvantage of contact method, i.e. corneal compression. In this technique, a small water bath or sclera shell is filled with saline and the probe immersed into the fluid. The shell is then placed between the patient's lids while being careful to avoid contact with cornea. Since there is no corneal compression, this technique is more accurate than the contact technique. In the immersion technique, six spikes are displayed rather than five. The probe and the cornea produce two separate spikes since they are not in contact with each other. However, some machines show five spikes (because the probe spike is shifted very far to the left and thus not seen on display). These five spikes represent the cornea, the anterior lens surface, the posterior lens surface, the retina, and the sclera. There are several advantages of the immersion technique:

- The technique does not involve corneal compression.
- There is display of a separate corneal spike which is absent in contact technique. This allows better alignment of the sound beam with visual axis and therefore more accurate measurements. The corneal spike is visible as a separate spike. Two peaks are produced: one corresponding to the epithelium and the other to the endothelium. The two spikes should be equally high. If not, the sound beam is not perpendicular to the corneal vertex. This allows one to check the alignment of sound beam to the visual axis.
- It is faster than contact technique and is also less operator-dependent.

Technique

The patient is positioned with the patient reclined. Topical anesthetic drops are instilled to anesthetize the cornea. The patient is asked to fixate at the target in primary gaze. The sclera shell is inserted between the lids and filled about two-thirds with methylcellulose while carefully avoiding air bubbles since this can interfere with measurements. The Prager shell (sclera shell) is also available for use. The examination is started with high gain setting and the probe is immersed into fluid just until the spikes are obtained. Once steep rising and highly reflective spikes are obtained, the gain setting is reduced to increase resolution. Measurement is taken when the spikes are distinct and at their maximum height.

Prager Shell

Immersion could be performed either with an open cylinder called Hansen shell (Hansen Shell, Iowa City, Iowa) or with a fixed immersion shell (Prager shell, ESI Inc, Plymouth, Minn.eyesurgin.com). Several models of Prager shell are available.

The Prager shell has two internal guide rings to maintain probe perpendicularity. All Prager models have a Leuer fitting on the side for connecting sterile tubing to the shell. A BSS (balanced salt saline) bottle or a syringe filled with BSS is attached to the tubing placed in a syringe. The Leuer connector contains a check valve system which acts as a one-way valve and does not allow regurgitation/backflow of contaminated fluid from the eye into the BSS source. The biometry probe is then inserted into the shell. The software of the biometry machine is such that it will capture scans only if the probe is at the "exact distance from the cornea" as specified by each ultrasound biometry manufacturer. The Prager shell possesses an "auto stop" feature that seats the probe at the manufacturer-specified distance from the cornea. This helps to ensure that the corneal gate of the scan is located on the anterior cornea. The perpendicularity of the probe is also assured.

A variety of other shells are available such as the Ossoinig sclera shell, the Hansen shell, and the Kohn shell.

Procedure

The patient is seated in a reclining fashion with the head positioned comfortably on the headrest. Topical anesthesia is instilled and the patient is provided with a fixation light. Place a sterile towel on patient's shoulder and rest the BSS bottle on the towel. Now, the patient is asked to look downward while the examiner simultaneously lifts the upper eyelid and inserts the flared rim under the lid. Next, the lower lid is pulled down to guide the lower part of shell into place in the lower fornix. To take the scans, pick up the BSS bottle or syringe and slowly inject the fluid into the shell. When the shell is filled sufficiently, the waveforms will be seen. The examiner can select the good scans while deleting the poor ones.

Potential Sources of Error with the Immersion Technique

- Presence of air bubbles in the fluid placed in the scleral shell is a potential source of error. These air bubbles lead to production of additional spikes on the echogram to the left of corneal spike. If these spikes are mistaken to be corneal spikes, the resultant AL measurement will be erroneously long. This error can be avoided by avoiding air bubbles in the fluid and also by correctly identifying the corneal spike. The corneal spike is double peaked. If too many air bubbles are present then the shell should be removed and reapplied after fresh instillation of methylcellulose.
- Improper gate placement (discussed above) can lead to error in ocular measurements.
- Selection of wrong eye type, e.g. selecting phakic mode for an aphakic eye will lead to errors.

DIFFICULT SITUATIONS IN BIOMETRY

Poor Patient Fixation

It is important to ensure good patient fixation during biometry examination. This can be achieved by making the patient comfortable and repeatedly encouraging the patient to fixate at the fixation target. Sometimes simply changing the head position is all that is required to solve the problem. However, in certain situations, it may be difficult to obtain patient fixation such as (1) strabismus, (2) one-eyed patients, (3) nystagmus (bilateral dense/mature cataract, and (4) marked blepharospasm. In case of unilateral squint, the patient can be asked to fixate with the straight eye and eye position adjusted in such a way as to bring the eye to be examined as near primary position as possible. In case of nystagmus and blepharospasm, repeated readings may need to be taken to obtain accurate results. An immersion scan is especially useful in such cases as it allows easy and more accurate measurements.

Use of Incorrect Sound Velocity Settings

Incorrect measurements will be obtained, if incorrect Vc is used. Therefore, it should be possible to change the Vc settings on the instrument. For example, in case of a silicon-oil filled eye, the Vc must be changed because sound travels much slower in silicon oil than in vitreous. In such cases, the "velocity conversion equation (VCE)" must be used.

Velocity Conversion Equation

In case, a wrong Vc was chosen during examination, a correct ocular measurement can be achieved by using the VCE. The correct measurement (corrected axial length or corrected AL) can be obtained by dividing correct Vc by the incorrect sound velocity used for measurement (Vm) and multiplying it with the measured AL. To obtain the corrected AL or total AL (TAL), divide the correct sound velocity or Vc by incorrect sound velocity used for measurement or Vm and then multiply with incorrect axial length (AAL).

$$TAL = Vc/Vm \times AAL$$

For example, for measurement in an aphakic eye a Vc of 1,532 m/sec must be used. If the measurement was performed using an incorrect Vc of 1,550 m/sec and an AL of 24.0 mm was obtained, the correct AL can be obtained by using the VCE as follows:

Correct AL = 1,532/1,550 m/sec × 24 mm

Therefore, correct AL = 23.72 mm.

Dense Cataract

This is a common scenario in developing countries where patients frequently present with even bilateral mature cataracts. Dense cataract causes attenuation of sound. This can significantly reduce the display of spikes. In such cases, maximum gain setting should be used to obtain spikes of adequate height from the posterior lens capsule and retina.

Severe corneal edema in cases of phacolytic glaucoma also poses a challenge. Similarly, dense calcification in crystalline lens causes severe sound attenuation and shadowing of the posterior ocular structures. In such cases, measurements must be obtained from the fellow eye for IOL power calculations.

Silicon Oil

There are several ways in which a silicon-filled eye differs from a normal phakic eye.

a. The velocity of sound in silicon oil is 1,040 m/sec (5,000 centistokes) and 980 m/sec (1,000 centistokes). This lower Vc must be taken into account while performing AL measurement in a silicon oil-filled eye.
b. Lower Vc also hampers with identification of retinal spike due to sound attenuation in a silicon oil-filled eye.
c. While measuring an oil-filled eye, it is better to have the patient seated upright. This is because the vitreous may not be completely filled with silicon oil. If AL measurements are taken with the patient lying down, the silicon oil being lighter than vitreous, may move up thus creating a fluid-filled space between the posterior surface of bubble and the retina. As a result, the spike produced by posterior surface of silicon oil may be confused with that of retina, leading to falsely low AL readings. When the patient is upright, the posterior surface of silicon oil is in contact with the retina.
d. In an oil filled eye, it is advisable to measure each component separately using the appropriate Vc and the appropriate gates (e.g. measure anterior chamber, lens, and vitreous cavity separately). Therefore one should measure anterior chamber, lens, and vitreous cavity separately by using appropriate velocity and appropriate gates. For this technique, one must be able to change the Vc on the machine. The values are then added together to obtain the AL.
e. If the instrument has only present value of Vc, the AL can be obtained by using the velocity conversion equation or VCE (explained above). To use VCE, perform the following steps with Vc preset at 1,532 m/sec:
   - Measure the ACD by placing the first gate on corneal spike and second gate on anterior lens capsule spike.
   - Measure the apparent lens thickness (LT) by placing the first gate at anterior capsule spike and second gate at posterior lens capsule spike.
   - Measure the apparent vitreous length by placing the first gate at posterior lens capsule spike and second gate at the retinal spike.
   - Apply the VCE as follows:
     - True LT = 1,641/1,532 m/sec × measured LT
     - True vitreous length = 1,041/1,532 m/sec × measured vitreous length.
f. To obtain the true AL, add ACD, LT, and vitreous length obtained as explained in step (e) above.
g. In case of emulsified silicon oil, ocular measurements are difficult to obtain. This is because emulsification of silicon oil results in the formation of tiny droplets of silicon oil throughout the vitreous cavity. These oil bubbles produce high reflective echoes and significant sound attenuation. The retinal spike may not be clear in such a situation. Therefore in such cases, measurements from the fellow eye must be used. Whenever possible, biometry should be performed prior to silicon oil injection.

Posterior Staphyloma

The presence of posterior staphyloma must be suspected in cases of high myopia. The presence of posterior staphyloma makes biometry examination difficult. This is because in posterior staphyloma, the ocular wall is enlarged posteriorly. This makes it difficult to obtain a distinct high retinal spike and can thus make AL measurement error-prone.

Anatomically the staphyloma may be located either in the peripapillary area or in the posterior pole. If the macula is eccentric to the area of maximum excavation of staphyloma, the AL measured is greater than the true AL along the visual axis. Also, in case the macula is situated along the slope of the staphyloma, an oblique sound beam is directed toward the macula. In such a situation, the localization of the macula and the display of a distinct high retinal spike can be very difficult.

As mentioned earlier, the presence of a staphyloma must be suspected in eyes with high myopia. It must also be suspected whenever it is difficult to display a high clear retinal spike. There are several steps one can take to obtain more accurate measurements in such a situation.

- B-scan ultrasound is very useful prior to A-scan to not only detect the presence of staphyloma but also to delineate its configuration as-well-as detect the position of macula relative to the staphyloma. The AL can also be measured on B-scan by using the immersion technique. Measurements can be made by two techniques—(1) by using electronic gates and (2) by superimposing a vector A-scan on the B-scan echography report.
- Immersion technique is very useful in such cases. However, in certain cases the retinal spike is indistinct and one may have to make do with a less distinct retinal spike.

- A combination of A-scan and B-scan may be used. The measurement of anterior chamber and LT is performed by A-scan (either contact or immersion technique) by appropriate placement of gates (described in previous section) and the measurement of vitreous cavity is undertaken by B-scan. For this, a horizontal axial B-scan ultrasound is done. Now, the first electronic caliper is placed on the posterior lens capsule and the second one on surface of macula as delineated on B-scan. The two measurements are now added together to obtain the final AL measurement.
- Always measure the fellow eye since staphylomas are usually bilateral. The AL of the fellow eye will usually be found greater than normal.
- Multiple measurements by multiple techniques may be obtained in order to arrive at the final values before IOL power calculation.

Macular Pathology

The presence of macular pathology can produce erroneous results on biometry examination. An elevated macular lesion can produce erroneous results in two ways: (1) it can interfere with the production of a good distinct retinal spike and (2) it can cause a shorter AL measurement than actual. Macular diseases which can cause such errors are macular edema and disciform lesions at macula. The presence of macular pathology must be suspected in the following situations:

- There is difficulty in obtaining a steep high retinal spike.
- The measured eye is 0.3 mm or more shorter than the fellow eye.
- There is increased distance between the retinal spike and the scleral spike.

Again in such a situation a B-scan may be useful to detect the presence of macular lesion or sometimes even establish the etiology.

Retinal Detachment

In such a situation the presence of RD must be confirmed on B-scan. Presence of RD involving macula will cause a shortening of AL. Also the distance between the retinal and the scleral spike is higher than normal.

Vitreous Abnormalities

Vitreous opacities and membranes may produce spikes on A-scan which may be confused with retinal spikes. This can result in false low AL measurement. The two most common vitreous lesions are asteroid hyalosis and vitreous hemorrhage. Asteroid hyalosis is particularly problematic because it produces medium to high spikes due to presence of calcium particles and these spikes may be confused with retinal spikes. Asteroid hyalosis must always be suspected in situations where abnormal spikes occur along vitreous baseline. B-scan can help in diagnosing asteroid hyalosis.

Retinochoroidal Coloboma

As with the presence of posterior staphyloma, the AL readings may be difficult to obtain and may be falsely long. Coloboma may also be an incidental finding in mature cataracts undergoing A-scan prior to cataract surgery. A B-scan is helpful in confirming the finding and a combined B- and A-scan (as described in posterior staphyloma) may yield more accurate AL measurements.

GUIDELINES FOR MINIMIZING ERRORS

- Always ensure the machine is set for correct velocity setting (e.g. cataract, aphakia, or pseudophakia). Ensure that the machine is properly calibrated.
- Obtain good echoes from cornea, anterior lens, posterior lens, and retina. The spikes should be clear, steeply rising and should be of good amplitude.
- It is both prudent and customary to measure AL in both the eyes. Always measure the AL to the nearest hundredth of a millimeter and record it carefully. An error of even 1 mm in AL measurement can cause an error of 2.5 D in IOL power calculation. Longer eyes are more forgiving whereas even small errors are serious in small eyes. Therefore, an error of 1 mm in AL can cause an error in IOL power calculation of approximately 1.75 D in an eye with AL of 30 mm and 3.75 D in an eye with AL of 20 mm. Therefore, greater care must be exerted in measuring shorter eyes.
- Always remeasure if:
  - There is >0.03 mm difference in both eyes.
  - Axial length is <22 mm or >25 mm in either eye.
  - Axial length does not correlate well with patient's spectacle correction.
  - There are problems in patient cooperation or patient fixation.
- Perform a B-scan to document the difference or to cross-check findings as and when required. B-scan is also essential to diagnose/confirm the presence and location of staphyloma in long eyes.
- Take care to avoid corneal compression, if using the contact method.
- Average the 5–10 most consistent results which give the lowest standard deviation (ideally <0.06 mm).
- Accurate keratometry and use of correct IOL power calculation formula are essential to obtain accurate results and desired postoperative refractive outcome.

BIOMETRY THROUGH DIFFERENT INTRAOCULAR LENS MATERIALS

There are several reasons why biometry may have to be performed on a pseudophakic eye. Most common reason is to compare the findings in both the eyes prior to cataract

Table 2: The velocity of sound through different IOL materials and the correction factor (CF).

IOL material	Speed of sound (m/s)	CF
PMMA	2,718	+0.4 mm
Acrylic	2,120	+0.2 mm
Silicone	980–1,107	−0.4–+0.8 mm

(IOL: intraocular lens; PMMA: polymethylmethacrylate)

surgery; one eye is phakic and the other pseudophakic. Other reasons are postoperative refractive surprise or in case a patient needs IOL exchange.

Biometry through a pseudophakic eye results in multiple reverberation echoes in the vitreous cavity which decrease from left to right of A-scan. The number and height of reverberations depends on the type of material of IOL. In such a case, gain setting can be reduced to reduce the spike amplifications due to the IOL.

The second most important thing is that knowledge of IOL material is essential to obtain an accurate scan since the velocity of sound through each material is different. Most of the currently available IOLs are made of either polymethylmethacrylate (PMMA) or acrylic or silicone. The velocity of sound through a pseudophakic eye is 1,532 m/sec plus the CF for the lens material. The velocity of sound through silicone is 980–1,107 m/sec (depending on the silicone used), acrylic is 2,120 m/sec and that through PMMA is 2,718 m/sec. If the biometer has only one pseudophakic setting then it will be accurate only for PMMA lenses because the machine belongs to the era when PMMA was the only IOL material available. In such a case, one must perform the measurements in "aphakic mode" at a Vc of 1,532 m/sec and then add the appropriate CF. The velocity of sound through different IOL materials and the CF to be used is shown in **Table 2**.

Thus, if the AL measurement is 22.54 mm in aphakic mode and the IOL is made of acrylic material, the correct AL is 22.74 mm. Problem may arise, if the material of IOL implanted is not known. In that case, the patient's IOL card can provide details of the IOL used. If that is not available, then the primary surgeon may have to be contacted. Lastly, the type of IOL reverberation pattern may provide some clue. PMMA produces the longest chain of reverberating echoes, followed by acrylic IOLs followed by silicone IOLs.

IMMERSION VECTOR A-/B-SCAN BIOMETRY

The immersion B-scan/vector A-/B-scan provides a two dimensional B-scan display along with superimposed vector A-scan. This has several advantages in ophthalmology but it is particularly advantageous in biometry. Since the instrument displays both the B-scan and the corresponding A-scan, A-scan vector can be adjusted to pass through the middle of cornea and anterior and posterior lens echoes and ensure that the vector lies on the retina in the region of fovea. This instrument also allows direct visualization of area being measured. Thus the examiner can direct the AL measurements so as to obtain the refractive AL rather than anatomic AL. This instrument is particularly helpful in detecting staphyloma or making measurements in a staphylomatous eye, particularly in the presence of mature cataract.

However, it is more expensive, requires a greater degree of skill to perform, and also takes a longer time to perform the measurements.

OPTIMAL CARE OF BIOMETRY EQUIPMENT

- The biometry machine must be stored properly in a designated storage place.
- Avoid dropping the probe. Any kind of impact must be avoided.
- Always inspect the probe and cable before each use.
- Avoid excessive stretching, bending, kinking, or pinching of the cable. Excessive stress on the cable can cause damage to the insulation and cause electric shock to the patient or examiner.
- Never use damaged or cracked probes. The cleaning or gel solution may leak into the transducer and can even cause electric shock.

CLEANING OF BIOMETRY EQUIPMENT

- Meticulously clean the probe with soft sponge or gauze pad to remove all residues and to make it clean before examining the next patient.
- One must strictly follow the instructions given by the manufacturer regarding cleaning and disinfection of transducers. Use only approved gels and cleaning solutions.
- Do not steam, heat autoclave, or use ethylene oxide gas on probes.
- After each session, disconnect the probe from the ultrasound console. Rinse the probe with warm soap-water solution. Air dry the probe before storing it.

CALIBRATION OF INSTRUMENT

A plastic test block is available for calibration with the biometry machine. There is a special mode to perform measurement on the test block and this should yield a specified measurement. This unit should be used regularly to calibrate the instrument.

INTRAOCULAR LENS POWER CALCULATION

Since the time Sir Harold Ridley implanted the first IOL in 1949 and experienced a postoperative refractive surprise of nearly 20 D, IOL power calculation has come a long way.

The target of cataract surgery is emmetropia in most cases and therefore, accurate IOL power calculation forms the backbone of cataract surgery.

Intraocular Lens Power Calculation Formulae

The first IOL power formula was published by Fyodorov and Kolonko in 1967. It was a theoretical formula and was based on Gaussian optics and Gullstrand schematic eye. First- and second-generation formulae, i.e. the theoretical and regression formulae are considered obsolete.

The third-generation formulae include the Hoffer Q, Holladay 1, and the SRK/T. They represent a merger of theoretical and regression formulae and require two variables: (1) AL and (2) keratometry along with one unique factor—the ACD constant for Hoffer Q, the A-constant for SRK/T and the "surgeon factor" for Holladay 1. The Hoffer Q formula utilizes AL, keratometry, and personalized A-constant for IOL power calculation.

The fourth-generation formulae are the Holladay 2, Haigis, Olsen, and Barrett Universal II (Barrett U 2). The fourth-generation formulae need more variable for IOL power calculation including the ELP (Effective Lens position, described above). The Holladay 2 formula requires seven variables to calculate ELP-AL, keratometry, white-to-white (WTW), preoperative refraction, ACD, LT, and patient's age in order of importance.

Few important IOL power calculation formulae are shown in **Table 3**.

Recently, Koch et al. suggested a new classification of IOL power formula based on: (1) method of calculating IOL power, and (2) the data used for these calculations.

- Historical/refraction based
- *Regression analysis based:* SRK and SRK-II
- Vergence formulae (based on Gaussian optics):
  - *Two variable:*
    - Holladay 1
    - SRK-T
    - Hoffer Q
  - *Three variable:*
    - Haigis
    - Ladas Super-formula
  - *Five variable:* Barrett U 2
  - *Seven variable:* Holladay 2
- *Artificial intelligence based:*
  - Hill-RBF (radial basis activation function)
  - Clarke neural network.
- *Ray tracing:*
  - Okulix
  - Phacooptics.

The Newer Intraocular Lens Power Calculation Formulae

The popular newer generation formulae include the Holladay 2, Barrett U 2, and the Hill-RBF. These formulae require more variables for IOL power calculation. The common factor in all these formulae (except the Hill-RBF) is the need to predict ELP. ELP is defined as the effective distance between the anterior surface of cornea and the lens plane, if the lens was infinitely thin. This is the only parameter that cannot be measured preoperatively since it is difficult to predict what will be the position of IOL or where the IOL will settle postoperatively. Both anatomical factors (keratometry value, AL, limbal WTW, preoperative ACD, and LT) and IOL related

Table 3: Important IOL power formulae at a glance.

Name of formula	*Generation of IOL power formula*	*Variables required*	*Comments*
SRK I and Binkhorst I	First generation	K and AL	Obsolete, high level of error, should not be used
SRK II and Binkhorst II	Second generation	K and AL	Obsolete, high level of error, should not be used
Holladay I	Third generation	K and AL	Trend toward better outcomes for eyes between 22.00 mm and 26.00 mm, compared to other third generation
SRK/T	Third generation	K and AL	Better outcomes for eyes >26.00 mm, compared to other 3rd generation formulae
Hoffer Q	Third generation	K and AL	Better outcomes for eyes <22.00 mm, compared to other third generation
Holladay 2	Fourth generation	K, AL, ACD, LT, horizontal WTW, age, and preoperative refraction	No data has been reported showing an advantage over an appropriately selected third generation formula
Olsen	Fourth generation	K, AL, ACD, LT, and horizontal WTW	There is evidence suggestive of improved performance over third generation formulae for eyes with AL 20.00–26.00 mm
Haigis	Fifth generation	K, AL, and ACD	Very good outcomes for eyes across the AL range and best reported outcomes for eyes > 28.00 mm. For best results, 3 IOL constants need to be optimized requiring data from at least 500 eyes

(ACD: anterior chamber depth; AL: axial length; IOL: intraocular lens; K: keratometry; LT: lens thickness; WTW: white-to-white)

Table 4: The various parameters required for the calculation of select IOL power formulae.

Parameter	*Haigis*	*Hoffer Q*	*SRK/T*	*Holladay 2*	*HILL-RBF*	*Barrett universal II*
AL	Yes	Yes	Yes	Yes	Yes	Yes
ACD	Yes	No	No	Yes	Yes	Yes
K	Yes	Yes	Yes	Yes	Yes	Yes
LT	No	No	No	Yes	Yes	Yes
WTW	No	No	No	No	Yes	Yes
Refraction (preoperative)	No	No	No	No	No	Yes

(ACD: anterior chamber depth; AL: axial length; IOL: intraocular lens; K: keratometry; LT: lens thickness; WTW: white-to-white)

factors (shape, length, flexibility, and anterior angulation if any, material of the haptic and shape and material of optic) affect ELP. ELP prediction is made by the IOL manufacturer in the form of "A-constant". The A-constant is an empirical value and is specific to IOL design. Advances in IOL power calculation formulae in the last 30 years are mostly due to advances in predictability of the variable called ELP.

The parameters required for the calculation of important IOL power formulae are depicted in **Table 4**.

Barrett Universal II

The formula is called universal because it is suitable for all types of eyes—short, medium, or long and also for different lens styles. This formula is based on a theoretical model of eye in which ACD is related to AL and K. In this formula, ELP is characterized by ACD and LF (lens factor). The LF is influenced by keratometry, AL, ACD, LT, and WTW in that order. This formula also takes into account the negative value of LF in calculating ELP in presence of negative-powered type of IOL. The Barrett U2 formula can be openly accessed on www.apacrs.org. Following are the features of Barrett U 2 formula:

- It is accurate for all eyes regardless of AL.
- Essential variables required for calculation are AL, keratometry, optical ACD, and desired postoperative refraction. Optional variables required are LT and WTW.
- Lens factor or "A-constant" of the selected IOL is required. If not available, ULIB "A constant" of SRK/T formula is recommended (ULIB is the User Group for Laser Interference Biometry).
- Axial length and keratometry data from optical biometer (e.g. IOLMaster and Lenstar) are required for calculation. However, applanation biometry data may also be used. Since optically measured AL is different from ultrasound measured AL, acoustic A-constant will fail to give optimum results when used with optical biometry. Therefore when AL obtained by US biometry is used in Barrett formula, an appropriate A-constant must be used (since an optically measured AL is different from US measured AL, IOL constants like the A-constant and ACD constant, will generally give poorer results when used in optical biometry. Therefore an individual optimization for a given IOL type is required. This requires pre- and postoperative clinical data and is done on a spreadsheet form in MS Excel format which can be downloaded from the ULIB website ocusoft.de/ulib/).
- Barrett U2 is able to predict for highly myopic eyes and negative powered IOLs without specialized constants or AL modification.

The refractive outcomes using Barrett U2 have been excellent.

Table 5: Nine types of eyes. Intraocular lens calculations are more accurate, if nine types of eyes are considered (not just short/medium/long eyes), with anterior segment size and AL as independent variables.

Large	Megalocornea + axial hyperopia (0%)	Megalocornea (2%)	Large eye buphthalmos megalocornea + axial myopia (10%)
Normal	Axial hyperopia (80%)	Normal (96%)	Axial myopia (90%)
Small	Small eye nanophthalmia (20%)	Microcornea (2%)	Microcornea + axial myopia (0%)
	Short	*Normal*	*Long*

Source: Holladay JT

Holladay 2

In 1993, Dr Holladay led a worldwide study involving 34 cataract surgeons to determine which of the seven variables were relevant as predictors of ELP. Surprisingly, horizontal WTW measurements emerged as the next most important variable after AL and keratometry. It was also proved that there is almost no correlation between AL and size of anterior segment in 80–90% of the eyes **(Table 5)**. This led to the concept of nine types of eyes—not just three (short, medium, or long).

These results led to the formulation of Holladay 2 formula, an easy-to-use program in which seven variables (AL, keratometry, ACD, LT, WTW, age of patient, and previous refraction) are inserted for calculation of ELP and appropriate IOL power.

This newer formula is a great choice for nearly every eye. It is a complete software package that not only allows IOL power calculation in many different types of eyes, but also honing of individual results by personalizing the A-constant. This formula is available as part of Holladay IOL consultant/surgical outcomes assessment program (HIC-SOAP, available at www.hicsoap.com). It is a paid software.

Hill-RBF on-Line Calculator

The new Hill-RBF method is an advanced, self-validating method for IOL power selection which employs pattern recognition, and sophisticated data interpolation. It was launched in 2016. It is purely "data driven", independent of ELP, and has no data bias. RBF method uses artificial intelligence-driven pattern recognition and sophisticated data interpolation. RBF algorithms are used globally in a variety of technologies like facial recognition software and thumbprint security scanners. Radial basis function IOL power selection performs the same for short, medium, and long eyes. It is entirely data-driven and free from calculation bias. A special feature is that it is the only IOL power calculation formula, which provides the user the reliability of result, i.e. the software can tell whether it is likely to be correct or whether it is unsure about the calculated IOL power. The older version of Hill-RBF online calculator used data from 3,400 eyes with a wide range of preoperative ocular parameters.

The Hill-RBF is the product of the efforts of Dr Warren Hill and his team which included engineers from MathWorks, and 39 investigators from over 17 countries. The Hill-RBF is incorporated in Lenstar Eye Suite and is also available to ophthalmologists globally as an open access web-based calculator (rbfcalculator.com/online). The uniqueness of Hill-RBF lies in the fact that greater the number of surgical outcomes that are fit into the model, greater the accuracy. In other words, the more the number of eyes added to database, the more accurate the calculator becomes.

However, the Hill-RBF has been optimized for biometry data from Lenstar LS900 optical biometer and for a particular IOL (Alcon SN60WF biconvex IOL). It may be used for other biconvex IOLs in the range of +6–+30 D. However, biometry data from other sources or other IOL models may lead to suboptimal results.

More information about the calculator can be obtained from Dr Hill at hill@doctor-hill.com and under "Online Tools" at ascrs.org.

Hill-RBF Calculator Version 2.0

The RBF calculator has been updated in 2017 (Hill-RBF Calculator Version 2.0) and includes data from 12,419 eyes. The data for normal eyes has been increased by about 7,000 eyes. 1,000 exceptionally short eyes and axial myopia with IOL power up to –5 D have now been included in the latest version. Version 2.0 of the Hill-RBF method was released as part of the Haag-Streit LENSTAR EyeSuite biometry software on January 25, 2018. It includes the following updates:

- It is now possible to enter target spherical equivalent similar to that in other popular vergence and ray tracing formulas.
- With the addition of more than 1,000 eyes with very short AL, the accuracy of calculation in high axial hyperopia is significantly increased.
- The range of calculations for high to extreme axial myopia has been greatly augmented by the addition of a large database of usual low power IOLs. This also includes calculations for meniscus design IOLs from +5.00 D to –5.00 D.

INTRAOCULAR LENS POWER CALCULATION IN HIGH-TO-EXTREME MYOPIA

High myopia is one of the most prevalent refractive conditions globally with a high risk of other associated eye conditions. Patients of axial myopia (AL > 25 mm) are at risk of suboptimal refractive outcome after cataract surgery. The single most important consideration in this setting is to avoid unanticipated postoperative hyperopia. Several authors have reported that AL measured by the optical biometry is more precise than ultrasound in an eye with posterior staphyloma. Secondly, the use of third-generation formulae may lead to incorrect IOL power calculation resulting in unsatisfied patient postoperatively.

In their landmark article, Wang et al. suggested that modification of AL is required to calculate IOL power with the SRK-T, Holladay 1 and 2, and Haigis and Hoffer Q formulas in eyes with AL > 25.2 mm. They looked at IOLs (IOL power that was required to be implanted) in two groups—power greater than 5 D and power 5 D or less. In both the groups, it was found that adjusting AL significantly reduced the incidence of postoperative hyperopia. The idea behind the AL modification is that when the original AL is fed into the Wang–Koch's formula **(Table 6)**, a value lower than the original AL value is calculated. When this lower AL value is reinserted into the formulae, an IOL power of higher dioptric value is obtained. This, in turn, eliminates the risk of postoperative hyperopia. However, the Wang–Koch

Table 6: Wang–Koch's formula for adjusting AL in eyes more than/equal to 25.2 mm.

Formula	*Modification*
Holladay 1 optimized AL	0.829 × IOLM AL + 4.27
Haigis optimized AL	0.929 × IOLM AL +1.56
SRK/T Optimized AL	0.854 × IOLM AL +3.72
Hoffer Q optimized AL	0.853 × IOLM AL +3.58

(AL: axial length; IOLM: intraocular lens master)

modification may be less accurate in very low power/ negative lenses.

Ghanem and Sayed found in their study that though SRK/T, Hoffer Q, Holladay 2, and Haigis work equally well in eyes with high myopia in low-plus powered IOL implantation, Haigis was better in cases requiring minus power IOL implantation. The study was conducted on 127 eyes of 87 patients with cataract and AL > 26 mm.

Newer formulae such as Barrett U2 and Holladay 2 have also been shown to be accurate in the setting of high myopia.

TORIC CALCULATORS

The correction of corneal astigmatism with toric IOLs has become a standard of care to improve refractive outcome after cataract surgery. Two components contribute to optimum correction of astigmatism—(1) accurate keratometry and (2) reliable method to calculate power of toric IOL. Choosing the correct toric IOL for a patient is more challenging than choosing a spherical IOL. Toric calculators are used to select the desired toric IOL for a given patient. An ideal toric calculator has the following characteristics:

- It is comprehensive, i.e. it can be used for preoperative planning, as well as for refractive surprises.
- Software should preferably be a part of the biometric device.
- It should be applicable to all IOL types.
- There should be dynamic display of variables (e.g. dynamic adjustment of astigmatic effects of phaco incision).
- It should be alert on axis-flip.
- It should take into account posterior corneal astigmatism (PCA).

Few generic toric calculators available online are "Assort Toric calculator" (www.assort.com) and "Holladay Toric calculator" (www.hicsoap.com). The Barrett Toric calculator contains Barrett U2 and Barrett Rx formula for lens exchange, piggyback IOLs or rotation of an existing toric IOL to correct for an unexpected refractive surprise. The Barrett Toric Calculator is available on the ASCRS (www.ascrs.org/barrett-toric-calculator) and APACRS (www.apacrs.org) websites.

FullMonte Intraocular Lens 2.0

The FullMonte IOL software system is a new adaptive, optimizing process based on Markov Chain Monte Carlo (MCMC) process. It is not a formula, rather a computing process which combines modern theoretical formulas (SRK/T, Holladay 1, Haigis, etc.) with surgeon's own postoperative refractive record to provide not a single value of IOL power for emmetropia, but expected refraction as a graph of probability distributions. The software continuously optimizes itself, adapting to several factors like short eye/ long eye, cases of unique anatomy, or postrefractive patients.

Kane Formula

This latest IOL power calculation formula is the Kane formula developed by Dr Jack Kane. It is a tool to enable the surgeon to select the most appropriate IOL for the patient.

The formula was arrived at by using data from 30,000 highly accurate cases. It is based on theoretical optics and utilizes both regression and artificial intelligence to arrive at a more accurate IOL power formula. The formula was created using "high-performance cloud-based computing" which uses the power of a cloud to create a virtual supercomputer which can perform several decades of computing in just a few days. One of the main aims of the formula was to reduce the error in IOL power calculation in extremes of ocular measurements. The formula requites the following data which are fed into the calculator:

- A constant
- Intraocular lens type
- Gender
- Target refraction
- Axial length
- K1 and K2
- Anterior chamber depth
- Lens thickness
- Central corneal thickness (CCT).

Compulsory fields are A-constant, AL, keratometry, ACD, and gender of the patient. Optional variables are LT and CCT. Thus, owners of older biometers can also use this formula. The "constants" page on the site has information about appropriate constants for different IOLs. However for better results, surgeons should use their own optimized A-constants for calculations.

A-SCAN FOR EVALUATION OF POSTERIOR SEGMENT DISEASE

Synchronized Vector A-scan

A-scan helps in studying the reflectivity of the structures along a given plane. Ophthalmic ultrasound scanners have a vector A-scan super imposed on the B-scan. It is important to direct the A-scan vector perpendicular to the structure whose reflectivity is to be measured. Thus the vector A-scan is an amplitude modulation scan.

Quantitative Echography

Quantitative echography is performed with A-scan. In A-scan biometry, a single parallel and thin sound beam is emitted from the tip of the USG probe at a frequency of 10 MHz. When the emitted sound beam strikes an interface between two medias of different densities and velocities, an echo is produced which bounces back to the probe tip. The echoes bouncing back to the USG probe tip from each of the ocular interfaces (corneal surface, aqueous/anterior lens surface, posterior lens capsule/anterior vitreous, the posterior vitreous face/retinal surface, and the choroid/anterior sclera surface) are converted by the biometer into spikes arising from the baseline **(Fig. 1)**.

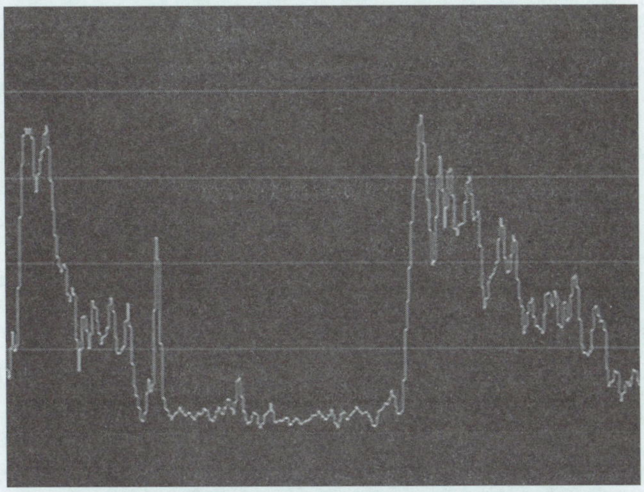

Fig. 1: High-quality contact A-scan of the phakic eye.

Contact A-scan of Normal Phakic Eye with Clear Lens

There are five high amplitude spikes: (1) Probe/cornea; (2) Anterior lens capsular; (3) Posterior lens capsule; (4) Sleepy rising retinal spike; and (5) Sclera spike. The orbital tissue spikes are of medium reflectivity and get progressively attenuated.

Thus by performing a quantitative echography, we can obtain an idea of the reflectivity (i.e. spike amplitude) of the tissue/lesion. The spike height is expressed as a percentage of the maximum height that can be displayed on the screen. Categorization of the lesion based on spike height percentage is given in **Table 1**. The greater the difference between the two medias on either side of an interface, the echo produced is stronger and hence the deflection from the baseline spike/ reflectivity is higher **(Figs. 2A and B)**.

If the difference between the two medias at the interface is not much, the echo bouncing back is likely to be weak and the spike displayed will be proportionately smaller [e.g. vitreous floaters following a posterior vitreous detachment (PVD)] **(Figs. 3A and B)**.

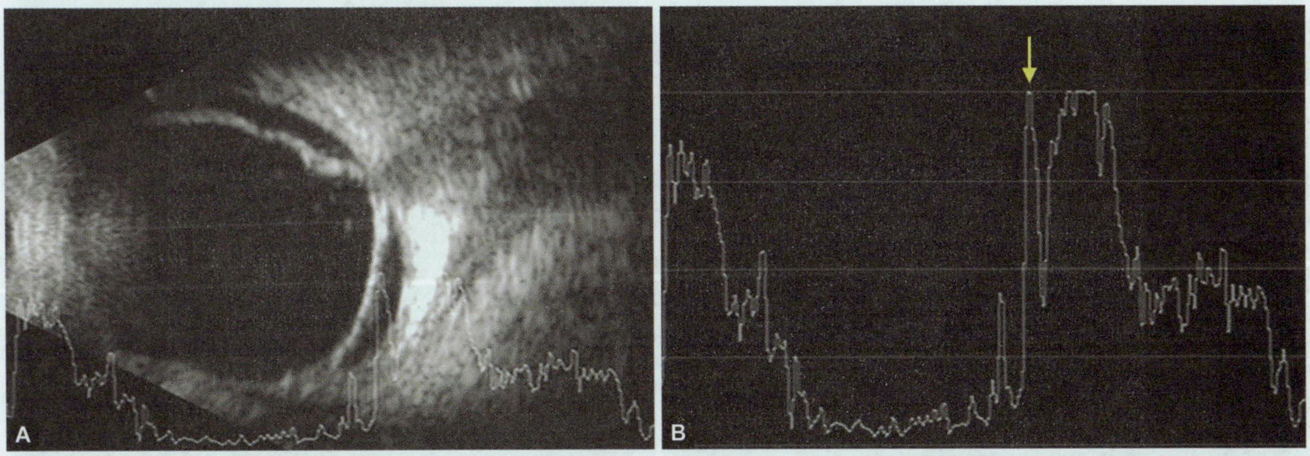

Figs. 2A and B: (A) Spike in a patient with retinal detachment; (B) High reflectivity spikes.

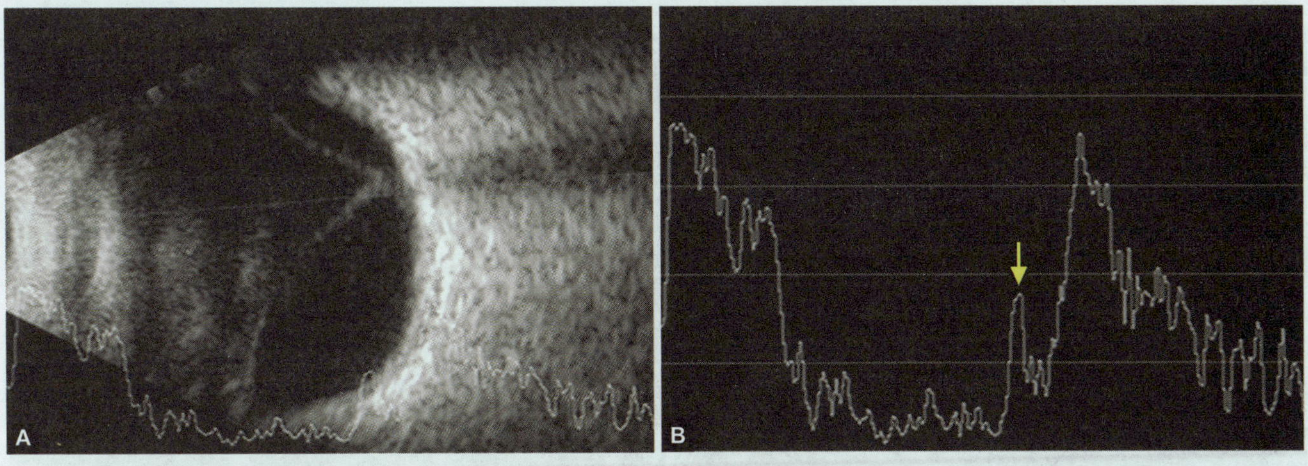

Figs. 3A and B: Medium reflective spikes in a patient of detached posterior hyaloid (A) and low reflective spikes in a patient with vitreous floaters (B).

When sound travels through two medias of identical densities, no echoes are produced at the interface, and hence the A-scan spike goes down to the baseline (e.g. normal vitreous and noncataractous lens in the young) **(Table 7)**.

The echo-poor vitreous acts as a natural contrast for ultrasonographic evaluation of the posterior segment of the eye. A-scan amplitude modulation scan produces a single dimensional display of multiple spikes on any plane through the eye. The plane is obtained by passing the vector A-scan on the B-scan image. The A-scan spikes represent amplitude/reflectivity of the echo from that plane.

The normal A-scan anatomy of the eye is obtained when the vector passes through the posterior capsule of the lens and the ocular coats near the optic disk.

Table 7: Characterization of lesion based on spike height percentage.

Spie height percentage	*Reflectivity*	*Lesion*
2–20%	Low	Vitreous floaters
10–60%	Low medium	Choroidal melanoma
20–80%	Medium	Vitreous membranes
80–100%	High	Asteroid hyalosis
100%	Very high	Retinal detachment

Evaluation of Posterior Segment Lesion using A-scan

- Vitreous floaters or vitreous syneresis is produced due to liquefaction of vitreous gel. This liquefaction could be secondary to vitreous degeneration due to old age, high myopia, following cataract surgery or may result from posterior segment inflammation or trauma. A-scan shows low reflectivity (20–25%) echoes as small up shoots from the baseline, best displayed at higher gain **(Figs. 4A and B)**.
- *Asteroid hyalosis:* Calcium soaps or calcium crystals may get deposited in the vitreous cavity following chronic degeneration of the vitreous and are called as asteroid hyalosis. On A-scan, asteroid hyalosis produces high reflectivity spikes due to presence of calcium deposits (50–100% reflectivity) **(Figs. 5A and B)**.
- *Vitritis and endophthalmitis:* Depending on the stage of development, vitritis may produce varying reflectivity. Low reflectivity echoes are observed in the early stages with a progressive increase in reflectivity as the vitreous debris and inflammatory cells get organized **(Fig. 6)**. The reflectivity of the ocular coats may be reduced due to the

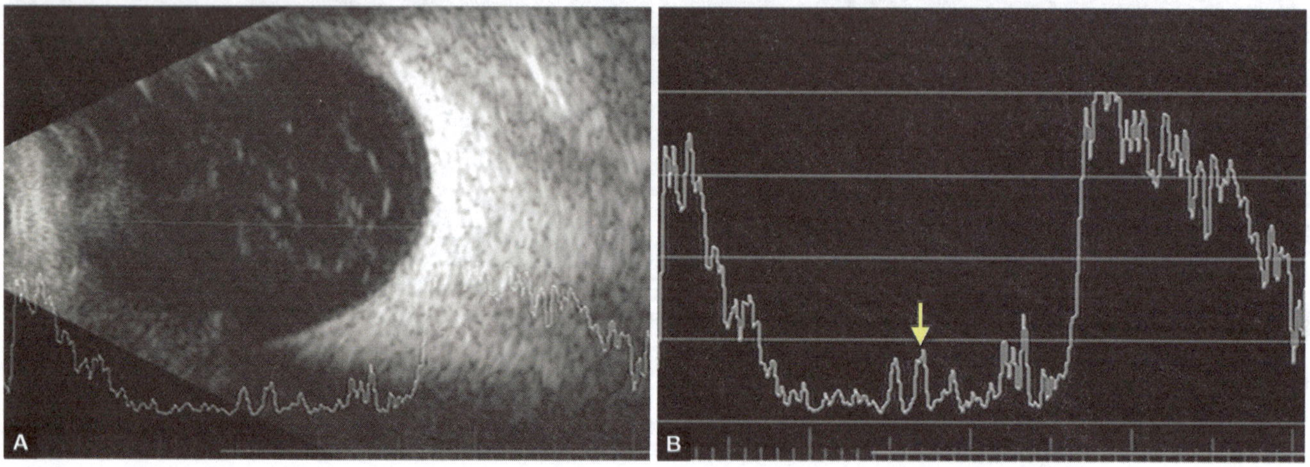

Figs. 4A and B: Vitreous floaters/vitreous syneresis A-scan shows low reflectivity (20–25%) echoes.

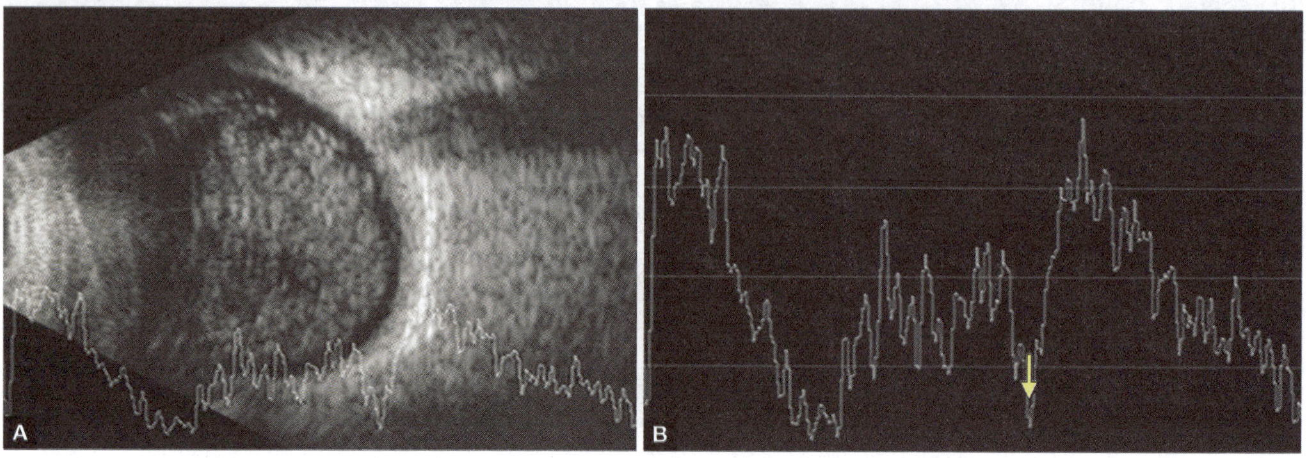

Figs. 5A and B: Asteroid hyalosis A-scan shows high reflectivity (50–100%) spikes due to presence of calcium deposits.

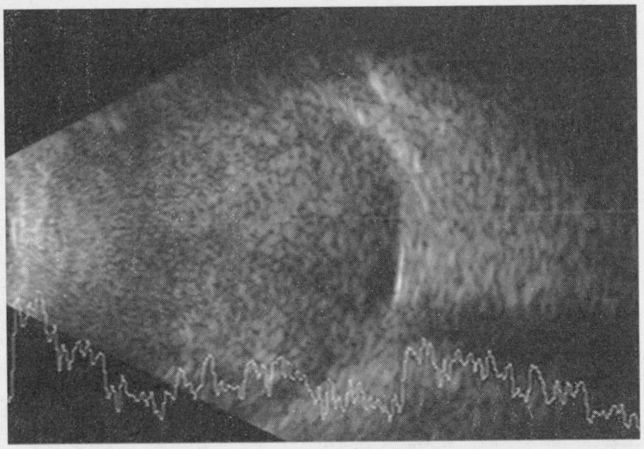

Fig. 6: *Endophthalmitis:* Low reflectivity echoes in early stages. The reflectivity of the ocular coats is reduced due to presence of edema and inflammatory exudates in the ocular coats.

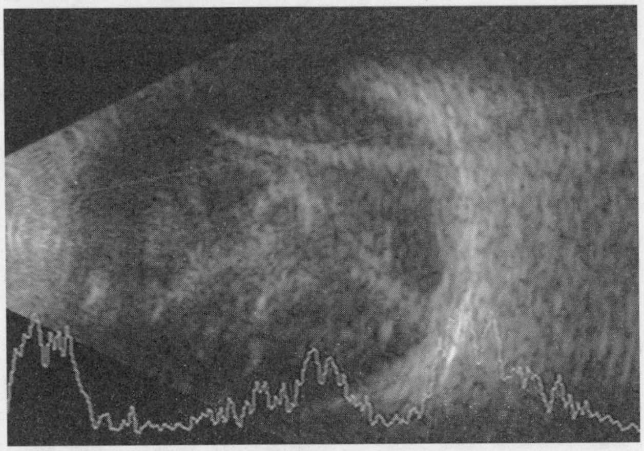

Fig. 8: Endophthalmitis with exudative choroidal detachment. The reflectivity of the choroidal detachment is low (60–70%) due to presence of exudates on either side of the choroidal detachment.

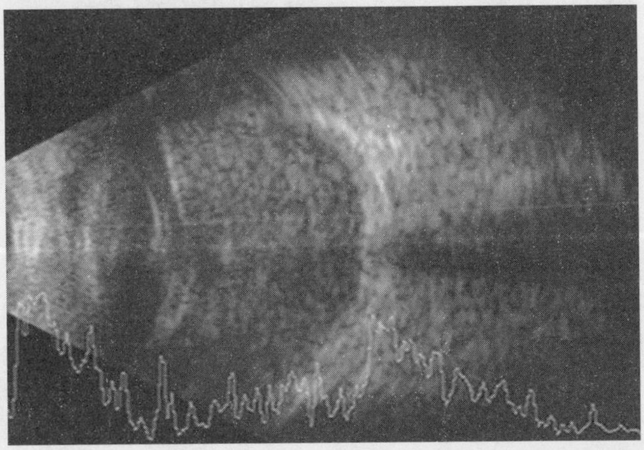

Fig. 7: Marked chorioretinal thickening in a patient with advanced and severe endophthalmitis. The reflectivity of chorioretinal layer is reduced due to edema.

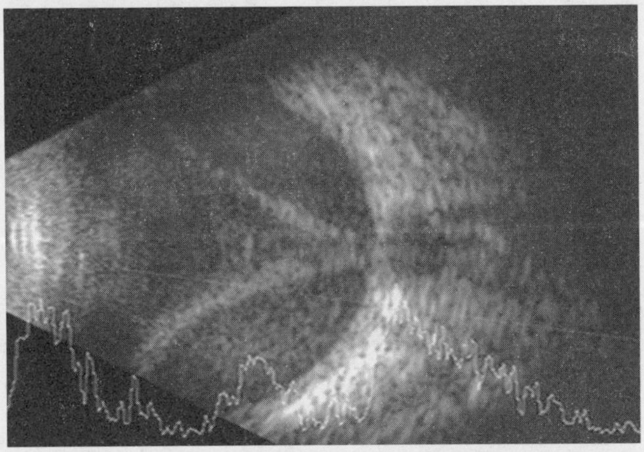

Fig. 9: Endophthalmitis with exudative retinal detachment showing an A-scan reflectivity of less than 80%.

presence of edema and inflammatory exudates in the ocular coats.

In advanced cases of endophthalmitis, the vitreous cavity becomes filled with dense-organized inflammatory exudates. There is a marked thickening of the chorioretinal layers and hence the reflectivity of the coats is reduced. The exact thickness of the ocular coats can be measured from the A-scan spikes.

Associated features include:

- Marked chorioretinal thickening **(Fig. 7)**
- *Associated serous or exudative choroidal detachment* **(Fig. 8)**: The choroidal detachment is usually shallow and will have multiple low intensity echoes in the suprachoroidal space due to exudates. The choroidal detachment is usually seen as low reflectivity spikes due to presence of exudates on both sides of the choroidal elevation.
- *Endophthalmitis with exudative RD:* Chronic endophthalmitis may lead to secondary exudative RD with reflectivity of less than 80% **(Fig. 9)**.
- *Panophthalmitis:* It occurs when the infection from the ocular coats extends into Tenon's and retro-ocular space. Infection in the Tenon's space is seen as irregular hypoechoic areas within the Tenon's space, which spreads over its entire extent leading to a semicircular **(Fig. 10)** hypoechoic rim with a reflectivity less than 50%.

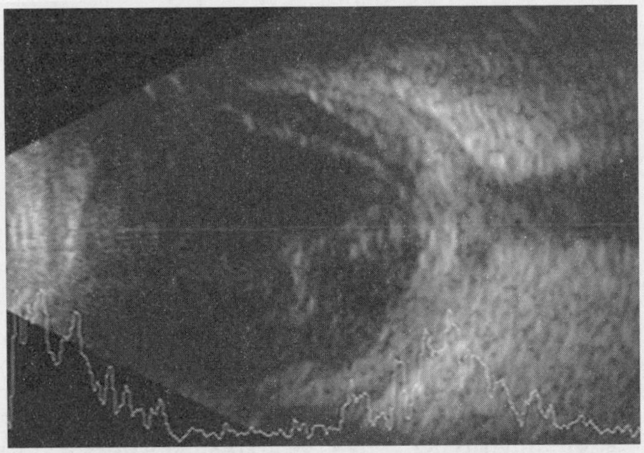

Fig. 10: Panophthalmitis with extension of infection into the sub-Tenon's space. In an A-scan, the reflectivity of the Tenon's space is less than 50%.

- *Phthisical eye following panophthalmitis:* Chronic endophthalmitis over a long period of time causes

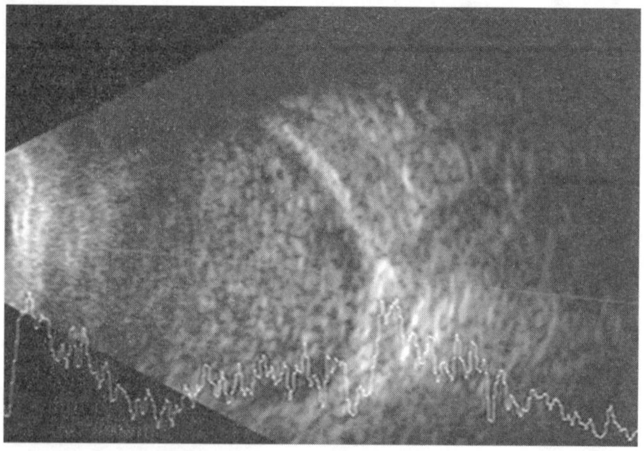

Fig. 11: Phthisis bulbi following panophthalmitis results in thickening of the ocular wall due to fibrosis and high reflectivity spikes from the ocular coats.

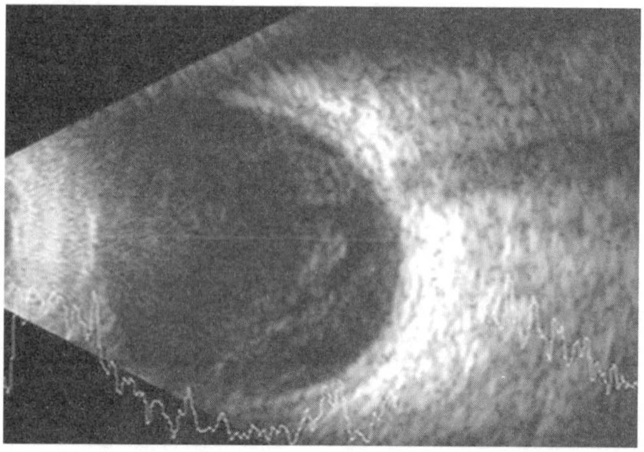

Fig. 12: Fresh vitreous hemorrhage producing low reflectivity echoes (<25%) in the vitreous cavity.

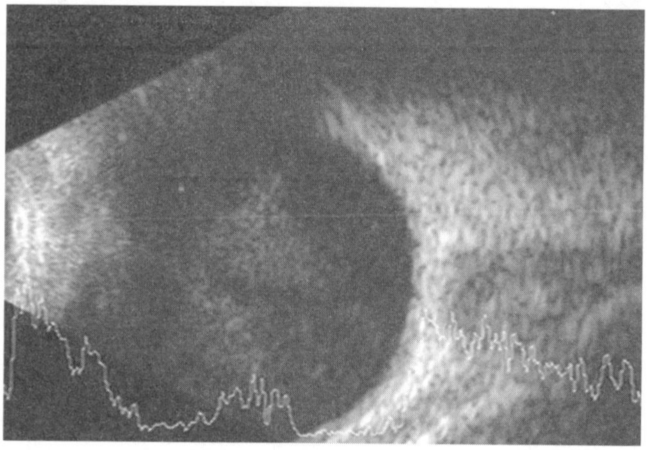

Fig. 13: Resolving vitreous hemorrhage producing moderate reflectivity echoes (40–60% reflectivity).

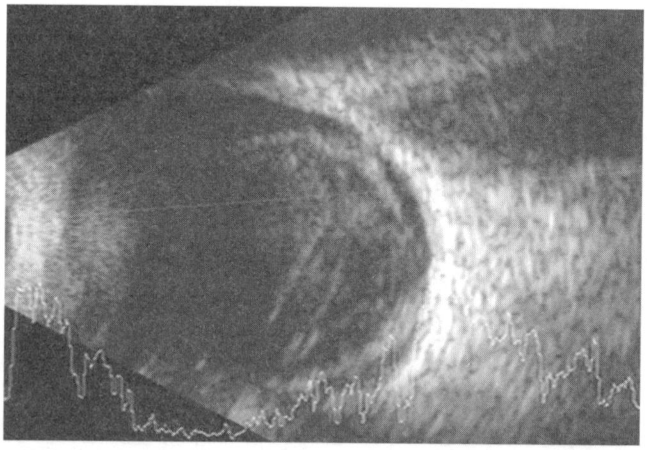

Fig. 14: Organized vitreous hemorrhage shows high (70–80%) reflectivity spikes due to fibrin content within the vitreous membranes.

fibrosis of the ocular wall, reduction in axial length and a loss of definition of ocular structures. A-scan spikes from the ocular coats show high reflectivity **(Fig. 11)**.

- *Vitreous hemorrhage:* It is the most common condition encountered on B-scan USG. The diagnostic USG criteria for vitreous hemorrhage depend on the stage of evolution of the hemorrhage whether fresh, resolving or organized. Fresh vitreous hemorrhage produces low reflectivity echoes (<25%) in the vitreous cavity **(Fig. 12)**.

  Resolving vitreous hemorrhage produces low-to-moderate reflectivity echoes (40–60%) **(Fig. 13)**.

  A-scan in eyes with organized vitreous hemorrhage shows high reflectivity (70–80%) spikes due to fibrin content within the vitreous membranes **(Fig. 14)**.

  Associated findings depend on the primary condition:
  - PVVH (postvitrectomy vitreous hemorrhage)—vitreous hemorrhage in a vitrectomized eye always remains in a fluid state and is uniformly distributed in the vitreous cavity and rarely leads to membrane formation. It is visualized as uniform low reflectivity (30–50%) echoes throughout the vitreous cavity **(Fig. 15)**.

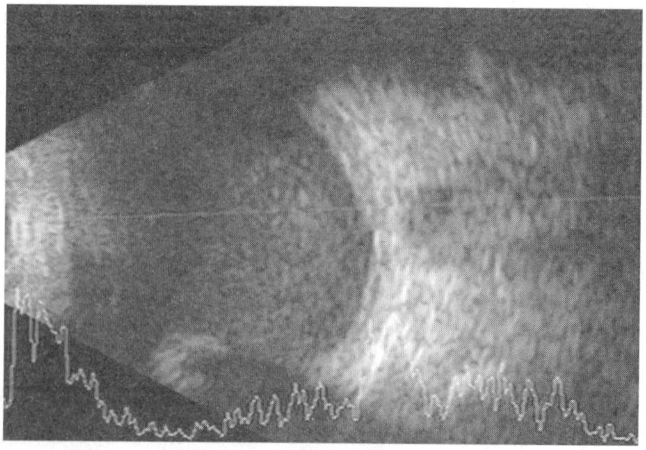

Fig. 15: *Postvitrectomy vitreous hemorrhage:* Producing low (30–50%) reflectivity spikes due to minimum interface.

  - Organized vitreous membranes (70–80% reflectivity spike).
  - Associated with asteroid hyalosis high (60–90% reflectivity irregular spike) **(Fig. 16)**.

  With retained intraocular foreign body (IOFB): Vitreous hemorrhage is invariably present in a severely

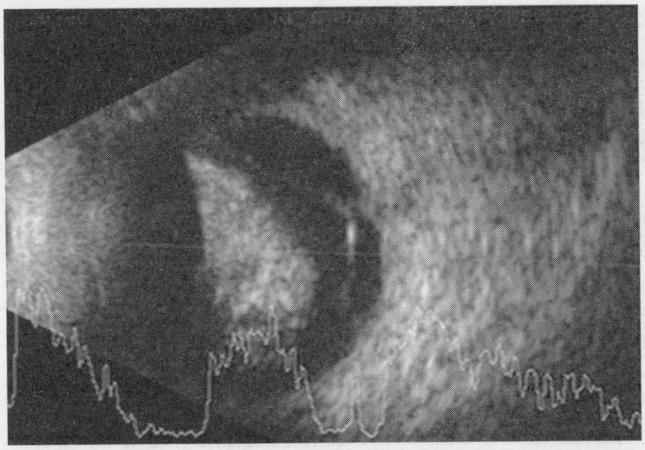

Fig. 16: Organized vitreous hemorrhage associated with asteroid hyalosis produces high irregular reflectivity spikes (60–90%) due to deposition of calcium.

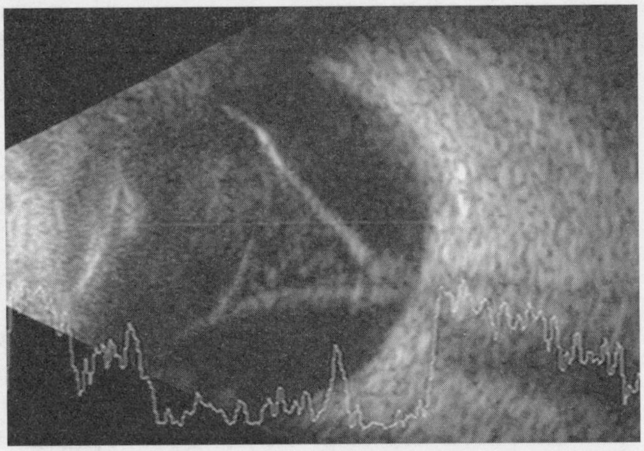

Fig. 18: Vitreous hemorrhage with retinal detachment produces A-scan reflectivity of 70% from the detached retina and 50–60% reflectivity echoes from the vitreous cavity.

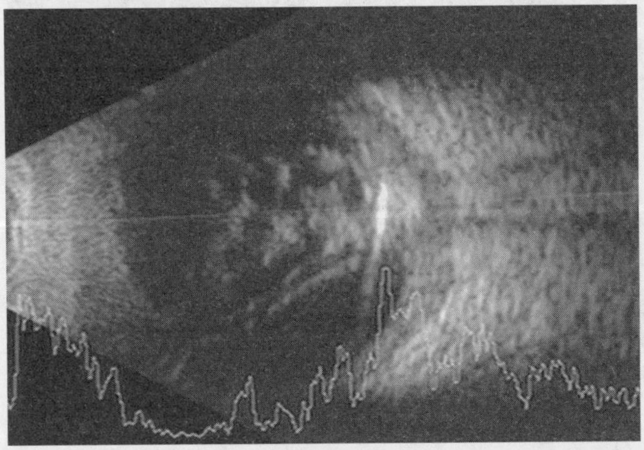

Fig. 17: Vitreous hemorrhage with intraocular foreign body producing 100% reflectivity spike for the retained foreign body and moderate reflectivity from the vitreous hemorrhage.

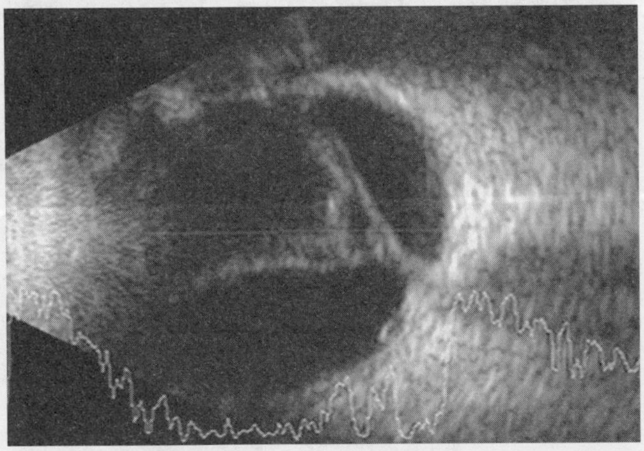

Fig. 19: Posterior vitreous detachment produces A-scan spikes of reflectivity less than 50%.

traumatized eye with retained IOFB. Traumatic vitreous hemorrhage is usually dense and leaves behind dense vitreous membranes on resolution. On A-scan, the reflectivity of traumatic vitreous hemorrhage is high (60–70%) and that of the IOFB is 100% **(Fig. 17)**.

- Associated RD **(Fig. 18)**
- *Posterior vitreous detachment:* ≤50% reflectivity spikes with maximum reflectivity near the optic disk with (50%) progressive decrease in reflectivity toward the periphery (25%) **(Fig. 19)**.

  Reflectivity is seen to progressively reduce toward the periphery.

  Posterior vitreous detachment with attachment to the optic disk should be differentiated from RD by its lower reflectivity (≤50%). The reflectivity of the A-scan spikes in PVD may reach up to 50–60% in cases, where the posterior hyaloids face has a layering of floaters or blood **(Fig. 20)**.

  The reflectivity of the echoes decrease when a long-standing PVD becomes contracted and attenuated (reflectivity is 40–50%).

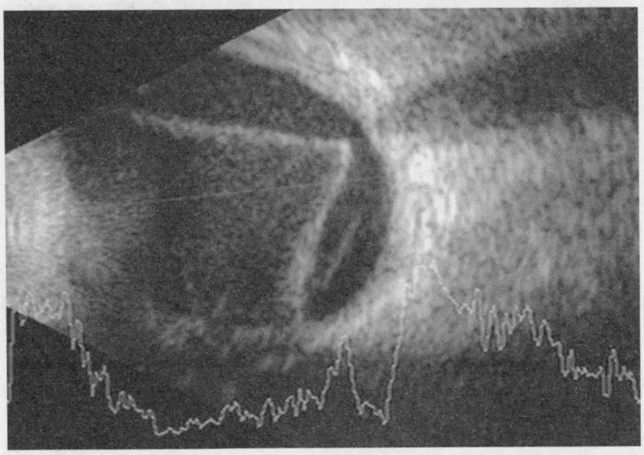

Fig. 20: Thick posterior vitreous detachment secondary to layering of vitreous hemorrhage producing A-scan spikes of 50–60% reflectivity.

- Subhyaloid hemorrhage on A-scan—the subhyaloid hemorrhage has a low reflectivity of around 20–30%. The elevated hyaloidal face over the hemorrhage has a reflectivity of 30–40% **(Figs. 21A and B)**.

• *Retinal detachment*: It has a single steeply rising, moderately thick spike of 80–100% reflectivity. It is

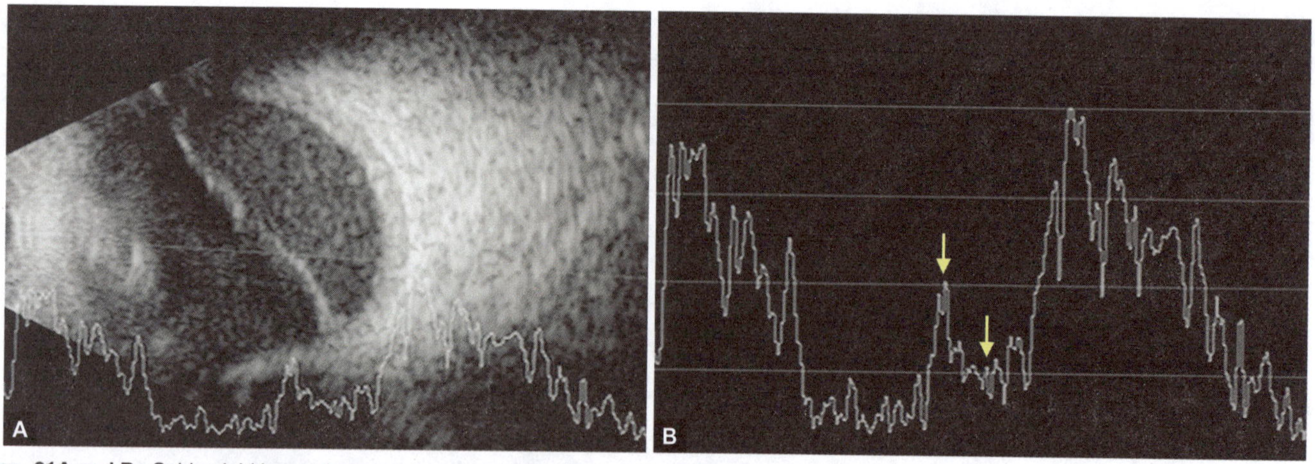

Figs. 21A and B: Subhyaloid hemorrhage on A-scan produces low reflectivity (20–30%) spikes. The associated PVD has a reflectivity of 30–40%.

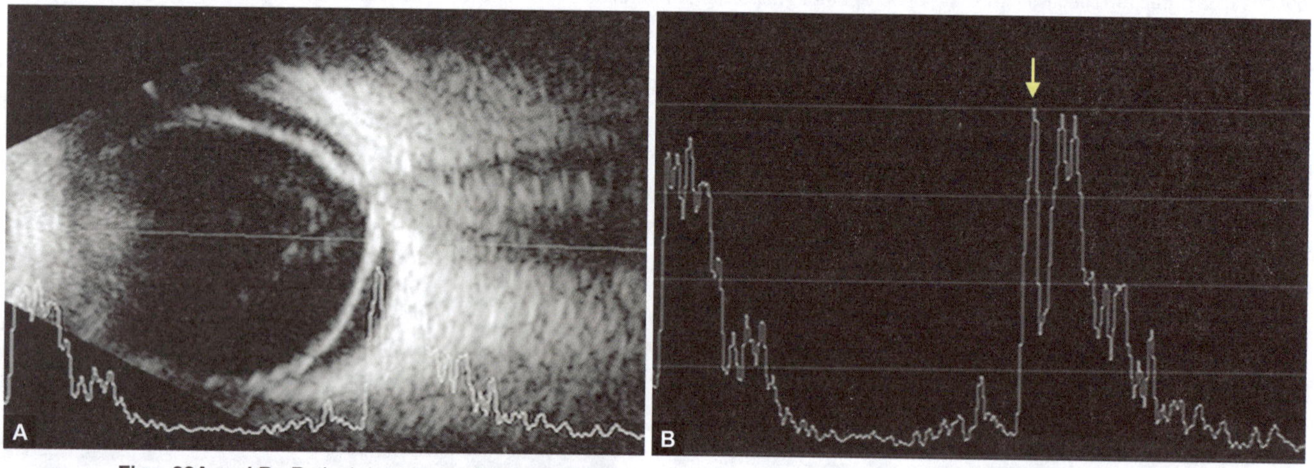

Figs. 22A and B: Retinal detachment (A) producing a steeply rising high reflectivity spike of 80–100% reflectivity (B).

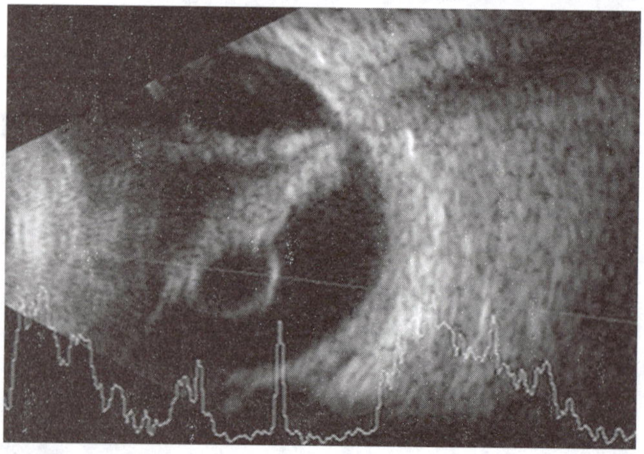

Fig. 23: Long-standing retinal detachment with dense proliferation producing a very high (100%) reflectivity and a broad base for the spike and an intraretinal cyst.

important to pass the A-scan vector at right angles to the membrane. The retinal reflectivity is consistently similar in the entire extent of the membrane **(Figs. 22A and B)**.

Secondary changes such as proliferative vitreoretinopathy (PVR) and intraretinal cyst formation may be associated with long-standing RD **(Fig. 23)**.

- *Exudative RD:* It may occur secondary to inflammatory diseases of the retina and choroid. They are usually shallow and show exudation into the subretinal space and are usually associated with a marked thickening of the retinochoroid due to choroidal edema and inflammation. On A-scan the reflectivity of an exudative detachment is 40–50% **(Fig. 24A)**.
- *Exudative RD:* Secondary to choroidal melanoma, metastasis or retinoblastoma. These detachments are shallow initially but may progress to complete RD. On A-scan, a choroidal melanoma shows a typical cascading reflectivity with low reflectivity for RD **(Fig. 24B)**.
- *Exudative retinal detachment due to choroidal hemangioma:* A-scan will show high reflectivity spikes for both choroidal hemangroma and RD **(Fig. 24C)**.
- Tractional RDs are dome-shaped with the traction bands attached to the highest elevation of the detachment.
- Retinoschisis has a reflectivity of 60–70% **(Fig. 25)**.

• *Conditions causing leukocoria:*
  - Retinoblastoma shows high irregular reflectivity on A-scan due to multiple interfaces produced by irregular distribution of tumor cells **(Figs. 26A and B)**.

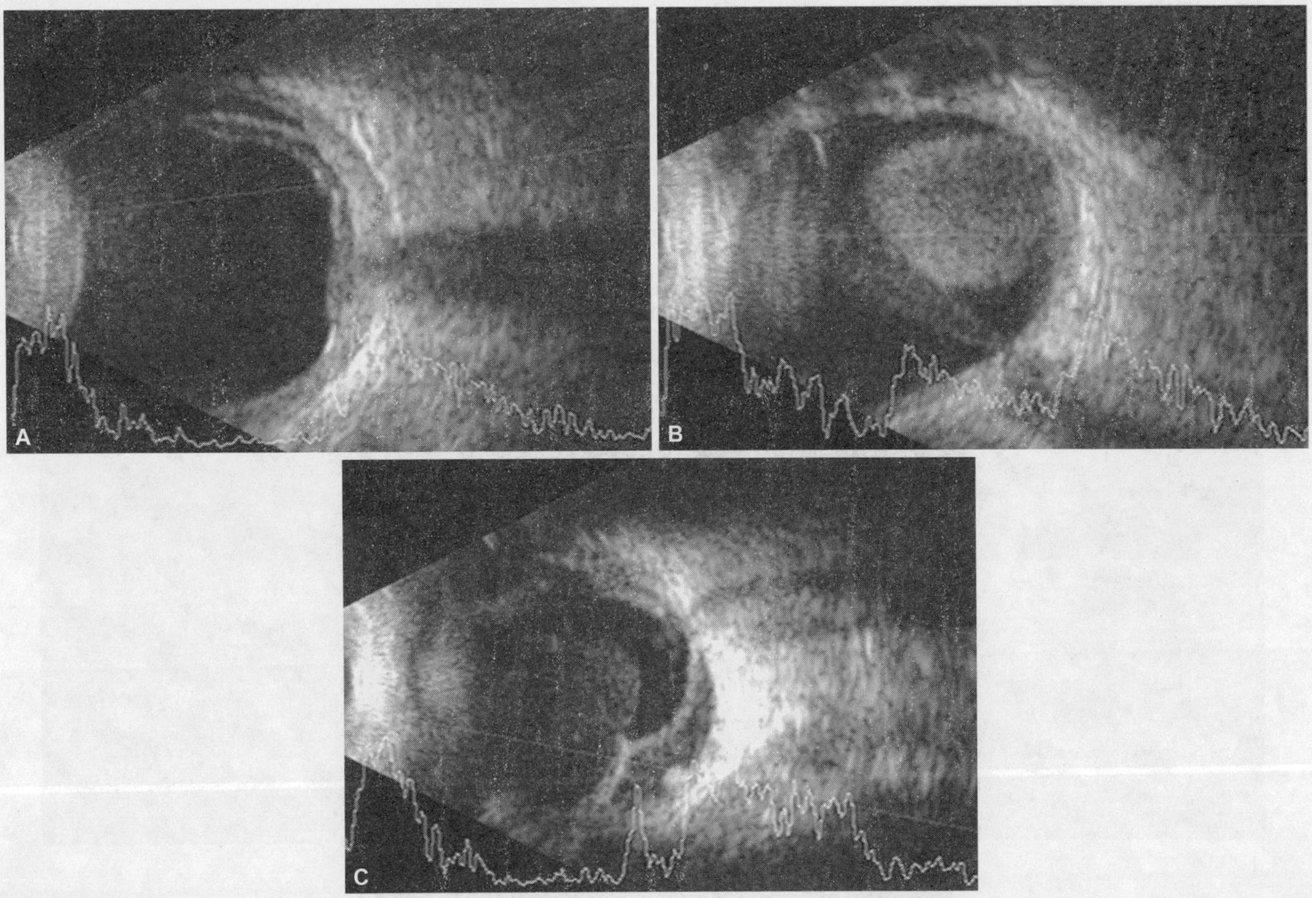

Figs. 24A to C: (A) Exudative retinal detachment secondary to inflammatory diseases of the uvea and sclera gives rise to a moderate reflectivity spike (40–50%) in A-scan and is associated with marked thickening of the chorioretinal layer; (B) Exudative retinal detachment secondary to choroidal tumors. Especially choroidal melanoma will show typical cascading reflectivity and a low reflectivity from retinal detachment; (C) Exudative retinal detachment secondary to with choroidal hemangioma: A-scan shows high reflectivity spike for both the retinal detachment as well as the tumor.

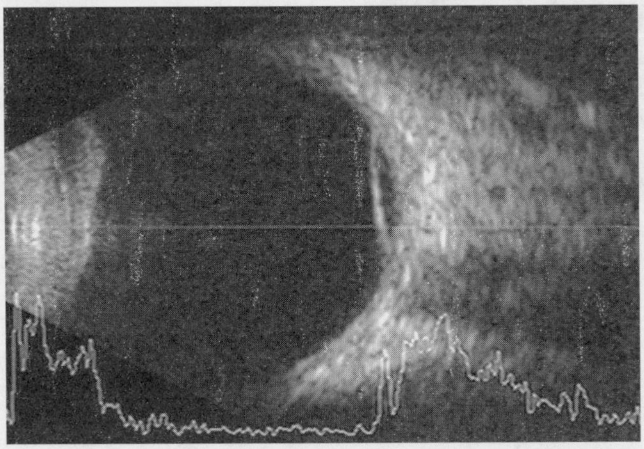

Fig. 25: Retinoschisis is visualized as a thin dome-shaped membrane not attached to the optic disk with 60–70% reflectivity.

When the vector A-scan passes through an area of calcification, there is a high reflectivity spike produced from the calcification with an echolucent area with absent reflectivity distal to it (distal shadowing) **(Figs. 26C and D)**.

Associated features:

- *Extrascleral extension of retinoblastoma:* Enlargement of the optic nerve and thickening of the ocular wall at the site of the tumor should raise the suspicion of extraocular extension. A-scan USG demonstrates a densely calcified mass lesion with absence of sclera spike. In presence of calcification in a lesion infiltrating the optic nerve, it is difficult to assess widening of optic nerve from B/A USG and hence performing a computed tomography (CT) scan is the best modality of imaging in these eyes **(Fig. 26E)**.
- Bilateral retinoblastoma
- Noncalcified lesion/fine nonshadowing calcification/calcification in the vitreous.

- *Persistent hyperplastic primary vitreous (PHPV):* Persistence of the primary hyaloid artery leads to PHPV producing unilateral leukocoria. Ultrasonographic evaluation shows a microphthalmic eye with a thick band extending between the posterior capsules of the lens anteriorly to the optic disk posteriorly. On the A-scan, PHPV shows 80–100% reflectivity due to presence of fibrous tissue. This reflectivity should be measured when the vector A-scan passes at right angles to the membrane **(Fig. 27)**.
- Coats' disease is a unilateral condition, commonly seen in boy in the first decade of life. The hall mark of

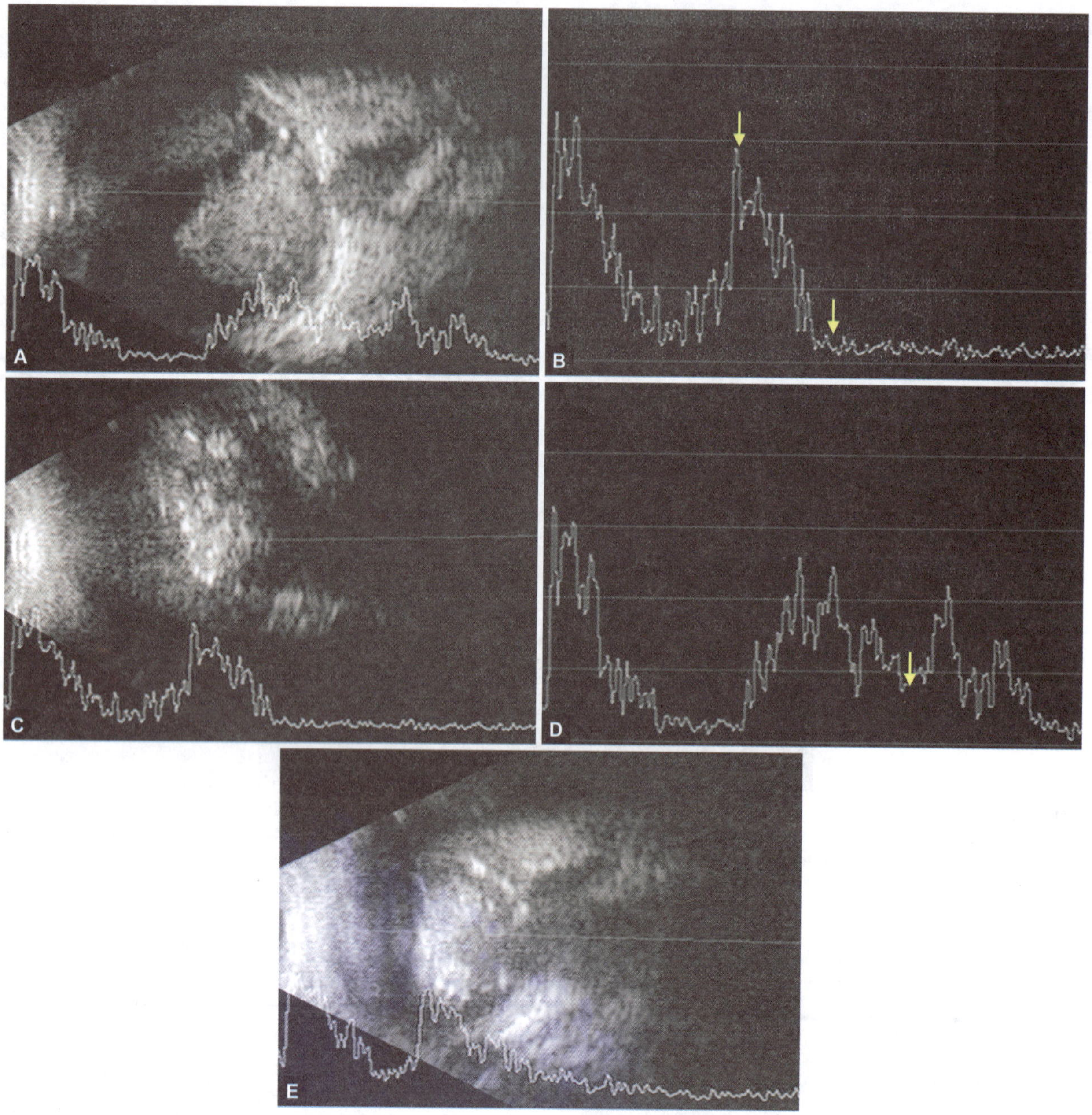

Figs. 26A to E: Retinoblastoma. (A and B) A-scan of the lesion showing high irregular reflectivity from the mass; (C and D) When the vector A-scan passes through an area of calcification, there is a high spike with no reflectivity distal to area of calcification (distal shadowing); (E) Extrascleral extension of a case of retinoblastoma with absent scleral spike.

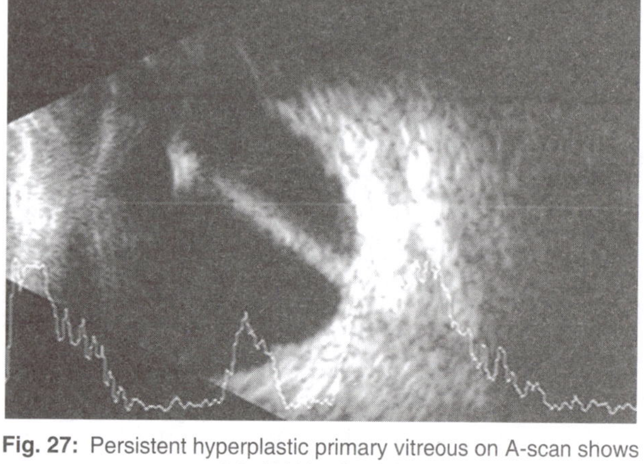

Fig. 27: Persistent hyperplastic primary vitreous on A-scan shows 80–100% reflectivity.

Coats' disease is exudative RD. On A-scan, the RD has 50–60% reflectivity and the subretinal exudation shows 20–30% reflectivity **(Fig. 28)**. The subretinal exudates may coalesce to form a dense echogenic opacification in the vitreous with 20–30% reflectivity. The overlying detached retina is seen as a dense echogenic membrane attached to the optic disk with 50–60% reflectivity. Calcification of the detached retina and other ocular tissues may be seen in chronic Coats' disease. The calcification in Coats' disease is dystrophic and occurs in the subretinal exudates and also in the choroid. These areas of dystrophic calcification are seen as high reflectivity spikes with distal shadowing.

- *Choroidal pathologies:*
  - Uveal malignant melanoma is the most common primary intraocular tumor in the adult age group. USG is necessary for diagnosis, assessment of volume calculation, and for follow-up of uveal melanomas. On A-scan, melanoma has a high anterior surface spike due to a large interface between the vitreous and the tumor. The internal reflectivity of the tumor is low to medium due to minimum interfaces between the tumor cells **(Fig. 29A to C)**. Since the melanoma is a highly cellular tumor, attenuation of the sound beam occurs during passage through the lesion causing a typical cascading internal reflectivity and acoustic hollowing at the base of the tumor.

    On A-scan the reflectivity of the acoustic hollowing in 20–30% **(Fig. 30A)**. Another feature though not characteristics of a choroidal melanoma is choroidal excavation, which is seen as an irregular hypoechoic curvilinear area at the base of the tumor. On A-scan the reflectivity of the excavation is less than 50% **(Fig. 30B)**. When hemorrhage or necrosis develops within a tumor, ultrasonographic evaluation will show a densely echogenic area with high irregular reflectivity. A choroidal melanoma may be associated with exudative detachment or vitreous hemorrhage.

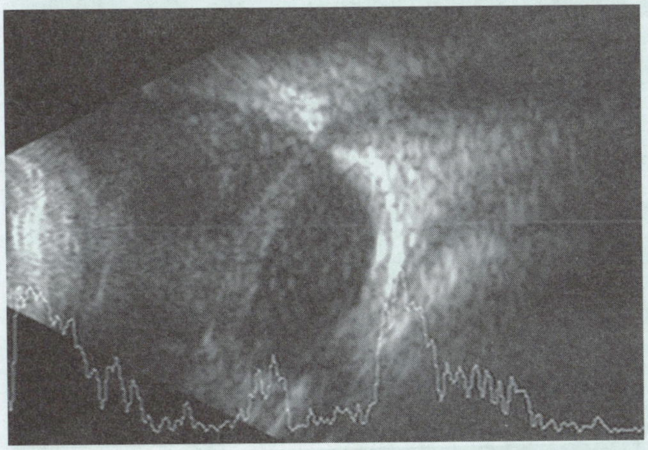

Fig. 28: Coats' disease on A-scan. The retinal detachment in Coats' disease has 50–60% reflectivity and the subretinal exudates show 20–30% reflectivity.

Ultrasonographic follow-up of choroidal melanoma: Early choroidal melanoma is seen as a small echogenic elevation arising from the choroid and may not have the characteristic sonographic appearance described earlier. On A-scan, there may be single or multiple high spikes. The role of B-scan in such cases is to measure the exact volume of the lesion and on follow-up scans to study its growth pattern. Increasing lesion size and demonstration of typical cascading reflectivity on follow-up indicates lesion growth **(Figs. 31A to C)**.

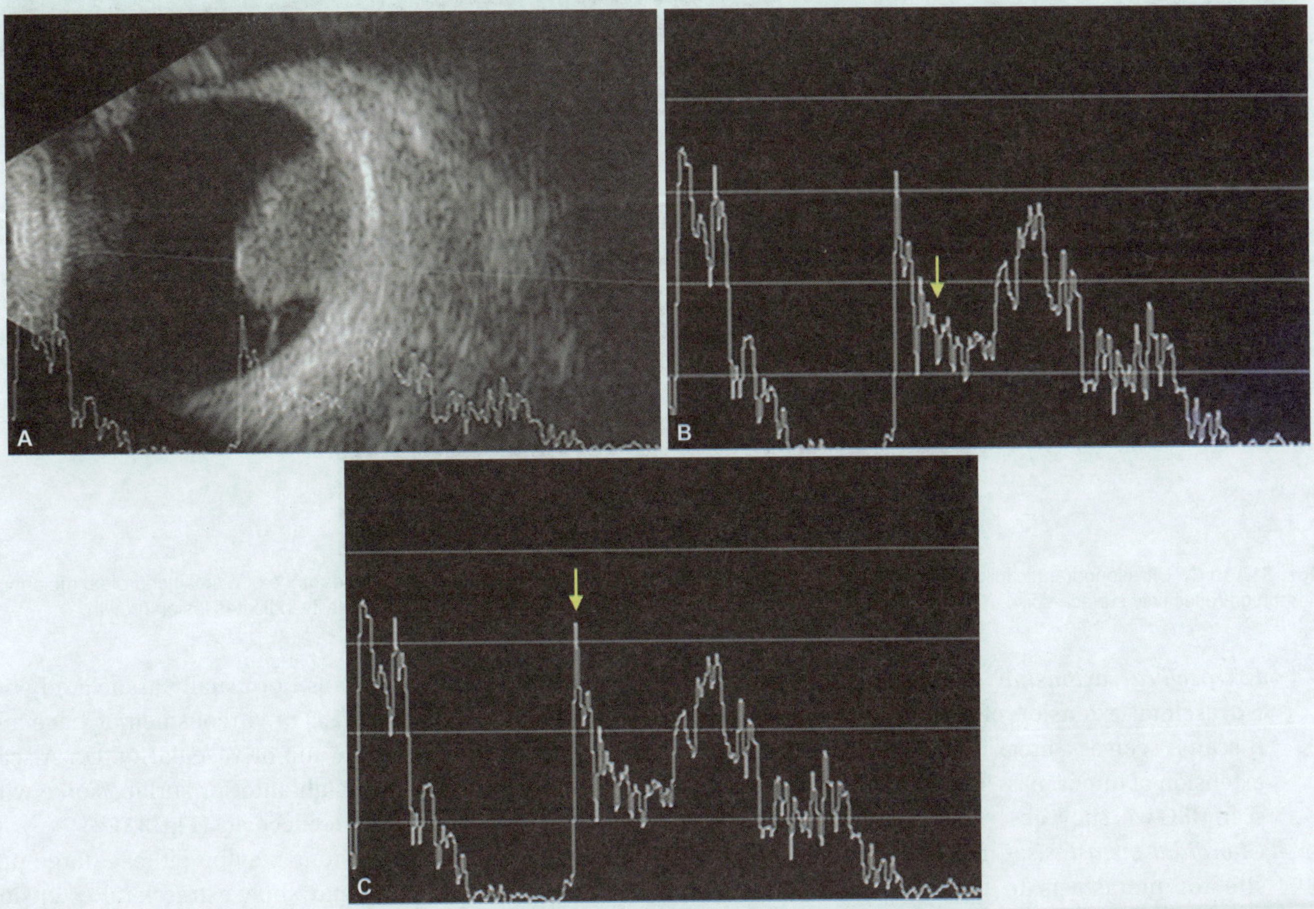

Fig. 29A to C: Choroidal melanoma demonstrating classic A-scan USG features of: (A) high reflectivity anterior surface spike; (B) Low-to-medium internal reflectivity; (C) Cascading internal reflectivity.

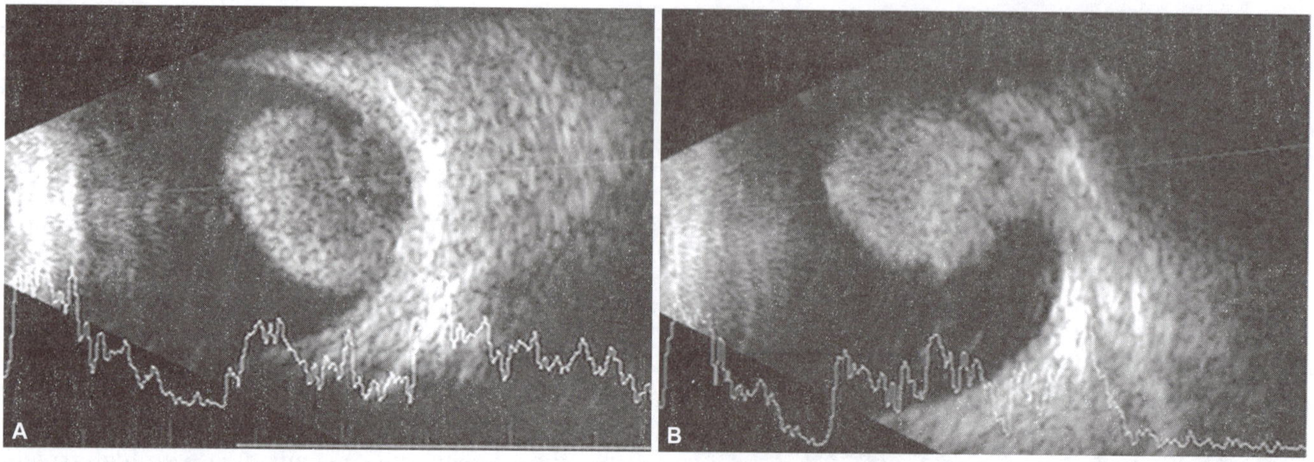

Figs. 30A and B: (A) Acoustic hollowing in a case of choroidal melanoma seen as a triangular hypoechoic area at the base of the melanoma with 20–30% reflectivity on A-scan; (B) Choroidal excavation seen as an irregular hypoechoic area at base of melanoma with A-scan reflectivity of <50%.

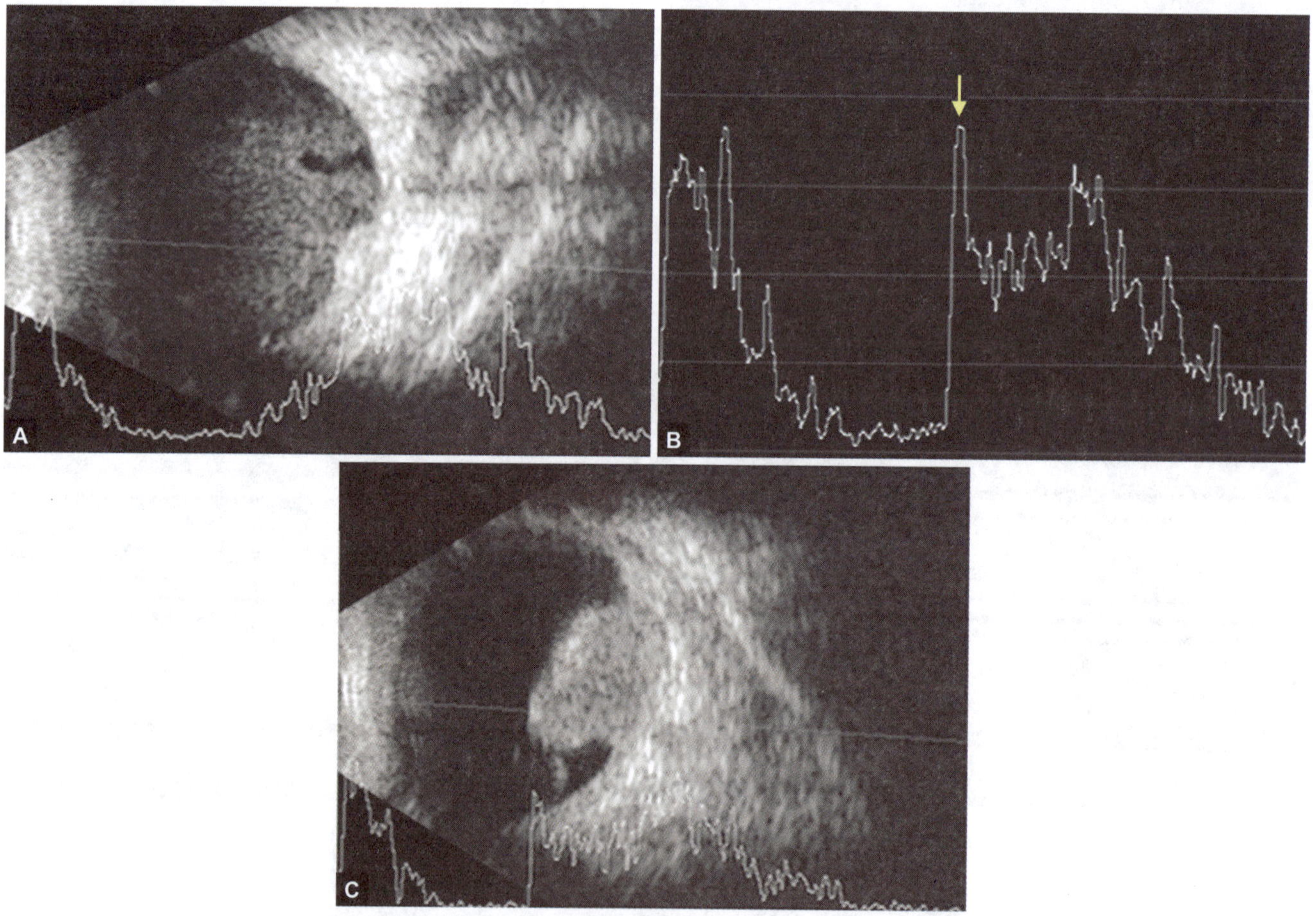

Figs. 31A to C: Ultrasonographic follow-up of choroidal melanoma. (A and B) A-scan ultrasonographic appearance of a small choroidal melanoma with a high reflectivity surface spike; (C) Increasing lesion size and demonstration of typical cascading reflectivity indicates lesion growth.

Extrascleral extension of choroidal melanomas: Extrascleral extension of a choroidal melanoma on B-scan is seen as a break in the scleral continuity with extension of tumor mass into the retro-ocular space. A scan USG will show absence of scleral spikes.

- *Choroidal metastasis:* Choroid is the most common site for metastasis to the eye due to its highly vascular nature. The most common primary tumor metastasizing to the choroid are from breast and lung. Choroidal metastasis is not usually associated with secondary exudative RD or vitreous hemorrhage and shows minimal or no tumor vascularity. On A-scan there is medium to high anterior surface spike with high irregular internal reflectivity **(Fig. 32)**.

The metastatic lesions may be either a large one or a flat lesion and may show extrascleral extension characterized by high irregular reflectivity in the extra-ocular space. Metastatic infiltrates from lymphoma

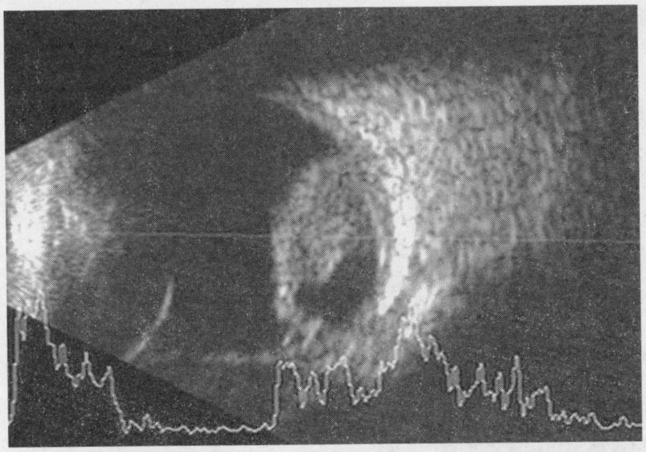

Fig. 32: Choroidal metastasis showing a medium-to-high reflectivity anterior lesion spike with high irregular internal reflectivity.

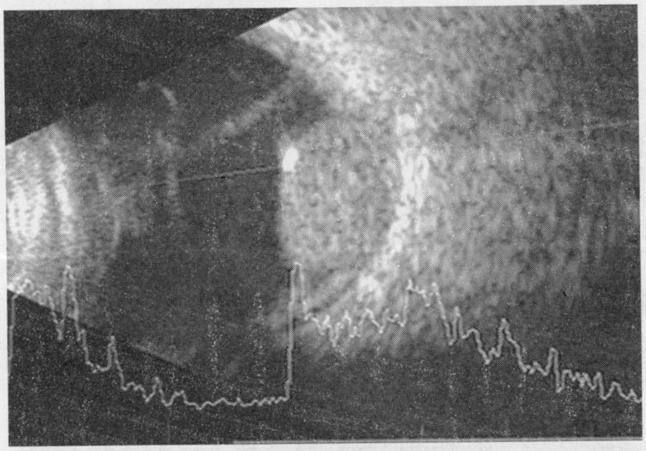

Fig. 33: Choroidal hemangioma exhibiting the characteristic features of highly reflective anterior lesion spike, with high irregular internal reflectivity.

and leukemia are highly cellular with a homogeneous texture and cascading internal reflectivity.

- *Choroidal hemangioma:* It may occur as a solitary lesion or as a part of Sturge–Weber syndrome. On A-scan USG, choroidal hemangiomas have a highly reflective anterior lesion spike due to a large interface between the vitreous cavity and the tumor. Due to multiple vascular interfaces within the tumor, choroidal hemangioma has a high and irregular internal reflectivity **(Fig. 33)**. It is very important to demonstrate a phlebolith in the choroidal mass lesion since its presence provides diagnostic confirmation. Hemangiomas associated with Sturge–Weber syndrome are seen as diffuse, flat echogenic choroidal masses with high reflectivity.

Bleeding into the vitreous cavity either spontaneously or following trauma may be seen in eyes with choroidal hemangiomas. The bleeding into the vitreous cavity may be dense enough to mask the tumor. Small choroidal hemangiomas may bleed into the subretinal space and may lead to hemorrhagic RD. On B-scan, the hemangioma is seen as an echogenic mass within:

- *Choroidal nevus:* These are small choroidal lesions with minimal elevation and are hence not detected during routine USG. Choroidal nevi with >2 mm elevation can be detected on B-scan as a small dome-shaped elevation with uniform echo texture. On A-scan USG, the internal reflectivity of choroidal nevus is around 50–60% with minimal cascading effect.

Elevated choroidal nevus cannot be differentiated from early choroidal melanoma or any other choroidal tumor. Hence USG has a definite role in monitoring rate of growth or change in echotexture of nevus to differentiate between early choroidal melanoma and choroidal nevus **(Figs. 34A to C)**.

A small choroidal nevus with medium reflectivity on A-scan, on serial follow-up may show (1) increase in size, (2) classical cascading reflectivity, and (3) presence of exudative RD indicating malignant transformation.

- *Choroidal osteoma:* These are relatively common benign tumors of the choroid, presenting as a localized and minimal elevation. It is important to differentiate choroidal osteoma from dystrophic calcification of the choroid, secondary to disuse atrophy is dense and irregular in outline and is associated with chronic RD or long-standing endophthalmitis. Areas of dystrophic calcification show high reflectivity **(Figs. 35A and B)**.
- *Choroidal calcification secondary to hypercalcemia:* It is uniform and regular in outline and is present over the entire extent of the choroid as a regular curvilinear shadow with high reflectivity and distal shadowing **(Figs. 36A and B)**.
- *Choroidal detachment*: It can occur spontaneously, or following trauma or surgery. The echotexture of the membrane is decided by the nature of the suprachoroidal contents namely blood, serous fluid, or exudates. Choroidal detachment is never attached to the optic disk.

In A-scan choroidal detachment produces 100% reflectivity at high gains **(Fig. 37)**. A double spike is seen when the detached choroid is thickened and folded on itself. When the choroidal detachment is associated with a RD, the detached retina is seen as a V-shaped membrane attached to the optic disk underneath which the choroidal detachment can be seen.

- *Suprachoroidal hemorrhage:* On A-scan, suprachoroidal hemorrhage produces high irregular reflectivity. The choroidal membrane may not produce a high spike due to the dense hemorrhage external to it. The reflectivity of the choroidal membrane is about 50%, which cannot be separated from the reflectivity of blood. In patients with fresh and extensive suprachoroidal hemorrhage, a triangular hypoechoes area anterior to the optic disk is seen in almost all

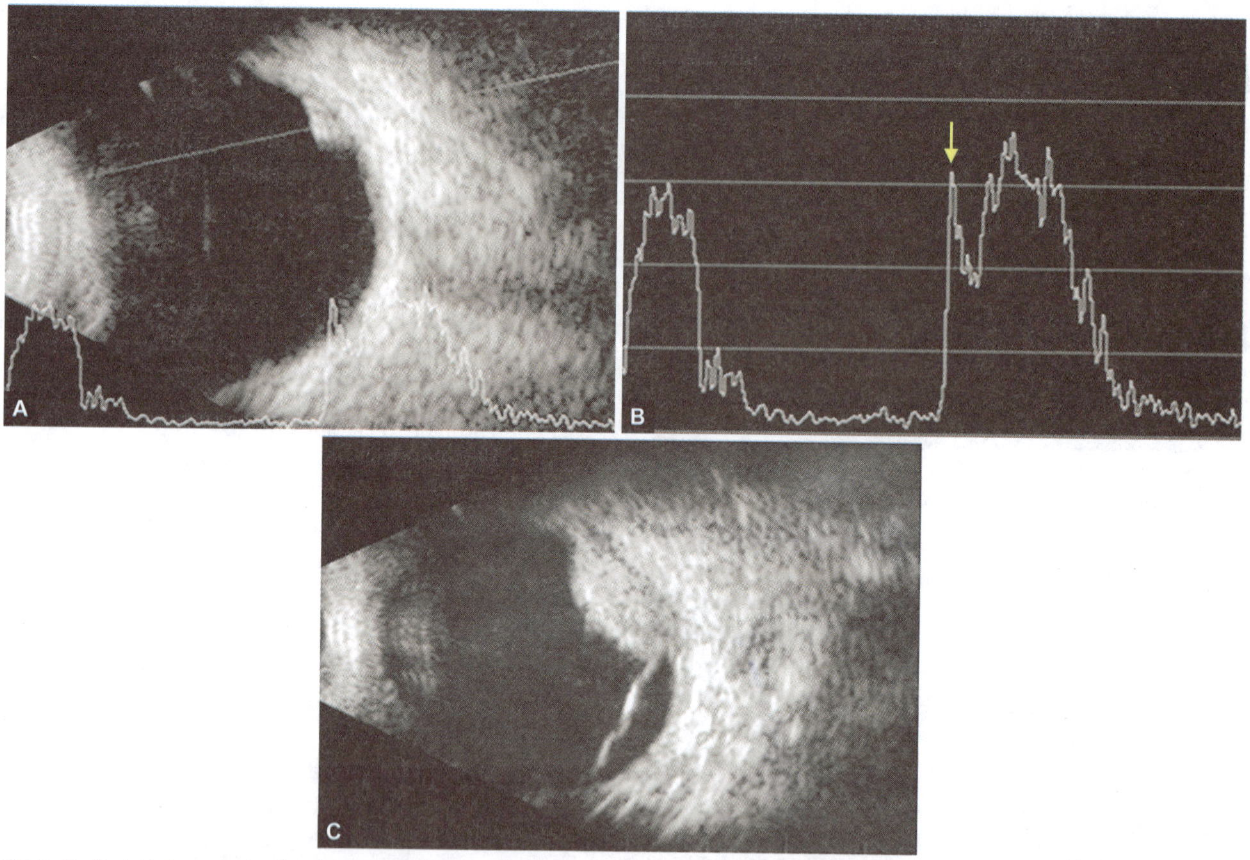

Figs. 34A to C: Serial follow-up of a choroidal nevus with ultrasonography. (A and B) A small choroidal nevus with medium reflectivity and nondescriptive feature; (C) Follow-up evaluation several years later shows increasing size, cascading reflectivity, and presence of exudative RD indicating a malignant transformation.

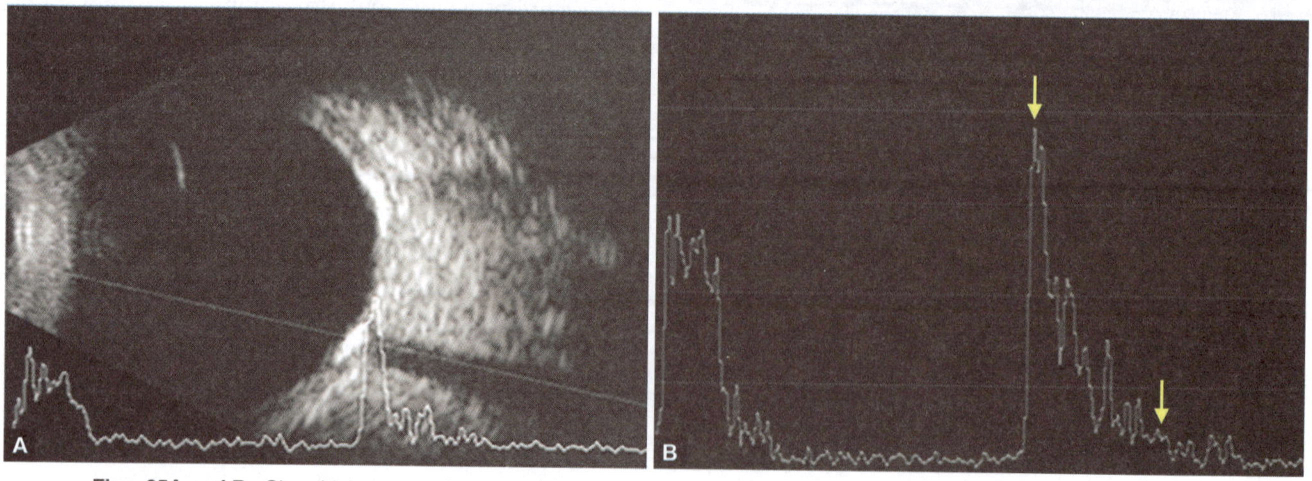

Figs. 35A and B: Choroidal osteoma demonstrating high reflectivity of the lesion on A-scan with orbital shadowing distally.

cases of extensive suprachoroidal hemorrhage. This hypoechoic area is the clear vitreous anterior to the optic disk as the choroidal detachment stops short of the optic disk. On A-scan, the suprachoroidal hemorrhage produces high irregular reflectivity, and in such situations, the reflectivity the choroidal membrane cannot be ascertained. It is possible to highlight and delineate choroidal detachment by using TF3 amplification to suppress the hemorrhage echoes **(Figs. 38A to C)**.

The role of USG in suprachoroidal hemorrhage is to identify the nature of the hemorrhage. The nature of the hemorrhage is an important criterion to determine the timing for surgical intervention. On serial follow-up of suprachoroidal hemorrhage, the echoes change their texture from echogenic to hypoechoic and finally anechoic texture. This change in texture is also associated with a reduction in the reflectivity of the hemorrhage, and indicates progressive liquefaction of the suprachoroidal blood and the optimum time for surgical intervention.

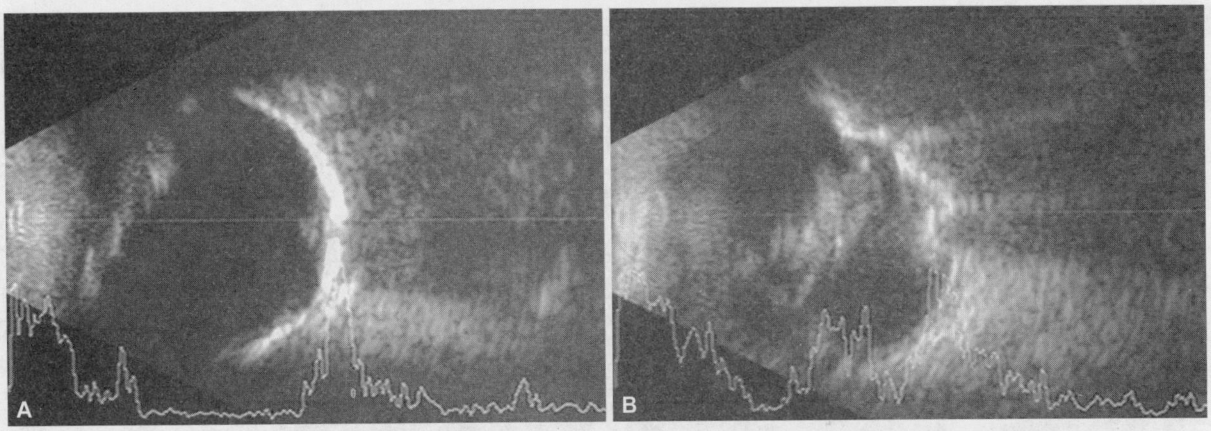

Figs. 36A and B: Choroidal calcification secondary to hypercalcemia; (B) dystrophic choroidal calcification.

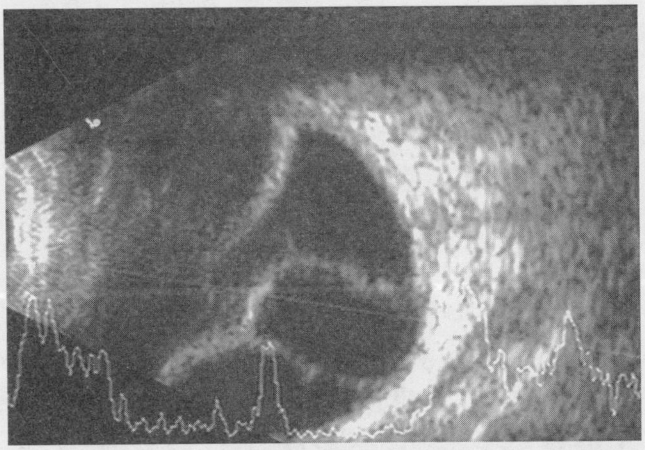

Fig. 37: Choroidal detachment producing 100% reflectivity at high gain.

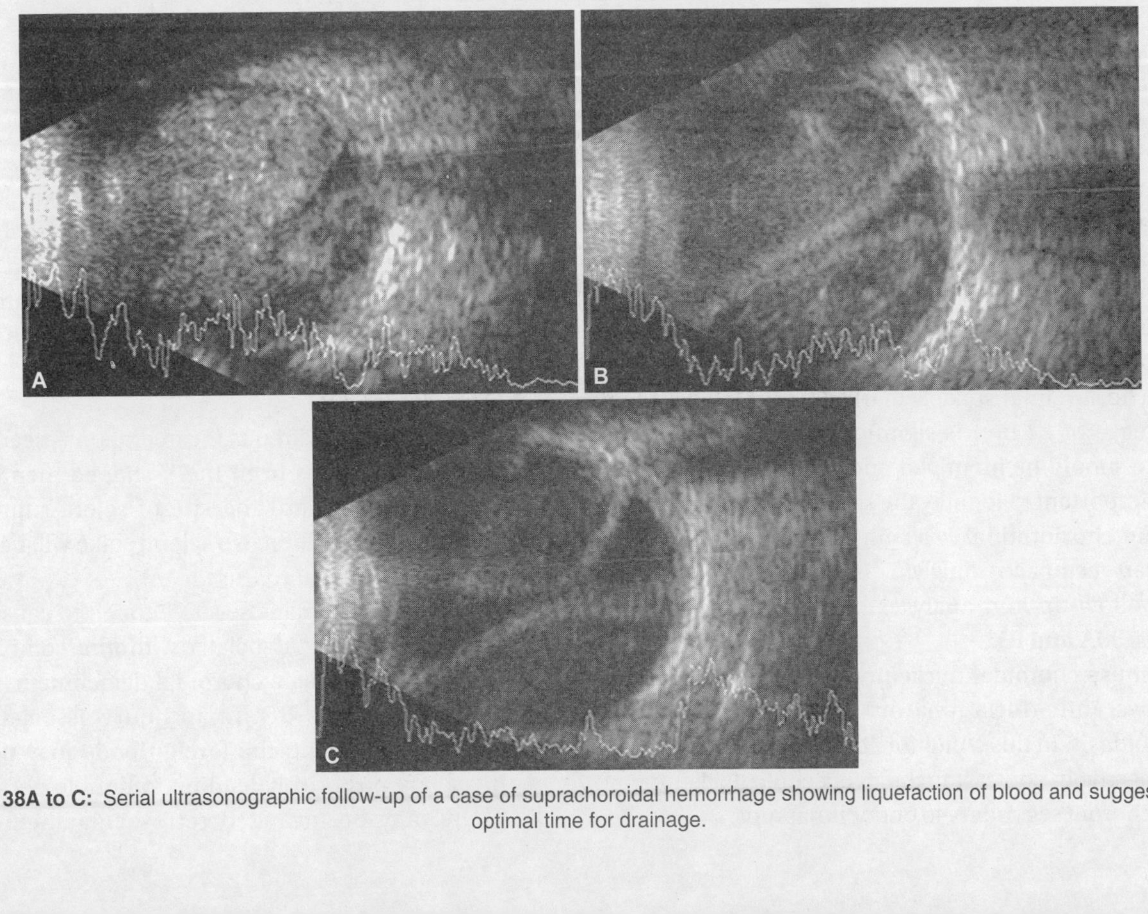

Figs. 38A to C: Serial ultrasonographic follow-up of a case of suprachoroidal hemorrhage showing liquefaction of blood and suggesting the optimal time for drainage.

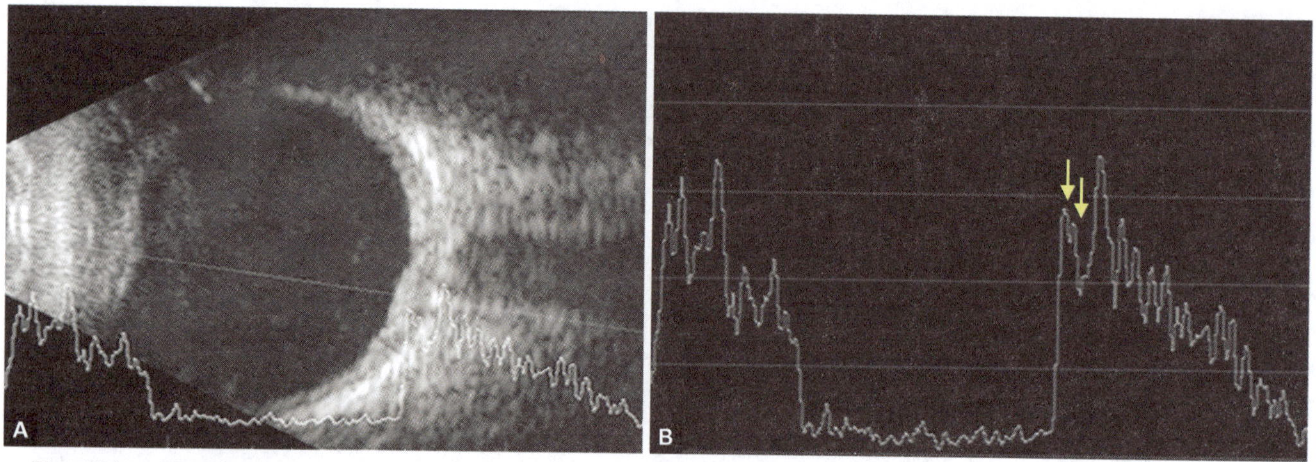

Figs. 39A and B: Chorioretinal thickening secondary to posterior uveitis. Note the marked separation of the retinal and choroidal spikes.

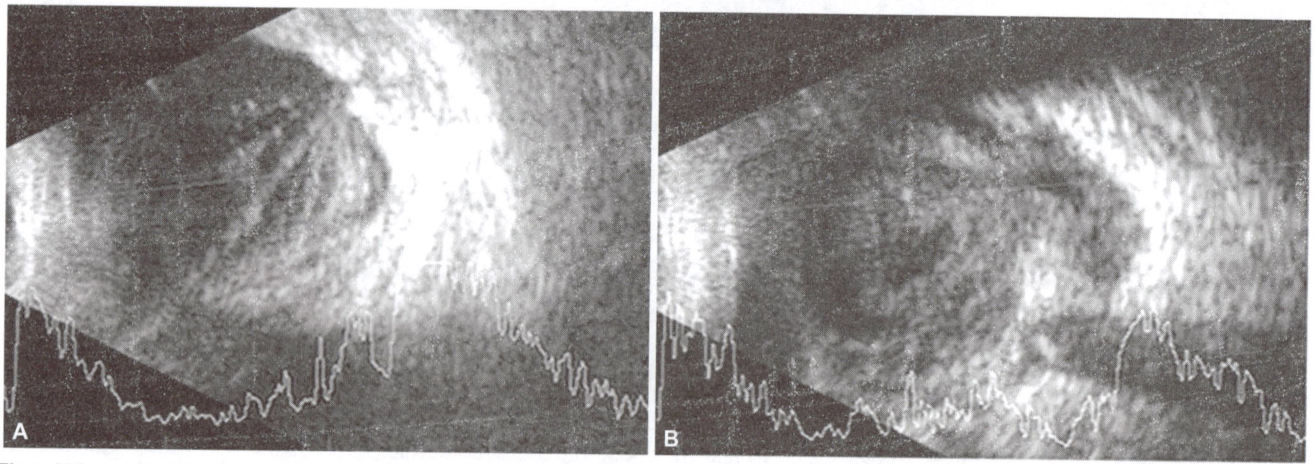

Figs. 40A and B: Occult scleral rupture with secondary signs to demonstrate site of rupture—vitreous incarceration, hemorrhage in the Tenon's space, thickened chorioretinal layer, discontinuity in the sclera.

- *Choroidal thickening:* It may occur secondary to posterior uveitis, endophthalmitis, VKH, lymphoid hyperplasia, or collagen disorders. In these conditions, there is focal or diffuse irregular thickening of the chorioretinal layer. The choroidal layer can be separated from the retina on reducing the gain due to excessive fluid accumulation in the choroid. Along with the choroidal thickening, multiple modules vitreous echoes may be noted. These echoes may be secondary to uveitis or endophthalmitis. On A-scan the chorioretinal spike is markedly separated and an increase of ≥2 mm is significant. The chorioretinal spike should be identified and accurately measured. It is important to identify the site of maximal thickness of the chorioretinal layer on B-scan and direct the A-scan vector accordingly. This measurement is useful for follow-up and analyses of response to therapy **(Figs. 39A and B)**.

Diffuse choroidal thickening may occur secondary to systemic inflammatory conditions such as sarcoidosis. In this condition, the thickened choroid in echogenic in contrast to the hypoechoic thickening of the choroid secondary to endophthalmitis.

- *Scleral pathologies:* Scleral rupture may occur following severe blunt or penetrating trauma. USG may not always be able to demonstrate this.
  - *Scleral rupture:* It may occur following severe blunt or penetrating trauma USG may not always be able to demonstrate a direct break in the sclera. However, secondary signs help to detect the site of rupture. The secondary signs of rupture are vitreous incarceration, hemorrhage in the Tenon's space, thickened chorioretinal layers, and a discontinuity in the sclera **(Figs. 40A and B)**.

  In the A-scan, vitreous incarceration is seen as high reflectivity echoes from the V-shaped membranous bands going toward the site of sclera rupture and vitreous incarceration. No scleral spike will be present at the site of scleral rupture.

  When the trauma is severe enough to cause scleral rupture, it is usually associated with other complications such as hemorrhagic choroidal detachment, vitreous hemorrhage, and RD. In an injury associated with an IOFB lodgment, the foreign body may perforate the sclera posteriorly leading to double perforation. There may be localized retro-ocular hemorrhage around the perforation and a retro-ocular high reflectivity foreign body with orbital shadowing distally **(Fig. 41)**.

- *Posterior scleritis:* It is an inflammatory condition of the sclera, which may extend into the choroid anteriorly and the retro-ocular space posteriorly and may be associated with an exudative RD. Posterior scleritis may be associated with a hyperechoic thickening of the sclera especially around the optic disk. With a hypoechoic rim due to inflammatory edema in the Tenon's space. The optic nerve shadow together with the hypoechoic Tenon's space produces the T sign which is pathognomonic of posterior scleritis **(Figs. 42A and B)**.

Table 8 summarizes the various posterior segment lesions and their characteristics.

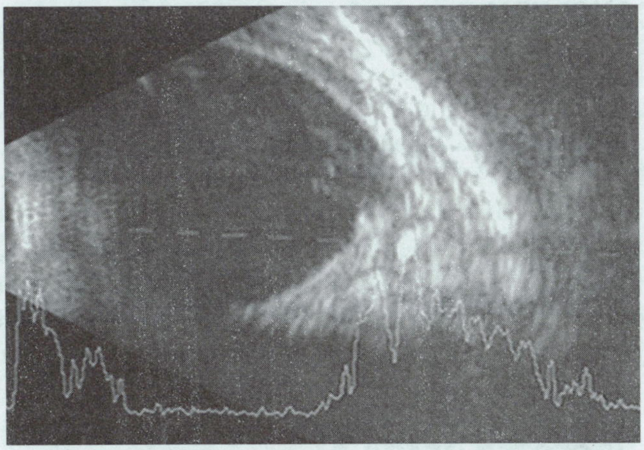

Fig. 41: Double perforation with retro-ocular hemorrhage and a high-reflectivity orbital foreign body.

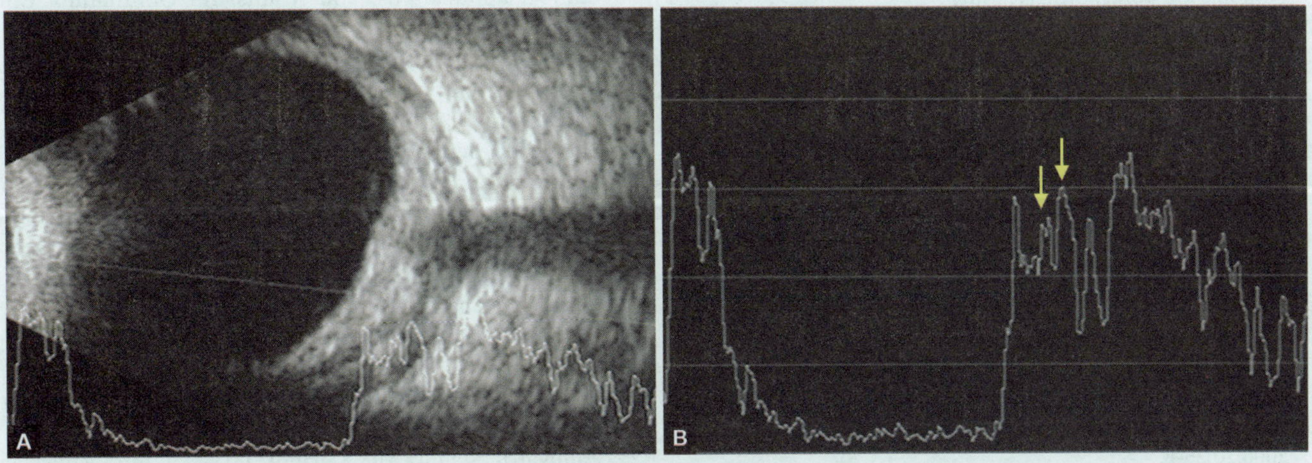

Figs. 42A and B: Posterior scleritis on A-scan produces high irregular scleral spikes associated with low reflectivity spikes from subtenous space (along with ON shadow constitute "T" sign).

Table 8: The various posterior segment lesions and their characteristics.

	Quantitative echography		***Kinetic echography***		
	Reflectivity	***Sound attenuation***	***Consistency (after months)***	***Vascularity***	***Others***
Point-like lesion echoes					
Senile vitreous degeneration	Low (2–20%)	Minimal	Marked		Few signals
Asteroid hyalosis	Medium (20–60%)	Minimal	Fast vertical		Preretinal vitreous uninvolved
Synchysis scintillans	High (80–100%)	Weak	Fast vertical		Preretinal vitreous uninvolved
IOFB	Extremely high (1,005)	Strong	Rare		
Membrane-like lesion					
Retinal detachment	Extremely high (100%)	Minimal	Minimal		Continuous surface thick
Choroidal detachment	100%	Minimal	Minimal		Typical location shape thick
PVD	40–100%	Minimal	Marked		
Well-defined mass lesions					
SRH	Low (10–60%)	Medium	Marked to slight	None	Usually flat
MM	Low (10–60%)	Medium	None (solid)	Slight to marked	Prominent, raised
Hemangioma	Mod high (60–80%)	Medium to strong	None solid	Marked	
Metastatic CA	High (80–100%)	Medium	None	None	
Retinoblastoma	Extremely high (80–100%)	Very strong	None	Marked	

(CA: carcinoma; IOFB: intraocular foreign body; MM: malignant melanoma; PVD: posterior vitreous detachment; SRH: subretinal hemorrhage)

CONCLUSION

Despite availability of more sophisticated imaging modalities for diagnosis and follow-up of ophthalmic pathologies, A-/B-scan USG has a definite role, which cannot be ignored. Measurement of axial length, biometry for IOL power calculation, and characterization of posterior segment pathology are the chief indications of A-scan. Combining different investigative modalities will definitely help in accurate characterization of the lesion under evaluation and hence A-scan USG should be used in conjunction with other imaging modalities.

SUGGESTED READING

1. Binkhorst RD. A Guide to the Author's Tl-58-59 IOL Power Module. Intraocular Lens Power Calculation Manual, 2nd edition. New York: Springer; 1981.
2. Binkhorst RD. The accuracy of ultrasonic measurement of the axial length of the eye. Ophthalmic Surg. 1981;12(5): 363-5.
3. Byrne SF, Green RL. Ultrasound of the Eye and Orbit, 2nd Edition. St Louis, MO: Mosby Inc; 2002.
4. Byrne SF. A-Scan Axial Length Measurements: A Handbook for IOL calculations. Mars Hill, NC: Grove Park Publishers; 1995.
5. Byrne SF. Improving A-scans. Ocul Surg News. 1994;12(6): 86-7.
6. Fielding JA. Ocular ultrasound. Clin Radiol. 1996;51(8): 533-44.
7. Fyodorov SN, Kolonko Al. Estimation of optical power of the intraocular lens. Vestn Ophthalmol (Moscow). 1967;4:27.
8. Gale RP, Saha N, Johnston RL. National Biometry Audit II. Eye. 2006;20:25-8.
9. Hoffer KJ. Biometry of 7,500 cataractous eyes. Am J Ophthalmol. 1980;90(3):360-8.
10. Hoffer KJ. The Hoffer Q formula: a comparison of theoretic and regression formulas. J Cataract Refract Surg. 1993;19(6): 700-12.
11. Holladay JT, Prager TC. Accurate ultrasonic biometry in pseudophakia. Am J Ophthalmol. 1989;107(2):189-90.
12. Kane JX, Van Heerdan A, Atik A, et al. Intraocular lens power formula accuracy: Comparison of 7 formulas. J Cataract Refract Surg. 2016;42:1490-500.
13. Kane JX, Van Heerdan A, Petsoglou C. Comparison of 10 Methods for IOL power calculation: results from over 3000 Eyes. RANZO. 2016. Free paper.
14. Kendall CJ. Ophthalmic echography. Thorofare, NJ: Slack Incorporated; 1990.
15. Nemeth J, Fekete O, Pesztenlehrer N. Optical and ultrasound measurement of axial length and anterior chamber depth for intraocular lens power calculation. J Cataract Refract Surg. 2003;29(1):85-8.
16. Ossoinig KC. Standardized echography: basic principles, clinical applications, and results. Int Ophthalmol Clin. 1979;19(4):127-210.
17. Retzlaff JA, Sanders DR, Kraff MC. Development of the SRK/T intraocular lens implant power calculation formula. J cataract refract Surg. 1990;16(3):333-40.
18. Shugar JK, de Juan E Jr, McCuen BW 2nd, et al. Ultrasonic examination of the silicone filled eye: theoretical and practical considerations. Graefes Arch Clin Exp ophthalmol. 1986;224(4):361-7.
19. Wang L, Shirayama M, Ma XJ, et al. Optimizing intraocular lens power calculations in eyes with axial length above 25.0 mm. J Cataract Refract Surg. 2011;37:2018-27.
20. Yang S, Lang A, Makker H, et al. Effect of silicone sound speed and intraocular lens thickness on pseudophakic axial length corrections. J Cataract Refract Surg. 1995;21(4):442-6.
21. Zaldivar R, Schultz MC, Davidorf JM, et al. Intraocular lens power calculations in patients with extreme myopia. J Cataract Refract Surg. 2000;26(5):668-74.

CHAPTER

18 B-scan Ultrasonography

Anand Rajendran, VSD Kiranmayi, RD Ravindran

INTRODUCTION

Ultrasound was first used in ophthalmology in 1956 by two American ophthalmologists, Mundt and Hughes. In 1958, Baum and Greenwood codeveloped the first two-dimensional B-scan ultrasound instrument for ophthalmology. Since then it has emerged as an indispensable tool in the diagnosis and management of various ocular and orbital abnormalities. Ultrasonography is mostly indicated in hazy media when the traditional optical evaluation is not possible. It is also of immense value in evaluation of intraocular space-occupying lesions.

OCULAR INDICATIONS FOR ULTRASOUND EVALUATION

Opaque Ocular Media

- Corneal opacification
- Hyphema
- Small pupil
- Cataract
- Vitreous hemorrhage or inflammation.

Clear Ocular Media

- Iris lesions
- Ciliary body lesions
- Intraocular tumors
- Retinal detachment (RD)
- Optic nerve abnormalities
- Evaluation of extraocular muscles and the orbit
- Intraocular foreign body (IOFB) detection and trauma evaluation.

PHYSICS OF ULTRASOUND

Ultrasound is an acoustic wave that consists of oscillations of particles within a medium. Ultrasound waves have frequencies greater than 20 kHz (20,000 oscillations/sec). Frequencies used in diagnostic ophthalmic ultrasound are in range of 8–10 MHz (1 MHz = 1,000,000 cycles/sec) which allow resolution of minute ocular and orbital structures.

Echoes are produced by acoustic interfaces created at the junction of two media with different acoustic impedance. The greater the difference in the acoustic impedance of the two interface media, the stronger the reflection of the sound wave (echo) **(Figs. 1A and B)**. The angle at

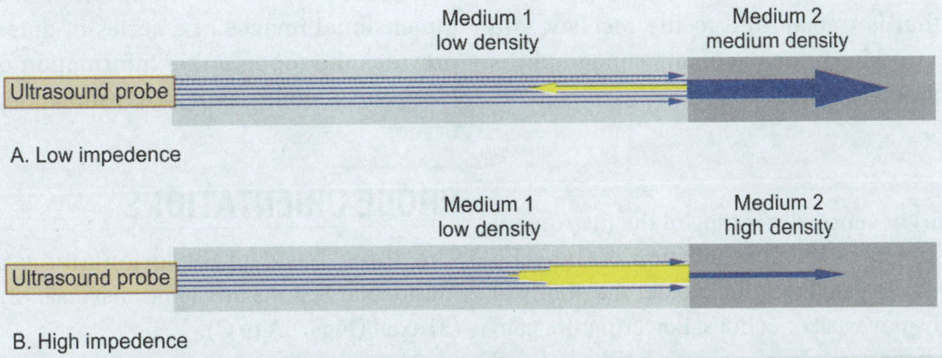

Figs. 1A and B: The effect of an interface between media of different densities on echo generation. (A) The difference in density is slight, with only little reflection; (B) There is a greater difference and the reflection is increased.

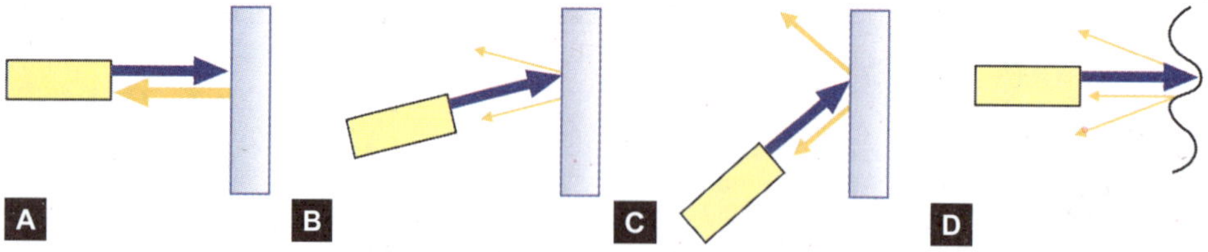

Figs. 2A to D: (A to C) The effect of probe positioning on the return of the echo. The greater the obliquity of the probe, the less echo returns; (D) The effect of an irregular interface on the echo—the strength of the returning echo is reduced.

Flowchart 1: Schematic diagram showing the working principle of the ultrasonography instrument.

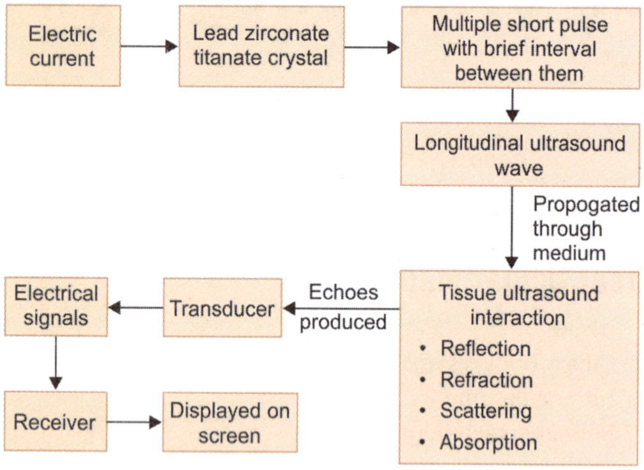

which the sound beam strikes an interface determines the strength of the returning echo. When the beam strikes an interface perpendicularly, it results in a stronger echo. If an incident beam strikes the interface at an oblique angle, some of the reflected energy is diverted away from the direction of its origin (refracted), resulting in a weaker echo **(Figs. 2A to D)**.

PROBE

The basis of the pulse echo system is the piezoelectric crystal located near the face of the probe, undergoes a mechanical vibration when stimulated by electrical energy. This vibration causes a longitudinal ultrasound wave (sound beam) to be propagated through the medium. A pause of several microseconds occurs, which allows the transducer time to receive returning echoes. Returning echoes strike the crystal and create mechanical vibration which in turn produces electrical energy that is transmitted to the receiver and display screen. The working principle of ultrasonography is shown schematically in **Flowchart 1**.

GAIN

Gain in decibels (db) or sensitivity setting of the instrument refers to the adjustment in the amplification of the echo signals. The higher is the gain level, the greater the ability of the instrument to display weaker echoes. Lowering the gain narrows the sound beam and thus improves both axial and lateral resolution. As the gain is lowered, only the stronger

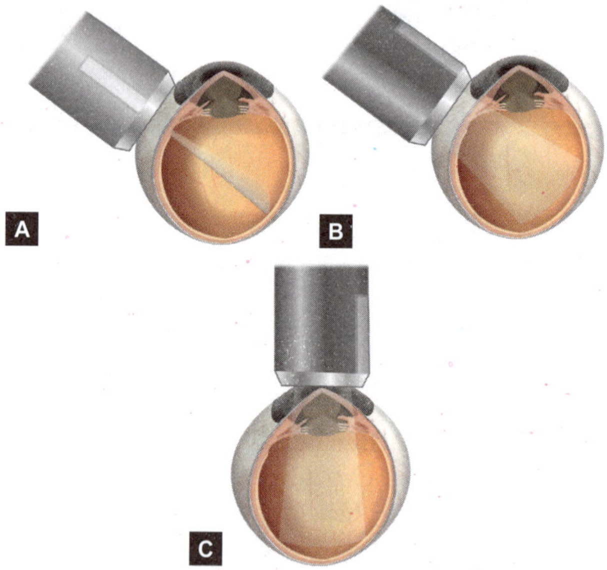

Figs. 3A to C: (A) Transverse scan; (B) Longitudinal scan; (C) Axial scan.

echoes are displayed. Time gain compensation allows greater amplification of the distant, weaker echoes than of the stronger echoes originating close to the transducer.

MODES

Ophthalmic ultrasonography commonly uses two modes of display—the A-scan and B-scan.

A-scan (amplitude modulation scan) provides one-dimensional image of vertical deflections from a base line. Spacing of the spikes is dependent on the time required for the sound beam to reach a given interface and for its echo to return to the probe.

B-scan (brightness modulation scan) provides two dimensional images of a series of dots and lines. B-scan provides the topographic information of shape, location, extension, mobility, and gross estimation of thickness of the tissue.

PROBE ORIENTATIONS

The three basic probe orientations used to evaluate intraocular lesions are: (1) transverse, (2) longitudinal, and (3) axial **(Figs. 3A to C)**.

The probe is placed on the globe opposite the area to be examined. The marker on the probe acts as the orientation point and corresponds to the upper portion of the echogram. The best detail of pathology is obtained in the central portion of the echogram.

Transverse Scan

The probe is placed on the globe so that the back and forth movement of the transducer occurs parallel to the limbus. To evaluate the superior and inferior fundus the marker is directed towards the nose (horizontal transverse), and to evaluate the nasal and temporal fundus, the marker is directed at 12 o'clock meridian (vertical transverse). Oblique transverse scans are performed with the marker directed upward **(Fig. 4)**.

Longitudinal Scan

The back and forth movement of the transducer is oriented perpendicular to the limbus **(Fig. 5)**. It defines the anteroposterior extent of a lesion. The optic disk is displayed on the lower portion of the screen. It is the best probe orientation for demonstrating the insertion of membranes into the optic disk.

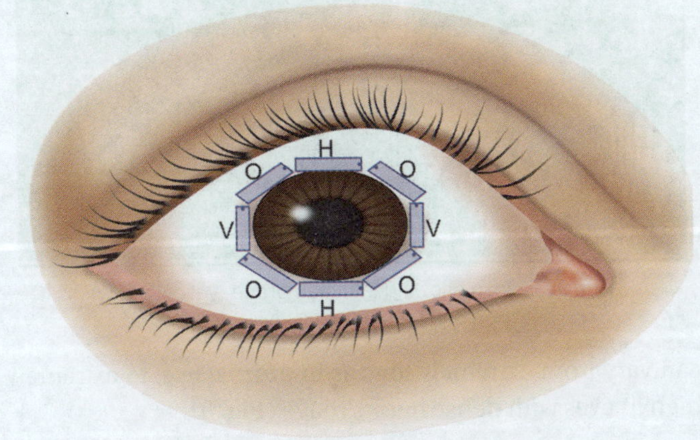

Fig. 4: Oblique transverse scans.

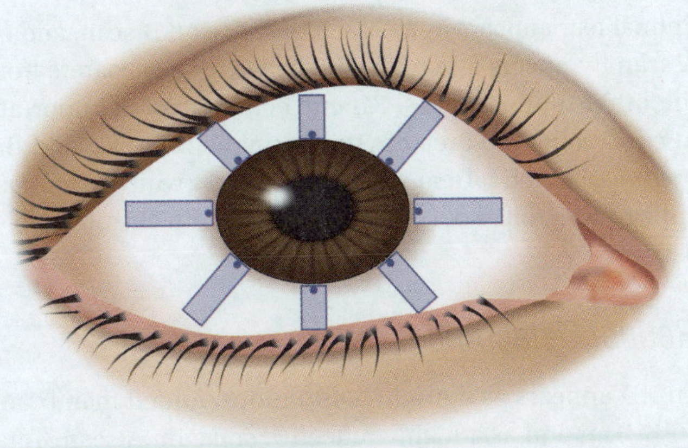

Fig. 5: Longitudinal scan.

Axial Scan

Axial scan is performed with the eye in primary gaze and the probe face is centered on the cornea. The optic nerve is displayed in the center of the echogram. It is useful for evaluating the macular region. The orientation of B-scan probe marker is shown in **Table 1**.

QUANTITATIVE ECHOGRAPHY

Quantitative echography is used to estimate reflectivity of all detected lesions. On A-scan, reflectivity is determined by estimating the height of a lesions spike from the baseline **(Table 2)**. On B-scan, the lesions signal brightness must be compared with that of either the normal highly reflective sclera or the very low reflective vitreous cavity.

KINETIC ECHOGRAPHY

Kinetic echography is used to dynamically assess the motion of or within a lesion.

- Aftermovement, indicative of mobility, is determined by observing motion of the lesion echoes following cessation of eye movement
- Vascularity (fast spontaneous motion of echoes) represents blood flow within vessels
- Convection movement (slow spontaneous movement of echoes) occurs due to convection currents of fine particles within a large cavity.

CLINICAL APPLICATION OF ULTRASOUND

Vitreous Body

Asteroid Hyalosis

Calcium soaps produce bright round signals on B-scan, and medium amplitude spikes in A-scan that move with

Table 1: Showing orientation of B-scan probe marker.

Probe position	*Direction of marker*
Transverse and axial scans	
Horizontal	Nasal
Vertical	Superior
Oblique	Superior
Longitudinal scan	Toward center of cornea and meridian being examined

Table 2: Showing height of a lesion from the baseline.

Category	*Spike height, %*
Extremely low	0–5
Low	5–40
Medium	40–60
Medium-high	60–80
High	80–100

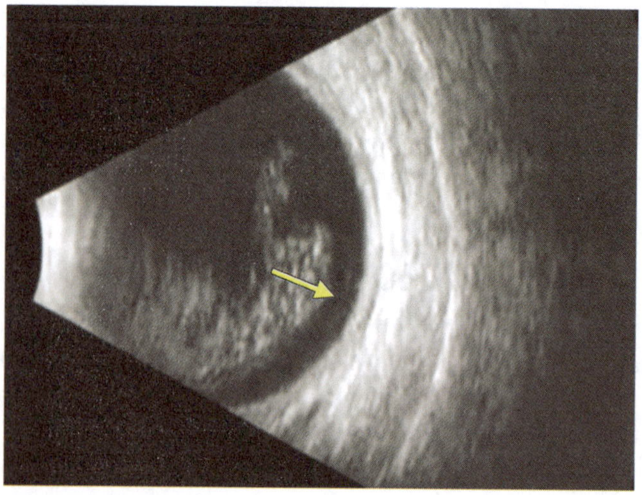

Fig. 6: Asteroid hyalosis. Dense opacities in the vitreous. Note the echolucent vitreous gel (yellow arrow) located between opacities and retina.

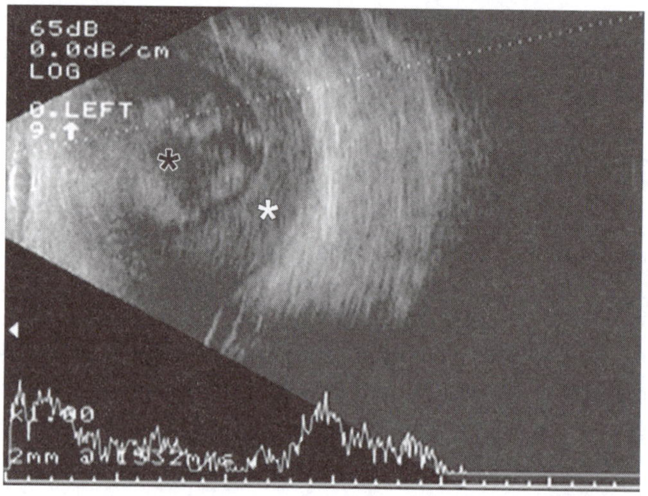

Fig. 8: Transverse B-scan showing medium reflective echoes in vitreous cavity suggestive of dense vitreous hemorrhage (black asterisk); low-to-medium reflective echoes in subvitreal space suggestive of subhyaloid hemorrhage (white asterisk).

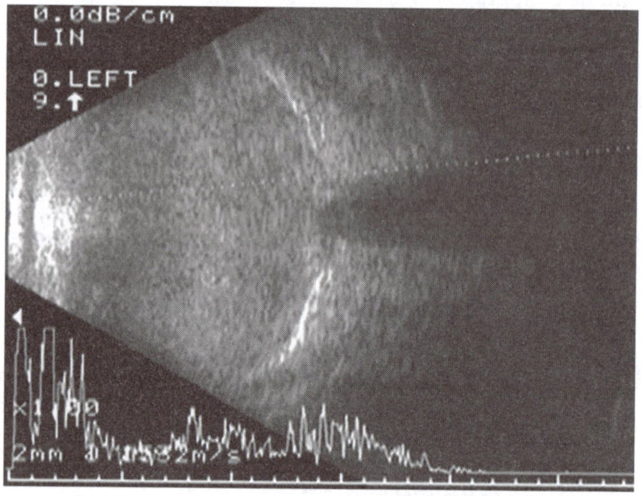

Fig. 7: Fresh vitreous hemorrhage seen as low reflective echoes in vitreous cavity.

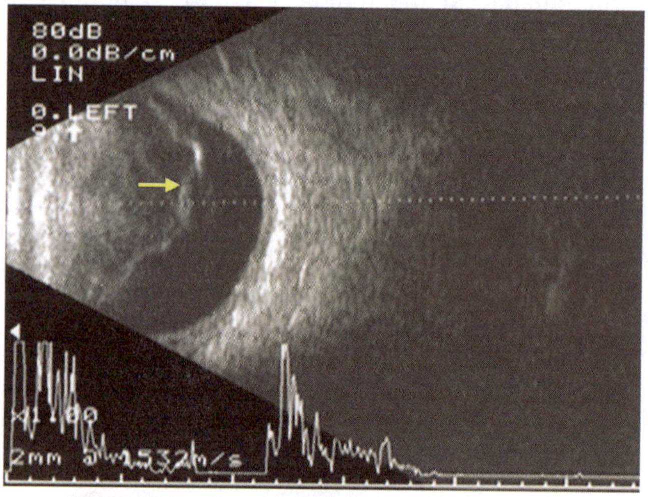

Fig. 9: B-scan showing thin membrane (yellow arrow) with medium reflectivity.

vitreous gel. An area of clear vitreous is present between the posterior boundary of the opacities and the posterior hyaloid **(Fig. 6)**.

Vitreous Hemorrhage

Fresh hemorrhage is seen as dots on B-scan, and a chain of low amplitude spikes is seen on A-scan. The more dense is the hemorrhage, the greater the number of opacities and higher the reflectivity **(Fig. 7)**. Vitreous hemorrhage can be associated with subhyaloid hemorrhage **(Fig. 8)**.

Posterior Vitreous Detachment

Posterior vitreous detachment (PVD) appears as an undulating membrane in front of the retinochoroidal layer that moves with movement of the eye. It may separate completely from the posterior pole or may remain attached to the optic disk. Kinetic echography shows undulating aftermovement of the PVD. On A-scan, the reflectivity of PVD can vary from extremely low, as in normal eye, to extremely high in eyes with dense hemorrhage **(Fig. 9)**.

Evaluation of Retina

Retinal Tear

Retinal tear appears as a breach of tissue on B-scan, and on A-scan it appears as a highly reflective tissue separate from the other fundus spikes. Kinetic echography is important in confirming the area of vitreoretinal adherence and the presence of a retinal tear. Giant retinal break with detachment appears as a rolled out tissue on B-scan with clear breach of tissue.

Retinal Detachment

An RD appears as a bright, continuous, folded membrane on B-scan and as a highly reflective spike on A-scan. Total RD is shown to insert into the optic disk posteriorly and the

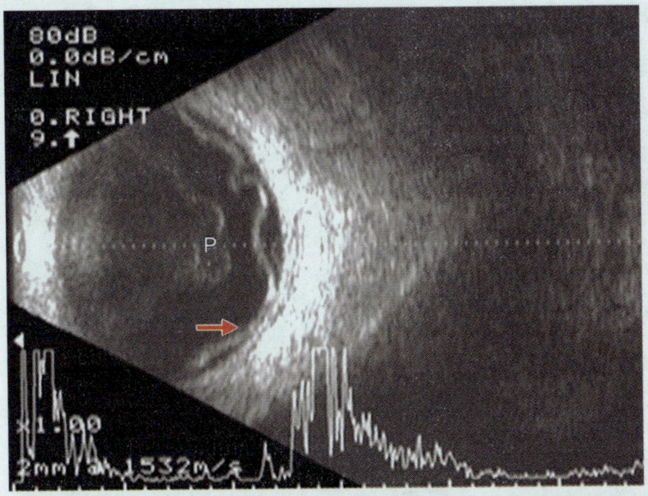

Fig. 10: B-scan echography showing low reflective posterior vitreous detachment (P) and high reflective membrane (red arrow) suggestive of retinal detachment.

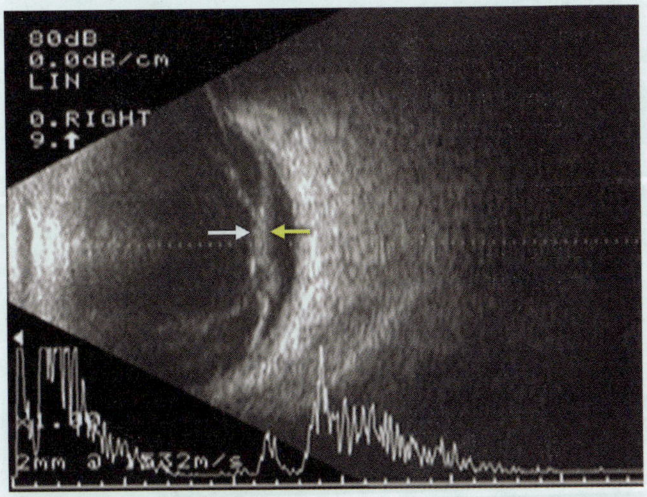

Fig. 11: Transverse B-scan echography showing posterior vitreous detachment with vitreoretinal adherence (white arrow) producing table top detachment of the retina (yellow arrow).

ora serrata peripherally. RD typically exhibits a tethered, restricted aftermovement that contrasts with the highly mobile undulating movement of PVD **(Fig. 10)**.

Detachments that are triangular or T-shaped, or that have fixed retinal folds, indicate proliferative vitreoretinopathy (PVR).

Longstanding RDs may develop retinal cysts and cholesterol crystals may accumulate in the subretinal space.

Traction retinal detachments: They have a tent-like or table-top configuration of the retina, with one or more points of traction and contraction **(Fig. 11)**. The detached retina appears to have a concave configuration, in contrast to the convex configuration of the rhegmatogenous RD.

Exudative retinal detachment: The configuration of the detachment is convex and bullous. It is usually secondary to tumors, inflammatory conditions [Vogt–Koyanagi–Harada (VKH)], or vascular disorders such as hypertensive choroidopathy, and toxemia of pregnancy. In VKH syndrome there is a diffuse choroidal thickening with low-to-medium echo reflectivity **(Figs. 12A and B)**.

Retinoschisis

More often involves the inferotemporal periphery and is usually bilateral. On B-scan, retinoschisis appears as smooth, thin, sharply demarcated, dome-shaped, and nonmobile membrane. On A-scan, 100% high, single peak spikes seen **(Fig. 13)**. After the membrane is localized with B-scan, scleral the space between the sclera and the retina flattens as the subretinal fluid is forced through the break into the vitreous cavity. Conversely, if the membrane represents retinoschisis, the space narrows but does not completely flatten.

Evaluation of Choroid

Choroid Thickening

Choroid thickening is seen in inflammatory conditions like VKH syndrome and sympathetic ophthalmia. On B-scan, the thickened choroid appears as an echolucent band, with low-to-medium reflectivity on A-scan.

Choroid Detachment

On B-scan a choroidal detachment appears as a smooth, dome-shaped, and thick membranous structure that does not insert to the optic nerve. The choroidal detachment can be localized, or involve the entire fundus (*kissing choroids*). On A-scan the thickened choroid appears as a series of high reflective spikes just behind the retinal spike. The detached choroid produces a 100% reflective, double-peaked spike (retina and choroid together). The kinetic evaluation shows little or no aftermovement with either A-scan or B-scan. The B-scan also can demonstrate the nature of suprachoroidal fluid; in serous detachment, the suprachoroidal space is echolucent, and in hemorrhagic detachment, the suprachoroidal space is echodense **(Fig. 14)**.

Evaluation in Ocular Trauma

Dislocated Lens

Dislocated lens appears as a round or oval globular structure in the posterior vitreous, and strands of vitreous might be attached to the dislocated lens **(Fig. 15)**.

Dislocated Intraocular Lens

A posteriorly dislocated intraocular lens (IOL) appears as a large, foreign body-like structure within vitreous cavity **(Fig. 16)**.

Posterior Scleral Rupture

On ultrasound, the sclera in the area of the rupture shows irregular contour, thickening and decreased reflectivity.

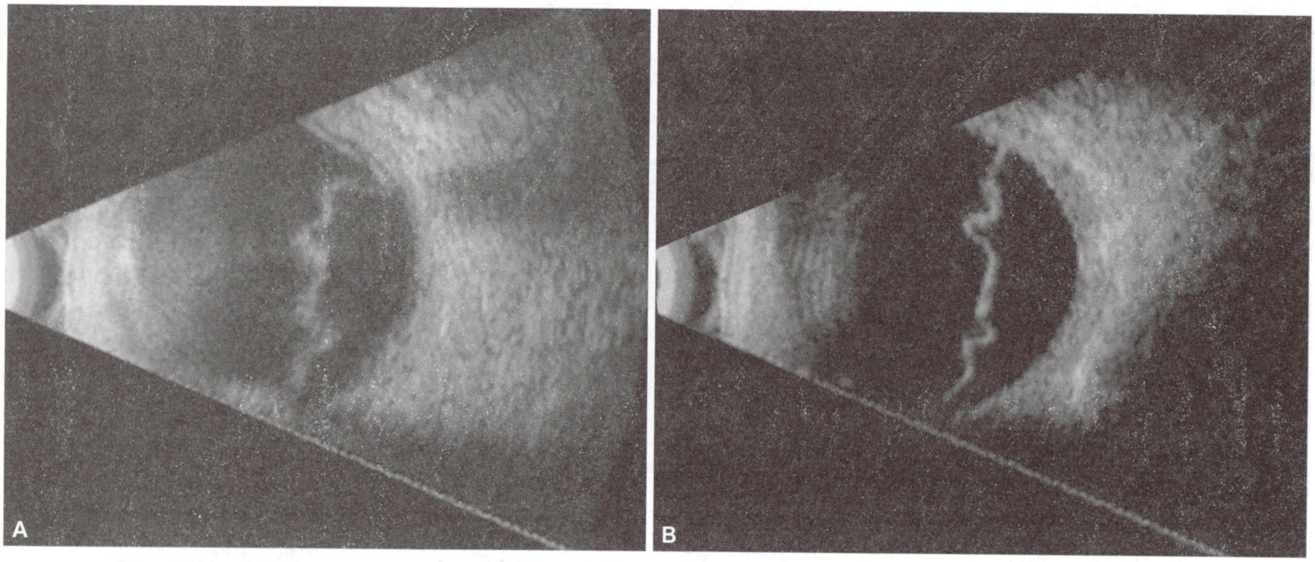

Figs. 12A and B: B-scan echography showing shifting of fluid between sitting (A) and supine (B) postures suggestive of exudative retinal detachment.

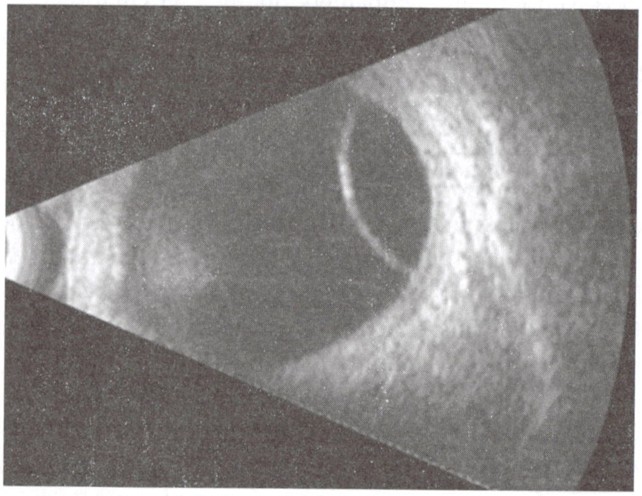

Fig. 13: Transverse B-scan echogram shows moderately elevated, thin, smooth, and dome-shaped membrane suggestive of retinoschisis.

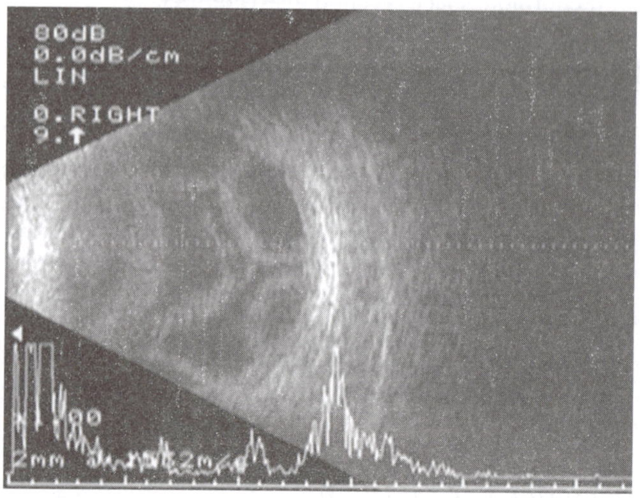

Fig. 14: Transverse B-scan echogram shows 360° bullous choroid detachment.

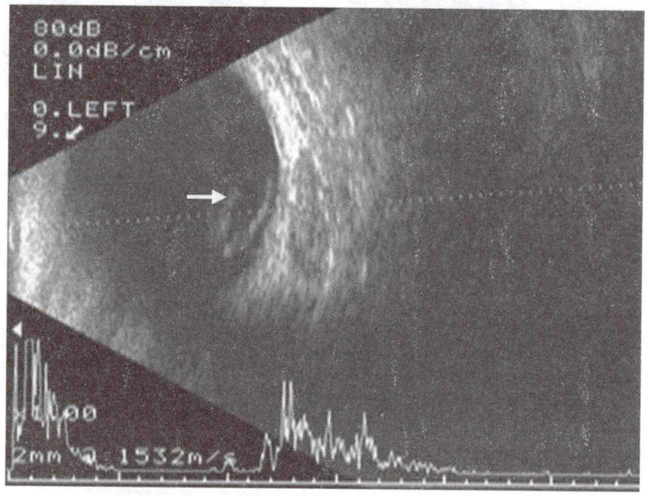

Fig. 15: Transverse B-scan echogram shows oval-shaped lens (white arrow) on surface of retina.

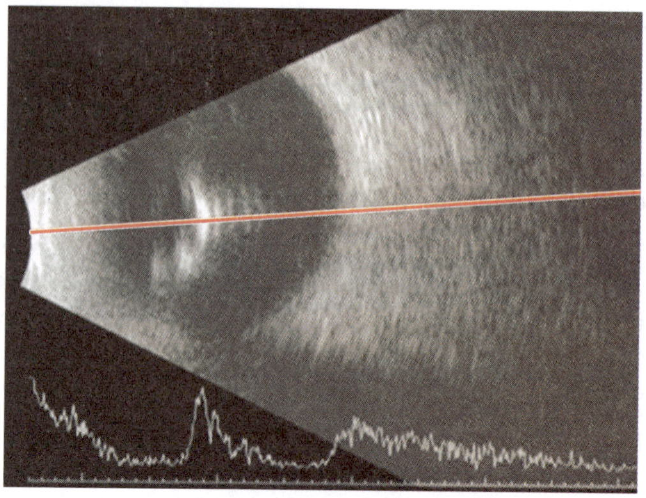

Fig. 16: Transverse B-scan shows echodense dislocated intraocular lens in mid-vitreous with reverberations posteriorly.

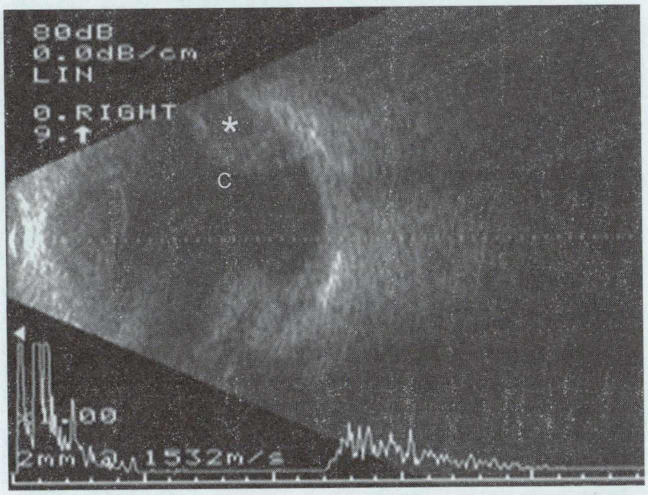

Fig. 17: B-scan echogram shows smooth convex appearance of choroid detachment (C) and opacities in suprachoroidal space (white asterisk).

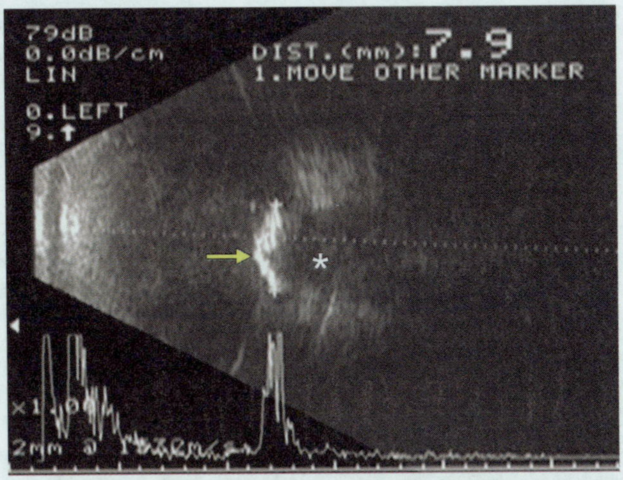

Fig. 18: B-scan echogram shows foreign body (yellow arrow) close to the surface of retina with shadowing (white asterisk); A-scan shows high reflective spike from foreign body.

Other features include: (1) vitreous incarceration associated with vitreous hemorrhage and PVD; (2) thickening or detachment of surrounding retina and/or choroid; and (3) hemorrhage in immediate episcleral space.

Avulsion of Optic Nerve

A B-scan may show a break in the sclera near the optic disk. In longstanding cases, there may be proliferative tissue at the optic disk.

Hemorrhagic Choroid Detachment

It is more common following a posterior scleral rupture. Traumatic hemorrhagic choroidal detachment may be localized or extensive reaching the edge of the optic disk **(Fig. 17)**.

Intraocular Foreign Body

- *Metallic foreign body*: It gives very echodense signal even at low gain, with marked shadowing of the ocular and orbital structures posterior to the foreign body. Metallic foreign body shows very high reflectivity on A-scan, regardless of the sound beam direction **(Fig. 18)**.
- *Glass foreign body*: When the sound beam strikes the long, smooth surface of a glass sliver in an oblique direction, most of the sound is reflected away from the probe, resulting in a weak echo. Only when the sound beam is directed perpendicular to the flat surface of the glass piece is a very echodense signal displayed that accurately indicates the presence of a foreign body. Small foreign bodies (<0.5 mm in diameter or thin wire) may not produce obvious shadowing even though they can be quiet echodense.

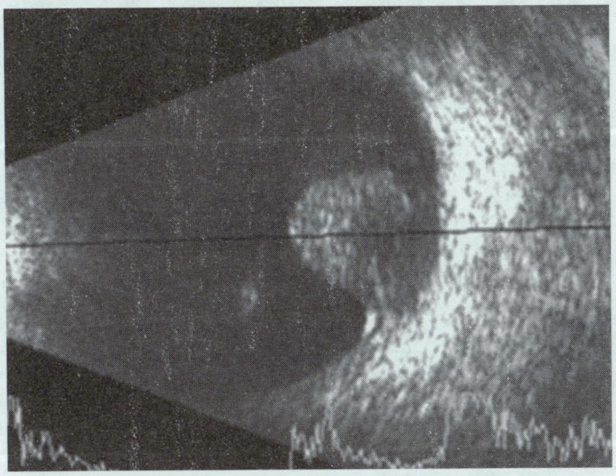

Fig. 19: Transverse B-scan shows typical collar button configuration; A-scan showing low-to-medium reflectivity that is typical of choroid melanoma.

INTRAOCULAR TUMORS

Ocular Melanoma

The cardinal features include: (1) solid consistency, (2) collar button (mushroom) shape, (3) low-to-medium internal reflectivity, (4) regular internal structure, and (5) internal blood flow vascularity. The collar button shape indicates that the tumor has broken through the Bruch's membrane. The cellular, homogenous histologic architecture of the tumor demonstrates regular medium internal reflectivity **(Fig. 19)**. Very large melanomas that contain hemorrhage and necrosis may exhibit atypical features like irregular and high internal reflectivity.

Choroid Metastasis

Metastatic carcinomas are mild to moderately elevated tumors with irregular, bumpy surface contour, and

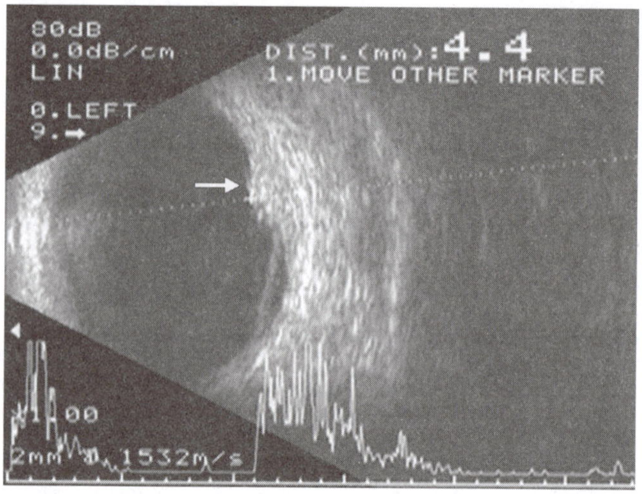

Fig. 20: Transverse B-scan shows dome-shaped lesion (white arrow); A-scan shows regular internal structure and high reflectivity typical of choroid hemangioma.

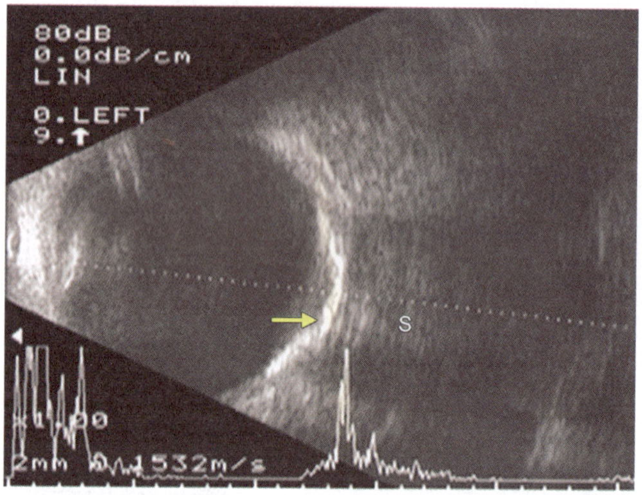

Fig. 21: Transverse B-scan shows irregular echodense plaque (yellow arrow) at level of retinochoroid layer and sclera (S) shadowing produced by calcification.

central excavation. They have an irregular internal structure and high internal reflectivity.

Choroid Hemangioma

They appear as dome-shaped lesions with high-internal reflectivity and regular internal structure **(Fig. 20)**. The high reflectivity is because of large interfaces formed by the vessel surfaces. By reducing the gain, the vascularity of the tumor can be better appreciated.

Choroidal Osteoma

A B-scan exhibits flat to mildly elevated lesions with extremely high reflectivity and marked shadowing of the orbital tissues posterior to the lesion **(Fig. 21)**.

Retinoblastoma

Echographically, retinoblastomas have a smooth and dome shape with irregular configuration. The internal reflectivity

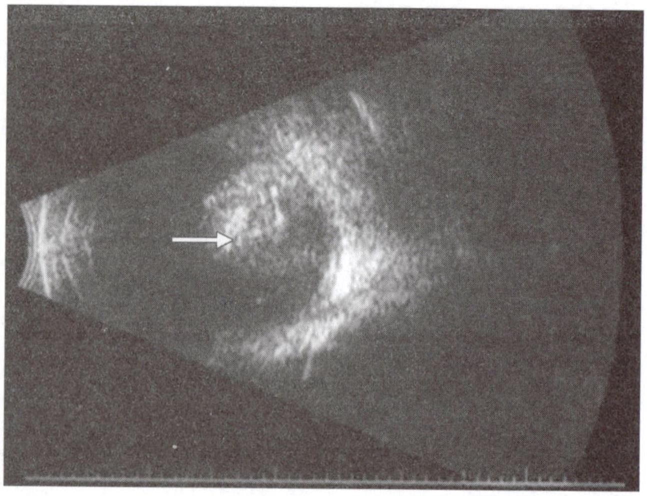

Fig. 22: B-scan echogram shows large bright mass within vitreous cavity showing multiple bright echoes (white arrow) corresponding to calcium within the lesion.

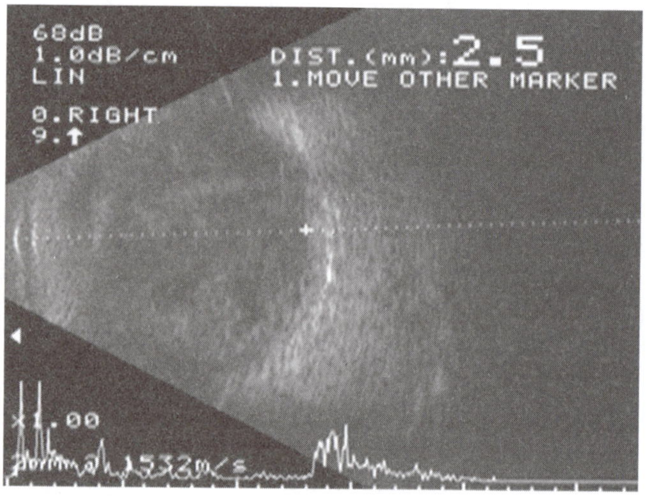

Fig. 23: Transverse B-scan shows low reflective spikes from within the vitreous cavity.

varies according to the degree of calcification within the lesion **(Fig. 22)**. Noncalcified tumors demonstrate low-to-medium reflectivity whereas calcium produces extremely high reflectivity. The axial length of the eye may be normal or increased in case the tumor invades the ocular wall. The increased is thus an important point in differentiating retinoblastoma from other conditions causing leukocoria.

INFLAMMATORY DISEASES OF THE EYE

Endophthalmitis

Ultrasonography of the eye with endophthalmitis depends on the degree and severity of infection and the extent of vitreous involvement. Generally opacities are noted, and membrane formation becomes apparent in severe cases. Choroidal thickening, choroidal detachment, RD, and retained IOFB are possible associated findings **(Fig. 23)**.

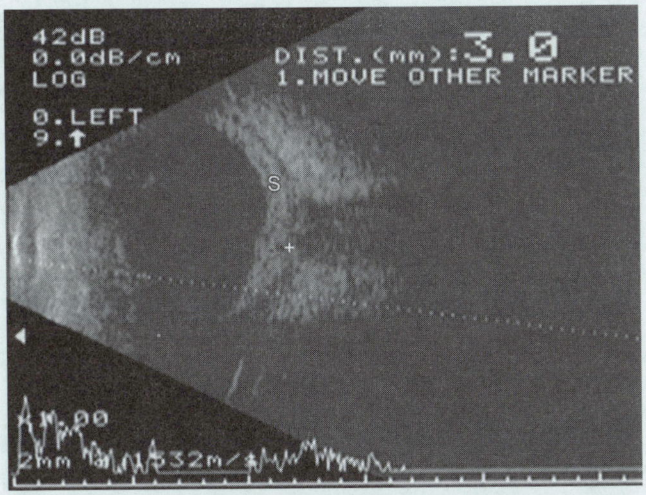

Fig. 24: Axial B-scan echogram shows diffuse thickening of retinochoroid layer and sclera (S); and edema of sub-Tenon's space (+).

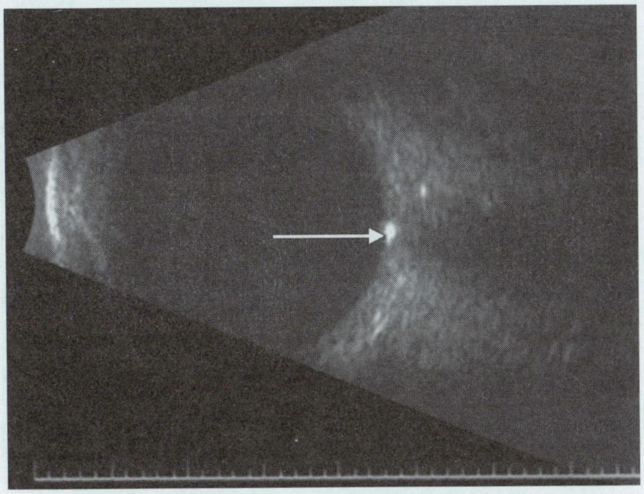

Fig. 26: Echogram shows elevated optic disk with calcification suggestive of drusen (white arrow).

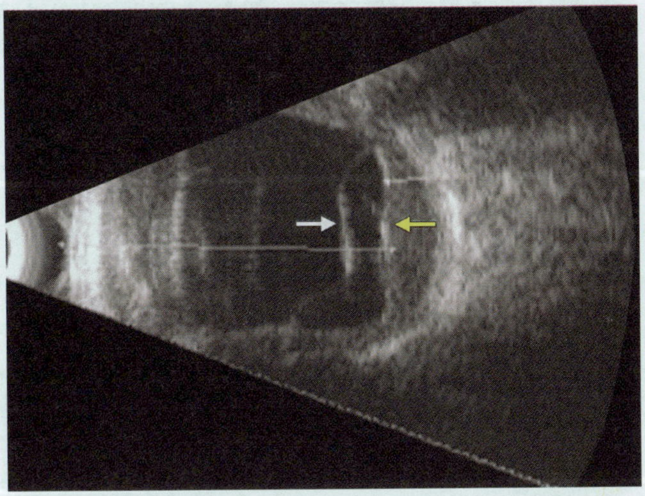

Fig. 25: Echogram displays diffuse thickening of choroid (yellow arrow) and shallow serous retinal detachment (white arrow).

Posterior Scleritis

The most important ultrasound feature is thickening of the sclera. The thickened sclera is usually highly reflective, with regular internal structure. In most cases there is an associated inflammatory reaction in the episcleral region, resulting in swelling of sub-Tenon's space. This fluid is the classically described "T-sign" on B-scan **(Fig. 24)**.

Vogt–Koyanagi–Harada Syndrome

Echography shows diffuse, low-to-medium reflective thickening of the choroid. The thickening is more pronounced in the peripapillary region. Other echographic features include serous RD, mild vitreous opacities, and thickening of sclera and/or episclera **(Fig. 25)**.

Sympathetic Ophthalmia

The clinical and echographic features for sympathetic ophthalmia resemble that of VKH. However, sympathetic ophthalmia occurs almost exclusively following penetrating ocular trauma or previous ocular surgery.

STRUCTURAL ANOMALIES OF EYE

Phthisis Bulbi

In phthisis bulbi the globe is smaller than normal with multiple echogenic vitreous opacities, choroidal thickening, and calcification of ocular coats, with resultant absence of high reflective orbital echo-spikes due to shadowing.

Atrophic Bulbi

Atrophic bulbi is characterized by a normal globe contour, and hence a normal axial length on A-scan with calcification of ocular coats.

Optic Disk Drusen

Optic nerve drusen are calcified nodules seen echographically to produce an echo of extremely high reflectivity at or within the optic nerve head **(Fig. 26)**. They are best seen with transverse and longitudinal B-scan approaches, which bypass the lens and demonstrate the calcified nodules better than the axial approach.

Posterior Staphyloma

Posterior staphyloma is seen as a shallow excavation of the posterior pole with smooth edges on sonographic evaluation of highly myopic eyes.

Choroidal Coloboma

Choroidal coloboma is seen as an excavation, usually involving the posterior pole **(Fig. 27)**; but in contrast to posterior staphyloma, its edges are sharp. Associated findings include microphthalmos and RD.

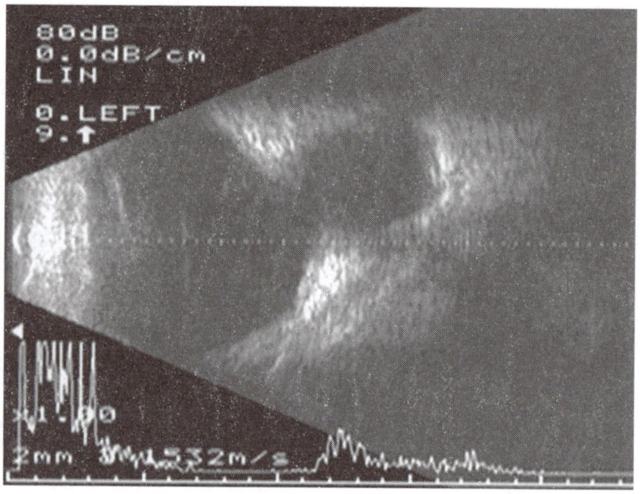

Fig. 27: Echogram showing deep excavation at posterior pole suggestive of coloboma.

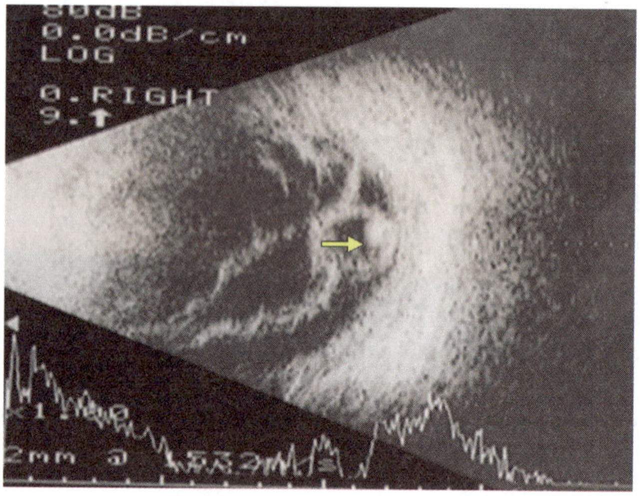

Fig. 28: Transverse B-scan shows subretinal cyst containing dense nodule (yellow arrow) corresponding to scolex of the organism.

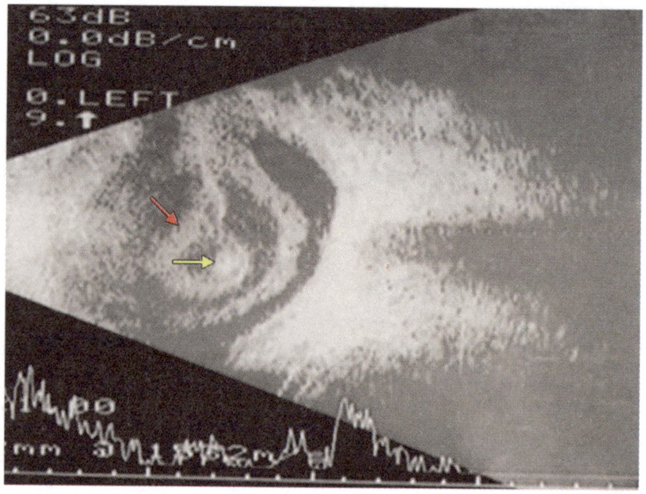

Fig. 29: Echogram showing cyst in vitreous cavity (red arrow) containing dense nodule (yellow arrow) suggestive of scolex.

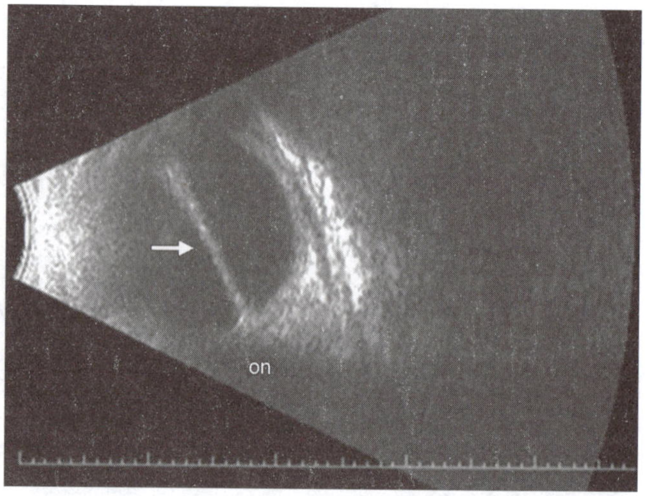

Fig. 30: Longitudinal B-scan shows thick echodense band (white arrow) extending from anterior aspect of eye to the optic nerve (on).

MISCELLANEOUS

Cysticercosis

Echography shows one or more well-outlined, oval-shaped cysts located in the subretinal space **(Fig. 28)** or vitreous cavity **(Fig. 29)**. The scolex of the parasite appears as a high reflective echodense nodule attached to the inner wall of the cyst.

Persistent Hyperplastic Primary Vitreous

In persistent hyperplastic primary vitreous (PHPV), a vitreous band (persistent hyaloid vessel) may be seen extending from the posterior lens capsule to the optic disk **(Fig. 30)**.

Nanophthalmos

Nanophthalmos is characterized by reduced axial length and a thickened posterior retino-choroido-scleral complex **(Fig. 31)**.

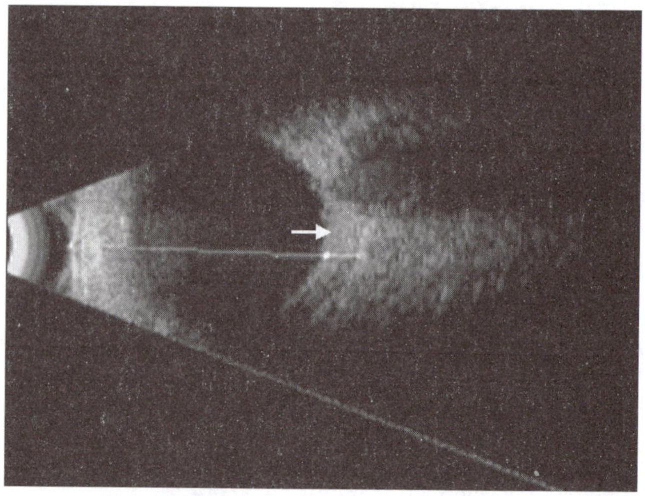

Fig. 31: Axial B-scan shows thickening of posterior retinochoroid layer and sclera (white arrow); axial length of the eye is 15.82 mm.

CONCLUSION

A B-scan ultrasonography plays an important role in the diagnosis of various intraocular and orbital diseases, especially when direct visualization of intraocular structures is not possible. Although it is an adjuvant to clinical assessment still the clinician may not be able to diagnose some of the ocular diseases without the help of this tool. The technique requires training, skill, and experience for proper interpretation of images.

SUGGESTED READING

1. AIOS (2011). Diagnostic Ultrasonography of the Eye: AIOS, CME series No. 24. [online] Available from: https://www.aios.org/cme/cmeseries24.pdf [Last accessed on November, 2019].
2. Byrne SF, Green RL. Ultrasound of the Eye and Orbit. St. Louis: Mosby; 2002.
3. Das T, Namperumalsamy P. Ocular ultrasound in preoperative evaluation of posterior segment of the eye. Indian J Ophthalmol. 1983;31:1022-4.
4. Das T, Vedantham V, Hussain A, et al. B-scan Ultrasonography. In: Nema HV, Nema N (Eds). Diagnostic Procedures in Ophthalmology, 3rd edition. New Delhi: Jaypee Brothers Medical Publishers; 2014.
5. DiBernardo CW, Greenberg EF. Ophthalmic ultrasound: a diagnostic atlas, 2nd edition. Germany: Thieme Medical Publishers; 2011.
6. Solarte CE, Shaikh A. Ultrasound techniques in ophthalmology. In: James B, Benjamin L (Eds). Ophthalmology Investigation and Examination techniques. Amsterdam, Netherlands: Elsevier; 2007.

CHAPTER

19 Ultrasound Biomicroscopy of the Eye

Sushmita Kaushik, Savleen Kaur

INTRODUCTION

Ultrasound biomicroscopy (UBM) dominated the field of anterior segment imaging after its introduction by Pavlin in 1991. It uses sound waves with a frequency (50–100 MHz) higher than conventional ultrasound (5–20 MHz). The use of a higher frequency transducer allows for a more detailed assessment of the anterior ocular structures than was available using conventional ultrasound. The standard UBM operating at 50 MHz has a depth of penetration about 4–5 mm only but provides lateral and axial physical resolutions of approximately 50 μm and 25 μm, respectively.

Ultrasound biomicroscopy provides an in vivo assessment of the anterior segment structures in a noninvasive manner. It can image through opaque media and even visualize the ciliary body or structures behind the iris, effectively, which may be beyond the scope of anterior segment optical coherence tomography (AS-OCT). Additionally, it provides qualitative and quantitative assessment of the pathophysiological changes involving anterior segment architecture.

APPARATUS

The transducer is the most important component converting the electric current to ultrasonic sound waves, which are transmitted to the ocular structures. It is housed in a handheld probe. The central processing unit processes the radio waves.

Scanning is usually performed in the supine position. A plastic eyecup of the appropriate size is inserted between the lids. The cup is filled with normal saline/methylcellulose as coupling medium. Recent generations of the UBM have balloon-like disposable probe covers, which contain distilled water that serves as a coupling medium between a UBM probe and the eye. It is much more convenient, comfortable and facilitates imaging even in the supine position.

SCOPE OF ULTRASOUND BIOMICROSCOPY

The UBM offers a real-time imaging of the anterior segment. While the OCT's light source is optimized for scanning the posterior segment and is now upgraded to image the anterior segment as well, only the surface of the iris can be visualized by the OCT. Thus the UBM is the solitary tool for scanning the structures behind the iris. The major drawback of the UBM is that it is a contact method which limits its use in open globe injuries or perforating corneal ulcers. It also requires a highly skilled operator with sufficient expertise to interpret the scans. The 50 MHz probes provide good resolution on UBM and better than the lower frequency probes. Higher frequency transducers provide finer resolution of more superficial structures, whereas lower frequency transducers provide greater depth of penetration with less resolution.

METHODOLOGY

The procedure can be carried out in an outpatient clinic under topical anesthesia. The white line on the side of the probe body indicates the direction of the linear movement of the transducer.

Types of Scans

Radial/Longitudinal Scan

Ultrasound biomicroscopy transducer is held over the area to be scanned and moved to and fro across the limbus, with the oscillations perpendicular to the limbus at the specific clock hour to be examined. It images the angle quite effectively. We have to ask the patient to look to the opposite side to image an angle.

Transverse Scan

The probe is held at 90° to a radial line at the limbus. It takes the cross section of the ciliary body when it is placed over it.

Sulcus-to-Sulcus Scan (Axial)

It scans two 180° opposite angles simultaneously if the patient is cooperative.

Imaging of Eye

The normal anterior segment can be imaged very well with the UBM. It has become an indispensable tool in qualitative and quantitative assessment of the anterior segment. On imaging the normal eye, cornea is a multilayered structure. Going from anterior to posterior, the first echogenic line structure is the corneal epithelium (a); The next is the Bowman's membrane (b); The stroma is minimally echogenic (c); and is then followed by another echogenic structure—the Descemet's membrane (d) **(Fig. 1)**.

The normal angle is seen as the junction between the cornea and sclera where the iris root inserts into the ciliary body **(Fig. 2)**. The junction between the relatively echolucent cornea and the highly reflective sclera marks the anterior Schwalbe's line (a); The anterior-most part of the junction between the sclera and the ciliary body band is the scleral spur (b). Identification of the scleral spur is critical to angle assessment using the UBM. The scleral spur is the only constant landmark allowing one to interpret UBM images in terms of the morphologic status of the anterior chamber angle and is the key for analyzing angle pathology. The area between the scleral spur and the anterior Schwalbe's line is the region identified as the trabecular meshwork (c) on the UBM.

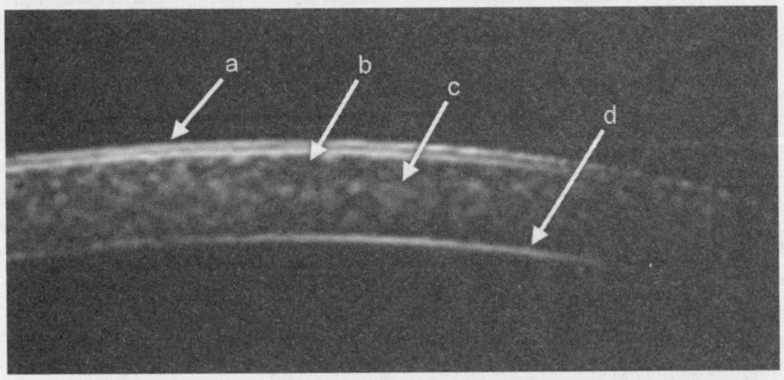

Fig. 1: Normal corneal epithelium as seen on ultrasound biomicroscopy.

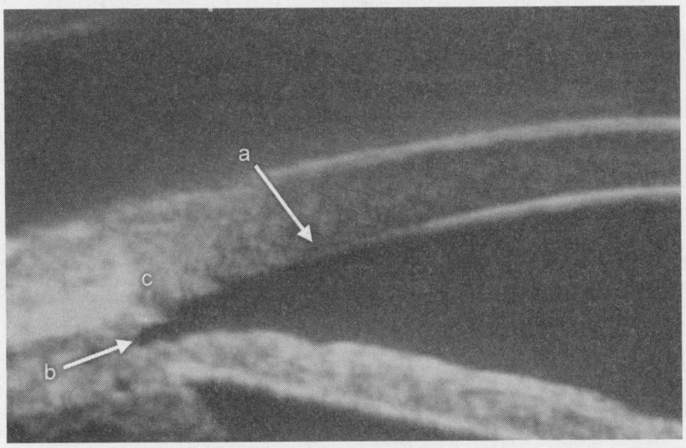

Fig. 2: Representative picture of the normal angle as seen on ultrasound biomicroscopy.

Generally, in the normal eye, the iris has a roughly planar configuration with slight anterior bowing, and the anterior chamber angle is wide and clear. However, since morphology of the anterior segment structures alter in response to a variety of physiologic stimuli such as accommodation and lighting, it is important to maintain a constant testing environment for longitudinal comparison. The normal depth of the anterior chamber is 2.5–3.0 mm **(Fig. 3)**.

The ciliary body is best visualized using the radial scan **(Fig. 4)**. It can be imaged for 360°. The ciliary processes may show a variable configuration and can be best seen with the transverse scan.

The area between the peripheral iris and above the ciliary processes is the ciliary sulcus. The zonules can be seen as a medium reflective line between the ciliary processes and the lens surface.

ULTRASOUND BIOMICROSCOPY IN GLAUCOMA

Quantifying the Angle

It is possible to use the UBM to quantify the width of the angle. Pavlin et al. established various quantitative measurement parameters as standards **(Fig. 5)**. The position of the scleral spur is used as a reference point for most of their parameters because this is the only landmark that can be distinguished consistently in the anterior chamber angle region.

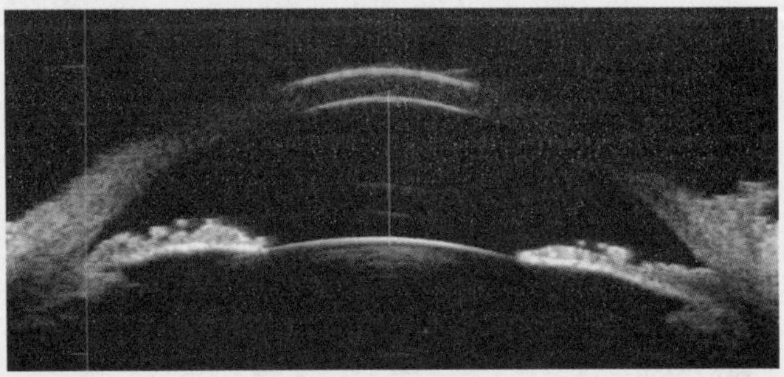

Fig. 3: A sulcus-to-sulcus scan on the ultrasound biomicroscopy depicting opposite angles with normal iris configuration and anterior chamber depth.

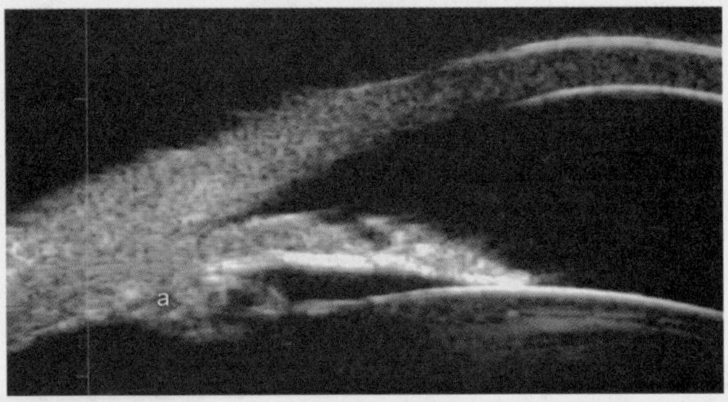

Fig. 4: Normal ciliary body visualized on the radial scan.

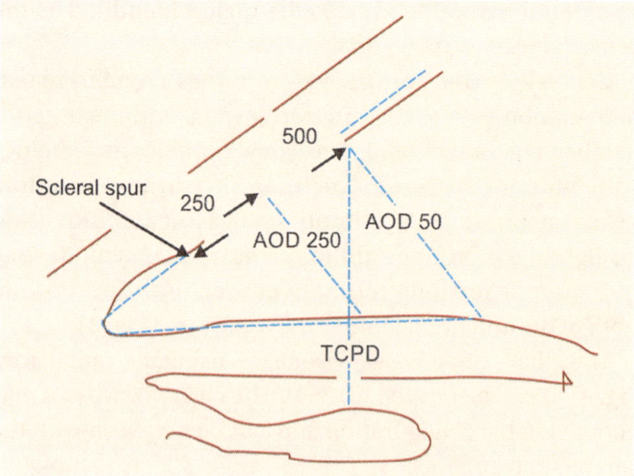

Fig. 5: Quantifying the angle on ultrasound biomicroscopy. (AOD: angle-opening-distance; TCPD: trabecular-ciliary process distance)

- The angle-opening-distance (AOD) is defined as the distance from the corneal endothelium to the anterior iris, perpendicular to a line drawn along the trabecular meshwork (TM), at a given distance from the scleral spur. This is measured at 250 μ (AOD 250), which consistently falls on the trabecular meshwork and 500 μ (AOD 500) from the scleral spur, which measures the angle opening anterior to the trabecular meshwork. The AOD reflects the amount of relative pupillary block in patients with occludable angles. The AOD 250 is a measure of the angle opening at the level of the posterior trabecular meshwork. AOD 500 is a measure of the angle opening at the level of the anterior Schwalbe's line.
- The trabecular-ciliary process distance (TCPD) is measured from a point on the trabecular meshwork, 500 μ anterior to the scleral spur, extended perpendicularly through the iris to the ciliary process. The TCPD defines the port through which the iris must traverse and has implications as to the potential maximal angle opening, and defines the space available between the trabecular meshwork and ciliary process. It is a typical feature in an individual eye. It is the sum of three segments—the angle opening 500 μ from the scleral spur, the thickness of the iris at that point, and the width of the ciliary sulcus. An anteriorly placed ciliary process can reduce the peripheral anterior chamber depth and make it susceptible to occlusion.

In a comparative study between UBM and gonioscopy, excellent correlation was found between gonioscopically quantified angles and those quantified by the UBM. There is actually no role of the UBM in quantifying the angle for diagnosing angle closure, but it is of immense help in qualifying the cause of a narrow angle.

Pupillary Block Glaucoma

Relative pupillary block with aqueous pooling behind the iris can be easily recognized on the UBM. Laser iridotomy is the treatment of choice and adequacy of treatment can be confirmed easily by UBM **(Figs. 6A and B)**.

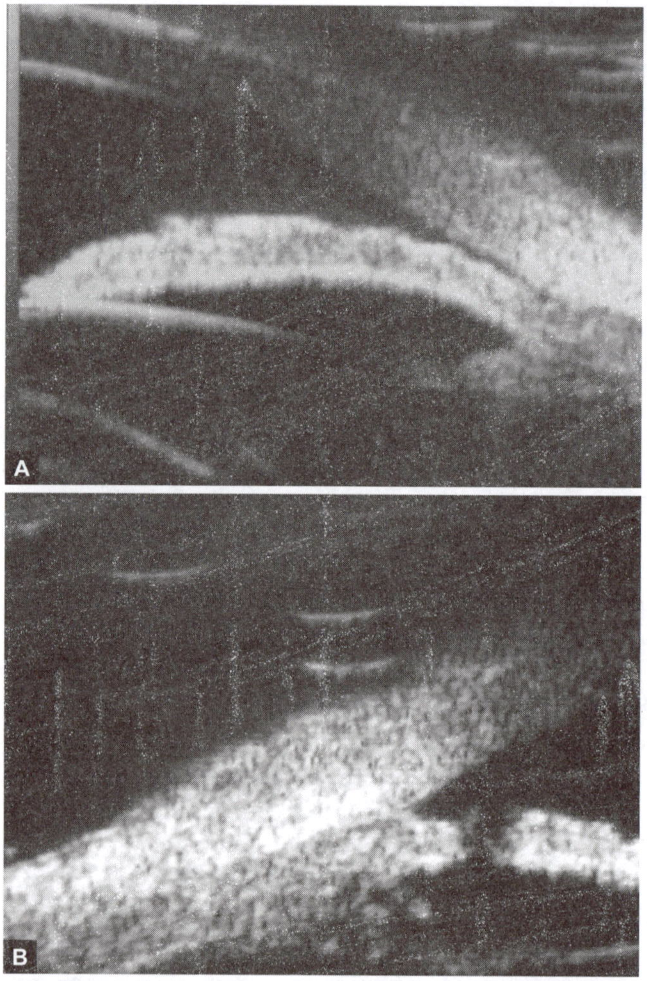

Figs. 6A and B: (A) Pupillary block angle closure; (B) Pupillary block angle closure with laser.

Iris Configuration

Plateau Iris

Often difficult to diagnose clinically, the typical gonioscopic features include a comparatively flat iris plane compared to an obvious convexity in pupillary block, and a sharp drop-off of the iris in the periphery. It is suspected when there is a persistency of symptoms or raised pressure despite a successful iridotomy. This entity can be beautifully diagnosed by UBM **(Figs. 7A to C)**.

In these cases, appropriate treatment is a laser peripheral iridoplasty. The UBM can show adequacy of treatment by demonstrating that the peripheral iris has been pulled away from the trabecular meshwork by the laser contraction burns.

Juvenile Open Angle Glaucoma

Ultrasound biomicroscopy can confirm the high insertion in juvenile open angle glaucoma **(Figs. 8A and B)**.

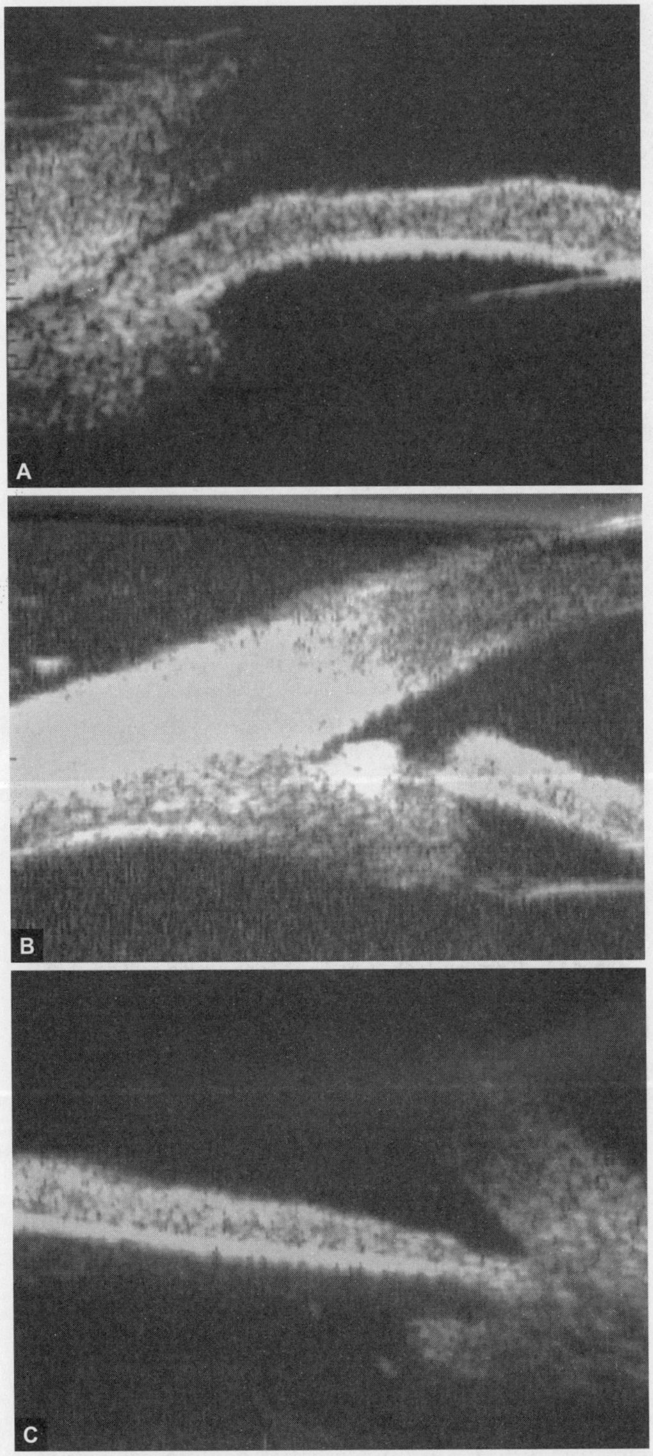

Figs. 7A to C: (A) Plateau iris with prominent ciliary process; (B) Plateau iris with patent but ineffective iridotomy; (C) Plateau after laser iridoplasty. Note the peripheral contraction burns.

Iris Cysts

Ultrasound biomicroscopy can identify cystic lesions of the iris and ciliary body which are not detected on slit-lamp examination. Well defined cysts with highly reflective wall and clear fluid are indicative of primary neuroepithelial cysts. These can be unifocal or multifocal **(Fig. 9)**. If these are present in iris midzone, in radial sections, they usually appear ovoid. If the pupil is dilated, they may be seen extending into the pupillary margin. In case they are iridociliary sulcus in origin, they are seen as spherical in shape. Elevation of the peripheral iris without iris involvement makes the diagnosis of an iridociliary cyst. If larger in size, they can often cause localized angle closure due to anterior bowing of the peripheral iris. In case of multifocal cysts, they can be seen in varying sizes in tangential sections also. The primary cysts are most commonly found in the horizontal meridians.

Sometimes we can find unilateral and unifocal cysts with thick walls and turbid intracavitary fluid. The walls are not as reflective as in primary cysts and the fluid turbidity can range from limited particles to prominent echoes. These are indicated of secondary implantation cysts. Secondary cysts can also be located adjacent to a tumor mass. Well defined spaces within a solid lesion indicate intratumoral cavitation. Ciliary body cysts are often missed on gonioscopy or slit-lamp examination but can be easily seen on UBM **(Fig. 10)**.

Pigmentary Glaucoma

In pigmentary glaucoma, the iris rubs against the ciliary processes and zonules resulting in pigment dispersion all over the anterior segment including the anterior lens surface, corneal endothelium and trabecular meshwork and a reverse pupillary block **(Figs. 11 and 12A)**. With time, this pigment clogs the trabecular meshwork and causes raised pressures and eventually optic nerve head damage. Laser peripheral iridotomy serves to reverse this pathology and the iris flattens, thus relieving the reverse pupillary block **(Fig. 12B)**.

Foreign Body in Iris

Ultrasound biomicroscopy is the key imaging modality for detecting occult foreign bodies in the angle and rest of the anterior chamber **(Figs. 13A and B)**.

Iridocorneal Endothelial Syndrome

This group is characterized by a membrane which grows on to the iris from the corneal endothelium, hence its name. The characteristic features include broad-based peripheral anterior synechiae, but the angle underlying is normal **(Figs. 14 and 15)**.

Bleb Morphology

After trabeculectomy surgery, bleb morphology can also be assessed on the UBM. Ultrasound biomicroscopy characterization of failed blebs appears to help in predicting the outcome of needle revision. In blebs where scleral route is obstructed, it may be better to plan a full bleb revision rather than needling alone. Ultrasound biomicroscopy may

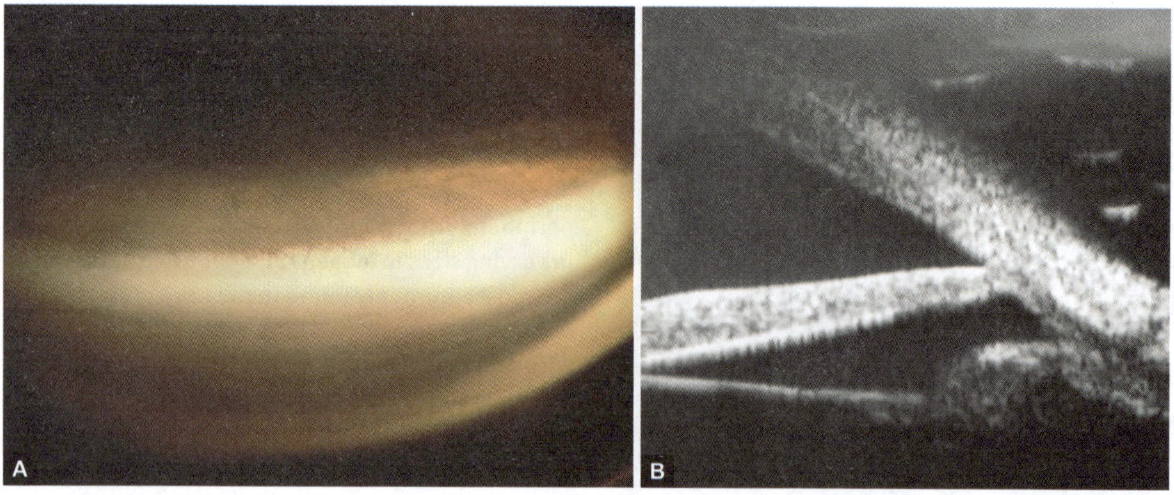

Figs. 8A and B: Gonioscopy picture with elongated iris processes and corresponding ultrasound biomicroscopy confirming the high iris insertion in JOAG.
(JOAG: juvenile open angle glaucoma)

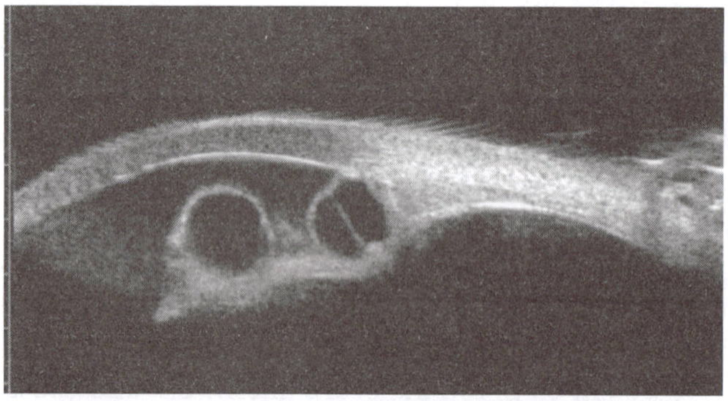

Fig. 9: Multifocal iris cysts causing secondary angle closure.

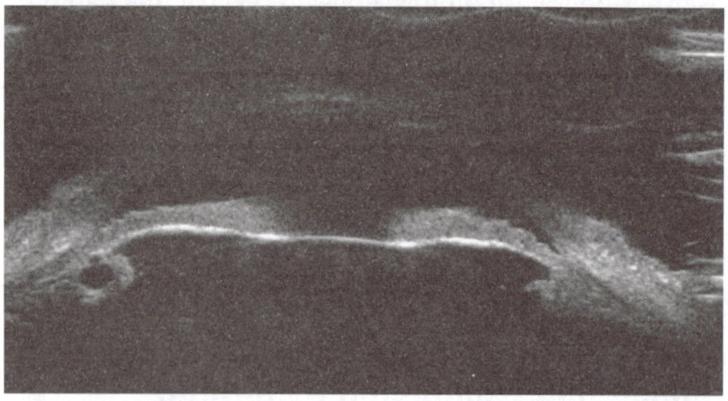

Fig. 10: Ciliary body cyst localized on ultrasound biomicroscopy which is often missed on gonioscopy.

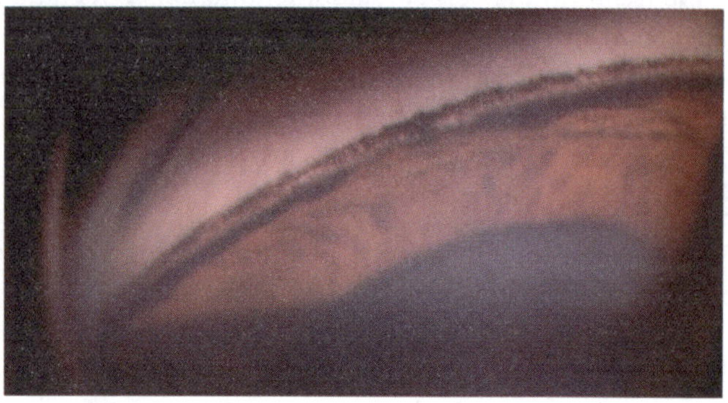

Fig. 11: Gonioscopy picture of a patient with pigment dispersion in angles.

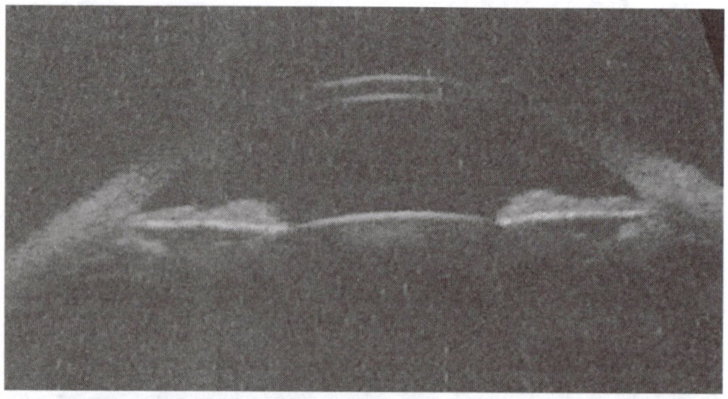

Fig. 12A: Pigmentary glaucoma with concave iris configuration.

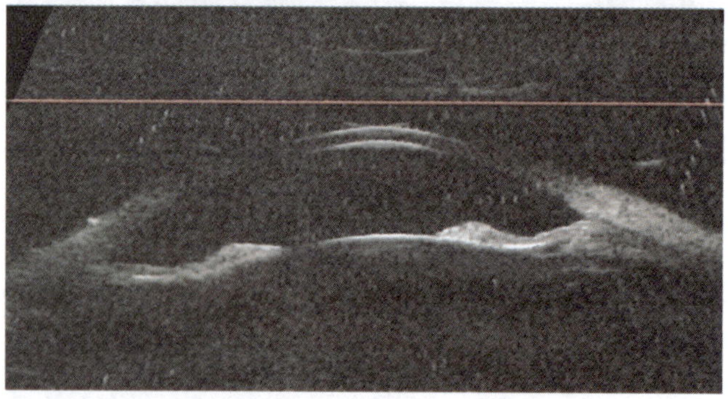

Fig. 12B: Pigmentary glaucoma after laser peripheral iridotomy. Note the flattened iris and resolution of reverse pupillary block.

help in avoiding an unnecessary needling procedure in blebs where it is likely to fail and detect aqueous flow under the scleral flap to plan needling **(Figs. 16A and B)**.

ULTRASOUND BIOMICROSCOPY IN STRABISMUS

Pavlin and Foster in 1995 first reported the use of UBM in detecting extraocular muscle (EOM) insertions. UBM can be used for localizing horizontal as well as vertical muscles as well as quantitatively measure the insertion from the limbus. The distance of EOM from the limbus is the major factor in

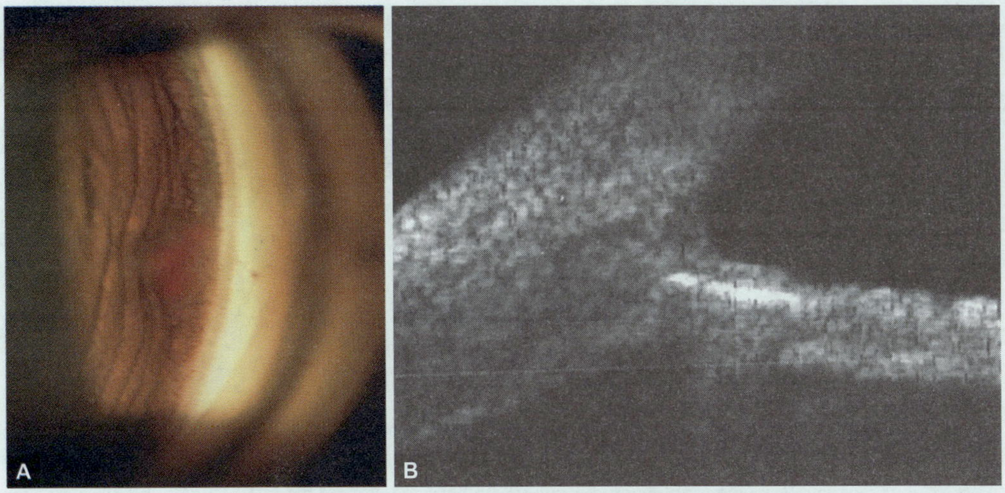

Figs. 13A and B: (A) Gonioscopy of the temporal angle in a patient with depression in the iris with localized blood; (B) Ultrasound biomicroscopy depicting foreign body embedded in the iris with high reflectivity.

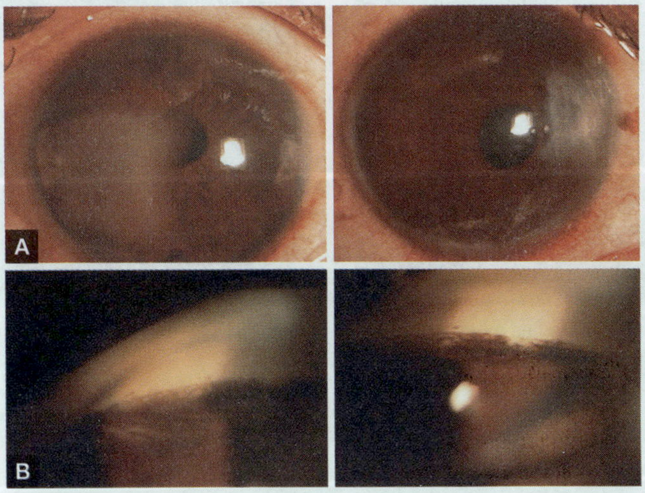

Figs. 14A and B: Clinical photograph and gonioscopy picture with suspected Chandler variety of iridocorneal endothelial syndrome.

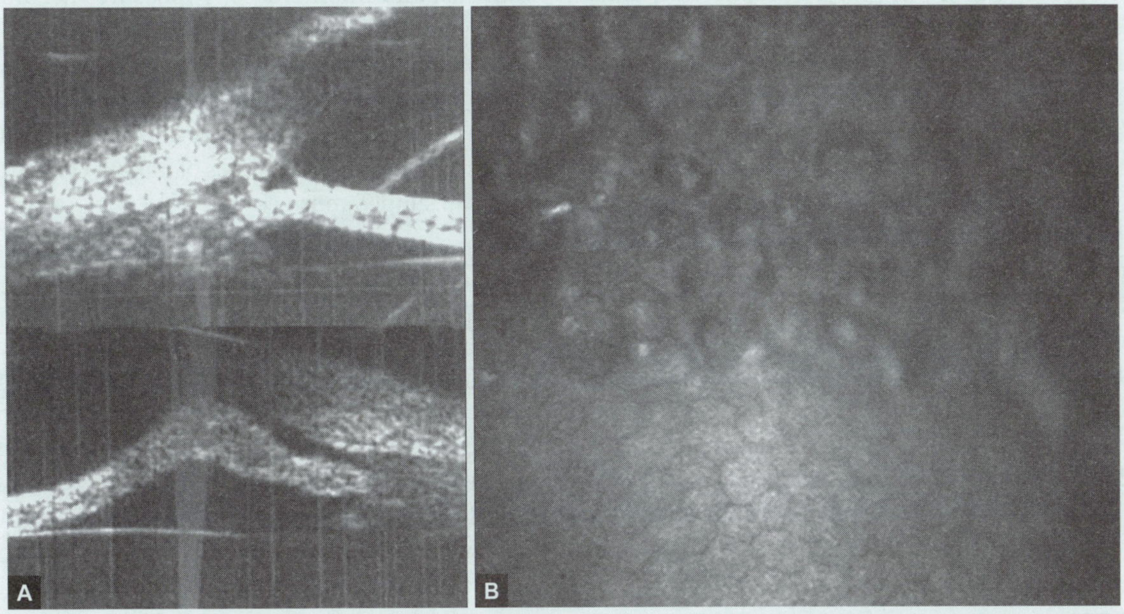

Figs. 15A and B: (A) Ultrasound biomicroscopy helps us in recognizing iridocorneal endothelial and distinguishing from other pathologies; (B) Confirmatory testing by confocal showing characteristic dark light reversal of endothelial cells.

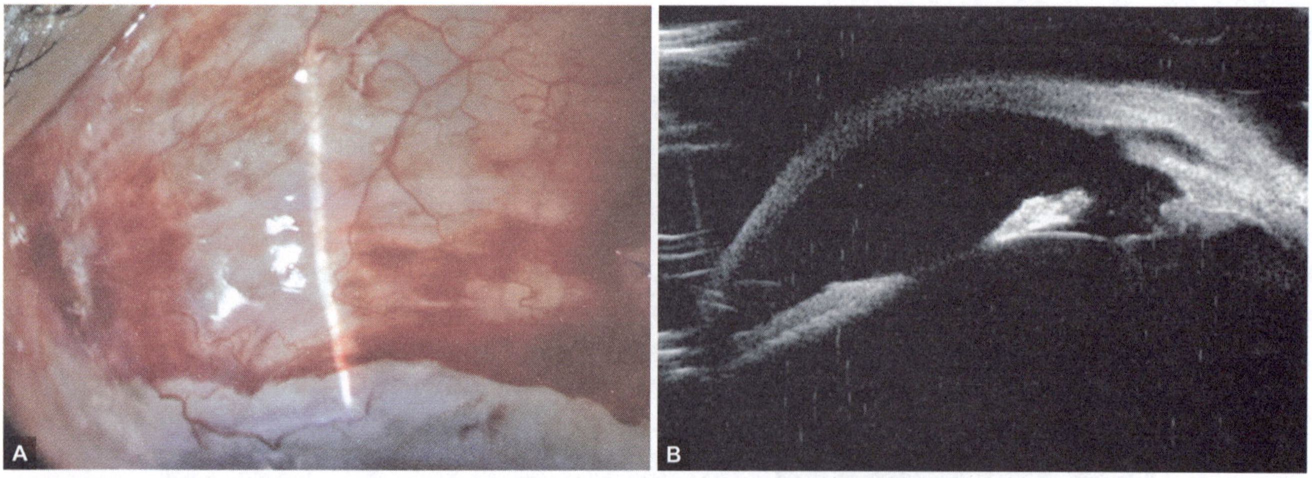

Figs. 16A and B: (A) A 47-year-old male 2 days after glaucoma surgery with flat vascularized bleb; (B) Ultrasound biomicroscopy picture depicting patent iridectomy with fluid under the bleb—an ideal candidate where needling might help.

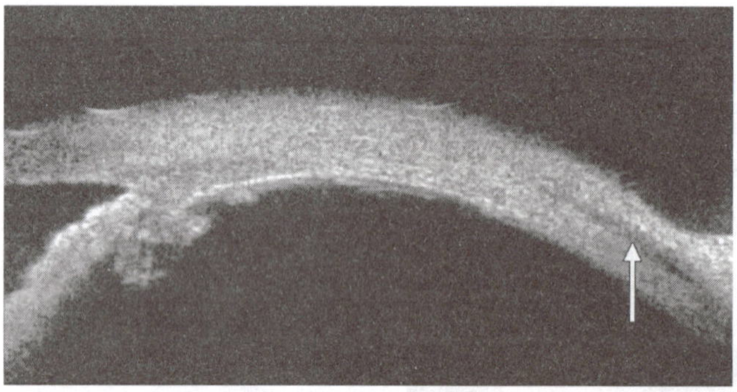

Fig. 17: The true muscle belly can be visualized as a hyporeflective area, which creates a distinct dark linear shadow (arrow).

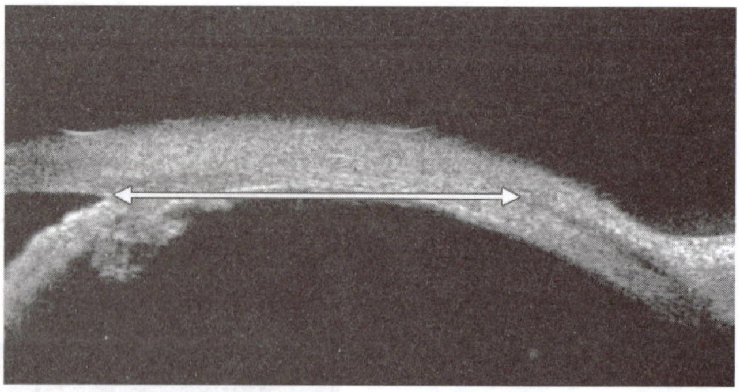

Fig. 18: The muscle insertion is delineated and its distance measured from the limbus using in-built caliper.

deciding the amount of recession or resection of the muscle to be performed during the squint surgery. Thus UBM may improve planning for surgical procedures subsequently needed. UBM can be used for muscle localization in cases of strabismus for preoperative planning, resurgeries, unwanted surgical results and in selective trauma cases.

Although conventional A and B scan ultrasound, computerized tomography, magnetic resonance imaging, and cine magnetic resonance imaging have all been used to define the size and location of the EOMs affected by disease or surgery; none of these techniques has been able to define the exact insertion of the muscles to the globe and the distance of the insertion from the limbus.

Normal imaging: UBM transducer is held tangentially over the muscle to be scanned and moved to and fro over the limbus, with the oscillations perpendicular to the limbus until a cross section of the muscle insertion is observed. The globe is held in abduction for the medial rectus muscle and in adduction for the lateral rectus muscle with a fixation forceps. The true muscle belly can be visualized by the UBM as a hyporeflective area, which is well delineated as shown in **Figures 17 and 18**, and creates a distinct dark linear shadow.

The muscle insertion is delineated and its distance is measured from the limbus using an in-built caliper in the UBM machine **(Fig. 18)**. Average of three readings is usually taken to determine the muscle insertion.

Ultrasound biomicroscopy measures accurately up to the 0.1 mm level as compared to a caliper which measures up to 0.5 mm.

Ultrasound biomicroscopy can pick up insertion of muscle in resurgery **(Figs. 19A to D)** where previous surgical records are not known, in cases of trauma **(Figs. 20A to E)** or to pick up slipped muscle.

ULTRASOUND BIOMICROSCOPY IN UVEITIS AND RETINAL DISEASES

While dealing in cases with uveitis, one must learn to examine the iris, ciliary body, pars plana, and peripheral retina. The UBM benefits most in cases with opaque media and hypotony.

Ultrasound biomicroscopy can identify thickening, atrophy or edema of the ciliary body. When there is hypotony we can look for supraciliary effusion which is seen as a hypoechoic space in the supraciliary area with medial

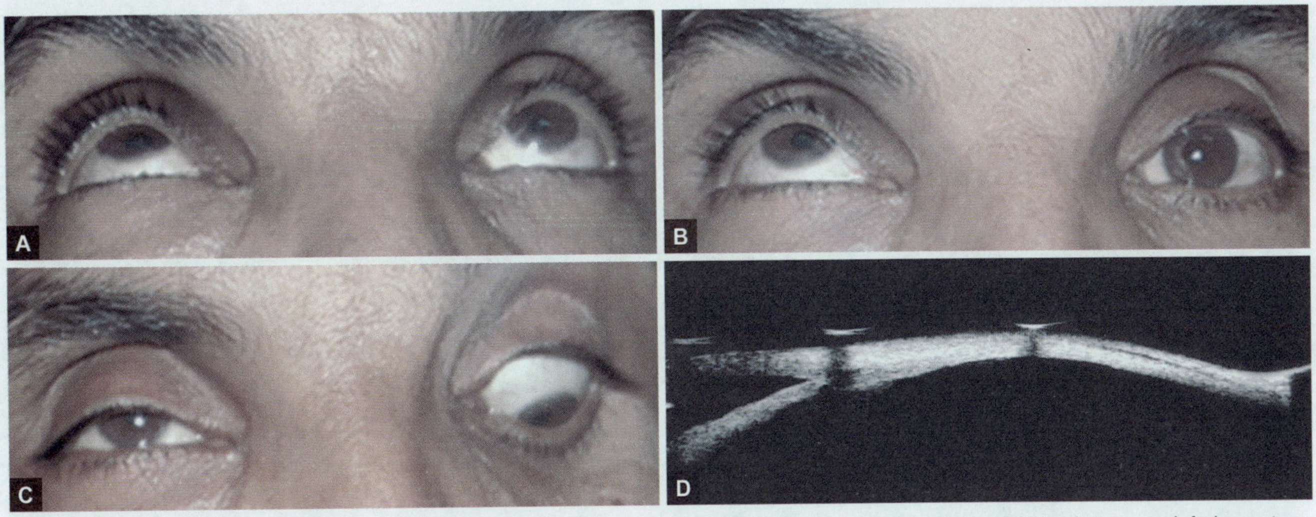

Figs. 19A to D: Suspected inferior rectus disinsertion post-trauma on clinical examination. On the ultrasound biomicroscopy, inferior rectus however could be traced at the normal insertion of 6 mm.

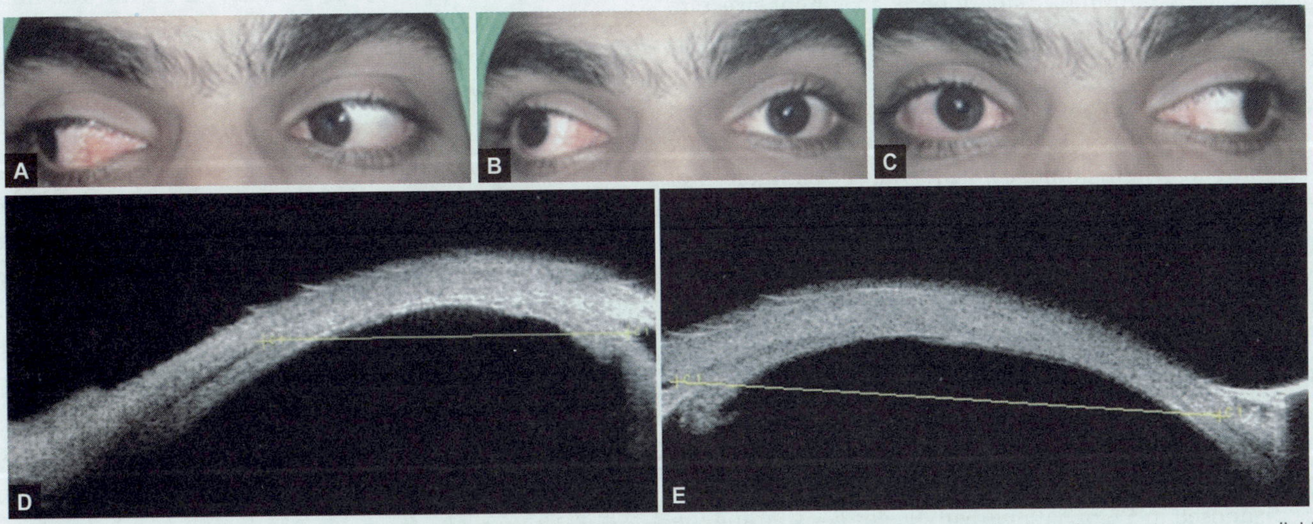

Figs. 20A to E: (A to C) A 24-year-old male presented 8 years after squint surgery in the right eye. No records of previous surgery were available. Due to deficient adduction in the right eye, ultrasound biomicroscopy was ordered. The medial rectus of the right eye was found at 5.5 mm and the lateral rectus recessed to about 11 mm from the limbus (D and E).

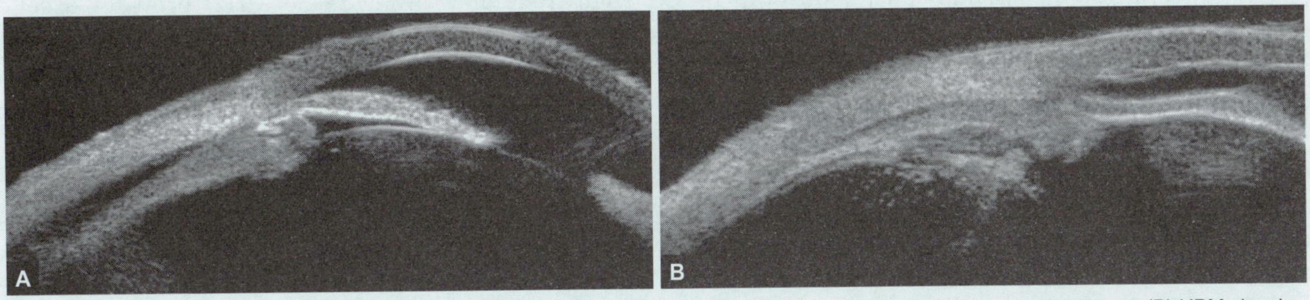

Figs. 21A and B: (A) Ultrasound biomicroscopy (UBM) picture depicting fluid in the supraciliary area causing angle closure; (B) UBM showing supraciliary effusion.

rotation of the ciliary body **(Fig. 21A)**. UBM can pick up even subclinical effusions **(Fig. 21B)**. Gradual resolution of exudates as well as swelling of the ciliary body in cases of acute anterior uveitis can be documented.

Preoperatively, in the presence of complicated cataract and hypotony, we can assess the ciliary body for the presence of tractional detachment of ciliary body. In cases of chronic iridocyclitis, cyclitic membranes with normal

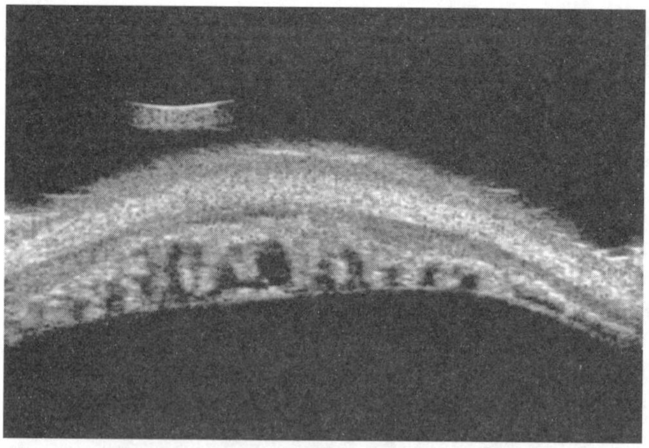

Fig. 22: Cyclitic membrane over the ciliary processes in a case of chronic uveitis.

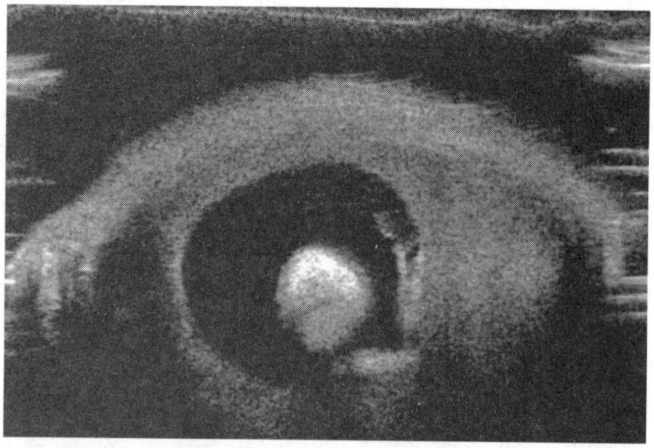

Fig. 23: Subconjunctival cysticercosis picked by the ultrasound biomicroscopy. Note the hyperechoic scolex in the hypoechoic lumen.

ciliary processes can be identified and removal of cyclitic membranes performed **(Fig. 22)**. Additional silicon oil tamponade is required if ciliary body atrophy is present. Cataract surgery can be deferred in such cases of atrophy as it will lead to phthisis.

Ultrasound biomicroscopy can confirm the disinsertion of ciliary body from the sclera spur and diagnose ciliary body detachment. Where gonioscopy precludes examination of the angle recess such as in cases of hyphema or retrocorneal membranes or hazy cornea, UBM can be helpful in diagnosing cyclodialysis cleft in cases of unexplained hypotony. UBM is especially useful even in cases where the cleft is not seen on gonioscopy. The extent of the cleft can also be noted on UBM. UBM delineation of cleft aids the precise identification and hence treatment.

Ultrasound biomicroscopy is an adjunct in detection and management of anterior segment tumors. Uveal melanomas are diagnosed in 5% of patients with uveitis constituting the masquerade syndromes. For undiagnosed causes of uveitis, especially in adult patients, one must look for melanomas. A solid mass in the iris, ciliary body or both with or without sclera infiltration with variable reflectivity indicate a melanoma. UBM can also be used to follow up these patients after brachytherapy. We can look for reduction in size and variation in the reflectivity.

Pars plana forms an important area to be visualized especially in eyes where there is miotic and/or seclusio-pupil with/without complicated cataract or dense vitritis. UBM can detect snow banking and typical pars plana deposits. It is seen as medium reflectivity in the area of pars plana. Pars plana condensation confirms the diagnosis of pars planitis. Authors have described grading of pars planitis by keeping a record of the number of cells and their echogenicity. We can hence monitor efficacy of our therapy even in patients with dense media.

Adnexal Diseases

Ultrasound biomicroscopy is a useful aid in examining any lesion over the surface of the eye. The depth of the tumor as well as the layer or origin can be studied. It can also be an aid in the diagnosis of conjunctival masses **(Fig. 23)**. Not only it helps identify the etiology but also gauge the depth of the lesion before surgical excision. Sclera inflammatory diseases can be diagnosed and monitored on UBM. Scleral nodules can be imaged and stratified according to the location. Even if visible clinically, the level of infiltration of the tumor can be studied. These usually appear as echogenic areas. Quantification of reduced sclera thickness with clinical regression of the nodule can also be documented on sequential scans. It also helps in differentiating cases of episcleritis from scleritis, early detection of sclera necrosis, and identification of nodular scleritis.

CONCLUSION

High frequency UBM (35–50 MHz) provides excellent tissue differentiation; resolution of 0.1 mm and penetrance of 5–7 mm of tissue depth. It provides a highly magnified image of the anterior segment along with a real-time imaging of the anterior structures in a noninvasive manner.

ACKNOWLEDGMENTS

We are very thankful to Dr Jaspreet Sukhija, Associate Professor (for **Figures 17 to 20**), Dr Ramandeep Singh, Additional Professor (for **Figures 21 to 23**) and Dr Pankaj Kataria, Senior Resident, Advanced eye center, PGIMER, Chandigarh.

SUGGESTED READING

1. Dorairaj S, Liebmann JM, Ritch R. Quantitative evaluation of anterior segment parameters in the era of imaging. Trans Am Ophthalmol Soc. 2007;105:99-110.
2. Ishikawa H. Anterior segment imaging for glaucoma: OCT or UBM? Br J Ophthalmol. 2007;91(11):1420-1.
3. Kaur S, Sukhija J. The accuracy of anterior segment optical coherence tomography (AS-OCT) in localizing extraocular rectus muscles insertions. J AAPOS. 2015;19(5):488-9.
4. Kaushik S, Ichhpujani P, Ramasubramanian A, et al. Occult intraocular foreign body: ultrasound biomicroscopy holds the key. Int Ophthalmol. 2008;28(1):71-3.
5. Kaushik S, Jain R, Pandav SS, et al. Evaluation of the anterior chamber angle in Asian Indian eyes by ultrasound biomicroscopy and gonioscopy. Indian J Ophthalmol. 2006;54(3):159-63.
6. Kaushik S, Kumar S, Jain R, et al. Ultrasound biomicroscopic quantification of the change in anterior chamber angle following laser peripheral iridotomy in early chronic primary angle closure glaucoma. Eye (Lond). 2007;21(6):735-41.
7. Li H, Leung CK, Cheung CY, et al. Repeatability and reproducibility of anterior chamber angle measurement with anterior segment optical coherence tomography. Br J Ophthalmol. 2007;91(11):1490-2.
8. Mundt GH Jr, Hughes WF Jr. Ultrasonics in ocular diagnosis. Am J Ophthalmol. 1956;41(3):488-98.
9. Pavlin CJ, Harasiewicz K, Foster FS. Ultrasound biomicroscopy of anterior segment structures in normal and glaucomatous eyes. Am J Ophthalmol. 1992;113(4):381-9.
10. Pavlin CJ, Harasiewicz K, Sherar MD, et al. Clinical use of ultrasound biomicroscopy. Ophthalmology. 1991;98(3): 287-95.
11. Pavlin CJ, Sherar MD, Foster FS. Subsurface ultrasound microscopic imaging of the intact eye. Ophthalmology. 1990;97(2):244-50.
12. Solarte CE, Smith DR, Buncic JR, et al. Evaluation of vertical rectus muscles using ultrasound biomicroscopy. J AAPOS. 2008;12(2):128-31.
13. Thakur N, Singh R, Kaur S, et al. Ultrasound biomicroscopy in strabismus surgery: efficacy in postoperative assessment of horizontal muscle insertions. Strabismus. 2015;23(2):73-9.
14. Watts P, Smith D, Mackeen L, et al. Evaluation of the ultrasound biomicroscope in strabismus surgery. J AAPOS. 2002;6(3): 187-90.

CHAPTER 20

Electrophysiological Tests for Visual Function Assessment

Subhadra Jalali, LS Mohan Ram, Garima Tyagi, Kallakuri Sumasri

VISUAL ELECTROPHYSIOLOGY TESTS

Visual electrophysiology is an extremely powerful tool to assess functional integrity of the visual pathway. Visual pathway starts from the photoreceptor and retinal pigment epithelial layer, proceeds through inner retinal layers, ganglion cell layer and then via optic nerve through the chiasma to the optic radiations in the brain, finally ending at the occipital cortex. This chapter aims to introduce some basic concepts of visual electrophysiological tests (VETs) with the help of some representative clinical cases.

Visual electrophysiological tests include the various types of electroretinogram (ERG), electrooculogram (EOG), and visual evoked potential (VEP). A patient may need some tests to ascertain the abnormality. Before ordering the tests a clear understanding of the nature of each of these is absolutely essential to derive a valid interpretation. A thorough clinical evaluation is a prerequisite before ordering any VET.

History

To understand how VETs reached its present status, some of the milestones are described here. Du Bois-Reymond of Berlin discovered standing potential of 6 millivolts in excised fish eyes and found that cornea was positive with respect to posterior pole of the eye in 1849. He thought that these signals originate in optic nerve. Holmgren showed electrical responses to light in excised frog and demonstrated that these to originate in the retina.

Dewar and McKendrick showed that electrical potentials could be recorded from intact animal eyes on illumination of the retina. In 1877, Dewar succeeded in recording ERG from the human eye but the resulting curves were not published.

The first human ERG was published by Kahn and Lowenstein.

Between 1933 and 1947 Ragnar Granit in Oxford did extensive studies with various chemical agents to analyze the origins of various phases of the ERG. American psychologist Lorrin Riggs and Gosta Karpe at the Karolinska Institute designed a contact lens electrode independently. The credit for taking the science of ERG from the laboratory to the clinic goes to Gosta Karpe who invited ophthalmologists to visit his clinic where routine diagnostic ERG was introduced.

Before ordering and interpreting these tests, a thorough understanding of the nature and limitations of each of test is a prerequisite to arrive at a valid interpretation and diagnosis.

The visual electrophysiology tests follow a hierarchal pathway along the various cell layers of the visual system. The EOG examines the function of the retinal pigment epithelium (RPE) and the interaction between the RPE and the rod photoreceptors. Following stimulation by light, the electrical responses from retinal photoreceptors and the inner retinal cells are assessed by the a- and b-wave components of the flash ERG, respectively. The macular photoreceptor function and the ganglion cells function is revealed and separated by the technique of pattern ERG recording. The integrity of the visual pathway from optic nerve via optic chiasma to the occipital cortex is assessed by various techniques of VEP recording.

For each of these recordings in the clinic, certain minimum standards have been laid down by the International Society for Clinical Electrophysiology of Vision (ISCEV pronounced as eyesev). These are available on the website *www.iscev.org*.

Importance of Electrophysiological Tests

Sometimes, the clinical examination of the eye cannot explain the exact cause of decrease in vision. These tests help to detect and categorize the site of lesion in the visual pathway.

In other cases, especially in retinal degenerations, these tests help to know the type and extent of disease and its prognosis. In vascular pathology, these tests can assess the extent of ischemia of the inner retinal layers. Other indications include detection of drug or metal toxicity, pediatric visual assessment, and cause of poor vision in infants. In a given situation, these tests prove invaluable in the proper management plan.

Side Effects and Precautions

Electrophysiology testing of the eye is very safe and there are no major side effects. VEP and EOG recording is done from skin and has no side effect. ERG testing very rarely leads to irritation and watering of the eyes for a few hours after the test and can be easily treated with lubricating eye drops. Rarely, patient can get infectious keratitis. The total test can take up to 3 hours. Alcohol or sedatives should not be taken for 24 hours before the tests as these can interfere with the results. Other medicines such as for diabetes, asthma, and hypertension can be continued. For VEP testing, the hair should be preferably washed and dried a night before so as to be free of oil and greasiness. The patient should be electrically isolated according to current standards for safety of clinical biologic recording systems in the user's country.

ELECTROOCULOGRAM

Electrooculogram examines the function of the RPE and the interaction between the RPE and the rod photoreceptors.[1] All vertebrate eyes are like a dipole, with a resting potential in which the cornea is positive with respect to the back of the eye. This creates a standing or resting potential of about 6 millivolts. This standing potential rises when the retina is illuminated to a steady light. EOG measures changes in the standing potential to light and dark conditions. Clinically, EOG measures the standing potential indirectly using the fact that the spatial orientation of a polarized eye is detected by skin electrodes placed nasal and temporal to the eye. Saccadic eye movements result in flow of current around orbit proportional to the magnitude of standing potential of each eye. Skin electrodes record these voltage changes.

Clinical Measurement

Geoffrey Arden and colleagues[2,3] described the indirect method of recording of clinical EOG. Skin electrodes are placed at the medial and lateral canthi to detect the amplitude of the signal between these two points. A ground electrode is fixed to the forehead. Pupils are dilated. A Ganzfeld is used to illuminate whole retina uniformly. Eye should not be exposed to too bright or too dim lights before EOG. After an initial 6 minutes of light adaptation, test is started. The patient makes fixed 30° lateral eye movements (using diode fixation lights) during a period of 20 minutes of dark adaptation, and then during a 12–15 minutes period of light adaptation. The eye movements are made every 1–2 seconds for approximately 15 seconds and a pause of 45 seconds, every minute. The dipole generated by the resting potential induces current flow in the skin electrodes upon shift of the eye position **(Figs. 1A to C)**. The changes in voltage are amplified and displayed on a computer data acquisition system **(Fig. 2)**. The changes in this indirectly measured potential, from darkness to light is the light-induced rise of the resting potential.[3] In the dark, the resting potential decreases while it slowly rises to a peak (slow oscillation of EOG) after the lights are switched on **(Fig. 2)**. The amplitude of the signal is recorded at its minimum during dark adaptation (the dark trough) and at its maximum during light adaptation (the light peak). The ISCEV has laid down standards for EOG testing.[4] The normal light peak occurs in conditions of normally functioning photoreceptors in contact with a normally functioning RPE, and is caused by progressive depolarization of the RPE basal membrane. The EOG is quantified by calculating the amplitude of the light peak in relation to the dark trough as a percentage, the *Arden index*.[3] A normal index would be >185% **(Fig. 2)**.

Clinical Uses

A normal ERG and abnormal EOG are classically seen in Bests' vitelliform macular dystrophy[5] **(Fig. 3)** even in very early stages of the disease with minimal fundus changes and in asymptomatic carriers. EOG abnormality is also seen in a variety of RPE and rod-photoreceptor disorders such as retinitis pigmentosa (RP), choroideremia, and age-related macular degeneration. EOG is also abnormal in choroidal melanomas and could be an adjunct tool to differentiate melanoma from nevi.[6] EOG is normal in isolated inner retinal cell dysfunction such as in congenital stationary night blindness (CSNB) where RPE and photoreceptors are normal. EOG can be used to study drug toxicity against RPE. One must remember that because light is used to provoke the voltage change in EOG, this test cannot separate the photoreceptor and RPE dysfunction. In recent years, Arden et al.[7] have shown that after intake of low doses of ethanol an EOG peak similar to the light-induced EOG peak can be recorded. This could test RPE layer function independent of its interaction with the photoreceptors.[7]

Limitations of Electrooculogram Recording

Patient cooperation and central fixation limit the clinical recording of EOG. Patients with poor central fixation or variable eccentric fixation, children, infants, and uncooperative adults cannot be tested satisfactorily. Many testing variables such as media opacities and illumination levels can influence the voltages. Therefore, borderline EOG abnormalities need to be interpreted with caution and test may have to be repeated for confirmation.[1]

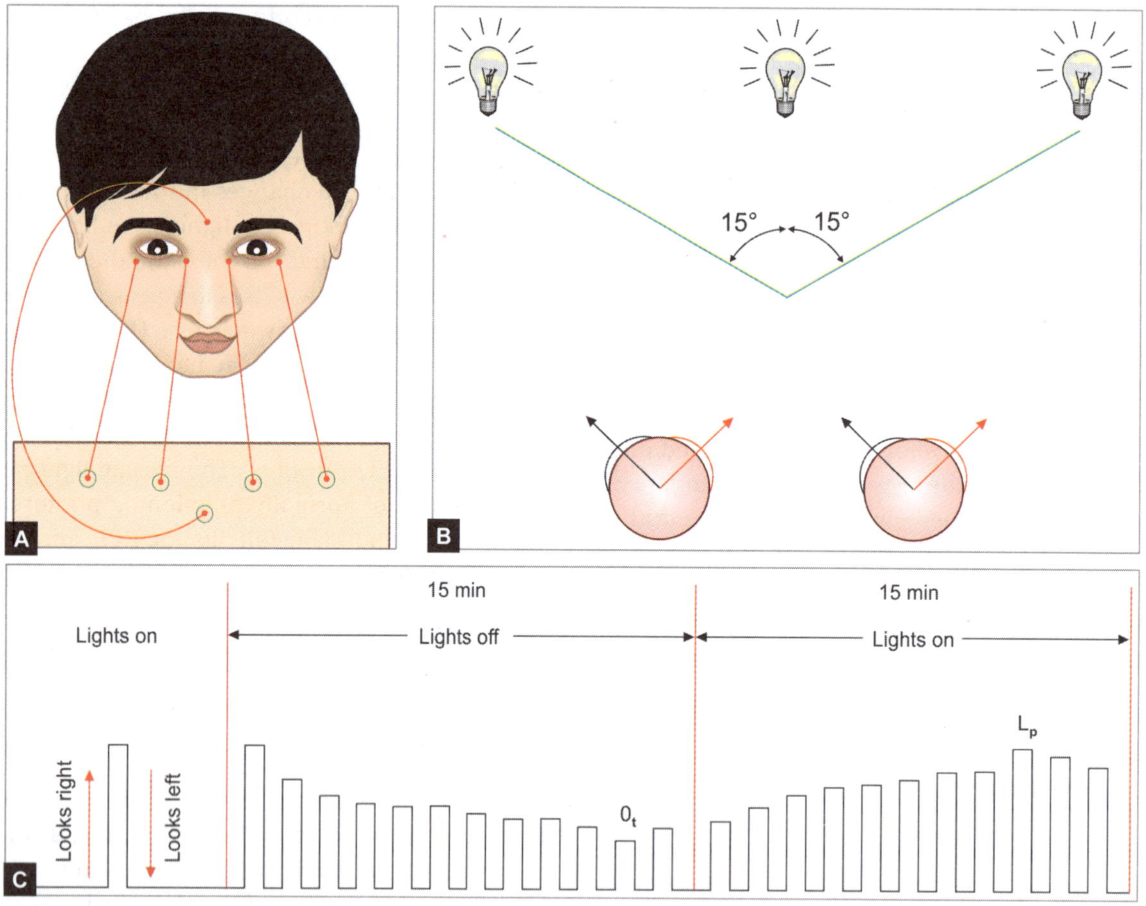

Figs. 1A to C: Electrooculogram recording procedure. (A) Skin electrode placement; (B) Ganzfeld fixating lights (light-emitting diode) 15° apart, with 30° excursion from right to left; (C) 16–20 sweeps per minute following a baseline recording of 6 minutes in white light. Recording is for 15 minutes in dark and 15 minutes in light.

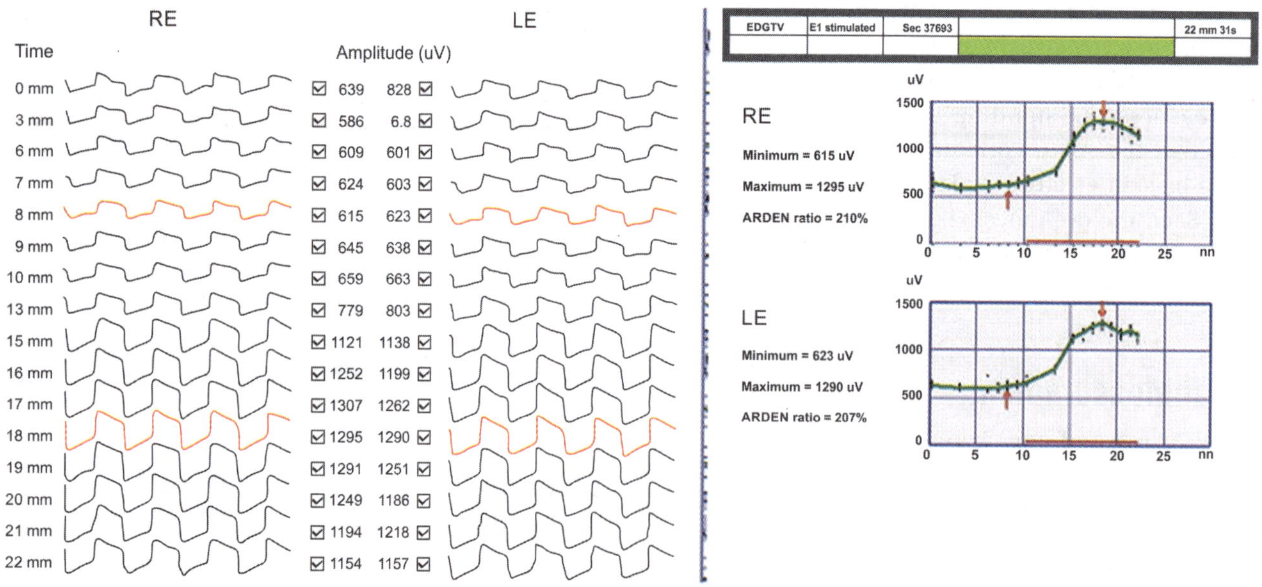

Fig. 2: Raw waveforms of the saccades (left) and the final EOG graph (right). Note the light rise and normal Arden ratio of >200% in each eye. (EOG: electrooculogram; LE: left eye; RE: right eye)

Fast oscillations of EOG: It was reported by Kolder et al.[8] that the EOG responses could be slow or fast, if the frequency of the light and dark periods for stimulation were altered. They found the "slow" oscillations were greatest with repeated light and dark periods of 12.5 minutes each, whereas, the greatest amplitude of "fast" oscillations of EOG were seen when the light and dark cycles were of 1.1 minute each. The amplitude of "fast" oscillations increased in dark

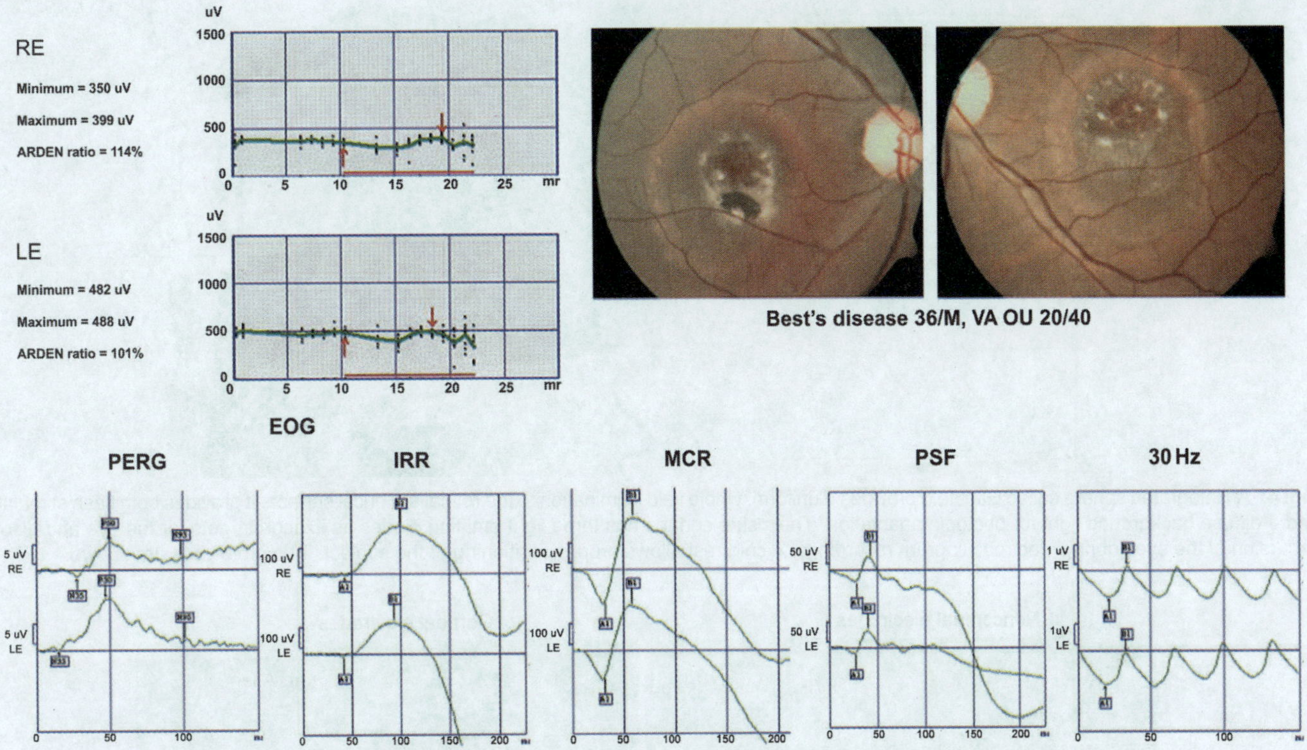

Fig. 3: Poor light rise on EOG in a patient with subnormal vision and bilateral macular lesions. ERG recordings including macular photoreceptors (PERG) was normal as shown in ERG results. (EOG: electrooculogram; ERG: electroretinogram; IRR: isolated rod response; LE: left eye; MCR: maximal combined response; PERG: pattern electroretinogram; PSF: photopic single flash; RE: right eye)

phase and reduced in light phase. The clinical value of these fast oscillations needs further study.

ELECTRORETINOGRAM

Due to selective transport of ions, the inside of the photoreceptor cells is more negative than the outside resulting in a standing membrane potential in the dark. Once light falls on the retina, it induces a change in the transmembrane movement of especially sodium and potassium ions, making the cells hyperpolarized, that is, they become more negative to the extracellular space than in the dark. These voltage changes are reflected in various ERG components.

Various techniques are in clinical use to assess the electrical response of retinal cells to light. The most common of these is the full-field flash ERG. Others are pattern ERG, focal ERG, and multifocal ERG (mfERG) **(Box 1)**.

The flash ERG is the mass response of the neural and non-neural retinal cells to a full-field luminance stimulation. This test reflects the function of the photoreceptors and inner nuclear layers of the retina in response to light stimulation. It is recorded by using stimuli delivered by an integrating sphere, called *Ganzfeld,* which provides a uniform whole field illumination to the retinal spherical surface.[9] The Ganzfeld provides both flash stimulation and a diffuse background for photopic adaptation besides fixation lights **(Fig. 4)**.

By varying the background illumination, the light- or dark-adapted state of the eye and the intensity of the stimulus flash, one can elicit and isolate response from different retinal cells. The ISCEV standard describes simple technical procedures that allow reproducible ERGs to be recorded under a few defined conditions, from patients of all ages including infants.[9,10] Details of the equipment standardization is beyond the scope of this chapter but is available in literature.[11]

Box 1: Specialized types of electroretinogram (ERG) [not covered by International Society for Clinical Electrophysiology of Vision (ISCEV) standard].[10]

- Macular or focal ERG
- Multifocal ERG
- Early receptor potential (ERP)
- Scotopic threshold response (STR)
- Direct-current ERG
- Long-duration flash ERG (on-off responses)
- Bright-flash ERG
- Double-flash ERG
- Chromatic stimulus ERG (including S-cone response)
- Dark and light adaptation of the ERG
- Stimulus intensity-response amplitude analysis (Naka-Rushton)
- Saturated a-wave slope analysis

Recording Electrode

The ERG is recorded using corneal or noncorneal electrodes **(Fig. 5)**. The closer the electrode is to the cornea, the higher the amplitude one gets, though latency will not change.

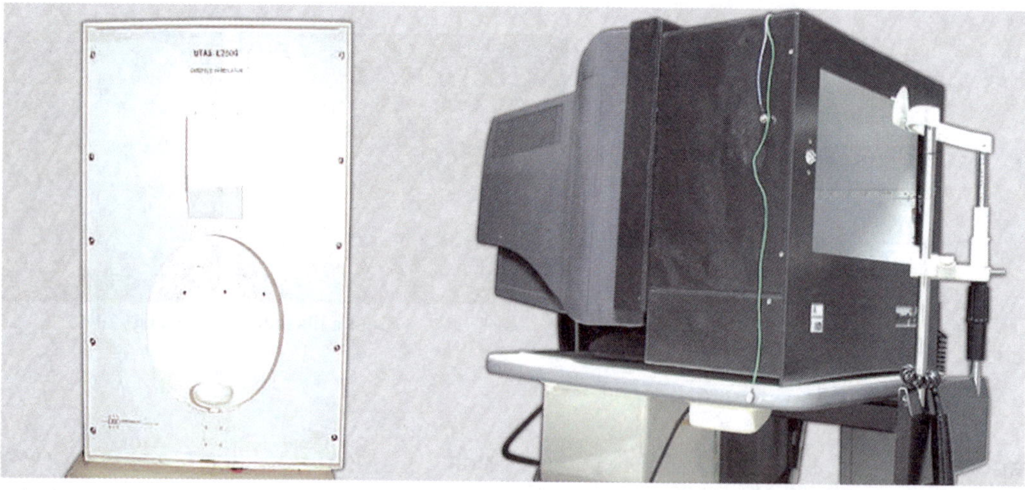

Fig. 4: An integrated sphere called Ganzfeld provides a uniform, whole field illumination to the retinal spherical surface. It provides both flash stimulation and a diffuse background light for photopic adaptation. The inside surface has three light emitting diodes as fixation targets for the eye and also for excursion of the eyes during electrooculogram recordings. A chin rest allows proper positioning of the subject. Two prototypes are shown.

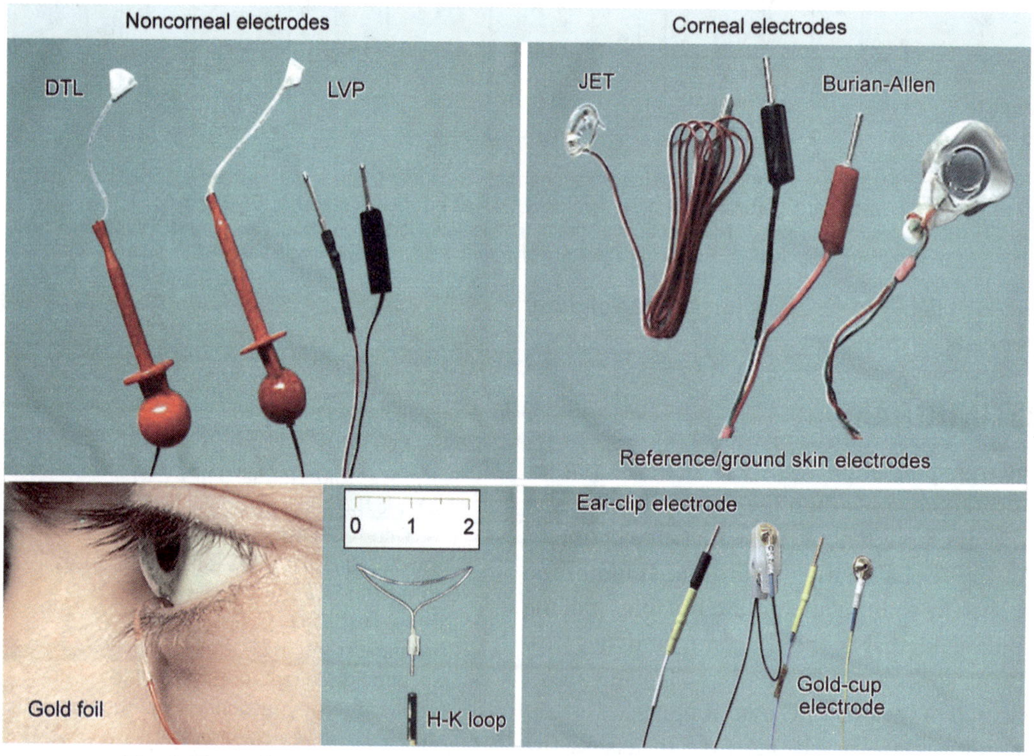

Fig. 5: Electrodes used in visual electrophysiology. Gold foil and H-K loop electrodes.
Courtesy: Dr G Holder, London
(DTL: Dawson-Trick-Litzkow)

Prototypes of corneal electrode are Burian-Allen and Jet electrodes. The corneal electrodes can be unipolar like the Jet-electrode or bipolar like the Burian-Allen electrode. The Burian-Allen electrode is centrally transparent with a large optical opening and incorporates a device to hold the lids apart. Topical anesthesia and a nonviscous solution like 0.5% methylcellulose are needed. More viscous solutions can attenuate signal amplitude. Corneal electrodes may be difficult to maintain due to a silver coating that needs resurfacing periodically, and are expensive and cause some discomfort besides rare possibility of corneal abrasion. The advantage, however, is that higher amplitudes are recordable due to proximity to the cornea. All reusable electrodes should be cleaned and sterilized after each use to prevent disease transmission.

The noncorneal electrodes include gold foil, the DTL-fiber (Dawson-Trick-Litzkow) and our own devised LVP-Zari electrode.[12-14] The LVP-Zari electrode is disposable, inexpensive, rigid and reliable and made from locally available Zari-embroidery thread. It has a core of nylon (traditionally had cotton thread core) covered with layers of silver copper and gold, making it a good conductor of

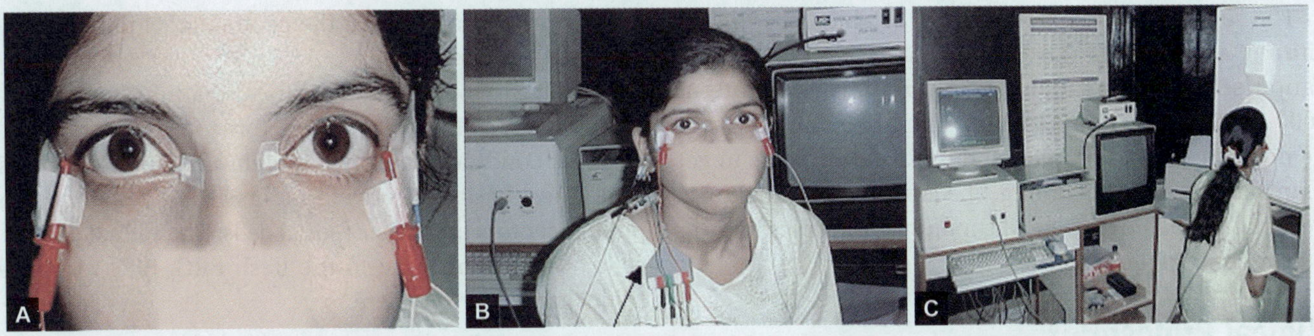

Figs. 6A to C: LVP electrode placement (A) and connections (B) to junction box (arrow); Electroretinogram in progress (C).

electric currents. Due to its nylon core, and multiple metallic coatings, the movement of the fiber across the limbus is minimal, making the recordings very reliable.

The recording electrodes, bipolar or nonbipolar are placed on the cornea. Topical anesthesia is necessary for contact lens electrodes but may not be required for other types of corneal and conjunctival electrodes. It is important to learn the technical requirements of a chosen electrode, to ensure good ocular contact, to ensure proper electrode impedance, to ensure that waveforms are comparable to standard responses, and to define both normal values and variability (which may be different with different electrodes) for their own laboratory.[9,10] Skin electrodes are in general not recommended as active ERG recording electrodes.

Reference electrodes: Reference electrodes may be incorporated into the contact lens-speculum assembly as in Burian-Allen **(Fig. 5)** or can be placed near each ipsilateral outer canthus as a reference for the corresponding eye. The forehead as a reference has a theoretical risk of signal contamination by ocular crossover or from cortical evoked potentials.

Ground electrode: A separate skin electrode, such as an ear clip **(Fig. 5)** should be attached to an indifferent point and connected to ground.

Electrode Placement

After topical anesthesia, corneal electrodes are filled with a mild viscous coupling solution such as 0.5% methylcellulose and inserted gently like a contact lens in the center of the cornea, with the lid speculum holding the lids apart simultaneously. The noncorneal electrode is placed in the lower fornix as close to the inferior limbus as possible. It should be stable, nonmobile, and not injure the cornea. The reference electrode is placed at the outer canthus. An ear clip electrode serves as a ground electrode. For all skin electrodes, good contact is essential with low impedance. To achieve this grease and dead cells on the skin are removed by rubbing with an abrasive and an alcohol pad. **Figure 6A** shows a subject with the LVP-Zari electrode in place, held across the fornix with a crocodile clip (red color) and the reference electrode (blue color) at the outer canthus. The ear clip ground electrode is also seen. All the electrodes are then connected to a junction box **(Fig. 6B)** which sends the signals through an interface box into the computerized amplifiers and recorders. Care should be taken to connect the electrodes to the correct site on the junction box. The outer canthal electrodes go to the positive and recording electrodes to the negative poles of the junction box.

Flash Stimulus Characteristics

The light stimulus should consist of flashes having a maximum of about 5 ms duration so that duration of each flash is considerably shorter than the integration time of any photoreceptor. These short white flashes obtained by stroboscopes and gas discharge tubes have a color temperature of 7,000 degrees K. A standard flash (SF) strength is defined as one that produces a stimulus strength (in luminous energy per square meter) at the surface of the Ganzfeld bowl of 1.5–4.5 photopic cd.s.m^{-2} (candela-seconds per meter squared).[10] In addition to producing flashes, the stimulator must be capable of producing a steady and uniformly even, white (colored in rare special situations) background luminance of 17–34 cd.m^{-2} across the full field. Prolonged-flash ERGs and chromatic lights are currently used for studying slow potentials and for separating on- and off-responses.

Technical Requirements

The system should be capable of attenuating the flash strength from SF over a range of at least 3 log units, either continuously or in steps of no more than 0.3 log unit. This attenuation should not change the wavelength. It is essential to periodically calibrate the stimulus and background illumination by integrated and nonintegrated photometers to achieve standard test conditions.[11]

The bandpass of the amplifier and preamplifier should include at least the range of 0.3–300 Hz and should be adjustable for oscillatory potential (OP) recordings and other specialized requirements. Amplifiers are generally alternating current (AC) coupled.

The recording equipment should be able to represent without attenuation the full amplifier bandpass. The computer digitizers should sample responses at rate of 1,000 Hz or higher. The observer should be able to watch the displays so as to monitor and make adjustments to get clean and less noisy recording. The computerized digitizers are usually capable of averaging multiple responses so as to remove some of the artifacts.

Clinical Protocol[9,10]

Electroretinogram is recorded after full pupillary dilatation so that all parts of retina get illuminated. Avoid any extra illumination (as in fluorescein angiography or fundus photography) but if these examinations have been performed, a period of dark adaptation of at least 1 hour is needed before scotopic recording.

The subject is placed in a completely dark room for 30 minutes. Next, the subject with electrodes in place is seated comfortably with the chin on the chin rest and eyes open with the face inside the Ganzfeld bowl **(Fig. 6C)**. The height of patient should be adjusted so that the neck and back muscles are not in a tensed-up position as this can induce muscle-generated artifacts. The cable from junction box is fixed to the shoulder at the subject's end and plugged into the interface box at the other end, sending the retinal signals into the amplifiers and computer analyzers. Patients are encouraged to fixate at the central target to reduce eye movement and artifacts.

The ISCEV standard describes[9,10] a minimum of five basic ERG response recordings, three in dark adapted or scotopic conditions and two in light-adapted or photopic state. These basic ERG waveforms are a mass response of the photoreceptors and inner retinal cells. The retinal ganglion cells do not contribute to the flash ERG. ERG responses **(Fig. 7)** are described here.

Isolated Rod Response

To isolate the signals from the rod system of photoreceptors, a dim white flash of strength 2.5 log units below the white SF is used. Serial responses are recorded with a minimum of 2 seconds interval between the flashes to allow the rods to return to dark-adapted state in between the flashes. A blue stimulus is equally appropriate if equated to the white standard. At this low intensity level, the cones are insensitive to the stimulus. The isolated rod response has almost no a-wave and a slowly rising, broad-peaked, b-wave. The b-wave in the isolated rod-response waveform is a postreceptor phenomenon, i.e. inner retinal cell response that is driven by only the rod photoreceptors. At this low luminance a-wave is not recordable due to poor photoactivation. There is progressive appearance and increasing amplitude of the a-wave as stimulus intensity

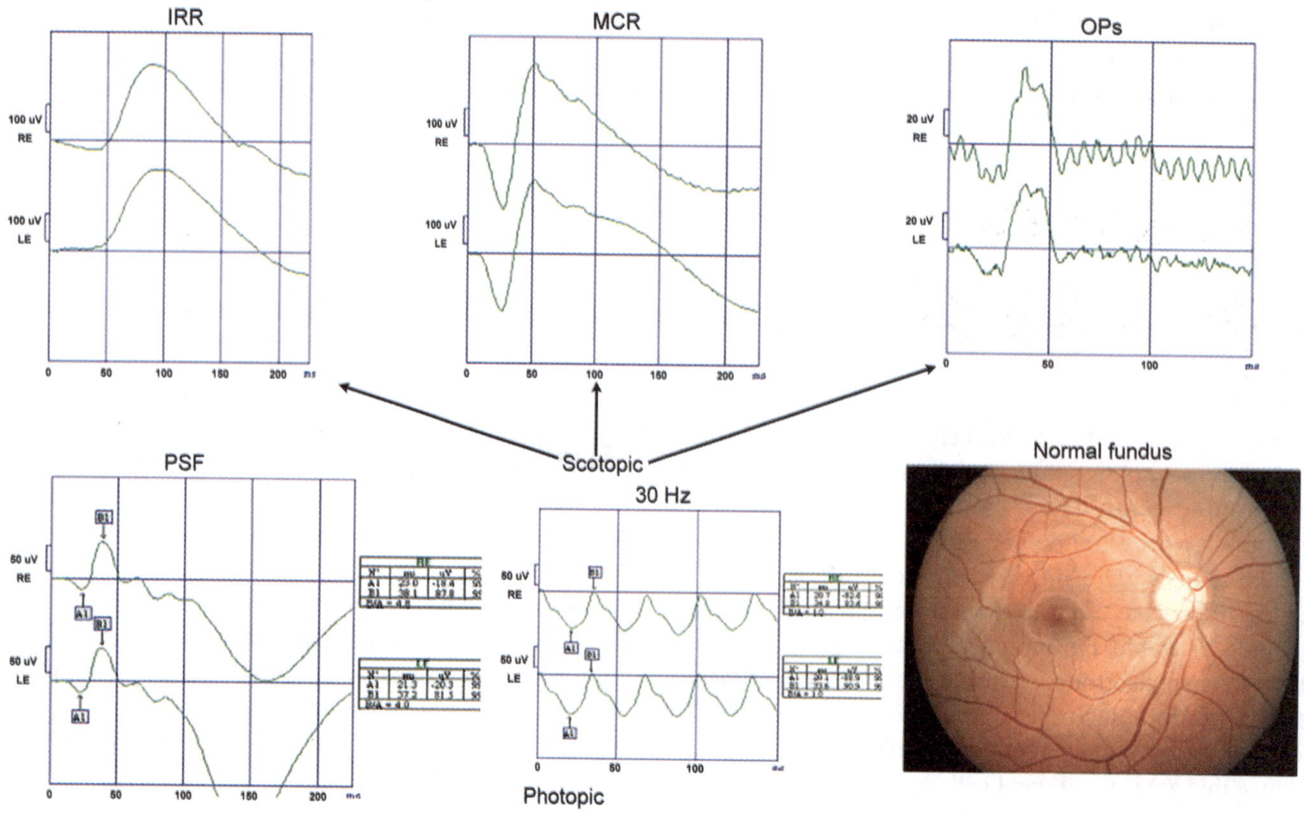

Fig. 7: Normal flash electroretinogram waveforms from a normal fundus. Under scotopic conditions, we can record the isolated rod response (IRR), the maximal combined response (MCR), and the scotopic oscillatory potentials (OPs). The photopic responses include the single flash for cones [photopic single flash (PSF)] and the 30 Hz flicker responses (30 Hz).

is increased from low level to the higher level of the SF (intensity response curve). As the a-wave starts appearing with increasing intensity of stimulus, it represents activity of the rod photoreceptors but with maximum flash intensity, the cones also start contributing to the a-wave as is seen in the maximal combined response.

Maximal Combined Response

The maximal response is dominated by rod responses but also has a small component of cone activity. The initial negative a-wave is generated by the photoreceptors, i.e. both rods and cones. The positive b-wave is generated postreceptoraly in relation to depolarization of the ON-bipolar cells.[15] Under scotopic conditions, flash ERG is obtained using the standard white flash which is 0 decibel attenuated. A sharp a-wave and a much larger, rapidly rising peaked b-wave which comes to baseline very slowly, are characteristic of this response. Duration between two flashes should be at least 10 seconds to remove effect of bleach of photoreceptors by the bright flash of light.

Oscillatory Potentials

The oscillatory potentials (OPs pronounced as opees) are small but high frequency oscillations on the ascending limb of the b-wave of the maximal combined response.

These are extracted and amplified to present the OPs as seen in **Figure 7**. They are generated in relation to amacrine cell activity in the middle and inner retinal cell layers. Under scotopic condition and using SF intensity as a stimulus, other wavelets are removed by resetting of the filters. The high-pass filter must be reset from the usual 0.3 Hz to 75 Hz, so that an overall bandpass of 75 at high end and 300 Hz at low end is achieved. The response varies with stimulus repetition rate and changes after the first stimulus. Flashes should be given 15 seconds apart to the dark-adapted eyes (1.5 seconds apart to light-adapted eyes), and only the second or subsequent responses should be retained or averaged.[9,10] Normal response is characterized by three major peaks followed by one to two smaller peaks. Comparison with normal individual laboratory values is often adequate to assess any abnormality.

Single-flash Cone Response

To record the photopic responses, the retina is exposed to 10 minutes of light adaptation by using the background light in the dome of 17–34 candelas per meter square of luminance (that saturates rods and makes them unresponsive). After this, the retina is exposed to an SF to obtain the photopic single flash (PSF) cone response. Inter-stimulus intervals should not be less than 0.5 seconds. This cone response is characterized by a small a-wave and a very sharply rising b-wave that rapidly returns to the baseline. Better localization of cone functions is seen with the single flash cone response than with the flicker response. The photopic cone a-wave has contribution from the hyperpolarizing (OFF) bipolar cells and also cone photoreceptors.[16] The cone b-wave probably reflects post-phototransduction activity. Separation of the cone ON (depolarizing bipolar cells) and OFF (hyperpolarizing bipolar cells) pathways is done by using a long duration stimulus with a photopic background.[17]

30 Hz Flicker Cone Response

Under the photopic condition repetitive SFs are presented at a frequency of 30 stimuli per second. Rods are suppressed by the photopic condition and are incapable of responding to the highly repetitive stimuli. The amplitude is measured from trough to peak of each response. The latency is measured as the distance between stimulus onset and time-to-peak. A vertical line in the trace should indicate the time of onset of the stimulus. The 30 Hz response is a sensitive measure of cone dysfunction, but is generated at an inner retinal level.[18] The response is affected in inner retinal ischemic states.

Electroretinogram Measurements and Recording

A typical flash ERG record is a double peak waveform. According to current convention, the amplitude of the initial cornea negative a-wave is measured from baseline to the trough, while b-wave amplitude is from the trough of a-wave to peak of cornea positive b-wave. Latency of each wave is measured from stimulus onset, marked by a vertical line across the baseline, to peak of the response **(Fig. 8)**. Both amplitude and implicit time should be measured for each

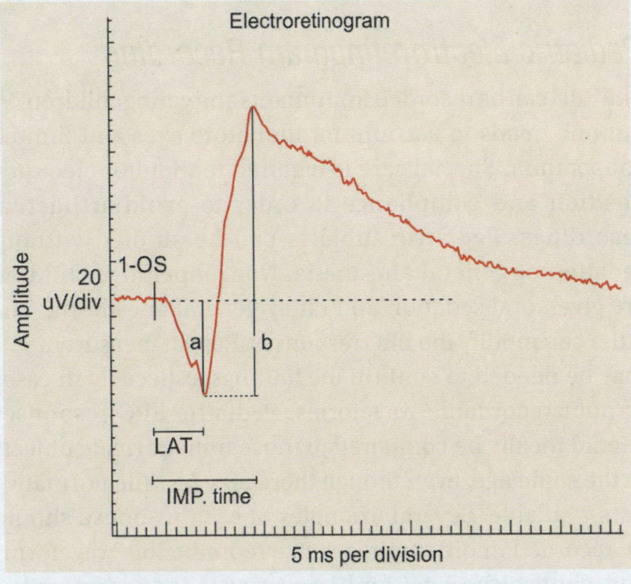

Fig. 8: Methodology of electroretinogram amplitudes and latency measurements (see text for details).

component of the waveform. For practical purposes, the variables most often measured are the b-wave amplitudes of the isolated rod response, maximal combined response and of single flash "cone response". The time-to-peak of the single flash 30 Hz flicker response and b-wave latency of maximal combined response is measured. Amplitudes and appearance of the OPs[9,10] are highly dependent upon stimulus conditions, adaptation, and amplifier filter characteristics, but most authors describe three major peaks often followed by a fourth smaller one. Comparison of the response to the laboratory normative wavelets may be adequate for many clinical purposes at our present state of knowledge. An overall index of OP amplitude can be obtained by adding up measurements of the three major peaks, preferably from lines spanning the bases of the adjacent troughs, but alternatively from the adjacent troughs directly (to allow use of measuring cursors with digitized systems). Some authors advise measurement of individual peaks.

Normal Values

Due to multiple variables that can affect the ERG waveforms, it is recommend that each laboratory should confirm normal values for its own equipment and patient population taking an appropriate sample size. All ERG reporting should include normal values and the limits of normal.

Reporting of the Electroretinogram

The reports or communications of ERG data should include two representative waveforms of each of the standard responses displayed with amplitude and time calibrations and labeled with respect to stimulus variables and the state of light or dark adaptation. Details of the standardized reporting conditions are available in the literature.[9,10]

Pediatric Electroretinogram Recording

The ERG can be recorded from infants and young children,[9,10] but one needs to account for immature eyes and limited cooperation. Special care is required to monitor electrode position and compliance in order to avoid artifactual recordings. Pediatric subjects can be studied without sedation or general anesthesia. Noncooperative children are given oral sedation and rarely general anesthesia. The latter can modify the ERG responses. Repeat measurements may be needed to confirm the findings, especially in cases of poor recordable waveforms. Pediatric ERG responses should ideally be compared to those from normal subjects of the same age, even though there may be little normative data available. Several examples of each response should be recorded in order to recognize reproducible waveforms and choose the best and largest of these reproducible responses.

Limitations of Electroretinogram

- Flash ERG is affected only if the retinal dysfunction is widespread. In localized conditions, even if they involve high-cell density area say of the macula, the flash ERG can be normal. This is seen in conditions like Stargardt's heredomacular degeneration and early stages of cone dystrophy or localized RP. Ganglion cell function is not reflected in flash ERG. Flash ERG does not correlate with visual acuity.
- Diurnal variation exists in rod-ERG b-wave amplitudes; therefore, it should be accounted in serial measurements or research protocols.
- A number of artifacts such as a blink reflex, muscular tension artifacts (photomyoclonic response) or improper electrode placement and contact can lead to erroneous results. The electrophysiologist should be aware of these and know how to get valid recordings.
- ERG recordings require a certain level of cooperation from the patient. Fixation is not critical in ERG recording but photophobia, claustrophobia, and excessive blinking and anxiety are known to alter the response.
- Hazy media and miotic pupils can cause erroneous results, as sufficient light does not reach the photoreceptors. Appropriate adjustments would be required to get meaningful data.
- Adjustments are also needed for age and high refractive error as these affect the ERG responses.

Pattern Electroretinogram

Some of the limitations of flash ERG can be overcome by more recent techniques of pattern electroretinogram (PERG) and mfERG. Pattern ERG is a contrast response driven by macular photoreceptors but originates in the ganglion cell layer of retina. It allows both a measure of central retinal function and retinal ganglion cell function. It is the only electrophysiological test that can provide direct assessment of the ganglion cells. PERG helps in improved interpretation of VEP abnormalities and helps to differentiate optic nerve pathology from the macular pathology.[19]

Recording Parameters and Measurement

The PERG is recorded **(Fig. 9A)** with refractive correction in place, without mydriasis, using noncontact lens electrodes.[12,13,19] Reference electrodes are placed on ipsilateral outer canthus, and not on forehead or ear, to avoid the contamination from the cortically generated VEP. Binocular stimulation and recording is usually preferred, except in cases of squint, so the better eye can maintain fixation and accommodation. It is a small response and may be difficult to record without stringent controls. Diurnal variation and test-retest variability may be important in longitudinal studies.

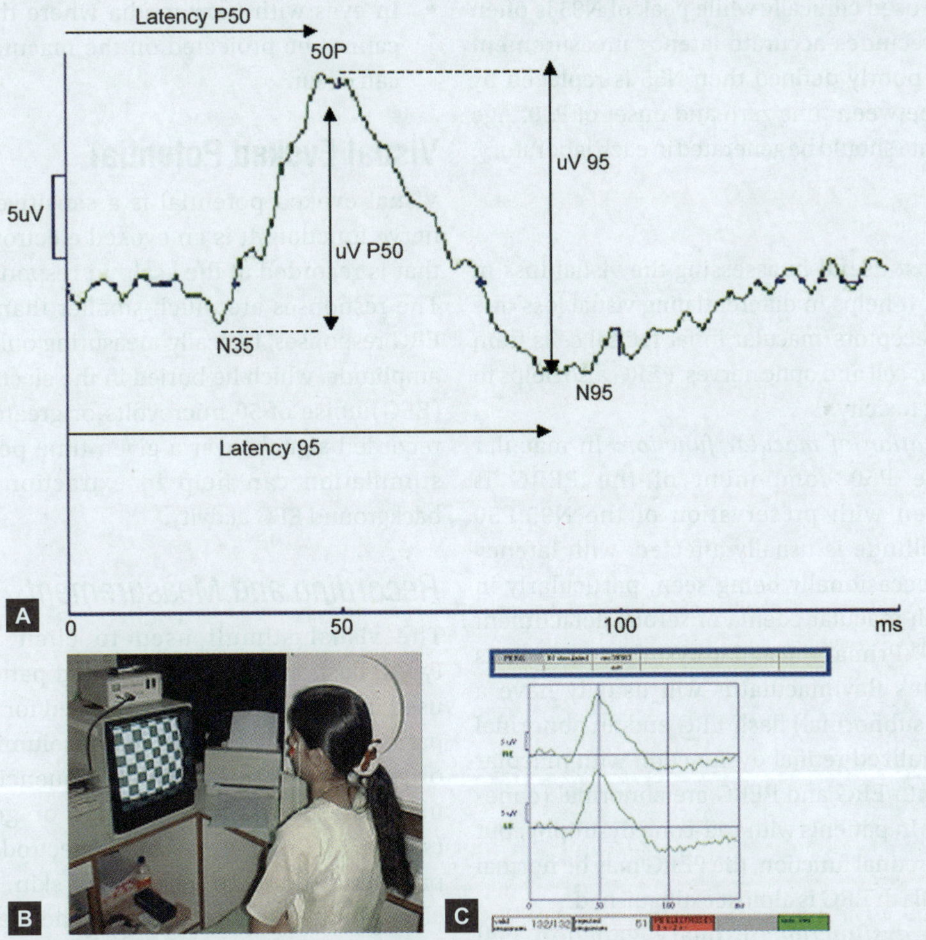

Figs. 9A to C: Pattern electroretinogram measurements (A); (B) Pattern electroretinogram (PERG) stimulus; (C) Actual recording of PERG from two eyes.

Pattern electroretinogram is measured as the electrical response to a pattern reversal checkerboard stimulus where the overall luminance is unchanged during pattern reversal. A high contrast (near 100%) black and white checkerboard pattern of 15- and 30-minute check size with pattern reversal method is recommended. Field size of stimulus should be between 10° and 16°, and the frame rate of the cathode ray tube (CRT) should be a minimum of 75 Hz or above. Stimulus strength of the white checks should be 80 cd m^{-2}. Steady fixation is very important because eye movement and blinking will cause severe artifacts. As the amplitudes of PERG signals are small, more averaging is needed. Often more than 150 responses are averaged to get each response. Sweep time of recording is about 150 ms. Computerized artifact rejection is essential and this should be set at no higher than 100 microvolts peak to peak. Background illumination should not be very bright or dim. Ordinary background room light suffices and should be kept constant for all recordings.

At a stimulus reversal rate of 16 reversals per second a sinusoidal waveform called steady-state PERG is obtained. This needs Fourier analysis to measure the amplitude and phase shift and is not often used clinically. At a slow rate of 1–3 Hz (2–6 reversals per second) pattern reversal, a transient PERG is obtained. Clinically, the transient PERG has two main components **(Fig. 9B)**. The P50 is an inner retinal component driven by the macular photoreceptors. N95 is the second component which is contrast related and is generated by the ganglion cells.[19] PERG P50 amplitudes can vary from 0.5 microvolts to 8 microvolts depending on stimulus characteristics such as the temporal frequency of the stimulus.[20] Bandpass filters of the AC coupled amplifiers are set from 1–100 Hz and notch filters should be switched off.

Three components are seen in PERG. There is an initial negative wave (N35) at 35 ms, a positive peak (P50) at 50 ms and a final negative N95 wave at 95 ms from stimulus onset. The P50 is an inner retinal component generated from ganglion cells but driven by the macular photoreceptors. N95 is the second component, which is contrast related, and is generated by the ganglion cells.

The P50 amplitude is measured form trough of N35 to the peak of P50, the N95 is measured from peak of P50 to the trough of N95 **(Fig. 9C)**. P50 latency is a more consistent measurement and used clinically while peak of N95 is often broad and this precludes accurate latency measurement for N95. If N35 is poorly defined then N35 is replaced by the average time between time zero and onset of P50. Age matched control data should be generated in each laboratory.

Clinical Uses

Pattern ERG is most useful in assessing the visual loss of unknown etiology. It helps in differentiating visual loss due to macular photoreceptors/macular inner retinal cells from diseases of ganglion cell and optic nerves. PERG also helps to monitor early drug toxicity.[21]

- *Primary evaluation of macular function*: In macular disorders, the P50 component of the PERG is abnormal, often with preservation of the N95:P50 ratio. P50 amplitude is usually affected, with latency changes only occasionally being seen, particularly in association with macular edema or serous detachment at the macula.[19] Primary macular dysfunction such as Stargardt-fundus flavimaculatus will usually have a normal (rarely subnormal) flash ERG and an abnormal PERG. In generalized retinal dysfunction with macular involvement both ERG and PERG are abnormal (cone-rod dystrophy). In patients with rod-cone dystrophy, but normal central retinal function, the PERG may be normal even when the flash ERG is almost extinguished.
- *Ganglion cell dysfunction*: Primary ganglion cell dysfunction is associated with marked N95 component loss, particularly Leber hereditary optic atrophy and advanced dominant optic atrophy.[19] Very severe optic nerve disease will also reduce P50 amplitude and P50 latency. Complete extinction of the PERG in relation to optic nerve disease rarely if ever occurs, providing at least one eye has enough vision to maintain fixation for binocular PERG recording. The PERG may still readily be detectable in an eye with no light perception.[19] It must be remembered that though pattern VEP is primarily used to detect optic nerve dysfunction, macular diseases can cause delayed VEP latency. PERG P50 defects associated with or without VEP abnormalities, point to macular dysfunction. Normal or a defect of only N95 component of PERG with an abnormal VEP suggests optic nerve/ganglion cell dysfunction.[19]

Limitations of Pattern Electroretinogram

- The PERG amplitudes are very small and so due to technical demands, not all laboratories record PERG as a routine. Stringent controls are required to avoid artifacts. The ISCEV standards are available for PERG recordings.[20]
- Patient cooperation is essential in recording PERG.
- All equipment for ocular electrophysiology do not have the capability to perform PERG.
- In eyes with hazy media where the pattern stimulus cannot be projected on the macula, erroneous results can occur.

Visual Evoked Potential

Visual evoked potential is a sensitive indicator of optic nerve function. It is an evoked electrophysiological signal that is recorded at the scalp in response to visual stimuli. The responses are much smaller than the full-field flash ERG responses, typically measuring only 5–10 microvolts in amplitude, which lie buried in the electroencephalographic (EEG) noise of 50 microvolts or greater. Averaging of the recorded signals over a given time period after repeated stimulation can help in extraction of VEP from the background EEG activity.

Recording and Measurement

The visual stimuli used to elicit VEP are of three types: flash, pattern-reversal, and pattern onset.[22] The SF used in ERG recording can be used for flash-VEP also. The pattern stimulus consists of an isoluminant checkerboard or grating of various spatial frequencies. Skin electrodes used are silver-silver chloride or gold-disk electrode (*see* **Fig. 5**). Good contact of the electrodes using conducting paste and thorough cleaning of skin, helps in obtaining clean and reliable recordings. The electrodes are placed on the scalp relative to bony landmarks in relation to the head size as per the international 10/20 system[23] **(Fig. 10)**. The anteroposterior midline measurements are based on the distance between the nasion, inion, and vertex. The active electrode is placed on the midline over the visual occipital cortex (OZ) while reference electrode at the frontal pole (FZ). The ground electrode is at the forehead or earlobe.

Recordings are done with refractive correction without mydriasis using monocular stimulation. Prechiasmal lesions are reliably detected by pattern-reversal stimulation while flash stimulus is used in difficult and uncooperative patients or those with dense media opacities and very poor vision. Pattern onset/offset stimulus is especially useful in malingerers and patients with nystagmus, due to short stimulus duration and inability of the subject to consciously defocus this stimulus. For chiasmal and postchiasmal lesions, multichannel recordings are required as a single midline channel with active electrode only over the occipital cortex can miss lesions. The VEP traces (two reproducible records of each) can be presented as positive upwards **(Fig. 11)** or negative upwards. The polarity convention and stimulus parameters used should be indicated in the report besides the amplitude and latency. Latency is measured from the stimulus onset to peak of the component measured. It must be remembered that interocular difference in the

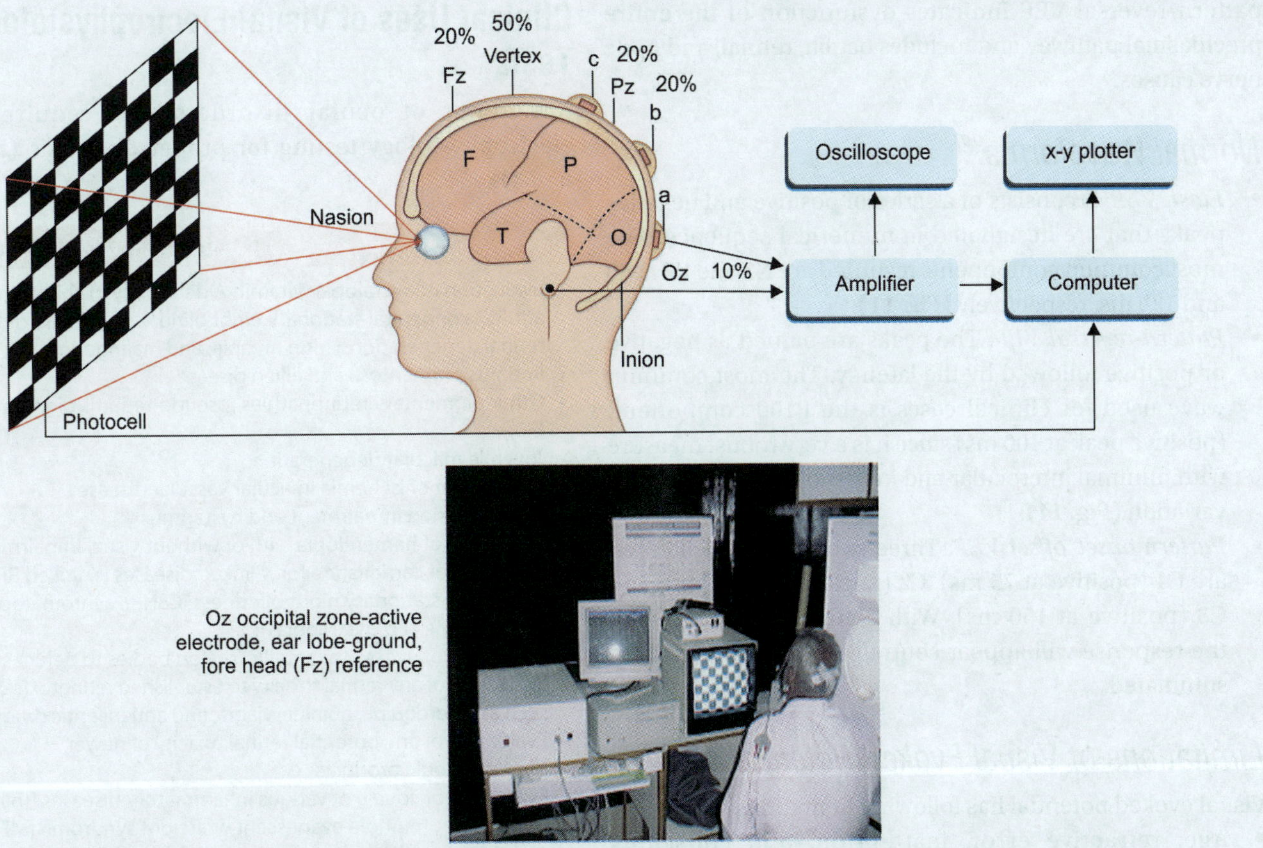

Fig. 10: The International 10/20 system of electrode placement for midline single channel visual evoked potential (VEP). Inset shows pattern VEP recording in progress.

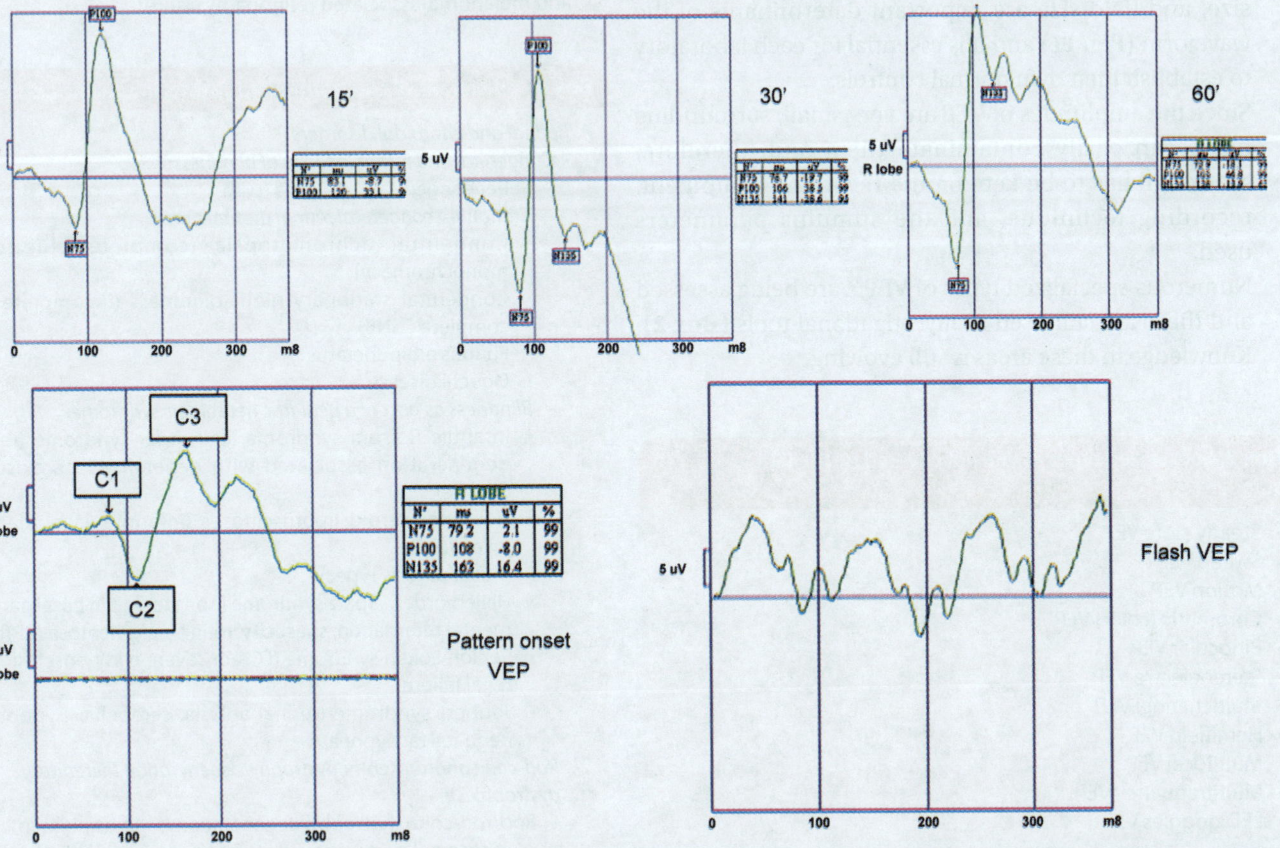

Fig. 11: Normal pattern reversal to three different check sizes (top—15, 30, and 60 minutes), pattern-onset (bottom left) and flash (bottom right) visual evoked potential (VEP).

pattern-reversal VEP indicates dysfunction of the entire prechiasmal pathway and includes ocular, retinal, and optic nerve causes.

Normal Waveforms[22]

- *Flash VEP*: It consists of a series of positive and negative peaks that are designated in numerical sequence. The most common components recorded are N2 and P2 at 90 and 120 ms, respectively **(Fig. 11)**.
- *Pattern-reversal VEP*: The peaks are named as negative or positive followed by the latency. The most common wave used for clinical cases is the P100 component, (positive peak at 100 ms) since it is a very robust measure with minimal interocular and intersubject measurement variation **(Fig. 11)**.
- *Pattern onset/offset VEP*: Three components described are C1 (positive at 75 ms), C2 (negative at 125 ms), and C3 (positive at 150 ms). With a stimulated hemifield, the response will appear contralateral to the hemifield stimulated.

Limitations of Visual Evoked Potential

Visual evoked potential has following limitations:

- Age, refractive error, inattention, and conscious defocusing of the pattern affect the VEP latency.
- Stimulus parameters such as contrast, luminance, check size, and field size are important determinants of the waveform **(Fig. 11)** and it is essential for each laboratory to establish their own normal controls.
- Since the amplitudes of VEP are very small, surrounding noise can easily contaminate them and, therefore, strict vigil has to be kept on the recording equipment, recording technique, and the stimulus parameters used.
- Numerous specialized types of VEP[22] are being assessed and these are still used as investigational tools **(Box 2)**. Knowledge in these areas is still evolving.

Box 2: Specialized types of VEP not covered by the ISCEV standard.[22]

- Steady state VEP
- Sweep VEP
- Motion VEP
- Chromatic (color) VEP
- Binocular VEP
- Stereoelectro VEP
- Multichannel VEP
- Hemifield VEP
- Multifocal VEP
- Multifrequency VEP
- LED goggles VEP

(ISCEV: International Society for Clinical Electrophysiology of Vision; LED: light-emitting diode; VEP: visual evoked potential)

Clinical Uses of Visual Electrophysiological Tests

A number of ocular disorders may require visual electrophysiology testing for proper diagnosis **(Boxes 3 and 4)**.

Box 3: Common indications for electroretinography.

- Evaluation of nyctalopia (vitamin A deficiency in children and adults), congenital stationary night blindness, primary diffuse retinal degenerations, high myopia, and malingering
- Retinitis pigmentosa and allied disease
- Other pigmentary retinopathies [pseudo-retinitis pigmentosa (RP)]
- Juvenile macular degeneration
- Assessment of ischemia in ocular vascular disease
- Infantile vision impairment and nystagmus
- Evaluation of hemerelopia with or without visual impairment
- Detection of carrier state for X-linked diseases [X-linked RP, congenital stationary night blindness (CSNB), achromatopsia, cone or cone-rod dystrophies)]
- Evaluation of eyes with metallic foreign bodies to detect siderosis
- Evaluation of any retinal toxicity to established retinotoxic drugs such as chloroquine, quinine, viagra, and antiepileptic drugs
- Evaluation of any potential retinal toxicity of newer pharmacologic products
- Evaluation of course of various inflammatory diseases [(birdshot retinopathy, multiple evanescent white dot syndrome (MEWDS), and acute zonal occult outer retinopathy (AZOOR)]
- Diagnosis of various malignancy induced autoimmune retinopathies [including cancer-associated retinopathy (CAR), and melanoma-associated retinopathy (MAR)]

Box 4: Indications of electrophysiology tests in specific diseases.

A. Retinal and choroidal disorders

- *Congenital and infantile forms of blindness*:
  - Leber congenital amaurosis (LCA)
  - *Stationary congenital retinal dysfunction*:
    - Congenital achromatopsia (complete blue cone monochromacy)
    - Congenital stationary night blindness (incomplete and complete CSNB)
    - Fundus albipunctatus
    - Oguchi disease
  - *Blindness as part of a pediatric neurologic syndrome*:
    - Infantile Refsum syndrome, Zellweger syndrome (retinal degeneration associated with generalized peroxisomal disease)
    - Neuronal ceroid lipofuscinoses (infantile, late infantile, juvenile)
    - Mucolipidosis type IV
    - Hallervorden–Spatz syndrome [iron storage in basal ganglia, mental retardation, spasticity, retinitis pigmentosa (RP)]
    - Senior–Loken syndrome (LCA or severe early-onset RP with renal failure)
    - Joubert syndrome (retinal aplasia, cerebellar hypoplasia, neonatal tachypnea)
- *Rod-cone photoreceptor dystrophy/degeneration (hereditary dystrophies)*:
  - Rod/rod-cone dystrophy/degeneration (retinitis pigmentosa)
    - Autosomal dominant, autosomal recessive, X-linked

Contd...

Contd...

- RP with slightly greater cone loss
- RP with electronegative electroretinogram ERG
– Cone and cone-rod dystrophies
- *Macular dystrophies*:
  – Peripherin/retinal degeneration slow type (RDS)
  – X-linked (juvenile) retinoschisis
  – Stargardt's macular dystrophy
  – Bests macular dystrophy
  – Pattern dystrophy

B. Choroidal dystrophies:
- Choroidal atrophy
- Gyrate atrophy of the choroid and retina
- Choroideremia—patients and carries
- Central areolar choroidal atrophy

C. Retinal dystrophies associated with other diseases:
- Usher syndrome (RP and congenital deafness)
- Bardet–Biedl syndrome (RP, hexadactyly, obesity, hypogenitalism, ± mental retardation)
- Kearns–Sayre syndrome [mitochondrial myopathy, chronic progressive external ophthalmoplegia (CPEO), RP, heart block]
- Chronic progressive external ophthalmoplegia plus (CPEO+)

D. Bruch's membrane disorders:
- Angioid streaks [pseudoxanthoma elasticum (PXE)]
- Dominant drusen

E. Hereditary vitreoretinal disorders:
- X-linked juvenile retinoschisis
- Goldmann–Favre syndrome
- Enhanced S-cone syndrome (ESCS)

F. Inflammatory conditions:
- Multiple evanescent white dot syndrome (MEWDS)
- Birdshot retinochoroidopathy
- Pars planitis
- Syphilis
- Pigmented paravenous retinochoroidal atrophy (PPRCA)
- Diffuse unilateral subacute neuroretinitis (DUSN)
- Rubella

G. Vascular disorders:
- Sickle-cell retinopathy
- Ophthalmic artery occlusion
- Central retinal artery occlusion
- Central retinal vein occlusion
- Carotid insufficiency (ocular ischemic syndrome)
- Diabetic retinopathy

H. Toxic disorders:
- Chloroquine and hydroxychloroquine
- Quinine
- Digoxin
- Thioridazine
- Chlorpromazine
- Indomethacin
- Methanol

I. Miscellaneous:
- Albinism
- High myopia
- *Acquired retinal dysfunction/degeneration*:
  – Vitamin A deficiency (malabsorption syndromes)
  – Autoimmune retinopathy, including cancer-associated retinopathy (CAR) and melanoma-associated retinopathy (MAR)
- Retinal (cone-rod) dystrophy with supernormal and delayed rod ERG b-waves

It must be remembered that ERG needs to be interpreted in the context of other clinical features and investigative reports to arrive at the correct diagnosis. One can be way off the true diagnosis if it is based on ERG recording alone.

Photoreceptor Dysfunction

In widespread genetic retinal photoreceptor disorders like RP or choroideremia, a profound reduction of ERG is seen even when retina looks apparently normal.

The diagnosis of RP is often obvious in patients with history of night blindness, progressive peripheral field constriction and typical retinal changes including equatorial pigment migration, arterial attenuation, RPE atrophy, and disk pallor as seen in this 40 years male with visual acuity of 20/50 and residual visual fields of 10° centrally **(Fig. 12A)** ERG has a limited role in diagnosis but helps to assess residual macular photoreceptor function. In the test ERG may not be recordable with routine testing using SF. With extensive filtering and averaging **(Fig. 12B)** response (arrow) can be elicited identifying residual cone function. PERG is a more reliable method of eliciting residual central macular function **(Fig. 13)**. Fields are also important in such cases to define legal blindness and functional disability in the patient. ERG, however, is essential in research studies to demonstrate diffuse, severe photoreceptor dysfunction that characterizes even early stages of RP. A normal ERG recorded beyond 6 years of age practically rules out possibility of developing RP in future. ERG helps to diagnose patients with atypical findings and helps in carrier detection. Flash ERG in RP **(Figs. 12 to 14)** can be either extinguished, or show a rod-cone or rarely a cone-rod or even a negative type of ERG dysfunction. All such types usually point to a progressive disease especially if implicit time abnormalities are present. True sector or localized central (restricted) disease **(Fig. 15)** may give amplitude reduction with no implicit time change, whereas diffuse or generalized disease is usually associated with abnormal implicit time.[24,25]

Localized Photoreceptor Loss with Pigmentary Retinal Dystrophy

In atypical retinal pigmentary dystrophies, ERG may help to confirm the diagnosis and differentiate various conditions. For example in a 65 years old female patient with best-corrected visual acuity (BCVA) of 20/80 in each eye, there was no history of night blindness or reduced dark adaptation but gradual progressive loss for reading since 5 years. Posterior pole showed RPE atrophy and mild pigment migration while the rest of the retina was normal **(Fig. 15)**. Retinal arteries showed attenuation and disk had temporal pallor. ERG was not extinguished or severely affected, excluding the diagnosis of typical RP. However, both scotopic and photopic responses showed 20–40% reduction in amplitudes with only

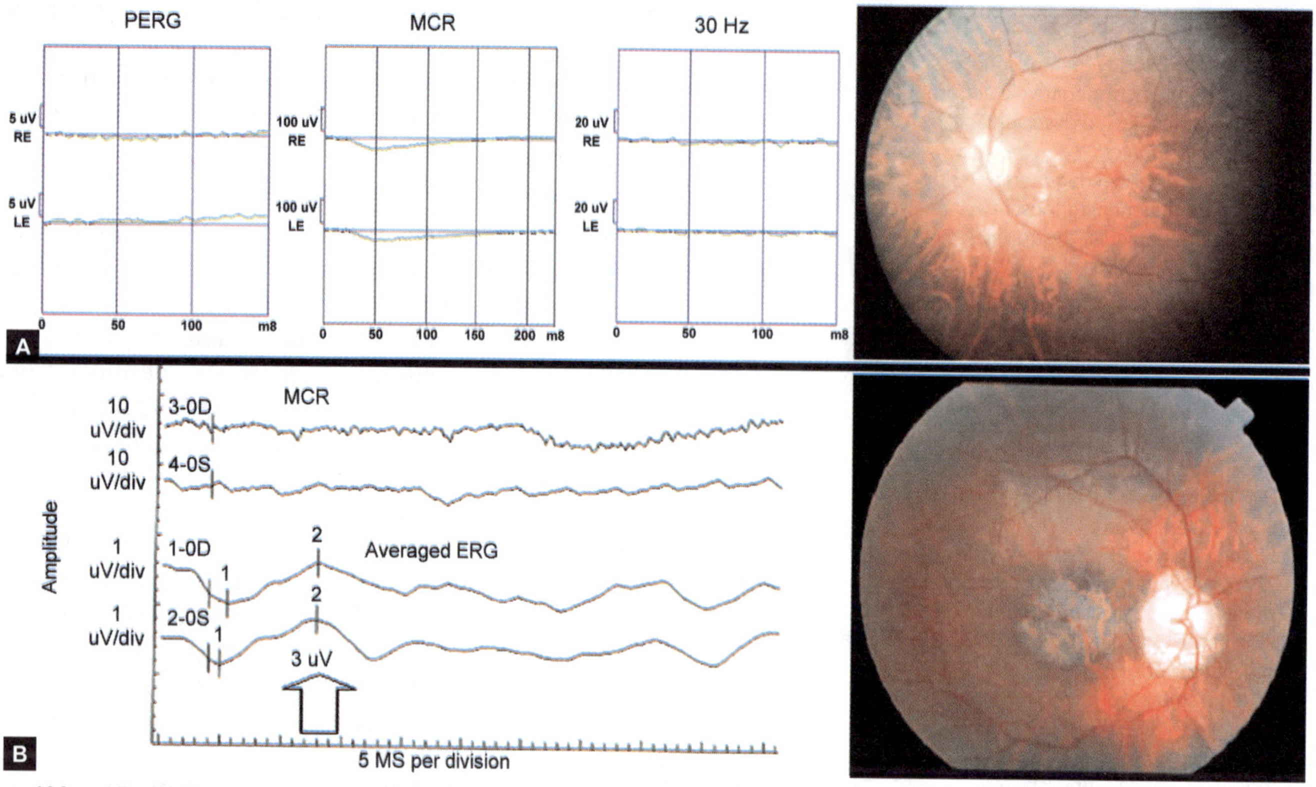

Figs. 12A and B: (A) Unrecordable PERG and flash ERG in advanced retinitis pigmentosa depicting macular involvement VA 20/80 OU, fields central 10°, night blindness present; (B) Extensive filtering and averaging of the MCR to elicit a microvolt ERG (arrow), outside ISCEV standard showing residual retinal function in patient of RP with visual acuity of 20/800 and macular atrophy.
(ERG: electroretinogram; ISCEV: International Society for Clinical Electrophysiology of Vision; MCR: maximal combined response; PERG: pattern electroretinogram)

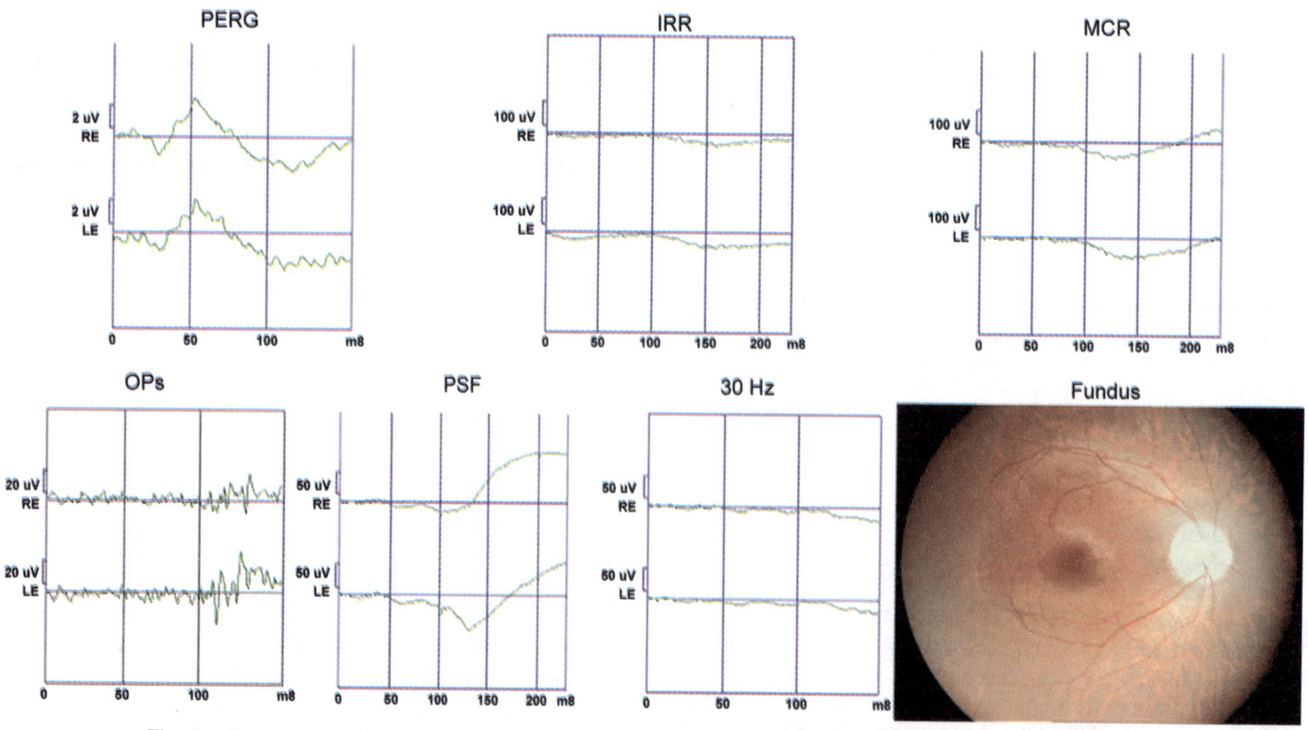

Fig. 13: Preserved PERG in a patient of RP with extinguished flash ERG responses showing macular sparing. Visual acuity of 25 years male was 20/25 and visual fields showed central island of 10°.
(ERG: electroretinogram; IRR: isolated rod response; MCR: maximal combined response; OPs: oscillatory potentials; PERG: pattern electroretinogram; PSF: photopic single flash; RP: retinitis pigmentosa)

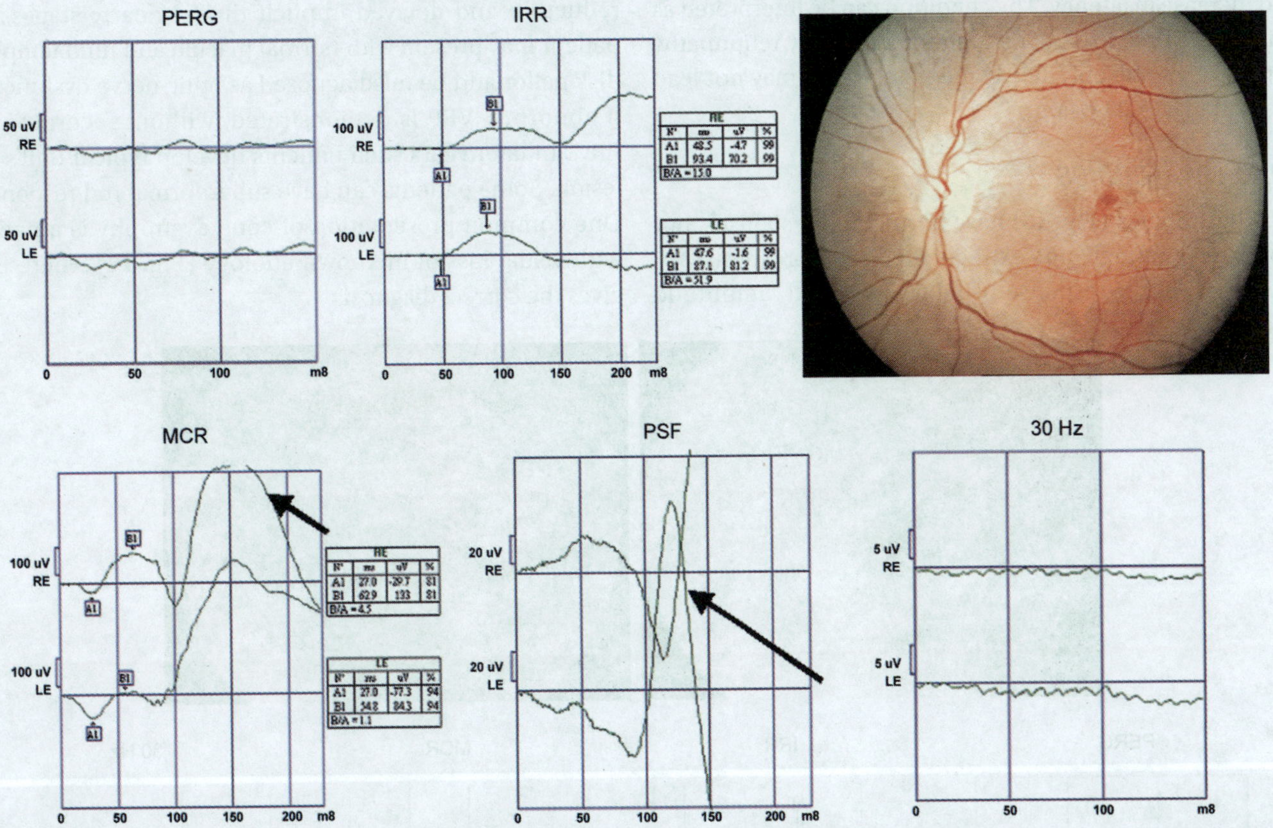

Fig. 14: *Cone-rod dystrophy*: Retinal dystrophy with macular bull's eye lesion, arterial narrowing, peripheral RPE degeneration and disk pallor. ERG showed absent cone functions with subnormal but recordable isolated rod response suggestive of cone-rod dystrophy in 29 years patient with VA 20/80. Note large blink artifacts towards end of recordings (arrows) that are not uncommon due to photophobia in these subjects.
(ERG: electroretinogram; IRR: isolated rod response; MCR: maximal combined response; PERG: pattern electroretinogram; PSF: photopic single flash)

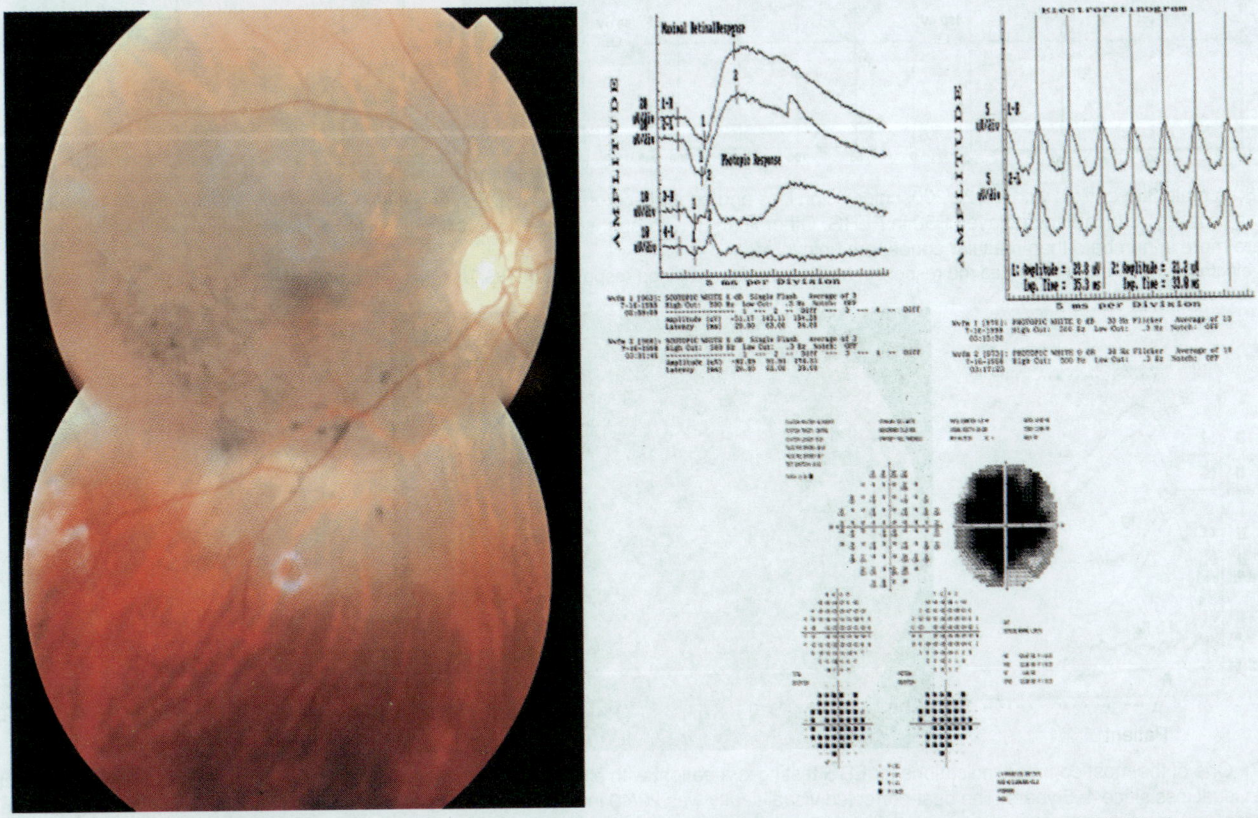

Fig. 15: Fundus photograph showing central location of pigmentary retinopathy with normal periphery. Electroretinogram (ERG) shows subnormal rod and cone functions and not extinguished ERG. The disease is likely to remain localized and minimally progressive. Visual acuity of patient 20/80, central scotoma on fields but with no night blindness.

mild increase in latency. The condition can be interpreted as an inverse RP/central RP or central pigmentary retinopathy that is likely to be only slowly progressive and may not lead to less than 20/400 vision.

Cone Dystrophies

Cone dystrophies **(Fig. 16)** have normal rod responses, but subnormal, though not extinguished, cone responses.[26] The 30 Hz flicker response usually shows both amplitude reduction and delayed implicit time. In early stages, the patient may present with normal macula and mild temporal disk pallor and be misdiagnosed as optic nerve dysfunction if abnormal VEP is demonstrated, without recording the ERG. In later years such patients develop typical Bull's eye lesion. Some patients can have supernormal rod responses. One common presentation of cone dystrophy is a patient with visual loss of unknown etiology **(Fig. 17)** where ERG gives the correct diagnosis.

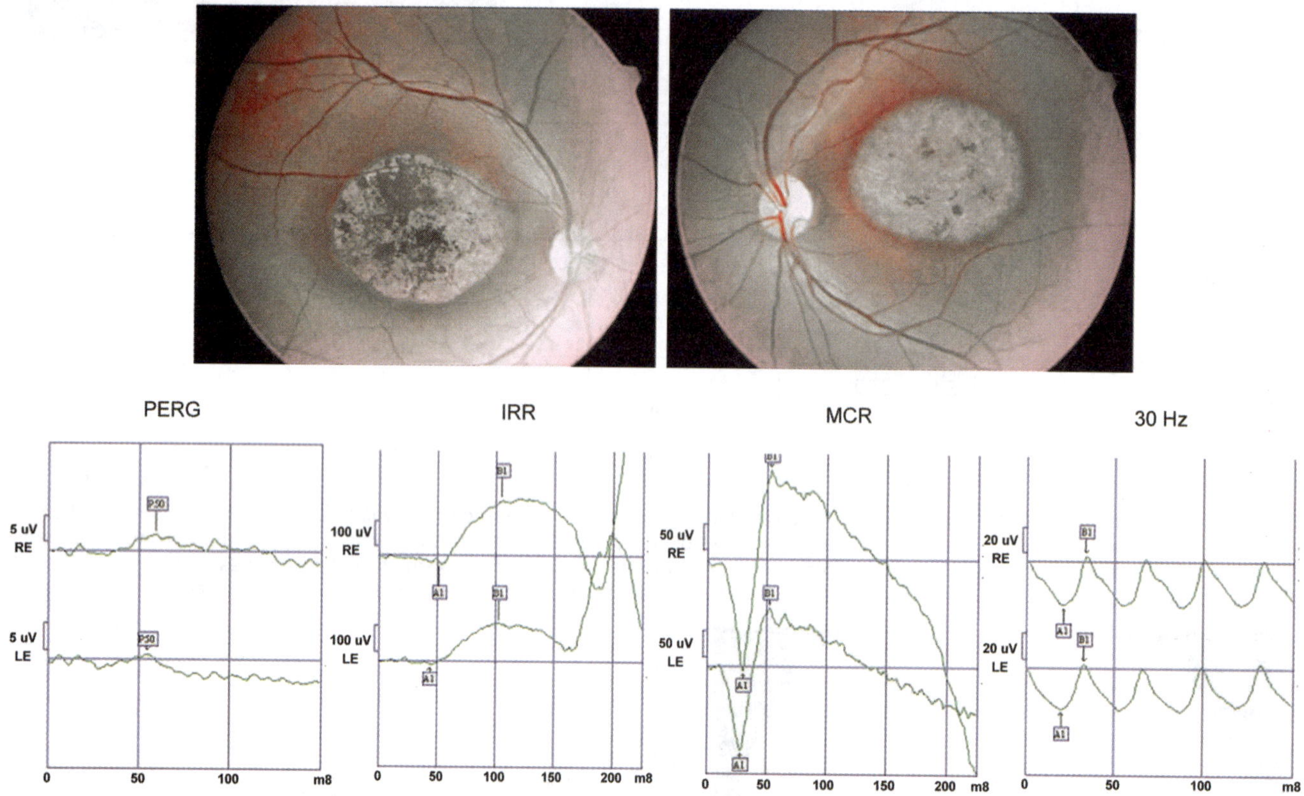

Fig. 16: A male 36-year-old with VA 20/200, color vision loss and central scotoma. Localized cone dystrophy involving only macular photoreceptors, it shows severely reduced and delayed P50 in PERG. Other flash ERG responses are normal including photopic responses as the peripheral cones (that are more in numbers than macular cones) are uninvolved.

(ERG: electroretinogram; IRR: isolated rod response; MCR: maximal combined response; PERG: pattern electroretinogram)

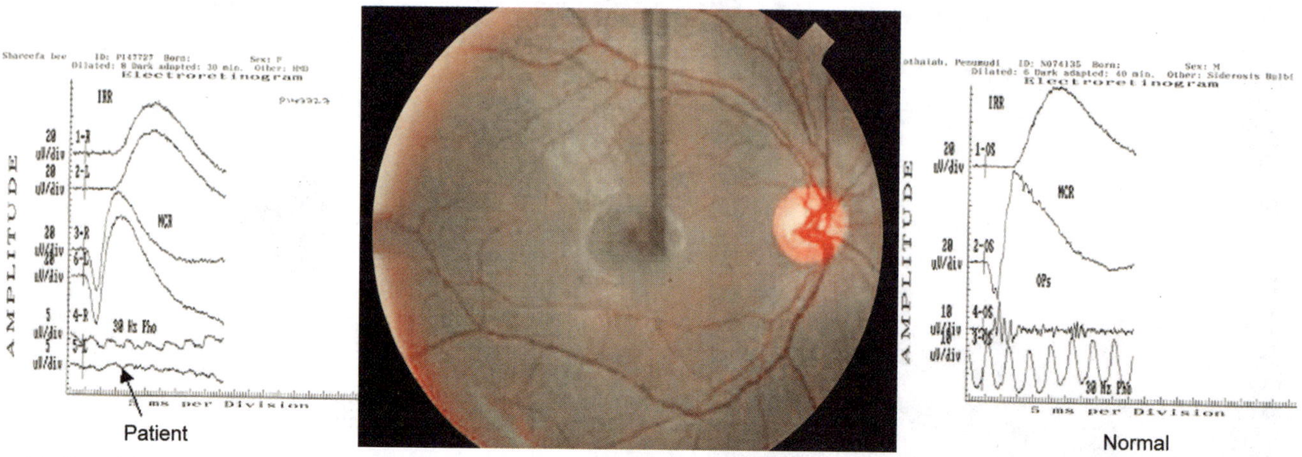

Fig. 17: One of the most common indications for ERG testing is a patient with a visual loss of unknown etiology. This 42-year-old female had history of mild visual loss since 4–5 years. The best-corrected visual acuity was 20/40 in each eye. Clinically, ocular examinations including detailed anterior and posterior segment evaluation were normal. Visual fields showed no abnormality. ERG showed markedly subnormal, but not absent, cone flicker response (arrow) with normal rod response suggestive of an early adult-onset cone dystrophy. The PSF is not depicted.

(ERG: electroretinogram; PSF: photopic single flash)

Inner Retinal Dysfunction: Negative Electroretinogram

A negative ERG is where the a-wave is unaffected but the b-wave in the scotopic maximal retinal response has a selective reduction of amplitude. It usually signifies diseases sparing the photoreceptors and involving the dysfunction of post-phototransduction and probably postreceptor cells in the middle retinal layers. In a majority of cases an etiology can be detected after correlating clinical and ERG findings, but in some cases the clinical entity cannot be labeled as specific.

Causes of negative ERG[27] include CSNB (complete and incomplete), fundus albipunctatus, Oguchi's disease **(Figs. 18 to 20)**,[28] X-linked retinoschisis,[29] quinine toxicity, melanoma-associated retinopathy (MAR),[30] Batten's disease, and occasionally in cone-rod dystrophy **(Box 5)**. Carcinoma-associated retinopathy (CAR) does not usually give a "negative" ERG but profound global ERG reduction in keeping with dysfunction at the level of the photoreceptor.[30] It occurs due to damage from circulating antibodies. Central retinal artery obstruction (CRAO) also has a negative ERG (*vide infra*). In patient of Oguchi's disease and increased amplitudes of responses in PERG and single flash cone ERG **(Fig. 19)** may occur after prolonged dark adaptation that also changes the golden metallic color of retina to a relatively normal color.

Ischemic Vascular Retinal Disorders

The ERG changes are profoundly helpful to detect inner retinal ischemia since fundus fluorescein angiography (FFA) or fundus appearance may not detect the true extent of retinal ischemia.[31,32] ERG is an indispensable and extremely powerful but unfortunately underutilized tool to differentiate ischemic from nonischemic obstruction of the central retinal vein **(Figs. 21 and 22)**. Reduced b-wave amplitude has 80-90% sensitivity and 70-80% specificity to detect inner retinal ischemia. An absolute increase of more than 37 ms in latency of the flicker ERG responses or a difference of more than 7 ms between affected and normal eye are almost pathognomonic of ischemic type of central retinal vein occlusion (CRVO) in a given clinical setting.

Reliable information from FFA may be available only in 50–60% cases of CRVO due to media haze, extensive hemorrhages, poor quality photographs, and inability to visualize peripheral retina. ERG circumvents all these limitations as it is global response from the whole retina and is not too much affected by media haze.

Other conditions like ocular ischemic syndrome[33] **(Fig. 23)**, central retinal artery occlusion (CRAO) **(Fig. 24)**, and ophthalmic artery occlusion (extinguished ERG)[34] are also very well detected on ERG. The "negative" ERG in CRAO[34] occurs due to the double blood supply of the retina. The RPE/photoreceptors (a wave) are spared as they are

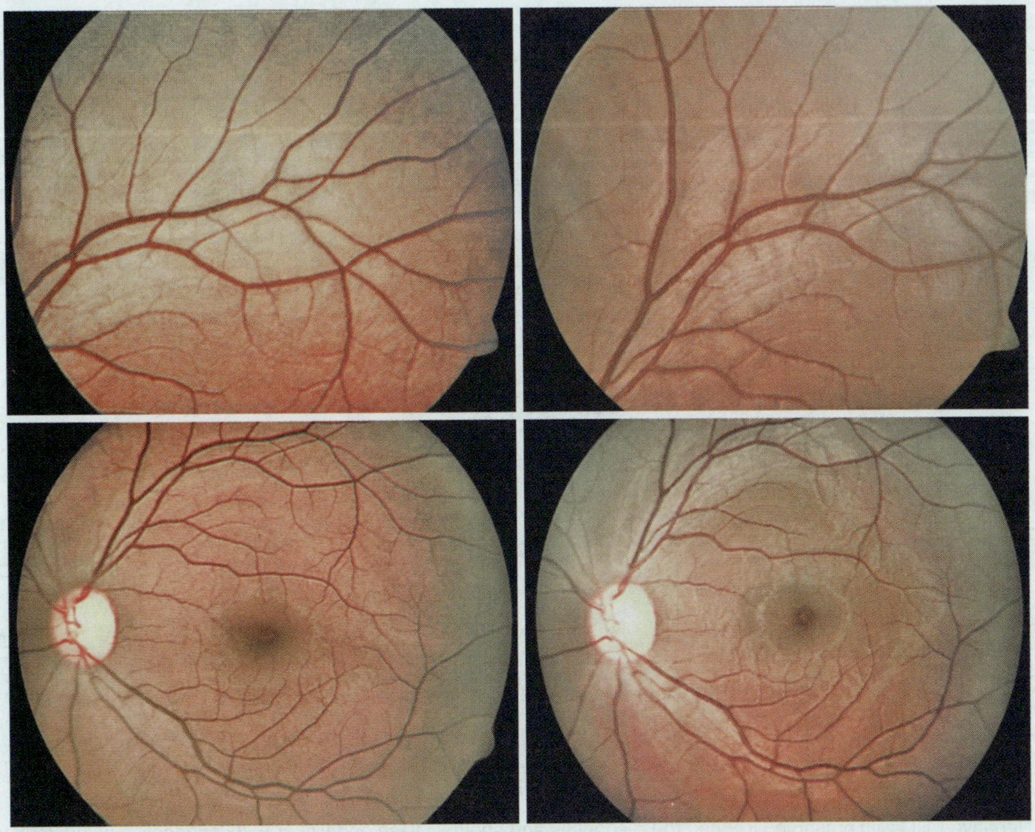

Fig. 18: Congenital stationary night blindness in Oguchi's disease. Fundus appearance before (left) and 2 hours after dark adaptation (right). Corresponding electroretinogram are shown in **Figure 19**.

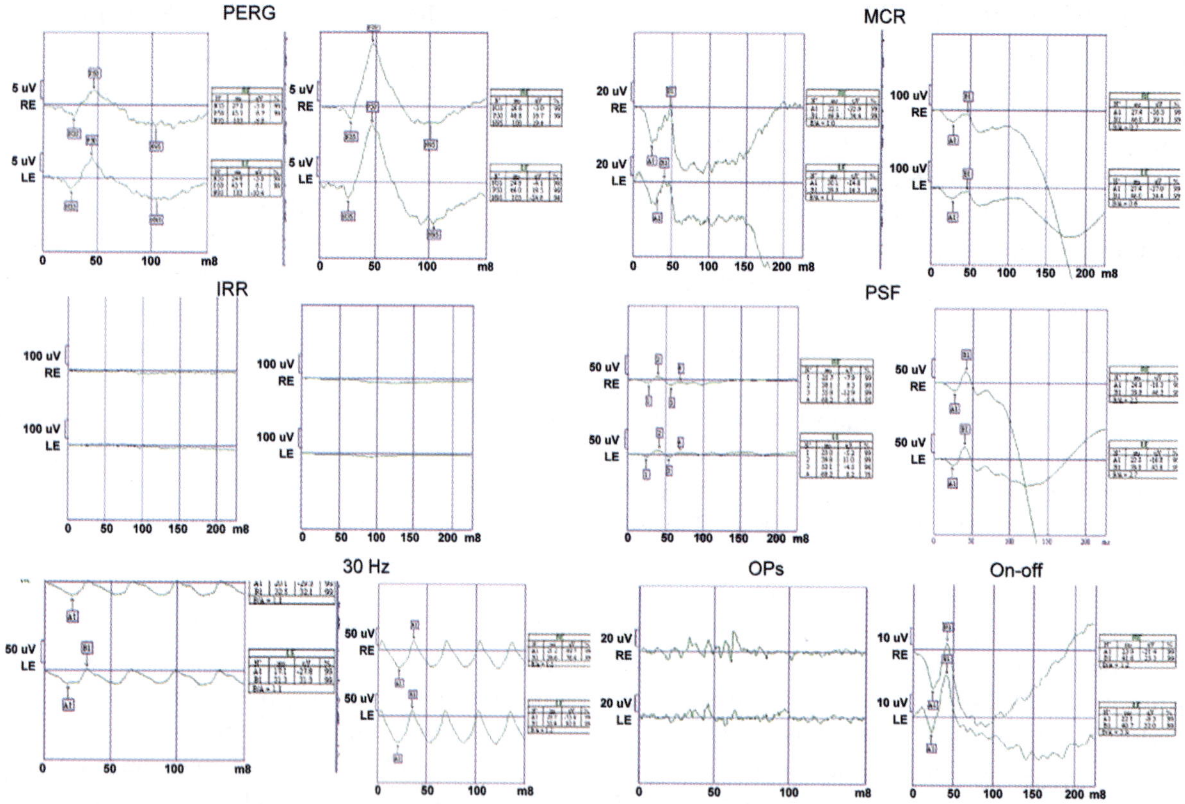

Fig. 19: Electroretinogram findings after 20 minutes and after 2 hours of dark adaptation in Oguchi's disease. In each case, the left graph is before and right graph is after the prolonged dark adaptation. The oscillatory potentials and on-off responses were recorded only once before prolonged dark adaptation and shows absence of off-response. Baseline findings are similar to those seen in complete forms of congenital stationary night blindness (CSNB) with normal fundus with the exception of a much smaller or nearly absent maximal combined response (MCR) b-wave in classical complete CSNB.

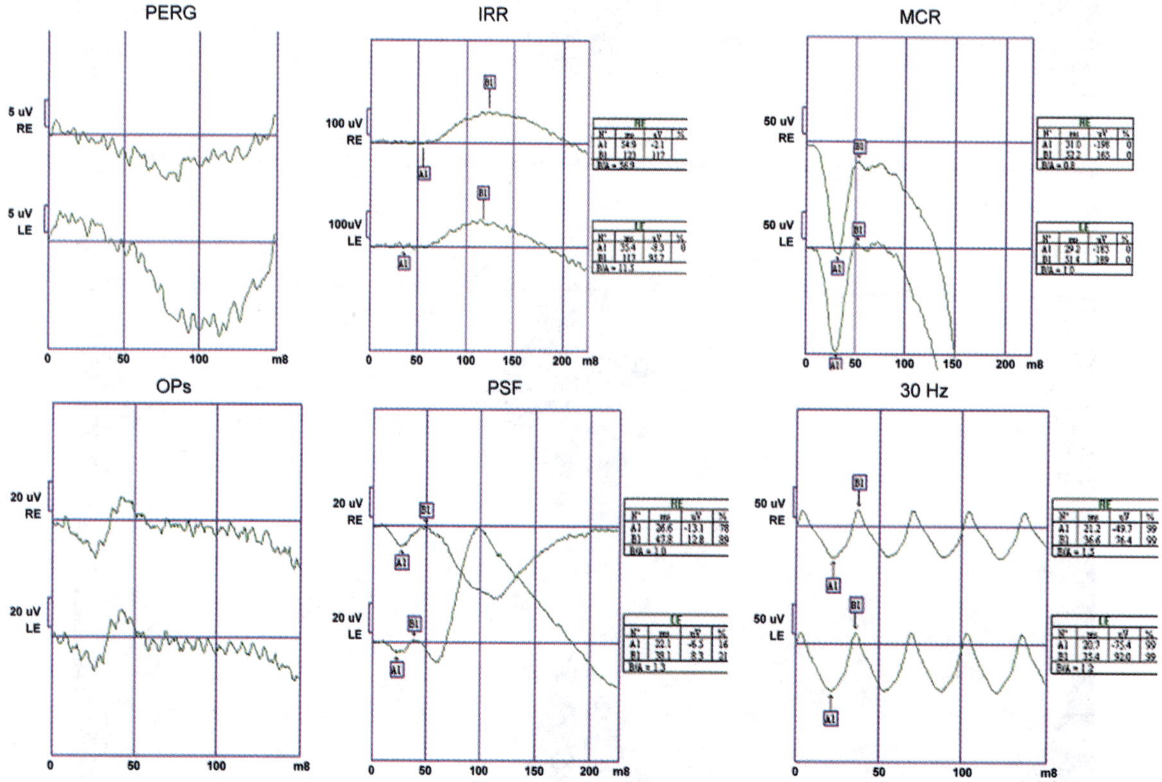

Fig. 20: Negative ERG with preserved isolated rod responses and photopic flash and flicker ERG suggestive of incomplete CSNB. (ERG: electroretinogram; IRR: isolated rod response; MCR: maximal combined response; OPs: oscillatory potentials; PERG: pattern electroretinogram; PSF: photopic single flash; CSNB: congenital stationary night blindness)

supplied via choroidal circulation, but bipolar cells and amacrine cells (b-wave and OPs) are affected as they are supplied via central retinal artery. In ophthalmic artery obstruction where both retinal and choroidal circulation are affected, the ERG is unrecordable as all retinal cell layers are involved.[34]

In ocular ischemic syndrome, ERG is extremely useful since clinical presentation of this under diagnosed clinical entity is variable.[35] In diabetic retinopathy[36] progressive abnormalities in ERG are seen with progression of the retinopathy. The OPs show profound reduction in case of new vessels on disk (NVD). The ERG can be subnormal even before clinical retinopathy, possibly due to metabolic effects on the retinal cells. ERG, however, cannot predict accurately the presence of PDR and is, therefore, not used clinically for monitoring diabetic retinopathy.

Box 5: Conditions associated with electronegative ERG.

- CSNB/Oguchi
- Juvenile retinoschisis
- CRAO and CRVO
- Familial optic atrophy
- Siderosis bulbi
- Quinine
- Some forms of RP and cone-rod dystrophy
- Melanoma-associated retinopathy and CAR
- Unclassified

(CAR: cancer-associated retinopathy; CRAO: central retinal artery obstruction; CRVO: central retinal vein occlusion; CSNB: congenital stationary night blindness; ERG: electroretinogram; RP: retinitis pigmentosa)

Drug Toxicity and Monitoring Health of Retina[25]

Electroretinogram helps to differentiate nyctalopia due to vitamin A deficiency from CSNB and RP. ERG is indicated particularly in adults such as those with alcoholic liver disease, chronic pancreatitis, or malabsorption syndromes. The rod responses are markedly affected and white flecks may be seen in the retina. Visual acuity is unaffected. Similarly, ERG abnormalities can be seen in drug toxicity especially with hydroxychloroquine, chloroquine, quinine, and thioridazine. VEP is useful to detect ethambutol toxicity **(Fig. 25)**.

Electroretinogram can detect and prognosticate siderotic changes in eyes with retained iron intraocular foreign body (IOFB).[30] Initially ERG has a subnormal b-wave on maximal combined scotopic response that can progress to a negative ERG with time and ultimately become extinguished. Removal of IOFB in eyes with recordable ERG, may lead to improvement in ERG changes and a stable outcome. In advanced siderosis, removal of IOFB will not stop progressive visual loss and sometimes phthisis bulbi develops.

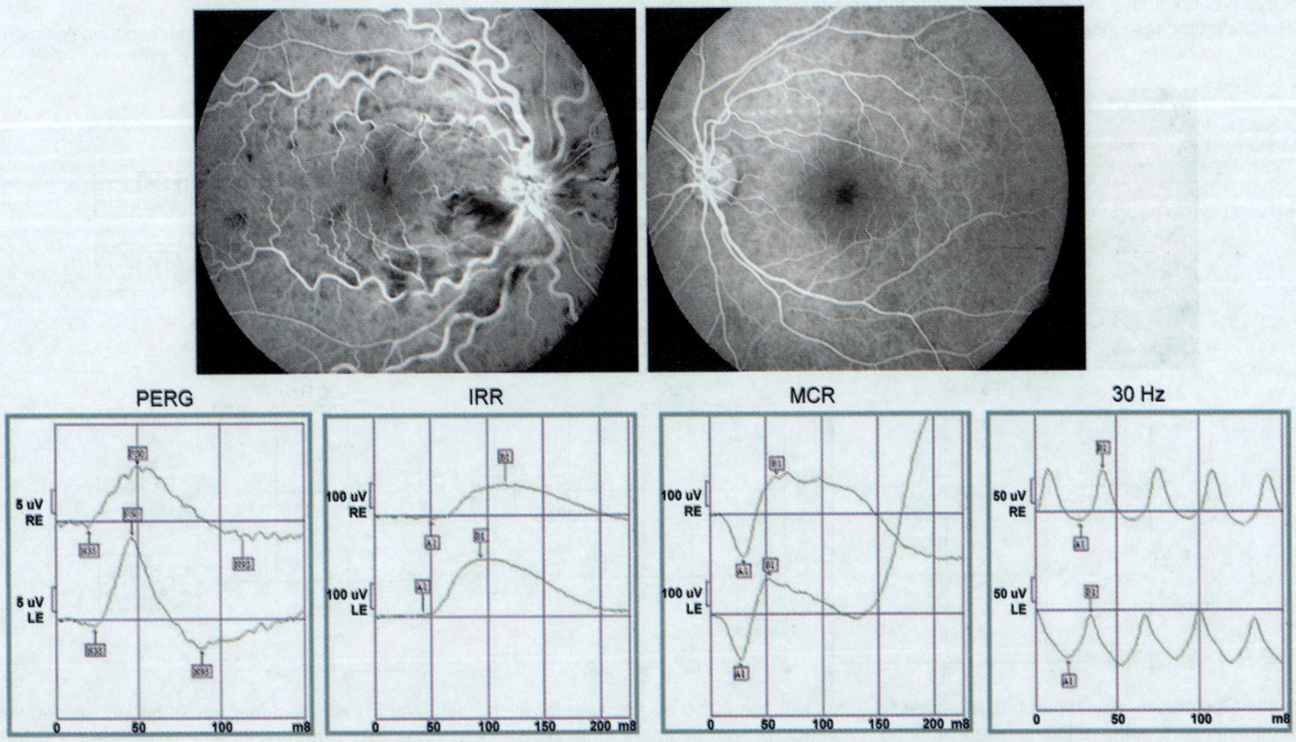

Fig. 21: This 28 years male had mild blurring of vision since 5 days due to CRVO with mild macular edema. The full-field ERG of right eye is very much comparable to the left eye; both of which are within normal limits suggestive of nonischemic CRVO. Note the PERG is showing reduced P50 amplitude in the right eye compared to left eye. Although the vision is same (20/20) in both eyes but the macular function of the right eye is not same as the left eye possibly due to macular edema leading to symptomatic reduced contrast sensitivity in the patient.
(CRVO: central retinal vein occlusion; ERG: electroretinogram; IRR: isolated rod response; MCR: maximal combined response; PERG: pattern electroretinogram)

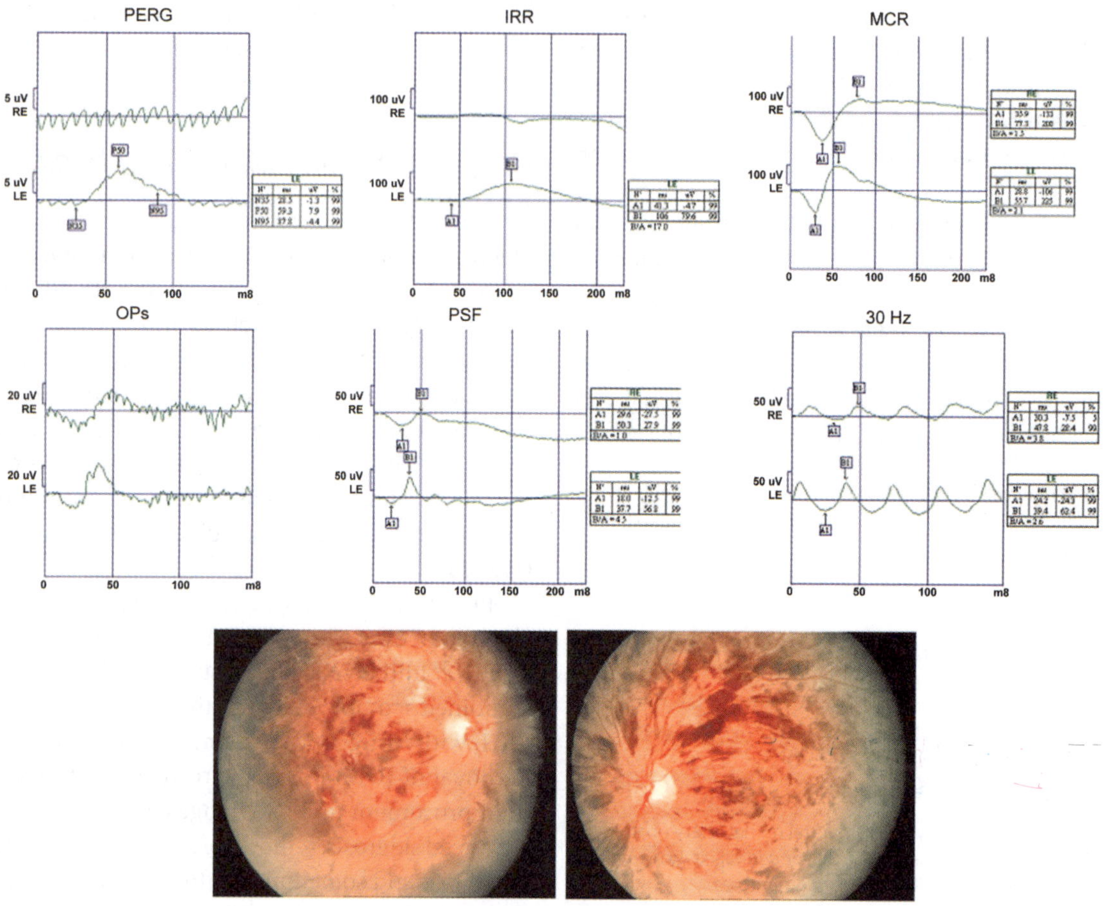

Fig. 22: Ischemic central retinal vein occlusion in right eye and nonischemic in left eye of a 40 years male. Right eye has reduced b/a-wave ratio and increased latency of b-wave in MCR; reduced amplitudes and delayed stimulus-to-peak time of 30 Hz flicker with absence of PERG, IRR, and OPs. Left eye has no delays in responses but reduced amplitudes of all waveforms.

(IRR: isolated rod response; MCR: maximal combined response; OPs: oscillatory potentials; PERG: pattern electroretinogram; PSF: photopic single flash)

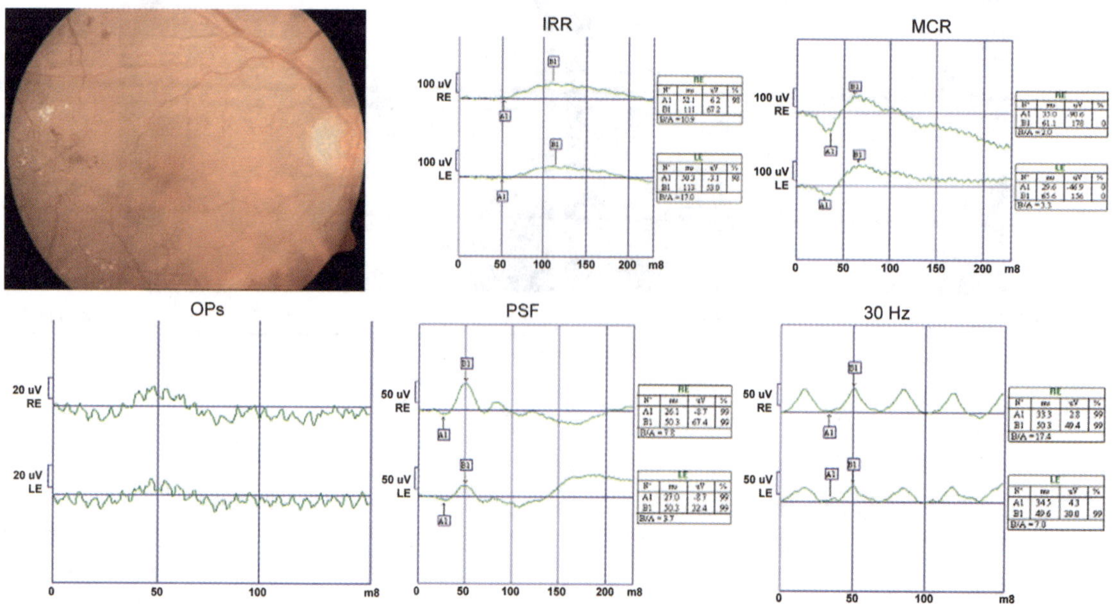

Fig. 23: Ocular ischemic syndrome. A female 68 years with VA 20/50 and early cataract in each eye. Fundus had features of NPDR, dilated veins and minimal disk pallor. ERG showed reduced amplitude of rod mediated inner retinal responses (IRR), and reduced b/a-wave ratio in MCR. The inner retinal ischemia was depicted by reduced amplitudes and poorly recordable oscillatory potentials, with delayed stimulus-to-peak time of 30-Hz flicker ERG. Carotid artery Doppler (not shown) showed moderate atheromatous changes. Patient developed neovascular glaucoma 6 months later without worsening of retinopathy in the right eye.

(ERG: electroretinogram; IRR: isolated rod response; MCR: maximal combined response; NPDR: nonproliferative diabetic retinopathy; OPs: oscillatory potentials; PERG: pattern electroretinogram; PSF: photopic single flash)

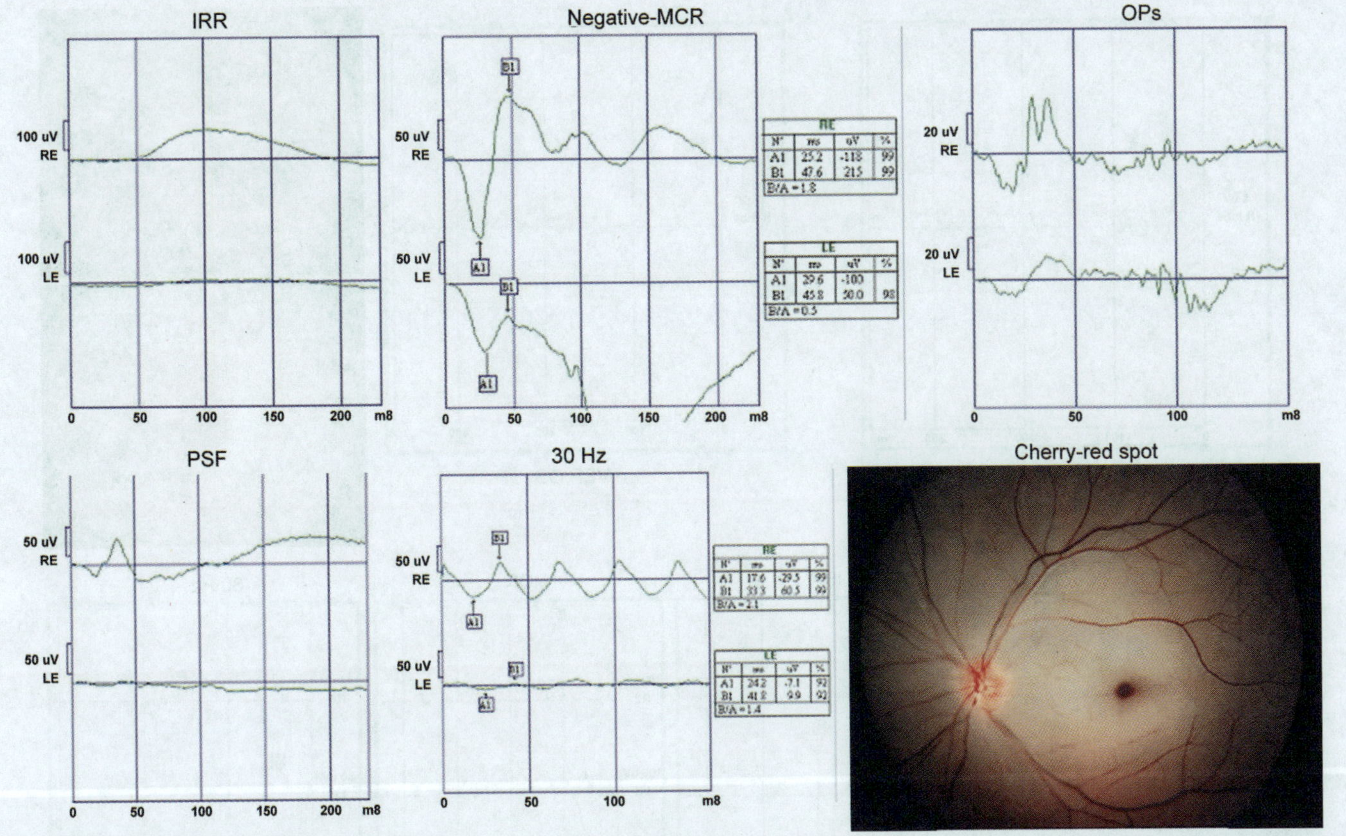

Fig. 24: Left eye with CRAO shows preserved a-wave and absent b-wave (negative ERG) in maximal combined response depicting preservation of outer retinal cell layers supplied by choroidal vasculature and ischemia in inner retinal layers supplied by central retinal artery. Right eye responses are normal.
(CRAO: central retinal artery obstruction; ERG: electroretinogram; IRR: isolated rod response; MCR: maximal combined response; OPs: oscillatory potentials; PSF: photopic single flash)

Pediatric Visual Impairment[37]

The ERG is indispensable in evaluating the cause of poor vision in children. Commonly seen conditions include Leber's congenital amaurosis (LCA), rod monochromatism **(Fig. 26)**, Stargardt's macular dystrophy, ocular albinism, and delayed visual maturation. Correct identification of the underlying dysfunction helps in proper counseling as regards risks to relatives, long-term prognosis, and sometimes identification of an underlying systemic disease such as abetalipoproteinemia, neuronal ceroid lipofuscinosis, mucopolysaccharidoses, and cystinosis.

Carrier Stage Detection

Electroretinogram can be helpful in detection of the carrier stage of certain X-linked conditions such as X-linked RP,[38] blue-cone monochromatism,[38] and X-linked cone dystrophy.

Optic Nerve and Visual Pathway

Optic nerve and visual dysfunction[39] include following condition:

- *Optic nerve demyelination*: The pattern VEP (PVEP) latency (P100) is usually delayed in optic nerve demyelination and the delay may be subclinical, i.e. it may occur with no signs or symptoms of optic nerve involvement.[40,41] This may significantly affect clinical management in a patient with spinal cord disease and possible multiple sclerosis (MS). The VEP is almost invariably delayed following symptomatic optic nerve involvement in MS, even when vision has returned to normal.
- *Papilledema*: In papilledema the VEP is normal unless secondary optic atrophy occurs.
- *Anterior ischemic optic neuropathy (AION)*: In AION, the PERG shows normal P50 amplitude and latency, elevation of N95, normal flash ERG, and reduced amplitude with normal P100 latency in VEP **(Fig. 27)**. Using multichannel VEP recordings, the chiasmal lesions, such as pituitary tumors, show a "crossed asymmetry" where there is an abnormal distribution over the two hemispheres which is in an opposite direction for the two eyes.[42] Stimulus parameters are crucial for accurate localization. In general, use of a large field, large check stimulus gives paradoxical lateralization[42] whereas a small field, small check stimulus gives anatomical lateralization. Retrochiasmal lesions give an "uncrossed" asymmetry where there is an abnormal distribution that is the same for the two eyes. Serial VEP recordings can help to detect

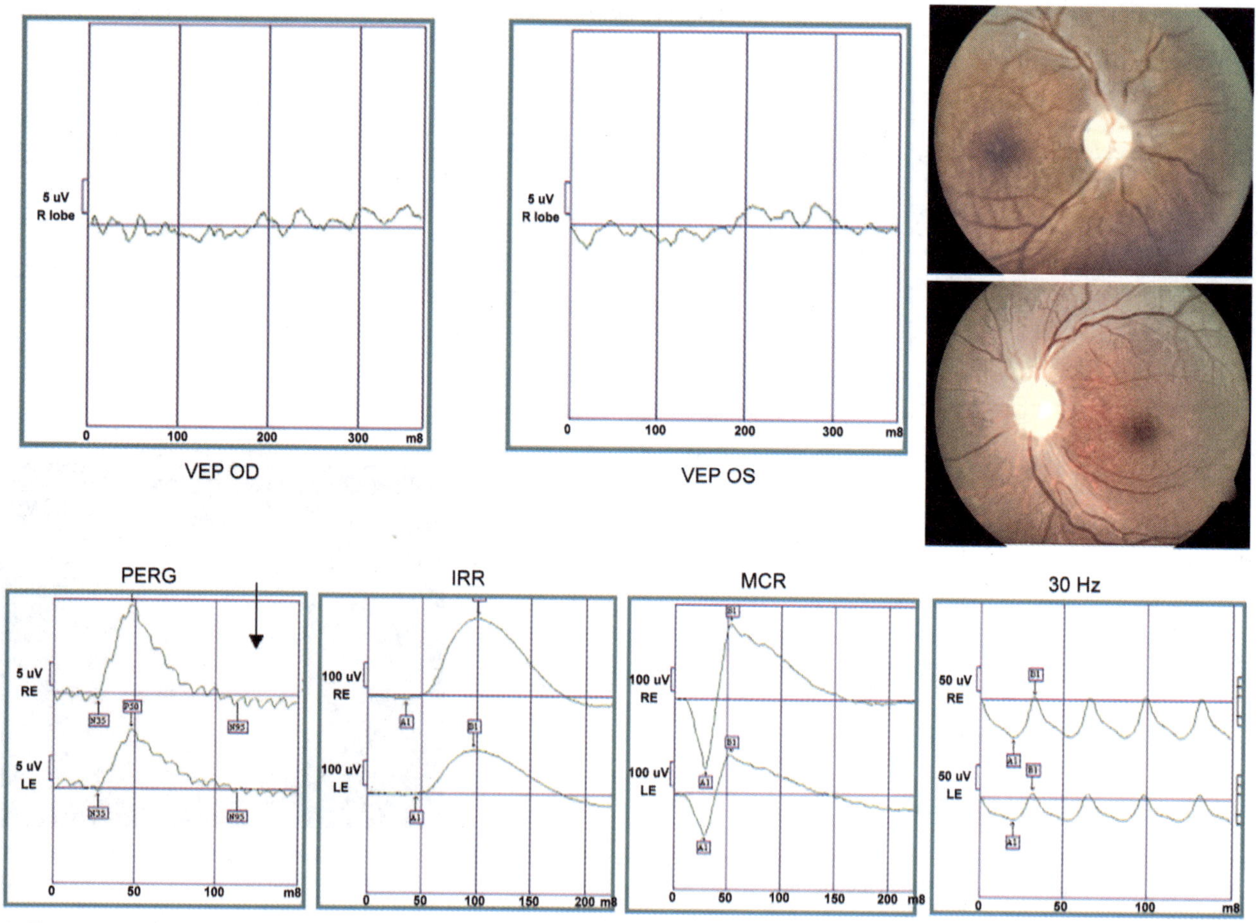

Fig. 25: This 18-year-old male has rapidly progressive, bilateral sequential loss of vision from 4 months (20/400). There was bilateral optic disk pallor with ill-sustained pupillary reactions but no RAPD. The pattern VEP was unrecordable. Flash ERG was normal. In PERG, the N95 was absent (arrow) and P50 was preserved confirming the patient to have bilateral optic neuropathy. Visual fields showed central 7° of scotoma in both eyes. History of antitubercular treatment in the past pointed to a diagnosis of possible ethambutol toxicity.
(ERG: electroretinogram; IRR: isolated rod response; MCR: maximal combined response; PERG: pattern electroretinogram; RAPD: relative afferent pupillary defect; VEP OD: visual evoked potential oculus dexter; VEP OS: visual evoked potential oculus sinister)

recurrences or nonresponsiveness to medical therapy as VEP abnormalities can occur before visual fields or visual acuity become abnormal.

- *Ocular albinism*: In some cases of ocular albinism, the condition may not be apparent in the absence of typical phenotypic expression of skin or iris, but child can have nystagmus and poor vision due to an albino genotype. All albinos, irrespective of genotype or phenotype exhibit misrouting. Heterozygote carriers do not demonstrate misrouting. The diagnosis of the intracranial misrouting of albinism, where the majority of optic nerve fibers from each eye do not decussate to the contralateral hemisphere, is readily demonstrated by multichannel VEP. Abnormalities may occur in response to either pattern appearance or diffuse flash stimulation, but the flash VEP appears to be more effective in infants and the pattern appearance VEP in adults.
- *Visual acuity assessment*: Objective assessment of visual acuity is performed with pattern appearance stimulation using a very brief appearance time in order to minimize the possibility of voluntary closure or defocusing.
- *Other optic nerve diseases*: Leber's hereditary optic neuropathy (LHON), toxic and nutritional optic neuropathies, and traumatic optic neuropathy show variable changes in amplitude and latency of VEP depending on extent of involvement.
- *Visual loss assessment in infants and children*: VEP is a useful tool along with ERG and other clinical assessments to differentiate various conditions such as cortical visual impairment, delayed visual maturation, and amblyopia.
- *Malingering*: Along with other tests, VEP helps to differentiate malingering from visual pathway lesions. Pattern onset is a useful technique as subjects cannot voluntarily blur this stimulus.

Recent Advances in Multimodal ERG[43,44] and Multifocal VEP[45]

Multifocal ERG technique developed initially by Bearse and Sutter[43] allows local ERG responses to be recorded simultaneously from many regions of the retina. The response is thought to originate from outer retina with relatively

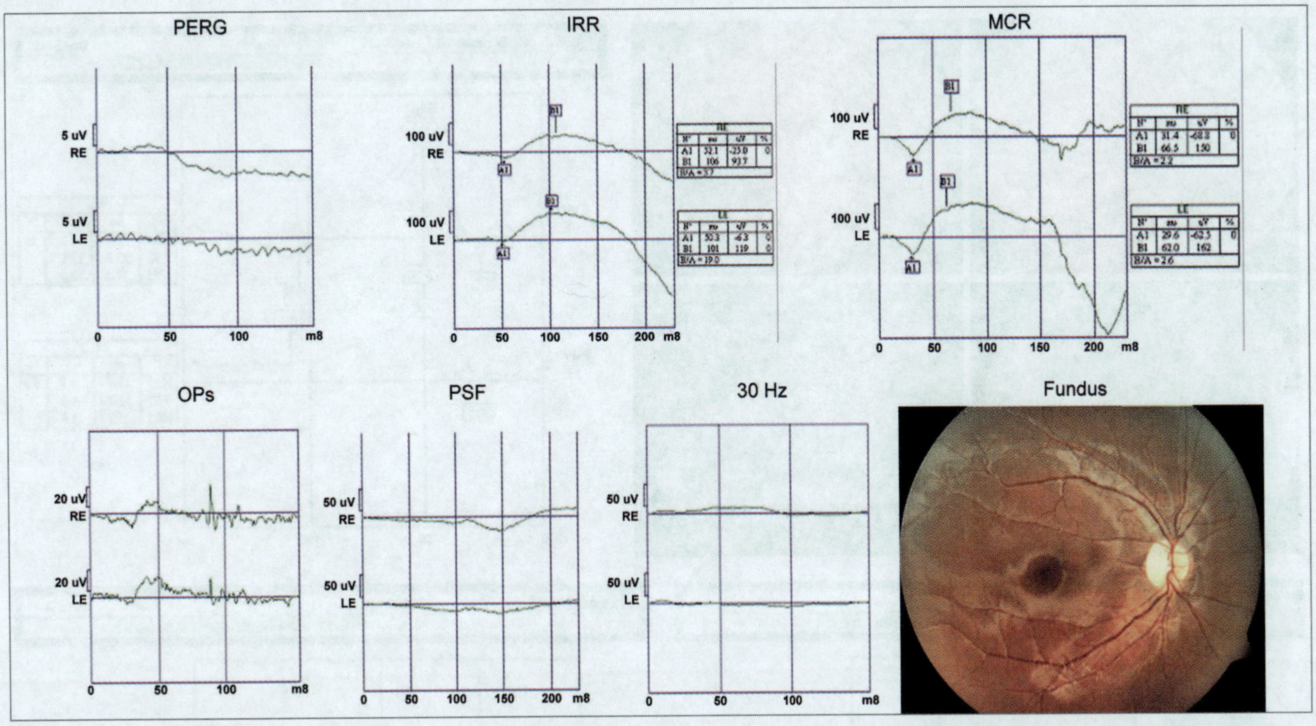

Fig. 26: Rod monochromatism. Showing poorly recordable PERG (due to nystagmus), and absent cone-mediated responses (PSF, 30 Hz) with normal scotopic rod-mediated responses (IRR and MCR). This child of 8 years had VA of 20/400, congenital nystagmus that had reduced with time and photophobia with complete achromatopsia.
(IRR: isolated rod response; MCR: maximal combined response; OPs: oscillatory potentials; PERG: pattern electroretinogram; PSF: photopic single flash; VA: visual acuity)

little contribution from the ganglion cells.[44] Responses are recorded to a scaled hexagonal pattern-reversal stimulus in photopic conditions **(Fig. 28)** although some laboratories are attempting to record scotopic mfERG also. MfERG helps to distinguish between diseases of the outer retina and of ganglion cells or optic nerves. Along with multifocal VEP (mfVEP), the mfERG helps to differentiate organic and nonorganic causes of visual loss.

There are some limitations of these techniques. Since, it is an evolving technology the recording parameters and interpretation are still not standardized, though guidelines have been formulated.[46] The techniques are still not widely available. Full-field ERG helps to evaluate the function of the retina as a whole. However, it cannot detect focal areas of abnormal function. mfERG is a new technique, it allows analysis of local ERG responses to assess focal retinal function. Basic technology is similar to full-field ERG in some aspects. In mfERG the recording, ground and reference electrodes and their placement close to or on the cornea, lateral canthus and ear lobe are similar as in routine ERG. Recording is done with dilated pupils with subject placed in ordinary room light for 15 minutes before testing.

Effect of Stimulus on Multifocal Electroretinogram[43,44]

Stimulus can be delivered by a CRT, i.e. monitor liquid-crystal display (LCD) projectors, light-emitting diode (LED) arrays or scanning laser ophthalmoscope. The most common frame frequency of the CRT is 75 Hz and should never be 50 or 60 Hz as this is similar to the line current frequency, which interferes as noise with the recordings. Stable fixation is essential to get reliable mfERG recordings and various fixation targets and monitoring devices may be used that do not interfere with the recordings.

The retina is stimulated with a black and white pattern of hexagonal elements each of which has a 50% chance of being illuminated every time the frame changes. The hexagonal pattern was designed to compensate for the local differences in signal density (and cone density) across the posterior retina. Thus, the central hexagons are smaller than the peripheral ones **(Fig. 28)**. Each hexagon element follows a fixed predetermined sequence called m-sequence that controls the order of flicker of the stimulus elements between light and dark. This sequence is designed in such a way that the overall luminance of the screen over the time of recording is relatively stable, i.e. equiluminant. The overall stimulus pattern should subtend a visual angle of 20–30° on either side of fixation. The stimulus region can be divided into different numbers of hexagons such as 61, 103 or 241. Duration of recording varies from 4–8 minutes depending on whether 61 or 103 elements are used. Various artifacts in mfERG recordings include electrical noise, movement errors due to fixation losses, eccentric fixation, shadowing errors due to edge of refraction lenses, and errors due to too much averaging.

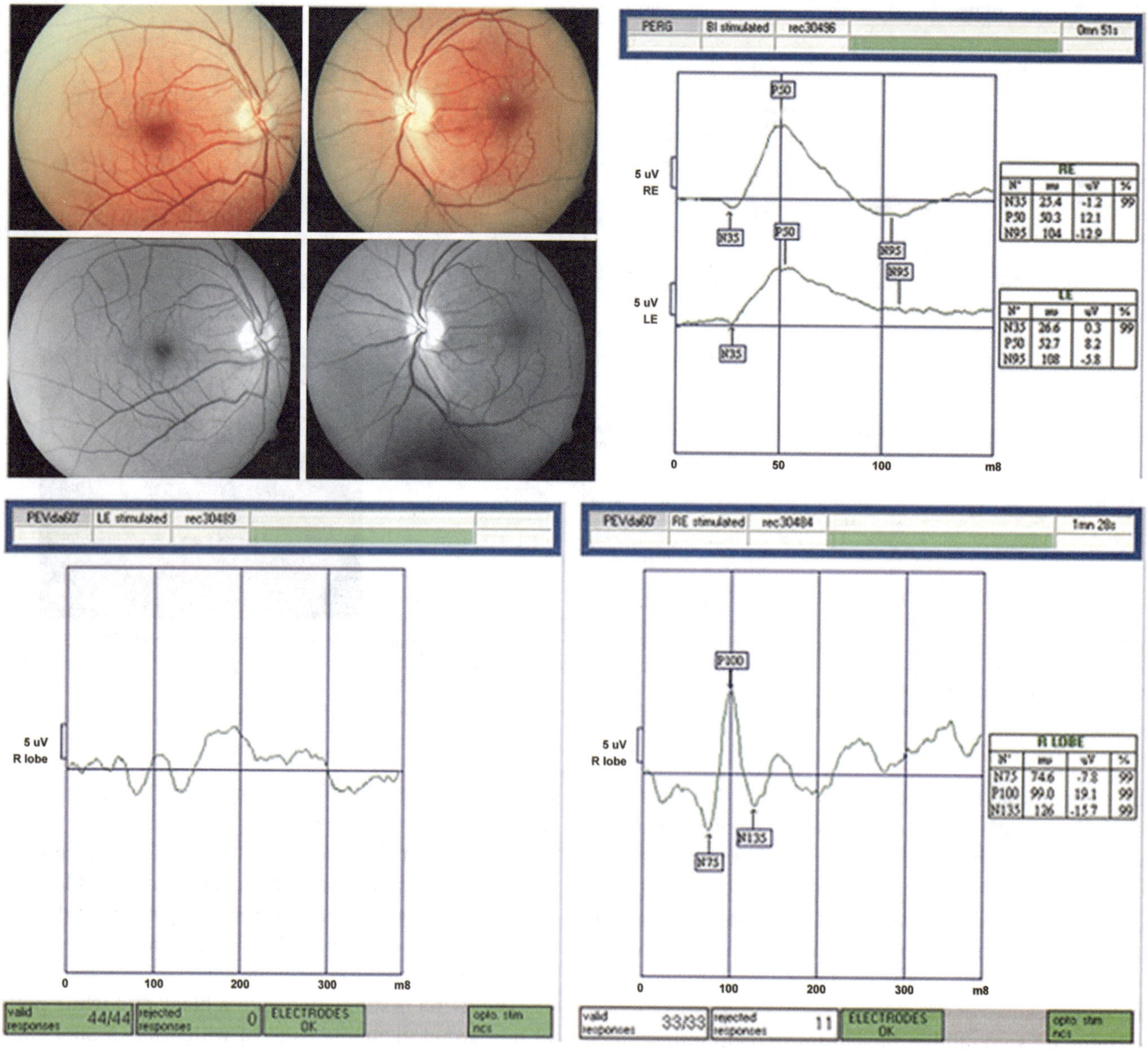

Fig. 27: *Anterior ischemic optic neuropathy*. A 48-year-old male had 1 month reduction of vision in the left eye. Visual acuity (VA) was 6/6 and 6/60 in the right and left eyes, respectively. Left eye showed diffuse field loss (not shown). Right eye color fundus (Top left) and red free photograph (Middle left) showed normal color of the disk with few RPE changes at macula. Color fundus photograph of the left eye (Top right) showed small disk with no cup and diffuse pallor. Red free photograph of left eye (Middle right) showed 3 quadrants disk pallor with sparing of inferotemporal segment. Pattern electroretinogram (ERG) showed normal P50 and N95 responses in right eye. Left eye had reduced amplitude and delayed latency of P50, with secondary elevation of N95 component, arrow (Extreme top right). The pattern visual evoked potential (VEP) had normal amplitude and latency in right eye (Bottom right) but was poorly recordable in the left eye (Bottom left).

Multifocal Electroretinogram Responses

By correlating the continuous ERG signal with the on or off phases of each stimulus element, the focal ERG signal associated with each element is calculated. The data obtained can be displayed in various ways; commonly as a topographic array, a three-dimensional plot or as group averages **(Fig. 28)**. The trace arrays are essential to display as they not only show the topographical variations due to focal pathology but also demonstrate the quality of the records. It is important to remember that the tracings of mfERG are not responses in the sense of direct electrical signals from a local region of the retina. The mfERG waveforms are a mathematical extraction of signals that correlate with the time that one portion of the screen is illuminated. The signals are hence influenced by adaptation effects from previous stimuli and by scattered light from other fundus areas.

The typical waveform of the primary mfERG (first order or first order kernel K1) is a biphasic wave. The initial negative deflection is called N1, which is followed by a positive deflection P1 and a second negative deflection called N2. The cellular origins of these responses are still under study

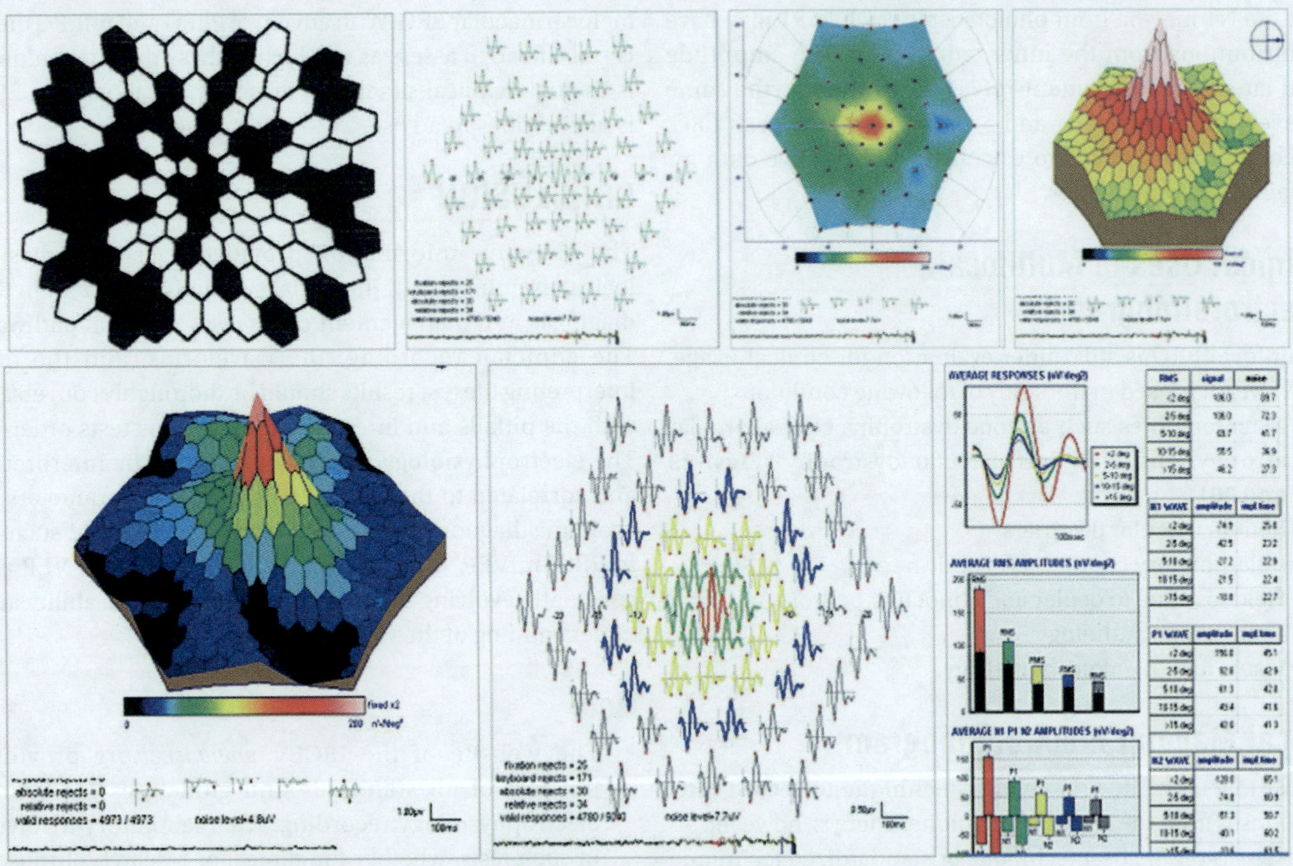

Fig. 28: Normal multifocal electroretinogram stimulus and variety of output display.

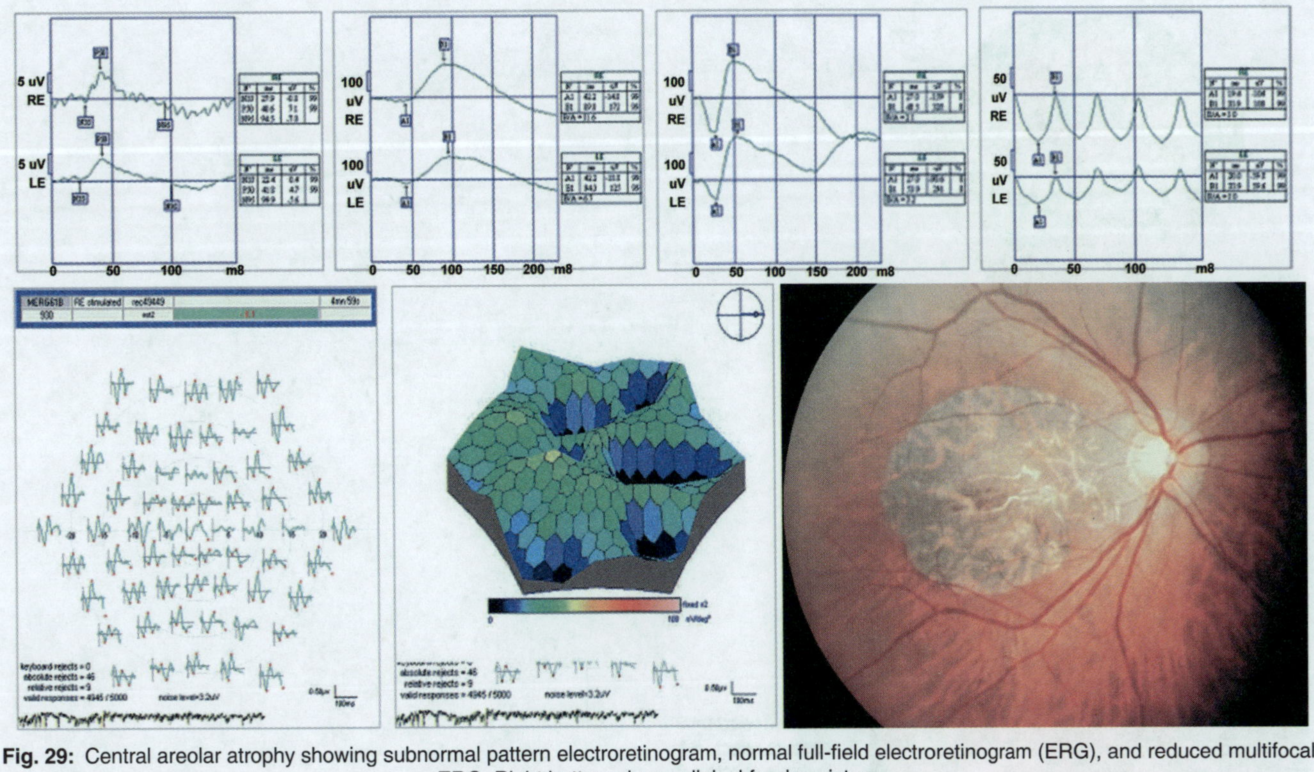

Fig. 29: Central areolar atrophy showing subnormal pattern electroretinogram, normal full-field electroretinogram (ERG), and reduced multifocal ERG. Right bottom shows clinical fundus picture.

but the N1 may be from photoreceptors while P1 may have contributions from the inner retinal cells. The amplitude and latency measurements of N1 and P1 follow the same convention as for the a- and b-waves of routine flash ERG. Each laboratory needs to establish its normative data for meaningful comparisons.

Clinical Uses of Multifocal Electroretinogram

Multifocal ERG is still under evaluation for clinical usage. However, it is used in the study of following conditions:

- Maculopathies such as cone dystrophy, central areolar atrophy, and Stargardt macular dystrophy **(Figs. 29 and 30)**
- Retinal vascular disorders
- Inflammatory conditions of optic nerve
- Field loss due to ocular and nonocular pathology
- Toxic retinal pathology
- Visual loss of unknown etiology.

Focal Macular Electroretinogram

Focal macular ERG[47] is another technique to record ERG responses from the macular area alone. There is, however, no consensus on the best technique or standardized technique for focal macular ERG. With advent of PERG and mfERG there is still a need to assess as to which of these three techniques is useful in clinical situations. Presently, focal macular ERG is not in widespread use.

CONCLUSION

The objective information provided by electrophysiological examination of the visual system is important in the diagnosis and management of diseases of visual pathway. The clinician recording, the waveforms, and the one interpreting the test results should be thoroughly conversant with the pitfalls and interrelation of various tests ordered. The electrophysiology results must always be interpreted and correlated to the clinical and other test parameters to avoid misdiagnosis. Newer techniques in this field such as mfERG, mfVEP, focal macular ERG, and motion VEP are constantly evolving that improve our diagnostic ability and understanding of the visual pathway.

Note

- The website of the ISCEV *www.iscev.org* provides full text of all standards and guidelines for ocular electrophysiology recording. Each laboratory involved in such tests, whether for clinical or research purposes,

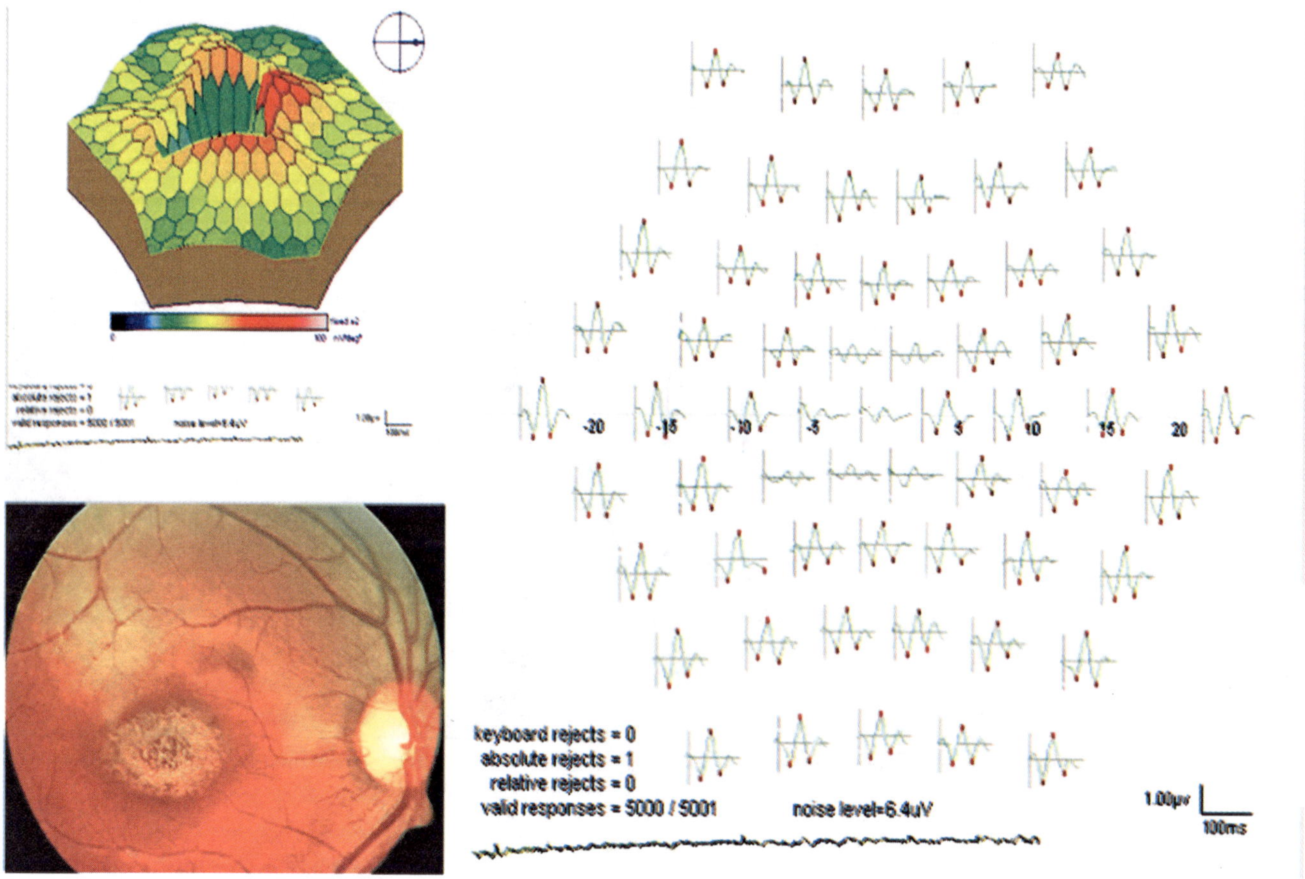

Fig. 30: Multifocal electroretinogram in Stargardt's heredomacular degeneration showing reduced central cone function.

Table 1: Normal values in the LVPEI laboratory using the metrovision system.

Response	*a-wave*		*b-wave*	
	Amplitude (microvolts)	*Latency (milliseconds)*	*Amplitude (microvolts)*	*Latency (milliseconds)*
Isolated rod response			130–160	90–110
Maximal retinal response	105–130	20.0–22.0	350–450	45.00 ± 4
Photopic cone 30 Hz flicker			120–180	27–31
			100–150	33–35

(LVPEI: LV Prasad Eye Institute)

must attempt to meet these standards so as to have meaningful international communications.

- The recordings shown in this chapter are on two types of electrophysiology recording systems (LKC UTAS-2000 and Metrovision). Due to space constraints only one waveform of each eye is shown instead of two reproducible waveforms. The normal values in our laboratory are given in **Table 1**.

REFERENCES

1. Welber RG, Eisner A. Retinal function and physiological studies. In: Newsome DA (Ed). Retinal Dystrophies and Degenerations. New York: Raven Press; 1988. pp. 44-69.
2. Arden GB, Barrada A, Kelsey JH. New clinical test of retinal function based on the standing potential of the eye. Br J Ophthalmol. 1962;46:449-67.
3. Arden GB, Fojas MR. Electrophysiological abnormalities in pigmentary degenerations of the retina. Arch Ophthalmol. 1962;68:369-89.
4. Marmor MF, Zrenner E. Standard for clinical electrooculography. Doc Ophthalmol. 1993;85:115-24.
5. Krill AE, Morse PA, Potts AM, et al. Hereditary vitelliruptive macular degeneration. Am J Ophthalmol. 1966;61:1405-15.
6. Brink HM, Pinckers AJ, Verbeek AM. The electrooculogram in uveal melanoma: a prospective study. Doc Ophthalmologica. 1990;75:329-34.
7. Arden GB, Wolf JE. The human electrooculogram: interaction of light and alcohol. Invest Ophth Vis Sci. 2000;41:2722-9.
8. Kolder H, Brecher GA. Fast oscillations of the corneoretinal potential in man. Arch Ophthalmol. 1966;75:232-7.
9. Marmor MF, Zrenner E. Standard for clinical electroretinography (1994 update). Doc Ophthalmol. 1995;89:199-210.
10. Marmor MF, Zrenner E. Standard for clinical electroretinography (1999 Update). Doc Ophthalmol. 1999;97:143-56.
11. Brigell M, Bach M, Barber C, et al. Guidelines for calibration of stimulus and recording parameters used in visual clinical electrophysiology. Doc Ophthalmol. 1998;95:1-14.
12. Dawson WW, Trick GL, Litzkow CA. Improved electrode for electroretinography. Invest Ophthalmol Vis Sci. 1979;18: 988-91.
13. Mohan Ram LS, Jalali S, Roopa Reddy PS, et al. Safety and efficacy evaluation of a new electrode (the LVP electrode) Part I. Pattern ERG pilot study. Doc Ophthalmol. 2003;107: 171-7.
14. Mohan Ram LS, Jalali S, Faheemuddin S, et al. Safety and efficacy evaluation of a new ERG electrode (the LVP electrode) Part II. Flash ERG pilot study. Doc Ophthalmol. 2003;107: 179-83.
15. Shiells RA, Falk G. Contribution of rod, on-bipolar and horizontal cell light responses to the ERG of dogfish retina. Vis Neurosci. 1999;16:503-11.
16. Bush RA, Sieving PA. A proximal retinal component in the primate photopic ERG a-wave. Invest Ophthalmol Vis Sci. 1994;35:635-45.
17. Bush RA, Sieving PA. Inner retinal contributions to the primate photopic fast flicker electroretinogram. J Opt Soc Am A. 1996;13:557-65.
18. Sieving PA. Photopic ON- and OFF-pathway abnormalities in retinal dystrophies. Trans Am Ophthalmol Soc. 1993;91: 701-73.
19. Holder GE. The pattern electroretinogram and an integrated approach to visual pathway diagnosis. Prog Retin Eye Res. 2001;20:531-61.
20. Bach M, Hawlina M, Holder GE, et al. Standard for pattern electroretinography. Doc Ophthalmol. 2000;101:11-8.
21. Neubauer AS, Steifelmyer S, Berninger T, et al. The multifocal pattern electroretinography in chloroquine retinopathy. Ophthal Res. 2004;36:106-13.
22. Odom JV, Bach M, Barber C, et al. For the International society for clinical electrophysiology of vision. Visual evoked Potential standard (2004). Doc Ophthalmol. 2004;108:115-23.
23. American Encephalographic Society. Guideline thirteen: Guidelines for Standard Electrode Placement Nomenclature. J Clin Neurophysiol. 1994;11:111-3.
24. Marmor MF. The electroretinogram in Retinitis pigmentosa. Arch Ophthalmol. 1979;97:1300-4.
25. Berson EL. Retinitis pigmentosa and allied diseases: Applications of electroretinographic testing. Int Ophthalmol. 1981;4:7-22.
26. Krill AE, Deutman AF, Fishman M. The cone degenerations. Doc Ophthalmol. 1973;35:1-80.
27. Koh AH, Hogg CR, Holder GE. The incidence of negative ERG in clinical practice. Doc Ophthalmol. 2001;102:19-30.
28. Miyake Y, Yagasaki K, Horiguchi M, et al. Congenital stationary night blindness with negative ERG: a new classification. Arch Ophthalmol. 1986;104:1013-20.
29. Tantri A, Vrabee TR, Cuunjieng A, et al. X-linked retinoschisis: a clinical and molecular genetics review. Surv Ophthalmol. 2004;49:214-30.
30. Scholl HP, Zrenner E. Electrophysiology in acquired retinal disorders. Surv Ophthalmol. 2000;45:29-47.
31. Hayreh SS, Klugna MR, Beri M, et al. Differentiation of ischemic from non-ischemic CRVO during the early acute phase. Graefes Arch Clinical and Exp Ophthalmol. 1990;228: 201-17.
32. Johnson MA, McPhee TJ. Electrophysiologic findings in iris neovascularization due to acute central retinal vein occlusion. Arch Ophthalmol. 1993;111:808-14.

33. Brown GC, Mgaragal LE. The ocular ischemic syndrome: clinical, fluorescein angiographic and carotid angiographic features. Int Ophthalmol. 1988;11:243-51.
34. Brown GC, Magaragal LE, Sergott R. Acute obstruction of the retinal and choroidal circulation. Ophthalmology. 1986; 93:1373-82.
35. Hussain N, Jalali S, Kaul S. Carotid artery diseases and ocular disorders. Ind J Ophthalmol. 2001;49:5-14.
36. Tzekov R, Arden GB. The electroretinogram in diabetic retinopathy. Surv Ophthalmol. 1999;44:53-60.
37. Kriss A, Jeffrey B, Taylor D. The electroretinogram in infants and young children. J Clin Neurophysiol. 1992;9:373-93.
38. Berson EL, Sandberg MA, Maguire A, et al. Electroretinograms in carriers of blue cone monochromatism. Am J Ophthalmol. 1986;105:254-61.
39. Heckenlively JR, Weleber RG, Arden GB. Testing levels of the visual system. In: Heckenlively JR, Arden GB (Eds). Principles and Practice of Clinical Electrophysiology of Vision. St Louis: Mosby; 1991. pp. 485-93.
40. Halliday AM, McDonald WI, Mushin J. Visual evoked response in the diagnosis of multiple sclerosis. Br Med J. 1973;4:661-4.
41. Holder GE. Multiple sclerosis. In: Heckenlively JR, Arden GB (Eds). Principles and Practice of Clinical Electrophysiology of Vision. St Louis: Mosby; 1991. pp. 797-805.
42. Holder GE. Chiasmal and retrochiasmal lesions. In: Heckenlively JR, Arden GB (Eds). Principles and Practice of Clinical Electrophysiology of Vision. St Louis: Mosby; 1991. pp. 557-64.
43. Bearse MA Jr, Sutter EE. Imaging localized retinal dysfunction with the multifocal ERG. J Opt Soc Am A. 1996;13:634-40.
44. Hood DC, Odel JG, Chen CS, et al. The multifocal ERG. J Neuroophthalmol. 2003;23:225-35.
45. Hood DC, Odel JG, Winn BJ. The multifocal VEP. J Neuroophthalmol. 2003;23:279-89.
46. Marmor MF, Hood DC, Keating D, et al. The International Society for Clinical Electrophysiology of Vision: Guidelines for basic multifocal ERG. Doc Ophthalmol. 2003;106:105-15.
47. Miyake Y. Focal macular electroretinography. Nagoya L Med Sci. 1998;61:79-89.

CHAPTER

21 Videonystagmography

Mihir Kothari

INTRODUCTION

Videonystagmography (VNG) or video electronystagmography (video ENG) is a technique of recording the eye movements using infrared light reflection technique. It is an essential tool for current day management of nystagmus.

VIDEONYSTAGMOGRAPHY SYSTEM

The VNG system typically includes an infrared light emitting diode. The light is directed to the eyes of the subject remotely from a distance of a meter. The reflected light from the iris is detected by the sensor. The unreflected light from the pupil is detected by the sensor as the area of signal void. The position and the movement of this signal void area is graphically recorded using an interface controller that converts a digital signal to a graphic analog signal. The VNG recording system can be a single channel system (30% less costly) or two channel system (both eyes recorded simultaneously). Recording of two eyes simultaneously is only needed in incomitant nystagmus or in the research setting.

For younger children, it is advantageous to have remote recording systems, which can allow the recording from a distance of approximately a meter. The remote recording systems are costlier (almost double the cost) but they process the image at higher sampling rate and they are Matlab™ software compatible which makes the image analysis and calculation of near expanded nystagmus acuity function (NAFX) easier.

All VNG machines can detect horizontal as well as vertical eye movements. Some instruments also record torsional (rotary) movements and other instruments have abnormal head rotation recorder to record the simultaneous recording of head rotations/head positions.

We use the single channel Intellinext VNG system made by Eye Dynamic Inc., CA, USA **(Fig. 1)**.

ADVANTAGES OF VIDEONYSTAGMOGRAPHY OVER ELECTRONYSTAGMOGRAPHY

- Less time consuming
- Direct recording of movements are available **(Fig. 2)**
- Less noise
- Real time recordings and adjustments can be made in patient position
- Otolithic function can be recorded

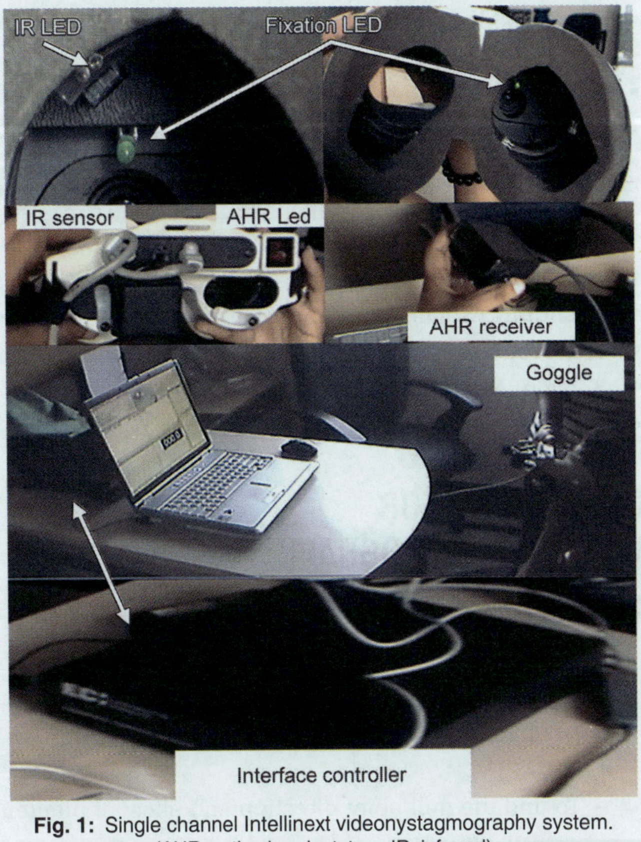

Fig. 1: Single channel Intellinext videonystagmography system. (AHR: active head rotatory; IR: infrared)

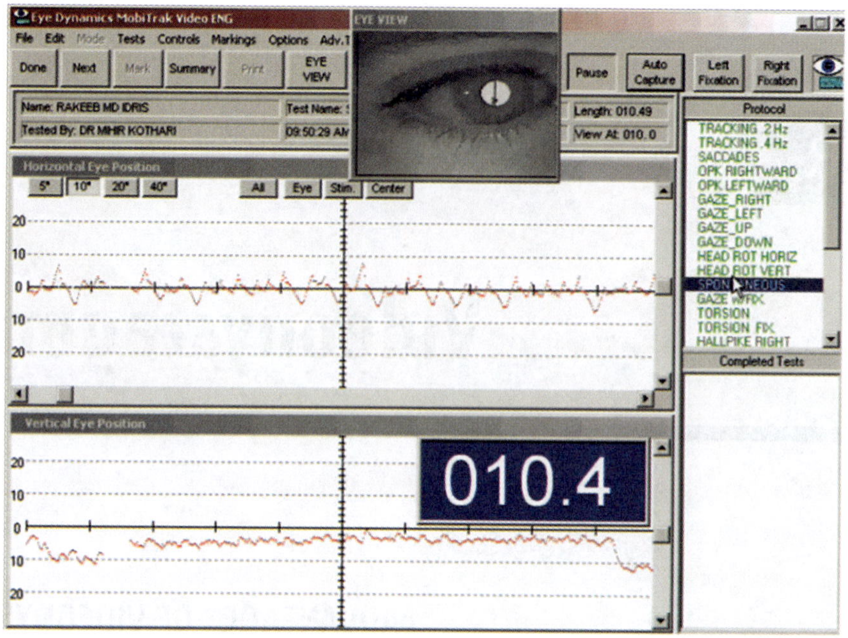

Fig. 2: Eye movement recording protocols available in VNG system.
(VNG: videonystagmography)

- Disjugate movements better appreciated as simultaneous recording is possible.

However, VNG technology is more expensive than an ENG.

Videonystagmography technology can also record:

- Eye tracking (pursuit) recording at various frequencies, e.g. 0.2 Hz, 0.4 Hz
- Saccades recording
- Recording of the optokinetic (OPK) nystagmus—rightward direction, leftward direction, downward, and upward directions
- Gaze recording (right, left, up, and down)
- Spontaneous recordings
- Recording with near fixation (gaze fixation)
- Head rotation recordings (vertical and horizontal)
- Torsion recording
- Hall pike and other vestibular function tests.

INDICATIONS FOR VIDEONYSTAGMOGRAPHY

- All the patients with nystagmus[1-19]
  - For appropriate classification of nystagmus
  - For objective documentation of the impact of treatment
  - For assessment of expanded nystagmus acuity function (NAFX) and automated nystagmus acuity function (ANAF)
  - To find the null point direction and effect of different gaze on nystagmus
  - To assess the intensity (frequency and amplitude) of nystagmus
  - To understand the evolution of nystagmus in an individual patient and for the understanding the neurology of nystagmus.
- *Squint*:[18]
  - Saccadic evaluation is useful for the detection of severity of paresis using saccadic velocity whether to do transposition or recess-resect procedure.
  - Optokinetic nystagmus evaluation is useful to differentiate infantile strabismus (infantile esotropia and infantile exotropia syndromes) from late onset strabismus.
- Neurological defects affecting ocular motility, e.g. Parkinson's disease and progressive supranuclear palsy.
- Psychiatric illnesses.[20]

HOW TO READ VIDEONYSTAGMOGRAPH?

In a VNG, following conventions are used **(Fig. 3)**.

X-axis = Time in seconds.

Y-axis = Amplitude in degrees (each gradation is usually 10°).

In horizontal recordings—upper segment shows right side of the patient and lower segment shows left side movement of the eye.

In vertical recordings—upper segment shows upside movement of the eye and lower segment shows left side movement of the eye.

First the frequency and amplitude of the nystagmus is noted **(Fig. 4)**.

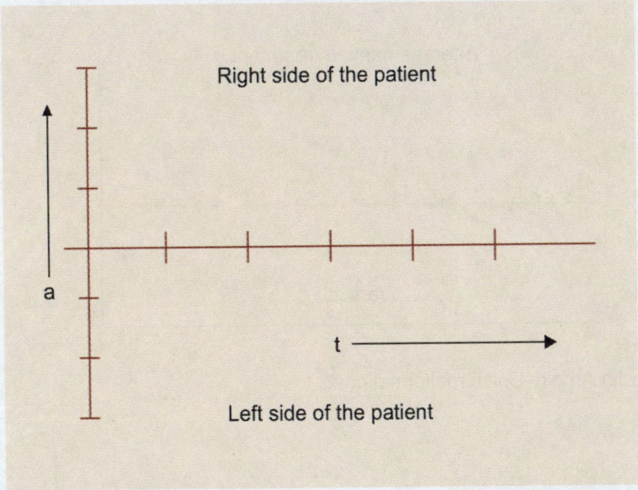

Fig. 3: Videonystagmograph convention.

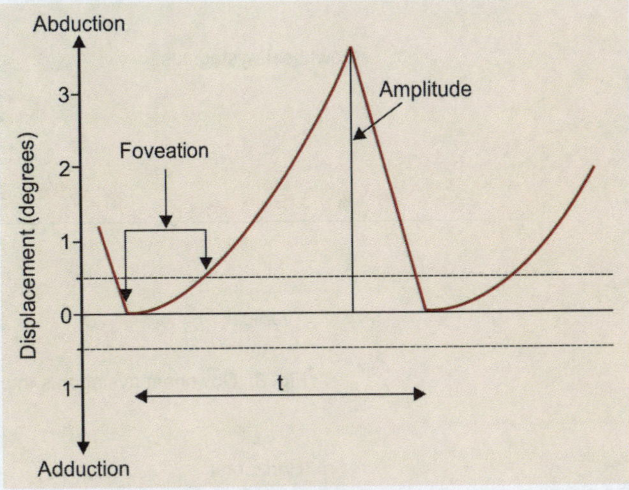

Fig. 6: Foveation analysis.

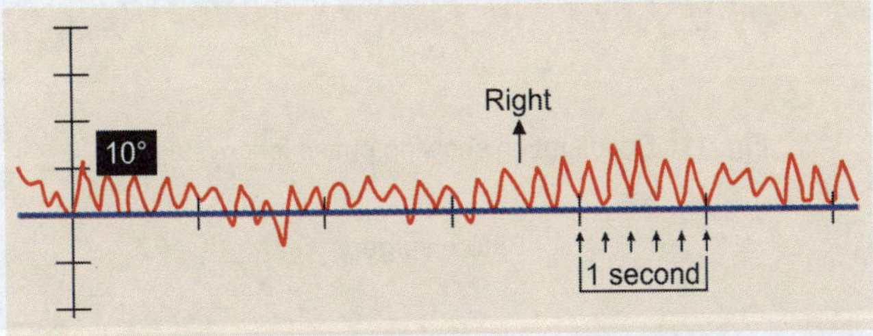

Fig. 4: Videonystagmograph of right beating 6 Hz 10° jerk nystagmus.

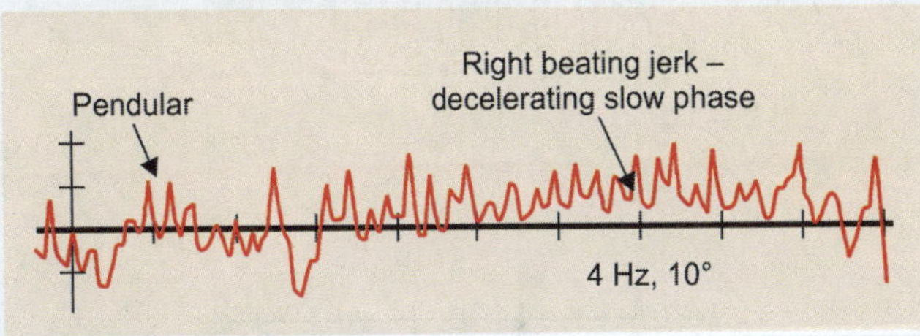

Fig. 7: Dimorphic (pendular with jerk nystagmus) in oculocutaneous albinism.

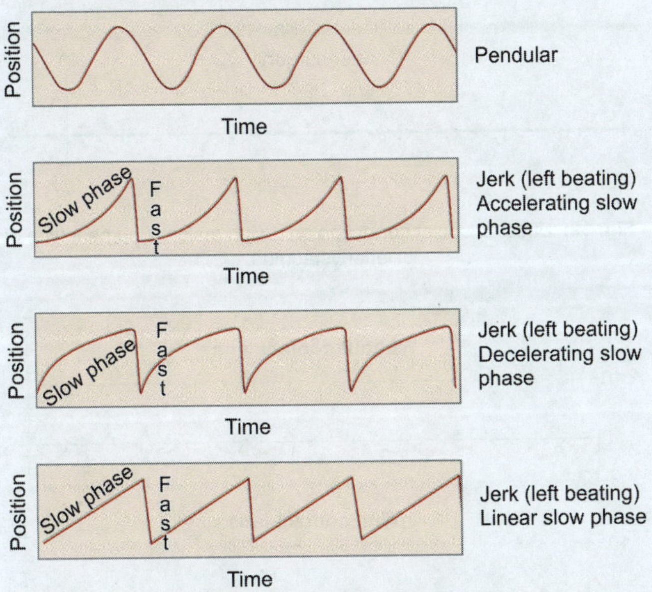

Fig. 5: Types of nystagmus.

Type of nystagmus is then identified, whether it is pendular or jerk and then whether it is increasing/decreasing or linear velocity slow phase and it is left beating or right beating or upbeating or downbeating **(Fig. 5)**.

The slow phase of nystagmus is identified as the phase having lesser slope (flatter curve).

The foveation time (NAFX/ANAF) is then calculated from the wavelet analysis **(Fig. 6)** (foveation time = foveation eye position <1° and eye velocity <4°/sec).

CLINICAL EXAMPLES

- Pendular waveforms with intermittent jerks (dimorphic nystagmus in patient with oculocutaneous albinism) **(Fig. 7)**.
- Downbeat nystagmus (4 Hz, 5° amplitude) in a patient treated with memantine 10 mg thrice a day due to Arnold-Chiari malformation type 2 **(Fig. 8)**.
- "Horizontal" nystagmus along with large vertical nystagmus in a patient with congenital optic atrophy. Presence of large vertical component in a horizontal nystagmus is indicative of associated sensory defect **(Fig. 9)**.
- Videonystagmography of a child with oculocutaneous albinism showing spontaneous, pursuit, and saccadic records **(Fig. 10)**.
- Videonystagmography of a patient with large exotropia, fusion maldevelopment nystagmus syndrome (latent nystagmus of previous years) and amblyopia **(Fig. 11)**.
- Decelerating slows phases typical of fusion maldevelopment nystagmus syndrome in patient with exotropia **(Fig. 12)**.
- Videonystagmography shows the effect of the plano bandage contact lens in INS in a patient experiencing 1 line logMAR improvement **(Fig. 13)**.
- Videonystagmography can show the convergence dampening in a patient with infantile nystagmus

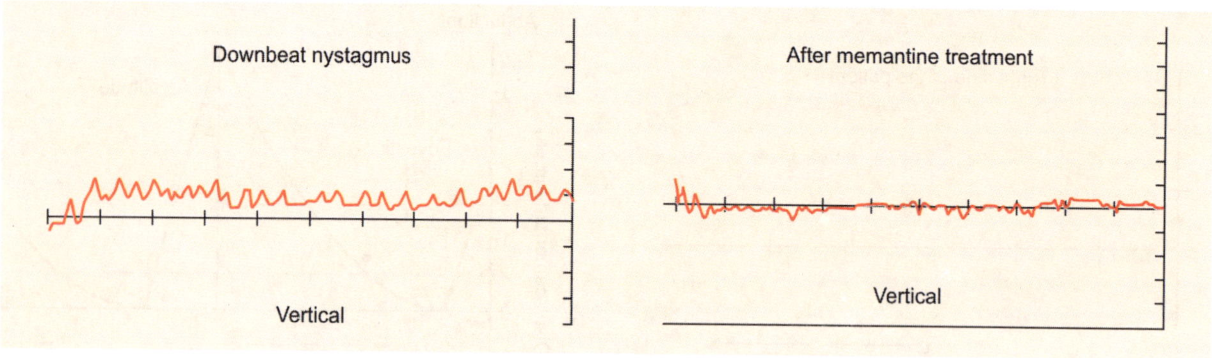

Fig. 8: Downbeat nystagmus in patient with Arnold–Chiari malformation-2.

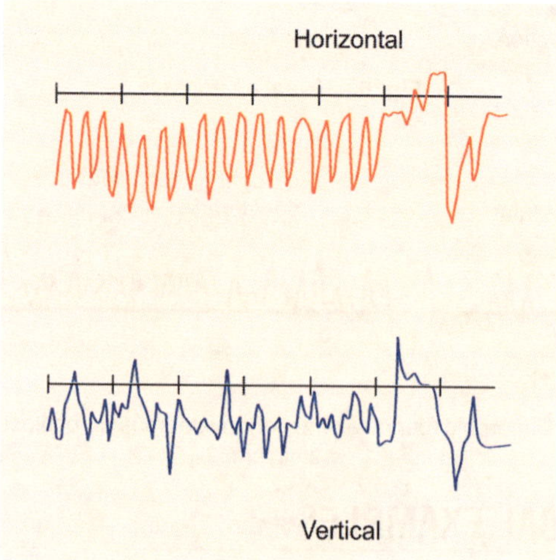

Fig. 9: Large vertical component in nystagmus indicating sensory defect.

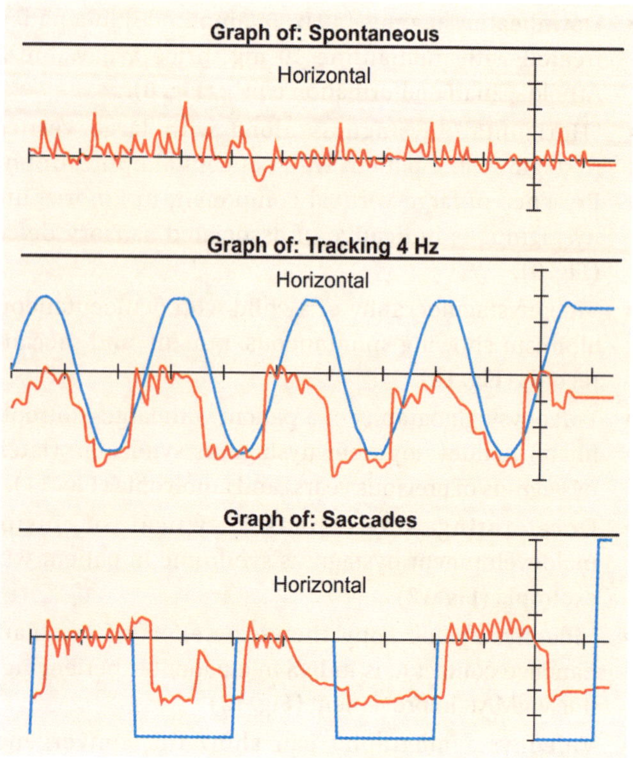

Fig. 10: Videonystagmographs showing records of spontaneous pursuits and saccades.

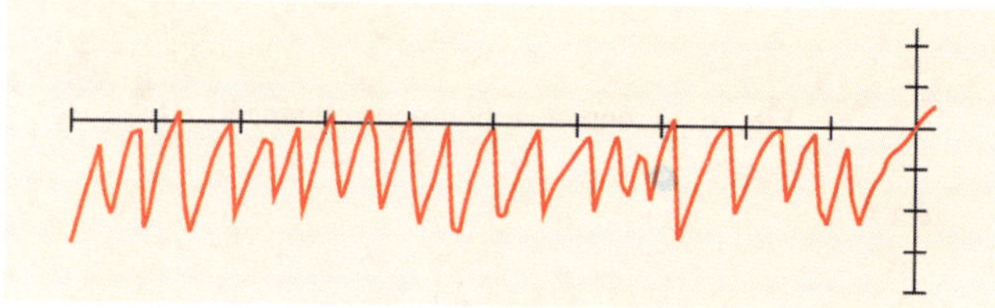

Fig. 11: Deceleration showing phase jerk nystagmus.

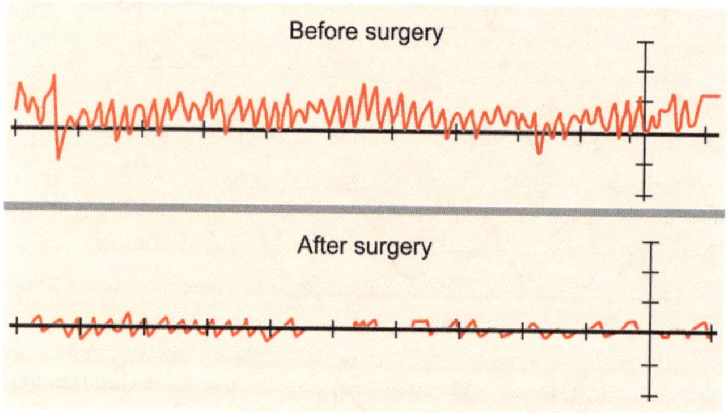

Fig. 12: Effect of squint correction on fusion maldevelopment type of jerk nystagmus.

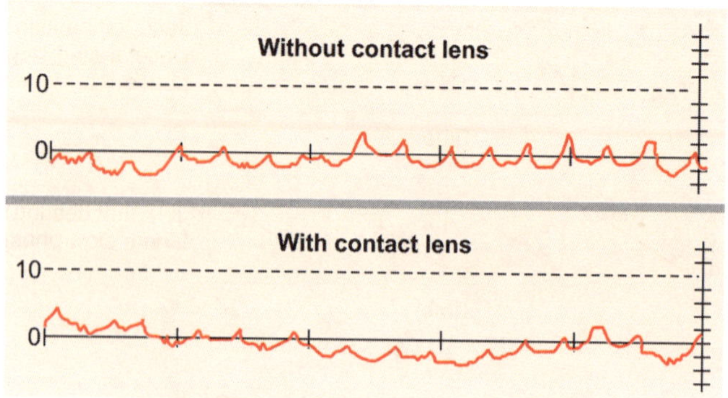

Fig. 13: Effect of contact lens on nystagmus.

syndrome who could be benefitted using artificial divergence surgery or base out prism therapy **(Fig. 14)**.

CONCLUSION

Videonystagmography acquires video images of eye movements, especially in nystagmus, and is very useful

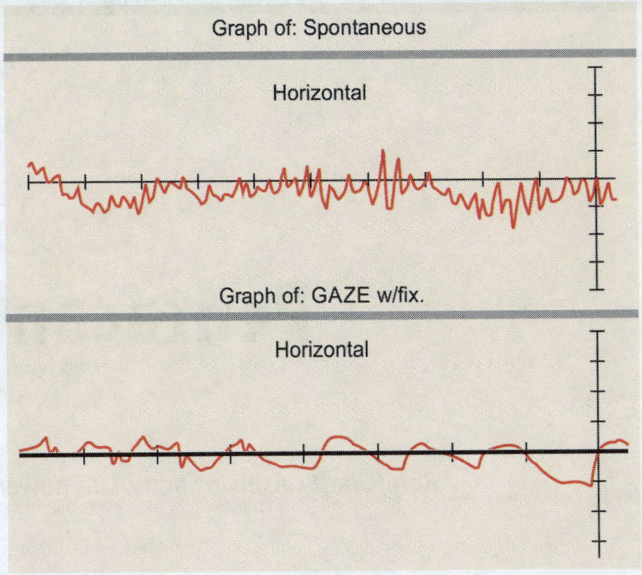

Fig. 14: Videonystagmography showing the dampening of nystagmus with contact lenses.

to clinicians in otorhinolaryngology, neurology, and ophthalmology. To critically interpret a patient's VNG results, it is essential to have reliable normative data because the results of VNG may be variable depending on the experience and expertise of the examiner. Ophthalmologists should more frequently order VNG in nystagmus, strabismus, and ocular degenerative disorders to obtain crucial information to enable them to plan management strategy.

REFERENCES

1. Hertle RW; National Eye Institute Sponsored Classification of Eye Movement Abnormalities and Strabismus Working Group. A next step in naming and classification of eye movement disorders and strabismus. J AAPOS. 2002;6(4):201-2.
2. Hertle RW, Maldanado VK, Maybodi M, et al. Clinical and ocular motor analysis of the infantile nystagmus syndrome in the first 6 months of life. Br J Ophthalmol. 2002;86(6):670-5.
3. Hertle RW, Dell'Osso LF. Clinical and ocular motor analysis of congenital nystagmus in infancy. J AAPOS. 1999;3(2):70-9.
4. Abadi RV, Bjerre A. Motor and sensory characteristics of infantile nystagmus. Br J Ophthalmol. 2002;86(10):1152-60.
5. Khanna S, Dell'Osso LF. The diagnosis and treatment of infantile nystagmus syndrome (INS). Scientific World J. 2006;6:1385-97.
6. Hertle RW, Anninger W, Yang D, et al. Effects of extraocular muscle surgery on 15 patients with oculo-cutaneous albinism (OCA) and infantile nystagmus syndrome (INS). Am J Ophthalmol. 2004;138(6):978-87.
7. Felius J, Fu VL, Birch EE, et al. Quantifying nystagmus in infants and young children: relation between foveation and visual acuity deficit. Invest Ophthalmol Vis Sci. 2011;52(12): 8724-31.
8. Hertle RW, Zhu X. Oculographic and clinical characterization of thirty-seven children with anomalous head postures, nystagmus, and strabismus: the basis of a clinical algorithm. J AAPOS. 2000;4(1):25-32.
9. Abel LA, Wang ZI, Dell'Osso LF. Wavelet analysis in infantile nystagmus syndrome: limitations and abilities. Invest Ophthalmol Vis Sci. 2008;49(8):3413-23.
10. Dorn L, Curković T, Dorn V. Foveation period and waveforms of congenital ocular nystagmus. Coll Antropol. 2005;29(Suppl 1):99-101.
11. Bagheri A, Aletaha M, Abrishami M. The effect of horizontal rectus muscle surgery on clinical and eye movement recording indices in infantile nystagmus syndrome. Strabismus. 2010;18(2):58-64.
12. Wang ZI, Dell'Osso LF. Eye-movement-based assessment of visual function in patients with infantile nystagmus syndrome. Optom Vis Sci. 2009;86(8):988-95.
13. Bifulco P, Cesarelli M, Loffredo L, et al. Eye movement baseline oscillation and variability of eye position during foveation in congenital nystagmus. Doc Ophthalmol. 2003;107(2): 131-6.
14. Yao JP, Tai Z, Yin ZQ. A new measure of nystagmus acuity. Int J Ophthalmol. 2014;7(1):95-9.
15. Tai Z, Hertle RW, Bilonick RA, et al. A new algorithm for automated nystagmus acuity function analysis. Br J Ophthalmol. 2011;95(6):832-6.
16. Taibbi G, Wang ZI, Dell'Osso LF. Infantile nystagmus syndrome: broadening the high-foveation-quality field with contact lenses. Clin Ophthalmol. 2008;2(3):585-9.
17. Jacobs JB, Dell'osso LF. Extending the eXpanded Nystagmus Acuity Function for vertical and multiplanar data. Vision Res. 2010;50(3):271-8.
18. Jacobs JB, Dell'Osso LF, Wang ZI, et al. Using the NAFX to measure the effectiveness over time of gene therapy in canine LCA. Invest Ophthalmol Vis Sci. 2009;50(10):4685-92.
19. Metz HS. Saccadic velocity measurements in strabismus. Trans Am Ophthalmol Soc. 1983;81:630-92.
20. Trillenberg P, Lencer R, Heide W. Eye movements and psychiatric disease. Curr Opin Neurol. 200;17(1):43-7.

CHAPTER 22

Pentacam

Rohit Shetty, Ashwin Shetty, Luci Kaweri

INTRODUCTION

Imaging is paying an increasingly important role in the decision-making process of the eye-care providers. There are several instruments for the diagnosis of eye diseases. A specific tool such as pachymeter or A-scan or B-scan ultrasound performs a specific task admirably well. However, in place of multiple instruments, there should be a comprehensive diagnostic tool that can image the entire anterior segment and present the data in an easy to interpret form. To some extent, Pentacam **(Fig. 1)** manufactured by Oculus Inc. is one of the tools that qualifies for this category.

BASIC PRINCIPLES

Scheimpflug Principle

In a normal camera, the film/sensor plane, lens plane, and the plane of sharp focus (imaginary surface positioned such that any object lying on it will be imaged sharply by the lens on the film plane) are all parallel to each other and do not intersect **(Fig. 2)**.

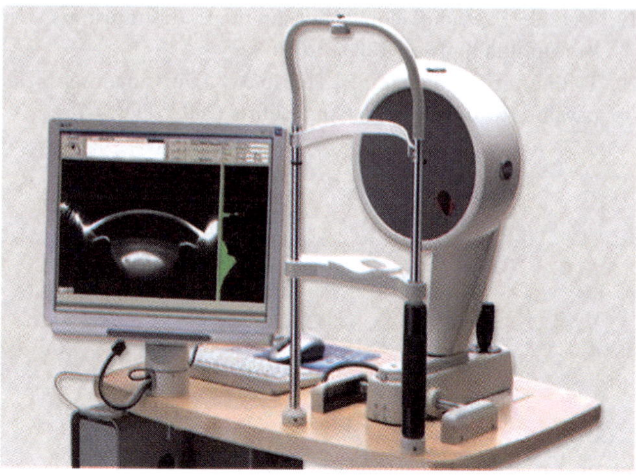

Fig. 1: The Pentacam HR workstation.

The Scheimpflug principle states that if a lens is tilted such that the lens plane intersects the film plane, the plane of sharp focus must also pass through that same line **(Fig. 3)**.[1]

Scheimpflug imaging differs from conventional techniques in that the object plane, lens plane, and image plane are not parallel to each other, but intersect in a common straight line **(Fig. 4)**. The major advantage of the Scheimpflug geometry is that a wide depth of focus is achieved allowing to obtain optical sections of the entire

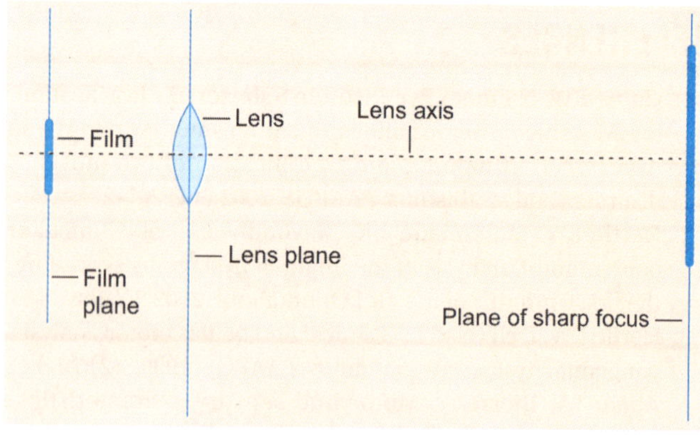

Fig. 2: Optics of a simple camera.

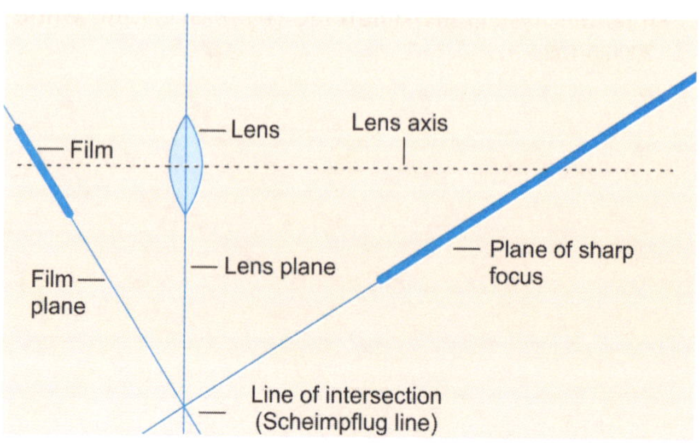

Fig. 3: The Scheimpflug principle.

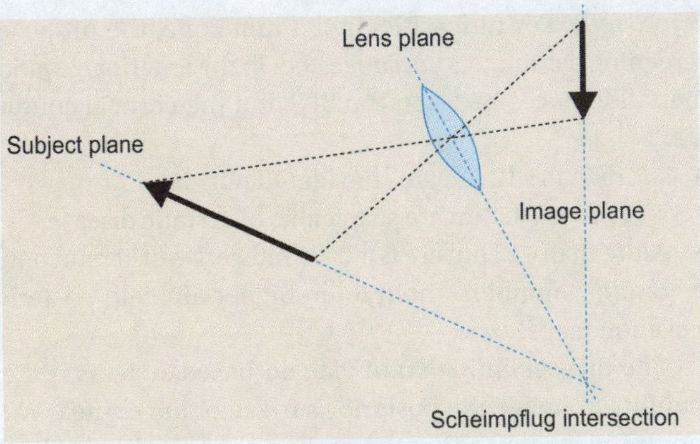

Fig. 4: The Scheimpflug camera—schematic diagram.

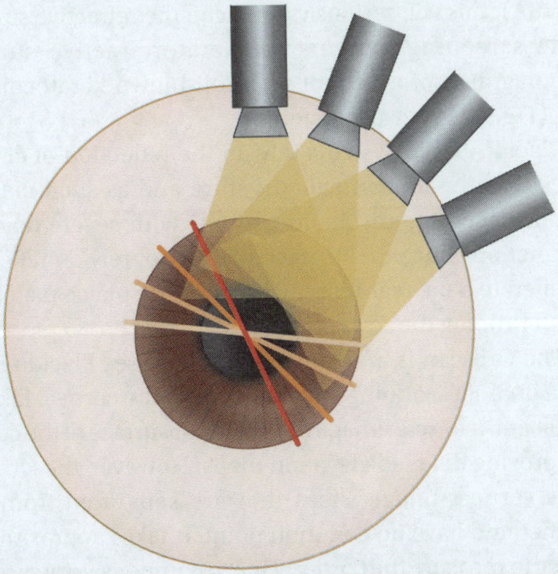

Fig. 5: Rotating Scheimpflug camera of the Pentacam.

anterior segment of the eye, from the anterior surface of the cornea to the posterior surface of the lens.[1]

The Pentacam system uses a rotating Scheimpflug camera **(Fig. 5)** to obtain 50 slit images within 2 seconds. It provides a comprehensive, three-dimensional (3D) scan of the anterior chamber from the anterior surface of the cornea up to the posterior surface of the crystalline lens. The image plane of the Scheimpflug camera is slanted at a 45° angle toward the optical axis of the camera optics. It performs a 360° rotating scan but captures the images only in the temporal 180° in order to avoid the nose shadow (for the right eye, it scans from approximately 130°–310°). During the scan, fixation control is achieved via a second camera focused on the pupil that monitors size and orientation; eye movements are corrected for automatically using a central registration after the scan is completed.[2]

OUTPUT

The raw data generated by the scans are then analyzed using highly sophisticated software and the following "maps" are generated.

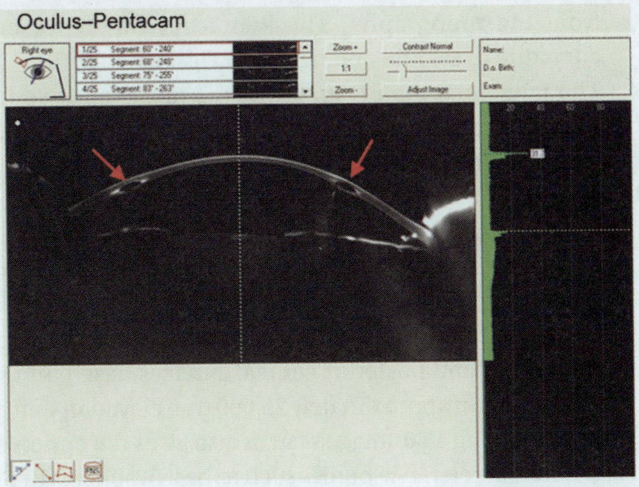

Fig. 6: Scheimpflug image of the anterior segment of right eye (up to posterior surface of the lens) two intracorneal ring segments (arrows) are seen.

Scheimpflug Images

A clear, sharp Scheimpflug image, depicting the entire anterior segment from the cornea to the posterior lens surface, including the angle area up to the most distal 100–150 μm is visualized **(Fig. 6)**. The image may be rotated to visualize any cross section. This image can also be reviewed with 3D animation.

This image may be used for:

- Localization of pathology within the cornea.
- Measuring the depth of implantation and stability of intracorneal ring segments.
- Measuring the white to white diameter for sizing of the implantable collamer lens (ICL).
- Verifying the central corneal thickness (CCT) and anterior chamber depth (ACD).
- Measurements in case the automated measurements are suspected.
- Measurement of lens thickness.

The Pentacam, however, cannot see beyond pigmented structures. Therefore, visualization of structures beyond the iris such as ciliary sulcus is not possible.[2]

TOPOGRAPHY

Before describing the topography features of the Pentacam, it would be useful to review a few basic definitions:

- *Corneal elevation* is the measurement of height between two different points at different elevations. The Pentacam uses elevation data as its primary data source.
- *Slope or the gradient* is commonly used to describe the measurement of the steepness incline or grade of a straight line from two points with different elevations. Slope is the primary data source for Placido-disk-based technology.
- *Curvature* is the rate of change of the slope. It is the second derivative of elevation and is calculated from slope data

from the topography. The Pentacam can represent curvature as sagittal or tangential **(Figs. 7A and B)**.

The tangential map **(Fig. 8A)** is the most sensitive for determining the geometry of the cornea. Sagittal map **(Fig. 8B)** or axial power map is the most common map used in topography and represents the axial power of the cornea at all points. Unlike the sagittal map, the tangential map curvatures are relative to the surface, not the axial center of the surface.

The Pentacam generates color-coded topography maps of the anterior and posterior corneal surfaces based on the measurements of approximately 25,000 true elevation points while performing a 50-image scan. It also gives the option of using different reference bodies such as best fit sphere (BFS), best fit ellipse, and best fit toric ellipsoid, to represent the elevation data. It measures the cornea from limbus to limbus thereby picking up pathologies in the corneal periphery that may be missed by Placido-based systems, which typically do not measure up to the limbus.

The Pentacam provides elevation and curvature (axial/tangential) data in the form of color-coded maps. Flatter areas (above BFS) are represented in "cooler" color (blue) and steeper areas (below the BFS) are shown in "warmer" color (red). For fitting BFS in a 9 mm zone, the proposed screening parameters are suggested. In the anterior elevation map differences between the BFS and the corneal contour are:[3]

- More than +12 µm are considered normal
- +12 µm to +15 µm are suspicious of ecstatic disease
- More than +15 µm are typically indicative of keratoconus.

Similar numbers about 5 µm higher apply to posterior elevation maps.

The biggest limitation of Placido-based systems is their inability to image the posterior surface of the cornea. With mounting evidence that the earliest topographic evidence of corneal ectasia is seen in the posterior corneal surface **(Fig. 9A)**, this will seriously handicap the refractive surgeon while screening patients for keratorefractive surgery. The diagnosis of a patient with full-blown keratoconus is easy **(Fig. 9B)** with any system.

Placido-based systems rely on the reflection of circular mires to estimate corneal curvature and as such may not produce accurate results in patients with severe tear film dysfunction. Since the Pentacam does not rely on reflection to generate data, tear film quality may not play a major role in determining the scan quality.

The Orbscan is a hybrid system that uses Placido mires and a dual slit scanning system to image the cornea. Like the Pentacam, it too can image the posterior surface of the cornea and provide detailed elevation maps. However, the Orbscan takes vertical image slices that are separated from one another and have no common point. It takes approximately 2.1 sec to measure the cornea. Due to compensatory saccadic movements by the eye to maintain fixation, the unit never knows exactly where the eye is during that 2.1 sec period. Therefore, the Orbscan cannot reregister the eye movements occurring during the process of capturing the images.

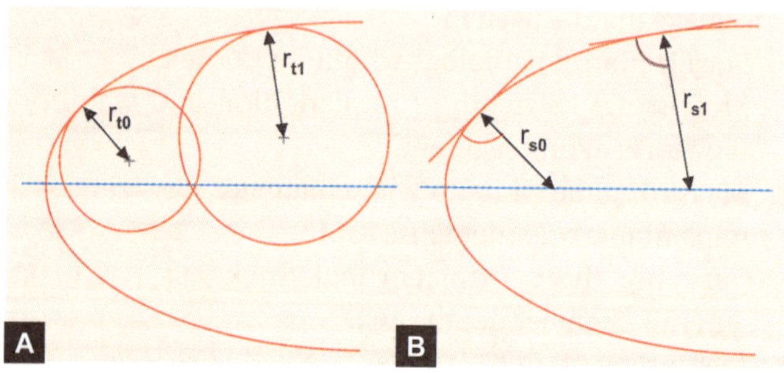

Figs. 7A and B: (A) Tangential curvature; (B) Sagittal curvature.

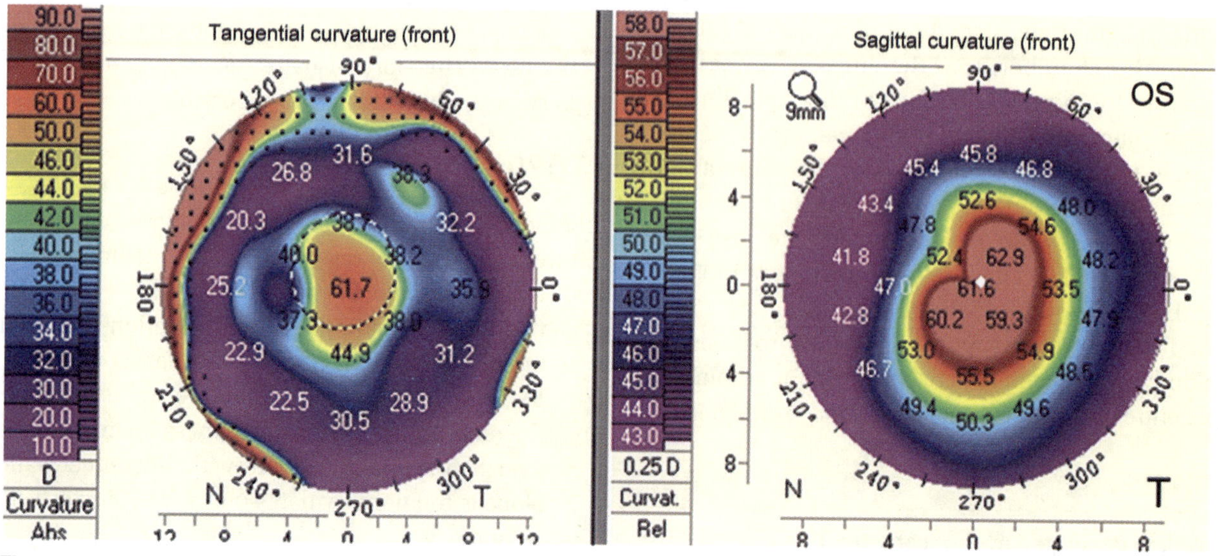

Figs. 8A and B: (A) The front tangential curvature map of the left eye of a patient with keratoconus; (B) Front sagittal curvature map.

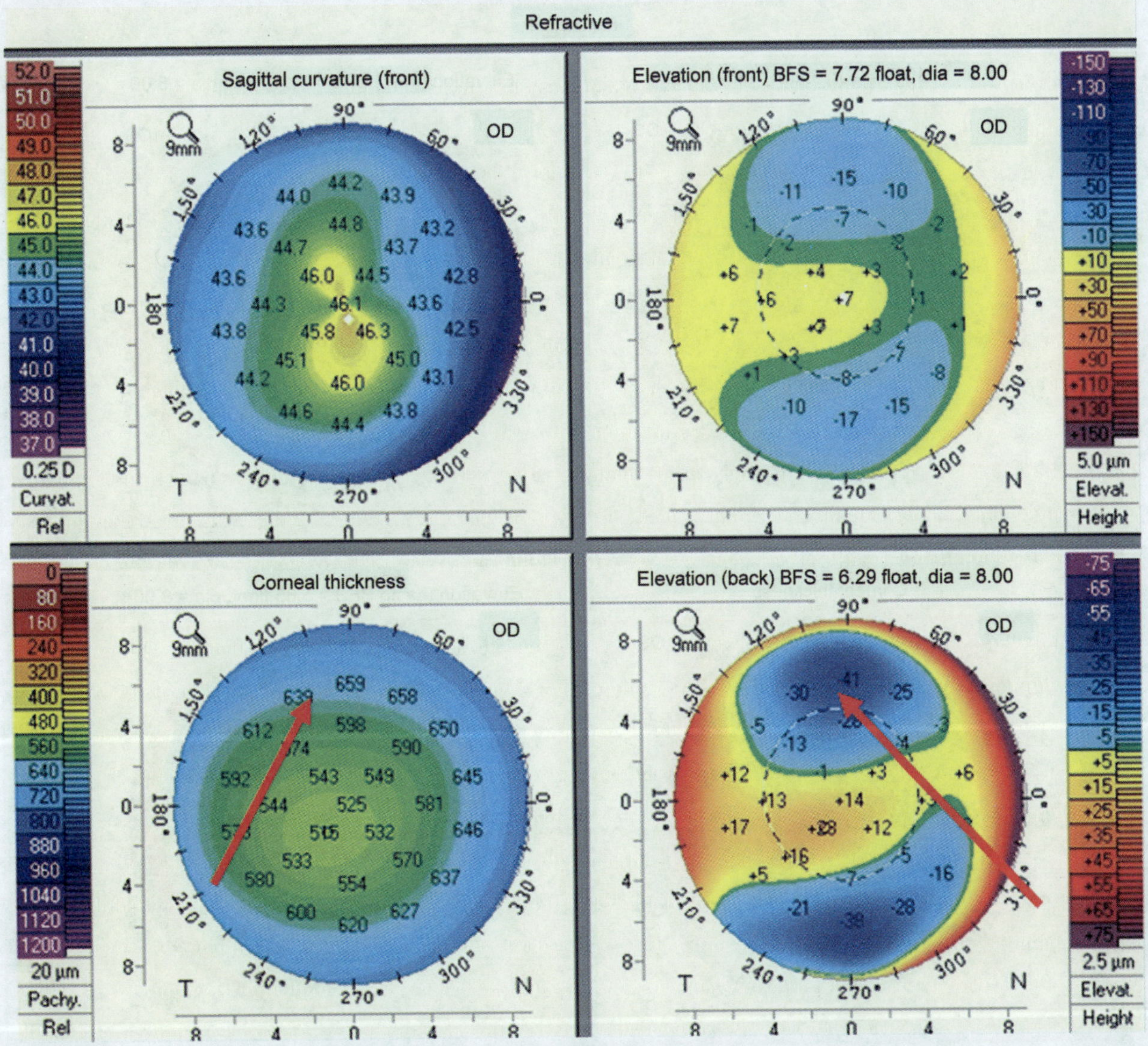

Fig. 9A: A typical 4-map refractive printout of the right eye of a patient. Note the relative normal appearing elevation values on the anterior elevation map. The posterior elevation map shows a maximal elevation of 28 μ (red arrow) which would be considered suspicious. The pachymetry map also shows a shifting of the thinnest point from the apex and it corresponds to the elevated area on the posterior curvature map (red arrow). A Placido-based system which only evaluates the anterior surface would miss the above.

The Pentacam maintains a fixed point on the vertex of the cornea and that acts as a reference point for image reconstruction while compensating for eye movements. This feature minimizes test-test variability and is extremely important as it allows reexamination of a particular area of interest in order to detect changes over time or response to therapy.

Specialized Maps

The Pentacam provides a corneal topographer with a host of additional features. As such, this tool will be used most often for screening patients and for planning refractive surgery. The biggest concern of the refractive surgeon today is picking up early ectasia in patients presenting for keratorefractive surgery. Along with the anterior and posterior elevations and curvature data, the Pentacam also provides a few specialized maps to aid in the diagnosis.

Belin-Ambrosio Enhanced Ectasia Display

Elevation maps are typically viewed by comparing the data to some standard reference surface thereby highlighting the differences in elevation. The most commonly used reference shape is the BFS. However, the BFS is itself influenced by any abnormal elevation of the cornea. In the case of keratoconus or ectasia, the apical protrusion will have the effect of steepening the BFS. This will minimize the elevation difference between the apex of the cone and the BFS making the cone less obvious while ideally we would like to see how the suspect area compares with the "normal" part of the patient's cornea. To do this, a reference surface is defined

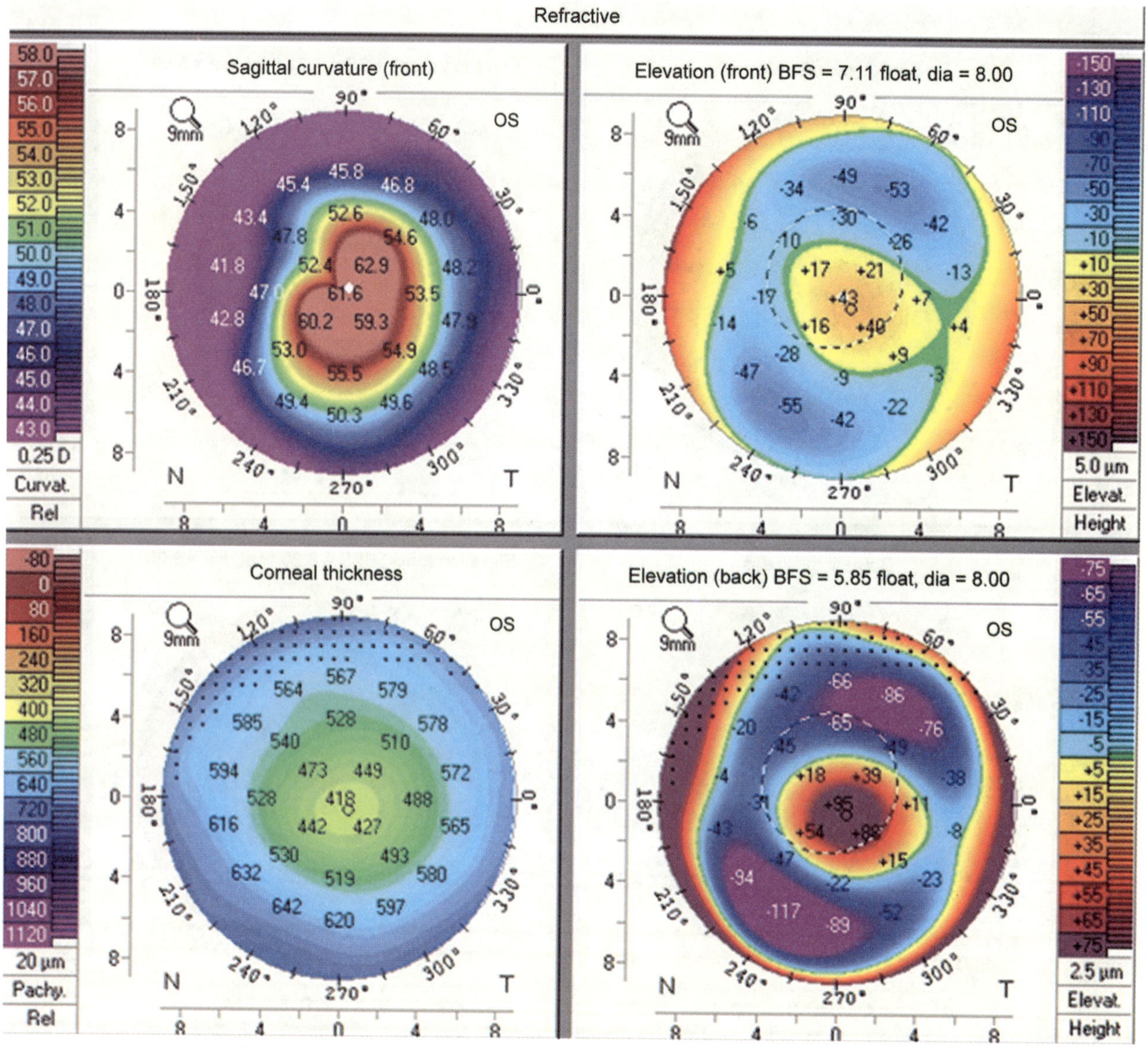

Fig. 9B: The left eye of the same patient shows full-blown pictures of keratoconus, not a candidate for keratorefractive surgery.

based on the individual's own cornea after excluding the ectatic region **(Fig. 10)**. A 4-mm optical zone centered on the thinnest portion of the cornea (exclusion zone) is excluded from the calculations for the new reference surface.

Then, the new "enhanced BFS" is defined by utilizing all the valid data from within the 9.0 mm central cornea with the exception of the exclusion zone.[4]

The printout of an enhanced ectasia display shows two segments—the topography segment on the left and the pachymetric section on the right **(Fig. 11)**.

The topography section comprises three rows of two maps each. The top row shows two elevation maps that display the baseline relative elevation of the anterior and posterior surface of the cornea of the BFS. Immediately below the standard anterior and posterior elevation maps are the anterior and posterior exclusion maps. These are generated by comparing the corneal elevation against an

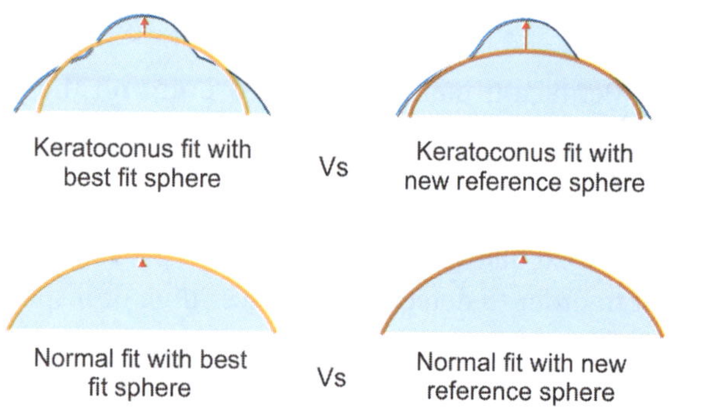

Fig. 10: Schematic diagrams to illustrate the effect of exclusion of the ectatic area on flattening the BFS. Also note the minimal or no effect on the BFS after removal of the exclusion zone in case of a normal cornea. (BFS: best fit sphere)

enhanced reference surface as described above. The location of the exclusion zone is indicated by a 4 mm red circle. The maps in the bottom row represent the elevation difference between the baseline and the exclusion maps. They contain only three colors, each one corresponding to the amount of elevation change. Green color represents a change in elevation of less than 6 microns on the anterior surface and 8 microns on the posterior surface of the cornea and is typically within the range seen in normal eyes. The yellow areas represent a change between 6 microns and 12 microns for the anterior surface and 8–20 microns for the back surface and are suspicious for ectasia. Red color represents areas where the elevation difference between the two maps is >12 microns anteriorly or >20 microns posteriorly typically seen in eyes with known keratoconus.[4]

The pachymetric section of the Belin-Ambrosio enhanced ectasia display will be dealt within the following segment on pachymetry.

The Holladay Equivalent Keratometry Reading for Postrefractive Surgery Intraocular Lens Power Calculation[5]

A significant number of patients who had undergone keratorefractive surgery [radial keratotomy (RK), photorefractive keratectomy (PRK), and laser in situ keratomileusis (LASIK)] in the past are now presenting with cataracts. Calculation of the intraocular lens (IOL) power in these patients is very difficult due to difficulty in estimation of the true central corneal power. Another factor compounding the problem is that most of these patients do not have their preoperative keratometry readings thereby making it impossible to use methods like the calculation history method. The need of the hour is for a system, which can accurately calculate the central corneal power in such patients without the need for preoperative data which may not be forthcoming.

Keratometers and Placido-based topographers calculate the refractive power of the cornea with the assumption that the ratio of radius of curvature between back and front of the cornea is 82% and constant. This leads to an overall average corneal refractive index of n = 1.3375; however, it does not hold good for eyes that have undergone keratorefractive surgery. For myopic treatment, the ratio decreases and for hyperopic treatments, it increases. Therefore, we have to consider the anterior and posterior curvatures to calculate the true corneal power, and specific refractive indices for cornea and for aqueous have to be used to convert curvature into refractive power. The equivalent keratometry readings (EKR) take in account all these effects.

Another consideration is that keratometers and Placido-based topographers have a blind spot in the center and, thus, is not directly measured. This area is interpolated assuming

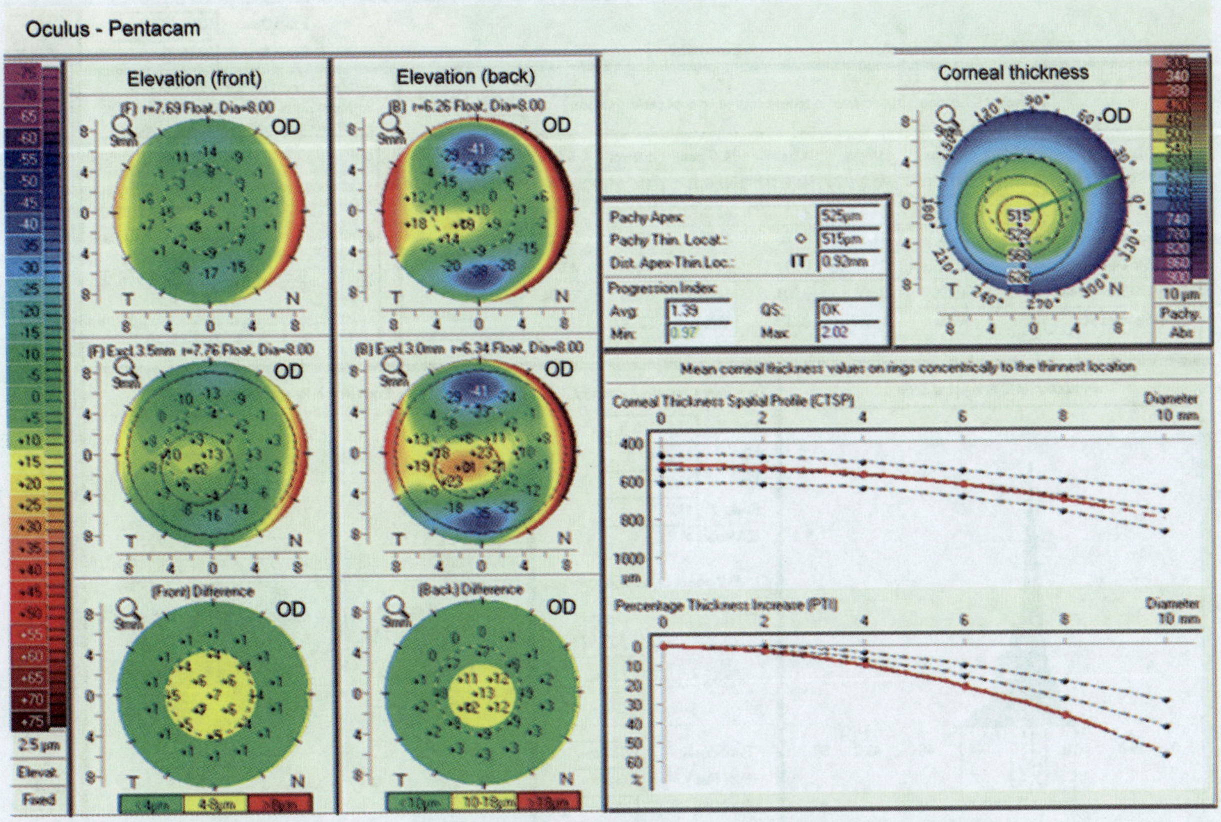

Fig. 11: The enhanced ectasia display of the right eye of the patient shown in **Figure 9A**.

a central steepening, which is accurate for untreated eyes but after myopic treatment, it is actually the opposite. This results in a wrong curvature and a wrong refractive central corneal power.

It is essential to measure the center for accurate corneal measurement, especially for the keratometry readings. The Pentacam's rotating camera measures the central cornea very precisely.

Equivalent Keratometry Reading Printouts

The table in the upper left displays the EKRs in different zones around the pupil center, which may be useful for patients with very large or small pupils. It also gives the number of points sampled in that zone **(Fig. 12A)**. The software typically defaults to the EKRs in the 4.5 mm zone as this has been found to be the most accurate by the developers of the software. However, the size of the zone may be varied according to the surgeon's preference. Some authors have found the 3 mm zone to be more accurate than the default measurements at the 4.5 mm zone.

The graph in the lower left displays the refractive power distribution of the EKRs in the selected zone. A small range of power evidenced by a tall peak is a good proponent for a good refractive outcome. Does this means that the cataract surgeon can sleep in peace...not quite. Although these values may be more precise than those obtained with other instruments, they can only be used to calculate the IOL power in formulas that are optimized for EKR, like the Borasio Edmondo Smith and Stevens (BESSt) or Holladay-2 formulas or if the American Society of Cataract and Refractive Surgery (ASCRS) postkeratorefractive IOL calculator is being used. Using these values directly will violate the assumptions contained in most third generation, two-variable formulas (SRK/T, Hoffer Q, and Holladay-1), affecting the estimation of the postoperative effective lens position (ELP), which determines the effective power of the implanted IOL. A few studies have also reported that the EKRs overestimate the corneal power and this effect increases with increasing flattening of the cornea[6] leading to underestimation of the IOL power and a consecutive postoperative hyperopia. Therefore, pending further refinement of the software, it may not be prudent to use only the EKR for IOL calculation after refractive surgery.

Pachymetry

The Pentacam provides a color-coded pachymetric map of the cornea **(Fig. 12B)** which shows thickness of the cornea from limbus to limbus. The measured values can be

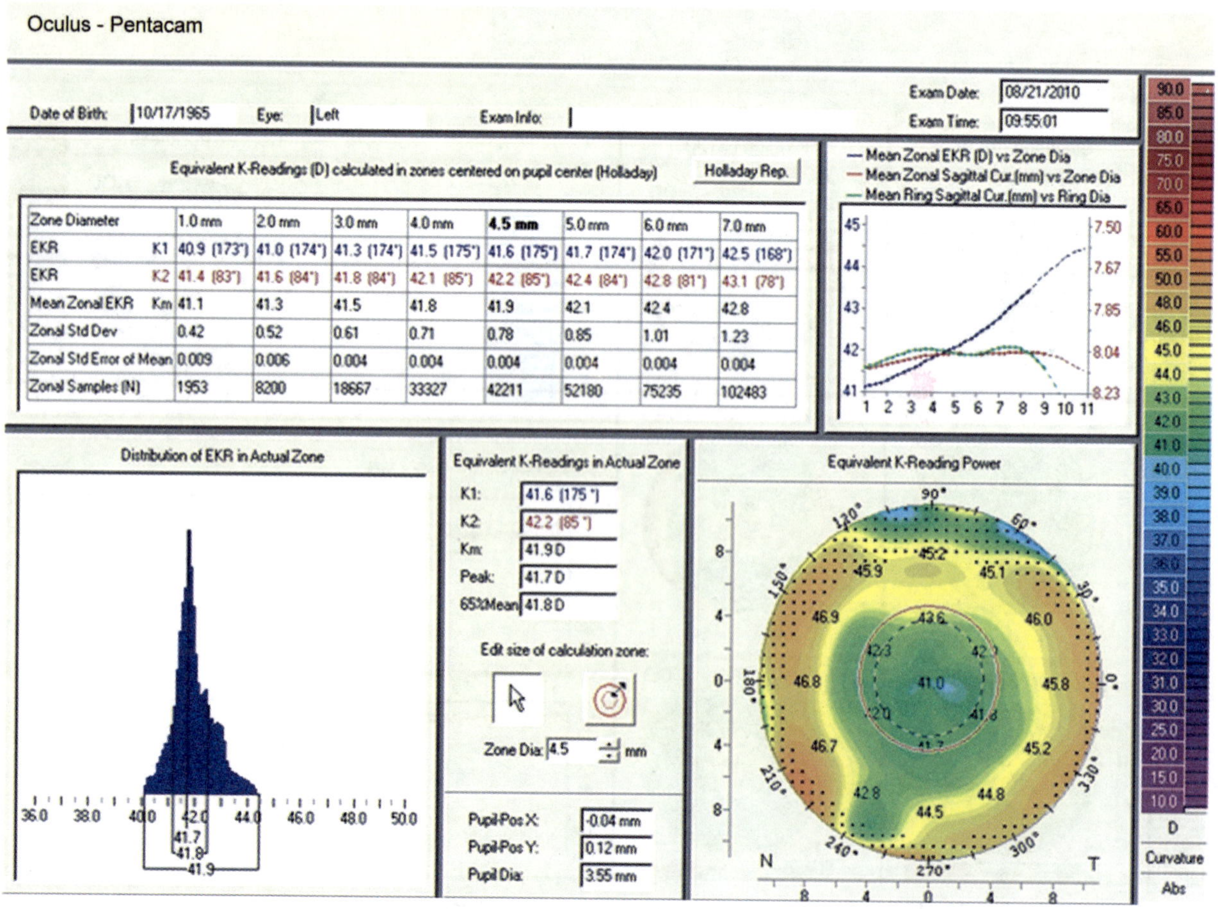

Fig. 12A: The Holladay EKR report.
(EKR: equivalent keratometry reading)

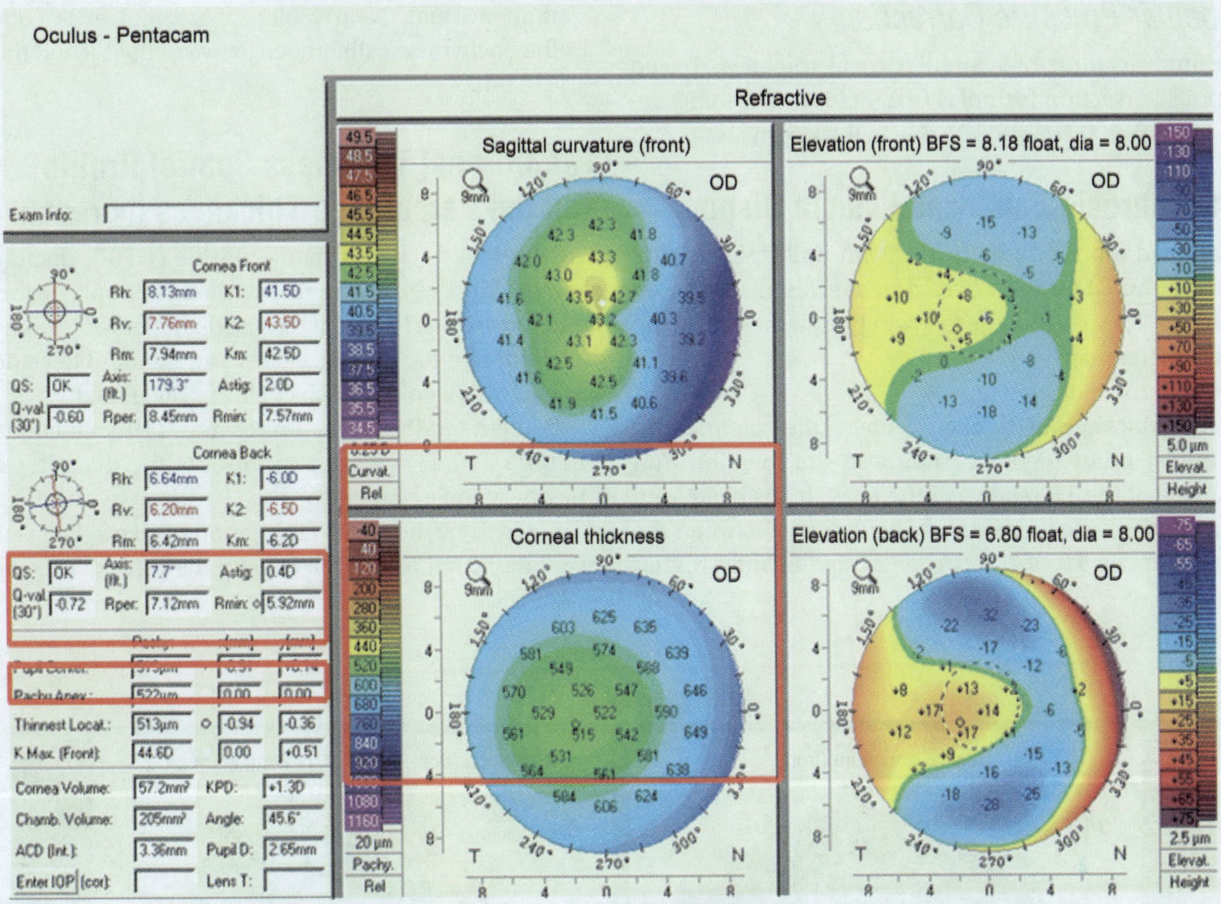

Fig. 12B: The pachymetric map and the pachymetric indices outlined in red.

displayed in a predetermined grid or represented manually at any point via mouse click.

The following readings are automatically provided in the lower left-hand corner of the quad map:

- Corneal thickness in the center of the pupil
- Corneal thickness in the apex
- The thinnest point (TP) of the cornea
- Corneal volume.

Applications

Presurgical Planning of Refractive Corneal Surgery

The high repeatability, interoperator reproducibility, and intra- and intersession repeatability[7] make the Pentacam an ideal tool for planning and following up cases for keratorefractive surgery. In cases, which are being considered for refractive surgery revision, the Pentacam gives very accurate values that can help rule out ectasia even in the presence of a LASIK flap.

Relative Pachymetry Map (Fig. 12C) for Early Keratoconus Detection

It gives the thickness of the cornea at a particular point as a percentage relative to the normal thickness at that point.

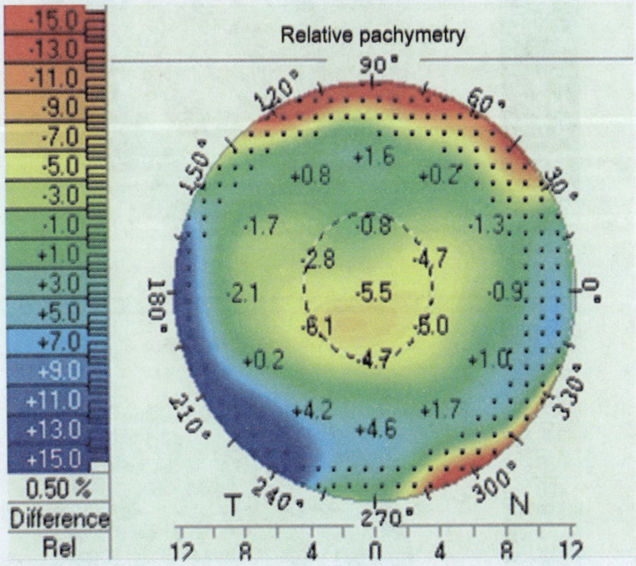

Fig. 12C: The relative pachymetric map of the patient discussed in Figure 9B. The point of maximum deviation (–6.1%) corresponds to the point of highest posterior elevation and the thinnest point on the pachymetry maps, respectively further increasing the sensitivity of the examination.

Thus, a normal map would be 0% at all points while any thinning would show a "–" value and thickening would show a "+" value. Relative pachymetry measurements that exceed –3.0% may be considered significant.

Intraocular Pressure Correction

Taking into account measured corneal thickness based on various correction formulas (e.g. Ehler or Dresden) are useful to rule out increased IOP due to thick corneas.

Belin-Ambrosio Enhanced Ectasia Display

As mentioned above, one-half of the Belin-Ambrosio displays **(Figs. 13A and B)** for early detection of ectasia is based on pachymetry. It consists of the following parameters:[4]

- Pachymetry map
- Pachymetric indices
- Corneal thickness at the apex (center of the examination)
- Thinnest point of the cornea and the location and distance of the TP relative to the apex. It has been seen that in eyes with keratoconus, the distance between the apex and the TP of the cornea is significantly higher than normal. Nearly 88% of normal eyes will have the pachymetric difference between the TP and the apex <10 μm.

The Corneal Thickness Spatial Profile and the Percentage Thickness Increase

The corneal thickness spatial profile (CTSP) displays the average thickness measurements along 22 concentric circles centered on the TP with increasing diameters of 0.4 mm steps. In addition to the average values, the standard deviations of the pachymetry along each circle are calculated.

Percentage thickness increase (PTI) is calculated by (CT@x - TP)/TP, where x represents the diameter of the imaginary circle centered on the TP with increased diameters as provided by the CTSP. Each graph displays the examined eye data in red and three broken dark lines. The top and

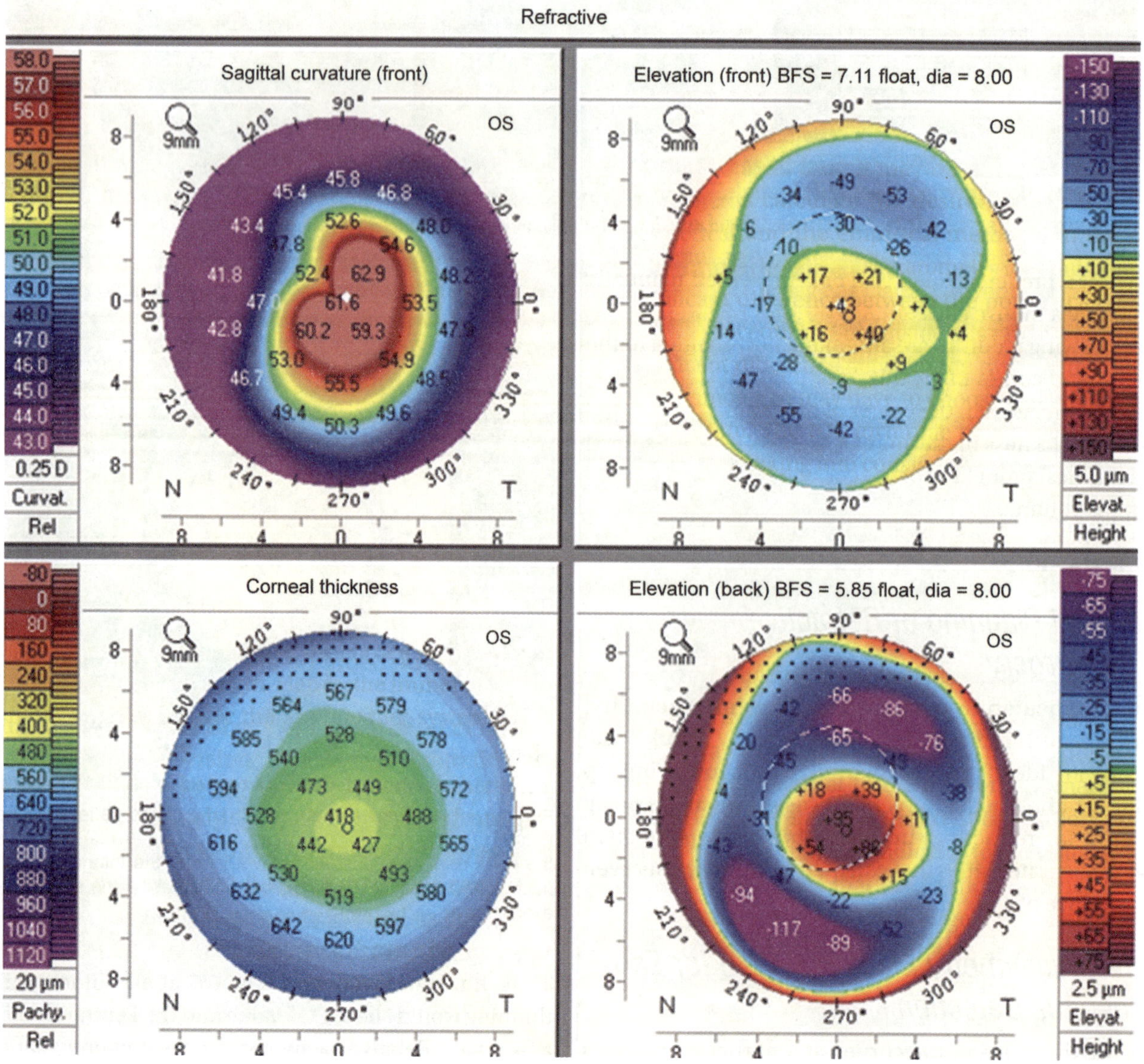

Fig. 13A

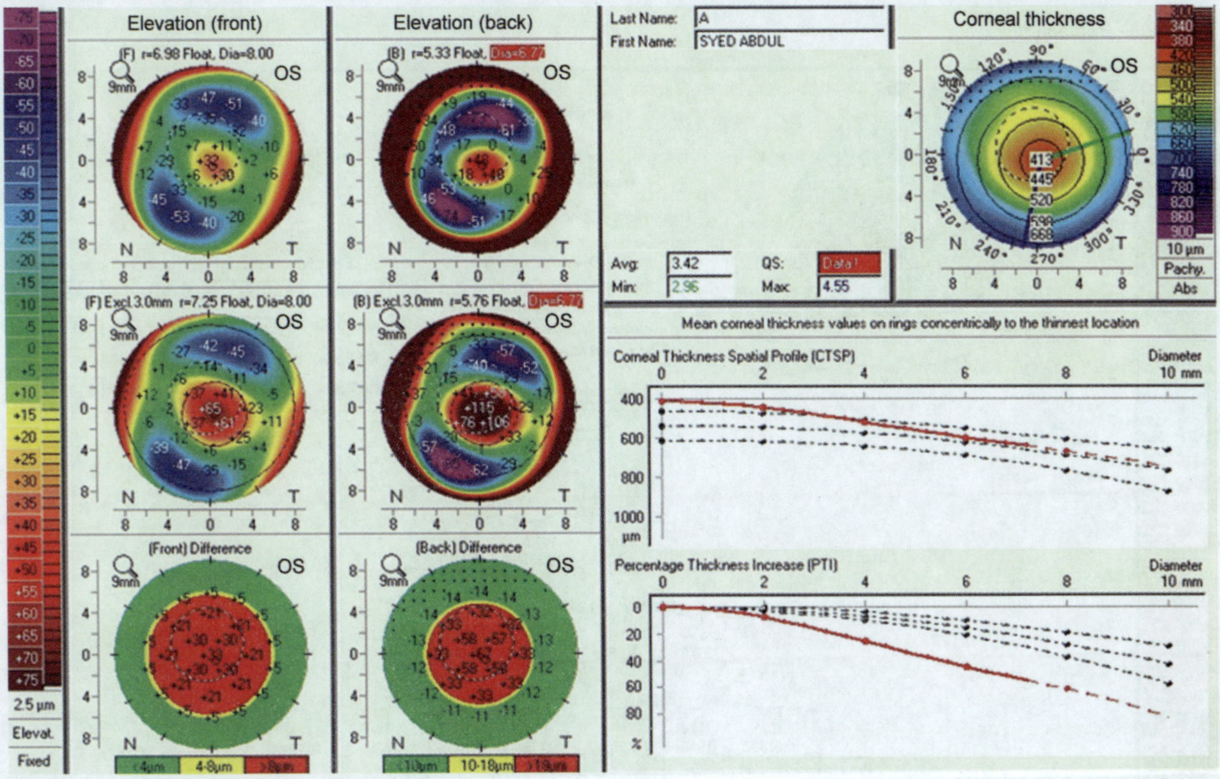

Fig. 13B

Figs. 13A and B: The Belin-Ambrosio enhanced ectasia display.

bottom lines represent the upper and lower double standard deviation, respectively (95% confidence interval) and the central line represents the average values from a normal population. Corneas with ectatic disease (e.g. keratoconus, post-LASIK ectasia) show a more rapid progression of thickening from the TP to the periphery or conversely. Ectatic corneas thin more rapidly than normal eyes going from the periphery to the thinnest part of the cornea.[8]

The CTSP and PTI graphs enable the rapid identification of early forms of ectasia, increasing sensitivity and specificity for screening candidates for refractive surgery. It also enables clinical differentiation of a normal thin cornea from an ectatic cornea, and a normal thick cornea from an edematous cornea.

Screening for Ectasia Using Pentacam

With the above background information on elevation, curvature and pachymetry outputs of a Pentacam, a few "rules of thumb" may be formulated to screen patients for ectasia. A cornea can be considered highly suspected for ectatic pathology if the following parameters are present:

- The highest curvature point and the TP on pachymetry coincide
- The highest curvature point coincides with the highest anterior and posterior elevation points
- The highest curvature point, the TP, and the highest anterior point and highest posterior point of the corneal surface all coincide to confirm the diagnosis of ectasia.

The above guidelines along with the enhanced ectasia display may help detect early ectasia and prevent the disastrous consequences of such corneas being subjected to keratorefractive surgery.

Three-dimensional Cataract Analysis

The lens densitometry program has shown good correlation with Lens Opacities Classification System III.[9] A good correlation has been also seen between Pentacam densitometry and total phaco energy used.[10]

Applications

Three-dimensional analysis can quantify objectively the density of lens opacities and has following applications:

- In evaluating risk factors for cataract development
- In assessing the efficacy of anticataractogenic drugs
- It can assist in predicting phacodynamics and adjusting machine parameters in phaco surgery.[10]

Three-dimensional Anterior Chamber Analysis

The Pentacam provides the following data on anterior chamber analysis:

- Anterior chamber depth—a key factor in deciding eligibility for phakic IOL (pIOL) implantation.
- The new Pentacam IOL-software module simulates the positioning of an iris fixated pIOL in the anterior

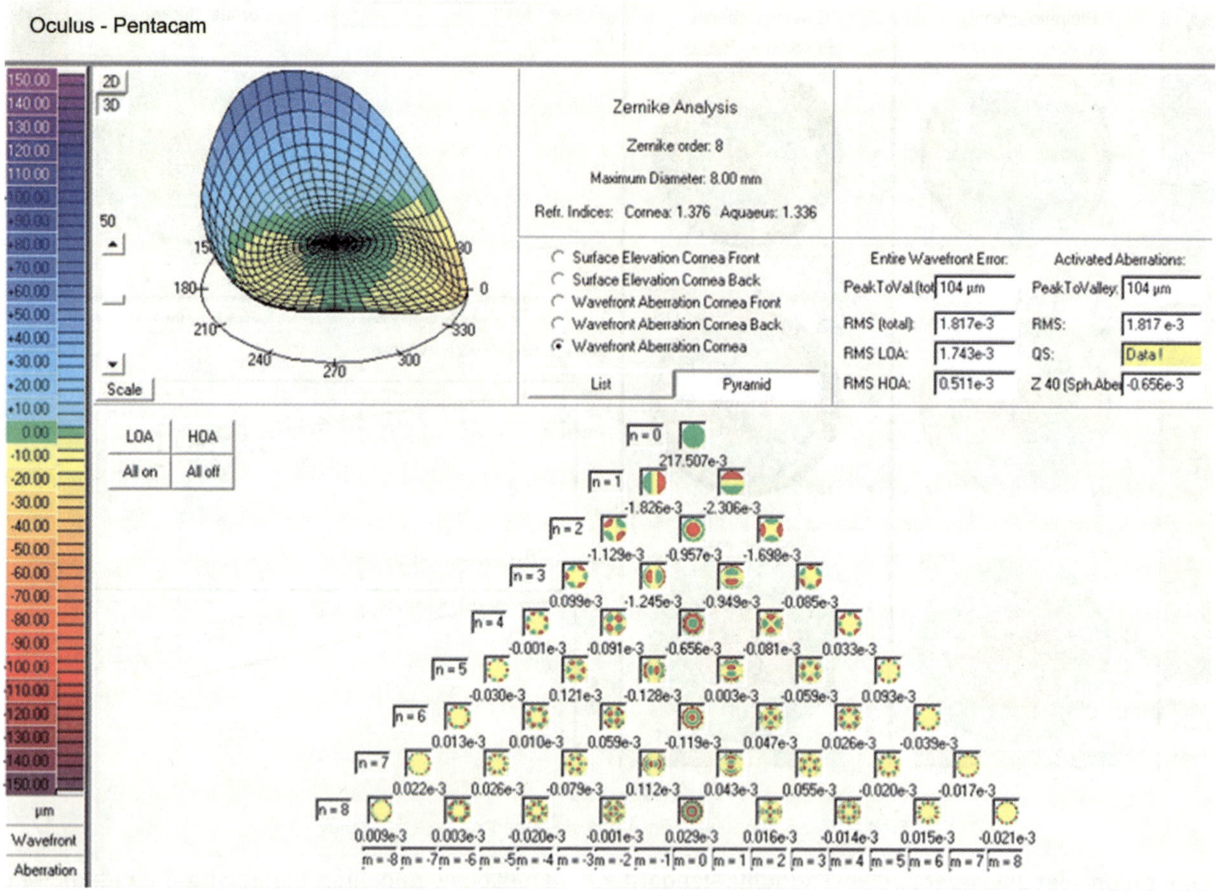

Fig. 14: Zernike analysis.

chamber 3D model. Distances to adjacent eye structures are calculated to each surface point three-dimensionally by the software.

It can also predict the changes in anterior chamber dimensions and the pIOL position up to 30 years in advance.

- Glaucoma screening.

Preoperative to postoperative comparison of changes in anterior chamber, e.g. after iridectomy or iridotomy:

- Colored ACD map
- Anterior chamber angle (ACA) in 360°
- Anterior chamber volume (ACV)
- Pupil diameter.

Anterior chamber depth measurements have shown excellent repeatability. However, dynamic measurements such as size and decentration of pupil, and the ACV have shown poorer repeatability.[7]

Corneal Wavefront Analysis

Applications

- Selection of aspheric IOLs for correction of corneal spherical aberrations (Z4.0); most eyes have positive anterior corneal spherical aberration and will do better with an aspheric IOL that adds negative spherical aberration (Tecnis-AMO/AcrySof IQ). However, in some cases, where the central cornea is quite steep, an aspheric IOL without the addition of negative spherical aberration is a better choice (Akreos AO).
- Patients with keratoconus or previous hyperopic LASIK (negative spherical aberration) may have improved postoperative contrast sensitivity following the implantation of a spherical IOL that adds a small amount of positive spherical aberration.
- Fitting of corneal rings in reference to the axis of the coma.
- Determination of low and high order aberrations.

The aberrometry function of the Pentacam can be performed with the help of Zernike analysis **(Fig. 14)**, however, it has shown poor repeatability.[11]

Contact Lens Fitting

Pentacam is very useful in fitting of contact lenses since it provides following information:

- It automatically displays all necessary measurement data for fitting contact lenses.
- It automatically suggests for contact lenses.
- It provides realistic fluorescein image simulation.
- It has integrated, expandable data bank with over 65,000 lens geometries.

The Pentacam is available in three models:

1. Basic
2. Classic
3. High resolution (HR).

The basic version can be upgraded to classic by a software upgrade. The HR version is a hardware upgrade and one cannot upgrade from a basic or a classic version. (For a full description of the capabilities of each version, one may refer to *www.pentacam.com.*)

REFERENCES

1. Merklinger HM (1992). The Scheimpflug Principle—Part I. Shutterbug. [online] Available from: http://www.trenholm.org/hmmerk/SHBG05.pdf. [Last accessed on November, 2019].
2. Pentacam HR. User manual. [online] Available from: https://www.pentacam.com/fileadmin/user_upload/pentacam.de/downloads/interpretations-leitfaden/interpretation_guideline_3rd_edition_0915.pdf. [Last accessed on November, 2019].
3. Holladay JT, Belin MW, Chayet AS, et al. Next generation technology for cataract and refractive surgeon. Cataract Refract Surg Today. 2005;35(Suppl 6):1-11.
4. Highlights in Ophthalmology. 2008;35(6). [online] Available from: http://www.ophthbooks.com/More.aspx?BID=1387. [Last accessed on November, 2019].
5. Belin MW, Holladay JT, Michelson MA, et al. The pentacam: precision, confidence, results, and accurate "KS!". Cataract Refract Surg Today. 2007;16:258.
6. Tang Q, Hoffer TJ, Olson MD, et al. Accuracy of Scheimpflug Holladay equivalent keratometry readings after corneal refractive surgery. J Cataract Refract Surg. 2009;35(7):1198-203.
7. Shankar H, Taranath D, Santhirathelagan CT, et al. Anterior segment biometry with the Pentacam: comprehensive assessment of repeatability of automated measurements. J Cataract Refract Surg. 2008;34(1):103-13.
8. Ambrósio R Jr, Alonso RS, Luz A, et al. Corneal-thickness spatial profile and corneal-volume distribution: tomographic indices to detect keratoconus. J Cataract Refract Surg. 2006;32(11):1851-9.
9. Grewal DS, Brar SP, Grewal SPS. Correlation of nuclear cataract lens density using Scheimpflug images with Lens Opacities Classification System III and visual function. Ophthalmology. 2009;116(8):1436-43.
10. Kim JS, Chung SH, Joo CK. Clinical application of a Scheimpflug system for lens density measurements in phacoemulsification. J Cataract Refract Surg. 2009;35(7):1204-9.
11. Piñero DP, Saenz González C, Alió JL. Intraobserver and interobserver repeatability of curvature and aberrometric measurements of the posterior corneal surface in normal eyes using Scheimpflug photography. J Cataract Refract Surg. 2009;35(1):113-20.

CHAPTER

23 Anterior Segment Optical Coherence Tomography

R Ramakrishnan, Arijit Mitra

INTRODUCTION

Imaging the ocular adnexae has evolved significantly since its conception. Until recently, there had been no reliable or useful method of imaging the anterior segment in cross section. Now ultrasound biomicroscope (UBM), anterior segment optical coherence tomography (ASOCT), or Pentacam (Scheimpflug imaging) provide detailed cross-sectional images of the cornea, anterior chamber (AC), angle, iris, and in the case of ultrasound, the lens.

Optical coherence tomography (OCT) is a cross-sectional, three-dimensional, and high-resolution imaging modality that uses low-coherence interferometry to achieve axial resolution in the range of 3–20 µm. Anterior segment imaging using OCT was first demonstrated in 1994 by Izatt et al. using light with a wavelength of 830 nm. However, it was not until Lübeck group described OCT imaging of laser thermokeratoplasty lesion in 1997 and Maldonado et al. reported imaging of laser in situ keratomileusis (LASIK) flap in 1998 that the anterior segment application of this technology was fully realized.

The OCT systems used in commercial retinal scanner thus far have used 830 nm wavelength, with image acquisition time of 1–5 seconds. The wavelength higher than 830 nm in posterior segment had more dissipation in vitreous hence was discarded from posterior segment use. However, that very property was useful in imaging the anterior segment using a higher intensity light beam but causing no damage to the retina due to the greater dissipation. Wavelength 1,310 nm allowed deeper penetration even through sclera and cross-sectional imaging of the AC, including visualization of the angle.

PRINCIPLE OF OPTICAL COHERENCE TOMOGRAPHY

The principle of OCT is based on Michelson's interferometry **(Fig. 1)**. The Michelson's interferometer was developed by Albert A Michelson in 1878. His theory was that—if a device could split a beam of light into two parts, then send the individual beams along perpendicular paths, and bring the beams back together again, the returned "echoes" could be measured to determine if their phase relationship had gotten "out of step". The amount of differentiation or "interference" would give a very accurate measure of distance.

The OCT contains an interferometer that resolves structures by measuring the echo delay time of light that is reflected and backscattered from different microstructural features in the tissue being studied. Posterior segment OCT uses a lower wavelength of light at 830 nm while the ASOCT uses a higher wavelength (1,310 nm) of light for the purpose of imaging.

This low-coherence infrared (1,310 nm) light coupled to a fiberoptic travels to a 50/50 beam splitter and is directed to a reference mirror on one side and to the tissue concerned on the other. Light passing through the tissue is reflected by structures in different tissue layers. The distance between the beam splitter and reference mirror is continuously varied. When the distance between the light source and tissue is equal to the distance between the light source and reference mirror, the reflected light from the tissue and reference mirror interacts to produce an interference pattern. The interference

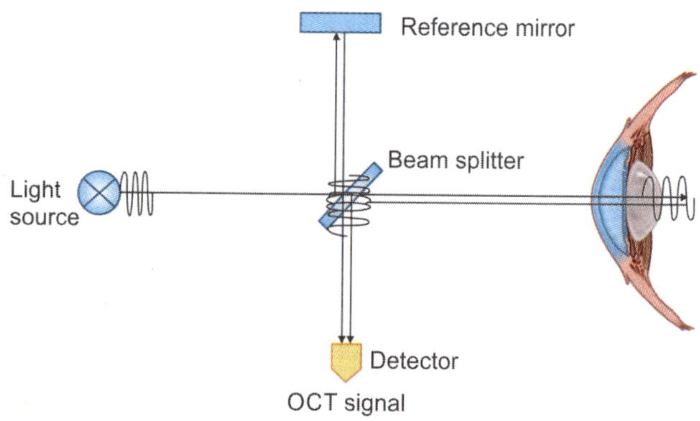

Fig. 1: Principle of optical coherence tomography (OCT).

pattern is detected and then processed into a signal. The signal is analogous to that obtained by A-scan ultrasonography using light as a source rather than sound. A two-dimensional image is built as the light source is moved across the tissue. One can think of the image as a series of stacked and aligned A-scans to produce a two-dimensional cross-sectional retinal image that resembles that of a histologic section. This imaging method thus can be considered a form of in vivo histology.

The ASOCT at 1,310 nm wavelength of light is better suited for AC angle imaging due to two important properties.

1. *Reduced scattering*: The scattering in tissue is lower at this wavelength. This in turn ensures better penetration through ocular structures like the sclera and the iris and hence a more detailed AC angle morphology can be visualized.
2. *More dissipation/absorption of the 1,310 nm wavelength light*: The 1,310 nm wavelength light is strongly absorbed by water in ocular media and therefore, only 10% of the light incident on the cornea reaches the retina. The reason for this is the unique phenomenon exhibited by light. For light, the absorption and scattering in most tissue constituents decreases with wavelength in the near-infrared spectrum whereas absorption in water, which is the primary constituent of vitreous humor, increases sharply, being approximately an order of magnitude higher at 1.3 µm than at 0.8 µm. The improved retinal protection allows for the use of high power illumination that, in turn, enables high-speed imaging.

The high-speed imaging helps in various ways:

- Reduces examination time
- Eliminates motion artifacts
- Enables imaging of dynamic ocular events
- Allows for rapid survey of relatively large areas.

Imaging Modes

The ASOCT has six imaging modes:

1. High-resolution cornea single
2. High-resolution cornea quad
3. Pachymetry
4. Anterior segment single
5. Anterior segment double
6. Anterior segment quad **(Figs. 2A to C)**.

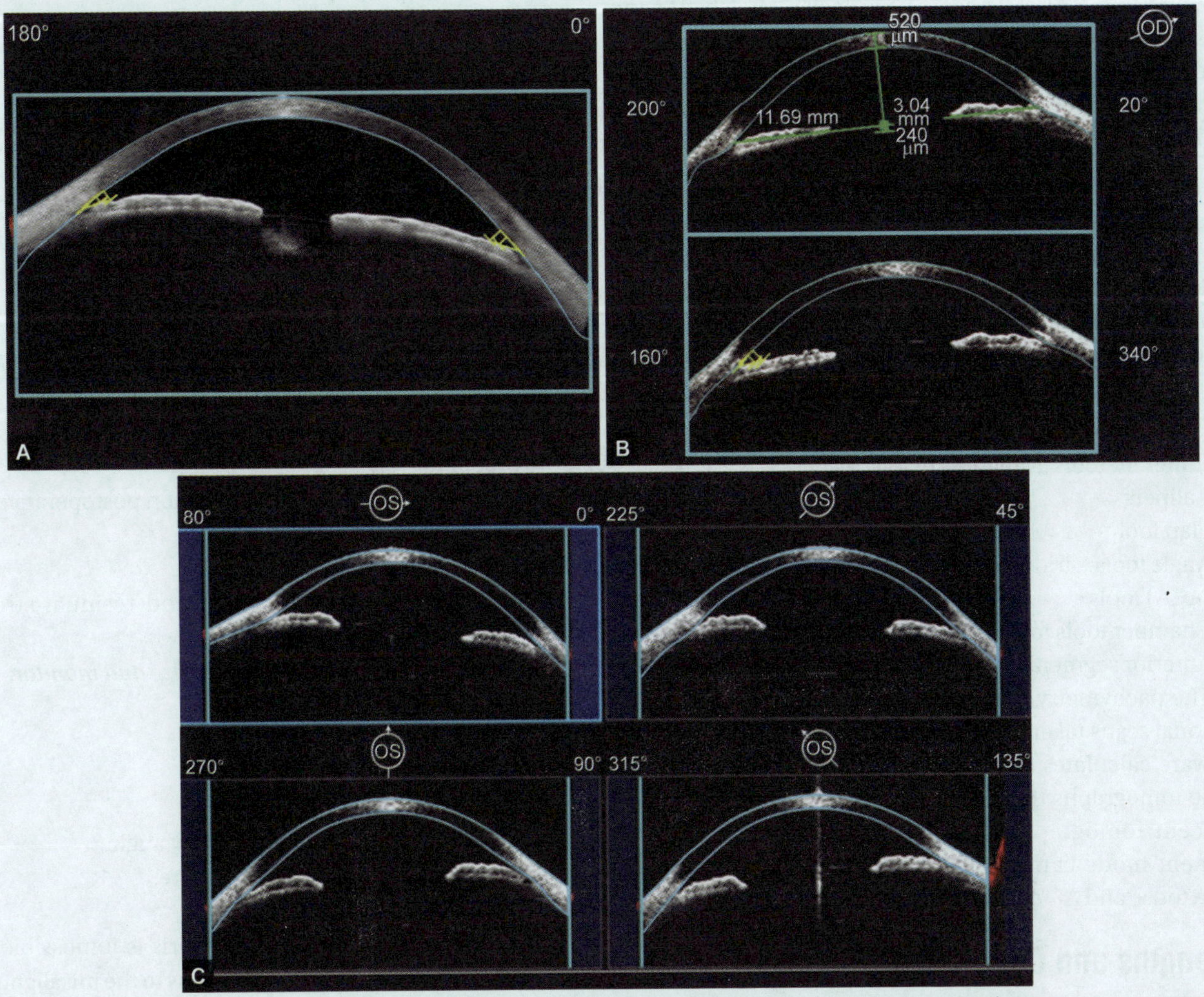

Figs. 2A to C: The types of scans: (A) The anterior segment single scan; (B) The anterior segment double scan; (C) The anterior segment quadruple scan.

Table 1: Two resolution modes of imaging.

Standard resolution imaging	*High/enhanced resolution imaging*
• Broader view of anterior segment 16 mm width/6 mm depth • *Full overview of anterior segment*: Cornea, anterior chamber, iris, and both angles 256 scans 0.125 seconds	• More detailed imaging 10 mm width/3 mm depth • Cornea and any segment needing detailed evaluation 512 scans 0.250 seconds

In the quad mode of both high-resolution cornea and anterior segment, four cross-sectional images are taken at 0°–180°, 45°–225°, 90°–270°, and 135°–315°, respectively. The anterior segment double OCT takes images at the preset angles of 20°–200° and 160°–340°. In the single mode, only a single image will be obtained at the desired angle. In all modes, the angle of image capture can be changed. In the double and quad modes, the preset angle separation will remain the same. Therefore, when manually changing the angle of image capture, all angles will rotate together. For example, if an image is being obtained in the anterior segment quad and the operator adjusts the angle by 15°, the new images will be captured at 15°–195°, 60°–240°, 105°–285°, and 150°–330°. All images have been rotated by 15° and are still separated by 90°. Two resolution modes of imaging are discussed in **Table 1**.

MEASUREMENT TOOLS

There are different tools available for measurement depending on which mode the image was captured in.[1] In any of the high-resolution cornea modes, you can apply thickness calipers, a flap tool, or annotation. The flap tool is composed of a caliper that automatically places itself on the boundaries delineating anterior/posterior surfaces of the cornea with a movable marker in between to be placed at the flap/stroma interface by the operator.

The different tools available are:

- Calipers
- Flap tool
- Angle tools—iridocorneal angle tool (ICAT) and AC angle (ACA) tools
- Chamber tools for AC depth and width measurements
- Anterior segment refractive tool set **(Figs. 3A to D)**.

The pachymetry map is generated from multiple cross-sectional scans taken at different angles. Again, the program software calculates or finds the anterior/posterior surface of the tomographs then interpolates the thickness between adjacent tomographs. Images captured in the anterior segment mode can be analyzed with thickness calipers, angle tools, and AC depth/width measurements.

Strengths and Clinical Applications

In its clinical application, the ASOCT is excellent at imaging the anterior segment. **Figures 4A and B** show Visante OCT 3.0 machine. **Figures 4C to E** show patients undergoing ASOCT. It is a simple, noncontact repeatable and reproducible procedure. **Figure 4F** shows some of the images of the anterior segment single map. **Figure 4G** shows the images of the printouts given to the patients. Primarily, it provides detailed examination of the structures anterior to the iris, with the following being a list of some of the strengths and clinical applications in which it provides useful information.

Advantages of Anterior Segment Optical Coherence Tomography

- Noncontact instrumentation
- Quick—no longer than 2 minutes from when the patient sits down
- Repeatable and reproducible
- *The ability to use measurement tools such as*:
  - Angle tools to measure any angle
  - The AC depth/width tool
  - Calipers to measure thickness
  - Flap tools to measure LASIK flaps and residual stromal beds.
- *Image through an opaque cornea*:
  - Useful in graft situations
  - Limited only by pigmented tissues.
- *Pachymetry*: The usefulness of pachymetry can be seen in the following situations:
  - Keratoconus
  - Fuchs' endothelial dystrophy
  - Glaucoma
  - Postoperative monitoring of corneal procedures.
- *Anterior chamber intraocular lens (IOLs) and phakic IOLs*:
  - Anterior chamber depth and width can be measured preoperatively
  - To monitor placement and position postoperatively.
- *Corneal refractive surgery*:
  - To measure corneal thickness
  - To assess the flap thickness and residual stromal bed.
- *Endothelial keratoplasty—to visualize and monitor*:
  - Attachment of graft
  - Placement of the graft
  - Swelling and resolution.
- *Narrow angles*:
  - Accurate measurement of narrow angle
  - Diagnostic images of angle closure.
- *Tilted IOLs implants*:
  - Although imaging through the iris is impossible, iris displacement gives information as to the misalignment of a posterior chamber IOLs.
- Patient education

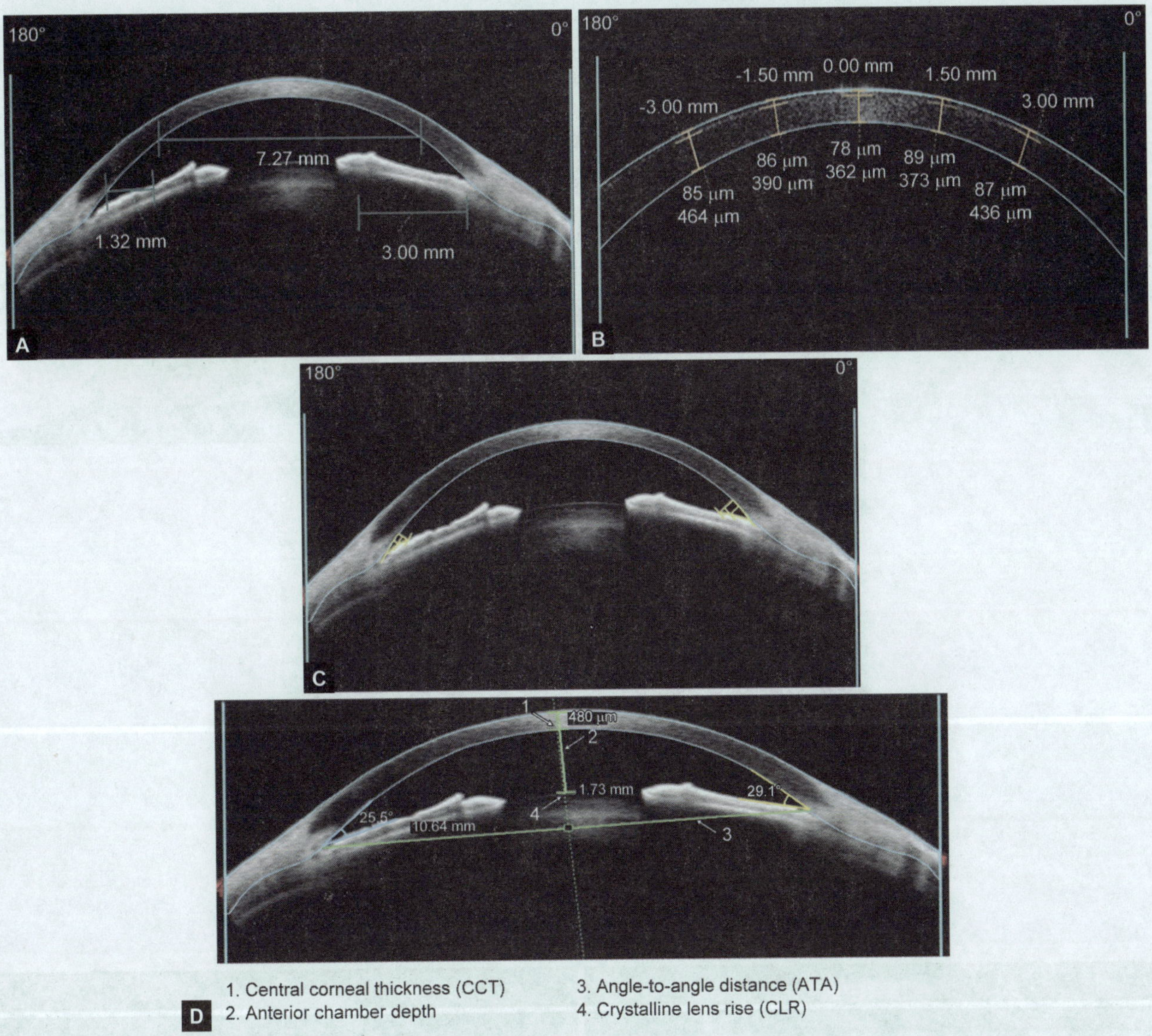

Figs. 3A to D: Some of the tools used by the ASOCT: (A) The caliper tool; (B) The flap tool; (C) The iridocorneal angle tool; (D) The chamber tools.
(ASOCT: anterior segment optical coherence tomography)

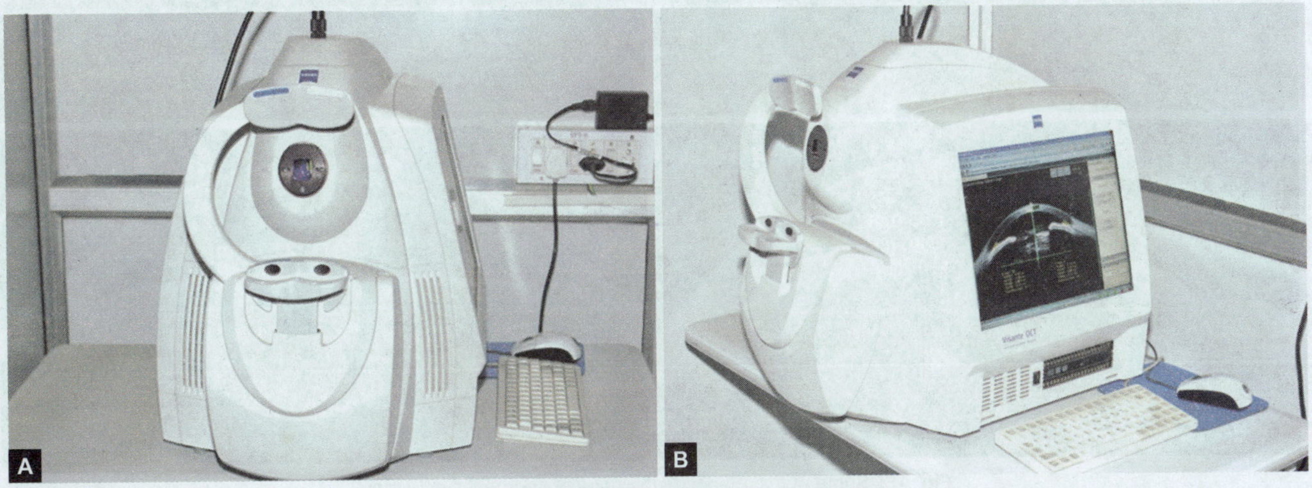

Figs. 4A and B: The Visante OCT 3.0 machine.
(OCT: optical coherence tomography)

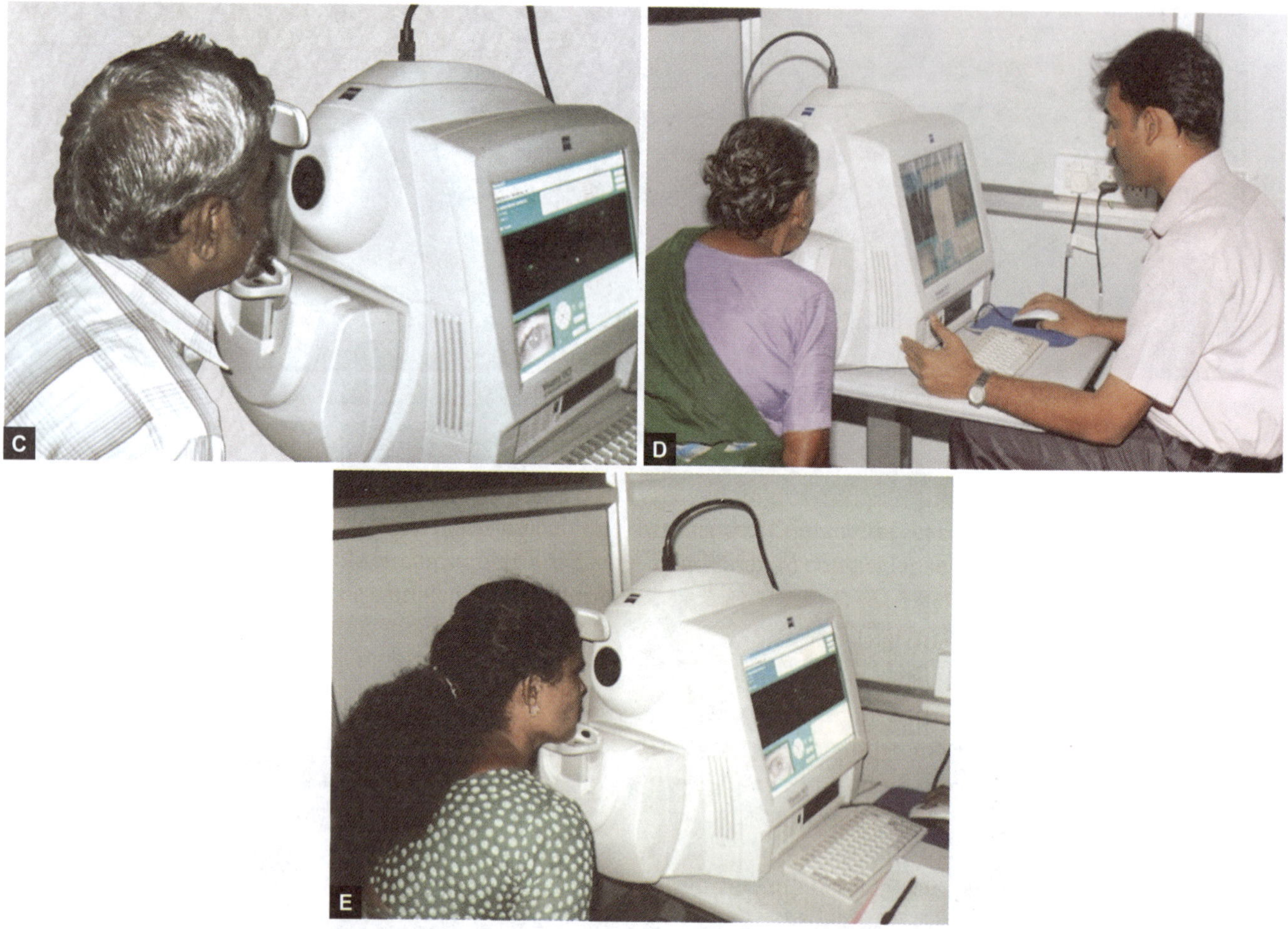

Figs. 4C to E: Patients undergoing anterior segment optical coherence tomography.

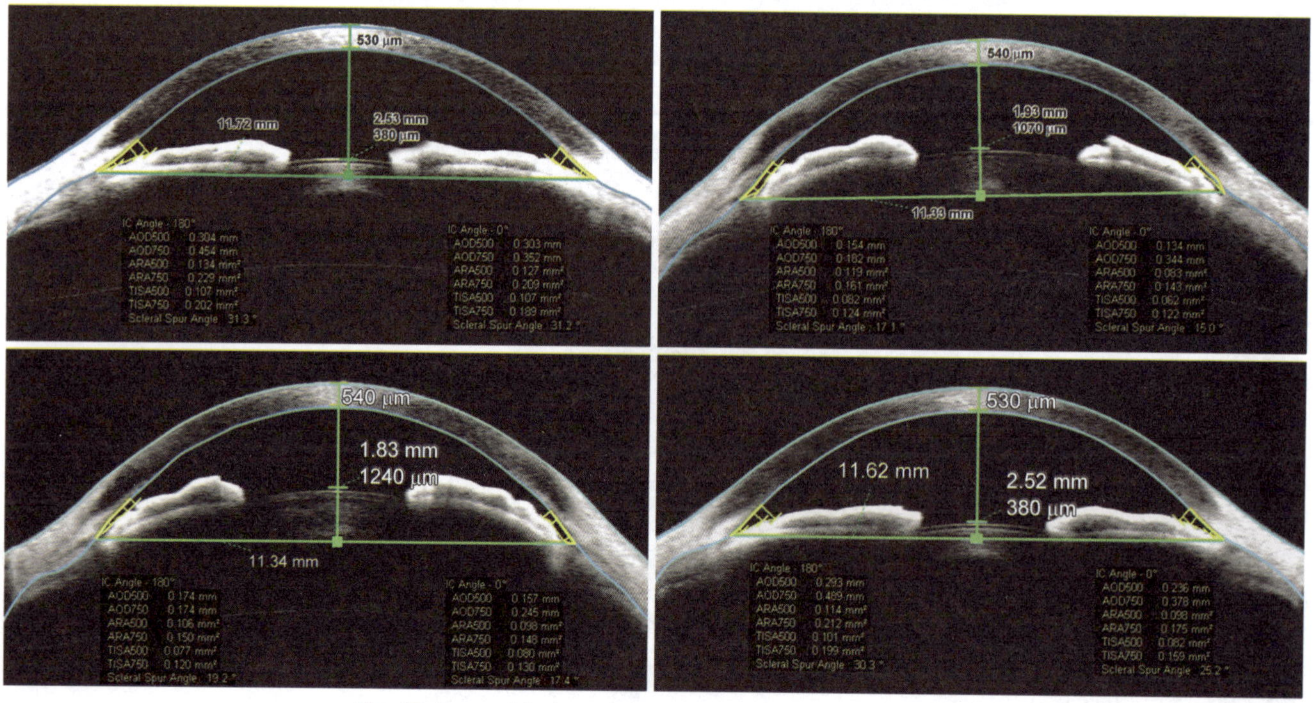

Fig. 4F: Some of the images of the anterior segment single map.

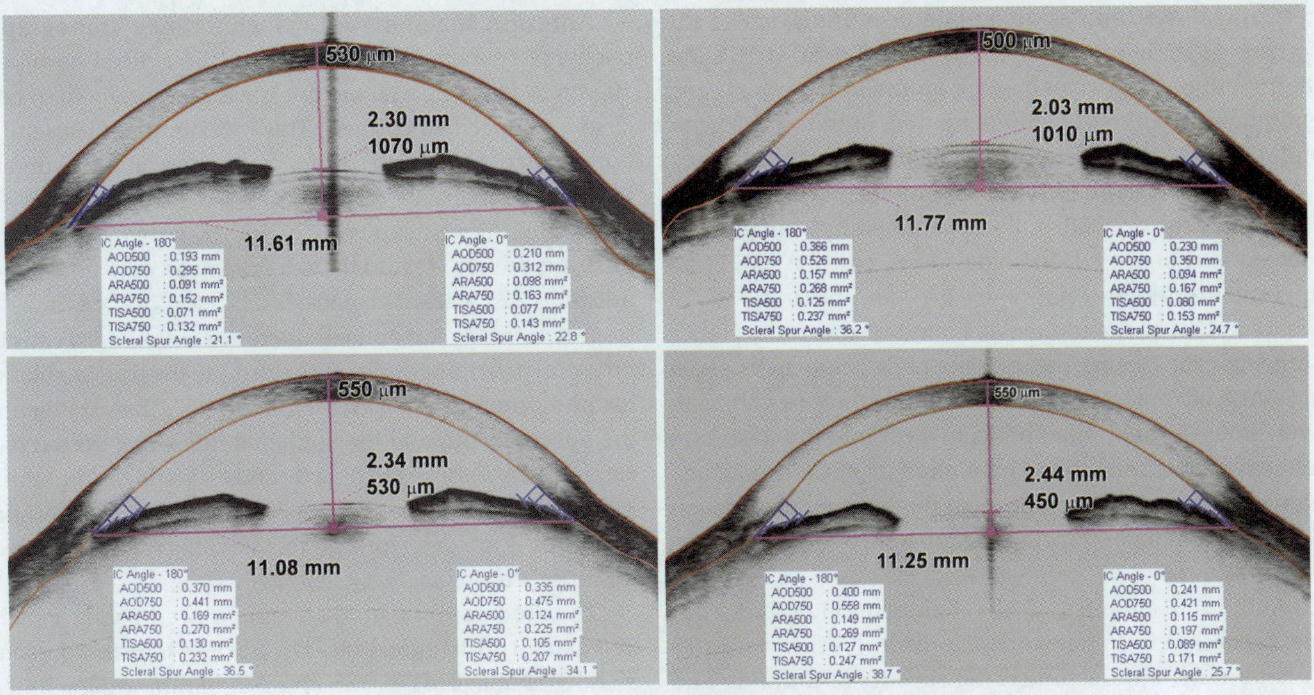

Fig. 4G: The printouts for the patients.

- *Research*:
  - The research that can be performed is only limited by the researcher's creativity, image resolution, and tool selection
  - Comparative studies of pachymetry.

LIMITATIONS

- *The Visante OCT uses 1,310-nm infrared wavelength light.*
  - Cannot penetrate through pigmented tissue
  - Cannot image anything past the posterior pigmented epithelium of the iris. It would be interesting to note the position of the posterior chamber IOLs and how it is truly affecting the iris rather than inducing the tilt from the iris displacement.
- *Seemingly slow rate of refresh*: Being a dynamic image, the computing software has to "catch up" at times, freezing the image on the operator's screen. This always seems to happen just when the operator wants to capture another image.
- *Software*:
  - The ASOCT software has a limited number of tools
  - There are no built-in analytical tools. It would be useful to have:
    - Software to analyze pachymetry maps
    - Software that automatically finds an angle measurement and indicates "narrow angles" to a technician
  - No keratometry/radius of curvature readings.
- Higher magnification would be helpful in the imaging and examination of epithelium, endothelium, and trabecular meshwork.

APPLICATIONS

The application of ASOCT is diverse but for the sake of discussion, it can be broadly grouped into applications in:

- Cornea
- Biometry and phakic IOL
- Glaucoma.

Applications in Cornea

- Laser in situ keratomileusis
- Descemet's stripping automated endothelial keratoplasty (DSAEK)
- Dystrophies and degenerations
- Corneal inflammatory and infiltrative disorders
- Keratoplasty
- Keratoconus
- Intacs
- Dry eye
- Descemet's detachment.

Anterior segment optical coherence tomography can assist in diagnosis and documentation of corneal conditions such as dystrophies and degenerations, as well as assorted inflammatory pathologies. It can be used to diagnose and manage corneal infiltrates, ulcers, dellen, or scars. The depth and extent as obtained by ASOCT is superior to that of anterior segment photography.[2] Monitoring of corneal infection is possible especially when deep, and aggressive infection occurs. Hypopyon and hyphema can also be monitored as a result of severe infection or trauma. ASOCT has the capability to determine the depth of a foreign body or the presence of residue once removed.

Corneal dystrophies affect one or more layers of the cornea.[2] High definition images obtained by ASOCT allow the practitioner to visualize the epithelium, stroma, and endothelium with clear differentiation. Monitoring Fuchs' endothelial dystrophy is another capability of this technology. Descemet's detachment, corneal guttata, corneal edema, Fuchs' dystrophy, and bullous keratopathy[3] can also be imaged and observed. In some severe cases, ASOCT can document corneal topography pre- and post-DSAEK in the treatment of pseudophakic bullous keratopathy (PBK). Surgeons can visualize the interface and document its depth in DSAEK patients. ASOCT can document thickness changes over time. Corneal inlay position with possible resultant refractive effect can also be monitored by ASOCT imaging.[4] **Figure 5** shows the monitoring of the inserted tissue post-DSAEK and changes from first postoperative day to 9 months postprocedure.

Anterior segment optical coherence tomography has the capability to image keratoconus and other ectastias to determine and document the severity of thinning and scarring. While moderate to severe keratoconus can be identified via slit-lamp examination and topography, subclinical or *form frusta* keratoconus and other thinning conditions can be recognized with pachymetry maps.[5] These cases are especially important to identify prior to refractive laser surgeries.[6] ASOCT images taken in a case of keratoconus clearly depict the area of eccentric thinning **(Fig. 6)**.

Anterior segment optical coherence tomography pachymetry maps scan areas from the central cornea to 10 mm, calculating a global thickness measurement in both clear and opacified corneas. This measurement is useful in both glaucoma workups and refractive or cataract surgery. Pachymetry maps allow the surgeon to create accurate and repeatable flap thicknesses in LASIK surgical planning. Postoperatively, residual bed thickness can be imaged utilizing these thickness maps.

Anterior segment optical coherence tomography can also be useful in helping surgeons determine the proper ablation for phototherapeutic keratectomy (PTK). By establishing the opacity depth and the epithelial thickness, the surgeon can properly remove the opacity and estimate the amount of induced refractive change.[5] It also allows him to determine if the scar is too deep for PTK to be as effective as with deep posterior stromal scars.[7]

The detachment of Descemet's membrane can be detected in postsurgical cases by ASOCT. **Figure 7** presents an ASOCT image of the Descemet's membrane detachment in a post small incision cataract surgery case.

Use of the Intralase laser (Abbott Medical Optics) as part of different corneal procedures is becoming more popular in the surgical arena.[8-11] ASOCT maps the cornea to determine the areas thick enough to create the channels for proper Intacs implantation. OCT imaging of corneal depth is also useful in Intralase-enabled keratoplasty (IEK) by determining the depth of ablation of the recipient tissue.

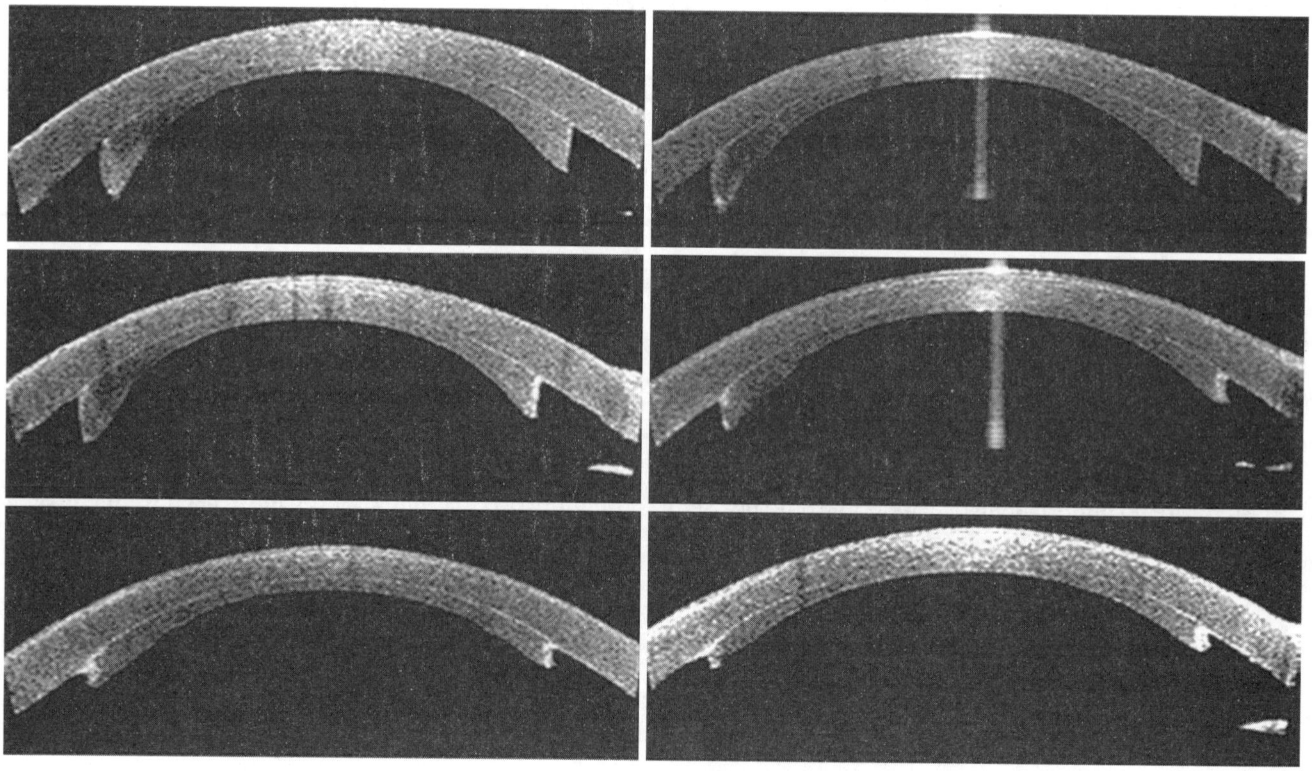

Fig. 5: Postoperative changes after Descemet's stripping automated endothelial keratoplasty.

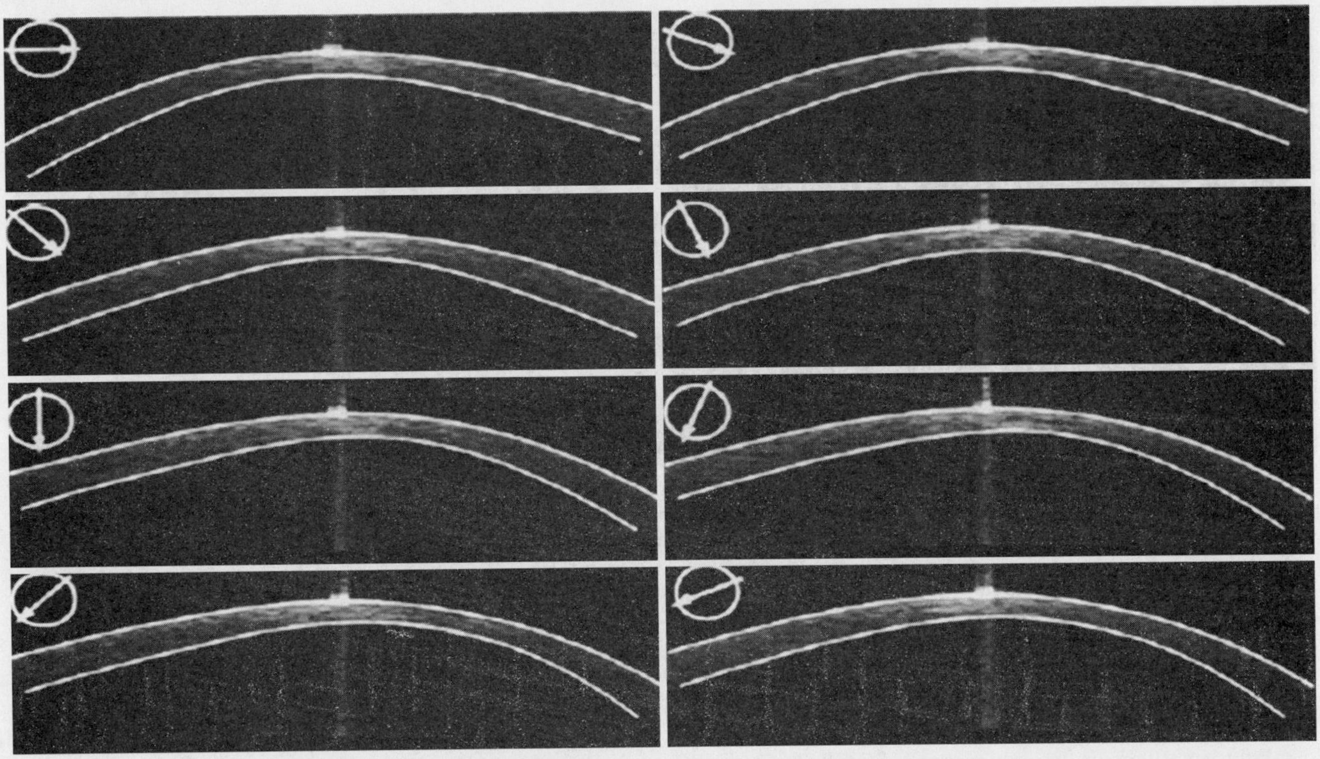

Fig. 6: Eccentric thinning seen in a case of keratoconus.

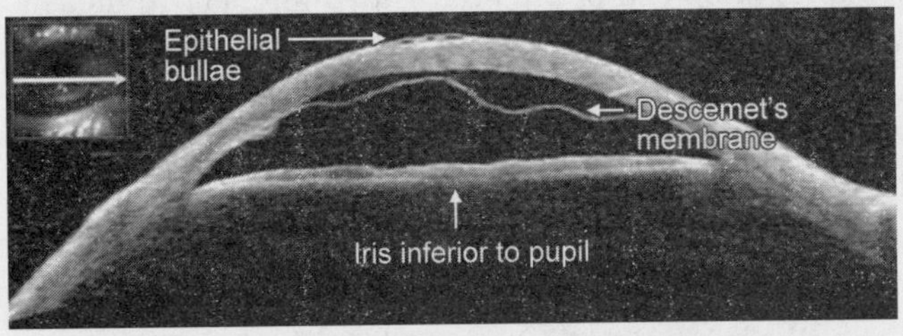

Fig. 7: An ASOCT image of the Descemet's membrane detachment. (ASOCT: anterior segment optical coherence tomography)

Anterior Segment Optical Coherence Tomography and Refractive Surgery

Refractive surgery has benefitted greatly from ASOCT technology. Preoperatively, patients can be scanned for any abnormalities. LASIK epithelial ingrowth can be monitored closely. Imaging of the corneal layers with high speed ASOCT provides useful information relevant to keratorefractive surgery. Many useful anatomic features can be identified in the image. Corneal flap thickness is an important parameter in LASIK because it determines the amount of residual stroma available for ablation. Currently, there is no technique that directly measures corneal flap thickness and it has been demonstrated that there are noteworthy discrepancies between intended and actual thickness values. By directly measuring corneal flap thickness intraoperatively, it can potentially improve the predictability of LASIK. It can also determine ablation rates, and factor causing variation in this parameter such as stromal hydration can be taken into account, thereby minimizing the differences between planned and actual ablation depths. Owing to superior resolution of morphological features, it can also be used for postoperative assessment of the anatomical correlates of the refractive outcome. It can also provide the comprehensive pachymetry map of the entire cornea and helps in the detection of normal from abnormally thin corneas in which subtractive refractive surgery like LASIK may need to be avoided.

Figure 8A shows the use of the "flap tool" in post-LASIK cases to measure the precise flap and bed thickness while **Figure 8B** shows the "global pachymetry map" which is formed from 16 modified high-resolution scans.

The following are the uses of ASOCT in LASIK cases:

- Comprehensive pachymetry map of the entire cornea can be derived.
- The thickness of the cornea from the individual scans as well as the global pachymetry map can be used to determine ablation rates.
- One of the major factors causing variation in this parameter is stromal hydration. The ASOCT can measure this hydration minimizing the differences between planned and actual ablation depths.
- Superior resolution of morphological features.
- Detection of normal from abnormally thin corneas in which subtractive refractive surgery like LASIK may need to be avoided.

The anterior surface reflection is strong at the perpendicular incidence and produces a vertical flare that marks the corneal apex. Finer features, such as the epithelial-Bowman and the flap lamellar boundaries, are best visualized with a slight off-normal beam incidence angle in the mid-periphery.

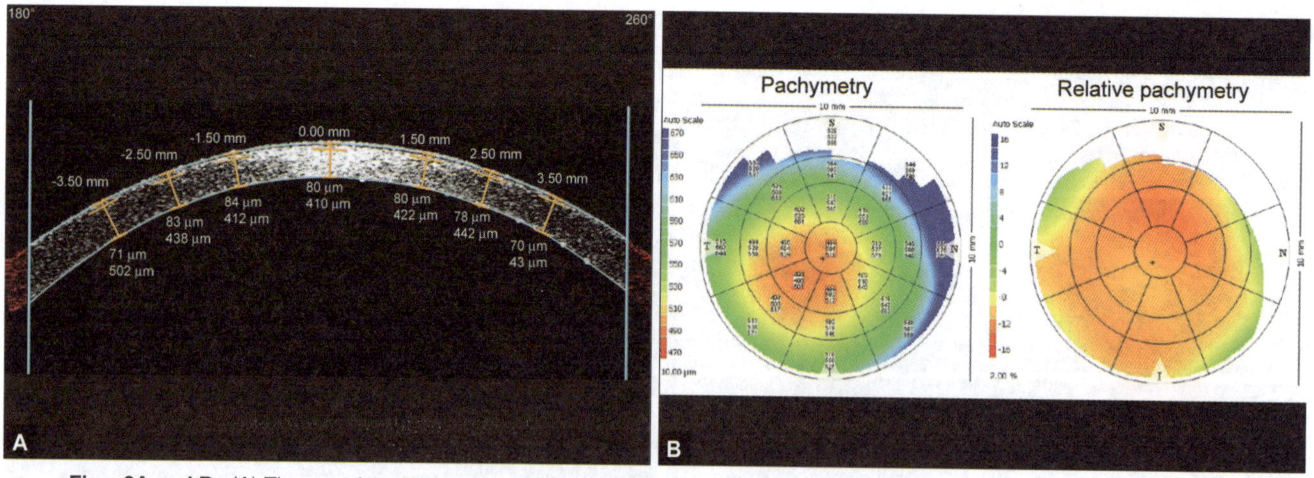

Figs. 8A and B: (A) The use of the "flap tool" in post-LASIK cases to measure the precise thickness; (B) The global pachymetry map which is formed from 16 modified high-resolution scans.
(LASIK: laser in situ keratomileusis)

Not all epithelial ingrowths need to be treated, therefore, measuring thickness of the epithelium and the LASIK flap help differentiate between the cases that must be treated by lifting the flap and those that can be monitored. A thinning flap due to epithelial ingrowth, especially centrally, warrants significant concern. ASOCT also images the architecture of the flap and the thickness of the residual corneal bed. When considering post-LASIK enhancement, proper assessment of the flap and residual bed thickness can easily be made with accurate measurement using the caliper tools.[7] Unexpected corneal ectasia postoperatively can also be assessed.

Anterior segment optical coherence tomography has been utilized in monitoring the epithelial healing progression under therapeutic contact lenses (TCL) following lamellar keratoplasty and epiLASIK.[12] Visualizing the epithelium postoperatively allows the surgeon to remove the TCL at the appropriate time without traumatizing the new epithelium or risking a secondary infection by leaving the TCL longer than necessary. ASOCT imaging of the anterior segment can also be beneficial in difficult rigid gas-permeable (RGP) fits. ASOCT can measure the curvature of the peripheral cornea and sclera, giving practitioners better insight to a successful fit.[13]

Biometry in Postrefractive Surgery Cases

Post-LASIK IOL power calculation has been a problem for quite some time. After LASIK the keratometry done routinely does not give the accurate picture of the corneal curvature details. Hence, the IOL power calculated on the basis of routine keratometry is flawed and inaccurate. In routine keratometry, the anterior curvature is measured and an extrapolation done to calculate the posterior corneal curvature. In post-LASIK cases, this extrapolation no longer works and thus the calculated keratometry reading becomes inaccurate. Resolution of this problem requires a method for accurately measuring the posterior corneal power or a technique for adjusting the IOL power after implantation. It is a perpetual problem and surgeons began performing multiple complex calculations to "guesstimate" the correct IOL power for patients who by their original decision to have photorefractive keratectomy (PRK) or LASIK had already demonstrated that they now have an average refractive demand. The need of the hour is two-fold: (1) To measure the posterior corneal curvature accurately, and (2) to develop an IOL power formula based on the ASOCT corneal power measurement. The breakthrough was achieved with the newer generation ASOCT that could image the posterior corneal surface with very high resolution, allowing it to measure corneal power precisely. Also the newer generation ASOCT uses a proprietary corneal segmentation algorithm that has been at least as effective, if not more effective, than other currently available methods for measuring corneal power.

Phakic Intraocular Lens

One of the areas of special interest for the use of ASOCT has been phakic IOLs **(Fig. 9)**. The ASOCT is looked upon with a great deal of optimism regarding its potential to guide the sizing of IOLs (phakic IOLs, specifically). Studies are currently ongoing with the use of Visian implantable collamer lens (ICL), STAAR Surgical Company, Monrovia, CA, where the authors are examining the safety issues and data that would potentially influence the choice of IOL size. The authors are measuring the AC depth, endothelial cell count, distance or dome of the cornea to the implant, pupil size, angle, and white-to-white (W2W) distance. The Visante OCT will not usually image to the ciliary sulcus; its power tends to be absorbed by the iris pigment epithelium. It will sometimes obtain a clear image of the sulcus in very light-colored eyes, but not routinely. When the Visante's AC measurements are compared to those of the IOL Master, the Visante's have been found to be slightly deeper. The measurements between the corneal endothelium and lens epithelium have also been

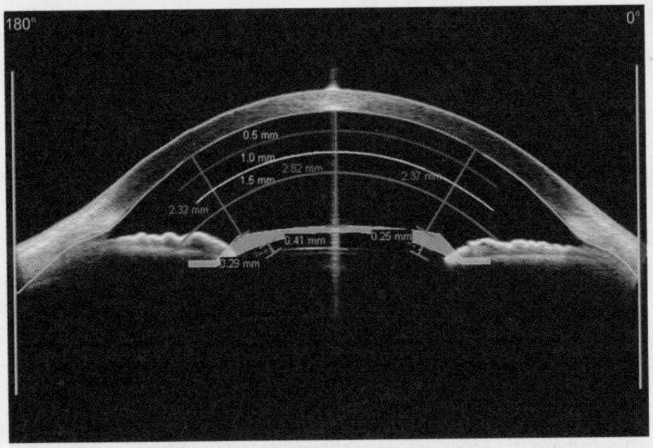

Fig. 9: Some of the phakic intraocular lens (IOL) tools. It shows the "RAINBOW" (0.5 mm, 1 mm, and 1.5 mm from the cornea), "SAFETY" (distance from cornea) at 180°, center and 0° and "VAULT" (distance between phakic IOL and crystalline lens) at 180°, center, and 0°.

found to differ greatly between the Orbscan and the Visante. The Visante seems more accurate, because at the slit lamp, we will get a different clinical sense of the chamber's depth compared with what the Orbscan reads. The ICL's sizing remains a challenge; "white-to-white" is imperfect and may be an understatement. However, ultrasound has been used to a practical advantage. Ultrasound measurements are technician-dependent, not always easily reproducible, and are fairly hard to perform on a routine basis because ultrasound is a very special application that requires at least 20 min. Luckily, the ICL has a fairly large range of acceptable vaulting, anywhere from 50 μm to 1,500 μm, probably due to poor sizing information.

The Sulcus

Based on UBM studies, the sulcus on an average has been found to be 0.21 mm more peripheral from one side to the other relative to the limbus or about 0.42 mm longer than a W2W measurement. In reality, the sulcus is highly variable in a given eye. Even just a few degrees away, it undulates in anatomy, and sometimes determining its location is difficult. These factors play no small part in the reason why ophthalmic surgeons have had difficulty making good correlations.

The ICL is designed to sit in the ciliary sulcus, although it does not always find the recess (sulcus). Measurements that would be helpful to know when implanting these lenses include the angle-to-angle (ATA) distance, the clearance involved, the chamber depth, and what is the width of the AC angle once the lens implant has been placed. A typical corneal vault would be 200 μm or a 40–50% vault. Minimal vaulting would leave very little appositional difference between the implant and the crystalline lens. With excessive vaulting, the angles would be unnecessarily narrowed, and the vault itself would be somewhat skewed and would tend to induce aberrations. Studies have shown that ATA and W2W measurements have a very poor correlation. So, when surgeons use the W2W measurement, they do not have a great deal of confidence that the ATA measurement will be the same. The question is whether the ATA measurement is better for ICL sizing and the answer appears to be "yes" in the light of the recent studies which strongly suggest that taking ATA gives a better fit than W2W.

Applications in Glaucoma

Anterior segment optical coherence tomography is used:

- To study the normal anatomy and physiology
- For screening of the spectrum of angle-closure glaucoma
- To study plateau iris syndrome (PIS)
- To study mechanism of malignant glaucoma
- To test the efficacy of laser peripheral iridotomy
- To test the patency of glaucoma drainage device.

Gonioscopy

Anterior segment optical coherence tomography provides direct visualization of the AC angle including the scleral spur (SS), ciliary body, and ciliary sulcus. Schlemm's canal can also be observed on some scans. Studies have shown ASOCT analysis of the angle is accurate, repeatable, and correlated to findings of traditional gonioscopy **(Figs. 10A and B)**.[14,15] Traditional gonioscopy suffers from artifact due to light and indentation errors.[16] Salient differences between ASOCT and gonioscopy are listed in **Table 2**. ASOCT allows the practitioner to view the anatomical angle features in both light and dark conditions, thereby allowing a better evaluation for possible angle-closure. ASOCT can identify the different mechanisms responsible for angle-closure glaucoma including pupillary block, plateau iris syndrome, and lens-related mechanisms. The SS insertion landmark is located where the less reflective ciliary muscle contacts the more reflective sclera. Identify the SS, and then the trabecular meshwork distance from it can be measured in addition to viewing the ciliary body's curvature and the depth of the AC.[16]

Gonioscopy, for those who perform it on a regular basis, is an easy procedure. However, physicians who do not practice it routinely can have difficulty ascertaining a confirmed diagnosis, such as with an open angle versus a narrow angle. The ASOCT can give a detailed view of the angle structures and help in ascertaining the presence or absence of angle-closure. It is noncontact and much less technically demanding than gonioscopy. Furthermore, the infrared light source does not stimulate pupil miosis and therefore, does not change angle anatomy.

Angle-closure

It is important to distinguish between appositional versus synechial closure, as the prognosis and management differ between these two types of glaucomas. **Figure 11** shows a very obvious case of synechiae where there is an alteration of the peripheral iris architecture. A more subtle case of synechial

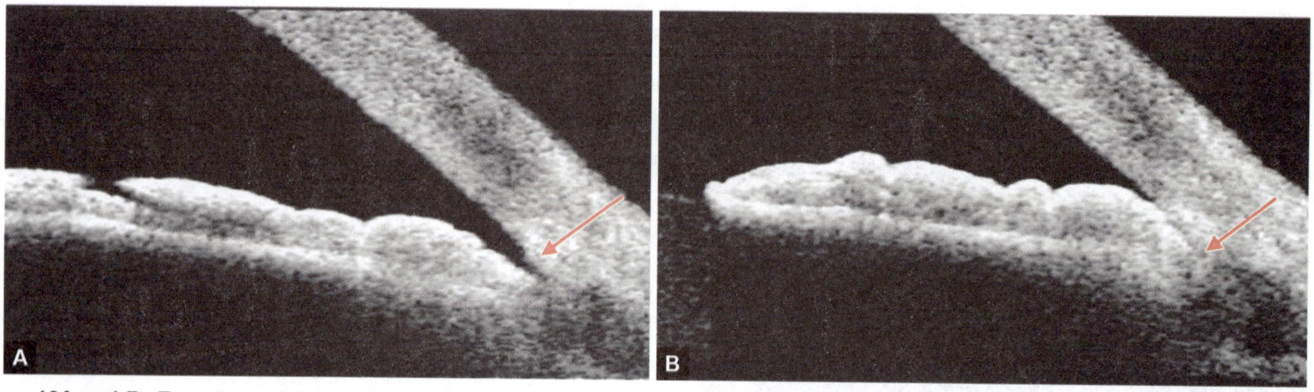

Figs. 10A and B: Two photographs of the same angle taken with the Visante ASOCT. The photograph on the left (A) was taken with the room lights on and it shows a clearly open angle. The one on the right (B) was taken after turning the lights off, which demonstrates iris–cornea apposition anterior to the scleral spur which is marked by the arrow.
(ASOCT: anterior segment optical coherence tomography)

Table 2: Differences between ASOCT of the angle and gonioscopy.

ASOCT of the angle	*Gonioscopy*
It is a nontechnical device	It requires technical skill
Objective test	Subjective test
Comfortable procedure	May be discomfortable
Noncontact procedure	Contact procedure
No light artifact	Light, indentation, and accommodation artifacts may be found
Control for focus is easy	More difficult procedure technically
Able to document the landmarks	Documentation is difficult
It is not a standardized procedure	Standardized procedure. Different grading systems and lenses are required
ASOCT is expensive	Goniolenses are inexpensive

(ASOCT: anterior segment optical coherence tomography)

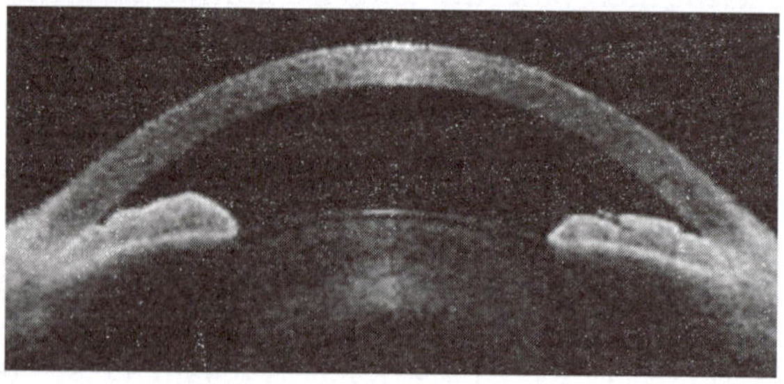

Fig. 11: A very obvious case of synechiae.

closure in an eye with a plateau iris is not uncommon **(Fig. 12)**. To make these determinations with the ASOCT, the surgeon uses evaluations much as those attempted with UBM, such as angle measures that include the angle opening distance (AOD) and angle recess area (ARA), to properly quantify and objectify the angle measurements.

Laser Iridotomy

Figures 13A and B show ASOCT images of an eye before and after undergoing laser iridotomy. The angle appears

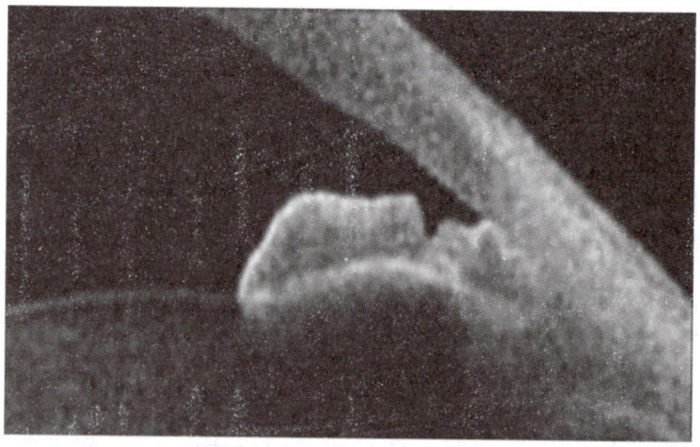

Fig. 12: A more subtle case of synechial closure in an eye with a plateau iris.

occludable before procedure, but it clearly demonstrates that the iridotomy has increased the angle's width. The amount of change can be documented as seen in **Figures 14A and B**. The patient may be followed up over a period of time with serial imaging to note the stability of the parameters during the follow-up. This instrument is exquisite in its ability to see significant deepening of the peripheral angle.

Properly identifying patients in need of an iridotomy is an important responsibility of eye-care practitioners. Iridotomy procedures have shown dramatic improvement of the angle structure when pupillary block mechanisms are present. However, when certain patients' angles do not improve as expected following iridotomy, nonpupillary block mechanisms (i.e. plateau iris, lens-related anterior rotation of the iris) can be easily identified. The characteristic iris configuration and thick profile in PIS are visualized by the ASOCT.[17] The eye surgeon can also observe blebs and implants by scanning the affected tissue. A limitation of the ASOCT during angle imaging is the inability to visualize pathology causing primary or secondary glaucoma including trabecular pigment or narrow bands of peripheral synechiae.[17]

In addition to AOD and ARA, which have been described previously in UBM studies, two new parameters—the

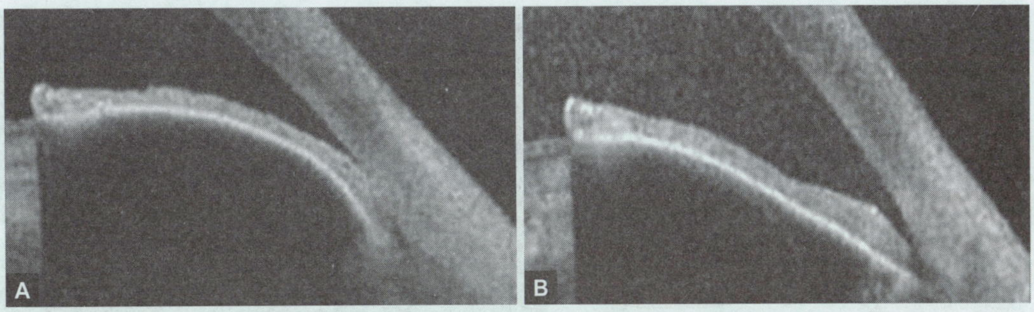

Figs. 13A and B: ASOCT images of an eye: (A) Before; and (B) After undergoing laser iridotomy. (ASOCT: anterior segment optical coherence tomography)

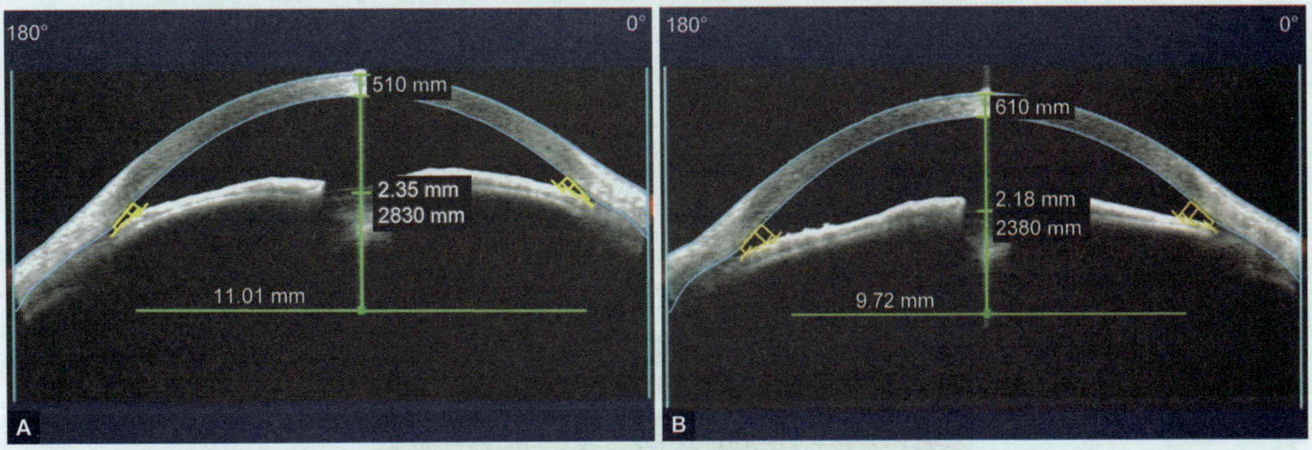

Figs. 14A and B: (A) The angle appears occludable before procedure; (B) The iridotomy has increased the angle's width.

trabecular-iris space area (TISA) and the trabecular-iris contact length (TICL)—are described for defining AC angle anatomy. The TISA differs from the ARA in that it only measures the filtering area in front of the sclera spur whereas the ARA also includes the nonfiltering angle recess. Thus, the ARA may be less sensitive in identifying a narrow angle in eyes with a relatively deep angle recess. In ASOCT imaging, another advantage of the TISA over the ARA is that identification of the SS is more reliable than the angle recess. This is because the SS is highly reflective and appears bright on the OCT image whereas the recess is less reflective and may be less precisely defined in some eyes.

Definitions

Angle Opening Distance

Angle opening distance (AOD_{500}) **(Fig. 15A)** is calculated as the perpendicular distance measured from the trabecular meshwork at 500 µm anterior to the SS to the anterior iris surface. AOD_{750} is calculated as the perpendicular distance measured from the trabecular meshwork at 750 µm anterior to the SS to the anterior iris surface.

Angle Recess Area

Angle recess area is measured as described by Ishikawa et al. The defining boundaries of this triangular area are the AOD_{500} or AOD_{750} (the base), the angle recess (the apex), and the iris surface and inner corneoscleral wall form sides of the triangle **(Fig. 15B)**.

The ARA is, theoretically, a better measurement parameter than the AOD because it takes into account the whole contour of the iris surface rather than measuring at a single point on the iris as is the case with the AOD. ARA may be less sensitive in identifying a narrow angle in eyes with a relatively deep angle recess.

Trabecular Iris Space Area

The defining boundaries of trabecular iris space area, a trapezoidal are as follows—anteriorly, the AOD_{500} or AOD_{750}; posteriorly, a line drawn from the SS perpendicular to the plane of the inner scleral wall to the opposing iris; superiorly, the inner corneoscleral wall; and inferiorly, the iris surface **(Fig. 15C)**. Studies have shown that this parameter represents the actual filtering area more accurately when compared with the ARA because the TISA excludes the nonfiltering region behind the SS.

Trabecular Iris Contact Length

Trabecular iris contact length is defined as the linear distance of iris contact with the corneoscleral surface beginning at the SS and extending anteriorly in an anatomically apposed or synechially closed-angle.

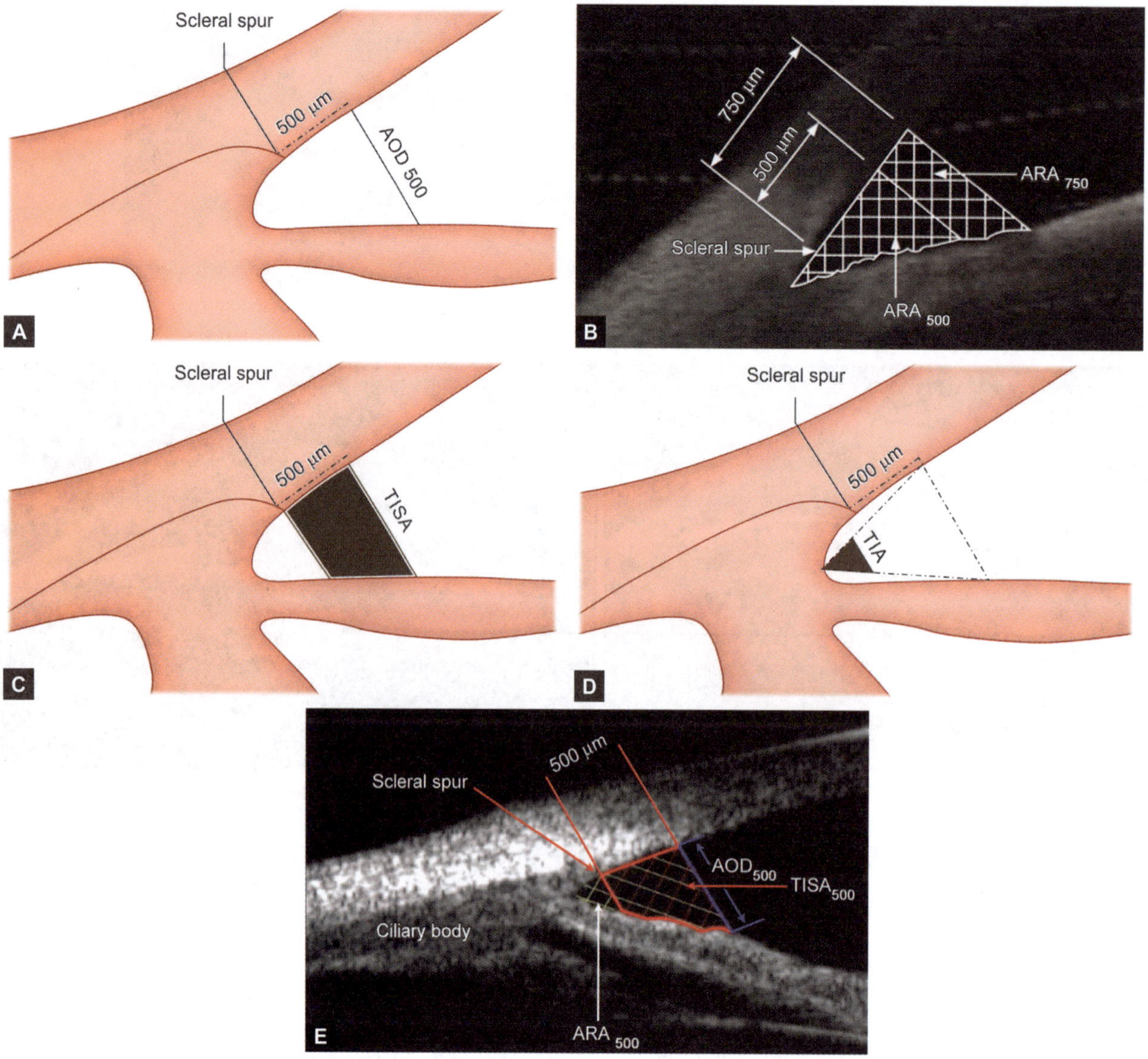

Figs. 15A to E: (A) Angle opening distance (AOD); (B) Angle recess area (ARA); (C) Trabecular-iris space area (TISA); (D) Trabecular-iris angle; (E) The composite image of all the parameters AOD, ARA, and TISA.

Trabecular Iris Angle

Trabecular iris angle **(Fig. 15D)** is defined as an angle measured with the apex in the iris recess and the arms of the angle passing through a point on the trabecular meshwork 500 µm from the SS and a point on the iris perpendicularly.

Scleral Spur Angle

Scleral spur angle is defined as an angle measured with the apex at the SS and the arms of the angle passing through a point on the trabecular meshwork 500 µm from the SS and a point on the iris perpendicular.

Figure 15E shows the composite image of all the parameters AOD, ARA and TISA.

Plateau Iris

Plateau iris configuration (PIC) is characterized by an appositional angle with a flat iris configuration, in contrast to an anterior bowing of the iris seen in a "typical" angle closure glaucoma in which there is a more crowded AC due to a hyperopic/short eye. **Figure 16A** shows the figurative images of a normal eye while **Figure 16B** shows an eye with plateau iris syndrome. ASOCT image of an eye with plateau iris is shown in **Figure 16C**. Classically with PIC, the iris configuration is planar and the depth of the AC is normal. In patients with PIC, the iris root is often short and inserted anteriorly on the ciliary face, causing a shallow and narrow angle.[18] With PIC there is a relative pupil block mechanism. PIS is due to an abnormal anterior position of the ciliary body. This anterior ciliary body displacement in turn alters the position of the peripheral iris in relation to the trabecular meshwork resulting in obstruction to aqueous outflow. PIS may be triggered by spontaneous pupillary dilation (e.g. in darkness), or in response to mydriatic agents. Slit-lamp evaluation of patients with PIC usually shows a normal AC depth and a flat iris plane.[19,20] A "double hump sign" on indentation gonioscopy is characteristically seen

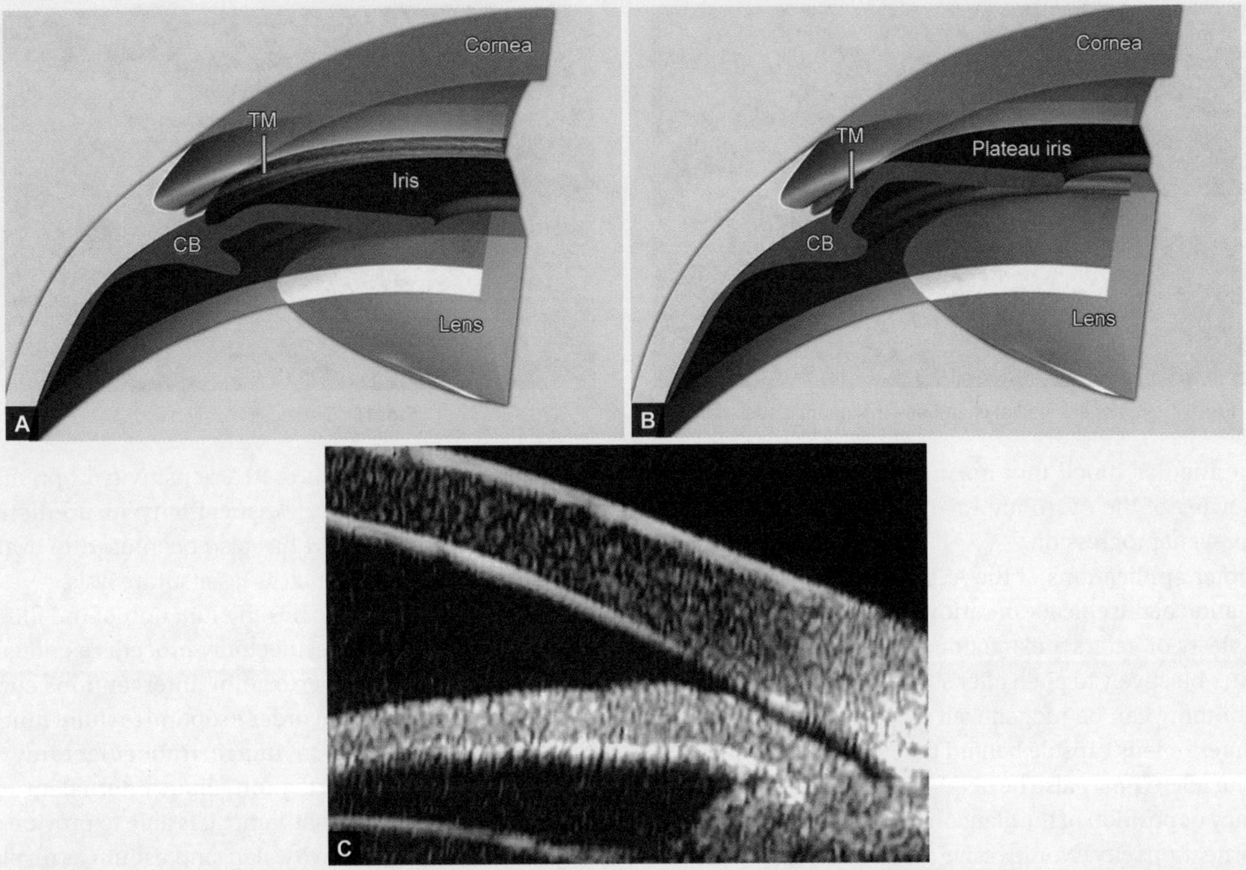

Figs. 16A to C: (A) The figurative images of a normal eye; (B) An eye with plateau iris syndrome; (C) ASOCT image of an eye with plateau iris. (ASOCT: anterior segment optical coherence tomography; CB: ciliary body; TM: trabecular meshwork)

in this condition. The peripheral "hump" on the iris is caused by the ciliary body propping up the iris root, whereas central "hump" represents the central third of the iris resting over the surface of the lens.[21] Though, plateau iris is believed to have a deep central chamber unlike a typical narrow angled individual who is hyperopic, UBM studies have found patients with plateau iris to have shallower AC. UBM is helpful in the diagnosis of PIC/PIS, as this modality can confirm the anatomic abnormalities of the ciliary body. However, UBM is cumbersome procedure as it needs the patient to lie down for a water bath over the eye and is a contact procedure. Many patients are not comfortable with the procedure. ASOCT has emerged as a tool, which can be quite effective in the diagnosis of plateau iris and at the same time, is a quick and easy procedure. By looking at the ARA and the iris thickness a diagnosis may be made. Studies are currently underway to further confirm it.

Malignant Glaucoma

Malignant glaucoma following filtration surgery remains one of the most challenging problems. It refers to a shallow or flat central and peripheral AC caused by the forward movement of the lens-iris and iris-hyaloid diaphragm accompanied by elevated IOP, in the presence of a patent peripheral iridectomy.[22] Using UBM, the configuration of the anterior segment structures has been visualized during the malignant glaucoma process. ASOCT findings were very similar to the acoustic features including iridocorneal touch, anterior displacement of the iris root, and appositional angle-closure. However, although ASOCT has a higher resolution than UBM, the visualization of lens, ciliary body, or anterior vitreous structures was limited because of absorption of infrared light by deeper scleral tissues and the pigment epithelium of the iris. This precluded imaging of anterior rotation of the ciliary body with apposition to the iris found with UBM. However, the UBM method has not yet been found to be useful in the management of the condition, and requires a coupling medium in an immersion bath, which restricts examinations in the immediate postoperative period.

Anterior segment OCT allows a noninvasive monitoring of the AC angle region for critical shallowing, and prompt initiation of medical or surgical treatment. The goal of the treatment for malignant glaucoma has been directed to restore the normal aqueous flow into the AC with resultant deepening. ASOCT has revealed to be helpful for the objective assessment of the therapeutic effects, and to recognize eyes that are unresponsive to medical or surgical management with a recurrent flat AC postoperatively **(Fig. 17)**. More importantly, since an important risk to develop malignant glaucoma is a chronic glaucoma with a narrow iridocorneal angle and an increased scleral thickness, ASOCT could be helpful in recognizing noninvasively the early stages of a

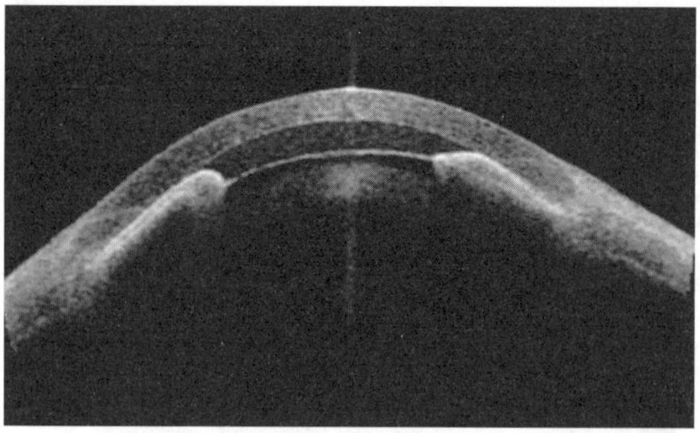

Fig. 17: Postoperative flat chamber—malignant glaucoma.

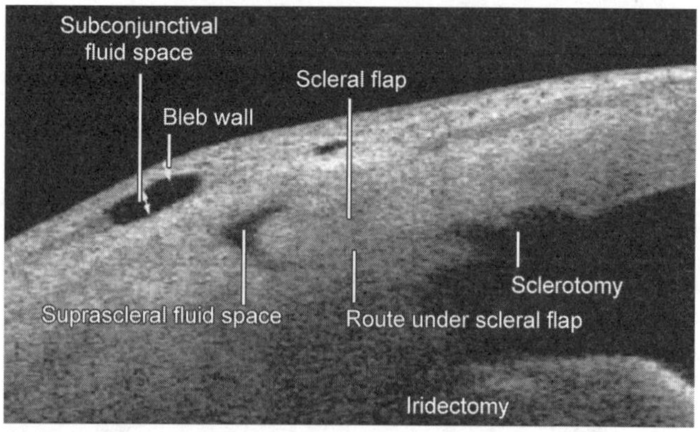

Fig. 18: Trabeculectomy bleb.

ciliolenticular block monitoring central and peripheral shallowing of the AC to improve therapeutic management and prevent progression.

Other applications of the ASOCT include its use in the evaluation of the efficacy of various treatments, such as laser iridoplasty or cataract extraction, where the angles may be shown objectively to open after such treatment. The patency of iridotomy can be judged well on the ASOCT by viewing the anterior lens capsule behind the full thickness PI.

The ASOCT may also be helpful in the assessment of tube patency or position of the glaucoma drainage device in cases of corneal opacity. Noninvasive nature of it allows its safe use in situations where ocular tissue has been lacerated or punctured and gonioscopy cannot be performed because of the danger of aqueous leak.

Imaging of Blebs

Bleb morphology after trabeculectomy is an important clinical parameter; it is an indicator of bleb function and a predictor of bleb-related complications such as bleb leak, blebitis, and bleb-related endophthalmitis. Blebs have been previously graded and classified by clinical, photographic, and imaging means. Early efforts at bleb classification featured inconsistent terminology and inexact assessments of the many aspects of bleb morphology. Subsequent bleb grading systems identified and incorporated a graded assessment of various bleb parameters such as vascularity, height, width, microcystic changes, encystment, and diffuse/demarcated zones with reference to clinical and photographic standards. Early postoperative morphologic features have also been described that predict late bleb failure. The three clinical bleb grading systems in current use include one developed by Picht and Grehn, the Indiana Bleb Appearance Grading Scale, and the Moorfields Bleb Grading System (MBGS). A recent study found generally good interobserver agreement between the latter two systems, but these systems are clinical and do not include imaging criteria. UBM has also been used in bleb assessment. One study classified blebs based on qualitative UBM features and found that bleb type was associated with intraocular pressure (IOP) control. UBM has been found to have 91% sensitivity in predicting a functioning bleb and 70% specificity in predicting a nonfunctioning bleb. UBM has also been used to evaluate blebs after interventions such as laser suture lysis.

Bleb morphology indicates the function of the filtration shunt created by the trabeculectomy procedure and guides the ophthalmologist in performing interventions such as needling and suture lysis in order to optimize shunt function. ASOCT has been used to image trabeculectomy bleb **(Fig. 18)** to provide information about internal structure that is not available at the slit-lamp. It is able to provide clear images of the bleb wall, cavity, flap, and ostium as displayed below. Successful blebs display conjunctival thickening as a hallmark of success, regardless of degree of bleb elevation. This reflects facility of transconjunctival aqueous flow. Highly elevated blebs sometimes display marked conjunctival thickening and only a small cavity. In failed blebs, ASOCT is particularly useful in imaging failed blebs to demonstrate the level of failure.

Ostial closure, flap fibrosis and presumed episcleral fibrosis in the absence of the former two situations are all clearly demonstrated. In the early postoperative period, a failing bleb with a closely apposed scleral flap may be resuscitated by suture lysis, resulting in a more expanded bleb.

Hence, ASOCT is a useful tool to image trabeculectomy blebs **(Fig. 18)** and may aid the clinician in postoperative bleb management. It can also image the intrascleral lake and implant used in nonpenetrating glaucoma surgery (deep sclerectomy) and glaucoma drainage devices.

SWEPT SOURCE OCT

Swept source ASOCT (SS-OCT, CASIA SS-1000, Tomey Corporation, Nagoya, Japan) is a variation of spectral-domain OCT that is specifically designed for anterior segment imaging using 1,310 nm wave width with a scan speed of 30,000 A-scans per second and an axial resolution of less than 10 μm. It is a non-contact, non-invasive three dimensional imaging swept source OCT system. The CASIA is indicated for cross-sectional imaging of the anterior segment components of the human eye, and also for dimension measurements such as curvature, length, area and volume by computed analysis. In the high-definition scan mode, both SS and Schwalbe's line can be identified. It can scan the anterior cornea to the posterior lens with just one image capture. It captures images around the angle as well in corneal topography mode and so it is possible to observe corneal topography, angle and IOL without switching measuring modes. It has better image penetration and thus can capture images through a cloudy cornea, sclera and conjunctiva.

FUTURE OF ANTERIOR SEGMENT OPTICAL COHERENCE TOMOGRAPHY

Anterior segment optical coherence tomography is currently being utilized in dry eye studies. Measuring tear meniscus height (TMH) and conjunctivochalasis are among some of the newer elements being studied utilizing ASOCT capabilities during diagnosis and management.[23,24] Using OCT imaging to determine effectiveness in dry eye treatment during clinical trials looks to be promising and encompasses another capability of this technology.

As post-LASIK patients age, determining proper corneal power for cataract surgery can be an issue. ASOCT measures both the anterior and posterior corneal curvature—the relationship affected by LASIK. Specific software for this measurement is being studied and released in some of the spectral domain optical coherence tomography (SDOCT) systems. SDOCT has dramatically increased speed acquisition and improved anatomical detail in both the posterior and anterior segment. Use of ASOCT has allowed for better and more efficient diagnosis, improved disease monitoring, enhanced surgical planning, and superior monitoring of response to treatment.

Future OCT technology includes imaging of microscopic structures and those located posterior to the iris. Achieving this result can someday result in biopsy-like images of corneal pathogens including protozoa and fungi. Future swept-source models with a longer wavelength allowing better penetrance of anterior segment tissue morphology may also enhance the role of OCT imaging on the eye-care profession.

REFERENCES

1. Kent C. Any way you slice it: a better anterior chamber view. Rev Ophthalmol. 2005;12:2.
2. Vajzovic LM, Karp CL, Haft P, et al. Ultra high-resolution anterior segment optical coherence tomography in the evaluation of anterior corneal dystrophies and degenerations. Ophthalmology. 2011;118(7):1291-6.
3. Ratanasit A, Gorovoy MS. Long-term results of Descemet stripping automated endothelial keratoplasty. Cornea. 2011;30(12):1414-8.
4. Esquenazi S, Rand W. Effect of the shape of the endothelial graft on the refractive results after Descemet's stripping with automated endothelial keratoplasty. Can J Ophthalmol. 2009;44(5):557-61.
5. Kent C. Making the most of anterior segment OCT. Rev Ophthalmol. 2011;18(4):39-46.
6. Ramos JL, Li Y, Huang D. Clinical and research applications of anterior segment optical coherence tomography: a review. Clin Exp Ophthalmol. 2009;37(1):81-9.
7. Dorairaj S, Lebmann JM, Ritch R. Quantitative evaluation of anterior segment parameters in the era of imaging. Trans Am Ophthalmol Soc. 2007;105:99-110.
8. Sansanayudh W, Bahar I, Kumar NL, et al. Intrastromal corneal ring segment SK implantation for moderate-to-severe keratoconus. J Cataract Refract Surg. 2010;36(1):110-3.
9. Piñero DP, Alio JL, El Kady B, et al. Refractive and aberrometric outcomes of intracorneal ring segments for keratoconus: mechanical versus femtosecond-assisted procedures. Ophthalmology. 2009;116(9):1675-87.
10. Slade SG. Applications for the femtosecond laser in corneal surgery. Curr Opin Ophthalmol. 2007;18(4):338-41.
11. Mashor RS, Rootman DB, Bahar I, et al. Outcomes of deep anterior lamellar keratoplasty versus intralase enabled penetrating keratoplasty in keratoconus. Can J Ophthalmol. 2011;46(5):403-7.
12. Pang CE, MV, Tan DT, et al. Evaluation of corneal epithelial healing under contact lens with spectral-domain anterior segment optical coherence tomography (SD-OCT). Open Ophthalmol J. 2011;5:51-4.
13. Sobara L, Maram J, Fonn D, et al. Metrics of the normal cornea: Anterior segment imaging with the Visante OCT. Clin Exp Optom. 2010;93(3):150-6.
14. Goldsmith JA, Li Y, Chalita MR, et al. Anterior chamber width measurement by high-speed optical coherence tomography. Ophthalmology. 2005;112(2):238-44.
15. Müller M, Dahmen G, Pörksen E, et al. Anterior chamber angle measurement with optical coherence tomography: Intraobserver and interobserver variability. J Cataract Refract Surg. 2006;32(11):1803-8.
16. Ahmed II, Teichman JC. OCT's applications for the cataract surgeon. Cataract Refract Surg Today (Suppl). 2007;7:3-5.
17. Dul MW. Glaucoma imaging: getting closer. Optometric Management. 2006;41(7):49-52,71.
18. Ritch R, Chang B, Liebmann JM. Angle closure in younger patients. Ophthalmology. 2003;110(10):1880-9. Review.
19. Diniz Filho A, Cronemberger S, Mérula RV, et al. Plateau iris. Arq Bras Oftalmol. 2008;71(5):752-8.
20. Wand M, Grant WM, Simmons RJ, et al. Plateau iris syndrome. Trans Sect Ophthalmol Am Acad Ophthalmol Otolaryngol. 1977;83(1):122-30.
21. Ritch R, Dorairaj S. Plateau iris syndrome in younger patients. Clin Exp Ophthalmol. 2007;35(5):399-400.
22. Johnson DH. Options in management of malignant glaucoma. Arch Ophthalmol. 1998;116(6):799-800.
23. Ibrahim OM, Dogru M, Takano Y, et al. Application of Visante optical coherence tomography tear meniscus height measurement in the diagnosis of dry eye disease. Ophthalmology. 2010;117(10):1923-9.
24. Veres A, Tapasztó B, Kosina-Hagyó K, et al. Imaging lid-parallel conjunctival folds with OCT and comparing its grading with the slit lamp classification in dry eye patients and normal subjects. Invest Ophthalmol Vis Sci. 2011;52(6):2945-51.

CHAPTER

24

Spectral Domain Optical Coherence Tomography

Sripathi Kamath, Rajeev R Pappuru

INTRODUCTION

Optical coherence tomography (OCT) is a new medical diagnostic technology, which can perform micron resolution tomographic cross-sectional imaging of biological tissues. The initial development of the technology was pioneered at the Massachusetts Institute of Technology in Boston, USA, and the first OCT machines became available for wide-spread clinical use around 10 years ago. After the first two generations of scanners, the latest type has been available on the market since 2002. Apart from its use in ophthalmology, OCT technology has also been applied in many other medical subspecialties such as urology, dermatology, and cardiology, and also in nonmedical fields such as engineering.[1]

PRINCIPLES

The OCT scanner uses low-coherence interferometry to create an image. An optical beam from a superluminescent diode laser emitting at 830 nm is directed onto an optical beam splitter, which functions as the interferometer. Half the beam is reflected from a reference mirror and the other is transmitted to the imaged tissue. The operation of the system can be understood qualitatively if one thinks of the light beam as being composed of short pulses of light. The pulse of light reflected from the reference mirror will only coincide with the pulse of light reflected from a given structure in the patient's eye if both pulses arrive at the same time. This will occur only if the distance that the light travels to and from the reference mirror precisely matches the distance that the light travels when it is reflected from a given structure in the patient's eye. When the two light pulses coincide, they produce a phenomenon known as interference, which is measured by a light-sensitive detector. To facilitate transmission of light, high-quality fiber optics and optical communications technology are used in the OCT setup. Successive longitudinal measurements at sequential transverse points (A-scans) are performed. As the light source moves across the retina, optical reflection and backscatter from retinal structures are detected. A two-dimensional set of data is collected and a cross-sectional map is obtained.[1,2]

Spectral domain optical coherence tomography (SD-OCT) allows us to visualize cross section, anterior segment, and three-dimensional (3D) views of the retina. This enables us to diagnose and monitor glaucoma and numerous retinal diseases and treatment efficacy. The data provided by SD-OCT are comparable to those obtained with ultrasound B examinations, but with some notable advantages. For example, ultrasound B has a resolution of about 150 μm, while time domain OCT has a resolution of 10 μm, and SD-OCT has a resolution of 5 μm. Retinal scans with SD-OCT are highly reproducible. The instrument is easy to operate, and the learning curve, even for 3D studies, is short. OCT allows the observation, measurement, and identification of structures not easily visible, such as the external limiting membrane (ELM), the junction between the internal segment and the external segment of the photoreceptors (IS/OS junction). It also shows various types of lesions with altered morphology, altered reflectivity and/or optically blank areas.

FUNCTIONS

- Measures retinal thickness
- Measures the retinal nerve fiber layer (RNFL)
- Measures the volume of the retina
- Creates retinal maps
- Isolates and creates maps of the internal limiting membrane (ILM) and the retinal pigment epithelium (RPE)

- Measures various parameters of the optic disk
- Displays 3D views
- Provides classic C-scan (en face) analyses, creating a section plane horizontally in the tissue
- Offers an RPE fit function, which provides a view of a tissue section.

APPLICATIONS

- Detect disease
- Evaluate treatment efficacy
- Quantify lesions and evaluate treatment efficacy
- Track progression and patient education.

ADVANTAGES OF OCT

- It has simple and short learning curve
- It is fast and reliable
- It is sensitive and reproducible
- It is noninvasive.

ADVANTAGES OF SD-OCT

Compared with time domain OCT, the spectral domain OCT offers a clearer view of pathology throughout the entire retina. It allows us to differentiate retinal layers, particularly the external retina, the photoreceptors and RPE, and to evaluate morphological variations.

It helps to study subtle histological structures that we may not be able to detect with time domain OCT. In addition, we can evaluate the intravitreal formations and delineate strands and particles formed in the vitreous and intravitreal membranes, as well as inflammation, hemorrhage or neovascularization. Vitreoretinal interface and hyaloid are more clearly visible with SD-OCT.

ANALYSIS OF OCT

Analysis of OCT can be divided into two components—qualitative and quantitative analyses **(Table 1)**.

Following a logical sequence is essential when analyzing an OCT scan. Initially, one must analyze each of the elements—hyperreflective lesions, hyporeflective lesions, anatomical changes, quantitative alterations, retinal thickness, and retinal map, to arrive at final interpretation.

Table 1: Qualitative and quantitative components of OCT.

Qualitative analysis	***Quantitative analysis***
Morphological alterations	Thickness
Anomalous structures	Volume
Reflectivity	Map
High reflectivity	
Low reflectivity	
Shadow zones	

Interpreting Colors on SD-OCT

Generally, it is preferable to study images in gray scale rather than conventional pseudocolors. It shows slight variations in the intensities of gray to distinguish details that are easy to miss. The SD-OCT software arbitrarily signs a color for each degree of reflectivity, allowing us to see marked differences in color where we would otherwise observe a gradual change in reflectivity **(Figs. 1 and 2)**.

Retinal Deformations

In cases of high myopia and especially posterior myopic staphyloma, OCT will show a marked concavity **(Fig. 3)**. Certain lesions in the sclera (staphyloma) contribute to a localized depression of the retina throughout its thickness.

In cases of serous detachment of the RPE, OCT often shows a convex shape. In rare instances, however, convexity may be due to subretinal cysts. In these cases, the convexity is less pronounced and includes the subretinal layers (the epithelium and choriocapillaris). In subretinal tumors, such as melanomas, the entire retina, including the RPE, is raised so that differentiating the tumor may be difficult.

Abnormal Retinal Profile

The normal retinal profile shows a regular, symmetrical foveal depression. OCT can detect following abnormalities:

- *Vitreoretinal traction:* The normal foveal depression deforms, becoming convex and irregular. This condition is associated with the formation of fissures or holes **(Fig. 4)**.[3]
- *Diffuse retinal edema:* The foveal depression may be reduced or disappear, and the retinal profile may become flat or slightly irregular. The absence of the foveal depression is a sign of clinically significant retinal edema **(Figs. 5A and B)**.
  - Complex vitreoretinal traction.
  - Retinal folds.
- *Macular pucker:* The retinal surface is deformed by waves and curled by traction caused by the epiretinal membrane (ERM) **(Fig. 6)**.
- Enlarged and irregular foveal depression.
- Macular pseudohole.

An enlarged foveal depression simulates a retinal macular hole. The presence of retinal tissue at all thicknesses above the RPE confirms the diagnosis of the pseudohole **(Fig. 7)**. In a true lamellar hole, we observe residual retinal tissue or some retinal layers above the RPE.

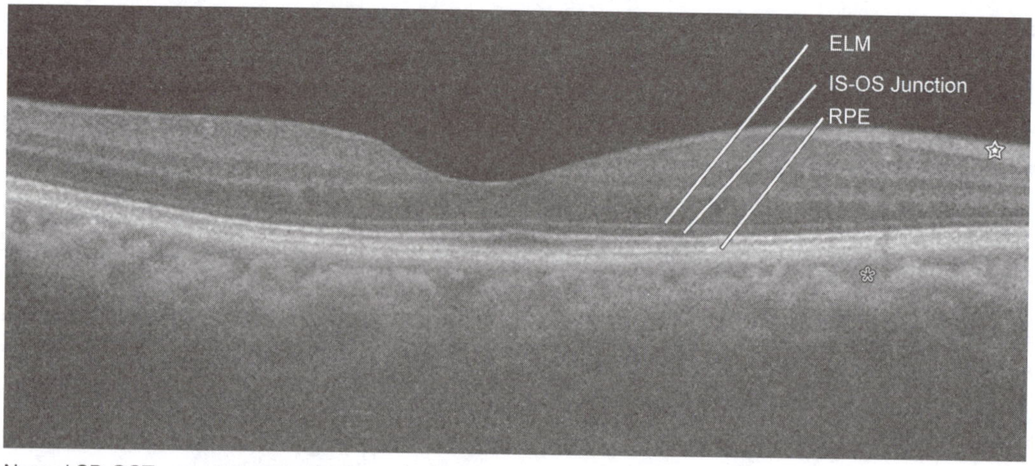

Fig. 1: Normal SD-OCT scan demonstrating the retinal layers. The external limiting membrane (ELM), inner and outer segment junction (IS/OS junction),* retinal nerve fiber layer,* choroid can also be imaged well with SD-OCT.
(OCT: optical coherence tomography; RPE: retinal pigment epithelium; SD-OCT: spectral domain optical coherence tomography)

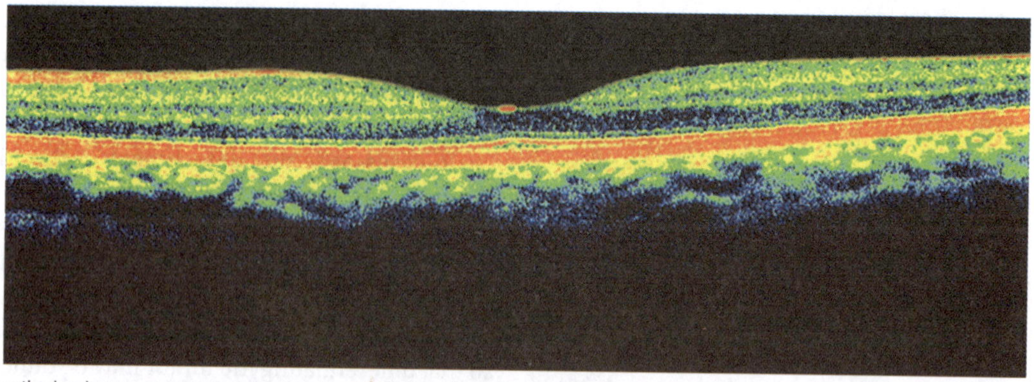

Fig. 2: Normal optical coherence tomography in color. Note that the retinal layer details are not appreciated well in color when compared to gray display, and gray display is better in identifying finer retinal details.

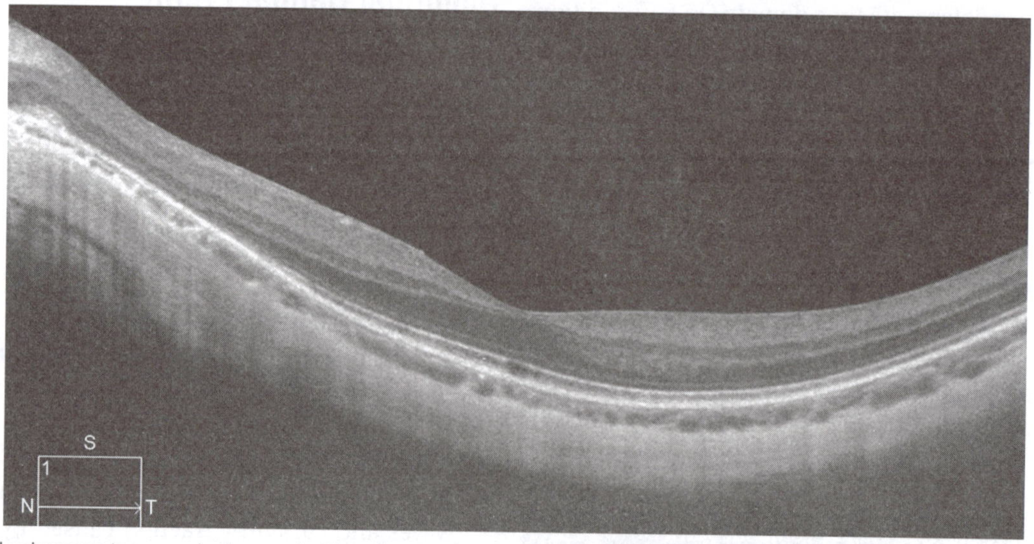

Fig. 3: Optical coherence tomography in myopia. Note the abnormal concave curvature of the retina and the presence of thinned out choroid.

Macular Hole

Optical coherence tomography facilitates identification, measurement, and classification of macular holes according to the Gass classifications.[4]

- *Stage 1*: The foveal depression disappears and a small optically blank area (cyst) forms above or below the retinal surface.
- *Stage 2*: Partial breaks of the internal retina are apparent, with operculum adhering to the margins of the hole, and slightly increased thickness.
- *Stage 3*: The hole penetrates to the RPE; the operculum no longer adheres to the retina; retinal edema is present, with increased thickness of the retina and a small detachment.

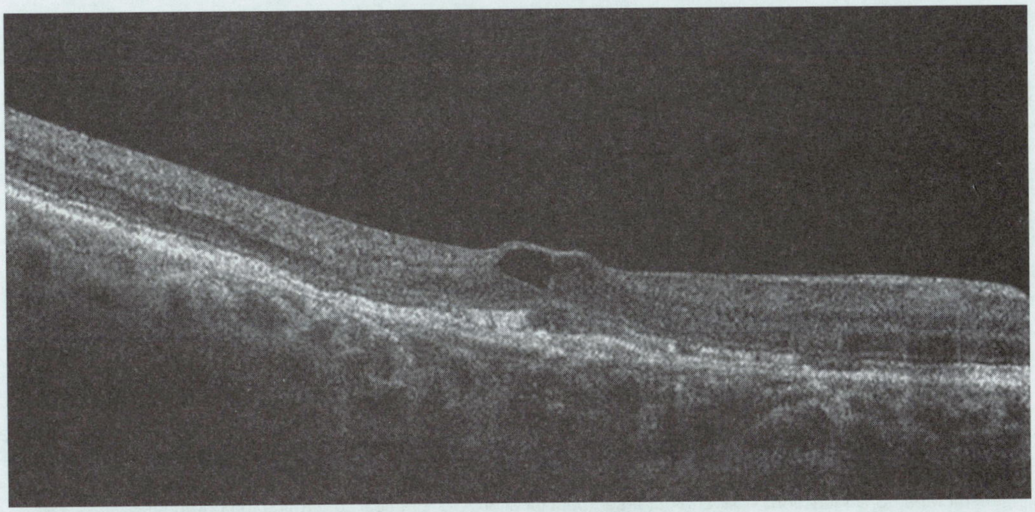

Fig. 4: Deformation of the retinal profile by vitreomacular traction. Partially adherent posterior hyaloid exerts traction on the retinal surface, causing the foveal depression to disappear.

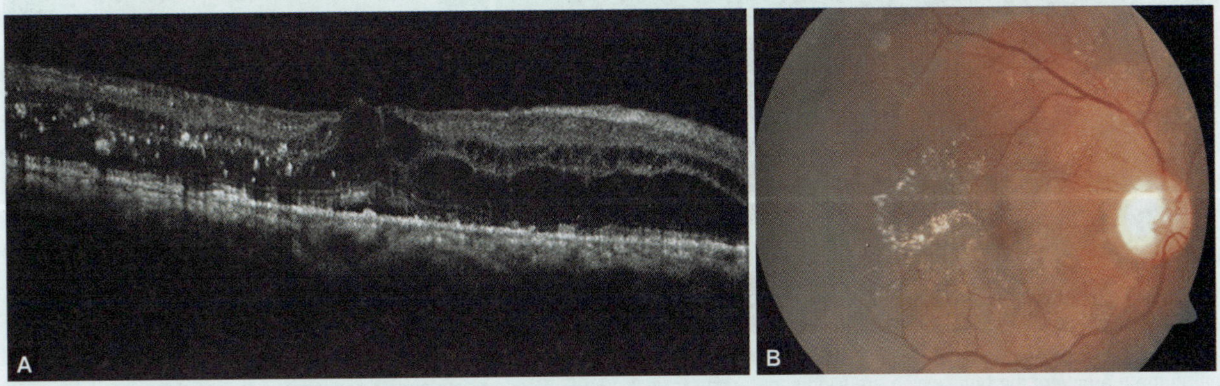

Figs. 5A and B: (A) Optical coherence tomography; (B) Fundus photograph in diabetic macular edema. The retinal thickness is increased due to macular edema. Note the presence of cystoid cavities in the outer retina, small neurosensory detachment and hyper-reflective spots suggesting the presence of hard exudates in diabetic macular edema.

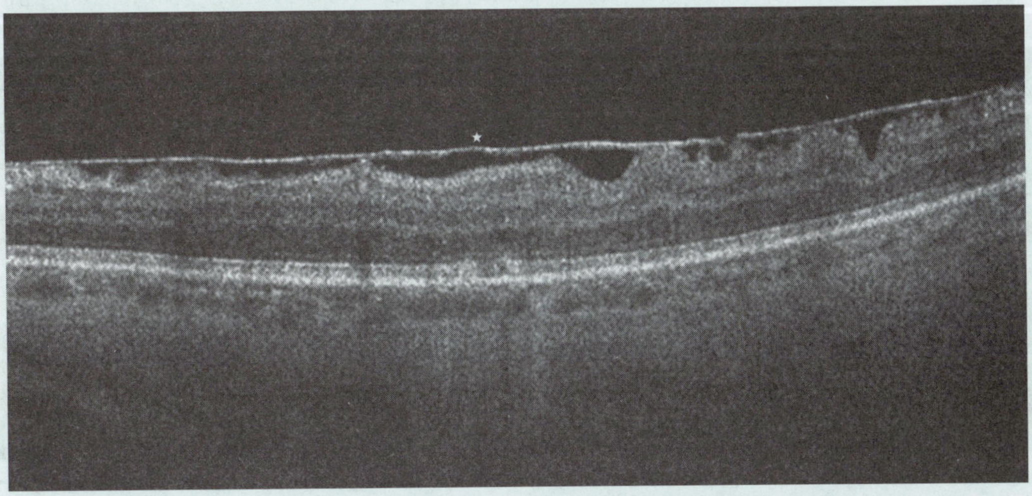

Fig. 6: Morphological alteration showing epiretinal membrane (ERM) and retinal folds. Partially adherent ERM exerts tangential traction on the retinal surface, causing folds on the internal limiting membrane.

- *Stage 4*: The hole penetrates entire thickness, with loss of retinal substance, retinal edema on the margins and detachment of the margins **(Fig. 8A)**.

Stage 1 macular hole may undergo spontaneous closure **(Fig. 8B)**.

Intraretinal Morphological Alterations

- *Posterior morphological alterations:* These anomalies, especially serous or hemorrhagic detachments, are observed at the RPE level. Serous RPE detachments

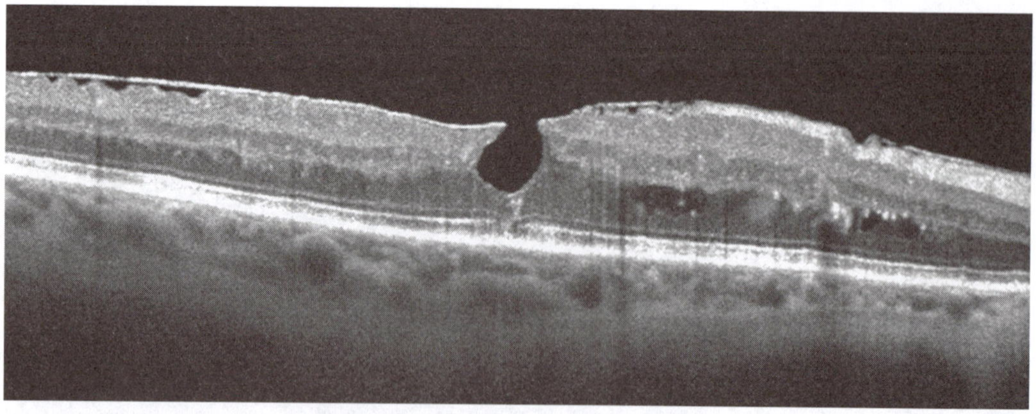

Fig. 7: Macular pseudohole. OCT demonstrates epiretinal membrane leading to tangential traction and causing macular pseudohole. There is no loss of retinal tissue at the fovea and hence it is pseudohole. Also note the disruption of ELM, IS/OS junction and also note the presence of high reflective spots suggestive of hard exudates, few cystoid spaces in the outer retina suggestive of macular edema.
(ELM: external limiting membrane; IS/OS junction: inner and outer segment junction; OCT: optical coherence tomography)

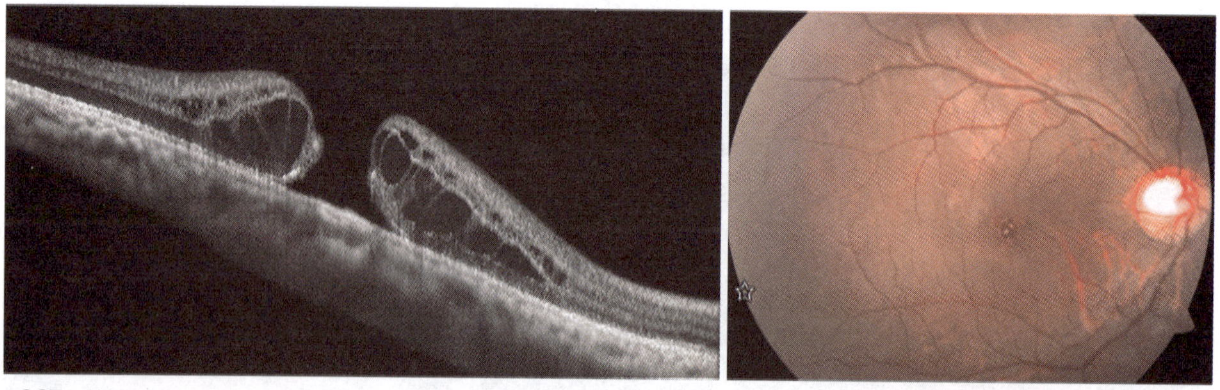

Fig. 8A: OCT and fundus photographs in macular hole. The hole penetrates all thicknesses, with only the RPE visible. Marked cystoid macular edema is thickening the margins of the hole, which are slightly detached from the RPE. These pseudocysts are located in the internal and external nuclear layers. It is important to measure all components of the hole and its dimensions at different levels to decide if surgical intervention is necessary and to follow progression. The ELM and the IS/OS junction are normal in the surrounding retina and slightly detached at the margins of the hole. They disappear around the fovea with the rest of the retinal tissue.
(ELM: external limiting membrane; IS/OS junction: inner and outer segment junction; OCT: optical coherence tomography; RPE: retinal pigment epithelium)

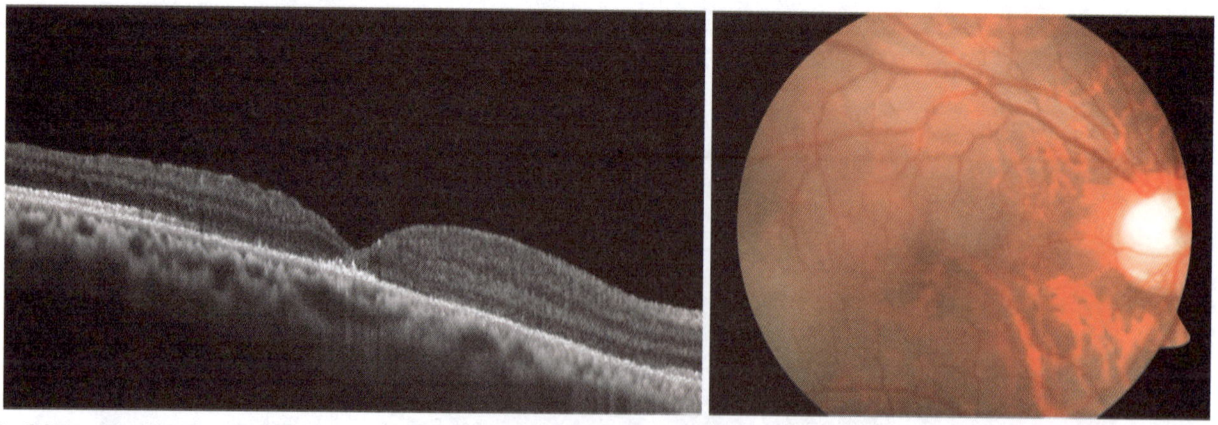

Fig. 8B: OCT and fundus photographs showing closure (type 1 closure) of the macular hole following surgery. The ELM/IS/OS junction appears to be broken despite closure of the macular hole.
(ELM: external limiting membrane; IS/OS junction: inner and outer segment junction; OCT: optical coherence tomography)

deform the posterior border of the retina and form an obtuse angle with Bruch's membrane and the choriocapillaris. Serous detachment of the neurosensory retina is less elevated and form acute angles with the RPE **(Figs. 9A and B)**.

- *Retinal pigment epithelium:* RPE thickness may be increased with a slightly irregular or diminished aspect. In general, in cases of atrophy, the epithelium atrophies and reveals Bruch's membrane. The RPE also can decrease irregularly, revealing one or more of the three

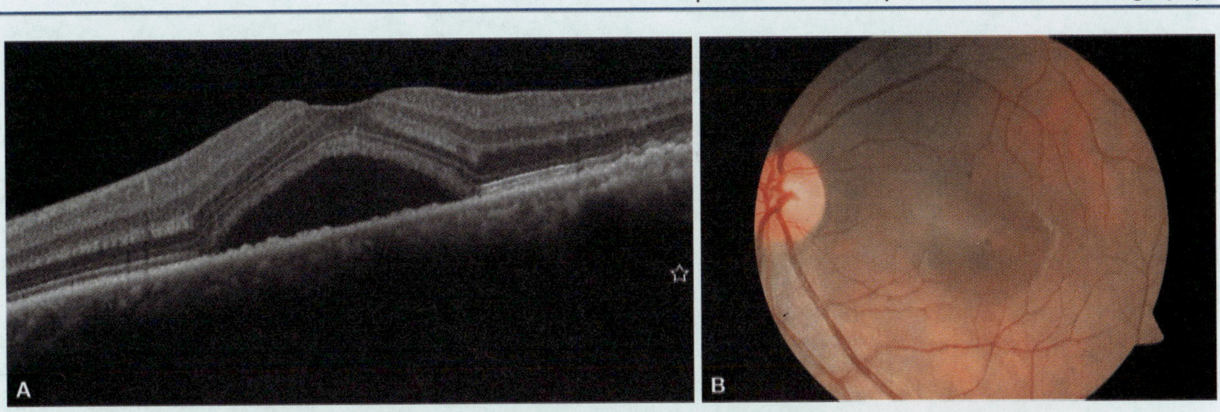

Figs. 9A and B: OCT and fundus photographs showing central serous chorioretinopathy. This OCT demonstrates the presence of normal inner retinal layers. There is a large neurosensory retinal detachment as demonstrated by the presence of convex-shaped hyporeflective space between the RPE and neurosensory retina indicating subretinal fluid. Also note the presence of few undulations in the RPE layer temporally.
(OCT: optical coherence tomography; RPE: retinal pigment epithelium)

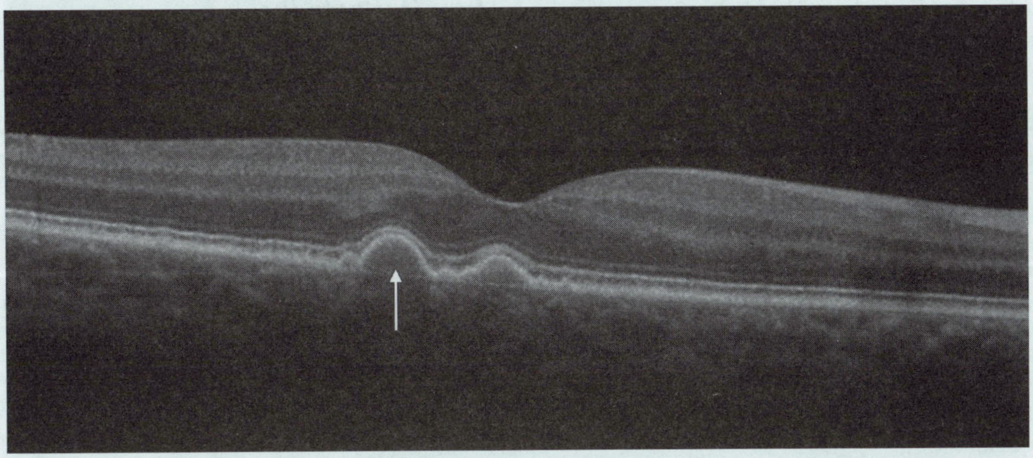

Fig. 10: OCT showing drusenoid PED. Note the presence of convex elevations along the RPE in the foveal region. The detachment shows homogeneous reflectivity suggestive of drusen.
(OCT: optical coherence tomography; PED: pigmented epithelium detachment; RPE: retinal pigment epithelium)

normal layers. In other cases, there can be more marked anomalies in these layers.

- In cases of atrophy or incipient neovascular membranes, we can observe dissociation and increased thickness of the RPE. Drusen are seen as irregular undulates with slightly hyperreflective content. They may be associated with drusenoid pigmented epithelium detachment (PED) **(Fig. 10)**. Serous detachment, on the other hand, often has an optically blank appearance. It is then possible to observe Bruch's membrane as a thin, rectilinear line.
- *Retinal outer nuclear layer (ONL)*: One must carefully observe the ONL because it gives essential information about the function of the photoreceptors. It can present as normal or of varied thickness in different pathologies affecting the outer retina. Any of these characteristics will indicate the integrity of the photoreceptors, especially when compared with other indications. We must be especially aware of the appearance of the junction of the internal and external segments of the photoreceptors (IS/OS junction) and the outer segments of the photoreceptors.
- *External limiting membrane*: The ELM is normally more resilient than the IS/OS junction. In fact, it can be observed after the IS/OS junction has disappeared. The ELM can be linear, broken in points, deformed by folds and RPE detachments, or altered in various ways. In some lesions, the ELM is absent or not visible.

Anomalous Structures

Because of increased scan density and higher resolution, SD-OCT can evaluate anomalous structures better than time domain OCT. The study of hyporeflective structures is easier, especially at the vitreous level and behind the RPE/choriocapillaris.

Pre- and Epiretinal Membrane

The density, thickness, and location of pre- and ERMs can be evaluated. The membrane may be adherent, fused with the ILM, or fully or partially detached. Its reflectivity, however, is greater than the normal reflectivity of the RNFL. They can be separate from the retina, in contact or adherent, or they can cause wrinkles in the retinal surface. The preretinal or ERM can be seen clearly as hyperreflective because of thickening of the fibroglial elements **(Fig. 6)**.

If detached, the posterior hyaloid presents on OCT as a slightly reflective image, often broken, thin but well delineated and adherent to the retina at some points.[5]

Macular Pucker

Retraction of the ILM is caused by a fibroglial proliferation causing tangential traction. The force of this action creates retinal folds, with resultant changes to the courses of blood vessels, which appear elongated when parallel to the folds and twisted when crossing them. The traction exerted perpendicularly on the vascular arcs, in turn, determines their distance from one another. Generally, retinal folds are transverse in the retina underlying the retracted membrane and radial to that outside the area of retraction **(Fig. 6)**.

Cotton Wool Spots

These hyperreflective spots are associated with ischemic lesions of the nerve fibers and are located at the periphery of the ischemic area.

Intraretinal anomalous structures such as hard exudates are localized in the posterior layers of the retina. They are formed from lipoproteins and can be isolated or part of the surrounding retina. They precipitate in the external plexiform layer at the boundary between the edematous area and the normal retina.

Classic neovascular membranes of wet age-related macular degeneration (AMD) are generally seen as fusiform, nodular, rounded and immediately anterior to the RPE. If active, they are accompanied by retinal edema or serous detachment of the neuroretina **(Fig. 11A)**. They often show improvement following intravitreal injection of anti-vascular endothelial growth factor (VEGF) injection **(Fig. 11B)**. Occult neovascular membranes are more difficult to distinguish, presenting as a thickening of the RPE/choriocapillaris complex. The active occult membranes are accompanied by diffuse or cystoid edema and localized serous detachments of the neuroretina.

The retinal scars in advanced macular degeneration or diabetic fibrovascular membrane present as thickened areas of hyperreflective fibrovascular tissue. They distort the profile of the retina and can cause the normal elements of the retina to disappear.[6-8]

Qualitative Analysis

High Reflectivity

The strength of the signal reflected from tissue depends on the following factors:

- The quantity of light when it arrives at a particular layer, having been partially absorbed by intervening tissues.
- The quantity of light reflected.
- The quantity of light reflected that reaches the detector after having been reabsorbed.
- Horizontal anatomical structures, such as the nerve fibers and the plexiform layers, are more reflective than vertical structures.

Increased reflectivity may be superficial, intraretinal or deep. Depending on its location, increased reflectivity may indicate the following lesions.

Superficial Increased Reflectivity

- Syndromes of the vitreoretinal interface, epiretinal or retinal fibrosis, macular pucker, pre- or ERMs.

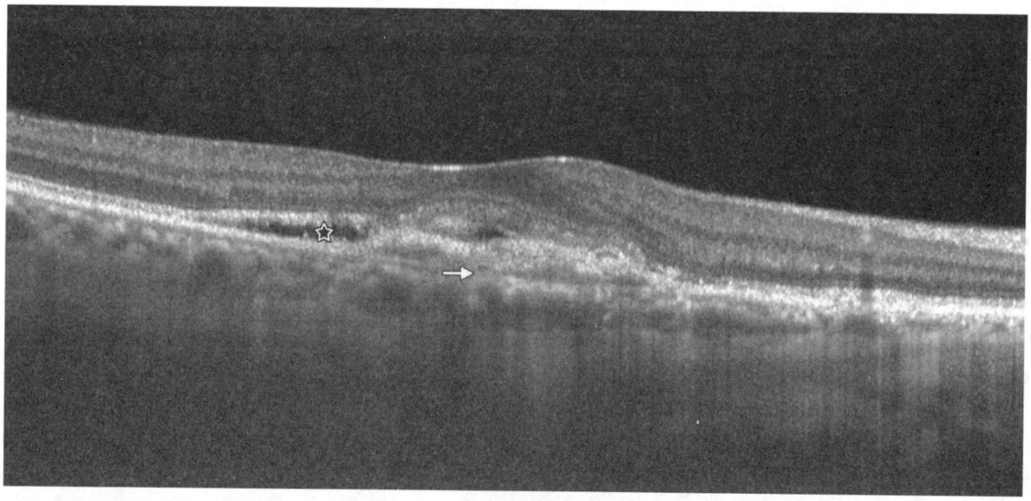

Fig. 11A: *OCT in wet AMD*: In this case of AMD, the neovascular membrane (arrow) is elongated, fusiform and located in front of the RPE. We can distinguish the lesions of the RPE and Bruch's membrane where it originated. Note the presence of subretinal fluid.
*In this case, pseudocystic cavities of edema do not appear. Edema and detachments of the neuroretina are always present with active nerve fiber membranes, whether classic or occult.
(AMD: age-related macular degeneration; OCT: optical coherence tomography; RPE: retinal pigment epithelium)

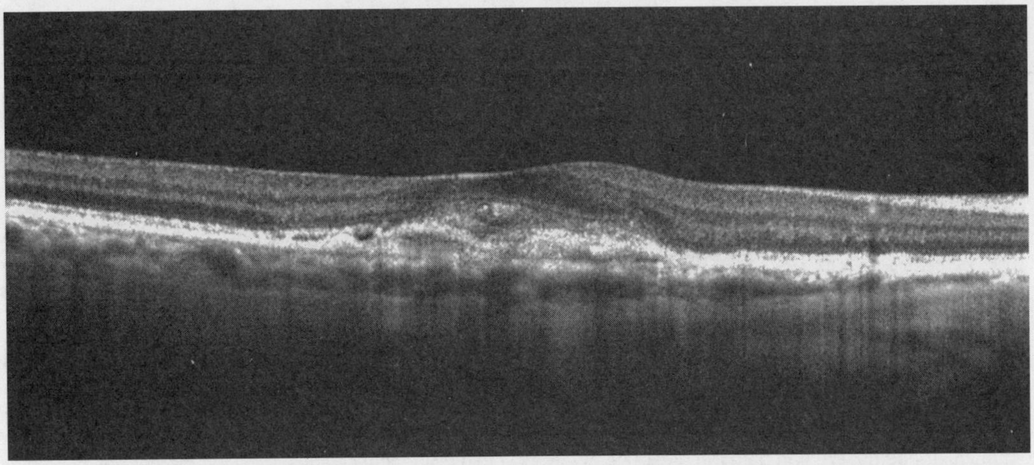

Fig. 11B: Note the disappearance of the subretinal fluid following intravitreal anti-VEGF injection. (VEGF: vascular endothelial growth factor)

- Superficial hemorrhage (dense with a screening effect), and cotton-wool spots (superficial with margins indistinct from the margins of the areas of recent ischemia).

Intraretinal Lesions

- *Lesions of the photoreceptors:* In these cases, the IS/OS junction shows irregularity, interruptions, and areas in which it is no longer visible. In cases of retinal atrophy, the ELM is more resistant and remains visible for a longer period.
- *Retinal serous detachments:* As in central serous chorioretinopathy (CSCR), the external segment of the photoreceptors, which can be thickened, irregular or have increased reflectivity, present granulations or flaking of the internal face of the detachment in the detached area.
- *Hemorrhage:* They are dense, with a shadow effect.
- *Hard exudates:* They are nodular, hyperreflective zones composed of lipoproteins at the boundary between the healthy retina and the edematous retina. They are generally located in deep layers **(Fig. 5)**.

Deep Lesions

- Drusen cause an undulation or localized increase in thickness of the RPE/choriocapillaris complex **(Fig. 10)**.
- Pre- and retroepithelial neovascular membranes that merge with the RPE complex: Bruch's membrane and choriocapillaris show increased reflectivity under a thin retina.
- Scars from choroiditis, traumatic lesions, retinal fibrosis, disciform degeneration: Recent laser impacts are seen as vertical, hyperreflective stripes leading from the RNFL to the RPE. Because of hyperpigmentation, those in the choroid appear as increased reflectivity in the RPE/choriocapillaris complex, and they cause a shadow zone. Increased retrodiffusion of light may indicate atrophy of the retina and RPE.

Low Reflectivity

Diminished reflectivity may be caused by less reflective tissue, such as atrophied RPE with less pigment. Collections of fluid may be seen as diffuse edema, cysts, cystic or pseudocystic areas, serous or hemorrhagic detachment of the neuroretina or RPE.[1]

Areas of low reflectivity may be minimal or extensive. They take on an important role in 3D studies and frontal scans.

- *Low intraretinal reflectivity:* It is seen in retinal edema, cystoid macular edema (CME) **(Fig. 12)**, cysts, microcysts, and impending hole.
- *Low subintraretinal reflectivity:* It is found in serous detachment of the neuroretina. The detachment forms an acute angle with the RPE.
- *Low reflectivity under the RPE:* It appears in the serous detachments of the RPE that has separated from Bruch's membrane. The fluid from the choriocapillaris accumulates in the subretinal space, creating an obtuse angle with the underlying layers. The area of the detachment or the cystic space can be optically blank in cases of serous detachment or more reflective in cases of inflammatory exudations or senile degeneration.
- *Hemorrhagic detachment:* The detachment shows areas that are not optically blank but may be shadowed by highly reflective areas.
- Diminution of the pigment in the area of atrophy of the pigment epithelium.

Shadow Zones

Dense, reflective tissue may create a shadow on posterior elements. The highly sensitive SD-OCT lends far more contrast to the shadow zones determined by the retinal blood vessels and intraretinal reflective formations. At the IS/OS junction and the ILM, the shadow of the retinal vessels obscures these structures and simulates lesions of the photoreceptors **(Fig. 13)**.

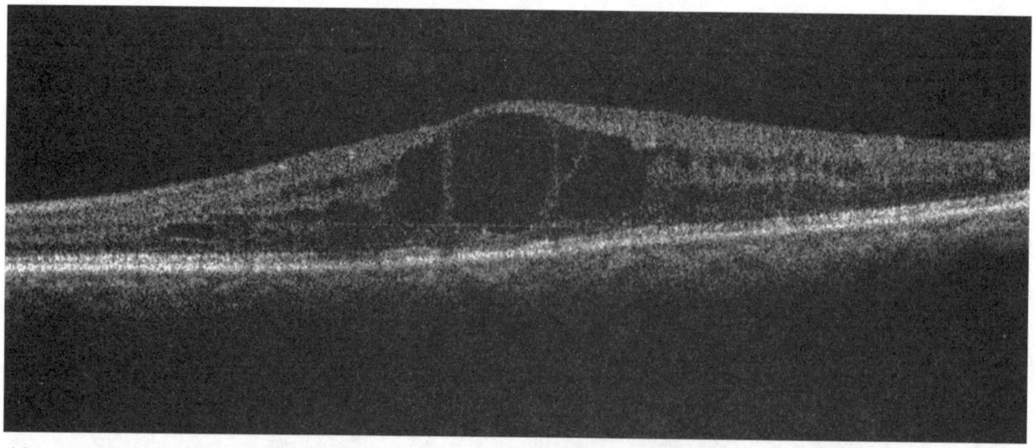

Fig. 12: Cystoid macular edema. We can note the presence of large cystoid cylindrical cavities involving the central fovea indicating chronic edema. Few hyperreflective spots are also noted in the inner retinal layers.

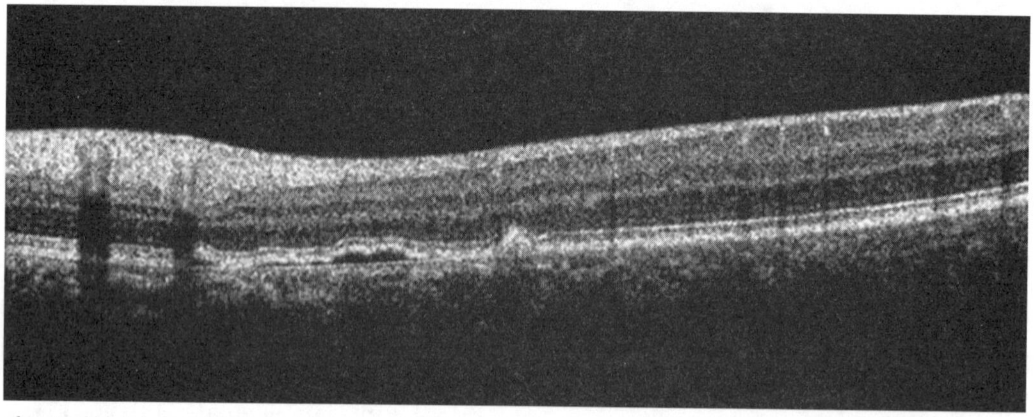

Fig. 13: Shadow of normal blood vessels in spectral domain OCT scans, the normal retinal blood vessels, which are difficult to observe in the RNFL, form vertical shadows that interrupt the underlying structures. It is important to recognize these to avoid confusing the interruptions of the ILM and the IS/OS junction with true alterations of the photoreceptors. Spectral domain OCT shows the blood vessel itself or its contents if the vessel is large. (ILM: internal limiting membrane; IS/OS junction: inner and outer segment junction; OCT: optical coherence tomography; RNFL: retinal nerve fiber layer)

The structures of the retina can be occluded at various levels—preretinal, intraretinal, and posterior. We have noted the following with regard to shadows apparent in SD-OCT studies.

Anterior level

The normal retinal blood vessels are difficult to distinguish, but they cast a cone of shadow that allows us to find them **(Fig. 13)**. Superficial or profound hemorrhage causes a cone of shadow as do cotton wool exudates.

Posterior level

Hard lipid exudates in the deep retinal layers cast a dense, inclined shadow. A screen of pigmented formations can appear with an inclined shadow. Hyperplasia and hypertrophy of the RPE are imaged as dense shadows.

Neovascularization of the choroid is detected by an increase in reflectivity in the RPE/Bruch's membrane complex and a slight increase in the thickness of this layer, with a shadow cast on the posterior layers. A dense, pigmented scar casts a shadow. Markedly hyperreflective subretinal neovascular membrane, if thick, can also cast a shadow.[9]

Quantitative Analysis

Quantification is an important aspect of an analytic examination. It allows comparison of numerical data in the natural course of a disease or its response to medical, laser or surgical therapy. With certain software, we can quantify the thickness of the retina or retinal elements (e.g. the RNFL in glaucoma), as well as the volume of the retina. SD-OCT gives us better definition and contrast between the retinal layers, allowing precise study and measurement of various layers.

In lesions of the internal retina, due to occlusions of the retinal venules or arterioles, there are marked variations of the nerve fibers, the ganglion layer, the internal plexiform layer, and the internal nuclear layer. In venous occlusions and recent arterial occlusions, there is an increase in thickness. In arterial occlusions, after a few weeks, a marked reduction in internal retinal thickness appears. The external nuclear layer is the most important layer of the external retina to evaluate because you can detect damage to the photoreceptors.[10]

Idiopathic polypoidal choroidal vasculopathy presents polypoidal choroidal vascular dilatations often associated with serosanguineous detachment of neurosensory retina

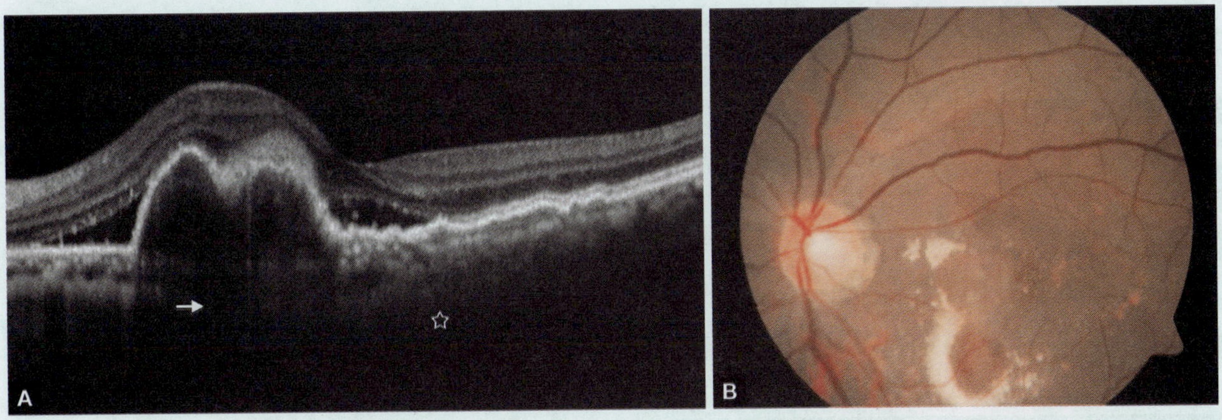

Figs. 14A and B: OCT and fundus photographs in idiopathic polypoidal choroidal vasculopathy. RPE detachment with detached neurosensory retina (arrow). The detachment* forms an obtuse angle with the portion of the RPE still being attached. Note the presence of non-homogeneous reflectivity along the inner side of RPE detachment suggesting hemorrhagic PED.
(PED: pigmented epithelium detachment; OCT: optical coherence tomography; RPE: retinal pigment epithelium)

and RPE. OCT can show polyps under the RPE associated with serous retinal detachment and hemorrhagic PED (**Figs. 14A and B**).

SD-OCT VS. TD-OCT

Time domain OCT automatically measures retinal thickness, showing the distance between the vitreoretinal interface and the anterior surface of the pigment epithelium, which varies from 275 µm to 200 µm. The foveal depression varies from 190 µm to 170 µm. At the fovea, the average thickness is approximately 170–190 µm; and the peripheral retina is 240 µm. The retinal fibers are thicker in the interpapillo-macular area. The nerve fibers form a slightly thickened arc of about 500 µm within the fovea, normally reaching 270 µm. The thickness is measured on single scans and over the retinal map. The normative database software enables us to compare variations to the normal eye. SD-OCT gives higher values for retinal thickness because it measures the RPE with more precision than time domain OCT, which confuses it with the IS/OS junction.

CONCLUSION

In summary, the introduction of OCT for the clinical examination of the macula has opened up several new avenues in the diagnosis and monitoring of macular diseases. This novel technique has become of particular importance in the assessment of diabetic macular edema and of macular edema associated both with age-related macular degeneration and with vitreomacular traction syndromes. It has added new diagnostic criteria as well as more objective data both to make informed therapeutic decisions and to monitor macular edema after treatment.

Novel technologies such as ultra-high resolution OCT, which uses a titanium-sapphire laser light source, may play an important role in the future by providing much needed increased image resolution of up to 3 µm. This technology will be particularly useful in the exact localization of the disease and better understanding of the pathology and pathogenesis.

REFERENCES

1. Fujimoto JG, Brezinski ME, Tearney GJ, et al. Optical biopsy and imaging using optical coherence tomography. Nat Med. 1995;1(9):970-2.
2. Hee MR, Izatt JA, Swanson EA, et al. Optical coherence tomography of the human retina. Arch Ophthalmol. 1995;113(3):325-32.
3. Gallemore RP, Jumper JM, McCuen BW 2nd, et al. Diagnosis of vitreoretinal adhesions in macular disease with optical coherence tomography. Retina. 2000;20(2):115-20.
4. Puliafito CA, Hee MR, Lin CP, et al. Imaging of macular diseases with optical coherence tomography. Ophthalmology. 1995;102(2):217-29.
5. Massin P, Allouch C, Haouchine B, et al. Optical coherence tomography of idiopathic macular epiretinal membranes before and after surgery. Am J Ophthalmol. 2000;130(6): 732-9.
6. Ting TD, Oh M, Cox TA, et al. Decreased visual acuity associated with cystoid macular edema in neovascular age-related macular degeneration. Arch Ophthalmol. 2002;120(6):731-7.
7. Otani T, Kishi S, Maruyama Y. Patterns of diabetic macular edema with optical coherence tomography. Am J Ophthalmol. 1999;127(6):688-93.
8. Nussenblatt RB, Kaufman SC, Palestine AG, et al. Macular thickening and visual acuity. Measurement in patients with cystoid macular edema. Ophthalmology. 1987;94(9):1134-9.
9. Hee MR, Baumal CR, Puliafito CA, et al. Optical coherence tomography of age-related macular degeneration and choroidal neovascularization. Ophthalmology. 1996;103(8): 1260-70.
10. Spaide RF, Lee JK, Klancnik JM Jr, et al. Optical coherence tomography of branch retinal vein occlusion. Retina. 2003;23(3):343-7.

CHAPTER

25

Intraocular Lens Power Calculation

Himanshu Shekhar, Rajesh Sinha, Jeewan S Titiyal

INTRODUCTION

Over the last 20 years, intraocular lens (IOL) power calculations have become a focal point of cataract surgery. The refractive power of the human eye depends on the power of the cornea and the lens, the position of the lens, and the length of the eye. Accurate assessment of these variables is essential in achieving optimal postoperative refractive results.

In 1977, the state-of-the-art for estimating IOL power for emmetropia was to simply add +19.0 D to the precataractous refraction. A decade later, being within ±1.00 D of the target refraction was still considered a reasonable standard. These days "benchmark" standard for refractive outcomes for normal eyes after cataract surgery should be within ±0.50 D for 55% of cases and within ±1.00 D for 85% of cases.[1]

Today, by carefully optimizing the individual component parts of IOL power calculations, combined with advanced surgical techniques, it is possible to be within ±0.50 D for better than 70% of surgeries and ±1.00 D for better than 90% of surgeries.[2]

As a result of heightened patient expectations, there is more than ever a need to accurately predict the correct IOL power. These demands have spurred the continued improvements in technology and refinements in biometry and IOL calculations.

Though IOL formulae have become increasingly accurate, there are many situations, mainly due to the structural and anatomical variations in the globe, where this accuracy may decrease.

INTRAOCULAR LENS POWER FORMULAS

Intraocular lens formulae can be divided into two major categories:

1. Theoretical formulae
2. Regression formulae

Theoretical Formulae

These formulae were calculated on the basis of a theoretical optical model of the eye. These formulae are all based on geometric optics, as applied to schematic eyes using theoretical constants. Some of the common formulae used are those of Fyodorov, Colenbrander, Hoffer, and Binkhorst **(Table 1)**.

- *Basic theoretical formulas*: These include Colenbrander's, Fyodorov's, Van-der-Heijde's formula and the Hoffer 1974-formula which yield approximately the same IOL powers. Binkhorst's formula yields 0.50 D stronger lens power.
- *Modified theoretical formulas*: These include Hoffer's 1983-formula, Shamman's fudged formula and Binkhorst's adjusted formula. These formulas are modification of Colenbrander's formula.
- *The modern formulas*: These include formulas of Holladay I and II, Hoffer Q, Sanders-Retzlaff-Kraff

Table 1: Emmetropic intraocular lens (IOL) power calculation.

For calculation of IOL power in emmetropes	
Colenbrander's formula	$P = \frac{1,336}{L-C-0.05} - \frac{1,336}{1,336-C-0.05} K$
Fyodorov's formula	$P = \frac{1,336-LK}{(L-C)} - \frac{1-CK}{1,336}$
Van der Heijde's formula	$P = \frac{1,336}{L-C} - \frac{1}{1-\frac{C}{K}1,336} K$
Binkhorst's formula	$P = \frac{1,336 \ (4R-L)}{(L-S)\ (4R-C)}$
Lin's S-formula (I)	$Z'P = \frac{1,336}{(L-S)} - \frac{1,336}{\frac{1,336-S}{DC}}$

(SRK)/T formula. The more recent formula is of Haigis using 3-constant optimization for all ranges of eye length and IOL types.

Disadvantages of basic theoretical formulae were:

- Theoretical simplistic assumptions were made about the optics of the eye, bringing forth the constant requirement for corrections in different situations.
- An assumed expected value of postoperative anterior chamber depth (ACD) had to be used in all these formulae.
- Practical inaccuracies often come in the way of axial length measurement, as one must know the exact values of the ultrasonography waves as it travels through the various structures of the eye. Because of the variations in the acoustical density of a cataract, these velocities cannot be known exactly. This velocity error may make the eye appear shorter or longer, thus adding to the unpredictability of the results in these formulas.
- It was observed by many surgeons using these formulae that the shorter the eye, the greater was the overcorrection produced by the lens implant calculated to achieve emmetropia.
- At the time when these formulae were developed, iris-supported lens were commonly used and many of these assumptions took this fact into consideration. With the increasing use of posterior chamber and anterior chamber IOLs, new estimates had to be made for the distance between the cornea and the implant (postoperative ACD).

Regression Formulae

These formulae are derived from empirical data based on retrospective analysis of postoperative refraction after IOL implantation. Unlike the theoretical formulae, no assumptions are made about the optics of the eye. Advantages of this type of formulae over the theoretical formulae were that as these equations are based on the statistical analysis of the actual results of many uncomplicated IOL implantations, they are more accurate.

These formulas are derived empirically from retrospective computer analysis of data of patients who have undergone surgery before. The factors on which IOL power calculation depends are:

- *Axial length measurement*: This is the most important step in calculation of lens power. The IOL master is a recent method using partial coherence interferometry (PCI) which gives high accuracy in measurement of axial length. An error of 1 mm affects the postoperative refraction by 1.2–2.5 D approximately. It is measured in millimeters (mm).
- *Corneal power*: It is measured either in diopters or in millimeters (radius of curvature). Keratometer measures the radius of curvature of the central part of anterior corneal surface (r_1) and given by:

$$K = 337.5/r_1.$$

$$Kc = 1.114K - C,$$

with C given by a mean value of 5.1 D, 5.5 D, or 6.5 D to count for the mean posterior surface power. The Lin's formula using the personalized $p - C = 41/r_1$ to count for the role of individual posterior corneal surface (r_2) which may deviate significantly from the commonly used mean value of 6.5 mm. As pointed out by Lin, each 1.0 D of corneal power would result in an error of about 1.3–1.6 D of IOL power calculation.

Postoperative Anterior Chamber Depth

It is least important factor in calculation of lens power. An error of 1 mm affects the postoperative refraction or IOL power by approximately 0.6–2.5 D depending on the ocular conditions.

The most popular of these regression formulae was the SRK formula which is:

$$P = A - 2.5L - 0.9K$$

Where,

P = Lens implant power (needed to produce emmetropia)

L = Axial length

K = Average keratometric reading

A = Specific constant for each lens type and manufacturer.

Although the ACD is not used in these formulae directly, it is incorporated into a constant called "A" constant which is derived empirically for each implant. If the A constant is greater, the closer the implant is to the retina.

Disadvantages of this type of formulae are:

- These equations are only as good as the accuracy of the data used to derive them.
- Though these formulae are based on evaluation of how the optical system changed after surgery rather than theoretical assumptions on how it would change, individual variations of eyes cannot be taken into account. The same IOL may rest more anteriorly in one eye than the other. Similarly, placement of the IOL in the sulcus or the bag or an IOL tilt may also affect the postoperative results.
  Flipping of planoconvex lenses (plane surface forward) decreases the effective power of the lens by about 0.75 D even if the position of the lens is unchanged. However, an additional 0.5 D loss may occur because the principal plane is usually displaced posteriorly in such cases. Similarly, if sutures have to be placed, they may cause some change in the postoperative corneal power. These changes in the postoperative eye may result in some deviation from the expected results based on these formulae.
- The SRK and other similar formulae are linear formulae describing a nonlinear system, hence beyond a certain

range, the values turn out to be inaccurate. Thus it underestimates the power of high-powered lenses and overestimates the power of the low-powered lenses. Certain modifications have been incorporated into this formula for very short and very long eyes, which goes by the name of the SRK II formulae. The modification is:

If the axial length is:

- *Less than 20 mm*: Add 3 D to the result
- *Greater than or equal to 20 mm but less than 21 mm*: Add 2D to the result
- *Greater than or equal to 21 mm but less than 22 mm*: Add 1 D to the result
- *Greater than or equal to 24.5 mm*: Subtract 0.5 D from the result.

- Errors (observer bias) while performing the preoperative keratometry and axial length measurements account for a significant source of inappropriate calculations.

  Holladay has given certain criteria where the preoperative measurements should probably be checked again to minimize these errors. These criteria are:
  - Axial length <22 mm or >25 mm.
  - Average corneal power <40 D or >47 D.
  - Calculated emmetropic implant power is more than 3D from the average for the specific style used.
  - The difference between the eyes in average corneal power is >1 D, in axial length is more than 0.3 mm and emmetropic implant power is >1 D. Hence, the other eye measurements should always be performed while taking measurements for one eye.
- Even without considering the observer bias, there are certain intrinsic problems that may arise while taking any measurement. Keratometry measures the radius of the anterior corneal surface, which is converted to an estimate of the refracting power of the cornea in diopters using the corneal refractive index of 1.37. This refractive index should, however, be used only if both the anterior and posterior corneal radii of curvature are known. As this is not the case, it can alter the calculation by about 0.75 D. Similarly indentation of the cornea by the A-scan tip may alter the axial length. Hence, the immersion bath system is preferred over the applanating system while performing biometry.
- Another factor to be considered is retinal thickness correction factor, which is the distance from the vitreoretinal interface to the photoreceptor layer. This is estimated to be about 0.15–0.5 mm. This can affect the accuracy of the IOL power calculated as the A-scan biometers measure the distance from the anterior surface of the cornea to the vitreoretinal interface while the light travels past the vitreoretinal interface to the retinal elements. Various formulas use correction factors to account for this.
  - The SRK/T formulae incorporate this factor by the following relationship:

    Retinal thickness correction factor = (0.65696 - 0.02029) axial length.

    The above formula is a theoretical formula that was optimized with regression techniques and is valid empirically. It indicates that the retinal thickness correction factor is larger in short eyes and smaller in long eyes. This formula has been reported to perform better in very long eyes (>28.4 mm) over the SRK II formula.
  - Similarly to the SRK/T formula, the Holladay formula adds 0.2 mm to the axial length. Both this and the SRK/T formulae perform the same in short, long and normal eye.
- The differing density of the cataract in the eyes where biometry is done may result in unequal placement of the ultrasound rays. This may result in an inappropriate calculated value of the implant. It has also been observed that the axial length may be underestimated in short eyes because the crystalline lens of a short eye occupies a greater percentage of the space between the retina and the cornea, and as sound travels faster in the lens as compared to the vitreous because of its higher refractive index, the axial length may be underestimated. Most instruments calculate the desired power by both the theoretical and the empirical methods. In the normal range of axial length and keratometry readings, there is no significant difference between the powers calculated by the two procedures. But outside this range, there may be a significant difference between the two and the attending ophthalmologist may have to choose what he finds more appropriate. The IOL formulae have been divided into generations taking into consideration the time when they were evolved and the corrections incorporated into them as human knowledge increased.

First Generation Formulae

Theoretical formulae:

- Fyodorov (the first formula given in 1967)
- Colenbrander
- Hoffer
- Binkhorst

Regression formulae:

- Sanders-Retzlaff-Kraff
- Lloyd and Gill

Second Generation Formulae

Theoretical formulae:

- Hoffer
- Binkhorst [determined a direct relation between the position of the PMMA (polymethyl methacrylate). PC

IOL (posterior chamber intraocular lens) and the axial length and presented a formula to better predict ACD].

Regression formulae: SRK II.

Third Generation Formulae

Theoretical Formulae

Holladay I formula: Holladay modified the Binkhorst's formula to incorporate the relation between the steepness of the cornea and the position of the IOL in his formula. This could predict the distance from the cornea to the iris plane and add to it the distance from the iris plane to the IOL, which he called the surgeon factor.

Theoretical formulae optimized with regression techniques: SRK/T.

Hoffer Q

In case of longer eyes, the SRK/T and the Holladay formulae have been seen to perform better while in case of shorter eyes (axial length <22 mm), the Hoffer Q formula has been seen to give better results.

Fourth Generation Formulae

Theoretical Formula

Holladay II formula: Holladay further calculated an estimated scaling factor which was a result of the ACD, the corneal thickness, the lens thickness, the refractive error, and the age of the patient to predict a more accurate implant power.

The New Generation Formulas

Formulas to be detailed in the following include: SRK (I, II), SRK/T, Hoffer Q, Holladay (I, II), Olsen and the more recently formulas of Haigis d-formula.

Sanders-Retzlaff-Kraff Formula

- *SRK I formula*: It is basic regression formula. It is given by:

  P = A – 0.9K – 2.5L,

  Where

  P = IOL power for emmetropia

  K = Keratometric power reading

  A = A constant

  L = Axial length in millimeter.

- *SRK II formula*: In this formula, the A constant is adjusted to different axial length ranges. It is given by:

  P = A1 – 0.9K – 2.5L

  Where,

  A1 = adjusted constant

  A1 = A + 3, if axial length (L) < 20 mm

  A1 = A + 2, if L is 20–21 mm

  A1 = A + 1, if L is 21–22 mm

  A1 = A, if L is 22–24.5 mm

  A1 = A – 0.5, if L > 24.5 mm

- *SRK/T formula*: Regression formula for ACD (or ELP) is used to calculate power based on Fyodorov's formula. This formula is more accurate than SRK I and II.

  ACD post = ACD – 3.336 + corneal height (H),

  where ACD is related to the manufacturer's A-constant by:

  ACD = 0.62467A – 68.747.

Hoffer Q Formula

The Hoffer Q formula[3] was published in 1993 and gives the IOL power:

P = f(A, K, Rx, pACD) which is a function of

A: Axial length

K: Average corneal refractive power (keratometry reading)

Rx: Refraction

pACD: Personalized ACD (ACD, constant)

Likewise, the Hoffer Q refractive error.

Rx = f(A, K, P, pACD), which depends on A, K, P and pACD.

For the calculations, K = 337.5 divided by the average radius of curvature of the cornea. The personalized ACD (pACD) is set equal to the manufacturer's ACD-constant, if the calculation was selected to be based on the ACD-constant. In case the A-constant was chosen, pACD is derived from the A-constant according to Holladay et al.[4]

pACD = ACD-const = 0.58357

x A-const-63.896

Personalization of the pACD is the process whereby one enters the IOL power actually used and the resultant spherical equivalent refractive result and back-calculate what ACD would have produced an error of zero. If one calculates this "perfect ACD" for a whole series of eyes (using same surgeon and IOL style), average the number and that becomes the personalized factor for that surgeon and IOL.

Holladay Formulas

The components of the three part Holladay system are:

- *Holladay (I) formula*:
  - Data screening criteria to identify improbable axial length and keratometric measurement.
  - The modified theoretical formula, which predicts the effective position of the IOL based on the axial length and the average corneal curvature.
  - Personalized surgeon factor (PSF) that adjusts for any consistent bias on surgeon from any source. It is an advance method, which requires patient refractions.

The initial formula uses the "basic surgeon factor". It can be calculated from the A-constant provided by lens manufacturer.

- *Holladay (II) formula*: The IOL power is calculated based on the Binkhorst's formula as in Holladay I.

Olsen Formula

Olsen proposed his regression formula for the predicted postoperative ACD as follows:

$$\text{ACD post} = \text{ACD mean} + 0.12H + 0.33\text{ACDpre} + 0.3T' + 0.1L - 5.18$$

Where H is the corneal height, T′ is the natural lens thickness. The above formula, however, can only apply to phakic eyes. For aphakic or pseudophakic eyes, the coefficients will change.

Haigis Formula

It uses three constants to set both the position and shape of a power prediction curve. The IOL calculation according to Haigis is based on the elementary IOL formula for thin lenses.

$$d = d = a_0 + (a_1 \times ACD) + (a_2 \times AL)$$

Where d = The effective (or optical) lens position

ACD = Measured anterior chamber depth of the eye

AL = Axial length of the eye

a_0 constant = Same as lens constants for the different formulas given before

a_1 constant = Tied to ACD

a_2 constant = Measured axial length

Thus the value for d is determined by a function rather than a single number.

The a_0, a_1, a_2 constants are derived by multivariable regression analysis. The Haigis formula IOL constants will appear different from normal as they interact with the ACD and the AL.

The conventional optimization based on one-constant (A-constant, surgeon's factor, ACD) which could only "parallel shift" the calculated curve to fit the measured data for a predicted mean zero error. Therefore, the validation range of the axial length is limited, where improvement for long eye results more errors for short eye, and vice versa. For example, SRK/T is accurate for long eye (L > 26 mm), but not for very short eye (L < 22 mm) which requires the Hoffer formula. Haigis 3-constant optimization allows the curve-fit by both parallel shift and rotation of the curve such that it covers wider range of axial length. However, the above Haigis formula also assumed thin-IOL and excludes the role of IOL configurations for different IOL types.

OPTICAL BIOMETRY

Since the introduction of IOL master **(Fig. 1)**, optical biometry has been gaining popularity due to the fact that it offers an easy, contact-free method to quickly and accurately assess the axial length. The axial length measured by optical biometry is not, however, directly comparable to ultrasound biometry. Ultrasound biometry measures the distance from the anterior corneal to the inner limiting membrane, while optical biometry measures from the cornea to the retinal pigment epithelium. Thus, the measured axial length obtained from ultrasound and optical biometry cannot be expected to yield the same values. Hitzenberger et al.[5] found that the axial lengths measured by optical biometry were 0.18 mm longer than those measured by the immersion technique and 0.47 mm longer than those measured by the applanation technique. Kiss et al.[6] reported a mean difference in the measured axial length obtained with optical biometry and immersion biometry of 0.22 mm (range—0.24 mm to +0.57 mm; R = 0.99, P < 0.05). In order to be able to continue to use the A-constants and other formula constants developed over the years with ultrasound biometry, readings taken with the IOL master were calibrated against the immersion ultrasound biometry. Haigis et al.[7] found that the postoperative refraction was predicted correctly within ±1 D in 86% and within ±2 D in 99% of all cases using the immersion biometry data. A similar result was obtained using optical biometry. Kiss et al.[6] also reported that the refractive outcome in cataract patients using optical biometry was comparable to that achieved with immersion biometry. Other investigators have demonstrated greater accuracy and reproducibility with the IOL master, as infrared laser-based measurement techniques using a 780-nm wavelength has an inherent advantage over a sound-based system with a frequency of 10 MHz and a resolution of 200 mm. Olsen[8] reported an average absolute IOL prediction error of 0.65 D with ultrasound and 0.43 D with optical biometry (P < 0.00001). Sixty-two percent of predictions using optical biometry were within ±0.5 D compared with 45% with ultrasound. Another report showed no significant difference in the axial length obtained using optical biometry between different operators.[7] Vogel et al.[9] reported intraobserver and interobserver variability (standard deviation) of ±25.6 mm

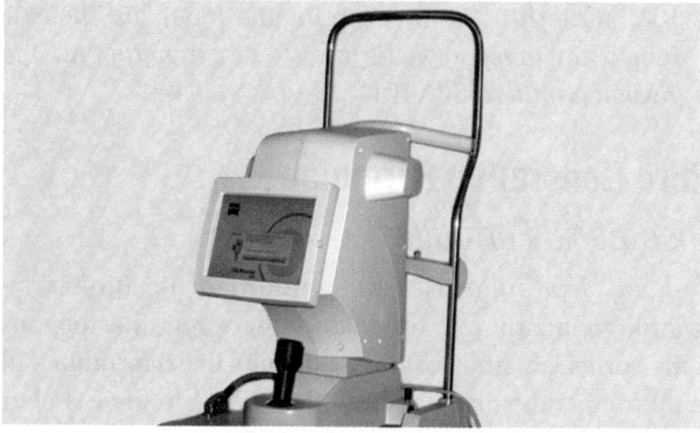

Fig. 1: Intraocular lens master.

and ±21.5 mm, respectively, for axial length measurements using the IOL master.

Optical biometry has several advantages over ultrasound biometry. One is that the axial length measurement is performed through the visual axis since the patient is asked to fixate into the laser spot. In highly myopic or staphylomatous eyes, this can be particularly advantageous because sometimes it may be difficult to measure the true axial length through the visual axis with an ultrasound probe. Optical biometry is also superior to ultrasound in the measurement of pseudophakic and silicone oil-filled eyes. For optical biometry, it is not as critical how the media change because the correction factor that must be applied is much smaller than in ultrasound biometry. The preoperative axial length measurement obtained with the IOL master was shown to be 0.07 mm longer than postoperative measurements ($P < 0.001$); this difference in axial length appears small, but statistically significant, correlated with the Lens Opacities Classification System III nuclear cataract score.[9-11]

Accurate measurements require that the infrared laser be able to pass through the eye and return to the interferometer. Therefore, opacities along the visual axis can block the infrared laser. Reliable measurements may not be obtained in eyes with tear film abnormalities, corneal pathology, mature and posterior subcapsular cataracts, vitreous opacities, maculopathy and retinal detachment. In addition, the patient must be able to maintain fixation. Various groups have reported that 8–20% of patients cannot be measured with optical biometry due to poor fixation, dense cataract or corneal pathology.[12-16] Freeman and Pesudovs[16] reported that posterior subcapsular cataract with a Lens Opacities Classification System III score of greater than 3.5 and mature cataracts accounted for 16% of measurement failures. Cortical and nuclear cataracts did not seem to affect measurements.

The new IOL master **(Fig. 1)** Advanced Technology software upgrade (version 5) is designed to enhance the signal-to-noise ratio in order to improve measurement of the axial length in eyes with media opacity. The new algorithm combines the individual measurement signals to form a composite signal. Peaks in each signal are combined, resulting in amplification of the signal, while random noise in the signal cancels each other out. The software then looks for the highest peak in this composite signal. Results of unpublished studies conducted by Warren Hill showed that the standard IOL master is capable of measuring 50–60% of patients for all classes of cortical density. With advanced technology, 87% of patients with cortical densities above 3.0 can be measured, 100% of patients with a nuclear color grading up to 3 can be measured, 93% of patients with a nuclear color grading above 3 can be measured, 100% of all eyes with a posterior subcapsular density up to grade 5 can be measured and 72% of eyes with a posterior subcapsular density above grade 5 can be measured.

INTRAOCULAR LENS POWER CALCULATION IN SPECIAL SITUATIONS

Polypseudophakia

When the calculated IOL power exceeds that available, and placement of a single IOL would result in an unacceptable refractive outcome, one option is for the surgeon to place two IOLs in the eye at the same operative session. The previous practice of stacking two acrylic lenses in the capsular bag has since been abandoned due to occasional problems with interlenticular opacification and reduced visual acuity. When primary polypseudophakia is indicated, the IOL calculation is carried out in six logical steps. First of all, the axial length should be measured as accurately as possible. Even a relatively small axial length error in extreme axial hyperopia can result in a significant postoperative refractive error. The axial length in this setting is best measured using the IOL master. Immersion 10-MHz A-scan biometry is a reasonable, but less accurate alternative.

Secondly, the total IOL power is calculated at the plane of the capsular bag. For IOL power calculations in the setting of extreme hyperopia, the Holladay II formula is recommended. Hoffer Q, or a fully optimized version of the Haigis formula (a_0, a_1, and a_2 optimized) is a reasonable alternative.

Then the residual IOL power is calculated followed by power adjustment for the anterior (ciliary sulcus) lens. The power of the anterior IOL is calculated followed by appropriate polypseudophakia lens pair selection.

Postkeratorefractive Surgery

Intraocular lens power calculations following keratorefractive surgery should not be carried out using standard keratometry combined with any one of several popular 2-variable third generation theoretic formulas, such as SRK/T without a special correction. A major shortcoming of most third generation, 2-variable formulas, such as SRK/T, is that they often assume that the anterior and posterior segments of the eye are mostly proportional and use only the axial length and keratometric corneal power to estimate the postoperative location of the IOL, known as the effective lens position (ELPo). Unless a specific correction is made for this situation, the artifact of centrally flattened Ks following keratorefractive surgery will have these formulas assume a falsely shallow postoperative ELPo. The end result is that without a special correction, following laser in situ keratomileusis (LASIK) these formulas will typically recommend less IOL power than is actually required. This is a second and little recognized source of unanticipated postoperative hyperopia following keratorefractive surgery

Table 2: Corneal power (Dc) calculation after refractive surgery.

Method	Formula
1. Clinical-history method	Dc = Kpre – RC RC = Refractive correction of LASIK
2. Contact lens method	Dc = B + P + Rw – Rno B = Base curve P = Power of CL Rw = Refractive error Rno = Bare refraction
3. Shammas method	Dc = 1.114 Kpost – 6.8
4. Maloney topography method	Dc = 1.114 Ktopo – 5.5
5. Koch method	Dc = 1.114 Ktopo – 6.1
6. Shammas refraction method	Dc = (1.114 Kpost – 6.8) – 0.23 (RC)
7. Hoffer mean-value method	Dc = 337.5 $(1/r_1 + 1/r_2)/2$
8. Lin Gaussian-optics (I)	Dc = 1.117 Kpost – $41/r_2$

(LASIK: laser in situ keratomileusis)

for myopia. Summary of IOL powers, generated by several forms for central corneal power estimation, has been shown in **Table 2**.

Silicone Oil-filled Eyes

Silicone oil is sometimes temporarily placed in the vitreous cavity for recurrent retinal detachments in eyes with proliferative vitreoretinopathy, proliferative diabetic retinopathy, cytomegalovirus retinitis, giant retinal tears, and following perforating injuries. An axial length measurement by ultrasound of an eye in which the vitreous cavity has been filled with silicone oil is an exercise with many potential pitfalls, especially if the silicone oil has become emulsified. The additional power that must be added to the original IOL calculation for a convex-plano IOL (with the plano side facing towards the vitreous cavity) is determined by the following relationship:[17]

- Ns = Refractive index of silicone oil (1.4034).
- Nv = Refractive index of vitreous (1.336).
- AL = Axial length in millimeter.
- ACD = Anterior chamber depth in millimeter.

Additional IOL power (diopters) = [(Ns – Nv)/(AL – ACD)] × 1,000.

For an eye of average dimensions and with the vitreous cavity filled with silicone oil, the additional power needed for a convex-plano PMMA intraocular lens is typically between +3.0 D and +3.5 D.

Another rather easy and reliable method is by using partial coherence interferometry with the IOL master.

Piggy Back Intraocular Lens

In 1993, Holladay[18] elegantly described a method for pseudophakic and aphakic intraocular lens power calculations, independent of axial length. When significant refractive deviations are seen, the refractive vergence formula is very helpful in understanding how much optical power must be added to, or subtracted from, an eye at the level of the anterior chamber, ciliary sulcus, or capsular bag. This formula also works well for the phakic and aphakic eye.

The power of the IOL to be implanted is determined by the following:

$$\text{IOLe} = \frac{1{,}336}{\dfrac{1{,}336}{\dfrac{1{,}000}{\dfrac{1{,}000}{\text{PreRx}} - \text{V}} + \text{Ko}} - \text{ELPo}} - \frac{1{,}336}{\dfrac{1{,}336}{\dfrac{1{,}000}{\dfrac{1{,}000}{\text{DPostRx}} - \text{V}} + \text{Ko}} - \text{ELPo}}$$

ELPo = Effective lens position
Ko = Net corneal power
IOLe = IOL power
V = Vertex distance
PreRx = Preoperative refraction
DPostRx = Desired postoperative refraction

Corneal Transplantation

There is presently no method that can be used to accurately carry out IOL power calculations prior to corneal transplantation combined with cataract removal and IOL implantation.

This is because it is impossible to know the central power of the donor graft prior to surgery. Simply basing preoperative calculations on a "best guess" of postoperative corneal power (such as 44.0 D) will quite often lead to an unpleasant postoperative refractive surprise.

It is a much better idea to instead carry out corneal transplantation with cataract removal, but without IOL implantation. The lens implantation would then be carried out at a later time, as a secondary procedure. After 4–8 months, when the corneal curvature has stabilized, and corneal astigmatism has been minimized, a careful aphakic refraction is performed and simulated keratometry by topography is used to estimate central corneal power.

Accuracy of Intraocular Lens Power Calculation

A second person should repeat the axial length measurements, keratometry readings and re-run the IOL power calculations for both eyes if:

- The IOL power for emmetropia is greater than 3.00 D different than anticipated.
- There is a difference in IOL power of greater than 1.00 D between the two eyes.
- If the patient has had prior excimer laser-based keratorefractive surgery and the calculated IOL power for standard phakoemulsification is less than +17.0 D or greater than +23.0 D.

CONCLUSION

With increasing patient expectations, the first step to obtain an accurate IOL power calculation is to be able to identify the patient's visual goals, especially if they have specific vocational or avocational needs. Using today's technology, it is possible to consistently have postoperative refractive outcomes within -0.25 D of the targeted refraction. In order to achieve these results, attention to proper patient selection, accurate keratometry and biometry, appropriate IOL power formula selection with optimized lens constant, and proper configuration of the capsulorhexis are required. Ultimately, the part with the highest variability and inaccuracy is going to determine the outcome. The accuracy of IOL biometry can be improved by implementing the following—minimizing variability and improving consistency by assigning a single properly calibrated instrument and experienced technician for the workup, repeating and verifying measurements by a second person when necessary, using the IOL master or immersion biometry rather than an applanation technique, using one of the newer IOL power calculation formulas and personalizing the lens constants for each formula, tracking your refractive outcomes, and optimizing your surgical technique by making the capsulorhexis round, centered and slightly smaller than the lens optic can all help to optimize your postoperative outcomes. By understanding the advantages and limitations of the current technology and following these guidelines, it is possible to consistently achieve highly accurate results.

REFERENCES

1. Gale RP, Saldana M, Johnston RL, et al. Benchmark standards for refractive outcomes after NHS cataract surgery. Eye (Lond). 2009;23(1):149-52.
2. Brandle J, Haigis W. IOL calculation in long and short eyes. In: Hoyos GA, Dementiev JE (Eds). Mastering the Techniques of IOL Power Calculations. New Delhi: Jaypee Brothers Medical Publishers; 2005.
3. Hoffer KJ. The Hoffer Q formula: A comparison of theoretic and regression formulas. J Cataract Refract Surg. 1993;19(6): 700-12.
4. Holladay JT, Prager TC, Chandler TY, et al. A three-part system for refining intraocular lens power calculations. J Cataract Refract Surg. 1988;14(1):17-24.
5. Hitzenberger CK, Drexler W, Dolezal C, et al. Measurement of the axial length of cataract eyes by laser Doppler interferometry. Invest Ophthalmol Vis Sci. 1993;34(6):1886-93.
6. Kiss B, Findl O, Menapace R, et al. Refractive outcome of cataract surgery using partial coherence interferometry and ultrasound biometry: Clinical feasibility study of a commercial prototype II. J Cataract Refract Surg. 2002;28(2):230-4.
7. Haigis W, Lege B, Miller N, et al. Comparison of immersion ultrasound biometry and partial coherence interferometry for intraocular lens calculation according to Haigis. Graefes Arch Clin Exp Ophthalmol. 2000;238(9):765-73.
8. Olsen T. Improved accuracy of intraocular lens power calculation with the Zeiss IOLMaster. Acta Ophthalmol Scand. 2007;85(1):84-7.
9. Vogel A, Dick HB, Krummenauer F. Reproducibility of optical biometry using partial coherence interferometry: intraobserver and interobserver reliability. J Cataract Refract Surg. 2001;27(12):1961-8.
10. Lam AK, Chan R, Pang PC. The repeatability and accuracy of axial length and anterior chamber depth measurements from the IOLMaster. Ophthalmic Physiol Opt. 2001;21(6): 477-83.
11. Chylack LT Jr, Wolfe JK, Singer DM, et al. The lens opacities classification system III: The Longitudinal Study of Cataract Study Group: Arch Ophthalmol. 1993;111(6):831-6.
12. Prinz A, Neumayer T, Buehl W, et al. Influence of severity of nuclear cataract on optical biometry. J Cataract Refract Surg. 2006;32(7):1161-5.
13. Connors R 3rd, Boseman P 3rd, Olsen RJ. Accuracy and reproducibility of biometry using partial coherence interferometry. J Cataract Refract Surg. 2002;28(2):235-8.
14. Kiss B, Findl O, Menapace R, et al. Biometry of cataractous eyes using partial coherence interferometry: clinical feasibility study of a commercial prototype I. J Cataract Refract Surg. 2002;28(2):224-9.
15. Rajan MS, Keilhorn I, Bell JA. Partial coherence laser interferometry vs conventional ultrasound biometry in intraocular lens power calculations. Eye (Lond). 2002;16(5): 552-6.
16. Freeman G, Pesudovs K. The impact of cataract severity on measurement acquisition with IOLMaster. Acta Ophthalmol Scand. 2005;83(4):439-42.
17. Shamnas HJ. IOL Lens Power Calculation: Ultra Sound Measurement of the Challenging Eye. Thorofare, NJ: Slack Incorporated; 2004. pp. 113-23.
18. Holladay JT. Refractive power calculations for intraocular lenses in the phakic eye. Am J Ophthalmol. 1993;116(1): 63-6.

CHAPTER 26

Diagnostic Procedures in Infectious Keratitis

Savitri Sharma, Sreedharan Athmanathan, Joveeta Joseph

INTRODUCTION

Microbial keratitis may be caused by bacteria, fungi, parasites or viruses and each of these may produce a spectrum of disease which may or may not have distinctive clinical appearance. Many a time it may not be possible to discriminate between infected or noninfected corneas. Introduction of in vivo confocal microscopy has helped confirm clinical diagnosis without laboratory aid, especially for *Acanthamoeba* and fungal keratitis although the high cost of the equipment remains a limitation.[1] Therefore, confirmation by laboratory methods continues to be the gold standard for the etiological diagnosis in microbial keratitis. Currently, molecular diagnostic methods have increased the sensitivity, specificity, and speed over the conventional microbiological techniques of microscopy and culture. To minimize morbidity that may develop secondary to delay in diagnosis and to achieve favorable outcome within a reasonable cost and time, laboratory investigations are indicated in patients with suspected microbial keratitis.

Two entirely different protocols are required to be followed while investigating viral and nonviral corneal ulcers, so determined on the basis of clinical features. A combination of the two protocols may be called for when a distinction of viral versus nonviral is not obvious clinically. In the interest of clarity, this chapter is divided in three parts to describe in vivo confocal microscopy, and microbiologic procedures required for workup of clinically nonviral and viral corneal ulcers.

Familiarity of ophthalmologists to the functions, limitations, and scope of microbiology laboratory is important for proper and meaningful interpretation of results. A well-equipped ocular microbiology laboratory with well-trained technical personnel has great advantages over a general microbiology laboratory, in handling and processing minute quantity of ocular samples, especially corneal samples. Special orientation toward processing and interpretation of results is of paramount importance.[2]

CORNEAL CONFOCAL MICROSCOPY

Confocal microscopy is a noninvasive technique that offers high image magnification and contrasts that allow visualization of corneal details in vivo. Repeated observations can be made which help in diagnosis and follow-up of cases with microbial keratitis.[3] Diagnostic accuracy of in vivo confocal microscopy in microbial keratitis has been studied extensively.[1,4] Hau et al. assessed confocal images on two occasions by four observers who were masked to the tissue diagnosis and calculated the diagnostic accuracy parameters.[4] They reported highest positive likelihood ratio of 2.94 and lowest negative likelihood ratio of 0.59 with agreement values fair to moderate and did not recommend stand-alone use of confocal microscopy for the diagnosis of microbial keratitis. On the other hand, Vaddavalli et al. compared inter and intraobserver variation in analysis and interpretation of confocal microscopy findings with conventional microbiology findings of the corneal scrapings from patients with *Acanthamoeba* or fungal keratitis and found high sensitivity (88.3%) and specificity (91.1%) of diagnosis by confocal microscopy.[1] **Figures 1A and B** show the typical branching fungal filaments with parallel walls: (A) and refractile cysts of *Acanthamoeba* (B) in the corneal stroma of patients. These authors recommended the use of confocal microscopy in fungal and *Acanthamoeba* keratitis, particularly when corneal infiltrates were deep seated or patients were on treatment or microbial keratitis developed after intracorneal implants such as intracorneal ring segments or refractive surgery.

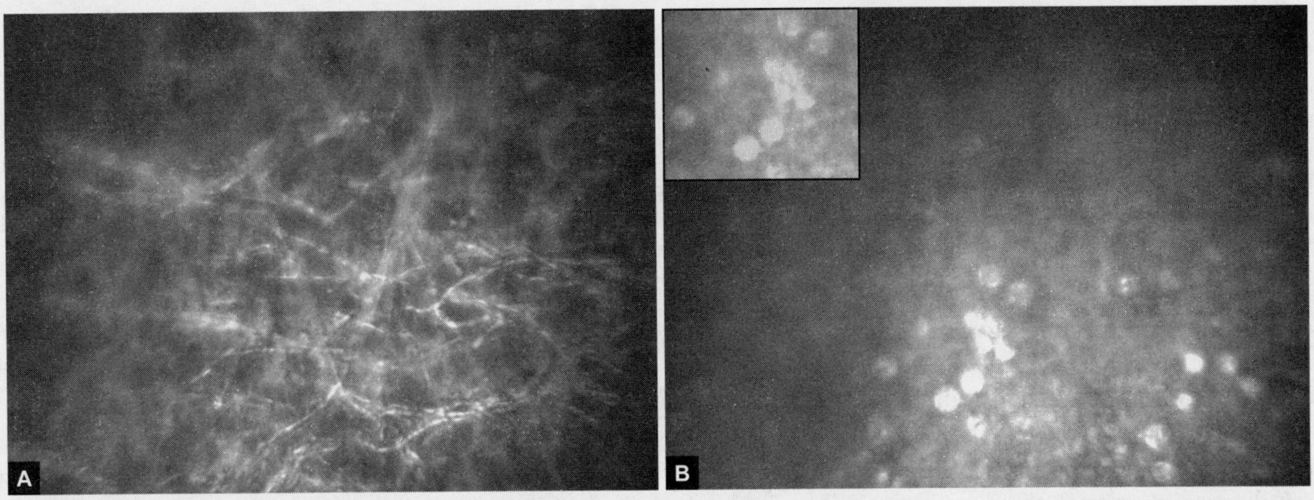

Figs. 1A and B: Confocal microscopy image using 40X Zeiss Achroplan lens imaged on the Confoscan 3 (Nidek) showing (A) Interlacing moderate-to-high reflective double-walled segmented filaments with a background of inflammatory cells suggestive of filamentous fungi; (B) A cluster of highly reflective *Acanthamoeba* cysts with low internal reflectivity.
Courtesy: Dr Pravin K Vaddavalli, LVPEI, Hyderabad.

Laboratory Methods for Nonviral Keratitis (Bacterial, Fungal, and *Acanthamoeba*)

Ideally, samples for the microbiologic investigations of a suspected microbial keratitis must be collected before the start of any antibiotic treatment. Treatment can be initiated based on the result of the smears and later if required, modified in accordance with the culture and sensitivity results. The protocol essentially consists of four steps: (1) Collection, (2) transport, (3) processing of the clinical samples, and (4) interpretation of the results.

Collection of Samples

Prior to collection of sample from the corneal ulcer itself, it is generally recommended to obtain a culture from the lids and conjunctiva of both the infected and the uninfected eye.[5] This procedure is purported to help in two ways; firstly, the organism(s) grown from the uninvolved eye (indicating normal flora) may be used for comparative purposes; secondly, in the absence of growth from the ulcer the organism(s) from the cul-de-sac of the involved eye may well be the causative organism(s).[5] Despite recommendation for this procedure in several textbooks, in our experience, samples from lids and conjunctiva have not yielded useful results in the management of corneal ulcers.[6] Similar observation has been made in the 1994 edition of "Laboratory Diagnosis of Ocular Infections" published by American Society of Microbiology,[7] which is a deviation from the earlier edition recommending collection and processing of samples from the eyelid margins and conjunctiva. Samples collected from the site of lesion, i.e. the infected corneal tissue are the most valuable for microbiological diagnosis of microbial keratitis. If available, any foreign body on the cornea, contact lens, contact lens case, or lens solutions may be collected.

Corneal samples can be collected using the slit lamp or operating microscope after instillation of topical anesthetic (4% lignocaine hydrochloride or 0.5% proparacaine hydrochloride). These anesthetic agents may have variable effect on the growth of organisms,[8] however, allowing some time interval between instillation of anesthetic agent and collection of sample would help reduce their effect, if any.

Cotton swabs are not recommended for collection of corneal samples, however, calcium alginate swabs, if available, may be used in cases of bacterial keratitis.[9] Platinum spatula, disposable blade (#15), bent needle, surgical knife, disposable cautery, have all been used for collection of corneal scrapings for microbiological processing. We routinely use blade no. 15 on Bard Parker handle. No difference was found by us in the quantitative yield of organisms from bacterial and mixed (fungal with bacterial) keratitis while comparing the use of calcium alginate swab with blade no. 15.[10] Although the yield of fungi was more with calcium alginate swab than with blade in this study we did not recommend replacing blade with swab. Swabs are likely to get contaminated by normal flora in the tear film and are less efficient in transferring clinical material onto slides and culture media. While collecting samples from the corneal ulcer the eyelids must be held wide apart to reduce inadvertent contamination by the lid margins or eye lashes. Adherent exudate on the surface of the ulcer may be removed using a sterile cotton swab prior to collection of scrapings.

The blade or spatula is scraped over the surface of the area of suppuration by a series of short, moderately firm strokes in one direction to sample both the central and peripheral margins of the infiltrated area on the cornea. Each scraping is used to inoculate one medium or to prepare one smear. Viable organisms may be present throughout the inflamed area or localized to the advancing margin or the ulcer crater.

In the absence of accessible corneal suppuration, a corneal biopsy can be done with a disposable skin punch, diamond knife or small corneal trephine.[11] Placed in a sterile petri dish the tissue specimen is minced with sterile blade and the pieces are used for making a smear for microscopy and inoculated into various media. Additional corneal scrapings can be obtained from the base of a partial-thickness corneal biopsy.

Collection of anterior-chamber exudates is advised only under exceptional circumstances owing to risk of inoculating organisms into the eye. The possible circumstances are deep stromal suppuration that cannot be sampled by an anterior approach and infections that have extended into the anterior chamber.[7]

Transport of Corneal Samples to the Microbiology Laboratory

Transportation of corneal scrapings in any transport medium is not recommended. The scrapings are plated directly onto culture media or smeared onto clean glass slides by the side of the patient in the clinic or operating room. It would help to maintain a corneal collection kit in the clinic or operating room containing a set of media, sterile slides (wrapped in foil), spatula/blades, glass marking pencil, swabs, etc. **(Fig. 2)** in case the microbiology laboratory cannot be reached and requested to provide the materials whenever required. One study has evaluated alternative use of Amies transport medium without charcoal. Amies medium was found as good as direct patient side processing of corneal scrapings for culture of bacteria and fungi after storage for 4 hours and 24 hours at room temperature.[12] However, corneal scrapings were smeared on slides at patient side, for microscopic examination.

Corneal biopsy tissue can be transported to the microbiology laboratory in a sterile dry petri-dish or in a sterile bottle. To prevent drying few drops of sterile saline may be added, however, this runs the risk of bacterial contamination especially with *Pseudomonas* spp. Aqueous humor is usually collected and transported in a tuberculin syringe. Exudates from the anterior chamber may also be directly plated on culture media and smeared on slides and sent to the laboratory. In case of contact lens associated microbial keratitis if the patient presents with contact lenses on the cornea the same may be collected aseptically with gloved fingers and placed in sterile petri-dish or bottle for transport. Contact lens cases may be sent to the laboratory in addition to contact lenses.

Processing of Corneal Scrapings

A complete microbiological workup of a nonviral corneal ulcer may require up to 10 corneal scrapings for a number of smears and culture media **(Table 1)**. In case of small ulcer, with limited material availability, high priority needs to be given to inoculation of blood agar (BA) or chocolate agar (CA) and to prepare only one or two smears. Preferred media may be selectively included based on clinical impression, e.g. nonnutrient agar (NNA) for a suspected *Acanthamoeba* keratitis patient. A schematic diagram to guide nonviral corneal ulcer workup is shown in **Figure 3**.

Direct Microscopic Examination Methods

Material is transferred from the blade/spatula to a glass slide over an area of a circle approximately 1 cm in diameter (marked on the reverse) to enable focused examination under the microscope. While the specimen is thinly spread

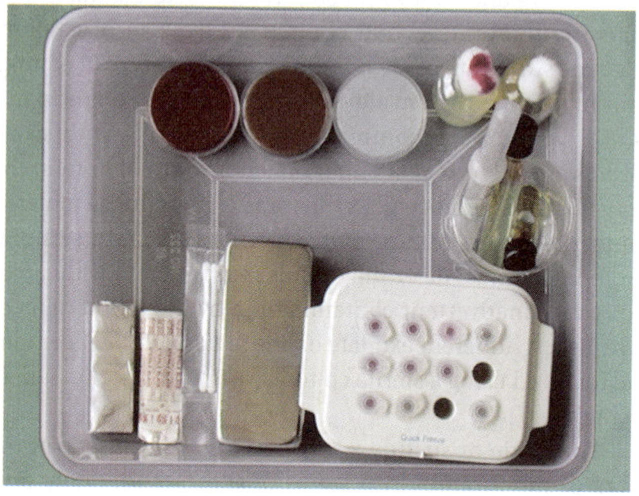

Fig. 2: Corneal scraping collection tray containing culture media, blades, glass slides marker pen, reagents, and coverslips.

Table 1: Sequence of smear preparation and culture media inoculation for the diagnosis of nonviral keratitis.

Smears	• Potassium hydroxide and/or calcofluor white • Gram stain • Giemsa stain
Media	• Blood agar—aerobic • Chocolate agar • Brain heart infusion broth • Thioglycollate broth • Robertson's cooked meat broth • Nonnutrient agar • Sabouraud dextrose agar
Optional Smears/media	• Blood agar—anaerobic • Potato dextrose agar • Lowenstein-Jensen medium • Brain heart infusion broth with antibiotic • Extra smear on slide

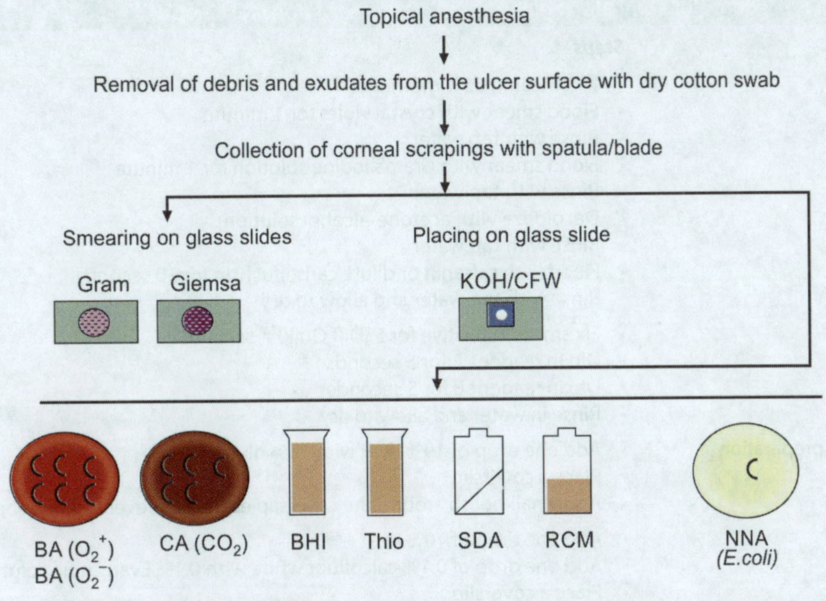

Fig. 3: Schematic diagram for microbiology processing of nonviral keratitis.
(BHI: brain heart infusion; CFW: calcofluor white; KOH: potassium hydroxide; RCM: Robertson's cooked meat; NNA: nonnutrient agar; SDA: sabouraud dextrose agar)

for dry smears (Gram, Giemsa, Gomori methenamine silver, etc.). it can be just placed within the circle for wet smears [potassium hydroxide (KOH), calcofluor white (CFW), lactophenol cotton blue (LPCB), etc.] under a coverslip. **Table 2** outlines the various staining procedures in brief.[11] At least two smears should be prepared. For several years, a combination of KOH+CFW, Gram, and Giemsa stained smears has provided a high sensitivity and specificity in our laboratory for the detection of bacteria, fungi, microsporidia, and *Acanthamoeba* in corneal scrapings. Common laboratory light microscope suffices in most instances for the examination of the smears except when fluorescent stains such as CFW or acridine orange are used which require a fluorescence microscope.

Culture Methods

Inoculation

Sheep BA and sheep blood CA plates are inoculated by lightly streaking both sides of the blade/spatula over a surface in a row of separate "C" shaped marks without penetrating the agar. This procedure helps distinguish valid growth from plate contaminants **(Fig. 4)**. Slopes of Sabouraud dextrose agar (SDA) or potato dextrose agar (PDA) in bottles are similarly inoculated by making a row of streaks from below upward. Liquid media such as brain heart infusion (BHI) broth is inoculated by agitating the blade/spatula directly in the broth. To facilitate this procedure without inviting contamination, the BHI or Robertson's cooked meat (RCM) should be available in screw capped tubes with the top level of the medium not below 1 cm from the brim of the tube. The inoculation of thioglycollate broth (thio) requires transfer of the scraped material onto a cotton or calcium alginate swab and insertion to the bottom of the tube to facilitate growth of anaerobic bacteria. It is a good practice to limit the inoculation of NNA with 1–2 strokes in the center of the plate with minimal disturbance of the surface of the medium. While inoculating the plates/bottles, care must be taken to minimize exposure of the medium to the atmosphere.

Corneal biopsy tissue can be cut into small fragments and inoculated into media or it can be emulsified in sterile saline using tissue homogenizer and then distributed in culture media, preferably under a biosafety laminar flow hood.

Aqueous fluid drops can be placed over agar plate surfaces as such without streaking and dropped directly into liquid media, preferably under a biosafety laminar flow hood.

Incubation

The inoculated culture media are placed in appropriate incubators. NNA (after sample inoculation) requires to be overlaid with few drops of heat killed or live *Escherichia coli* suspension prior to incubation. While BA (aerobic), BHI broth, RCM broth, thio broth, NNA, SDA, and PDA are incubated under normal atmospheric conditions, CA is incubated in a candle jar which provides 5% CO_2, and one BA (anaerobic) is incubated in anaerobic jar or cabinet, if available. All media are incubated at 35°C (±1) except SDA and PDA which are kept at 27°C (±1) in BOD incubator. Petri dishes are incubated with lids facing downward to prevent condensed moisture from dripping onto the medium. Broth tubes are held upright in racks. Early growth may

Table 2: Common staining procedures for corneal scrapings in the diagnosis of nonviral keratitis.

Method	*Steps*
Gram stain	• Fix smear in 95% methanol • Flood smear with crystal violet for 1 minute • Rinse with tap water • Flood smear with Gram's iodine solution for 1 minute • Rinse with tap water • Decolorize with acetone-alcohol solution • Rinse with tap water • Flood with safranin or dilute carbolfuchsin for 30 seconds • Rinse with tap water and allow to dry
Giemsa stain	• Fix smear in fixative for 5 (Diff Quik)™ seconds • Dip in reagent A for 5 seconds • Dip in reagent B for 5 seconds • Rinse in water and allow to dry
Potassium hydroxide (KOH) preparation	• Add one drop of 10% KOH with 10% glycerol • Place a coverslip • Apply nail polish around the coverslip edges to prevent drying (optional)
KOH + calcofluor white	• Add one drop of 10% KOH • Add one drop of 0.1% calcofluor white with 0.1% Evans blue solution • Place a coverslip • Examine under ultraviolet (UV) light (fluorescence microscope)
Zn acid-fast stain	• Flood fixed smear with hot (steaming) strong carbolfuchsin and leave for 5 minutes • Rinse with water • Decolorize with 20% H_2SO_4 for 1–2 minutes • Rinse with water • Flood with methylene blue counterstain for 2 minutes • Rinse with water and allow to dry
Kinyoun's modification of acid-fast stain	• Flood fixed smear with strong carbolfuchsin for 2 minutes • Rinse with water • Decolorize with 1% H_2SO_4 • Rinse with water • Flood with methylene blue counterstain for 2 minutes • Rinse with water and allow to dry
Lactophenol cotton blue (LPCB)	• Mix specimen colony in a drop of LPCB • Apply coverslip • Apply nail polish around edges of coverslip to prevent drying (optional)
Acridine orange	• Mix specimen in 0.01% of acridine orange • Apply coverslip • Examine under UV light (fluorescence microscope)

be detected on culture plates in most instances within 24–48 hours of incubation, however, media such as BA (aerobic), CA, thio and BHI that show no growth, should be incubated until at least 7 days before discarding. In case of no growth BA (anaerobic), SDA, PDA and NNA may be incubated until 2 weeks. Incubation beyond 2 weeks, in our experience, has not resulted in increased positivity. Instead, incubation longer than 2 weeks may lead to drying of media, and growth of contaminants due to repeated opening of plates for observation. We prefer to take reading of plates under laminar flow hood which reduces contamination due to exposure.

Observation

On solid agar plates growth on inoculation marks ("C" streaks) are regarded important while growth outside the inoculation marks are disregarded as contaminants **(Fig. 4)**. All culture media [except BA (anaerobic) in

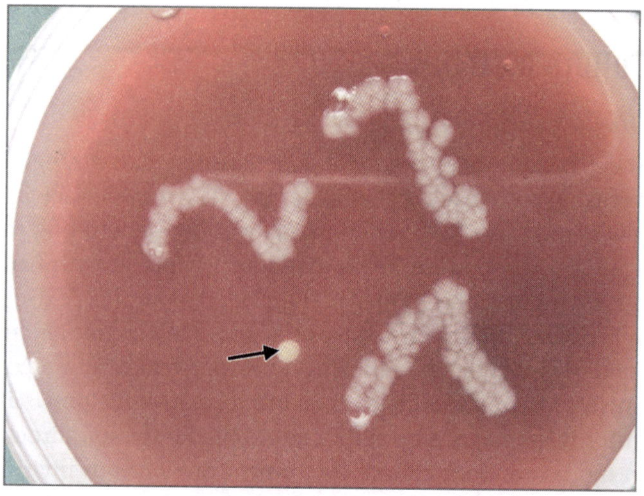

Fig. 4: Blood agar, inoculated with corneal scraping and incubated at 35°C for 48 hours, showing confluent gray, moist colonies (*Pseudomonas aeruginosa*) on the inoculum ("C" streaks) and a contaminant colony away from the inoculation marks (arrow).

anaerobic jar/cabinet] must be examined daily for detection of any growth. BA (anaerobic) may be examined at intervals of 2–3 days for 2 weeks.

Size, color, texture, consistency, and number of colonies on the inoculation marks are counted and recorded. Ten or more colonies are considered confluent. While bacterial and fungal colonies are examined with unaided eyes, the observation of *Acanthamoeba* growth requires use of microscope. NNA plates (with lid on to avoid contamination) are placed under 4× objective lens of the microscope and presence of trophozoites is looked for in the vicinity of the inoculation mark on the surface of the medium. No colonies are formed by *Acanthamoeba*. Suspected growth will require confirmation at higher magnification and examination with open lid.

Growth in liquid media appears as turbidity which requires to be subcultured and Gram-stained for identification.

Identification

Microbiological identification details of various organisms that may be isolated from cases of nonviral keratitis are neither the intent nor the scope of this chapter. Bacterial colonies are usually Gram-stained and identified after consideration of colony characteristics, gram reaction, morphology, and results of biochemical tests. Conventional procedures may be adopted for biochemical tests or commercial kits from a number of companies (bioMérieux, France; Lachema, Czech Republic; Organon Technika, USA, etc.)[13] may be obtained.

Identification of fungal species requires observation of rate of growth, color, consistency and texture of the colony and characteristic microscopic features. Though most species are identified easily more than 20% of filamentous fungal isolates may remain unidentified because of the lack of characteristic spores. Biochemical tests for identification are needed only in case of yeast or yeast-like fungal growth. Helpful hints for identification are available from several sources.[14]

Presence of characteristic cysts and trophozoites on the surface of NNA **(Fig. 5)** helps to identify *Acanthamoeba* genus. Speciation of this genus is presently not in the realm of a clinical ocular microbiology laboratory.[15]

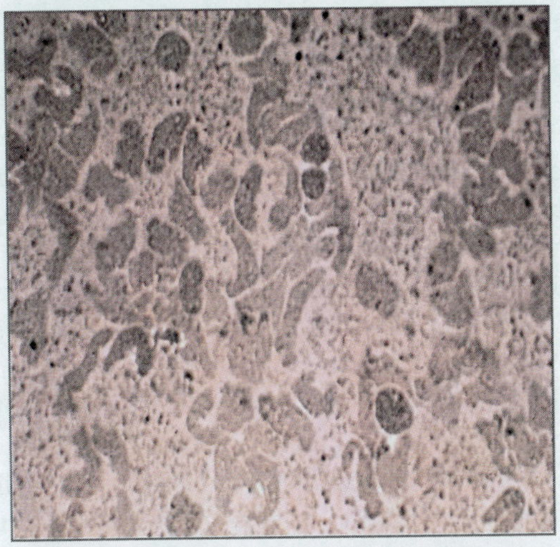

Fig. 5: *Acanthamoeba trophozoites* (irregular, vacuolated) on the surface of nonnutrient agar with *Escherichia coli* (original magnification ×500).

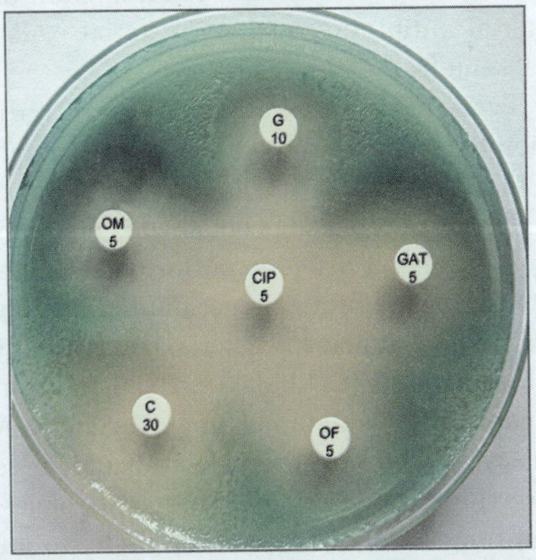

Fig. 6: Antibiotic susceptibility test on Mueller-Hinton agar for *Pseudomonas aeruginosa* isolated from corneal ulcer. The diameter of zone of inhibition around antibiotic disks is measured and reported as sensitive, intermediate, or resistant (disk diffusion test). Note the greenish pigmentation produced by the organism in the medium.

Antimicrobial Susceptibility Testing

Antimicrobial susceptibility testing is done in vitro to identify the response of an organism to a panel of selected drugs. Commercially available panels for Gram-positive and Gram-negative bacteria are used to determine sensitivity by disk-diffusion method. In this method (Kirby-Bauer) the bacteria is cultured on Mueller-Hinton agar (MHA), and antibiotic impregnated disks are applied. Antibiotic susceptibility testing of fastidious organisms such as *Streptococcus pneumoniae* requires MHA with 5% sheep blood. After incubation, the diameter of the zone of inhibition around each disk gives an approximation of susceptibility or resistance of the organism **(Fig. 6)**. Commercially available kits provide a zone size interpretative chart to facilitate interpretation. Slow-growing bacteria and anaerobes cannot be reliably tested with disk-diffusion method. Susceptibility of bacterial isolates to antibiotics is well standardized by Clinical Laboratory Standards Institute and guidelines are available for disk diffusion assay (CLSI M02-A10, 2009) as well as for broth dilution and agar dilution methods (CLSI M07-A8, 2009) for determination of minimum inhibitory concentration (MIC) of antibacterial agents. Estimating the MIC of antibiotics may provide a more useful information than labeling organisms as sensitive or resistant[7] especially because the results of disk-diffusion tests relate to levels of drug achievable in serum and do not relate directly to concentration of drug produced in the preocular tear film and ocular tissues by standard routes of administration.

For the dilution methods to determine MIC, the antibiotic is serially diluted and added to tubes with broth or wells of a microtiter plate or incorporated into agar plates. A standard suspension of the organism is then inoculated. The MIC is recorded as the lowest concentration with no visible growth. The tubes or wells with inhibited growth can be subcultured and the lowest concentration with no growth is recorded as minimum bactericidal concentration. A simple method of MIC determination has become available in the form of E-test, which is a commercially available quantitative antimicrobial susceptibility test based on diffusion. It combines the simplicity and flexibility of disk diffusion test with the ability to determine MICs of up to five antibiotics at one time. Availability of this technique has made it possible to test bacterial isolates for MIC of antibiotics on a routine basis. Large number of publications are available where E-test has been used for determination of MIC of antibacterial antibiotics against bacterial isolates from microbial keratitis.[16,17]

The availability of antifungal and antiamebic susceptibility testing is limited. In vitro test methods are diverse for fungi[18] and *Acanthamoeba*[19] and clinically predictive value of the results obtained is not known. MIC testing of antifungal drugs is performed for yeasts and filamentous fungi by broth or agar dilution methods. Disk diffusion method similar to bacterial susceptibility testing is available for yeasts (CLSI M44-A, 2009) and some of the nondermatophyte filamentous fungi (CLSI M51-A, 2010). E-test of several antifungals is also available for yeast and filamentous fungi. However, unlike bacterial isolates, routine testing of fungal isolates for susceptibility to antifungal drugs is yet to become common place in microbiology laboratories.

Molecular Methods

Molecular techniques are extremely sensitive, specific, and ideal for detection of organisms that are difficult to culture such as viruses, microsporidia, *Propionibacterium acnes, Toxoplasma gondii*, etc. or that take long time to grow, such as *Mycobacterium tuberculosis.* Their application in the diagnosis of nonviral keratitis is limited as the conventional techniques are easier to employ, are cost-effective, and have reasonable sensitivity and specificity. Several studies[20-22] have compared the most commonly used molecular method of polymerase chain reaction (PCR) with conventional methods of diagnosis of fungal keratitis. A higher positivity and good correlation has been reported with PCR compared to conventional methods. However, as of now, all studies recommend the use of PCR as an adjunct to conventional techniques and not as a replacement. Comparison of three different panfungal primers for the diagnosis of fungal keratitis has shown the sensitivity of PCR using internal transcribed spacer (ITS) primers to be significantly higher than 18S rDNA and 28S rDNA primers.[23] ITS region is also ideal to determine DNA sequence-based identification of different species of fungi. DNA technology in the form of DNA chip has been developed by Xcyton Diagnostics Ltd., Bangalore, India which provides a platform to apply multiplex PCR and hybridization for simultaneous diagnosis of bacterial, fungal, and viral eye infections.[24] Sequencing of DNA fragments of organisms often helps identify organisms that are difficult to identify by conventional methods resulting in recognition of novel organisms. After reporting the first case of microsporidial keratoconjunctivitis from India we found that this infection is common in India.[25] Since microsporidia are obligate intracellular organisms (phylogenetically related to fungi) that require tissue culture for growth, PCR-based confirmation of the smear findings is recommended.[26] Although PCR-based diagnosis of *Acanthamoeba* keratitis have been published[27,28] we believe that the sensitivity of PCR is similar to conventional method while specificity, positive predictive value, and negative predictive value are marginally higher.[29] Kim et al. compared PCR to microbial culture for the detection and identification of bacterial and fungal pathogens in microbial keratitis and found that PCR identifies potentially pathogenic organisms.[30] They reported higher yield and concordance with fungal than bacterial, however, concluded that the practical utility of PCR for the diagnosis of nonviral microbial keratitis is limited by artifactual amplification of nonpathogenic or commensal organisms likely to be present on ocular surface. In a well-conducted study on fungal keratitis, where PCR has been compared with conventional microbiology methods, Vengayil et al. have similarly recommended application of PCR as an adjunct rather than primary tool for diagnosis.[22] Quantitative PCR (real-time PCR) detects and quantitates number of organisms in a clinical sample and the test has begun to be applied to the diagnosis of bacterial and fungal keratitis.[31] While clinical validation of many of these recently available tests are awaited, there is no doubt that molecular techniques have a great role to play in identification of otherwise unidentifiable organisms that can cause microbial keratitis.

Interpretation of Microbiology Results

Microscopy

Commonly used stains for microscopic evaluation of smears and the organisms that are visualized are listed in **Table 2**. The results of smear examination form the basis for provisional diagnosis and initial choice of an antimicrobial agent.

Though reported to be useful in the detection of bacteria in corneal scrapings,[32] we do not have much experience with acridine orange. However, we have used CFW for several years and find the stain very useful in the detection of fungi, *Acanthamoeba,* and microsporidia in corneal scrapings **(Figs. 7A to C)**. The Gram stain is useful in identifying bacteria, fungi, as well as *Acanthamoeba* cysts and microsporidia spores **(Figs. 8A to E)**. Precipitated stain, carbon, salt crystals, and necrotic debris can lead to troublesome artifacts in Gram-stained smears. It is easier to detect Gram-positive bacteria (especially *S. pneumoniae*) than Gram-negative bacteria. Gram variable bacteria may sometimes be seen.[33] Fungal hyphae and *Acanthamoeba* cysts stain variably since their cell walls do not stain well and may often be seen as negative outlines **(Figs. 8A to E)**. Presence of partially stained or unstained bacilli in Gram-stained smear is suggestive of mycobacteria and the same smear restained (after decolorization) with Ziehl-Neelsen stain (20% H_2SO_4) would show the acid fast bacilli **(Figs. 9A and B)**.[34] Trophozoites of *Acanthamoeba* are difficult to recognize owing to their irregular morphology and similarity to macrophages.[35] Giemsa-stained smear serves as a supportive smear. Cytological details are seen well and bacteria, fungi as well as *Acanthamoeba* cysts can be seen.

Arbitrary quantitation of bacteria per high power field may help determine the significance as bacteria comprising the indigenous microflora of the conjunctiva and tear film may be detected in small numbers. Smears with more than 10 organisms are more determinate. However, detection of bacteria in smears often needs to be correlated with corresponding bacterial growth in culture for determining significance. Failure of an organism, seen in smears, to grow in culture would indicate either nonviable organisms or sample variation. Sampling error must always be ruled out in case of discrepant results.

Presence of partially stained or unstained bacilli in Gram- or Giemsa-stained smears has often indicated

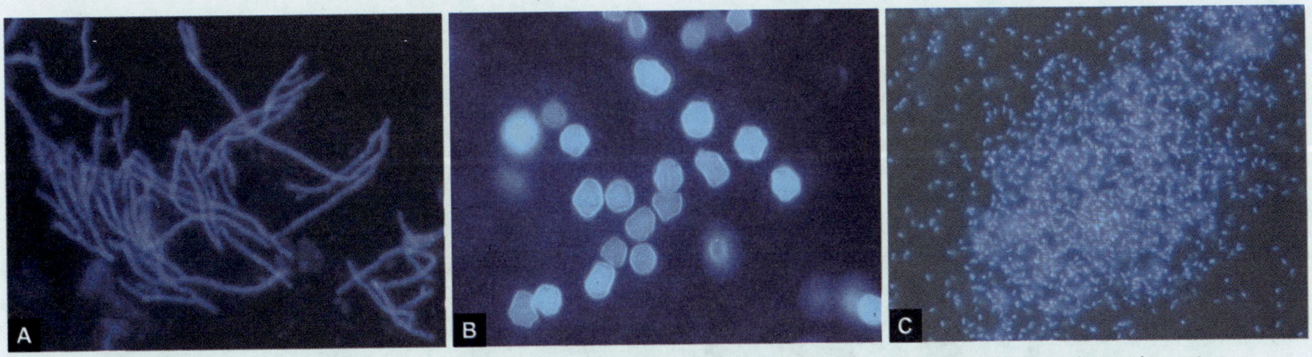

Figs. 7A to C: Corneal scrapings stained with KOH+CFW showing (A) Septate fungal filaments; (B) *Acanthamoeba* cysts; (C) Microsporidia spores under fluorescence microscope (original magnification for all, ×500). (CFW: calcofluor white; KOH: potassium hydroxide)

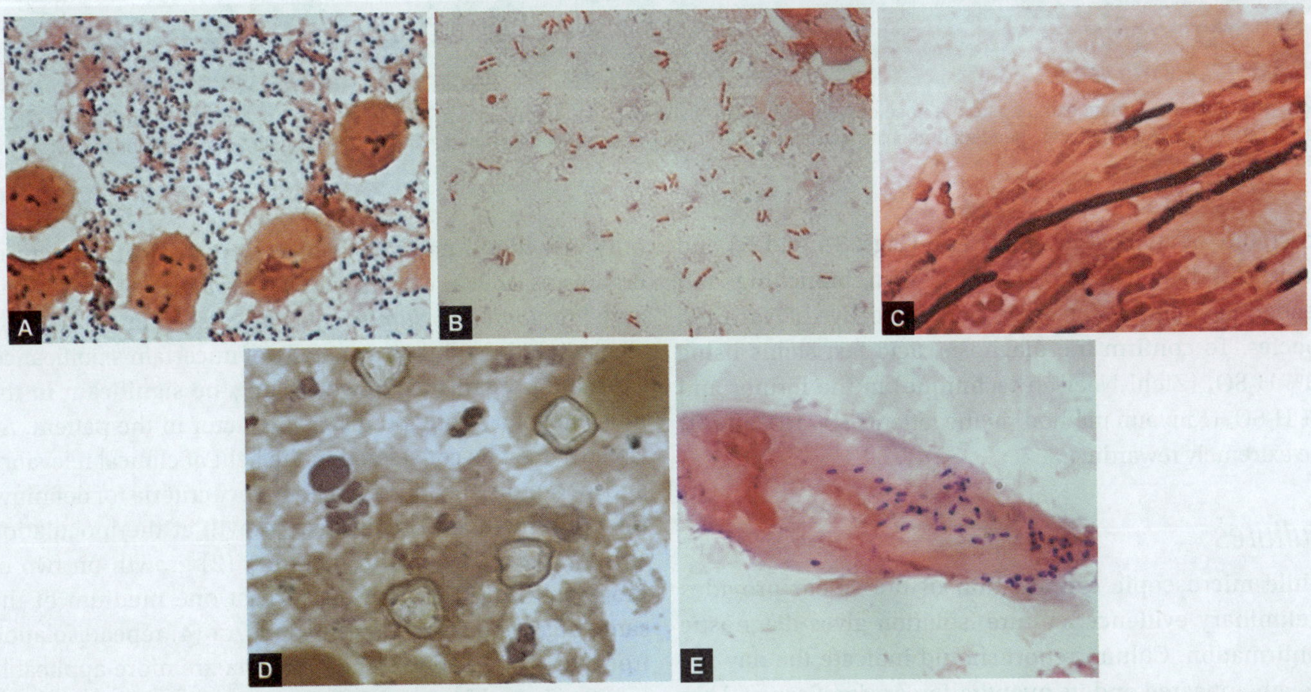

Figs. 8A to E: Corneal scrapings stained with Gram stain showing (A) Gram-positive cocci in pairs (×1000); (B) Gram-negative bacilli (×1000); (C) Septate fungal filaments (×1000); (D) *Acanthamoeba* cysts (×1000); (E) Microsporidia spores (×500).

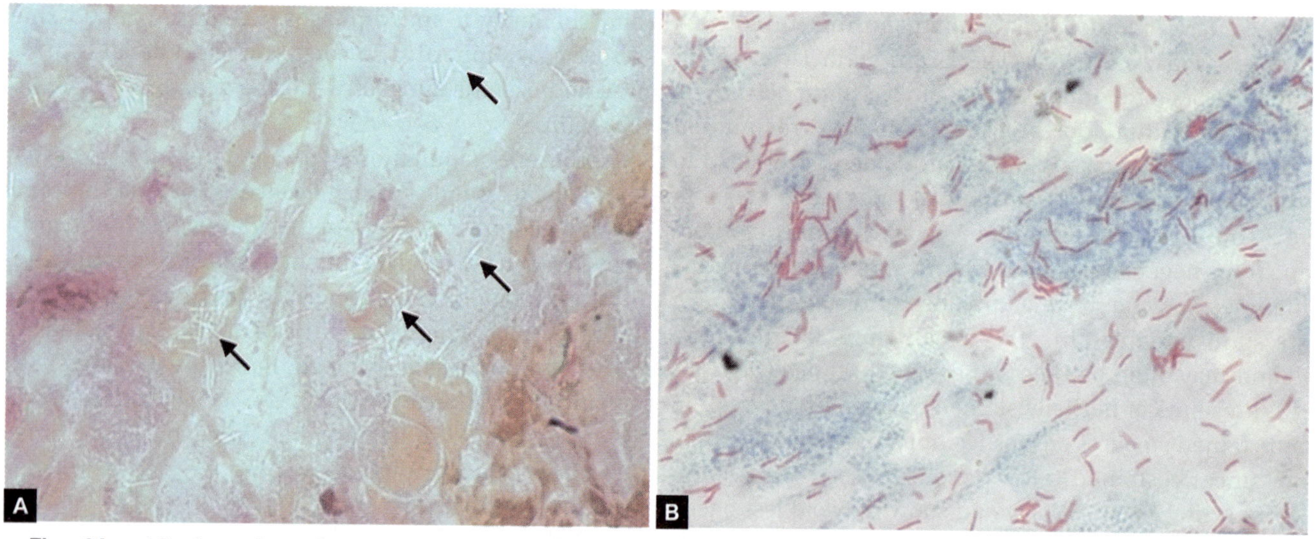

Figs. 9A and B: Corneal scraping from a case of *Mycobacterium chelonae* keratitis (post-LASIK surgery) showing (A) Unstained slender long bacilli in Gram stain (arrows); (B) Acid-fast bacilli in Ziehl–Neelsen staining (20% H_2SO_4) (original magnification ×1000).
(LASIK: Laser in situ keratomileusis)

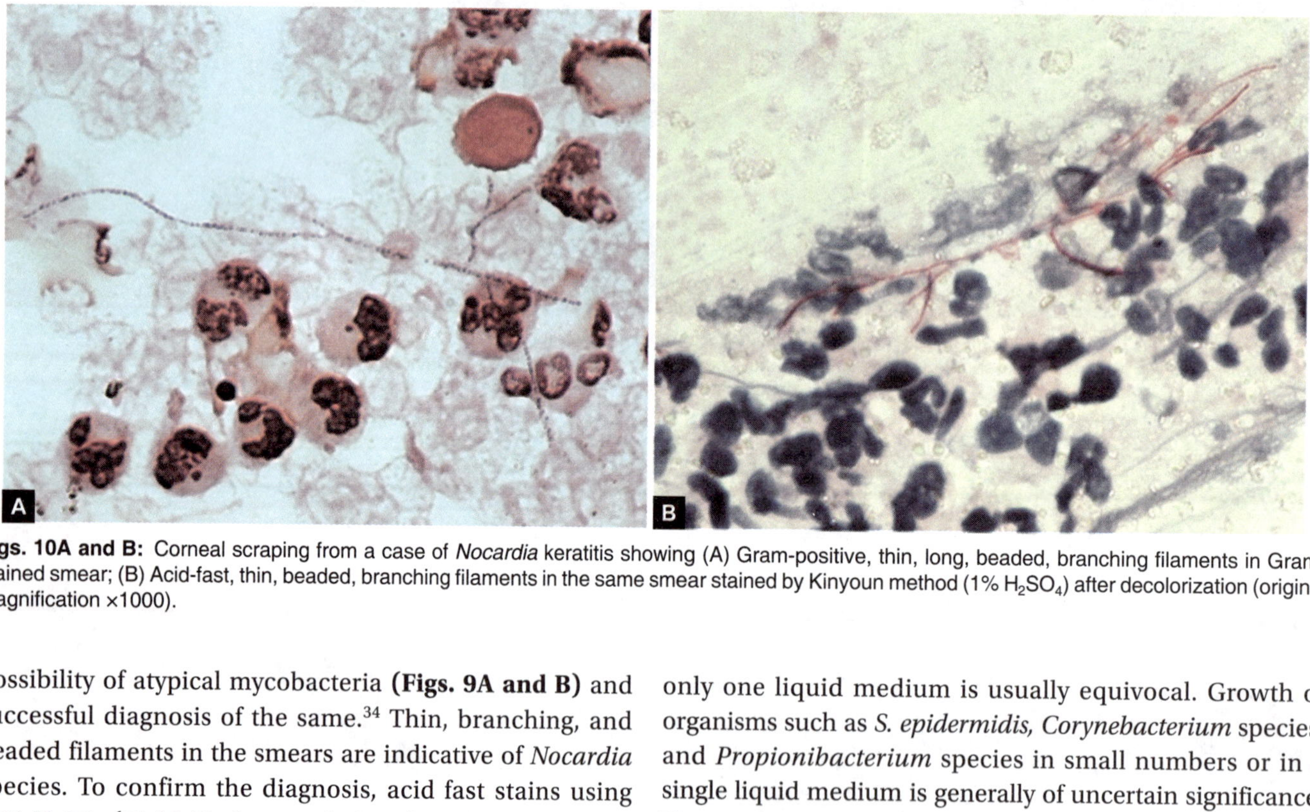

Figs. 10A and B: Corneal scraping from a case of *Nocardia* keratitis showing (A) Gram-positive, thin, long, beaded, branching filaments in Gram-stained smear; (B) Acid-fast, thin, beaded, branching filaments in the same smear stained by Kinyoun method (1% H_2SO_4) after decolorization (original magnification ×1000).

possibility of atypical mycobacteria **(Figs. 9A and B)** and successful diagnosis of the same.[34] Thin, branching, and beaded filaments in the smears are indicative of *Nocardia* species. To confirm the diagnosis, acid fast stains using 20% H_2SO_4 (Ziehl-Neelsen technique) in the former and 1% H_2SO_4 (Kinyoun method) in the latter **(Figs. 10A and B)** are extremely rewarding.

Cultures

While microscopic examination of the smear provides preliminary evidence, culture isolation gives diagnostic confirmation. Culture report should indicate the day the growth appeared and its quantitation or significance. Less than 10 colonies on only one solid medium or growth in only one liquid medium is usually equivocal. Growth of organisms such as *S. epidermidis, Corynebacterium* species, and *Propionibacterium* species in small numbers or in a single liquid medium is generally of uncertain significance. The same organisms, however, may be significant in the presence of a strong predisposing factor in the patient. All isolates must be considered in the light of clinical relevance and laboratory significance. Laboratory criteria for definitive infection include (1) confluent growth at the inoculation site on at least one solid medium; (2) growth on two or more media; (3) growth on at least one medium of the same organism seen in smears; and/or (4) repeat isolation from the same patient. These criteria are more applicable to bacteria and fungus than *Acanthamoeba* as it is neither a normal commensal nor a laboratory contaminant.

Antibiotic Susceptibility

Interpretation of agar disk diffusion test (for bacterial susceptibility) that relate to levels of drug in serum is often controversial. However, since higher antibiotic concentrations can be achieved in the cornea by topical administration of antibiotics, an organism labeled as resistant or intermediate in sensitivity by this test may respond to the drug in vivo. The reverse is unlikely to be the case.

The quantitative MIC can be compared to the antibiotic concentration expected at the site of infection. Although resistance breakpoints for ocular isolates have not been determined and there are no generally accepted cutoff points, results of disk diffusion test have been reported to correlate with MIC at least in *Pseudomonas* keratitis.[36] For antifungal susceptibility testing MIC cutoff points available in CLSI guidelines for most drugs is similarly based on serum levels. Cutoff point for most commonly used antifungal agent in fungal keratitis, natamycin, is not available in CLSI guidelines; however, recent studies have considered MIC greater than 16 μg/mL as sensitive.[37,38]

MOLECULAR METHODS

The results of PCR on corneal scrapings are usually as good as the choice of primers (oligonucleotide sequence for a particular gene of a particular organism) and the stringent performance of the test. Being a highly sensitive test, instances of false positives can be high if PCR test is not handled carefully. Any laboratory that undertakes molecular diagnostics must comply with all requirements to contain amplicon contamination, use appropriate controls and provide reliable results. The PCR results are best viewed in conjunction with the clinical impression and, if possible, with another supporting laboratory evidence toward the diagnosis.

PROTOCOL FOR VIRAL KERATITIS

The advancement made in the field of laboratory techniques for the diagnosis of viral infections in the past decade has been enormous with the introduction of newer techniques and improvisation of earlier techniques. These techniques have been extensively employed for the diagnosis of viral keratitis, especially in advanced countries. However, owing to the cost constraints, the techniques are yet to become a routine in most laboratories in India, including large university laboratories. Several factors may need to be considered before a laboratory chooses to adopt laboratory techniques for the diagnosis of viral keratitis or in fact any viral disease. These factors include information regarding the prevalence of the particular viral infection, need of screening for the same in a given population, cost of the technique, availability of the infrastructure, and whether a rapid diagnosis can be provided. An ideal technique would be cost-effective, provide a rapid diagnosis in a reasonable time frame, easy to perform and interpret and adaptable in routine microbiology laboratories.

As pertinent in nonviral keratitis, the collection, transport, and processing of corneal samples for the diagnosis of viral keratitis have a distinct protocol which may be combined with the former in case of clinical uncertainty.

Collection of Samples

A variety of samples including corneal scrapings, corneal swabs, corneal impression smear, and corneal button may be submitted for viral diagnosis. In addition or instead of corneal samples, conjunctival scrapings/swabs or aqueous humor may also be helpful in some situations. As is true for most diseases, collection of clinical sample early in the disease prior to administration of antimicrobial agents, is most useful for laboratory diagnosis.

Transport of Samples

Unlike the banishment for transport of corneal scrapings (in a transport medium to the laboratory) in the protocol for nonviral corneal ulcer diagnosis, the sample for viral diagnosis always needs to be collected in an appropriate transport medium (except the smears) and sent to the laboratory. Methods of transport would vary according to the type of sample collected. **Box 1** outlines the methods of transportation of samples to the virology laboratory.

Box 1: Methods of transportation of specimens to the virology laboratory for investigation of viral keratitis.

- *Corneal scrapings*:
  - Smear on glass slide, air dry and send for staining/IF/IP
  - Transfer in a vial (0.5–1 mL) of viral transport medium (VTM) and send for culture. It can be stored at 4°C without freezing
  - Transfer on a cellulose acetate membrane, air dry, fix in acetone/methanol and send for staining/IF/IP
  - Transfer in 1 mL of PBS/MEM/HBSS and send for PCR
- *Corneal impression smear on glass slide or cellulose acetate membrane*: Air dry, fix in acetone/methanol/15 minutes and send for staining/IF/IP
- *Corneal/conjunctival swab*:
  - Use cotton swab to collect material and transfer in VTM and send for culture. It can be stored at 4°C without freezing
  - Dry swab and calcium alginate swabs are unacceptable
- *Corneal button*:
  - Place in VTM and send for culture
  - Place in 10% buffered formalin and send for histopathology
  - Place in PBS/MEM/HBSS and send for PCR
- *Aqueous humor*:
  - Place few drops in VTM and send for culture
  - Place in sterile tube/eppendorf and send for PCR or staining/IF/IP

(HBSS: Hank's balanced salt solution; IF: indirect immunofluorescence; IP: indirect immunoperoxidase; MEM: minimum essential medium; PBS: phosphate buffered saline; PCR: polymerase chain reaction)

Processing of Samples

Samples received in a virology laboratory may be processed using a variety of techniques. The choice of technique would depend on the type of sample and the specific virus that is being looked for. Most of the procedures can be performed in a moderately equipped laboratory. The procedures standardized and adopted by us for the diagnosis of herpes simplex virus (HSV) keratitis are outlined in **Box 2**. Of all available laboratory techniques for diagnosis of viral infections only a few can be adopted in a particular laboratory. The choice is made based on the advantages, disadvantages, and cost-effectiveness of the techniques and their overall utility.

Direct Microscopic Examination (Cytology)

A rapid diagnosis of viral keratitis can be established by observing stained smears of corneal scrapings, conjunctival scrapings/swabs, or centrifuged deposits of aqueous humor (cytospin).[39] This may be accomplished using nonspecific staining techniques such as Giemsa, Papanicolaou, and Hematoxylin-Eosin stain. These techniques help visualize multinucleated giant cells **(Fig. 11)** which is a nonspecific finding in cytology smears, usually associated with viral infections,[40] koilocytic changes, and intranuclear/intracytoplasmic inclusions, and various inflammatory cells which are predominantly lymphocytes. Koilocytic changes are characteristic perinuclear clearing (halo) with increase in density of surrounding rim of cytoplasm, classically described in human papilloma virus infected squamous epithelial cells of the cervix. Intranuclear inclusions are more efficiently seen in Papanicolaou stain than Giemsa-stained smears; however, Giemsa stain is good for enumerating cell types. Though these staining techniques have the advantage of being rapid and inexpensive they are often nonspecific and offer low sensitivity in the diagnosis of viral infection. For example, these stains cannot differentiate the intranuclear inclusions of HSV from that of varicella zoster virus (VZV).

Box 2: Methods for laboratory diagnosis of viral keratitis at LV Prasad Eye Institute.

- *Nonspecific smear examination (cytology) methods*:
  - Papanicolaou stain
  - Giemsa stain
- *Cell-associated antigen detection methods*:
  - Direct/Indirect immunofluorescence (IF) assay
  - Indirect immunoperoxidase (IP) assay
- *Virus isolation (tissue culture) methods*:
  - Conventional tissue culture
  - Shell-vial technique
- *Molecular virology method*: Polymerase chain reaction

Specific cytology techniques used for viral diagnosis are techniques that indirectly suggest the presence of viral antigen in the clinical sample. Detection of cell-associated viral antigen in a corneal scraping, impression cytology or conjunctival scraping is very useful in the diagnosis of viral keratitis.[41,42] We have been routinely using direct and indirect immunofluorescence (IF) **(Fig. 12)** and indirect immunoperoxidase (IP) **(Fig. 13)** assays in the diagnosis of HSV, VZV keratitis, and adenoviral keratoconjunctivitis. Both these tests are rapid, specific and sensitive when suitable monoclonal or purified polyclonal antibodies are used in the test system. Relatively higher sensitivity and lower specificity is achieved with purified polyclonal antibodies while monoclonal antibodies show high specificity but lose out on sensitivity. IP assay has distinct advantages over IF assay. The former provides a permanent preparation for records and utilizes an ordinary light microscope while the latter has the inherent problem of quenching (fading) of fluorescence and requires a sophisticated and expensive fluorescence microscope. In addition, the IP technique can be used on paraffin-embedded tissue while the IF technique provides better results with frozen tissue sections.

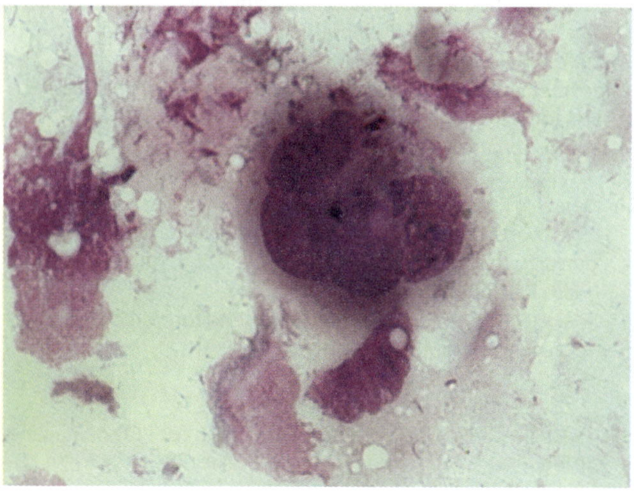

Fig. 11: Corneal scrapings from a case of herpes simplex virus keratitis showing multinucleated giant cell (Giemsa stain, original magnification ×1000).

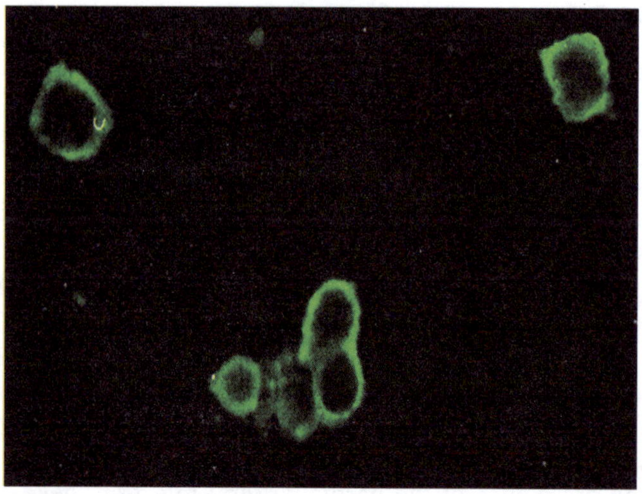

Fig. 12: Corneal scraping from a case of herpes simplex virus (HSV) keratitis showing presence of HSV-1 antigen in the epithelial cells (indirect immunofluorescence assay, original magnification ×250).

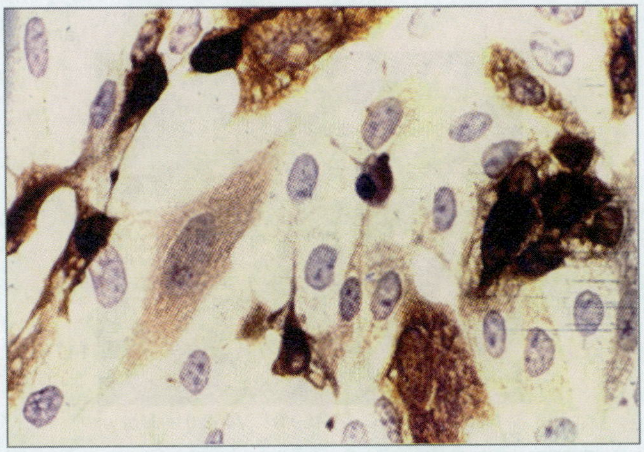

Fig. 13: Corneal scraping from the same patient of herpes simplex virus (HSV) keratitis **(Fig. 12)** showing presence of HSV-1 antigen (stained brown) in epithelial cells (indirect immunoperoxidase assay, original magnification ×500).

Table 3: Rapid diagnostic tests for viral keratitis.

Type of test	*Time*	*Viruses detected*
• *Less than 1 hour*:		
– Giemsa stain (Diff Quik)™	5 minutes	HSV 1/2, VZV, adenovirus
– Papanicolaou stain	45 minutes	HSV 1/2, VZV, adenovirus
– HSV test kit (Sure Cell Herpes)(R)	20 minutes	HSV 1/2
– Latex agglutination (Virogen)(R)	35 minutes	HSV 1/2
• *Between 1 hour and 6 hours*:		
– Immunofluorescence	2–3 hours	HSV 1/2, VZV, adenovirus
– Immunoperoxidase	4–5 hours	HSV 1/2, VZV, adenovirus
– HSV antigen detection (Herp check)(R)	5 hours	HSV-1
– ELISA	3–4 hours	HSV ½

(ELISA: enzyme-linked immunosorbent assay; HSV: herpes simplex virus; VZV: varicella zoster virus)

Detection of soluble viral antigens in corneal scrapings collected in buffer and body fluids including tears, aqueous, and vitreous, have been described using enzyme-linked immunosorbent assay (ELISA),[43] latex agglutination,[44] and radioimmunoassay (RIA). Results obtained by ELISA and RIA are more objective compared to IF and IP assays (which tend to be subjective); however, we do not have experience using these techniques for the diagnosis of viral keratitis. Some of the rapid methods of antigen detection in viral keratitis are described in **Table 3**.

Tissue Culture Methods

Classically described techniques of virus isolation have been embryonated eggs and animal inoculation, which are not favored by most virology laboratories for routine diagnostic purposes. Much favored technique is that of tissue culture, especially cell cultures. Established cell lines such as HeLa, Vero, HEp 2, MRC-5, etc. have been used for isolation of HSV from corneal scrapings.[45] We have recently succeeded in using immortalized human corneal epithelial cell line[46] for isolation of HSV.

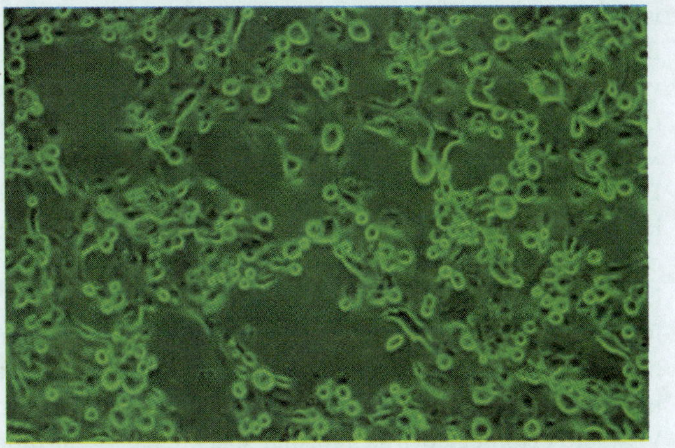

Fig. 14: Monolayer of vero cell line showing cytopathic effect caused by herpes simplex virus-1 indicating growth of the virus in the cells (tube culture, phase contrast, original magnification ×200).

Growth of virus in the cell lines can be determined either by characteristic cellular changes or cytopathic effect (CPE) as shown in **Figure 14** or by IF or IP techniques, which detect viral antigens in the infected cell lines (described above). Appearance of CPE may take several days but antigens can be detected even before CPE occurs, thereby rendering the latter a more rapid method. Viruses may be cultured in cell lines maintained in tubes (tube culture) or on coverslips in vials (shell vial).[47] Shell vial technique is a modification of conventional tissue culture technique wherein entry of virus into the monolayer of susceptible cells (on a coverslip in a vial) is facilitated by centrifugation of the vial containing cells and the clinical sample (spin amplification).[48] The virus growth occurs in a shorter period (18–72 hours) by this method and additionally, both IF and IP techniques can be performed easily on the coverslips retrieved from the vials for antigen detection. Both these factors are responsible for increased sensitivity of shell vial technique in isolation of viruses.

Molecular Methods

As mentioned earlier, more than any other infection, molecular methods are most suited for the diagnosis of viral infections. PCR technique has been employed extensively for the detection of viral DNA in clinical samples which is one of the best indications for diagnostic use of this technique.[49] By virtue of being extremely sensitive and specific and at the same time simple and rapid. PCR is presently the most sought-after technique for viral diagnosis. In our experience, combination of cytology coupled with antigen detection by IF or IP techniques and viral DNA detection by PCR may obviate the role of cumbersome procedures of viral isolation by tissue culture, in the diagnosis of viral keratitis.[50] By cost considerations, setting up and running a molecular virology laboratory may be less expensive than tissue culture laboratory. Diagnosis of atypical herpetic epithelial keratitis using primers for 142 base pair segments of the DNA polymerase gene of the HSV genome by PCR have been reported.[51,52] A variety of primers for PCR diagnosis of HSV type 1/2 and VZV infections of the eye (other than keratitis) have been described and they can be adapted for the diagnosis of keratitis.[53,54] A nested PCR for stromal herpetic keratitis diagnosis has also been described.[55] We have designed a multiplex PCR for the detection of HSV-1, VZV, and cytomegalovirus in ocular specimens.[56] Real-time PCR is being increasingly used for viral load estimation in various tissues including corneal tissue. Rapid diagnosis of adenoviral keratoconjunctivitis has been reported using fully automated real-time PCR.[57] Apart from diagnosis, a wide range of utility of real-time PCR has been reported such as assessment of prevalence and clinical consequence of HSV type-1,[58] and quantitation in tear fluid and aqueous humor.[59] In case of typical herpetic epithelial keratitis usually a large number of HSV DNA copies are detected compared to stromal keratitis.[60]

As has been mentioned in the protocol for nonviral keratitis guarding against false positives in PCR-based test is a great challenge to a molecular virology laboratory. Top-of-the-line quality control, appropriate controls, and good laboratory practices are mandatory to obtain reliable laboratory reports.

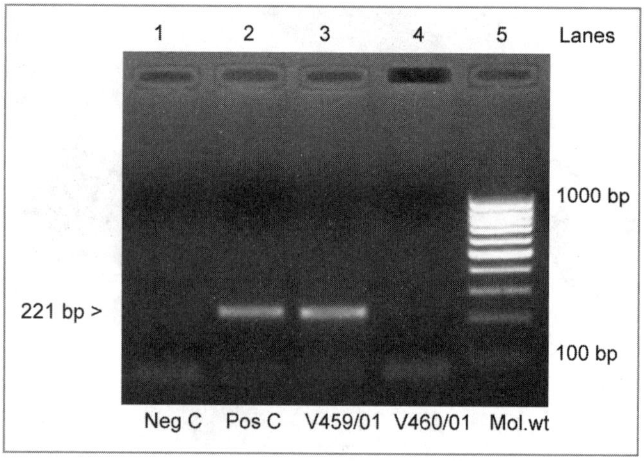

Fig. 15: Detection of HSV-1 by PCR in a corneal scraping from a case of HSV keratitis. Agarose gel electrophoresis (Ethidium Bromide stained) showing negative control (lane 1), positive control (lane 2), test samples (lanes 3, 4), and molecular weight marker (lane 5). Note the band of 221 bp size (HSV-1, glycoprotein D gene specific) in lane 2 and 3. Sample V 459/01 is positive and V460/01 is negative for HSV-1 DNA.
(HSV: herpes simplex virus; PCR: polymerase chain reaction)

Interpretation of Virology Results

As indicated in **Box 2**, our laboratory routinely performs a variety of techniques for the laboratory diagnosis of viral keratitis which includes cytology by Giemsa stain, antigen detection by IF/IP techniques, and PCR **(Fig. 15)**. In an analysis of 170 clinically suspected cases of HSV keratitis whose corneal scrapings were tested by PCR, antigen detection by IF, and cytology by Giemsa stain, the sensitivity of the tests was 100%, 85.7%, and 57.1%, respectively.[50] A laboratory diagnosis of HSV keratitis was offered when HSV-1 antigen was detected and/or HSV DNA was detected by PCR with or without cellular changes in Giemsa-stained smear. PCR results were interpreted with caution when this test alone was positive. It was always correlated with clinical findings and with the results of other tests. False positives were avoided by using a different primer set and adopting a reduced sensitivity PCR.[61]

It is evident from our observations that adopting a single technique alone may result in underdiagnosis. Giemsa stain, though less sensitive than others, is a valuable test. Presence of multinucleated giant cells, intranuclear inclusions, and koilocytic changes are indicative of HSV/VZV infection. Initiation of antiviral therapy is indicated based on these smear findings coupled with positive antigen detection by IF or IP assays. Both IF and IP assays detect viral proteins in the absence of viable virions when cultures would be negative. We have often been more successful in detecting the viral antigen than isolating the virus. We recommend that antigen detection assays and Giemsa or Papanicolaou staining be done in the laboratory diagnosis of viral keratitis where facilities for culture and PCR are unavailable.

REFERENCES

1. Vaddavalli PK, Garg P, Sharma S, et al. Role of confocal microscopy in the diagnosis of fungal and *Acanthamoeba* keratitis. Ophthalmology. 2011;118(1):29-35.
2. Agarwal V, Biswas J, Madhavan HN, et al. Current perspectives in infectious keratitis. Indian J Ophthalmol. 1994;42(4):171-92.
3. Kaufman SC, Musch DC, Belin MW, et al. Ophthalmic Technology Assessment Committee Cornea Panel. Confocal Microscopy: a report by the American Academy of Ophthalmology. Ophthalmology. 2004;111(2):396-406.
4. Hau SC, Dart JKG, Vesaluoma M, et al. Diagnostic accuracy of microbial keratitis with in vivo scanning laser confocal microscopy. Br J Ophthalmol. 2010;94(8):982-7.
5. Burd EM. Bacterial keratitis and conjunctivitis. In: Smolin G, Thoft RA (Eds). The Cornea: Scientific Foundations and Clinical Practice. Boston: Little Brown and Co; 1994.
6. Sharma S, Sankaridurg PR, Ramachandran L, et al. Is the conjunctival flora a reflection of the pathogenic bacteria causing corneal ulceration? Invest Ophthalmol Vis Sci. 1994;35(Suppl 4):1947.
7. Wilhelmus KR, Liesegang TJ, Osato MS, et al. Cumitech 13A, Laboratory diagnosis of ocular infections. In: Specter SC (Ed). CUMITECH. Washington, DC: American Society for Microbiology; 1994. p. 15.
8. Badenoch PR, Coster DJ. Antimicrobial activity of topical anaesthetic preparations. Br J Ophthalmol. 1982;66(6):364-7.

9. Benson WH, Lanier JD. Comparison of techniques for culturing corneal ulcers. Ophthalmology. 1992;99(5):800-4.
10. Jacob P, Gopinathan U, Sharma S, et al. Calcium alginate swab versus Bard Parker blade in the diagnosis of microbial keratitis. Cornea. 1995;14(4):360-4.
11. Sharma S. Diagnostic methods in ocular microbiology. In: LC Dutta (Ed). Modern Ophthalmology, 2nd edition. New Delhi: Jaypee Brothers Medical Publishers; 1999. pp. 216-24.
12. McLeod SD, Kumar A, Cevallos V, et al. Reliability of transport medium in the laboratory evaluation of corneal ulcers. Am J Ophthalmol. 2005;140(6):1027-31.
13. Murray PR, Baron EJ, Pfaller MA, et al. Manual of Clinical Microbiology, 6th edition. Washington DC: American Society of Microbiology; 1995.
14. Larone DH. Medically Important Fungi: A Guide to Identification, 3rd edition. Washington DC: ASM Press; 1995.
15. Gast RJ, Ledee DR, Fuerst PA, et al. Subgenus systematics of Acanthamoeba: Four nuclear 18S rDNA sequence types. J Eukaryot Microbiol. 1996;43(6):498-504.
16. Duggirala A, Joseph J, Sharma S, et al. Activity of newer fluoroquinolones against gram-positive and gram-negative bacteria isolated from ocular infections: an in vitro comparison. Indian J Ophthalmol. 2007;55(1):15-9.
17. Reddy AK, Garg P, Babu KH, et al. In vitro antibiotic susceptibility of rapidly growing nontuberculous mycobacteria isolated from patients with microbial keratitis. Curr Eye Res. 2010;35(3):225-9.
18. Thomas PA. Mycotic keratitis—an underestimated mycosis. J Medi Vet Mycol. 1994;32(4):235-56.
19. Saunders PP, Proctor EM, Rollins DF, et al. Enhanced killing of Acanthamoeba cysts in vitro using dimethylsulfoxide. Ophthalmology. 1992;99(8):1197-200.
20. Embong Z, Wan Hitam WH, Yean CY, et al. Specific detection of fungal pathogens by 18S rRNA gene PCR in microbial keratitis. BMC Ophthalmol. 2008;8:7.
21. Ferrer C, Colom F, Frasés S, et al. Detection and identification of fungal pathogens by PCR and by ITS2 and 5.8S ribosomal DNA typing in ocular infections. J Clin Microbiol. 2001;39(8):2873-9.
22. Vengayil S, Panda A, Satpathy G. et al. Polymerase chain reaction-guided diagnosis of mycotic keratitis: a prospective evaluation of its efficacy and limitations. Invest Ophthalmol Vis Sci. 2009;50(1):152-6.
23. Balne PK, Reddy AK, Kodiganti M, et al. Evaluation of three PCR assays for the detection of fungi in patients with mycotic keratitis. Br J Ophthalmol. 2012;96(6):911-2.
24. Basu S, Sharma S, Kar S, et al. DNA chip-assisted diagnosis of a previously unknown etiology of intermediate uveitis-*Toxoplasma gondii*. Indian J Ophthalmol. 2010;58(6): 535-7.
25. Das S, Sharma S, Sahu SK, et al. New microbial spectrum of epidemic keratoconjunctivitis: clinical and laboratory aspects of an outbreak. Br J Ophthalmol. 2008;92(6):861-2.
26. Sharma S, Das S, Joseph J, et al. Microsporidial keratitis: need for increased awareness. Surv Ophthalmol. 2011;56(1):1-22.
27. Mathers WD, Nelson SE, Lane JL, et al. Confirmation of confocal microscopy diagnosis of Acanthamoeba keratitis using polymerase chain reaction analysis. Arch Ophthalmol. 2000;118(2):178-83.
28. Lehmann OJ, Green SM, Morlet N, et al. Polymerase chain reaction analysis of corneal epithelial and tear samples in the diagnosis of Acanthamoeba keratitis. Invest Ophthalmol Vis Sci. 1998;39(7):1261-5.
29. Pasricha G, Sharma S, Garg P, et al. Use of 18S rRNA gene-based PCR assay for diagnosis of Acanthamoeba keratitis in non-contact lens wearers in India. J Clin Microbiol. 2003;41(7):3206-11.
30. Kim E, Chidambaram JD, Srinivasan M, et al. Prospective comparison of microbial culture and polymerase chain reaction in the diagnosis of corneal ulcer. Am J Ophthalmol. 2008;146(5):714-23.e1.
31. Itahashi M, Higaki S, Fukuda M, et al. Detection and quantification of pathogenic bacteria and fungi using real-time polymerase chain reaction by cycling probe in patients with corneal ulcer. Arch Ophthalmol. 2010;128(5):535-40.
32. Groden LR, Rodnite J, Brinser JH, et al. Acridine orange and Gram stains in infectious keratitis. Cornea. 1990;9(2):122-4.
33. Choudhury K, Sharma S, Garg P, et al. Clinical and Microbiological profile of Bacillus keratitis. Cornea. 2000; 19(3):301-6.
34. Garg P, Bansal AK, Sharma S, et al. Bilateral infectious keratitis following after laser in situ keratomileusis: a case report and review of the literature. Ophthalmology. 2001;108(1):121-5.
35. Sharma S, Srinivasan M, George G. Acanthamoeba keratitis in non-contact lens wearers. Arch Ophthalmol. 1990;108(5): 676-8.
36. Garg P, Sharma S, Rao GN. Ciprofloxacin-resistant *Pseudomonas* keratitis. Ophthalmology. 1999;106(7):1319-23.
37. Pradhan L, Sharma S, Nalamada S, et al. Natamycin in the treatment of keratomycosis: correlation of treatment outcome and in vitro susceptibility of fungal isolates. Indian J Ophthalmol. 2011;59(6):512-4.
38. Lalitha P, Vijaykumar R, Prajna NV, et al. In vitro natamycin susceptibility of ocular isolates of *Fusarium* and *Aspergillus* species: comparison of commercially formulated natamycin eye drops to pharmaceutical-grade powder. J Clin Microbiol. 2008;46(10):3477-8.
39. Jack I, Marmion BP. Direct virus diagnosis. In: Collee JG, Duguid JP, Fraser AG, Marmion BP (Eds). Mackie and McCartney Practical Medical Microbiology, 13th edition. Edinburgh: Churchill Livingstone; 1989.
40. Athmanathan S, Pranesh VM, Pasricha G, et al. Atypical herpes simplex keratitis (HSK) presenting as a perforating corneal ulcer with a large infiltrate in a contact lens wearer: multinucleated giant cells in the Giemsa smear offered a clue to the diagnosis. BMC Ophthalmol. 2001;1:1.
41. Athmanathan S, Sridhar MS, Anand R, et al. Herpes simplex virus bullous keratitis misdiagnosed as a case of pseudophakic bullous keratopathy with secondary glaucoma: An unusual presentation. BMC Ophthalmol. 2001;1:2.
42. Athmanathan S, Bandlapally SR, Rao GN. Collection of corneal impression cytology directly on a sterile glass slide for the detection of viral antigen: An inexpensive and simple technique for the diagnosis of HSV epithelial keratitis: a pilot study. BMC Ophthalmol. 2001;1:3.
43. Kowalski RP, Gordon YJ, Romanowski EG, et al. A comparison of enzyme immunoassay and polymerase chain reaction with the clinical examination for diagnosing ocular herpetic disease. Ophthalmology. 1993;100(4):530-3.

44. Kowalski RP, Gordon YJ. Evaluation of immunologic tests for the detection of ocular herpes simplex virus. Ophthalmology. 1989;96(11):1583-6.
45. Simon MW, Miller D, Pflugfelder SC, et al. Comparison of immunocytology to tissue culture for diagnosis of presumed herpes virus dendritic epithelial keratitis. Ophthalmology. 1992;99(9):1408-13.
46. Athmanathan S, Bandlapally SR, Nutheti R, et al. Comparison of an immortalized human corneal epithelial cell line with Vero cells in the isolation of herpes simplex virus-1 for the laboratory diagnosis of Herpes Simplex Keratitis. BMC Ophthalmol. 2002;2:3.
47. Athmanathan S, Bandlapally S, Rao GN. Comparison of the sensitivity of a 24 h-shell vial assay, and conventional tube culture, in the isolation of Herpes simplex virus-1 from corneal scrapings. BMC Clin Pathol. 2002;2(1):1.
48. Johnson FB, Luker G, Chow C. Comparison of shell vial culture and the suspension-infection method for the rapid detection of herpes simplex viruses. Diagn Microbiol Infect Dis. 1993;16(1):61-6.
49. Podzorski RP, Persing DH. Molecular detection and identification of microorganisms. Chapter 13. In: Murray PR, Baron EJ, Pfaller MA (Eds). Manual of Clinical Microbiology, 6th edition. Washington DC: American Society of Microbiology; 1995.
50. Subhan S, Jose RJ, Duggirala A, et al. Diagnosis of herpes simplex virus-1 keratitis: comparison of Giemsa stain, immunofluorescence assay and polymerase chain reaction. Curr Eye Res. 2004;29(2-3):209-13.
51. Tei M, Nishida K, Kinoshita S. Polymerase chain reaction detection of Herpes simplex virus in tear fluid from atypical herpetic epithelial keratitis after penetrating keratoplasty. Am J Ophthalmol. 1996;122(5):732-5.
52. Koizumi N, Nishida K, Adachi W, et al. Detection of herpes simplex virus DNA in atypical epithelial keratitis using polymerase chain reaction. Br J Ophthalmol. 1999;83(8):957-60.
53. Yamamoto S, Pavan-Langston D, Kinoshita S, et al. Detecting herpes virus DNA in uveitis using polymerase chain reaction. Br J Ophthalmol. 1996;80(5):465-8.
54. Cunningham ET Jr, Short GA, Irvine AR, et al. Acquired immunodeficiency syndrome—associated herpes simplex virus retinitis. Clinical description and use of a polymerase chain reaction—based assay as a diagnostic tool. Arch Ophthalmol. 1996;114(7):834-40.
55. Kudo E, Shiota H, Kinouchi Y, et al. Detection of herpes simplex virus DNA in tear fluid of stromal herpetic keratitis patients by nested polymerase chain reaction. Jpn J Ophthalmol. 1996;40(3):390-6.
56. Chichili GR, Athmanathan S, Farhatullah S, et al. Multiplex polymerase chain reaction for the detection of Herpes simplex virus, Varicella-Zoster virus and cytomegalovirus in ocular specimens. Curr Eye Res. 2003;27(2):85-90.
57. Koidl C, Bozic M, Mossböck G, et al. Rapid diagnosis of adenoviral keratoconjunctivitis by a fully automated molecular assay. Ophthalmology. 2005;112(9):1521-8.
58. Remeijer L, Duan R, van Dun JM, et al. Prevalence and clinical consequence of herpes simplex virus type 1 DNA in human cornea tissues. J Infect Dis. 2009;200(1):11-9.
59. Fukuda M, Deai T, Higaki S, et al. Presence of a large amount of herpes simplex virus genome in tear fluid of herpetic stromal keratitis and persistent epithelial defect patients. Semin Ophthalmol. 2008;23(4):217-20.
60. Kakimaru-Hasegawa A, Kuo CH, Komatsu K, et al. Clinical application of real-time polymerase chain reaction for diagnosis of herpetic diseases of the anterior segment of the eye. Jpn J Ophthalmol. 2008;52(1):24-31.
61. Yamamoto S, Shimomura Y, Kinoshita S, et al. Detection of Herpes simplex virus DNA in human tear film by the polymerase chain reaction. Am J Ophthalmol. 1994;117(2):160-3.

CHAPTER

27 Diagnostic Procedures in Uveitis

Jyotirmay Biswas, Reesha KR, Ranju Kharel (Sitaula)

INTRODUCTION

Uveitis encompasses entities of varying duration, severity, location, and above all a vast plethora of possible etiologies with quite similar and overlapping presentations. Examination of a patient with uveitis needs to be meticulous as the incidence of association with systemic diseases is high. Uveitis is often diagnosed based on clinical features alone (e.g. Fuchs' heterochromic iridocyclitis and serpiginous choroiditis) with the help of ancillary tests [fundus fluorescein angiography (FFA), indocyanine green angiography (ICG), optical coherence tomography (OCT)] or with the help of laboratory tests (sarcoid, tuberculous, and syphilitic uveitis). The importance and role of biopsy is significant in masquerade syndromes, intraocular inflammation, infections, intraocular tumors, and metastasis.[1]

Characteristic features displayed on one or more of the ocular imaging tools have made it possible to discern a number of specific uveitic entities. Sophisticated imaging modalities have also provided an insight into the pathogenesis of several uveitic entities. The diagnostic procedures used in uveitis can be broadly divided in two groups.

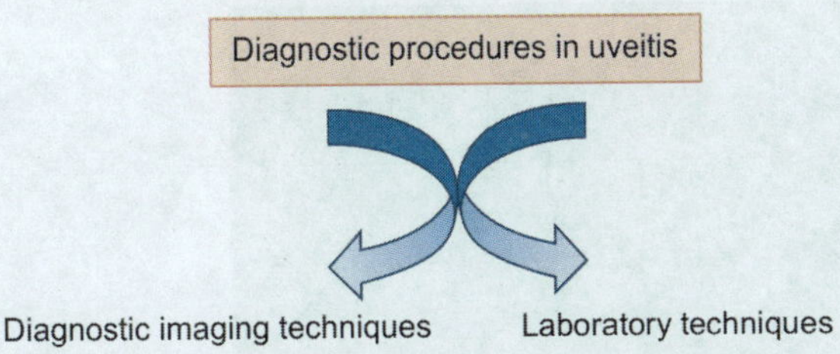

DIAGNOSTIC IMAGING PROCEDURES

Advances in the field of ocular imaging techniques have revolutionized the accurate diagnosis of the uveitic disorders and monitor its progression or regression in a better way. The following is the list of imaging procedures performed in uveitides:

- Ultrasonography
- Ultrasound biomicroscopy (UBM)
- Fundus autofluorescence (FAF)
- Fundus fluorescein angiography
- Indocyanine angiography
- Wide field angiography (WFA)
- Optical coherence tomography.

Ultrasonography

Ophthalmic ultrasonography is a noninvasive, safe, dynamic, and simple imaging technique for the evaluation of posterior segment structures in eyes with or without media opacities. It is a useful adjunctive tool that has an important role for the differential diagnosis and follow-up of inflammatory and noninflammatory pathologies of the posterior segment.

The sound wave transmitted from a probe into the eye travels in ocular media of different densities. In the normal eye, the vitreous is echolucent and the vitreoretinal interface produces a high spike. Inflammatory cellular infiltration of the vitreous cavity produces low reflects mobile echoes with diffuse distribution. Intravitreal hemorrhage produces higher reflective echoes. Posterior vitreous detachment is common in eyes with uveitis and appears as a mobile low reflective thin line whereas retinal detachment has high reflective spike with no after-movement. Focal retinochoroidal infiltrates or granulomas can also be imaged by ultrasonography in the form of localized thickening of the posterior layers and/or focal elevations toward the vitreous cavity.

In cases of choroiditis, choroidal thickness is increased and appears as low-to-medium reflectivity. The posterior scleritis shows high reflective thickening of the posterior wall of the globe. Fluid accumulating in the Tenon's space in posterior scleritis causes an echolucent zone posterior to the thickened wall continuous with the optic nerve giving rise to a characteristic T-sign image sign. Malignant or nonmalignant intraocular tumors mostly have ultrasonographic characteristics that differentiate them from inflammatory lesions.

Ultrasound Biomicroscopy

Ultrasound biomicroscopy is a qualitative investigation to study the pathology of iris, ciliary body, pars plana, and anterior portion of posterior segment of eye. In UBM, a high frequency transducer (50–100 MHz) is incorporated into a B-scan ultrasound so the resolution is better but penetration of ocular tissues is only up to the level of pars plana.

Ultrasound biomicroscopy is considered useful in uveitis for the evaluation of thickness of pars plana region, detection of ciliochoroidal effusion, supraciliary effusion, and foreign body at the angle. UBM can show pars planitis and pars plana membrane at the ciliary process **(Fig. 1)**. It also detects exudates around the pars plana, vitreous base, and peripheral retina. UBM is capable of identifying the presence of cells in the anterior and posterior chambers and anterior vitreous cavity in case of media opacity. It has proven to be most useful in imaging morphologic abnormalities in eyes with hypotony.[2]

Fundus Autofluorescence

It is also a noninvasive tool that allows in vivo imaging of retinal pigment epithelium (RPE) and outer retinal pathologies without the use of dye. FAF imaging is based on the autofluorescence phenomenon associated with lipofuscin granules in the RPE cells. Lipofuscin accumulation in the RPE cells is associated with photoreceptor outer segment turnover and renewal. In the normal eye, the FAF signal at the fovea is reduced because of the absorption by luteal pigment. The uses of FAF imaging in uveitis could be in inflammatory posterior uveitis like toxoplasmosis, serpiginous choroiditis, multifocal choroiditis with panuveitis, intraocular lymphoma, acute posterior multifocal placoid pigment epitheliopathy (APMPPE), birdshot chorioretinopathy, serous retinal detachment, cystoid macular edema, and secondary choroidal neovascular membrane.[2] It can distinguish between active chorioretinal lesion and scar because an active lesion will appear hyperfluorescence and scar will appear hypofluorescence. Hence, in suspected case of reactivation of posterior fundus lesion, the hypofluorescence lesion will be surrounded by hyperfluorescence **(Fig. 2)**.

Fundus Fluorescein Angiography

An understanding of fluorescein angiography and the ability to interpret fluorescein angiograms are essential to accurately evaluate, diagnose, and treat patients with retinal vascular and macular disease.[3] In uveitis, fluorescein angiography is

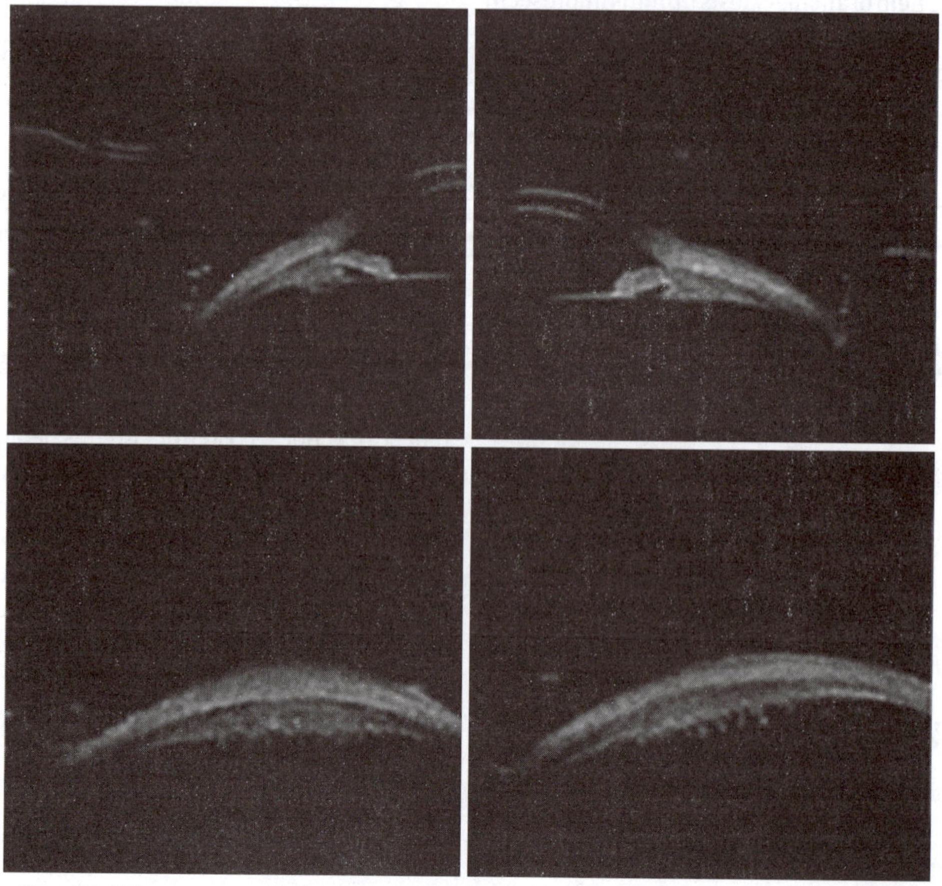

Fig. 1: Ultrasound biomicroscopy of a 48-year-old female of pars planitis showing 360 hypodense ciliary body with thin pars plana membrane at the ciliary process.

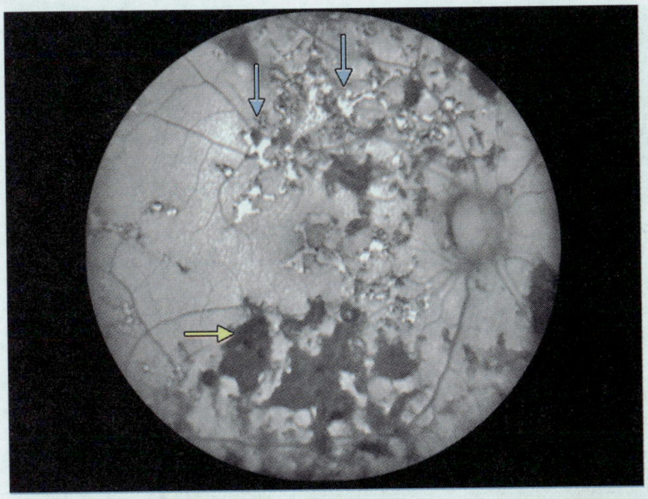

Fig. 2: Fundus autofluorescence angiography of a 54 years female with serpiginous choroiditis showing hyperfluorescence areas (blue arrow) suggesting of active lesions along with hypofluorescence areas of inactivity (yellow arrow).

Table 1: Pattern of FFA in some uveitic diseases.

Disease	*FFA (Early phase)*	*FFA (Late phase)*
Acute multifocal posterior placoid pigment epitheliopathy	Early hypofluorescent	Late hyperfluorescent
Vogt-Koyanagi-Harada disease/ Sympathetic ophthalmia	Pinpoint RPE leaks	Late pooling of dye in the subretinal space
Active toxoplasmic/ Serpiginous choroiditis	Early hypofluorescence	Late fuzzy staining of active leading edge of lesion
Posterior scleritis	Pinpoint RPE leaks	Late pooling of dye in the subretinal space
Multiple evanescent white dot syndrome	Stippled early hyperfluorescence	Hyperfluorescence persists in late phase
Cystoid macular edema	Progressive leakage and accumulation of dye in the cystoids spaces surrounding fovea	Petalloid pattern of parafoveal hyperfluorescence

(FFA: fundus fluorescein angiography; RPE: retinal pigment epithelium)

useful for the evaluation of optic disk inflammation, macular edema, occlusive and nonocclusive retinal vasculitis, neovascularizations, retinal pigment epithelial changes, and exudative retinal detachment.[2]

Inflammation of the retinal capillaries can be detected by FFA even in its early stage. Hence, FFA is an essential imaging study in all uveitic entities where retinal vasculature is primarily involved, such as Behçet's uveitis, Eales disease, and intermediate uveitis. Occlusive versus nonocclusive nature of retinal vasculitis can be identified by FFA.

Abnormal patterns of FFA appear either as hypofluorescence or hyperfluorescence areas. Fluorescein angiography is essential to make this distinction and to guide treatment. Pattern of FFA in some uveitic diseases is shown in **Table 1**.

Indocyanine Green Angiography

It is an invasive technique to analyze the inflammatory choroidal pathologies of choriocapillaris and the choroidal stroma. Choroidal impregnation by ICG fluorescence is disturbed in chorioretinal inflammatory disorders causing areas of altered fluorescence, hence making it a very useful adjunctive tool in chorioretinal inflammatory diseases.[4]

Hypofluorescent spots appearing as dark dots have been described as an ICG sign of active choroidal inflammation **(Fig. 3)** and they disappear after treatment. In ICG type 1 pattern, choriocapillaris nonperfusion shows patchy/ geographic deposition in the early and intermediate phase persisting in the late frames, whereas stromal choroiditis shows regular dots with an even distribution in the early phase.[5] In type 2 pattern, choroidal vasculitis may be seen as early stromal vessel hyperfluorescence, but it is best appreciated as fuzziness of choroidal vessels in the intermediate phase ICGA (Indocyanine green angiography). Numerous late phase pinpoints hyperfluorescence on ICGA is indicative of granulomatous disease.

Hypofluorescent dots are best appreciated in the intermediate phase and tend to have a uniform size and distribution in Vogt-Koyanagi-Harada (VKH) disease, sympathetic ophthalmia and birdshot chorioretinopathy but may have random distribution in sarcoidosis and tuberculosis.[2] In ocular toxoplasmosis, dark dots are typically seen only around the focus of retinochoroiditis. Pattern of ICGA in some uveitic diseases is summarized in **Table 2**.

Thus ICGA may reveal essential diagnostic information, especially when funduscopy and FFA fail to explain visual loss in patients with inflammatory choroidal diseases, such as acute posterior multifocal placoid pigmentary epitheliopathy **(Fig. 3)**, multiple evanescent white dot syndrome (MEWDS), multifocal choroiditis, early birdshot chorioretinopathy, and acute idiopathic blind spot enlargement syndrome.[2]

Wide Field Angiography

Wide field angiography helps in visualizing significant retinal findings which are likely to be missed by conventional 60° FFA. The newer WFA so called as ultrawide field angiogram discloses the true extent, nature, and severity of retinal vasculitis which can thereby help to formulate the plan on laser photocoagulation and use of corticosteroid with or without immunosuppressant. It also allows the clear visualization of the areas of neovascularizations and peripheral nonperfusion **(Fig. 4)** which thereby enhanced the correct documentation of disease activity, progression and outcome of laser photocoagulation.[6]

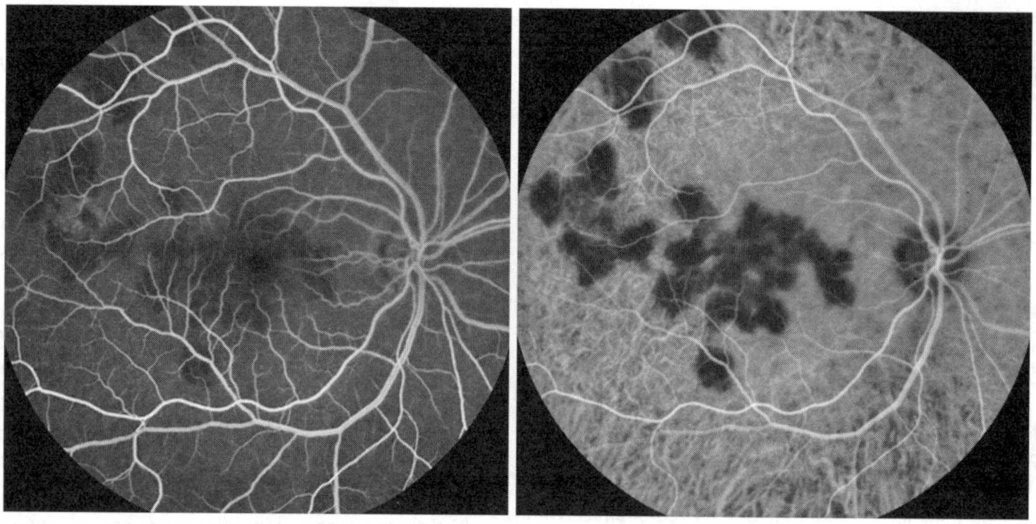

Fig. 3: Case of acute posterior multifocal placoid pigmentary epitheliopathy with hypofluorescence areas in fundus fluorescence angiography (left) and indocyanine green angiography.

Table 2: Pattern of ICGA in some uveitic diseases.

Type of uveitis	*ICG findings*
Serpiginous choroiditis	Hypofluorescent spots in early, intermediate, and late phases
Multifocal choroiditis	Large hypofluorescent spots all over the retina with much number of spots as compared to FFA and late homogeneous background fluorescence
Acute multifocal posterior placoid pigment epitheliopathy	Well demarcated, irregularly sharp hypofluorescence in all phases
Ampiginous choroiditis	Hypofluorescence in early and intermediate phases with heterogeneous background hyperfluorescence in late phases
Vogt-Koyanagi-Harada syndrome	Hypofluorescent spots scattered throughout the fundus becoming hyperfluorescence in the late stage of the study with confluent areas of hypofluorescence
Presumed tubercular choroiditis	Extensive patchy hypofluorescence in the posterior pole with ring of hyperfluorescence around hypofluorescence in late stages
Multiple evanescent white dot syndrome	Hypofluorescent spots around the disk and posterior pole in intermediate and late ICGA phases which was not apparent on FFA

(FFA: fundus fluorescein angiography; ICGA: indocyanine green angiography)

Optical Coherence Tomography

Optical coherence tomography imaging is identical to ultrasound, except that it uses light instead of sound to acquire high-resolution images of ocular structures as it relies on optical property rather than acoustic properties of ocular tissue thereby help in better understanding the pathologies and structural changes of the retinal disorders.

The currently available spectral domain optical coherence tomography (SD-OCT) instruments allow improved visualization of 4 lines in the sensory retina, which represent the external limiting membrane (ELM), the photoreceptor inner and outer segment junction (IS/OS), the interdigitation of the photoreceptor outer segments (OS) and the RPE, and the RPE-choriocapillaris complex.[3]

Optical coherence tomography is suitable for detecting and monitoring uveitic macular edema and provides important information about the fluid distribution in eyes with macular edema and the morphology of the vitreoretinal interface. The loss of the IS/OS junction on OCT in eyes with uveitic macular edema may be associated with poor visual acuity.[2]

Concurrent vitreoretinal traction in the form of an epiretinal membrane (ERM) appears as a hyperreflective line adhering to the retinal layer. ERM is found to be associated with macular thickness.

Optical coherence tomography reveals characteristic findings in VKH and SO where there are areas of serous retinal detachment in the outer segment demarcated by the ELM and RPE line, hyperreflective bands indicating fibrinous septae within the serous detachment, disruption of the continuity of the RPE and IS/OS junction, and undulations and bumps on the RPE surface adjacent to the serous retinal detachment.[2]

Optical coherence tomography findings in APMPPE appear has mild hyperreflective area above the RPE in the photoreceptor layer in the early phase of the disease and nodular hyperreflective lesion on the plane of the RPE with mild underlying backscattering in the later phase.[2] In serpiginous choroiditis, OCT shows increased reflectance of the choroid and deeper retinal layers, along with disruption of the photoreceptor IS/OS junction in both active and inactive lesions. The OCT can be even used to visualize the anterior chamber (AC) cells and angle structures in eyes with corneal haze.

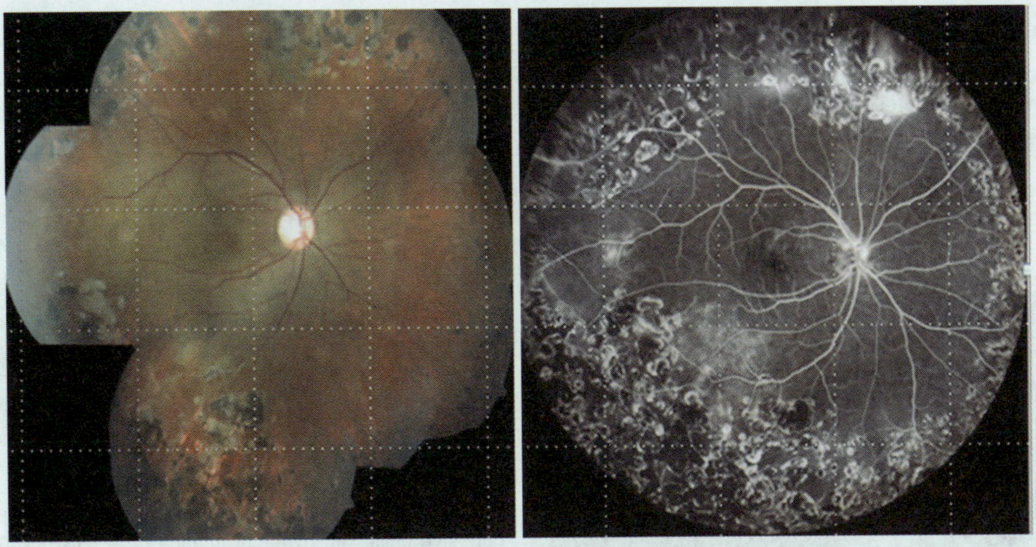

Fig. 4: Montage right eye showing laser marks in the peripheral retina in a case of retinal vasculitis and the wide field fundus angiography showing laser scars with an active neovascular frond in superonasal quadrant.

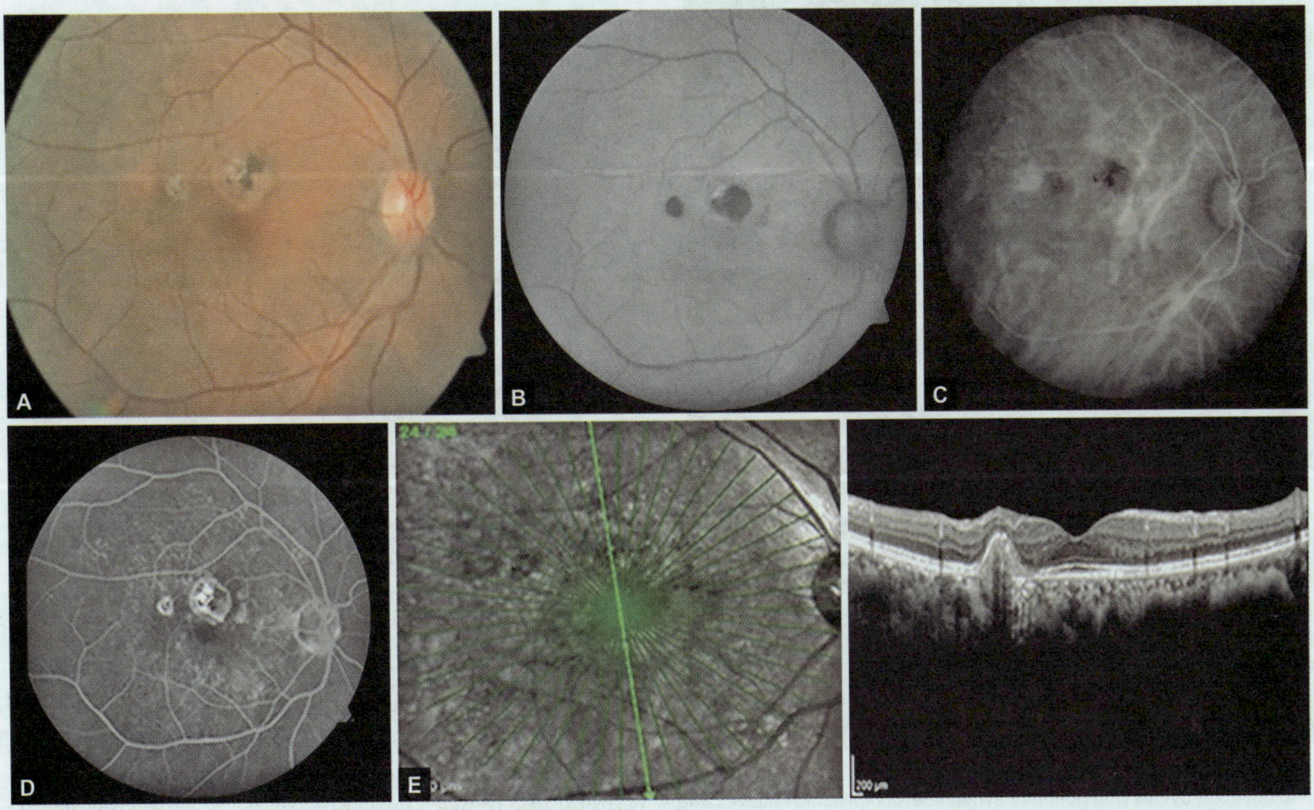

Figs. 5A to E: Multimodality imaging of a 49-year-old female with ocular toxoplasmosis. (A) Color fundus photograph showing retinochoroidal lesion at the macula with a satellite lesion; (B) Fundus autofluorescence angiogram showing hypofluorescence lesion with no activity; (C) Indocyanine green angiogram showing mid-phase hypofluorescence at the lesion site; (D) Fundus fluorescent angiogram showing retinochoroidal lesions with sharply demarcated margin which is staining without leakage; (E) Optical coherence tomography shows normal foveal counter with retinochoroidal scar adjacent to the foveal zone.

The recent advances have led to development of multimodal imaging where the FFA, ICGA, FAF, and OCT can be done from a single device at one time **(Figs. 5A to E)**.

INVASIVE PROCEDURES IN UVEITIS

With advancing surgical techniques and instrumentations, the biopsy procedures **(Box 1)** have become safe to arrive at a correct diagnosis, thereby guiding appropriate treatment and also providing insights into the disease.

Anterior Chamber Paracentesis

Anterior chamber paracentesis is a valuable procedure in the diagnosis of uveitis, particularly in diagnosing infective causes.[7] Various methods for performing AC paracentesis

Box 1: Various types of biopsy procedures used in uveitis.

Biopsy procedures in uveitis:
- Anterior chamber paracentesis
- Vitreous tap and diagnostic vitrectomy
- Iris and ciliary body biopsy
- Choroidal and retinochoroidal biopsy
- Fine needle aspiration biopsy

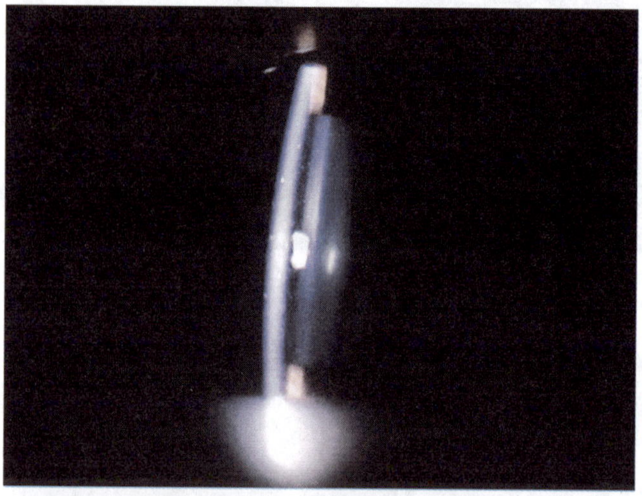

Fig. 6: An 8-year-old girl with persistent hypopyon uveitis, not responding to topical and systemic steroid.

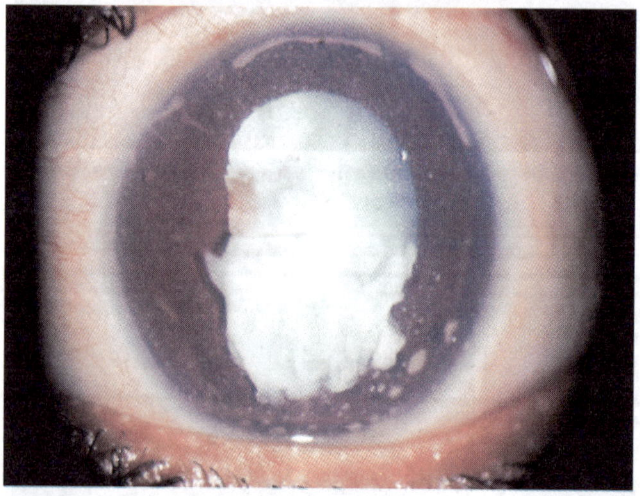

Fig. 7: A 14-year-old girl with finger nail injury, on examination showed granulomatous uveitis with posterior synechiae, complicated cataract and ruptured anterior capsule of lens.

have been described.[8,9] We describe herein a simple and safe technique, which can be performed in an outpatient department (OPD) setting, taking adequate aseptic precautions. The indication for an AC paracentesis may be many, but some of the difficult situations are in patients with masquerade syndromes with persistent hypopyon **(Fig. 6)**, and lens-induced uveitis **(Fig. 7)**. When paracentesis is performed, the diagnosis can be confirmed on the cytopathologic evidence **(Figs. 8 and 9)**.

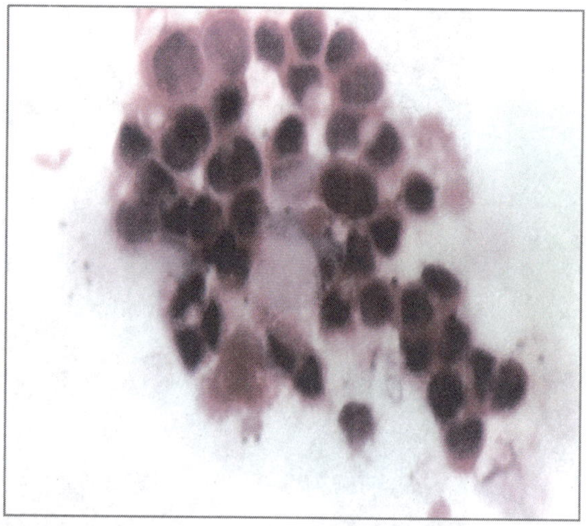

Fig. 8: Aqueous aspirate of the patient in **Figure 7** showing basophilic cohesive cells with hyperchromatic nuclei (H&E, ×400) suggestive of malignancy.

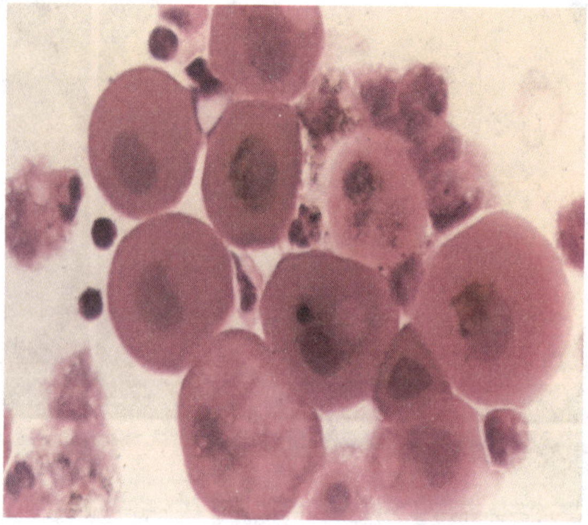

Fig. 9: Aqueous aspirate of the patient in **Figure 7** showing macrophages with engulfed lens matter (H&E, ×400).

Procedure

After using local antibiotic drops and a local anesthetic, a tuberculin or 2 mL syringe with a 27–30 gauge needle is used. In the presence of fibrin or granulomatous uveitis, it is preferable to use a large bore of 25–26 gauge needles. The needle entry into the AC is oblique through the stroma via the lower limbus. This acts as a valvular self-sealing paracentesis wound on withdrawal of the needle. One should avoid touching the corneal endothelium and particularly the lens in phakic patients and should stay over the peripheral iris at all times. Obtain a 0.1–0.3 mL of aqueous, and on withdrawal external pressure is applied to the entrance with sterile cotton tipped applicator. A drop of antibiotic is instilled in the conjunctival sac and the eye is patched for half-an-hour after which the patient is re-examined to ensure AC reformation.

The procedure is quite safe. In case of infectious uveitis and endophthalmitis, a portion of the material should be

Table 3: Cytopathological findings in aqueous aspirate in uveitis.

Diagnosis	*Cytopathologic findings*
Lens-induced uveitis	Macrophages engulfing lens particles, acute and chronic inflammatory cells
Masquerade syndrome (Retinoblastoma, leukemia)	Malignant cells, e.g. retinoblastoma cells and leukemic cells
Parasitic uveitis	Eosinophils, polymorphs and sometimes the parasite
Postoperative endophthalmitis	Bacteria or fungus and inflammatory cells

Table 4: Cytological findings in vitreous biopsy.

Diagnosis	*Findings*
Phacoanaphylactic uveitis	Lens fragments surrounded by polymorphs, epitheloid cells and giant cells
Large cell lymphoma (Reticulum cell sarcoma)	Large pleomorphic cells with prominent round or oval nuclei and scanty cytoplasm, micronuclei are not present in such cells
Endophthalmitis	Acute and chronic inflammatory cells and causative organisms on appropriate stain
Uveitis	Heterogeneous lymphocytic infiltrate

sent to microbiology for direct smear and culture for bacteria, fungus and mycobacteria and polymerase chain reaction (PCR). Remaining fluid should undergo cytospin study to obtain better cell recovery for microscopic examination.

The authenticity of aqueous humor analysis has been reported following analysis of samples using smears, cultures, PCR, and real-time PCR. Van der and Rothova et al.[8] have reported the usefulness of AC tap in isolation of infection in posterior uveitis. Tran et al.[10] had also supported the utility of PCR analysis of aqueous humor samples in necrotizing retinitis. Cytopathologic features of aqueous aspirate[11] help in the diagnosis of lens-induced uveitis, masquerade syndrome, delayed endophthalmitis, parasitic uveitis, to name a few **(Table 3)**. Complications that can occur following AC tap are rare; nevertheless, one needs to be aware of the possibility of wound leak, hyphema, iritis, and endophthalmitis.

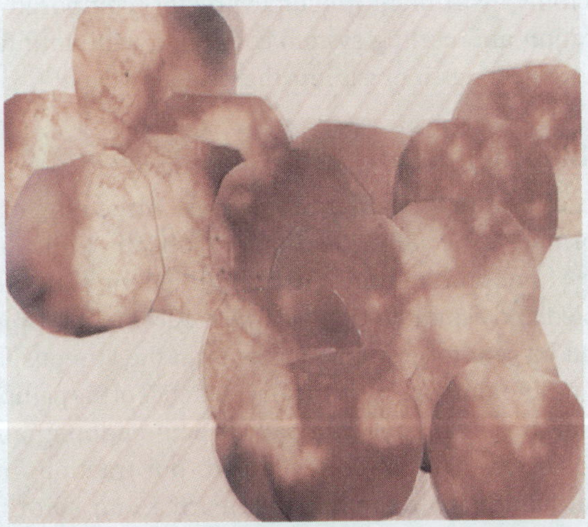

Fig. 10: Montage fundus photograph showing a subretinal mass in a case of intraocular lymphoma.

Vitreous Tap and Diagnostic Vitrectomy

Vitreous biopsy can be vitreous tap or diagnostic vitrectomy. Such vitreous biopsy is required in infective posterior uveitis, recalcitrant posterior uveitis, suspected large cell lymphoma particularly, in the elderly population. Material obtained from such procedures should be evaluated cytologically, and also subjected it to PCR, detection of intraocular antibodies [by enzyme-linked immunosorbent assay (ELISA)], flow cytometry (FCM) and culture.[12-14] Obtaining vitreous samples by tap is easier and can be done in the OPD,[15] however, material obtained is small. A diagnostic vitrectomy when performed provides large amount of material (though diluted), but needs to be done always in an operation theater. A cytologic analysis of vitreous aspirate can be of conclusive evidence in phacoanaphylactic uveitis, endophthalmitis and in specific large cell lymphoma **(Fig. 10)**. Cytological findings in vitreous biopsy in uveitic diseases are shown in **Table 4**.

Technique of Vitreous Tap

When performed in the OPD, the technique is similar to that of AC paracentesis. As the perforation of the sclera is more painful than performing a keratocentesis, subconjunctival injection of 0.1 mL of 2% lidocaine can be given at the site of scleral perforation and entry into the vitreous space, 3.5–4 mm posterior to the limbus in phakic and 3.0–3.5 mm posterior to the limbus in aphakic/pseudophakic patients. It should be better done in the operation theater under aseptic precautions.

The vitreous sampling is done using 25–23 gauge needles. Most eyes with long-standing intraocular inflammation have liquefied vitreous or fluid pockets within the vitreous. In such a situation, fine bored 25-guage needle can be used. When organization of vitreous is seen, 23-gauge needle is preferred. The needle is inserted in the vitreous cavity under direct visualization with slit lamp. The empty syringe withdraws the vitreous, and manipulating the stopcock, a similar quantity of antibiotic is injected into the vitreous cavity. After the injection the needle is slowly withdrawn from the eye. Complications with vitreous tap are vitreous hemorrhage, endophthalmitis, lens injury, retinal tears, and secondary glaucoma.

Technique of Vitreous Sampling and Biopsy

For analysis of the vitreous, it is essential to obtain undiluted vitreous specimen under sterile conditions intraoperatively. Newer techniques using vitrectomy with attachments and pneumovitrector have been described. Doft et al.[16] obtained vitreous samples in eyes with endophthalmitis by directly connecting a syringe to the aspiration tube of the vitreous cutter. Others have used a collecting bottle with openings at both sides integrated into the aspiration system. Smiddy et al.[17] obtained vitreous samples through a three-way stopcock through a manual aspiration. Scholda et al.[18] have developed a new technique, in which a metal device is integrated into the aspiration system of the vitrectomy unit, which fits on standard laboratory plastic containers with integrated caps. Peyman has devised a full functional vitrectomy instrument (pneumovitrector) composed of an aspiration and cutting system combined with an infusion line for injecting air or gas into the vitreous cavity.[19]

Vitrectomy

A more thorough standard three-port vitrectomy can be performed, especially when therapeutically indicated in cases of endophthalmitis. The undiluted vitreous can be sampled and aspirated via a side-port. All vitreous aspirated should be sent for examination as even the vitreous in the infusion line and vitrector can carry evidence of the pathology. Suction of the vitreous in a patient with endophthalmitis is very tricky. The vitreous tends to put traction on the retina, leading to unanticipated tearing and splitting of the retina and ultimately retinal detachment. To minimize traction on the retina caused by vitreous condensation and fibrous tissue formations, it is best to aspirate vitreous in the operating room under sterile conditions and under the controlled suction and cutting with vitreous instrument. This is highly preferable to the unstable "sucking only" of a large-bore needle aspiration at the pars plana. The cutting rate of the vitrectomy instrument should be turned up higher than 300 cuts per minute, which further serves to minimize tractional forces. Too much cutting of the vitreous, however, disturbs, disrupts, contorts, and destroys the cellular elements of vitreous. The optimal degree of vitreous surgery should include aspiration with a minimum of cutting of cellular elements, but with enough rapid cutting so as not to prolong tractional forces. Such a vitreous sample diluted by the irrigating solution is then passed through a disposable membrane filter system. Adequate sterile technique must be maintained. The procedure for obtaining the vitreous includes a stop-cock assembly somewhere in the line before the machine receptacle is encountered by the sterile line. This varies with each machine used, but some forethought to the system allows for sterile maintenance of the fluid.

Handling and Testing of Aqueous and Vitreous Specimen

The specimen should be handled in such a way as to allow the maximum number of tests to be performed based on the clinical diagnosis. To maximize the chance of detecting the offending agents, the aqueous humor and vitreous specimen obtained should be divided in two equal volumes. One half of the specimen is used for the following tests.

Microbiology

The samples should be immediately inoculated into blood agar, chocolate agar, brain-heart-infusion-broth (BHIB), thioglycollate fluid (maintained at body temperature), Sabouraud's agar, Brucella agar, and BHIB with gentamicin (maintained at room temperature for fungal isolation).

Polymerase Chain Reaction

The PCR is a powerful method to amplify specific sequences of DNA from a large complex mixture of DNA. For example, one can design PCR primers to amplify a single locus from an entire genome. PCR done on these samples particularly, the vitreous sample can be a significant indicator of the presence of the organism. A minimum volume of 0.05 mL should be reserved for this test especially when *Propionibacterium acnes*, fungal endophthalmitis, and uveitis of viral etiology are suspected.

The other half of the original sample can be processed for the following tests.

Nested Polymerase Chain Reaction

Nested PCR means that two pairs of PCR primers were used for a single locus. The logic behind this strategy is that if the wrong locus were amplified by mistake, the probability is very low that it would also be amplified a second time by a second pair of primers.

Real-time Polymerase Chain Reaction

In molecular biology, real-time PCR, also called quantitative real-time PCR (Q-PCR/qPCR/qrt-PCR) or kinetic polymerase chain reaction (KPCR), is a laboratory technique which is an evolution of PCR. In this technique, both evidence and quantification are done simultaneously and hence this investigation has the advantage of quantifying the load of the pathogen.

Cytology

The entire sample can be spin down, the supernatant transpipetted and the pellet resuspended in formalin or glutaraldehyde. These pellets are passed through two or more millipore filters and a number of specific staining methods including immunohistochemistry are carried out to identify the infiltrating cell types.[20] The other technique includes cytocentrifuge by cytospin method (about 1,000 revolutions for 5 minutes). Cytopathologic findings of vitreous aspirate are given in **Table 4**.

Antibodies

The supernatant obtained after spinning down the cellular components within the aqueous humor should be subjected to ELISA. The local production of specific antibodies within the ocular fluids is an important indication for the possible etiology especially when toxocara or toxoplasma is suspected.[21]

In Europe, the estimation of the Goldmann Witmer coefficient is done as given below:

Titer of antibody in aqueous concentration of serum globulin × Titer of antibody in serum concentration of aqueous globulin = Goldmann Witmer coefficient.

Significance

- 0.5–2 = No intraocular antibody production
- 2–4 = Suggestive of intraocular antibody production
- 4 = Diagnostic of intraocular antibody production.

FLOW CYTOMETRIC ANALYSIS

Flow cytometry measures the physical and chemical properties of individual particle or cell moving in a single file in a fluid stream. The most clearly defined application of FCM is in diagnostic surgical pathology.[1] It is an adjunct to histologic examination in the diagnosis of lymphoproliferative and leukemic processes. FCM is applied to the study of uveal melanomas, retinoblastomas, and ocular lymphoid proliferations, especially masquerade syndrome. It is now also being used to provide valuable information regarding the ratio between the cytotoxic and helper T-cells, an indication for the immunologic events taking place during the course of the ocular disease.

In a recent study, Davis et al.[22] showed patient with intraocular lymphoma, the positive predictive value (PPV) of cytology was 100%, but the negative predictive value (NPV) was 60.9%. For infection, PPV for bacterial and fungal culture was 100% and NPV was 94.9%. CD 22 +ve B lymphocyte ≥20% of total cells on cytofluorographic analysis had a PPV of 88% for lymphoma.

Iris and Ciliary Body Biopsy

Biopsy is usually performed in suspected tumors of iris and ciliary body. These lesions include glioneuromas, medulloepitheliomas, iridociliary cysts, leiomyomas, malignant melanomas, and nematode granulomas.[23] Indications of iris and ciliary body biopsy in uveitic conditions are:

- Metastatic lesions to the iris and ciliary body masquerading as uveitis.
- Ruptured iris cysts mimicking anterior uveitis.

Iris and ciliary body nodules secondary to granulomatous conditions like tuberculosis and sarcoidosis. Moorthy et al. reported three patients with coccidioidomycosis iridocyclitis diagnosed by biopsy of iris nodules.[24]

Choroidal and Retinochoroidal Biopsy

Lesions within the choroid can be difficult to differentiate clinically, although technological advances in noninvasive imaging have helped to monitor the size and the growth. The ophthalmologist has to consider the option of performing a choroidal or retinochoroidal biopsy. With advances in instrumentation and microsurgical techniques, endoretinal biopsy and chorioretinal biopsy can be performed easily and safely. Although the diagnosis of intraocular lymphoma can usually be made on the basis of diagnostic vitrectomy alone, sometimes it requires a more aggressive approach with choroidal biopsy, when pars plana vitrectomy and extensive medical examination fails to confirm the diagnosis.

Trans-scleral Choroidal Biopsy

After conjunctival recession and hemostasis, the area of sclera overlying the lesion is marked. A half-thickness scleral trapdoor hinged posteriorly is created. 7-0 preplaced vicryl sutures are placed to allow rapid closure. Diathermy is applied to the circumference of the biopsy site. An opening of smaller dimension is made into the suprachoroidal space within the floor of the lamellar scleral dissection. This opening is enlarged to expose the choroid which is excised using Vannas scissors taking care to avoid perforation of the retina. The scleral trap door is then sutured.[25]

Internal Approach for Retinal, Subretinal or Chorioretinal Biopsy

A vitreous biopsy is obtained at the beginning of the procedure before starting infusion.[26] The biopsy site in case of detached retina is selected at the junction of involved and normal retina. Unimanual bipolar endocautery is used at the margin of the proposed biopsy site. A biopsy specimen of at least 2 × 2 mm is then cut with 20-gauge vertical cutting scissors. The specimen is left attached at one corner and an intraocular forceps is used to remove it from the eye. After reattaching the retina, endolaser is applied to the biopsy site and long-acting gas or silicone oil tamponade is used. In case of attached retina, combined retinal and choroidal biopsy is obtained. Intense endo-diode laser is first applied around the margin of the biopsy site. Two minutes later a 2 × 2 mm biopsy specimen is cut within the margins of the laser burns with vertically cutting intraocular scissors until sclera is visible.

Fine Needle Aspiration Biopsy

Fine needle aspiration biopsy had been first described as early as 1847, though the first report was published in 1930.[1] Jakobiec et al. proposed fine needle aspiration biopsy (FNAB) for intraocular tumors in 1979. FNAB offers a histopathologic correlation to the clinical diagnosis in the case of atypical presentation of intraocular tumors. It aids in effective planning and management, and enables histopathological diagnosis without sacrificing the eye or having to resort to open biopsy methods.

Fine needle aspiration biopsy has been recommended in following conditions:

- Cases of suspected infectious subretinal lesions (abscess or tuberculoma) mimicking as choroidal tumors. Gregor et al. diagnosed a *Nocardia* asteroides subretinal abscess following a transvitreal FNAB.[27]
- Cases where diagnosis is difficult, distinction between benign and malignant lesion is not clear, all ancillary tests are inconclusive and where therapeutic decisions will be made on the basis of cytological findings, like metastatic disease of the choroid, but with no primary and cases where patient refuses recommended therapy until histopathological confirmation is obtained.

Technique of Fine Needle Aspiration Biopsy

Approaches

- Limbal route is used to approach anterior uveal lesions.[28] For example, iris lesions or in aphakic patients for posterior ciliary body lesions
- In the posterior segment lesions pars plana transvitreal approach is used.

In this approach, the needle is passed from the pars plana region (3.5 mm from the limbus) in the quadrant opposite to the lesion, through the vitreous gel. For some of the eyes with tumors located posteriorly, a vitrectomy needs to be performed before aspiration biopsy.

Corneolimbal approach

This approach through the zonules prevents dissemination of the tumor mass through the needle track. This approach is used in patients with retinoblastoma, a highly friable tumor, as the chance of needle track dissemination is extremely high. Through a corneolimbal approach the needle passes through multiple planes, thus wiping out the tumor cells as the needle is removed from the eye.

Subretinal fine needle aspiration biopsy

This can be done in cases of subretinal abscesses and tuberculomas, considering the site is approachable.

Complications

- The most common complication of FNAB is bleeding from the site of the needle track.
- Orbital dissemination of tumor cells and distant metastatic spread caused by tumor implantation along the needle track have been reported which are rare now.
- Iatrogenic retinal perforations are unavoidable by the indirect needle approach to the choroidal lesions and can theoretically cause a retinal detachment after FNAB.

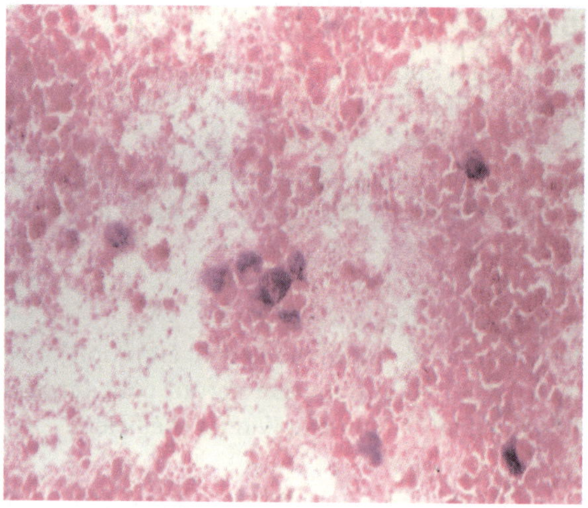

Fig. 11: Fine needle aspiration biopsy showing pleomorphic malignant cells in necrotic background (H&E, ×400).

Biopsy of Intraocular Lymphoma

Steroids should be stopped before diagnostic procedures to increase the diagnostic yield in suspected lymphoma cases. Samples should be obtained from the densest part of the infiltrate.[29] It is worthy to note that lymphoma cells undergo apoptosis 90–100 μ from their blood supply. If a distinct subretinal mass is present, a direct subretinal biopsy is better than a vitreous tap. The cells of lymphoma are fragile **(Fig. 11)**. Due to the associated presence of inflammatory cytokines, they may degenerate and also the DNA degrades resulting in false negative results.[30] Samples may be placed in cell culture media to improve viability of cells. Interleukin 10 (IL-10) levels have been found to be elevated in serum and vitreous of patients with non-Hodgkin's lymphoma while interleukin 6 (IL-6) levels are elevated in the vitreous of patients with intraocular inflammation. Whitcup, et al. found in a study that IL-10 levels exceeded the IL-6 levels in all 5 of studied patients with primary central nervous system lymphoma involving the eye but in none of 13 patients with uveitis.[31]

Biopsy in Vasculitis

Biopsy of the temporal arteries is often performed for suspected inflammatory bowel disease (Crohn's disease and ulcerative colitis) which can present with uveitis both anterior nongranulomatous or posterior type. Frequent biopsies are taken to assess the activity of disease and to assess changes that precede malignancy. The FNAB has a sensitivity and specificity rate of 84% and 98%, respectively.[32]

CONCLUSION

In the future, newer association with infection, systemic disease, and genetic patterns in uveitis will arise and needs to be explored further, focusing on the pathogenesis of the underlying ocular inflammation. However, while translating these research findings into clinical application, several points like cost-effectiveness will have to be considered. The different immunological hypotheses of etiology of uveitis needs to be verified, and adopted or rejected and management done accordingly. Biopsy pathology in ocular inflammation has no doubt a well defined place in the investigation protocol especially considering the rarity of certain types and the overlapping features that may coexist in the same patient. The most important consideration is that biopsy-proven pathogenesis and etiology is reliable and treatment can be instituted based on the histopathological outcome.

REFERENCES

1. Biswas J, Annamalai R, Krishnaraj V. Biopsy pathology in uveitis. Middle East Afr J Ophthalmol. 2011;18(4):261-7.
2. Foster CS, Vitale A. Diagnosis and Treatment of Uveitis. Philadelphia: WB Saunders Company; 2002. pp. 31-812, 264-72, 315-32, 710-25.
3. Ryan SJ, Sadda SR. Ryan's Retinal Imaging and Diagnostics, 1st edition. Elsevier; 2013. pp. 28-81.
4. Agrawal RV, Biswas J, Gunasekaran D. Indocyanine green angiography in posterior uveitis. Indian J Ophthalmol. 2013;61(4):148-59.
5. Gupta V, Gupta A. Ancillary investigations in uveitis. Indian J Ophthalmol. 2013;61(6):263-8.
6. Kaines A, Oliver S, Reddy S, et al. Ultrawide angle angiography for the detection and management of diabetic retinopathy. Int Ophthalmol Clin. 2009;49(2):53-9.
7. de Boer JH, Luyendijk L, Rothova A, et al. Analysis of ocular fluids for local antibody production in uveitis. Br J Ophthalmol. 1995;79(6):610-6.
8. Van der Lelij A, Rothova A. Diagnostic anterior chamber paracentesis in uveitis: a safe procedure? Br J Ophthalmol. 1997;81(11):976-9.
9. May DR, Noll FG. An improved approach to aqueous paracentesis. Ophthalmic Surg. 1988;19(11):821-2.
10. Tran T, Rozenberg F, Cassoux N, et al. Polymerase chain reaction analysis of aqueous humor samples in necrotising retinitis. Br J Ophthalmol. 2003;87(1):79-83.
11. Biswas J. Pathology of uveitis. Afro-Asian J Ophthalmol. 1995;11:205-8.
12. Priem H, Verbraeken H, de Laey JJ. Diagnostic problems in chronic vitreous inflammation. Graefes Arch Clin Exp Ophthalmol. 1993;231(8):453-6.
13. Palexas GN, Green WR, Goldberg MF, et al. Diagnostic pars plana vitrectomy report of a 21-year retrospective study. Trans Am Ophthalmol Soc. 1995;93:281-314.
14. Verbraeken H. Diagnostic vitrectomy and chronic uveitis. Graefes Arch Clin Exp Ophthalmol. 1996;234(Suppl 1):S2-7.
15. Liu K, Klintworth GK, Dodd LG. Cytologic findings in vitreous fluids. Analysis of 74 specimens. Acta Cytol. 1999;43(2):201-6.
16. Doft BH, Donnelly K. A single sclerotomy vitreous biopsy technique in endophthalmitis. Arch Ophthalmol. 1991;109(4):465.
17. Smiddy WE, Michels RG, de Bustros S, et al. Histopathology of tissue removed during vitrectomy for impending idiopathic macular holes. Am J Ophthalmol. 1989;108(4):360-4.
18. Scholda CD, Egger SF, Lakits A, et al. A system for obtaining undiluted intraoperative vitreous biopsy samples. Arch Ophthalmol. 1996;114(10):1271-2.
19. Peyman GA. A pneumovitrector for the diagnostic biopsy of the vitreous. Ophthalmic Surg Lasers. 1996;27(3):246-7.
20. Ben Erza D. Diagnostic intraocular interventions. In: Ben Erza D (Ed). Ocular Inflammation: Basic and Clinical Concepts. Martin Dunitz Ltd. 1999. pp. 83-9.
21. Joynson DH, Payne RA, Rawal BK. Potential role of IgG avidity for diagnosing toxoplasmosis. J Clin Pathol. 1990;43(12):1032-3.
22. Davis JL. Diagnosis of intraocular lymphoma. Ocul Immunol Inflamm. 2004;12(1):7-16.
23. Johnston RL, Tufail A, Lightman S, et al. Retinal and choroidal biopsies are helpful in unclear uveitis of suspected infectious or malignant origin. Ophthalmology. 2004;111(3):522-8.
24. Moorthy RS, Rao NA, Sidikaro Y, et al. Coccidioidomycosis iridocyclitis. Ophthalmology. 1994;101(12):1923-8.
25. Foulds WS. The uses and limitations of intraocular biopsy. Eye (Lond). 1992;6(Pt 1):11-27.
26. Rutzen AR, Ortega-Larrocea G, Dugel PU, et al. Retinal and choroidal biopsy in intraocular inflammation: a clinico-pathologi study. Trans Am Ophthalmol Soc. 1994;92:431-58.
27. Gregor RJ, Chong CA, Augsburger JJ, et al. Endogenous Nocardia asteroides subretinal abcess diagnosed by transvitreal fine-needle aspiration biopsy. Retina. 1989;9(2):118-21.
28. Shanmugam MP, Biswas J. Fine needle aspiration biopsy in the diagnosis of intraocular mass lesions. Indian J Ophthalmol. 1997;45(2):105-8.
29. Zaldivar RA, Martin DF, Holden JT, et al. Primary intraocular lymphoma: clinical, cytologic, and flow cytometric analysis. Ophthalmology. 2004;111(9):1762-7.
30. Murray P, Hoekzema R, van Haren MA, et al. Aqueous humor interleukin-6 levels in uveitis. Invest Ophthalmol Vis Sci. 1990;31(5):917-20.
31. Whitcup SM, Stark-Vancs V, Wittes RE, et al. Association of interleukin 10 in the vitreous and cerebrospinal fluid and primary central nervous system lymphoma. Arch Ophthalmol. 1997;115(9):1157-60.
32. Midena E, Bonaldi L, Parrozzani R, et al. In vivo detection of monosomy 3 in eyes with medium-sized uveal melanoma using transscleral fine needle aspiration biopsy. Eur J Ophthalmol. 2006;16(3):422-5.

CHAPTER

28 Diagnostic Procedures in Retinopathy of Prematurity

Yog Raj Sharma, Parijat Chandra, Rajni Sharma, Rajvardhan Azad

INTRODUCTION

Retinopathy of prematurity (ROP) is a vasoproliferative disorder of retina and is an important cause of childhood blindness in preterm infants. There are multiple risk factors[1] that are associated with the development and severity of ROP like low birth weight, early gestational age, multiple birth, hyperoxia, hypoxemia, hypercarbia, hypocarbia, respiratory distress syndrome, apnea, blood transfusions, sepsis, intraventricular hemorrhage (IVH), prolonged parenteral nutrition, etc.

With improvement in neonatal care, smaller babies continue to survive, and the incidence of ROP is on the rise, especially in developing countries like India.[2] This is compounded by the lack of awareness about ROP among pediatricians and ophthalmologists, which leads to late presentation of these babies with advanced disease, thereby causing blindness. The timely diagnosis of ROP is important to prevent the progression of disease, and to treat it in a timely manner to prevent blindness.

The understanding of pathogenesis, screening, and management of ROP has markedly changed since Terry first described it. Guided initially by the Multicenter Trial of Cryotherapy for Retinopathy of Prematurity (Cryo-ROP)[3] and now the Early Treatment Retinopathy of Prematurity (ETROP)[4] study—there are now clear national and international guidelines for screening and treatment of ROP.

RETINOPATHY OF PREMATURITY CLASSIFICATION

During normal retinal development, the retinal vessels start to develop at the optic disk at approximately 16 weeks of gestation and migrate toward the ora serrata. They reach nasal ora serrata by 36 weeks of gestation and the temporal ora serrata by 39–41 weeks of gestation. The interruption of this normal vasculogenesis leads to ROP. The retinal ischemia in avascular retina leads to development of neovascularization at the junction, which can advance to retinal detachment in advanced stages of ROP.

The International Classification of Retinopathy of Prematurity (ICROP)[5] was devised by an international group of ROP experts. This classification divided the ROP presentation by zones and stages, and thereby helped in communication between ophthalmologists and neonatologists.

Zones: The coordinated developmental sequence permits the retina to be subdivided into three concentric zones.

- *Zone I*: Circle from center of disk with radius of twice distance from disk to macula
- *Zone II*: From nasal edge of zone I to ora nasally and up to equator temporally
- *Zone III*: From temporal crescent of retina anterior to zone II **(Fig. 1)**.

Stages: The different stages described by ICROP are as follows:

- *Stage 1: Demarcation line:* Earliest feature of ROP in a premature baby is the development of a flat white line at the junction of vascularized and avascular retina.

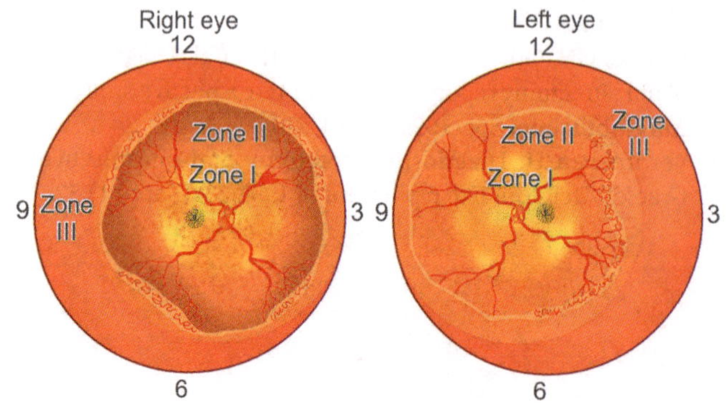

Fig. 1: Zones of retinopathy of prematurity.

The demarcation line can develop in any zone depending upon the level of prematurity **(Fig. 2)**.

- *Stage 2: Demarcation ridge:* The demarcation line gains height and width and progresses to a ridge which is pink or white elevation of the thickened tissue. Some neovascular tufts can be seen posterior to this ridge **(Fig. 3)**.
- *Stage 3: Extraretinal fibrovascular proliferation:* Neovascular growth occurs into and above the ridge. The vessels also grow into the vitreous and can lead to vitreous hemorrhage **(Fig. 4)**.
- *Stage 4: Partial retinal detachment:* With progressive growth into the vitreous, contraction of the fibrovascular proliferation exerts traction on the retina, leading to partial retinal detachment (Stage 4 ROP), either without foveal involvement (Stage 4a) or with foveal involvement (Stage 4b) **(Fig. 5)**.
- *Stage 5: Total retinal detachment:* These retinal detachments are mostly funnel-shaped and their configuration can further be described as open and closed anteriorly and open or closed posteriorly **(Fig. 6)**.

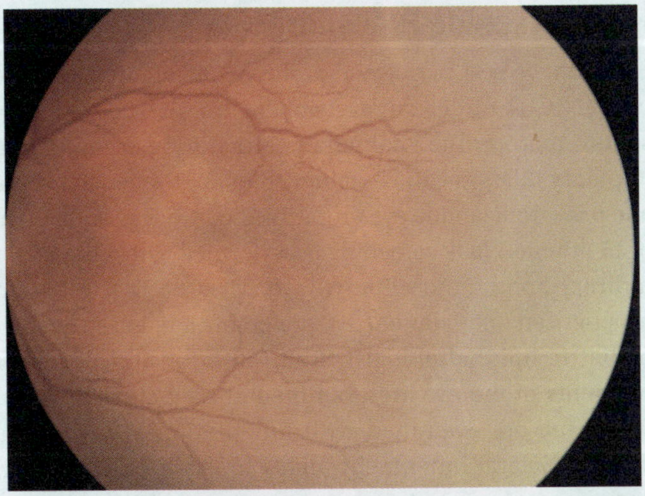

Fig. 2: Stage 1 retinopathy of prematurity—demarcation line.

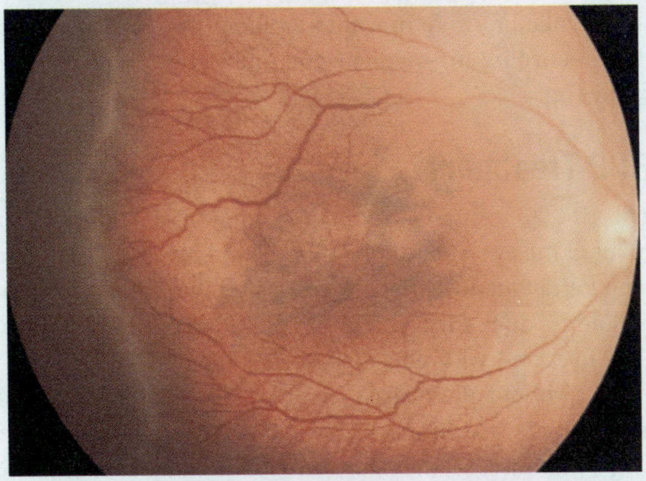

Fig. 3: Stage 2 retinopathy of prematurity—demarcation ridge.

Some other important terminologies associated with ROP are:

- *Plus disease:* It is defined as dilated and tortuous blood vessels at the posterior pole along with pupillary rigidity

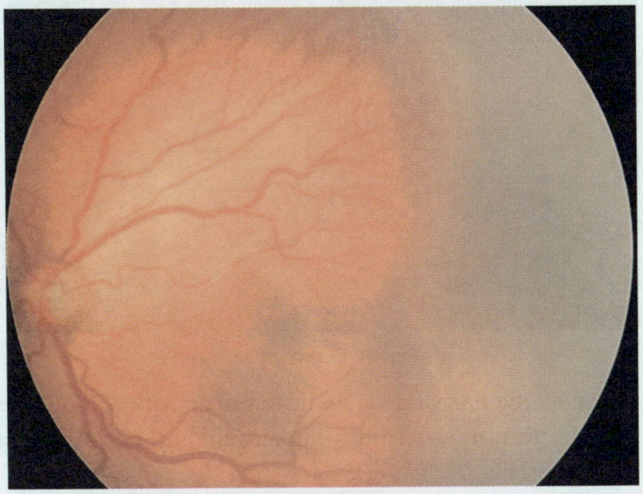

Fig. 4: Stage 3 retinopathy of prematurity—extraretinal neovascularization.

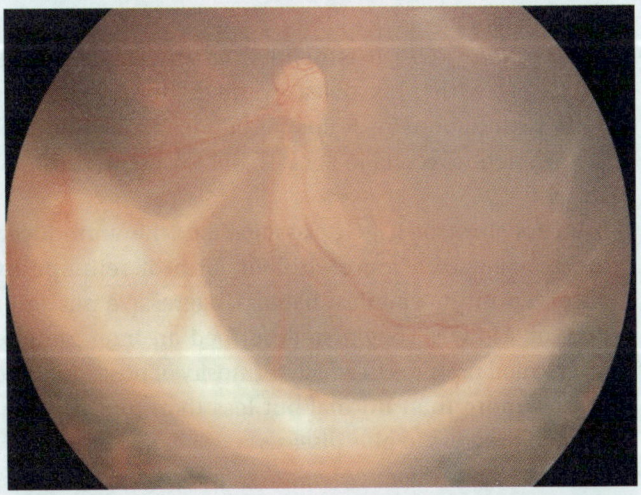

Fig. 5: Stage 4 retinopathy of prematurity—subtotal retinal detachment.

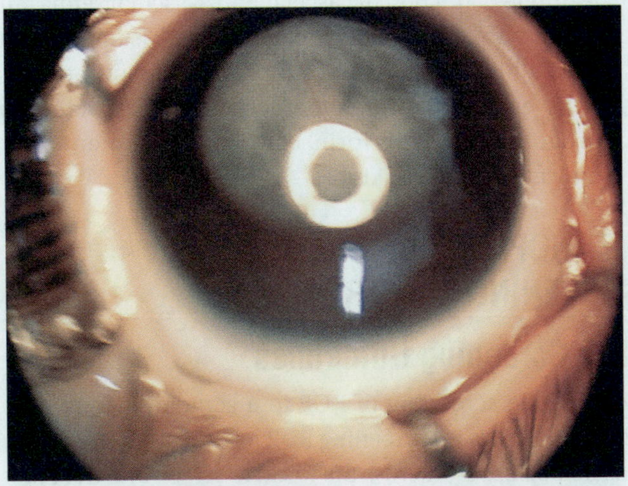

Fig. 6: Stage 5 retinopathy of prematurity—total retinal detachment.

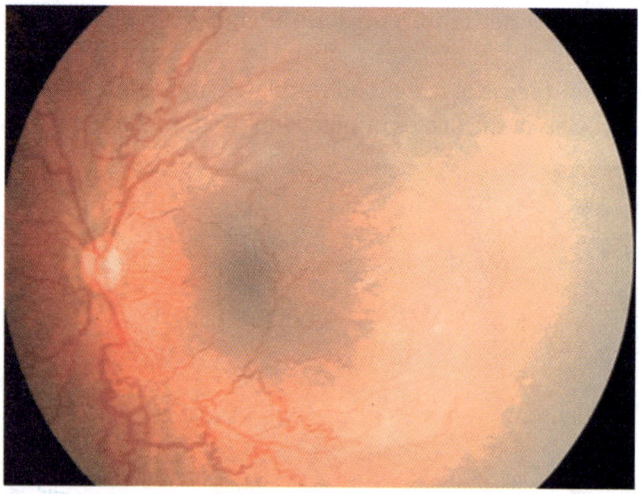

Fig. 7: Plus disease.

and media haze. It is an indicator of activity of ROP, and an important criterion for treatment and regression of disease **(Fig. 7)**.

- *Threshold ROP*: It is defined as Stage 3 + ROP in zone-I or II, or zone I any stage with no plus, occupying at least 5 contiguous clock hours or 8 noncontiguous clock hours of retina.
- *Prethreshold ROP:* It is defined as any stage of ROP in zone-I with plus disease and ROP stage 3 plus with 3 contiguous or 5 noncontiguous clock hours of involvement of retina in zone-II, but less than threshold stage.

  In an update of the ICROP classification,[6] they introduced the concept of a more virulent form of retinopathy observed in the smallest babies—aggressive posterior ROP or APROP. They also described an intermediate level called pre-plus in which tortuosity of posterior pole vessels more than normal but less than plus disease. It could progress to plus disease.
- *Aggressive posterior retinopathy of prematurity:* It is a severe form of ROP which is characterized by posterior zone, severe plus disease, fast progression to stage 5, a featureless junction of vascular and avascular retina, and a high rate of progression to blindness. It is important to have a high index of suspicion for aggressive posterior ROP, ensure its timely detection by ROP screening programs, and perform complete treatment when indicated at the earliest.

RETINOPATHY OF PREMATURITY: SCREENING AND TREATMENT

ROP Screening Guidelines

To facilitate screening of ROP in a standardized manner, clear guidelines for screening ROP have been devised which has helped experts across the world to screen and treat these babies in time. The American guidelines[7] suggest we should screen all babies <30 weeks gestational age and <1,500 g birth weight, or higher if the attending neonatologist believes the child is high-risk to develop ROP. The first screening of all babies should be done at 31 weeks postconceptional age or 4 weeks after birth whichever was later.

However, in developing countries like India due to poor neonatal care even larger babies are developing severe ROP.[8] To address this issue of screening bigger babies, Rashtriya Bal Suraksha Karyakram (RBSK), Ministry of Health, Government of India released national ROP screening guidelines[9] which suggests that ROP screening should be performed in all preterm neonates who are <34 weeks gestation age and/or < 2,000 g birth weight. Larger babies between 34 weeks and 36 weeks gestational age or birth weight more than 2,000 g can also be screened if they have risk factors for ROP. The first screening should be performed not later than 4 weeks of age. However, in very small infants born <28 weeks or <1,200 g birth weight, they can be screened as early as 2–3 weeks of age, for early detection of APROP.

ROP Screening Procedure

Screening is best performed at the neonatal intensive care unit (NICU) under supervision of trained neonatology staff to monitor the vital parameters during examination. Pupillary dilation can be achieved by 2.5% phenylephrine and 0.5% tropicamide eye drops instilled twice at an interval of 15 minutes. ROP screening is performed with a binocular indirect ophthalmoscope with a 28 D/20 D lens by an experienced ophthalmologist, preferably a retina specialist/ pediatric ophthalmologist. Both anterior and posterior segments of the eye are examined and all clock hours of the retina are examined with indentation to detect the disease. Scleral indentation helps to examine the retinal periphery, to rotate the eye to see areas of interest, and contrast structures by gentle indentation. It is necessary to record all the screening findings accurately and correctly in a detailed form to prevent ambiguity and ensure correct data recording for medical documentation, referral, and follow-up.

ROP Treatment

The ETROP group[4] gave clear guidelines for laser treatment of the avascular retina in ROP and classified ROP into type I and type II ROP. They suggested that laser treatment should be done for type I ROP defined as: (1) Any stage of ROP in zone-I with plus disease, (2) Stage 3 ROP in zone-I with or without plus disease, and (3) Stage 2/3 ROP in zone-II with plus disease. In cases of type II ROP, based on the zone, stage, plus disease, the babies are followed up at an interval of 1–2 weeks.

Anti-vascular endothelial growth factor (VEGF) drugs like Ranibizumab/Bevacizumab have emerged as useful adjuncts to laser treatment in progressive disease, and is now commonly used as first line treatment for zone I APROP, but its safety profile still needs to be established.[10] Stages 4–5 ROP are advanced stages of disease and need vitreoretinal surgery. The surgical outcomes in stage 4 ROP are good as only subtotal retinal detachment has occurred[11] but the surgical results in stage 5 ROP are poor[12] as complete retinal detachment is difficult to operate and is often associated with secondary glaucoma, corneal opacity, etc.

There are various diagnostic modalities which are helpful in understanding the disease process of ROP and improving its outcomes such as wide-field retinal screening, fluorescein angiography, ultrasound biomicroscopy, B-scan ultrasound, handheld optical coherence tomography (OCT), etc. Let us elaborate the role of some of these modalities.

WIDE-FIELD RETINAL SCREENING

Wide-field pediatric retinal imaging systems are useful to screen the eyes of preterm babies for ROP. RetCam (Natus Medical Inc., USA) is a popular tool that offers a quicker and faster way to examine these babies with less stress compared to indirect ophthalmoscopy. In fact, it is possible to document the entire retina in as few as five images. The second-generation ROP lens provides a wide-angle view of the retina with a field of 130°. It has several interchangeable lenses to capture images in different magnifications. A coupling medium is required and the handheld camera is placed directly over the cornea, changing the focus and brightness using the foot switch to record high-quality images. It allows real-time imaging, storage, and image retrieval, and allows easy access of patient data and images for review, opinion, and teaching.

RetCam 3 is the latest version with benefits like flat monitor, frame-by-frame video review, 20-second video capture and is especially useful for performing fluorescein angiography. It is a useful tool for training residents, counseling parents and can be performed by a trained technician or nurse in any location like the neonatal ICU or the operation theater, if needed.

A major role of wide-field imaging has been for telescreening purposes. RetCam examination performed by technicians can be transmitted to a central reading center where ROP experts can review the images and advice necessary action. Development of ROP specific mobile applications allows images to be reviewed by ROP experts on their mobile phones anywhere in the world. Digital photography has a high degree of specificity and sensitivity for detecting referral warranted ROP is a very cost-effective option. Stanford University Network for Diagnosis of Retinopathy of Prematurity (SUNDROP)[13] and KIDROP[14] program in Karnataka are examples of successful telescreening models.

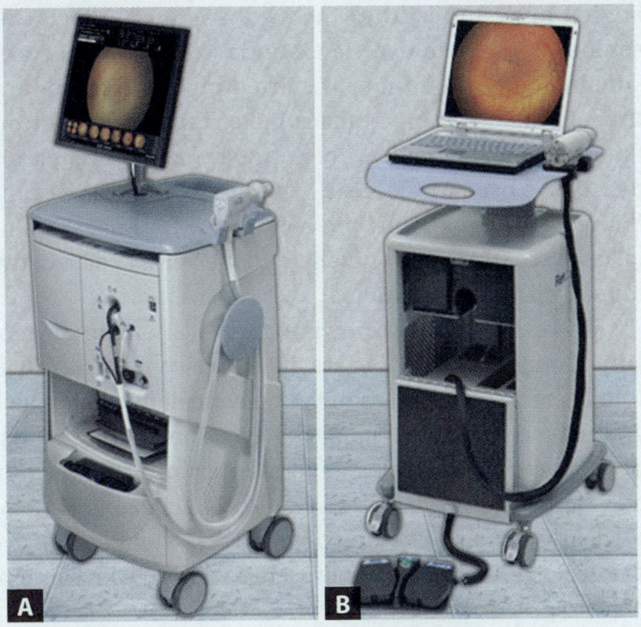

Figs. 8A and B: (A) RetCam 3; (B) RetCam Shuttle.

A major limitation of the RetCam is that it is very expensive. The growing popularity of wide-field imaging has led to development of many cheaper wide-field indigenous cameras like 3nethra Neo (Forus Health Pvt. Ltd.), which have similar specifications, yet are more portable and cheaper. Some have even tried ultra wide-field imaging for ROP using Optos imaging equipment providing 200° field of view by noncontact mechanism using flying baby technique, but this is difficult to perform in preterm babies.[15]

Tele-screening is expected to become mainstream in the coming years to meet the ROP screening needs of the growing number of NICUs, and neonatologists might take a lead to conduct ROP screening in future **(Figs. 8A and B)**.[16]

FLUORESCEIN ANGIOGRAPHY

Fluorescein angiography is a very useful tool[17,18] to study in detail the vascular status of ROP eyes. Fluorescein angiography is performed with the help of the fluorescein angiography module of the RetCam. Before performing fluorescein angiography, it is essential to take informed consent from the parents. The vital monitoring is done by the attending neonatologist.

The RetCam is prepared by switching to the blue light source, the barrier filter is inserted into the camera hand piece, and the timer is set when the procedure is to be started. An intravenous cannula is inserted in the baby, flushed with saline, and prepared before dye injection. The child's eye is topically anesthetized with proparacaine eye drops, then the lid speculum is inserted, and the coupling gel media is poured over the cornea. To start the fluorescein angiography procedure, the neonatologist injects the sodium fluorescein dye via the intravenous cannula, and simultaneously the timer is started on the RetCam, and the handheld camera is placed over the cornea and the fluorescein angiography is performed. Sodium fluorescein dye 20% is used in the dose of 4 mg/kg. All phases of the fluorescein angiography are recorded, with images being taken every 10 seconds initially, and then every consecutive minute till about 10 minutes.

Fluorescein angiography is especially useful in diagnosis and management of cases of aggressive posterior ROP. It helps to visualize areas of flat neovascularization, which are not seen easily by the naked eye. Though these areas may appear as featureless, and the demarcation junction may be difficult to visualize, fluorescein angiography helps to clearly visualize the junction and also shows extensive dye leakage in areas of neovascularization, which might help experts make early decision for treatment.

Sometimes there are vascular loops which confuse residents regarding the posterior extent of laser treatment. Incomplete laser treatment sparing a large area of posterior retina, will eventually lead to ROP progression. Thus, detecting avascular areas behind these vascular loops, and treating these areas completely with the laser is essential; and fluorescein angiography provides a clear visualization of these areas helping residents perform complete laser treatment. This is also useful after anti-VEGF injection to look for macular vascularization, vascular growth/arrest and early recurrence.

Even with ROP experts managing cases of aggressive posterior ROP, sometimes the plus disease persists despite the best of laser treatment. Fluorescein angiography helps to detect skip areas of treatment, or identify new areas of avascular retina which were not visible to the naked eye earlier, thereby ensuring that complete laser treatment is performed and prevent ROP sequelae such as macular dragging.

However, fluorescein angiography has some limitations. In nondilating pupils, not much information can be elicited. In cases of aggressive posterior ROP, with severe plus disease, the dye may leak quickly into the anterior chamber and vitreous chamber, making visualization very difficult. Therefore, there is a small window of time to record all the useful information from fluorescein angiography. In some cases, the dye takes a long time to transit across the eye leading to the late venous filling. While in other cases, there may be early dye wash out, making the late phase information of not much use **(Fig. 9)**.

ULTRASOUND BIOMICROSCOPY

Ultrasound biomicroscopy (UBM) is a very useful tool[19] to study the lens, ciliary body, anterior vitreous, and pars plana in babies with ROP. UBM is helpful particularly in cases of advanced stage 5 ROP which requires complex vitreoretinal surgery.

Since advanced cases of ROP are associated with extensive anterior vitreoretinal traction and retrolental membranes—there is little space behind the lens and in anterior vitreous for surgical instrument entry and movement. The UBM helps determine the anterior surgical space in all quadrants, and finds the maximum space where it will be easier to insert the surgical instruments, without trauma and associated complications. UBM in ROP babies is also a useful tool for decision-making for lensectomy in surgery for stage 5 ROP. UBM can clearly define landmarks related to the lens, tractional retina, vitreous membranes, ciliary body, and adjacent spaces.

Performing UBM examination in preterm babies is difficult. Although the UBM settings are mostly same,

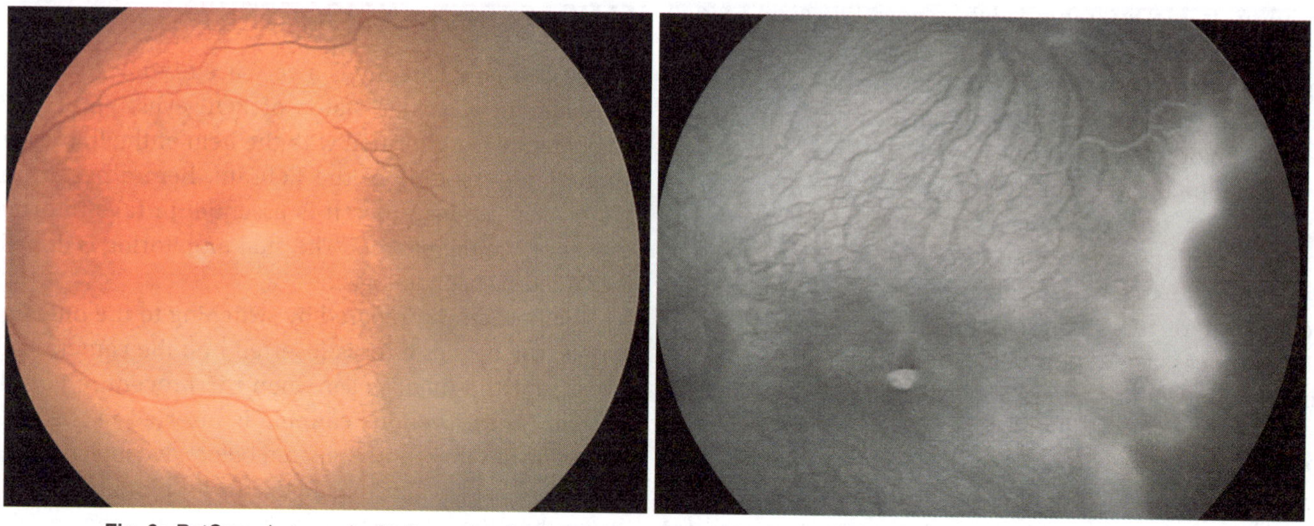

Fig. 9: RetCam photograph of left eye showing faint ridge, which leaks heavily on fluorescein angiography suggestive of extensive neovascularization.

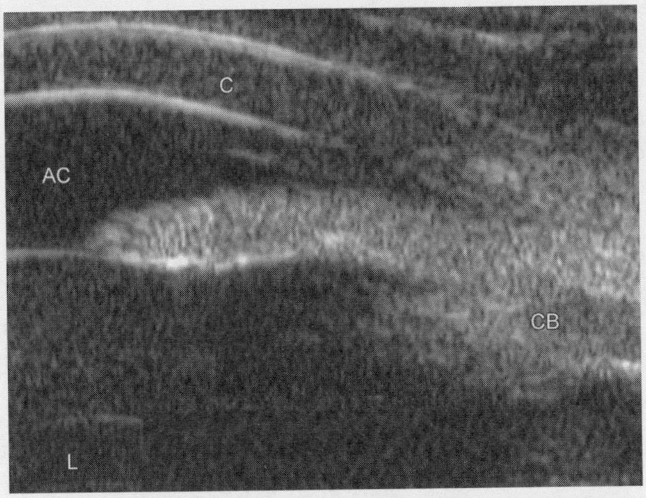

Fig. 10: Ultrasound biomicroscopy showing area of surgical access in stage 5 ROP.
(AC: anterior chamber; C: cornea; CB: ciliary body; L: lens; ROP: retinopathy of prematurity)

children are difficult to cooperate for the procedure. After topical anesthesia, lid speculum is inserted followed by a UBM cup to hold the viscous gel. Sometimes, the eyes are so small that there is no space to insert a UBM cup, and in such cases, it might be useful to create small well using cotton and then pour the coupling medium inside the cotton well. Since these children constantly move their eyes, performing UBM examination is not easy, and areas of interest are difficult to capture.

Interpreting UBM images requires a thorough understanding of the pathoanatomy of ROP, its development and progression through different stages. Reviewing the UBM images before surgery for advanced ROP can provide useful information for the surgeon **(Fig. 10)**.

ULTRASONOGRAPHY

Ultrasound examination is a useful investigative tool for the examination of cases with advanced ROP, especially in stage 5 ROP.[20] Usually these cases carry a very poor prognosis for surgical intervention, and B-scan ultrasound helps to examine the posterior segment of the eye, when the anterior segment limits visibility of the fundus—in cases with shallow anterior chamber, posterior synechiae, cataract, dense retrolental fibrovascular proliferation, etc.

From a surgical point of view, ultrasound helps to determine the funnel configuration of the tractional retinal detachment in stage 5 ROP and it can be divided into various categories like open-open, narrow-narrow, open-narrow, and narrow-open funnel configurations. Based on the funnel configuration, the surgeon gets a good idea about the posterior segment and then decides whether to operate or not, or plan the surgical steps, and advise the parents regarding the prognosis of the case and the possible outcomes **(Fig. 11)**.

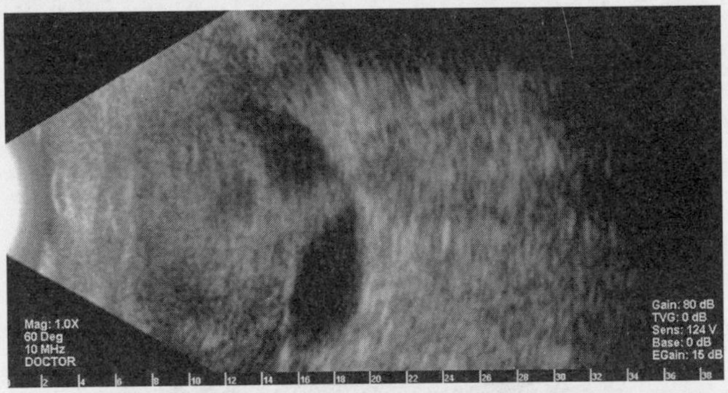

Fig. 11: Ultrasound showing anterior-open and posterior-closed funnel retinal detachment in stage 5 retinopathy of prematurity.

OPTICAL COHERENCE TOMOGRAPHY

Recently, OCT technology is also found to be useful in the management of preterm babies with ROP. Using OCT, it has been reported that the choroidal thickness decreases, and cystoid macular edema (CME) increases with severity of ROP,[21,22] while total retinal thickness is often increased in preterm babies.[23] While many studies have been conducted to see the effect of ROP and prematurity on the retinal structure using the standard OCT, this can be performed only in bigger children who are cooperative or can be performed in younger children under sedation with proper positioning.

However, the main advantage of OCT in preterm babies is using the handheld OCT, which allows rapid high-resolution imaging of the retina in premature babies to detect retinal structural anomalies. Much like the wide-field imaging systems, the handheld OCT system is much easier to use in preterm babies. It is possible to get real-time images and full 3D volumetric data analysis of the retina, which is useful to assess retinal changes and compare it with visual outcomes after ROP regression, laser or surgical management.

Leica Envisu C-Class OCT is one such handheld OCT equipment which captures high-resolution images till 3 μm, allows acquisitions of 22,000 scans per second, thereby compensating for pediatric eye movements, and uses various interchangeable lenses. General retina lens has 70° field of view, while other lenses allow variable field of view. Performing OCT in preterm babies with small eyes under topical anesthesia is challenging and requires considerable experience to effectively perform this procedure, as well as interpret the observed changes **(Figs. 12 and 13)**. With advent of the handheld swept-source optical coherence tomography angiography (SS-OCTA), retinal microvascular imaging in preterm babies will reach a new level.[24]

CONCLUSION

Retinopathy of prematurity is becoming an important cause of childhood blindness worldwide because of the improved survival of very low-birth-weight babies developing ROP, compounded with lack of facilities for ROP screening

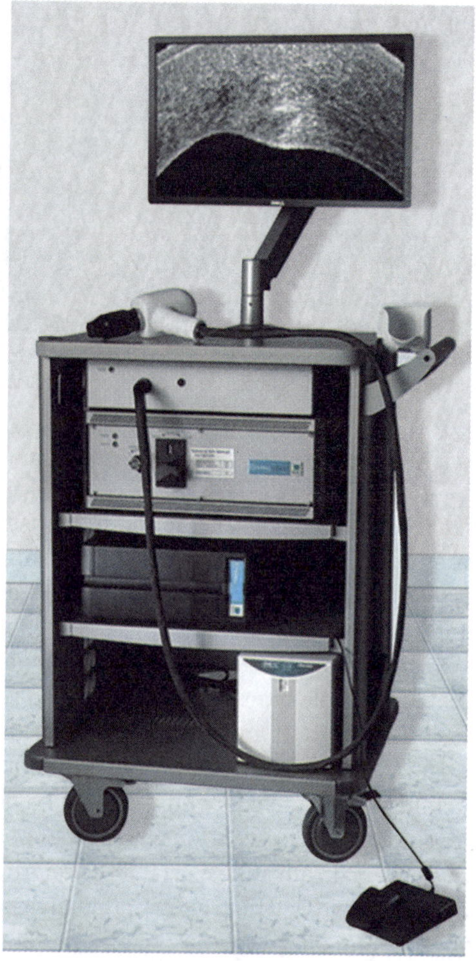

Fig. 12: Leica Envisu C-Class optical coherence tomography.

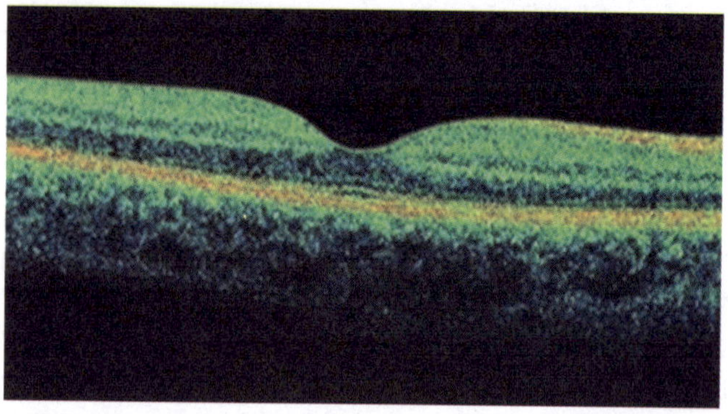

Fig. 13: OCT macular line scan of a preterm baby with ROP. (OCT: optical coherence tomography; ROP: retinopathy of prematurity)

and management. Wide-angle imaging systems like the RetCam have revolutionized the way we screen and follow-up cases of ROP, and with development of cheaper and portable cameras, community ROP telescreening models will soon become common. Artificial intelligence and deep learning are rapidly integrating with these tools to improve predictability of development of severe ROP and treatment outcomes.[25] Prediction algorithmic models like WINROP are getting better to predict the occurrence of severe ROP even before it develops.[26] Newer diagnostic imaging tools like fluorescein angiography UBM, ultrasound, and OCT help in better understanding of ROP, leading to optimized management strategies and better outcomes. There is an urgent need to spread awareness about ROP among ophthalmologists and neonatologists in developing countries for timely referral and management to prevent childhood blindness due to ROP.

REFERENCES

1. Kumar P, Sankar MJ, Deorari A, et al. Risk factors for severe retinopathy of prematurity in preterm low birth weight neonates. Indian J Pediatr. 2011;78(7):812-6.
2. Blencowe H, Lawn JE, Vazquez T, et al. Preterm-associated visual impairment and estimates of retinopathy of prematurity at regional and global levels for 2010. Pediatr Res. 2013;74 (Suppl 1):35-49.
3. Cryotherapy for Retinopathy of Prematurity Cooperative Group. Multicenter trial of cryotherapy for retinopathy of prematurity: ophthalmological outcomes at 10 years. Arch Ophthalmol. 2001;119(8):1110-8.
4. Good WV; Early Treatment for Retinopathy of Prematurity Cooperative Group. Final results of the Early Treatment for Retinopathy of Prematurity (ETROP) randomized trial. Trans Am Ophthalmol Soc. 2004;102:233-50.
5. An international classification of retinopathy of prematurity. The Committee for the Classification of Retinopathy of Prematurity. Arch Ophthalmol. 1984;102(8):1130-4.
6. International Committee for the Classification of Retinopathy of Prematurity. The International Classification of Retinopathy of Prematurity revisited. Arch Ophthalmol. 2005;123(7):991-9.
7. Fierson WM; American Academy of Pediatrics Section on Ophthalmology; American Academy of Ophthalmology; American Association for Pediatric Ophthalmology and Strabismus; American Association of Certified Orthoptists. Screening examination of premature infants for retinopathy of prematurity. Pediatrics. 2013;131(1):189-95.
8. Vinekar A, Dogra MR, Sangtam T, et al. Retinopathy of prematurity in Asian Indian babies weighing greater than 1250 grams at birth: Ten year data from a tertiary care center in a developing country. Indian J Ophthalmol. 2007;55(5):331-6.
9. Guidelines for Universal Eye Screening in Newborns Including Retinopathy of Prematurity. Rashtriya Bal Swasthya Karyakram. [online] Available from: https://www.nhm.gov.in/images/pdf/programmes/RBSK/Resource_Documents/Revised_ROP_Guidelines-Web_Optimized.pdf [Last accessed February, 2021].
10. Sankar MJ, Sankar J, Chandra P. Anti-vascular endothelial growth factor (VEGF) drugs for treatment of retinopathy of prematurity. Cochrane Database Syst Rev. 2018;1:CD009734.
11. Chandra P, Kumawat D, Tewari R, et al. Surgical outcomes of immediate sequential bilateral vitreoretinal surgery for advancing retinopathy of prematurity. Indian J Ophthalmol. 2019;67(6):903-7.
12. Gopal L, Sharma T, Shanmugam M, et al. Surgery for stage 5 retinopathy of prematurity: the learning curve and evolving technique. Indian J Ophthalmol. 2000;48(2):101-6.
13. Wang SK, Callaway NF, Wallenstein MB, et al. SUNDROP: Six years of screening for retinopathy of prematurity with telemedicine. Can J Ophthalmol. 2015;50(2):101-6.

14. Vinekar A, Jayadev C, Mangalesh S, et al. Role of tele-medicine in retinopathy of prematurity screening in rural outreach centers in India: a report of 20,214 imaging sessions in the KIDROP program. Semin Fetal Neonatal Med. 2015;20(5): 335-45.
15. Patel CK, Fung TH, Muqit MM, et al. Non-contact ultra-wide field imaging of retinopathy of prematurity using the Optos dual wavelength scanning laser ophthalmoscope. Eye (Lond). 2013;27(5):589-96.
16. Gilbert C, Wormald R, Fielder A, et al. Potential for a paradigm change in the detection of retinopathy of prematurity requiring treatment. Arch Dis Child Fetal Neonatal Ed. 2016; 101(1):6-9.
17. Azad R, Chandra P, Khan MA, et al. Role of intravenous fluorescein angiography in early detection and regression of retinopathy of prematurity. J Pediatr Ophthalmol Strabismus. 2008;45(1):36-9.
18. Lepore D, Molle F, Pagliara MM, et al. Atlas of fluorescein angiographic findings in eyes undergoing laser for retinopathy of prematurity. Ophthalmology. 2011;118(1):168-75.
19. Azad R, Mannan R, Chandra P. Role of ultrasound biomicroscopy in management of eyes with stage 5 retinopathy of prematurity. Ophthalmic Surg Lasers Imaging. 2010;41(2): 196-200.
20. Muslubas IS, Karacorlu M, Hocaoglu M, et al. Ultrasonography findings in eyes with stage 5 retinopathy of prematurity. Ophthalmic Surg Lasers Imaging Retina. 2015;46(10): 1035-40.
21. Erol MK, Coban DT, Ozdemir O, et al. Choroidal thickness in infants with retinopathy of prematurity. Retina. 2016; 36(6):1191-8.
22. Erol MK, Ozdemir O, Turgut Coban D, et al. Macular findings obtained by spectral domain optical coherence tomography in retinopathy of prematurity. J Ophthalmol. 2014;2014: 468653.
23. Park KA, Oh SY. Analysis of spectral-domain optical coherence tomography in preterm children: retinal layer thickness and choroidal thickness profiles. Invest Ophthalmol Vis Sci. 2012;53(11):7201-7.
24. Moshiri Y, Legocki AT, Zhou K, et al. Handheld swept-source optical coherence tomography with angiography in awake premature neonates. Quant Imaging Med Surg. 2019;9(9): 1495-502.
25. Gupta K, Campbell JP, Taylor S, et al. Imaging and informatics in retinopathy of prematurity consortium: a quantitative severity scale for retinopathy of prematurity using deep learning to monitor disease regression after treatment. JAMA Ophthalmol. 2019;137(9):1029-36.
26. Sanghi G, Narang A, Narula S, et al. WINROP algorithm for prediction of sight-threatening retinopathy of prematurity: initial experience in Indian preterm infants. Indian J Ophthalmol. 2018;66(1):110-3.

CHAPTER

29 Localization of Intraocular Foreign Body

Lingam Gopal, Su Xinyi

INTRODUCTION

Intraocular foreign body (IOFB) refers to unintended presence of foreign material in the eye that has gained access to the interior of the eye. In contrast, deliberate introduction of foreign material into the eye is often performed with therapeutic intent. These include: (1) Intraocular lens (IOL); (2) Slow-release devices such as fluocinolone acetonide (Iluvien) which leaves behind permanent residues in the vitreous cavity; (3) Implanted refillable reservoirs for intermittent injection of anti-vascular endothelial growth factor (anti-VEGF) agents as in "port delivery system" being developed by Roche. Unintended IOFBs are associated with penetrating injury to the globe and hence more commonly seen in younger age group[1] and in manual workers. About 18–41% of all open globe injuries are associated with IOFB in various studies.[2]

The most common type of injury associated with IOFB is metal-on-metal injury exemplified by hammering activity (60–80%).[3-5] Power machine tools contribute to 18–25% of IOFBs and weapon-related injuries contribute to about 19%. About 70–90% of IOFBs are metallic and 80% of these are magnetic. This has a significant bearing on the management and the ease with which the foreign body (FB) can be extracted from the eye.

This chapter deals with suspecting and localizing of the IOFB. It does not cover the management of IOFB.

TYPES OF INTRAOCULAR FOREIGN BODIES

Intraocular foreign bodies can be metallic or nonmetallic. Metals can be magnetic or nonmagnetic. Although nickel and cobalt are also magnetic in addition to iron, in the circumstances of ocular injuries, it is iron and its alloys that are important. Among the nonmagnetic metallic IOFBs, lead FBs seen in bullets are important. Brass and other metals can be seen in explosive injuries such as bomb blasts. Common nonmetallic IOFBs include wood, vegetable matter (thorns of plants), plastic, glass, etc.

CIRCUMSTANCES OF INJURY

The circumstances of injury often throw light on the type of IOFB that is likely to be encountered. Work-related trauma is often associated with metallic (mostly iron) FB. This is especially true of injuries caused while using hammer and chisel. Injuries caused by blast injuries can produce miscellaneous varieties of FB in the eye including gravel, metal, etc. Injuries in the rural setup are often caused by thorns and plant twigs and often associated with endophthalmitis, especially of fungal origin. Glass FB is often associated with vehicular accidents where in the pieces of windscreen or spectacle glass can find their way into the eye.[6]

IMPORTANCE OF FOREIGN BODY IN OVERALL MANAGEMENT OF THE EYE

Presence of FB complicates the management of an injured eye. In addition to the damage caused by the injury and passage of the FB into the eye, the physical presence of FB can cause further damage to the structures of the eye—physically as well as due to the nature of the FB. Metals such as iron and copper are associated with liberation of the ions that incite toxic reaction acutely (with copper) or chronically (with iron). The FB can take with it a bolus of infective organisms that can incite acute or chronic intraocular infection.

Hence, removal of IOFB is important in the overall management of the eye. However, there could be circumstances when FBs are left behind if they are considered inert and not causing physical trauma to the sensitive structures. Inert FBs include glass of certain varieties (not photochromatic glass), gold, etc.

Considering the importance of removal of IOFB in the overall management of the traumatized eye, suspecting its presence is the first step before attempts are made to localize the FB. The type of injury often provides the first clue. Work related injuries should always be evaluated for possibility of IOFB.

LOCALIZATION OF INTRAOCULAR FOREIGN BODY

The fundamental prerequisite to removal of IOFB is its localization in relation to the anatomy of the eye. Physical examination aided by appropriate investigations help the clinician in identifying the presence of IOFB, its location and possibly its nature.

Direct Examination

Foreign bodies may be detectable by direct techniques of ocular examination. This presupposes sufficient clarity of media to permit visualization of the FB.

Slit-lamp Examination

Cornea: Foreign bodies on the cornea and in anterior chamber are often detectable by slit-lamp examination. The location of the corneal scar often guides the surgeon to the possible location of FB. A small glass piece lying in the inferior angle of the eye can be missed even after a careful examination. Localized corneal edema at 6 o'clock position can be the first clue to this possibility. Large corneal wounds are associated with correspondingly large IOFBs or no IOFB (if the injuring agent has lacerated the cornea but dropped out or was plucked out).

One should understand that the size of the corneal scar does not always correspond to the actual size of the IOFB. The elastic stretch of the cornea at time of impact enables a FB to enter the eye through a corneal wound that ultimately appears smaller.

Iris

Presence of iris hole is a very important clue to the presence of the IOFB. The relationship between the location of the iris hole and the corneal scar also indicates the direction in which the FB was traveling and the quadrant of fundus where it is likely to be present. However, on occasions, iris hole can be hidden under a dense arcus senilis.

Presence of siderosis bulbi may be evident on slit-lamp examination of the iris and lens. The rusty brownish hue is striking.

Lens

On occasions the tell-tale track of the FB may be evident in the lens. However, in most cases lens opacity rapidly becomes total. Intactness of posterior capsule can be assessed sometime clinically and if this is not possible by slit-lamp examination, ultrasound evaluation is recommended. If the vitreous is perceived to be clear and the posterior capsule is intact despite lens injury, one can presume that the FB is located in the anterior segment. On occasions, FB can traverse across the zonule of the lens without disrupting the lens. Hence, corneal wound with presence of intact posterior capsule does not necessarily exclude the possibility of posterior segment FB. Intralenticular FB can be obvious on slit-lamp examination provided the lens fibers anterior to the FB are clear. Intralenticular FBs can be surprisingly tolerated for a long time without reaction.[7,8]

Caveats

- Glass IOFB in anterior chamber can be particularly difficult to see even on slit-lamp examination.
- Gonioscopy may be the only way to identify a small FB in the angle.
- Foreign body located in the ciliary body area is difficult to identify by both slit-lamp evaluation and fundus examination.

Fundus Examination

The importance of evaluation of fundus using indirect ophthalmoscopy cannot be overemphasized. Since the injury is likely to produce vitreous hemorrhage and vitritis, the visualization of fundus details may deteriorate very rapidly. Therefore, the initial fundus examination should be as thorough as possible. The documentation of fundus findings made by the first examiner is often valuable for the subsequent ophthalmologist who may be called upon to manage the case. Binocular indirect ophthalmoscopy with scleral indentation may detect IOFB **(Fig. 1)**, if the media are clear enough. In delayed cases, the IOFB may be surrounded by fibrous capsule and could be missed. In case of iron FBs that are present on the retina for significant period of time, one may find tell-tale signs

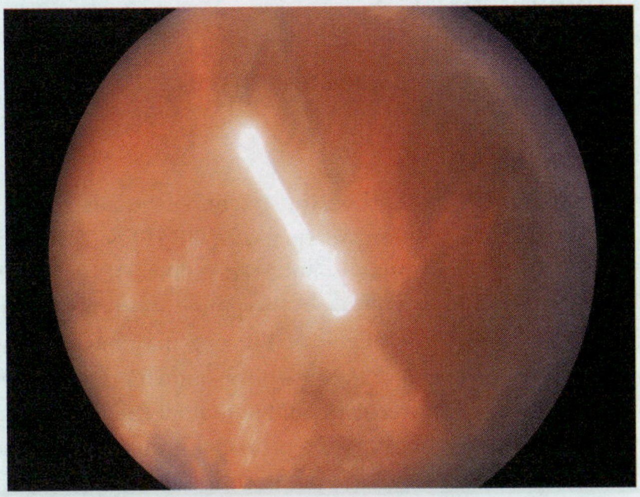

Fig. 1: A large metal foreign body on the retina.

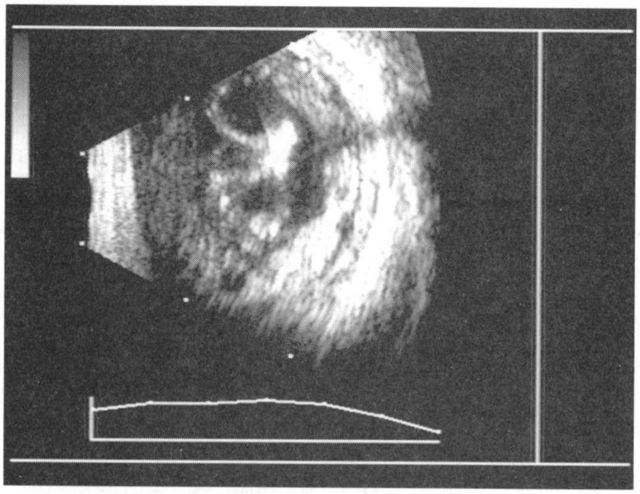

Fig. 2: Ultrasound B-scan showing metallic IOFB near the retinal surface.
(IOFB: intraocular foreign body)

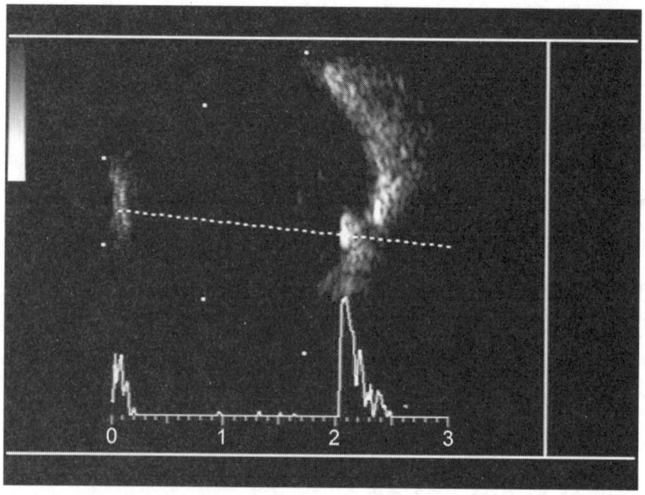

Fig. 3: Ultrasound B-scan showing large piece of metallic IOFB with orbital shadowing.

of localized siderosis bulbi. Even large glass pieces may evade clinical detection with ophthalmoscopy, if they are embedded in the peripheral opaque vitreous (hemorrhage/ exudates).

Signs in the Fundus that may Facilitate Localization of Foreign Body

Vitreous track formed by blood may point to the location of FB.

Intraretinal hemorrhage may indicate the site of impaction of FB. On occasion, the FB may hit the retina and ricochet to another location or fall down to the inferior periphery. Therefore, inferior periphery should be inspected carefully if FB is not located at the site of retinal hemorrhage. Signs of double perforation of globe indicate the presence of FB in the ocular coats posteriorly or even behind the eye in the orbit.

Investigational Aids to Localize Intraocular Foreign Body

Studies have shown that <45.6% of IOFBs are detected clinically while CT scan can detect up to 94.9%.[9]

Ultrasonography

A combined B-scan and vector A-scan is the easiest way of evaluating the eye for presence of IOFB (**Figs. 2 and 3**). A 10-MHz probe is routinely employed. A 20-MHz probe can give higher resolution but lacks the penetration of 10-MHz probe. For anteriorly located IOFB, one may have to use immersion scan or standoff, or use ultrasound biomicroscopy (UBM). Since the injured eye could potentially have a wound that can open on pressure, the ultrasonography should be done very gently. For the same reason, ultrasonography is done over closed lids.[10] Where it is felt that performance of ultrasonography could be damaging, it is best to depend entirely on radiological evaluation.

Features

Foreign bodies are characterized by a high echogenicity. They are seen as dense white spots on grayscale display and persist even at low gain. It is important to lower the gain to detect the FBs against the backdrop of multiple echogenic structures in an injured eye. Depending on the size, reverberating echoes may also be seen. Metal and stone have a high echogenicity, more than any other normal structure except bone. Echoes from wood and vegetable matters are only of intermediate amplitude.

Caveats

- Very large FBs can cause shadowing and can be surprisingly difficult to infer on their characteristics on ultrasonography.
- *Reverberation artifacts*: The movement back and forth of the ultrasound beam between two parallel surfaces can result in multiple echoes one behind the other but equally spaced. If the reverberating echoes are very closely spaced, it produces a near continuous echogenic streak that appears posterior to the FB (comet-tail or ring down artifact).[11]
- Linear glass FBs can sometimes produce misleadingly low amplitude echoes due to the ultrasound beam not being perpendicular to the surface of the FB.
- *Foreign bodies in the eye wall/close to eye wall*: It may be difficult to be certain whether the FB is closer to the vitreous cavity or scleral surface. The shadowing caused by the FB can also make it difficult to assess the integrity of the coats of eyeball.
- Very anteriorly located FBs can be missed by routine ultrasonography and would need UBM (see below).

- Small FBs entrapped in dense vitreous hemorrhage can be missed by routine ultrasonography as is often seen in blast injuries.
- Air bubble in the vitreous cavity can mimic IOFB due to the high reflectivity. However, air tends to float in the vitreous cavity and hence is located in the nondependent position.
- Multiple FBs can present bizarre echo patterns. FB with irregular surface can give the impression of multiple FBs.
- Degradation of FB with time can make it difficult to detect the FB when patient presents late. Even in eyes with frank siderosis bulbi, one may find no FB to remove, since it has completely degraded with time.

In addition to the identification of FB, ultrasonography serves as an important tool to evaluate the collateral damage to the structures of the eye. One should look for the presence or absence of choroidal detachment (hemorrhagic or serous), retinal detachment, and vitreous detachment. Vitreous incarceration in the posterior coat of the eye indicates possible site of double perforation.

Ultrasound biomicroscopy

Using a 50-MHz probe, the resolution is increased but at the expense of depth of penetrance. FBs located in the anterior segment and in ciliary body/pars plana area are easily detectable. Since the investigation can only be done in contact with the globe, it is obviously contraindicated in eyes with open globes or precariously approximated wounds. IOFB such as caterpillar hair can only be picked up with UBM.[12]

Radiological Investigations

By far, radiological investigations give the best tool for identifying the presence of IOFB as well as to localize it. Plain X-ray evaluation along with aids such as limbal rings, opaque contact lenses, and Sweet's method[13] have been pushed to the status of historical methods, with the advent of computerized tomography and magnetic resonance imaging (MRI).

Computer tomographic scan: The advantages of computerized tomography (CT) scan evaluation are that:

- It is noninvasive to the eye and hence safe in an open globe situation.
- It enables evaluation of entire eyeball and orbit.
- Multiple FBs can also be detected easily.
- The location of the FB vis-à-vis the coats of the eye is better delineated.
- Associated damage to orbital structures and brain can also be detected.
- Presence of suspected magnetic foreign bodies is not a contraindication.

Chacko et al. have identified that there is 100% detection by CT scan if the FB is larger than 0.06 mm^3.[14] CT scans are however, notorious for missing nonmetallic FBs—especially wooden FBs. **Figures 4 to 6** illustrate examples of CT scan with IOFBs.

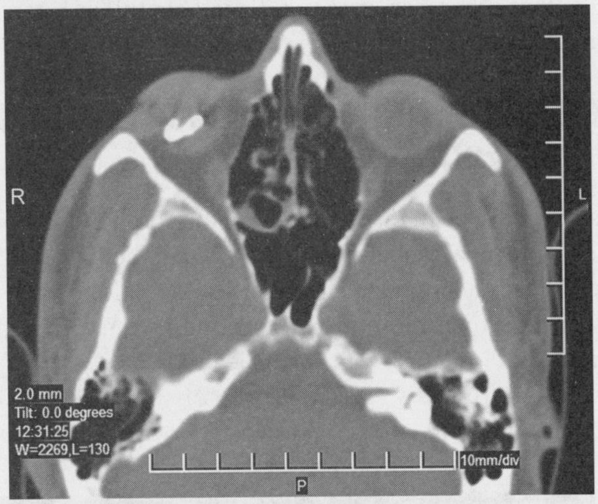

Fig. 4: CT scan showing a piece of metallic wire within the vitreous cavity.

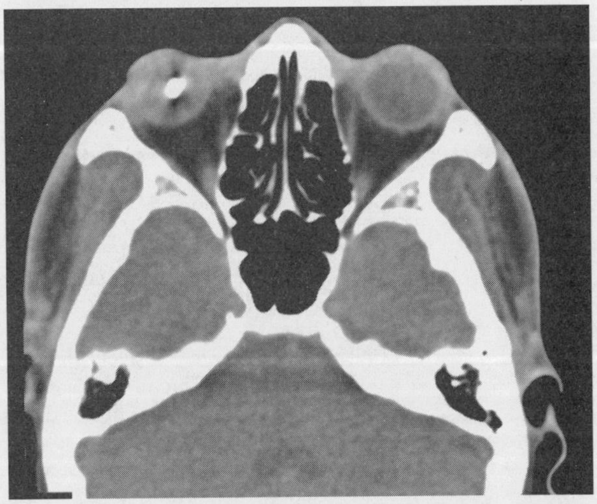

Fig. 5: CT scan showing metallic IOFB within mid-vitreous cavity.

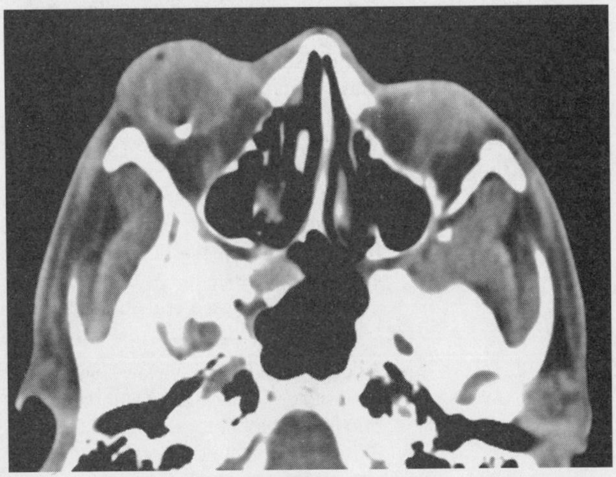

Fig. 6: CT scan showing a metallic IOFB within the ocular coats with retinal detachment.

Magnetic resonance imaging: In general, one avoids using MRI in the milieu of suspected IOFB for fear of inducing movement of a potentially magnetic IOFB that can cause additional trauma to the structures of the eye.[15] However, Zhang et al. have used MRI to detect tiny ferromagnetic IOFBs that otherwise were not detectable (plain X-ray/CT scan/ultrasonography).[16]

DIFFERENTIATING THE CHARACTERISTICS OF IOFBS WITH IMAGING

Attempts have been made to identify the composition of the FB using its imaging characteristics. Modjtahedi et al. have investigated the imaging characteristics of various types of FBs by inserting them into enucleated eyes and imaging them.[17] **Table 1** details some of the features.

Similar studies were done by Moisseiev et al. using CT scan and MRI and a wide variety of potential IOFB materials.[18] They could detect more materials by MRI compared to CT scan. The apparent size on MRI was increased (magnification) by a factor of about 1.5 with substances such as bottle glass, windshield glass, porcelain, gravel stone, concrete, thorn and graphite, while plastic, spectacle plastic, and wood had a minification.

These authors have derived an algorithm for identifying the material of FB based on the imaging characteristics on CT scan and MRI for nonmagnetic objects.[19]

Table 1: Characteristics of IOFBs with imaging.

Sr no.	*Imaging tool*	*Features*
1.	Plain X-ray	• All metallic FBs, windshield glass, bottle glass, and slate are radiopaque and nondistinguishable from each other • Aluminum is moderately radiopaque • PVC is minimally radiopaque • Dry and wet wood and spectacle plastic are not detected
2.	Ultrasound	• Spectacle plastic less echogenic than surrounding retina/choroid • Other FBs have higher echogenicity than surrounding choroid/retina but to various degrees • All metallic FBs and windshield glass have ring down artifacts; broad (headlight type) in case of lead and windshield glass and narrow (flash-light type) in case of aluminum with others falling in between • No ring down artifact with wood, PVC and spectacle plastic
3.	CT scan	• Bottle glass, windshield glass, PVC, slate, and aluminum were high density objects without surrounding artifact • Brass, copper, and steel show high-density and shadow artifact • Wet and dry wood show low attenuation and no scatter artifact • Metals except aluminum had attenuation coefficient of >3,000 Hounsfield units (HU) • PVC and spectacle plastic have attenuation coefficient of 484 and 123 HU respectively • Wood has negative attenuation coefficient (–102 to –371 HU)
4.	MRI	• All nonmetallic FBs have low signal intensity on T1 and T2, surrounded by a thin film of high intensity • Blooming artifact was more pronounced with slate and windshield glass

(CT: computed tomography; FBs: foreign bodies; MRI: magnetic resonance imaging; PVC: polyvinyl chloride)

The summary of the algorithm is as follows (for nonmetallic objects):

- If FB is detected on CT scan and T1/T2 MRI shows signal void—it is more likely to be glass material. The shape is likely to be smoother with bottle glass and irregular in case of windshield glass.
- If FB is detected on CT scan and T1/T2 MRI shows signal void with hyperintense rim around—it is more likely to be stone material.
- If FB is not detected on CT scan and T1/T2 MRI shows signal void—it is likely to be plastic/spectacle plastic.
- If FB is not detected on CT scan and T1/T2 MRI has signal void with hyperintense rim around—it is likely to be wood material.

INTRAOPERATIVE LOCALIZATION

Most FBs can be easily identified during vitreoretinal surgery, once the medial opacities are cleared. However, there are occasions when the identification of the FB intraoperatively can pose issues.

Associated endophthalmitis: In the presence of extensive vitreous exudation, the FB can be hidden in the peripheral opaque vitreous. Since aggressive vitrectomy can increase the risk of retinal tears in an edematous retina, one has to be selective in debulking the vitreous in the quadrants, where it is expected to be present (based on the preoperative evaluation). In cases of magnetic FB, placement of the intraocular magnet can sometimes retrieve the hidden FB.

Foreign body covered by capsule: It is surprising how quickly a capsule can form around the FB hiding its true colors. If the FB is magnetic, placement of intraocular magnet over the capsule will show some movement beneath. If the FB is buried in the ocular coats, the movement is not elicitable. Careful incision on the capsule should expose the internal end of the FB.

Foreign body deeply embedded in eye wall but not outside the eye: On occasion, one finds that the FB is deeply embedded in the eye wall when it makes it easier to deliver it externally rather than tear it through the tissues/fibrosis that are overlying the FB. Here precise localization of the FB is done on the sclera using indirect ophthalmoscopy (similar to how a retinal break is localized during repair of retinal detachments). A cut-down performed in this area should expose the FB for its external removal.

Foreign body that is mostly outside the eye after double perforation: Since the FB is attached to the eye wall, CT and ultrasonography may not clearly delineate how much of the FB is inside the eye. On occasion, one finds that most of FB has gone outside the eye and only a small part is lodged in the deepest of the choroid and scleral layers. Very often the site of posterior perforation is covered by clot/fibrosis depending on the duration. Deep exploration of the wound may not yield the FB. It is best in such cases to plug the sclerotomies and explore the orbit in the corresponding quadrant. The extraocular portion is also not always easily identified, since this is also covered by inflammatory fibrous capsule. Careful dissection aided if necessary, by disinsertion of the extraocular muscle can expose the FB.

Foreign body in the ciliary body: Foreign body that entered the eye through the sclera beyond the limbus can sometimes lodge itself in the ciliary body, if the velocity was not enough to carry it inside the eye. Very often placement of external magnet over the site of scleral perforation can bring the FB out. The exit can be aided by slightly enlarging the scleral wound.

REFERENCES

1. Punnonen E, Laatikainen L. Prognosis of perforating eye injuries with intraocular foreign bodies. Acta Ophthalmol (Copenh). 1989;67(5):483-91.
2. Shock JP, Adams D. Long-term visual acuity results after penetrating and perforating injuries. Am J Ophthalmol. 1985;100(5):714-8.
3. Roper-Hall MJ. Review of 555 cases of intra-ocular foreign body with special reference to prognosis. Br J Ophthalmol. 1954;38(2):65-99.
4. Williams DF, Mieler WF, Abrams GW, et al. Results and prognostic factors in penetrating ocular injuries with retained intraocular foreign bodies. Ophthalmology. 1988;95(7): 911-6.
5. Percival SP. A decade of intraocular foreign bodies. Br J Ophthalmol. 1972;56(6):454-61.
6. Gopal L, Banker AS, Deb N, et al. Management of glass intraocular foreign bodies. Retina. 1998;18(3):213-20.
7. Chang YS, Jeong YC, Ko BY. A case of an asymptomatic intralenticular foreign body. Korean J Ophthalmol. 2008;22(4):272-5.
8. Dubey D, Karkhur S, Sen A. Retained gold intralenticular foreign body. Indian J Ophthalmol. 2019;67(8):1341.
9. Patel SN, Langer PD, Zarbin MA, et al. Diagnostic value of clinical examination and radiographic imaging in identification of intraocular foreign bodies in open globe injury. Eur J Ophthalmol. 2012;22:259-68.
10. Bhende M, Gopal S, Gogi A, Sharma T, Gopal L, Gopal L, Sen P, Menon S (Eds). The Sankara Nethralaya: Atlas of Ophthalmic Ultrasound. New Delhi: Jaypee Brothers Medical Publishers; 2006. pp. 61-8.
11. Feldman MK, Katyal S, Blackwood MS. US artifacts. Radiographics. 2009;29:1179-89.
12. Bhende M, Biswas J, Sharma T, et al. Ultrasound biomicroscopy in the diagnosis and management of pars planitis caused by caterpillar hairs. Am J Ophthalmol. 2000;130(1):125-6.
13. Duke-Elder S. Mechanical Injuries: Intraocular Foreign Bodies. In: Duke-Elder S (Ed). System of Ophthalmology. London: Henry Kimpton; 1972. pp. 570-611.
14. Chacko JG, Figueroa RE, Johnson MH, et al. Detection and localization of steel intraocular foreign bodies using computed tomography. A comparison of helical and conventional axial scanning. Ophthalmology. 1997;104(2):319-23.
15. Ta CN, Bowman RW. Hyphema caused by a metallic intraocular foreign body during magnetic resonance imaging. AM J Ophthalmol. 2000;129(4):533-4.
16. Zhang Y, Cheng J, Bai J, et al. Tiny ferromagnetic intraocular foreign bodies detected by magnetic resonance imaging: a report of two cases. J Magn Reson Imaging. 2009;29:704-7.
17. Modjtahedi BS, Rong A, Bobinski M, et al. Imaging characteristics of intraocular foreign bodies: a comparative study of plain film X-ray, computed tomography, ultrasound, and magnetic resonance imaging. Retina. 2015;35(1):95-104.
18. Moisseiev E, Last D, Goez D, et al. Magnetic resonance imaging and computed tomography for the detection and characterization of non-metallic intraocular foreign bodies. Retina. 2015;35(1):82-94.
19. Moisseiev E, Barequet D, Zunz E, et al. Validation of an algorithm for nonmetallic intraocular foreign bodies' composition identification based on computed tomography and magnetic resonance imaging. Retina. 2015;35(9): 1898-904.

CHAPTER

30 Concomitant Strabismus: Diagnostic Methods

Digvijay Singh, Harinder Singh Sethi, Pradeep Sharma

INTRODUCTION

Terms strabismus and squint are in use synonymously. Strabismus is often a perplexing case for the general ophthalmology practitioner. If the amount of deviation is equal in all gazes (absence of motility limitation), the strabismus is classified as concomitant; with unequal deviation, it is called an incomitant squint. Most of the cases of strabismus can be clearly distinguished as either of the two; there are some cases of overlap. Long-standing concomitant squints can turn incomitant while incomitant squints may develop spread of comitance. A careful history and examination can differentiate these two scenarios. This chapter focuses on the workup and diagnosis of a case of concomitant strabismus.

Features of Concomitant Strabismus

Cases of concomitant strabismus present following characteristic features:

- Onset in early childhood though not present at birth ("often labeled as infantile")
- Absence of diplopia (except acute concomitant esotropia or a manifest intermittent exotropia)
- Normal ocular motility (no limitation)
- Constant angle between axes of the eyes in all directions of gaze
- Both eyes have full movements, if tested monocularly (sometimes a pseudolimitation seen on testing binocularly).

Terminology and Notation in Concomitant Strabismus

- *Convergent strabismus:*
  - Latent—esophoria (E)
  - Manifest constant—esotropia (ET)
  - Manifest intermittent—esotropia [E(T)]
- *Divergent strabismus:*
  - Latent—exophoria (X)
  - Manifest constant—exotropia (XT)
  - Manifest intermittent—[X(T)]
- *Vertical strabismus:*
  - If right eye higher—right hypertropia (RHT)
  - If left eye higher—left hypertropia (LHT)
- *Patterned strabismus—vertically incomitant horizontally comitant strabismus:*
  - A esotropia or exotropia
  - V esotropia or exotropia
  - X, Y or lambda (λ).

DIAGNOSTIC METHODS[1,2]

History Taking

Clinical history is an integral part of a strabismus workup. The clinician needs to enquire about which eye mostly deviates, the onset of deviation, precipitating factor, duration, whether the strabismus is constant or variable, and presence of any additional complaint such as asthenopia or diplopia. History of any previous surgical intervention or other therapy should be taken as well.

In concomitant esotropias, typically the strabismus is present since early childhood (usually from 4 months to 6 months of age in infantile esotropia) and has a fixed large angle in the absence of diplopia. If one eye is constantly deviated inward then amblyopia may develop over time.

Exotropias usually develop at a later age and are often associated with a precipitating event such as an illness or trauma. The patient has a fixed (but sometimes increasing) angle of deviation, which may be intermittent or constant and almost never associated with strabismic amblyopia.

The concomitant strabismus may be congenital but is more often of sudden onset at an adult age, and may show

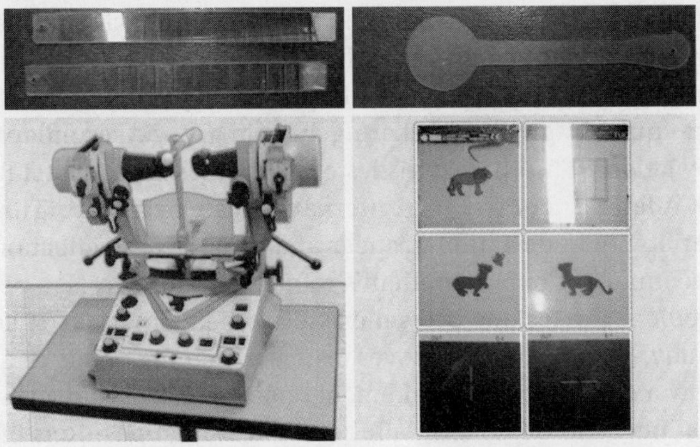

Fig. 1: Essential equipment needed for the diagnosis of strabismus. Clockwise from left top: Prism bars, Spielman occlude, synoptophore, and synoptophore slides.

slow improvement or worsening and often have associated diplopia.

A detailed history directs ophthalmologist toward the nature of the strabismus and helps decide the examination and investigations.

Essential Equipment

The examination of strabismus requires some essential equipment **(Fig. 1)**. These include prism bars [horizontal and vertical prism bars and loose prisms set (at least 30Δ and 45Δ)], an occluder, fixation targets (for distance and near to control the accommodation as desired), refraction trial set with prisms of 1–8Δ, Bagolini striated glasses, red and green goggles, double Maddox rod set, Snellen chart with letters and E in rows and also a single letter E chart, protractor with a foot ruler, ophthalmoscope, stereotest (Randot or TNO).

Examination

A case of strabismus requires examination of:
- The motor status
- The sensory status.

Examination of Motor Status

The examination of the motor status entails looking for:
- Head posture
- Ocular deviation
- Limitation of movements or the extent of the versions
- Fusional vergences.

Head Posture

Observation of head posture starts at the first glance of the patient, as he enters the clinic. He must not be made conscious of the keen observation since much of information is lost after the patient becomes conscious and corrects his head posture. Head posture has three components:
1. Chin elevation or depression (vertical)
2. Face turn to right or left side (horizontal)
3. Head tilt to right or left shoulder (torsional).

Head posture may be quantified in terms of degrees by using a cephalometer or a protractor with foot ruler. This is important as it may help in the surgical decision.[3]

Measurement of Interpupillary Distance

Interpupillary distance (IPD) is the distance between pupils of the two eyes. A narrow IPD simulates and accentuates esotropia and may predispose to it. A wide IPD gives an impression of exotropia but it is also a common feature of this type of deviation. IPD can be measured either by an ordinary millimeter rule or by using the Pulzone-Hardy rule or by using the synoptophore.

Ocular Deviation

The examination of ocular deviation is the most important aspect of strabismus examination because it not only establishes squint but also quantifies it. Further, it is very important to differentiate the true from the apparent squint (pseudosquint).

QUALITATIVE TESTS

Detection of Strabismus

A cover-uncover test is required to confirm the diagnosis of squint and to differentiate it from pseudostrabismus. It is necessary to perform this test when the corneal reflections are unequal, or if the history suggests a squint. It is an objective test, which is a cornerstone of the strabismus diagnosis and management. It has two components, cover and uncover, each of which requires separate observations and provides different information.

A cover test requires a central fixation and an accommodative target. The target may be a figure or letter of size 6/9 of Snellen chart for distance. This is to control the accommodation and prevent any false deviation. A fixation achieved by a torchlight is not desirable. Lang fixation stick that has very small figures is very useful for young children and reduced Snellen letters or numbers are ideal for the adults and older children for near and distance testing. The subject is asked to fixate on the target at the requisite distance and an observation is made. The examiner notes whether both eyes appear to fixate (no apparent squint) or one appears to fixate as the other deviates (apparent squint).

- *The cover test* (observation made during covering): The next step is to cover the apparently fixating eye and observe what happens to the other (apparently deviating) eye. If that moves to take up fixation, it confirms the presence of a manifest or true strabismus (heterotropia). However, if both the eyes appear to fixate in the first instance, the examiner attempts to cover either of the eyes to observe the behavior of the contralateral eye. If it moves, it implies a heterotropia—it would imply a true squint masked by appearance.

- *The uncover test (observations made during uncovering)*: The second part, uncover, is helpful in unmasking the latent strabismus (heterophoria) which presents with both eyes appearing to fixate the target. One of the eyes is covered, which breaks the fusion, and if there is any heterophoria (tendency for squint) the eye behind cover deviates (in/out/up/down). The examiner then observes the behavior of this eye as he removes the cover. If it remains deviated it confirms a latent squint with poor fusion (poor recovery) and if it recovers, the examiner observes the speed of recovery. The speed of recovery indicates the strength of fusion and is an important prognostic sign.

Another observation can be that on uncovering the eye, the uncovered eye reassumed fixation as the other eye deviates. This indicates the presence of a strabismus with the "uncovered" eye being dominant. This also indicates that the visual acuity is probably unequal in the two eyes. A free alternation of fixation between the two eyes indicates equal vision in the two eyes. The correction of a ptosis of a hypotropic eye, when this eye fixates implies that it is a pseudoptosis.

Alternate Cover Test

In the alternate cover test, the eyes are rapidly and alternately occluded from one eye to the other and then back again. Essentially, it is a repeated cover-uncover test for both the eyes alternately. This procedure causes breakdown of the binocular fusion mechanism and will reveal refixation movements of each eye at the moment of uncovering. The cover-uncover test is less dissociating than alternate cover test. In the absence of a manifest strabismus, such a strabismus implies a latent squint. The test can be combined with a prism bar for the prism bar cover test.

Prerequisites of Cover–Uncover Test

The cover-uncover test requires the following prerequisites:

- Ability of both eyes to fixate the target
- Ability of both eyes to have central fixation
- Ability of both eyes to have no gross/severe motility defect.

Thus, in the presence of one eye being blind or having markedly subnormal vision or a severe limitation of movement or an eccentric fixation, all of which may prevent refixation, and the cover-uncover test may be fallacious. For infants who would not allow an occluder or a hand close to their face, the examiner can use indirect occlusion test or distant cover test. Here the fixation light or target is obstructed for one eye by an occluder at some distance away from the child.

Both the cover-uncover test and the alternate cover test provide valuable information to the ophthalmologist. The test helps to confirm a true manifest or latent strabismus along with its type such as exodeviation, esodeviation, or vertical deviations. It also indicates the visual dominance or the presence of amblyopia. It also identifies comitance of the squint by grossly comparing the primary and secondary deviations. The characteristics of strabismus like unilateral or bilateral, constant or alternating can be noted. The variability in deviation for near and distance, the effect of accommodation and patient's refractive error can also be studied. The test uncovers the associated latent nystagmus, if any. A good cover-uncover test pays rich dividends and only a quantitative measurement remains. A cover-uncover test needs to be done in all the nine cardinal positions of gaze, as also for near and distance fixation. With experience, the examiner can detect even small angle squints with the exception of microtropia of less than 5Δ deviation.

QUANTITATIVE TESTS

Measurement of Ocular Deviation

Deviations can be measured by two methods—objective and subjective. Both require the cooperation of the patient, but in subjective tests, the patient's subjective response is also required. The objective tests depend on the observations by the examiner of the patient's fixation pattern. This is based on neutralizing the movement of the deviating eye as it takes up the fixation.

Prism Bar Cover Test

The simple and best way to measure deviation is by using prisms or prism bar along with the cover test known as prism bar cover test (PBCT). In fact, it is the cover-uncover with the addition of neutralization of deviation by the prisms.

For neutralizing esodeviations, prisms are placed base out and for exodeviations they are placed base in. A simple rule to remember is that the apex of the prism should point toward deviation. Thus, in a vertical deviation, base down prism is used in front of the hypertrophic eye. In combination of horizontal and vertical deviation, the prisms are placed horizontally in front of one eye and vertically in front of the other eye. For large deviations, a combination of loose prism of 30Δ or 45Δ in front of one eye and prism bar in front of the other eye can be used. The plastic prisms are placed in the frontal position, parallel to the infraorbital margin while the glass prisms are placed in the Prentice position, posterior face of the prism being perpendicular to the visual axis.

It may be reiterated that the fixation distance (both for near and distance), the fixation target (6/9 Snellen size for accommodative control), and proper dissociation of the two eyes should be ensured.

It is important to understand that the deviation to be measured is to be static deviation and should be free of the dynamic factors of accommodation and fusion. It is the static angle that requires surgical correction whereas the dynamic deviation of accommodation should be corrected by glasses.

Measurement of Deviations

To determine the various aspects of strabismus, deviations should be measured in following ways:

- Deviation with distance and near fixation should be determined with its nature such as esotropia—basic/convergence excess divergence insufficiency and exotropia—basic/convergence insufficiency/divergence excess.
- Deviation in nine different cardinal positions of gaze to determine any incomitance (paralytic, restrictive, or spastic element).
- Deviation in up gaze of 25° and down gaze of 35° for determining A-V patterns.
- Deviations with right and left eye fixating alternately to determine primary and secondary deviations in case of paralytic squint.
- Deviations with subjective method and objective method to determine the type of retinal correspondence (normal or anomalous).
- Deviations after prolonged cover to differentiate a true divergence excess type from the simulated divergence excess exotropia as also to determine the fully dissociated deviation.

Precautions for Prism Bar Cover Test

- It is essential to prevent fusion by continuous use of alternate cover test.
- It is essential to control accommodation by use of an accommodative target.
- A high-powered prism reduces the clarity of vision, often impairs fixation if placed in front of an amblyopic eye. Therefore, it should preferably be placed in front of a better eye.
- Children can cooperate for a short time only so it is preferable to start with approximately the correct prism rather than to work up from much lower strength.
- In cases with combined vertical and horizontal squint, it is preferable to use square prisms as they can be easily held together between thumb and the finger.

Synoptophore

Synoptophore is a basic orthoptic instrument based on the haploscopic principle. It is also known as amblyoscope (Major, Curpax-Major) and troposcope. It consists of a chin rest and forehead rest with two tubes carrying the targets seen through an angled eyepiece. The tubes are placed horizontally and are movable in the horizontal and vertical planes. The distance between the two tubes can also be adjusted with the subject's IPD. The targets in the tubes are illuminated slides, which can be raised up or down and be tilted to test for vertical and torsional deviations. All these adjustments can be read on the scales in degrees and prism diopters. The tubes can be locked individually or both with respect to each other. The illumination of each target can be increased or decreased and flashes can be given if desired. Additional devices like Haidinger brushes can be attached to synoptophore. The targets are placed at a fixed distance from the eyepiece which are of +6.0 D or +6.5 D, so that the targets are at optical infinity. This should theoretically not stimulate accommodation. However, in reality proximal convergence does come into play distorting the deviations. This factor has significantly reduced the applicability of the synoptophore as a reliable instrument to measure deviations, especially horizontal ones.

Uses of Synoptophore

In cyclovertical strabismus, the synoptophore is a useful instrument to measure torsion. It is also useful for studying accommodation-convergence relationship and for imparting orthoptic exercises.

The synoptiscope of Curpax-Major is a modification that uses semitransparent mirrors in place of opaque mirrors in front of eyes. This allows the subject to view a distant object superimposed on the targets in slide holders. The synoptometer (oculus) is a modification that allows measurement of deviations in peripheral positions with the help of mirrors.

Corneal Reflection Tests

If a light is shone on an orthophoric patient's eyes, the corneal reflex of both eyes falls at the center of the cornea and is symmetrical. However, in strabismic eyes, the reflex will fall at the center of the cornea of the fixing eyes but eccentrically on the cornea of the deviating eye. Strabismus can be roughly quantitated on the basis of the displacement of this corneal reflex from the center. Methods using corneal reflections give approximate values but are useful when PBCT cannot be done for young children, uncooperative patients and patients with poor vision or fixation. Deviations of less than 10Δ may not be measured by this test.

Hirschberg Test

The test estimates the deviation of corneal light reflex from the center of the pupil and provides a rough measurement of degree of strabismus. A light is shone simultaneously on both the eyes and the corneal light reflex is seen. The corneal reflections, even normally are not exactly centered because of angle kappa, but are symmetrical in the absence of a squint. The reflection is asymmetrical in cases of squint.

In case of esodeviation, the corneal reflection falls more temporally and in exodeviation, falls nasally. Roughly, a 1 mm shift signifies a 5° deviation (earlier thought to be 7°). Thus, if the reflex falls on the nasal pupillary margin it is 15° (30Δ) of squint while if it falls on the limbus, the exodeviation is 30° (approximately 60Δ). This test can be used in infants, who are not very cooperative or in cases of eccentric fixation or nonfixation (blind eyes).

Krimsky Test

In the Krimsky test (or prism reflex test), a prism bar is utilized to quantify the deviation with the aid of the corneal reflections. It is preferable to place the prism bar on the fixating eye and to increase or decrease the power of prisms, so that the light reflex gets centered in the deviating eye (nonfixating). The power of prism required indicates the amount of squint present.

Synoptophore

A foveal-sized slide is placed in front of the fixing eye and the position of the corneal reflections is noted whilst the amblyoscope tubes are at zero. The tube in front of the fixing eye is moved along the eye in such a way that reflection in the squinting eye moves into the normal position (comparable with that in other eye). The angle can be recorded in degree or prism diopter.

Subjective Tests of Deviation

These tests utilize the subject's perception of the deviation. When there is misalignment, the subject perceives diplopia and the separation between the two images indicates the subjective deviation. This is the diplopia principle. Here the single physical location is perceived by the subject as two perceptual localizations. Diplopia testing with the red-green goggles is based on this principle. Measurement of deviation on Maddox tangent scale with the help of Maddox rod is also based on it. Subjective tests can be performed on the haploscopic principle, where two "physical locations" are used to have one "perceptual localization." It can be tested subjectively on the Hess or Lees screen **(Fig. 2)**.

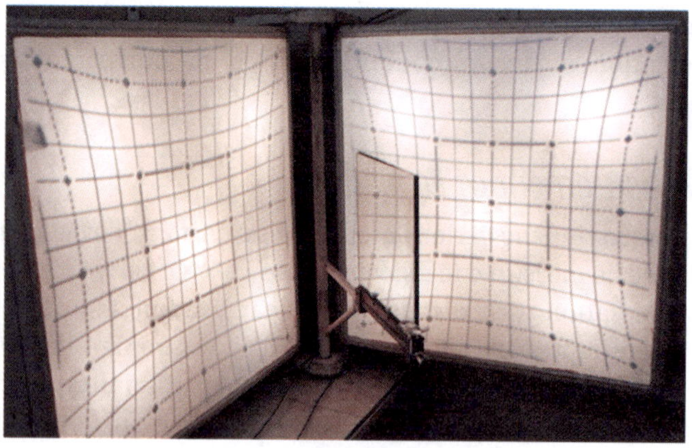

Fig. 2: Lees screen.

Ocular Movements

In addition to measuring the ocular deviations, it is valuable to note the limitations of movements. In restrictive strabismus, the limitation of movements is marked compared to the ocular deviation which is small. In contrast in the paralytic squint, the two collaborate with each other. Both the ductions and the versions should be noted and documented. Usually a subjective assessment is made on a scale of 7 points (+3 to -3) or 9 points (+4 to -4). This is usually helpful in follow-up of cases of incomitant strabismus. It should be noted that due to variations in the adnexal structures, these cannot be foolproof method of assessing such excursions. Normally adduction is considered normal when the nasal one-third cornea crosses the lower lacrimal punctum. Less than this is considered to be limited. For abduction to be considered normal, the temporal limbus should touch the lateral canthus. Vertical movements are difficult to assess due to variable palpebral aperture. This is even more so for the obliques.

The overaction of the obliques can be assessed in following manner:

- *Mild overaction:* If vertical deviation is appreciable only in sursum adduction or deorsum adduction
- *Moderate over action:* If it is appreciable in adduction also
- *Severe overaction:* If there is hypertropia or hypotropia in primary position itself.

Measurement of Vergences

In actual practice, the manifestation of a strabismus (heterotropia) only occurs if the latent tendency for the strabismus (heterophoria) is not overcome by the fusional vergences. Thus, the measurement of vergences is very important as it determines the capability of the motor system to cope with an induced misalignment of visual axes. If vergence amplitudes are large, even a large angle squint remains asymptomatic but with a small vergence amplitude, even a small angle squint manifests or intermittent and remains symptomatic.

Vergences are tested in the three planes:

1. Horizontal vergences—convergence and divergence
2. Vertical vergences—sursumvergence and deorsumvergence
3. Torsional vergences—incyclovergence and excyclovergence.

In principle, to measure the vergences, the axes are misaligned artificially with prisms or synoptophore. The horizontal and vertical vergences only can be measured by prisms in this manner but the prisms cannot induce a torsional misalignment.

Near Point of Convergence

The simplest way to measure the convergence is to bring a line drawn on a paper (or any other linear target) closer to the eyes, till the point, it becomes double. This determines the near point of convergence (NPC). It is important to note that the line should appear to be double, not blurred. The point at which it is blurred would determine the near point of accommodation (NPA). It is best tested with number 9 near vision target. The test is done with each eye separately (monocular) and also with both eyes together (binocular). For testing NPC in presbyopic eyes or ametropic eyes, suitable glasses should be used by the subject. Normally NPC is 8–10 cm. NPC of 10 cm or more is considered as convergence insufficiency. Apart from the patient describing the diplopia, an objective assessment is made by the examiner by seeing one of the eyes deviating out. Near point ruler, Royal Air Force binocular gauge and Livingstone gauge are instruments which may be used to measure NPC and NPA. Normal vergence amplitudes measured with prisms are shown in **Table 1**.

Examination of Sensory Status

The evaluation of sensory status of a patient with strabismus is aimed at establishing the following facts:

- Presence of binocularity
- The presence of confusion and diplopia
- Presence of suppression, its extent and depth
- Presence of amblyopia and its degree
- Type of retinal correspondence
- Presence of stereopsis and its grade.

Binocularity and Diplopia

Presence of binocular diplopia indicates binocularity. The presence of true diplopia should be established by differentiating it from false impression of diplopia due to blurring or elongation of an image due to astigmatism. It is also necessary to establish binocular nature of diplopia by closing one eye. If it disappears, it is suggestive of binocular diplopia. In long-standing cases of squint even of adult onset, patient may learn to ignore the other image. In such cases use of dissociating mechanisms like red-green goggles, Bagolini glasses, and single or double Maddox rod are helpful in visualization of diplopia.

In cases of squint without diplopia or in cases without squint, dissociation test are helpful in detecting the presence of binocular perception.

Table 1: Normal vergence amplitudes measured with prisms.

	Near (Δ)	*Distance (Δ)*
Convergence	30–40	15–20
Divergence	6–10	15–20
Vertical	2–4	2–4
Cyclovergence	8°–12°	8°–12°

Suppression

Suppression is a sensory adaptation to squint in children, which only occurs when the eyes are open. It is a temporary phenomenon. As soon as the fixating eye is covered, deviated eye takes up the fixation. It occurs from the active cortical inhibition of disparate and confusing retinal images originating from the retina of the deviating eye. The stimulus for suppression is diplopia, confusion, or a blurred image resulting from astigmatism/anisometropia.

Clinically, suppression can be classified into three types:

1. *Central or peripheral*: In central suppression, the image from the fovea of the deviating eye is inhibited to avoid confusion. In peripheral suppression, image forming on the peripheral retina is inhibited to eradicate diplopia.
2. Facultative suppression occurs only during binocular conditions and obligatory occurs during monocular conditions.
3. Suppression may be present in one eye (unilateral) or it may alternate between two eyes (alternating).

Suppression can be detected using dissociating tests like Bagolini striated glasses, polarized glasses, red-green glasses, Maddox rod test, Worth four dot test, synoptophore, and afterimage test.

Test for Binocularity

Bagolini Striated Glasses

Bagolini striated glasses **(Fig. 3A)** test is the most physiological method to test for dissociation of eyes. It entails the use of striated glasses, which cause a point source of light to appear as a line each perpendicular to the striations on the glass. Since the striations are at 45° and 135°, the lines in orthophoric patients should be perpendicular to each other. In suppression, two types of response can be seen:

1. *Single line response:* If only one line is seen, it is suggestive of other eye scotoma, i.e. suppression response.
2. *Cross response with central gap in one:* It is suggestive of central suppression scotoma in that line, i.e. eye.

Polaroid Glasses

Polaroid glasses are also a physiological means of dissociating the two eyes and can be used along with an appropriate polaroid picture or screen to document suppression.

Red-green Glasses

Red-green glasses **(Fig. 3B)** are a stronger dissociating tool where the red and green glass is in front of either eye.

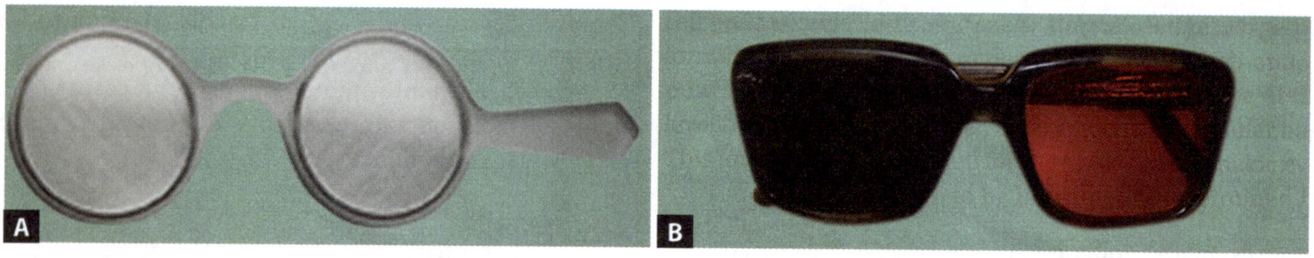

Figs. 3A and B: (A) Bagolini striated glasses; (B) red-green glasses.

If there is suppression of any of the eye, the patient will not appreciate that color when looking at a light source.

Maddox Rod Test

Maddox rod test involves the use of two Maddox rods in an orientation perpendicular to each other and a point source of light to demonstrate suppression.

Synoptophore

Synoptophore is a maximally dissociating test whereby the two eyes see totally different slides and suppression can be detected even in the milder cases. The synoptophore has the advantage of using a flickering light to help the patient appreciate both images.

Afterimage Test

Afterimage test is also a maximally dissociating test where an afterimage is created in each eye after prolonged exposure to a streak of two perpendicular lights in front of either eye.

Retinal Correspondence

Investigation of state of retinal correspondence is indicated in all cases of constant squint. A bifoveal correspondence is called normal retinal correspondence (NRC). A correspondence between fovea of one eye and extrafoveal point of the other eye (deviating eye) is called anomalous retinal correspondence. It is an acquired binocular functional sensory adaptation to squint at the cortical level. Suppression precedes the development of anomalous retinal correspondence (ARC). At the cortical level, there is a change in synaptic connections from the foveo-foveal to the foveo-extrafoveal. The extrafoveal point should have good visual potential in order to have an association with the fovea of the fixing eye.

Diagnosis of Anomalous Retinal Correspondence

To diagnose ARC, it is necessary to measure the angle of deviation by subjective and objective methods. ARC is present when there is difference in the subjective and objective deviations. In NRC, objective and subjective angles are equal. If the subjective angle is zero, i.e. no subjective squint, in the presence of objective angle showing a squint, it is termed as harmonious ARC. If the subjective angle is not zero but less than the objective angle of deviation, it is nonharmonious ARC. The difference between objective and subjective angle is the angle of anomaly. Hence, in harmonious ARC, subjective angle is zero and objective angle is equal to angle of anomaly. In unharmonious ARC, objective angle is greater than subjective angle and hence angle of anomaly. In NRC, objective and subjective angles are same and angle of anomaly is zero.

The objective angle of deviation can be measured by PBCT or by cover-uncover test, on the synoptophore with alternate on-off method.

The subjective angle of deviation can be measured by various methods depending on the method used for dissociation. In order of decreasing dissociation, they are as follows:

- Afterimage test
- Synoptophore
- Worth four dot test
- Maddox rod or red filter test
- Polaroid dissociation
- Phase difference haploscope
- Bagolini striated glasses.

The use of these modalities has been described briefly above. Here, we describe the use of the two most commonly used methods for detecting retinal correspondence.

Worth Four Dot Test

This test is performed after dissociating the two eyes with red-green glasses. The patient is then asked to view four backlit circles—one is red, two are green, and one is white. In the presence of normal retinal correspondence, the individual would see two red or three green depending on the dominant eye or may see both together. In the presence of squint, this response would indicate harmonious ARC. In the presence of unharmonious ARC, the patient will see two red and three green similar to the diplopia response as shown in **Figure 4**. Suppression of either eye will prevent the patient from seeing dots of that color. Thus, the Worth four

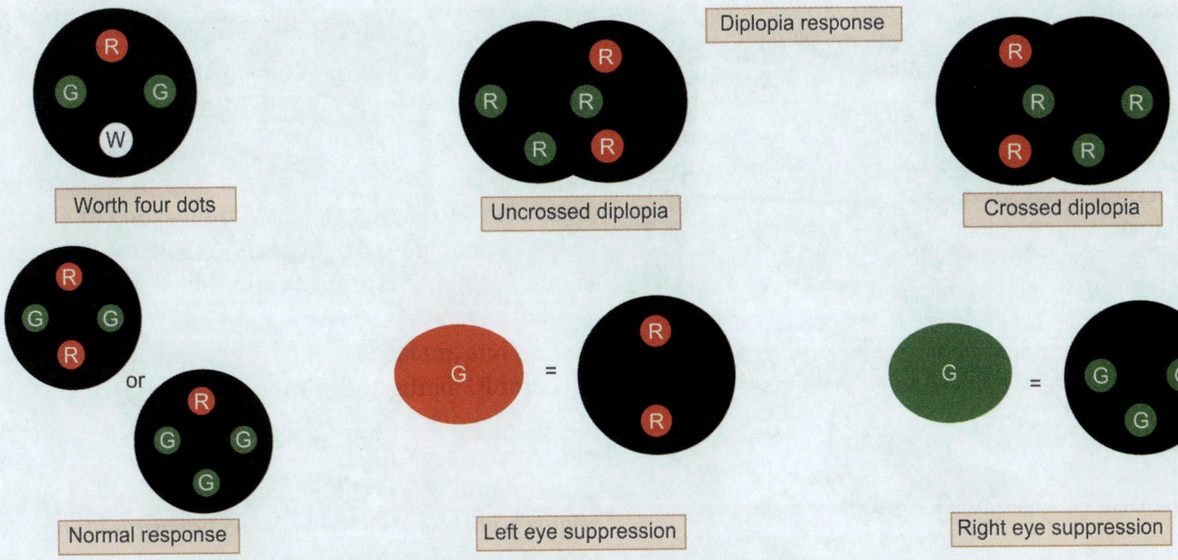

Fig. 4: Interpretation of Worth four dot test.

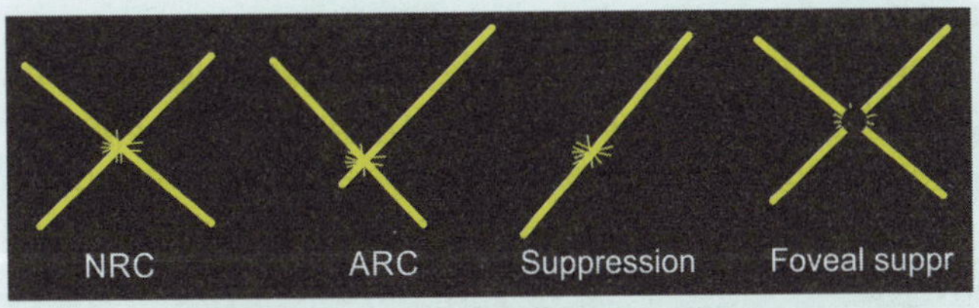

Fig. 5: Interpretation of Bagolini striated glasses. (ARC: abnormal retinal correspondence; NRC: normal retinal correspondence; Suppr: suppression)

dot test can effectively deduce the retinal correspondence status of the individual **(Fig. 4)**.

Bagolini Striated Glasses

The patient with strabismus is first evaluated with cover-uncover test and objective angle is measured with PBCT. Next with the squint manifested, the patient looks through the Bagolini striated glasses. If he sees a cross response (as seen by person with NRC with no squint) in the presence of manifest squint, it implies a harmonious ARC. If the patient does not see a cross response, i.e. X, the prisms are added to get X cross response. The prism power required is the subjective angle of deviation and it is termed nonharmonious ARC. In presence of squint with NRC, patient sees two oblique lines crossing asymmetrically to form a V or A instead of X response. In the presence of suppression, patient sees only one line, other line of the other eye which is suppressed is not seen **(Fig. 5)**. In case of central scotoma, the eye with the scotoma sees a line with a break in the center. Treatment to overcome ARC is contraindicated due to development of intractable diplopia, and nonrestoration of binocular single vision. Many patients with ARC have useful and symptom-free binocular single fusion. ARC allows the patient to maintain binocular single vision (BSV), often some stereopsis. In many cases, binocular vision is sufficiently stable to maintain the eyes in a cosmetically satisfactory position.

Stereoacuity

Stereopsis refers to our ability to appreciate depth that is the ability to distinguish the relative distance of objects with an apparent physical displacement between the objects. Assessment of stereoacuity is important as a detectable stereoacuity indicates the presence of orthophoria, heterophoria or in cases with subnormal stereoacuity, an intermittent squint. The distance stereoacuity has also been used to assess the need for surgical intervention in intermittent exotropia.[4-6]

Stereopsis can be tested by following methods:

- Synoptophore—with stereopsis slides
- Randot stereotest and Titmus fly stereotest—with polaroid spectacles
- TNO test—with red-green goggles
- Frisby and Lang stereotest—without using glasses
- Special 3D pictures.

Randot Stereotest

Randot stereotest **(Figs. 6A to D)** is the most popular clinical test that has replaced the earlier popular Titmus fly test. It uses Julesz' random dot background to mask the monocular cues which are there with the animal tests and Wirt's circle test. Geometric figures like square, circle, triangle, star, etc. are also presented devoid of any monocular clues. But, the latter type figures, though a better test, are usually not appreciated by small children.

The test requires polaroid glasses to be worn by the patient. It is used at a distance of 40 cm and thus tests near

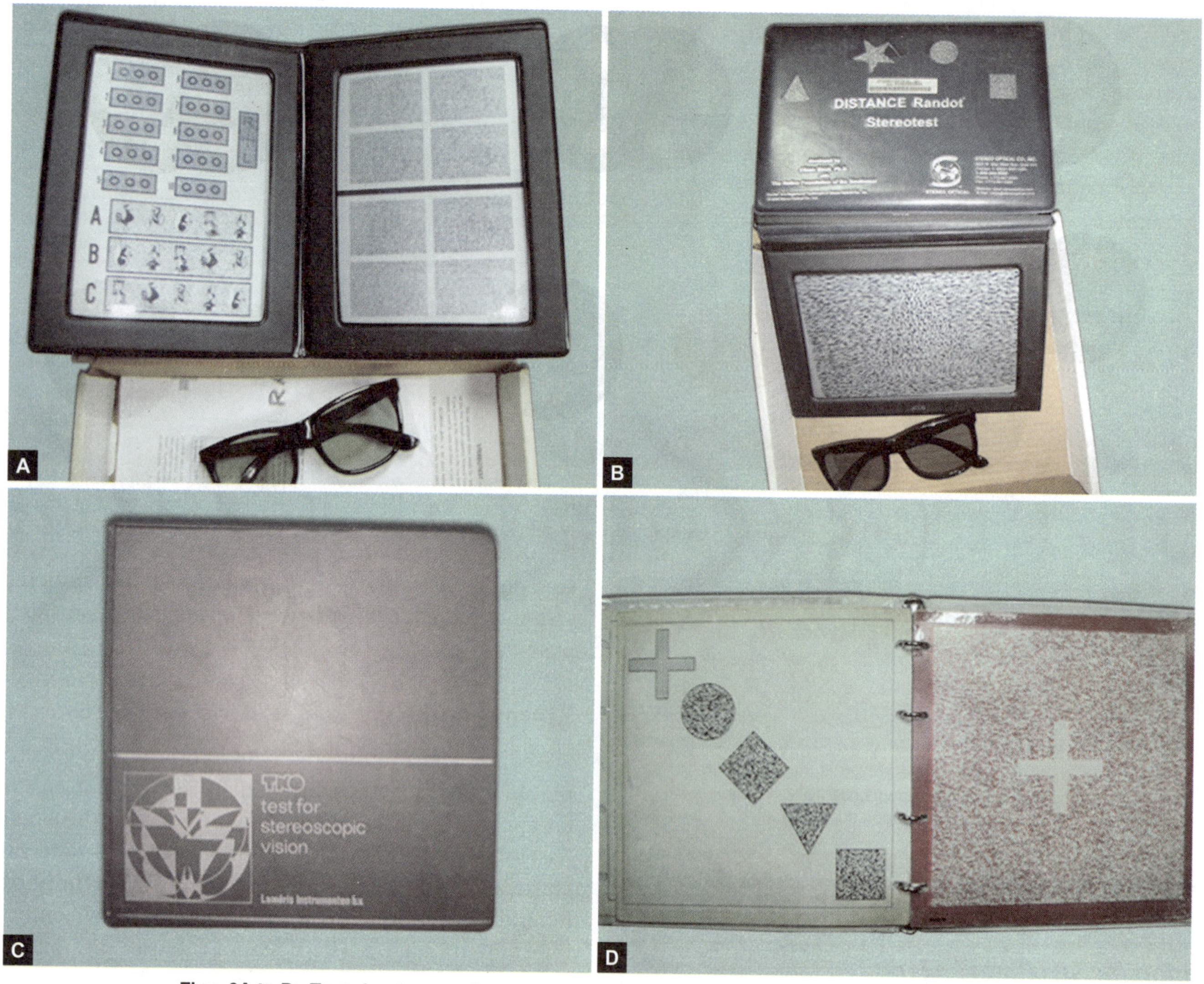

Figs. 6A to D: Tests for stereoacuity measurement. (A) Near Randot test; (B) Distance Randot test; (C) TNO stereotest; (D) Inner leaflets of TNO stereotest.

binocular vision, therefore, the myopes up to 3 diopters can be missed in the screening test. The Wirt's circles 1–10 test the stereoacuity from 400 arcseconds to 20 arcseconds.

TNO Test

TNO test **(Figs. 6A to D)** is another popular stereotest which uses red-green glasses and is more dissociating and possibly reliable. It measures from 400 arcseconds to 40 arcseconds.

Distance Stereotests

Stereotests can be performed for distance also and this is often useful in planning when to operate a case of intermittent divergent squint. The various tests that may be used for this are distant Randot and the Frisby Davis distance test.

Normal Stereoacuity

Adults are capable of appreciating stereopsis with disparities as fine as 15–20 arcseconds. The adult-norm is 40 arcseconds. For children, 3–5 years old, the norm is 70 arcseconds, and for 5–7 years, it is 50 arcseconds. Children above 8 years have the adult-norm.

Gross Stereopsis: Lang Two Pencil Test

In the absence of fine stereotest, a gross estimation of stereopsis can be made by a bedside test—two pencil test popularized by Lang. A pencil is held in the examiner's hand horizontally and the child is asked to touch the tip with the tip of another pencil rapidly, coming from one side. Care should be taken to avoid giving the end on view of the pencil, as that can be accomplished even monocularly; therefore, horizontal pencils are better, as they do not allow an end-on view. Always compare the binocular task with monocular task. The test is a gross-stereopsis test of about 400 arcseconds disparity.

Amblyopia

Amblyopia is a condition with unilateral or bilateral decrease of visual functions caused by form vision deprivation and/

or abnormal binocular interaction that cannot be explained by a disorder of ocular media or visual pathways. It is a condition caused by abnormal visual experience during early childhood, the critical period of visual development. In appropriate cases, it is reversible by therapeutic measures.

Classification of Amblyopia

- Strabismic amblyopia
- *Anisometropic amblyopia (unilateral or asymmetric)*:
  - Anisohyperopic
  - Anisomyopic
- *Vision deprivation amblyopia (unilateral or bilateral)*:
  - Stimulus deprivation amblyopia or amblyopia ex anopsia due to ptosis covering pupil, media opacities, unilateral occlusion or penalization
  - *Ametropic amblyopia (uncorrected bilateral high refractive error)*:
    - Hyperopia
    - Myopia
    - Astigmatism (meridional amblyopia)
  - Nystagmus related amblyopia
  - *Organic amblyopia*:
    - Subclinical macular damage
    - Malorientation of cones
    - Cone deficiency syndrome.

Clinical Features[7]

Amblyopia is a disorder of visual perception, only one of which is the visual acuity on the standard vision charts (Snellen acuity); but there are other visual functions too that are affected. The amblyopia syndrome shows the following abnormalities:

- Decreased visual acuity (Snellen's)
- Decreased grating acuity (Teller's)
- Decreased vernier acuity
- Decreased or lost stereoacuity
- Decreased contrast sensitivity
- Decreased brightness perception
- Abnormal contour interaction
- Increased perception and reaction times
- Nasotemporal asymmetries in resolution of vertical gratings
- Motility defects in pursuit, saccades, and fixation.

Amblyopia of various types is often associated with strabismus and it is very important to diagnose and manage amblyopia as a part of strabismus management.

CONCLUSION

Concomitant squint is the most common form of strabismus faced by ophthalmologists. Though it may seem perplexing, a step-by-step workup will lead to a comprehensive assessment and enable an accurate diagnosis and management. A good workup done is half the battle won.

REFERENCES

1. Sharma P. Strabismus Simplified, 2nd edition. New Delhi: CBS Publishers and Distributors; 2013.
2. van Noorden GK, Campos EC. Binocular Vision and Ocular Motility: theory and Management of Strabismus, 6th edition. St. Louis: Mosby Inc.; 2002.
3. Kim DS, Coats DK, McCreery KM, et al. Accuracy of clinical estimation of abnormal head postures. Binocul Vis Strabismus Q. 2004;19(1):21-4.
4. Leske DA, Holmes JM. Maximum angle of horizontal strabismus consistent with true stereopsis. J AAPOS. 2004; 8(1):28-34.
5. Sharma P, Saxena R, Narvekar M, et al. Evaluation of distance and near stereoacuity and fusional vergence in intermittent exotropia. Indian J Ophthalmol. 2008;56(2):121-5.
6. Holmes JM, Birch EE, Leske DA, et al. New tests of distance stereoacuity and their role in evaluating intermittent exotropia. Ophthalmology. 2007;114(6):1215-20.
7. Kanonidou E. Amblyopia: a mini review of the literature. Int Ophthalmol. 2011;31(3):249-56.

CHAPTER

31

Incomitant Strabismus: Diagnostic Procedures

P Vijayalakshmi, P Vrushali, R Muralidhar

INTRODUCTION

By definition, incomitant strabismus refers to strabismus in which the deviation changes in different gazes and may also be different with either eye fixing. Differences between incomitant strabismus and comitant strabismus are tabulated in **Table 1**. The incomitant strabismus is usually of two types: paralytic strabismus and restrictive strabismus. This chapter covers the basic steps involved in examination, diagnosis, and differential diagnosis of both categories of strabismus.

Table 1: Differences between comitant and incomitant strabismus.

Features	*Incomitant squint*	*Comitant squint*
Type of onset	Often sudden	Usually gradual
Age of onset	Any age	Usually during childhood
History of head trauma	Common	Uncommon
Diplopia	Common	Uncommon
Severe amblyopia	Uncommon	Common
Comitance	Only in late stages	Common
Abnormal head posture	Commonly present	Rarely present
Systemic association	May be present	Usually absent but present in syndromes
Past pointing	Common with recent paralysis	Rare
Ocular movements	Limited in the direction of action of paralyzed muscle	Usually full
Primary vs. secondary deviation	Secondary > primary	Secondary = primary

PARALYTIC STRABISMUS

Paralytic strabismus is caused by weakness of one or more extraocular muscles due to the paralysis of either third/ fourth/or sixth cranial nerve. When there is complete absence of movement in one or more positions of gaze, it is called as paralysis, if some movement is possible, known as paresis. Paresis is more common than paralysis. The more general term palsy is often used to include both conditions. Usually only one eye is affected but bilateral palsies also occur.

Paralytic squint can be present at birth (congenital) or it can be acquired at any age. Acquired palsies usually occur later in life as a result of disease or injury and give rise to diplopia. Sixth nerve palsy is more often seen followed by 4th nerve palsy then 3rd nerve palsy. Patients with congenital ocular muscle palsy are less likely to complain of diplopia. They may present in childhood with the head tilt or in adult life with diplopia due to decompensation of fusion mechanism.

Palsy of any one of the muscles results in a series of changes in other related ocular muscles and this is called muscle sequelae. Using right lateral rectus palsy as an example (defective abduction right eye), the possible muscle sequelae are as follows:[1-3]

- There will be overaction of the contralateral synergist of the affected muscle, which is the left medical rectus. This is explained by Herring's law. The paretic right lateral rectus requires more innervation to act and equal innervation goes to the normal left medical rectus, which is more than it's requirement causing it to overact.
- The right medial rectus, which is the antagonist of the right lateral rectus, may overact in time. This is explained by Sherrington's law, which ensures that as a muscle contracts its antagonist relaxes so that smooth movement can occur. When the right lateral rectus is not

Table 2: Common features of paralytic strabismus (right eye).

Muscle	*Main action*	*Secondary action*	*Eye position*	*Diplopia*	*Muscle sequelae*	*A or V*	*Compensatory head posture*
Lateral rectus	Abduction	Nil	Esotropia Distance > Near	Uncrossed maximum to right may fuse for near	o/a LMR o/a RMR u/a LLR	Nil	Face turn right
Medial rectus (very rare, suspect INO)	Adduction	Nil	Exotropia near > distance	Crossed maximum to left	o/a LLR o/a RLR u/a LMR	Nil	Face turn left
Superior oblique	Depression on adduction	Intorsion abduction	Hypertropia Extorsion Esotropia	Vertical near > distance right image is intorted (if recent onset)	o/a LIR o/a RIO u/a LSR	V Pattern especially in bilateral so palsies	Head tilt left, face turn left, chin depressed
Inferior oblique	Elevation on adduction	Extorsion abduction	Hypotropia Intorsion Esotropia	Vertical, right image is extorted	o/a LSR o/a RSO u/a LIR	A (loss of abduction on elevation)	Head tilt right face turn left, chin elevation
Superior rectus	Elevation on abduction	Adduction, slight intorsion on adduction	Hypotropia Exotropia	Vertical, right image is intorted	o/a LIO o/a RIR u/a LSO	V (loss of adduction on elevation + o/a IO)	Face turn right chin elevated (eyes down left)
Inferior rectus	Depression on abduction	Adduction, slight extorsion on adduction	Hypertropia Exotropia	Vertical, right image is extorted	o/a LSO o/a RSR u/a LIO	A (loss of adduction on depression)	Face turn right chin depressed (eyes up left)

(o/a: over action; u/a: under action; INO: internuclear ophthalmoplegia; LIO: left interior oblique; LIR: left inferior rectus; LLR: left lateral rectus; LMR: left medial rectus; LSR: left superior rectus; RIR: right inferior rectus; RLR: right lateral rectus; RMR: right medial rectus)

functioning (absent relaxation), the antagonist medial rectus remains contracted, causing it to overact.

- Because the right medical rectus is contracted, it requires less innervation to bring about adduction. The same less innervations therefore goes to its contralateral synergist, the left lateral rectus, which is sufficient to bring about enough abduction, resulting in underaction of this muscle. This is explained by Herring's law.

Overaction of the left medial rectus would occur at the onset of the palsy, but the remaining sequelae take time to develop. These changes do not follow a definitive rule and may take weeks to months. Common features of paralytic squint are summed up in **Table 2**.

Evaluation

Each case of incomitant strabismus is subjected to following procedures:

- History taking
- Examination
- Special tests
- Investigations.

History Taking

History of onset of symptoms, manifestation age, type of onset, precipitating factors, and congenital or acquired are noted. The congenital palsies present mainly for the compensatory head posture, strabismus and rarely with the decompensation resulting in double vision. Differences between old congenital and recent acquired palsies are summed up in **Table 3**.

Table 3: Old congenital vs. recent acquired paralytic strabismus.

Features	*Congenital*	*Acquired*
Diplopia	Rare	Usually present, may be limited to paretic field
Amblyopia	May be present	Absent
Comitance	Spread comitance obscures original paresis	Characteristically incomitant
Head posture	May or may not be present	Disappears on covering paretic eye
Orbital/facial/skull asymmetry	Common	Absent
Contracture of antagonist with positive forced duction test	May be present	Absent
Past pointing	Absent	Present
Old photographs	May show head posture	No head posture
Secondary deviation	Slight primary deviation	Marked primary deviation

Diplopia is the main complaint in almost all acquired palsies and is more marked in the direction of action of the paralyzed muscle. Diplopia results from the same image forming on noncorresponding points. It can be crossed or uncrossed. Diplopia can be horizontal (horizontal muscle palsy), vertical (vertical muscle palsy), or tilted (oblique muscle palsy). When fixing with the paretic eye, false localization and past pointing (overshooting) results from increased innervation required to move the paretic eye into fixation. Diplopia and false localization might result in nausea and vertigo. Confusion, which results from different objects being projected on the fovea is rarely reported.

Duration of complaints, worsening/improving symptoms, diurnal variation in the deviation (myasthenia gravis), past similar episodes, history of ocular, sinus, neurosurgery, raised intracranial pressure, hemiplegic attack, diabetes, hypertension, and trauma, are of great significance and should also be recorded.

Examination

- General examination of eyes
- Orthoptic evaluation including special tests
- General systemic examination
- Neurological examination.

Examination of eyes: Apart from estimating the visual acuity, refraction, fundus examination, the following points to be noted including position of the globe (in/out/down/upward), presence of enophthalmos (blow out fractures, Duane's syndrome), status of the palpebral fissure (narrowing or widening), position of the lids (ptosis or retraction, lagophthalmos, lid lag), any abnormal eye/lid movements, size and reaction of the pupil should be noted. When fundus is examined, an associated torsion should be looked for in cases of suspected oblique muscle involvement.

Orthoptic evaluation

Inspection: Presence of anomaly of skull and facial asymmetry gives a clue towards congenital etiology.

Compensatory head posture: It is a common feature of incomitant squint. It is achieved to avoid diplopia. Hence, the eyes are turned away from the action of paralyzed muscle and are placed in the direction of least deviation so that binocular single vision is maintained in that position. A patient with left lateral rectus palsy will keep his face turned to the left, i.e. he will have a right gaze.

Components of head posture

Face turn: Horizontal muscle palsy causes face turn towards the action of paretic muscle. In right lateral rectus (LR) palsy, face turns to right side. But in cyclovertical muscle palsy, face turn is such that the eyes are brought away from the field in which muscle has its greatest vertical effect. Superior rectus (SR) and inferior rectus (IR) have maximal vertical effect in abduction, therefore in their palsy face will be turned towards the affected side while the opposite is true for the obliques.[1,2]

Head tilt: In oblique muscle palsy, head tilt occurs to compensate the torsion caused by the direct antagonist of paralyzed muscle. In left superior oblique (SO) palsy, head tilt occurs towards right to compensate for the extorsion caused by the right inferior oblique (IO). In other words, a patient with left SO palsy will have a head tilt to the right **(Figs. 1A to C)** to compensate for extorsion. In vertical muscle palsy, head tilt occurs to compensate the torsion caused by contralateral agonist of paralyzed muscle. In right SR palsy, head will tilt to right, to compensate for extorsion of left eye caused by overacting left IO.

Chin elevation or depression: It occurs in paresis of elevators or depressors, respectively, so that involved eye is brought out of the field of action of paretic muscle. A patient with double elevator palsy will have a chin elevation to keep the eyes in down gaze. Presence of a head posture definitely gives a clue to the involved muscle, but it can be absent in case of suppression of any one image or in cases with poor vision in one eye **(Figs. 1A to C)**.

Examinations of ocular movements

The direction of restricted ocular motility readily suggests the diagnosis. On occasion this could be rather subtle, and one has to fall back on evaluating the deviations in different gazes and other suggestive clinical features. It is always better to use a fixation target while examining the ocular movements. Both versions and ductions should be tested. Versions are important to compare the movements of the two eyes apart from noting the muscle sequelae such as over and under actions **(Figs. 2A to D)**. Ductions are important to diagnose true restriction. The saccades should also be tested; presence of slow saccades implies reduced muscle strength.

Corneal reflex test: It determines the degree of manifest strabismus and is an approximate measure of the deviation fixing either eye.

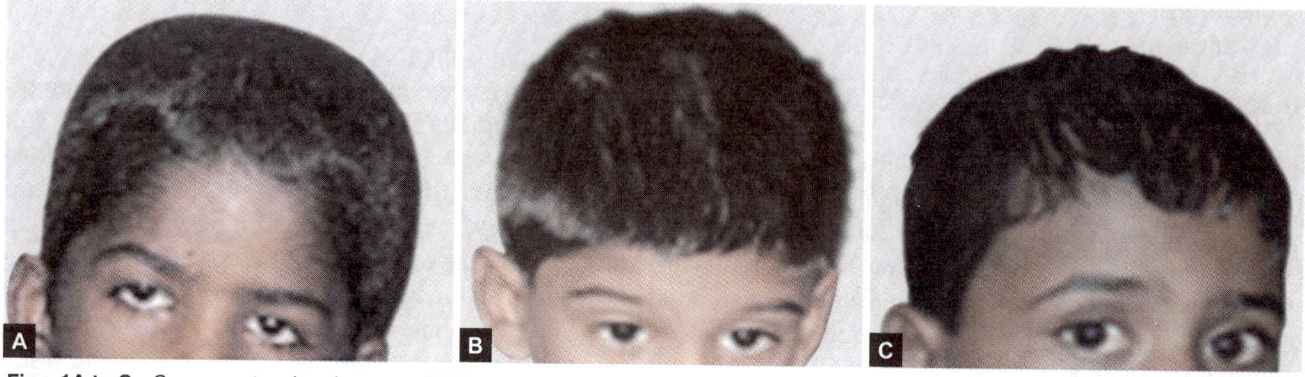

Figs. 1A to C: *Compensatory head posture*: (A) Right superior oblique palsy; (B) Bilateral superior oblique palsy; (C) Left lateral rectus palsy.

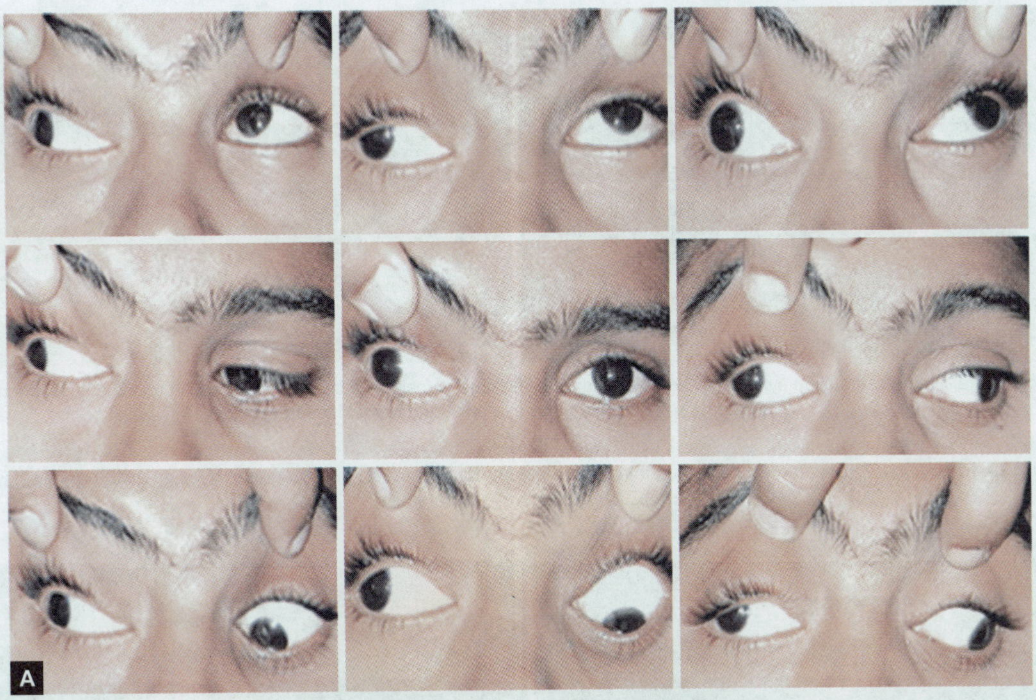

Note: Right exotropia, limitation of adduction, elevation and depression.

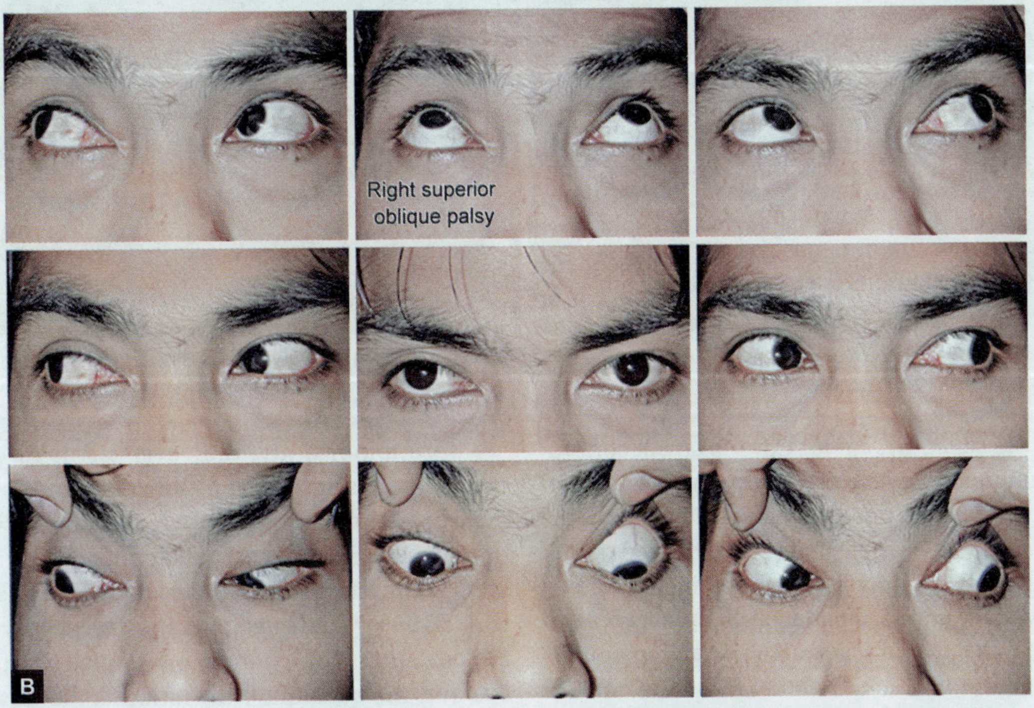

Note: Right hypertropia in primary position, right superior oblique underaction, right inferior oblique overaction and left inferior rectus overaction.

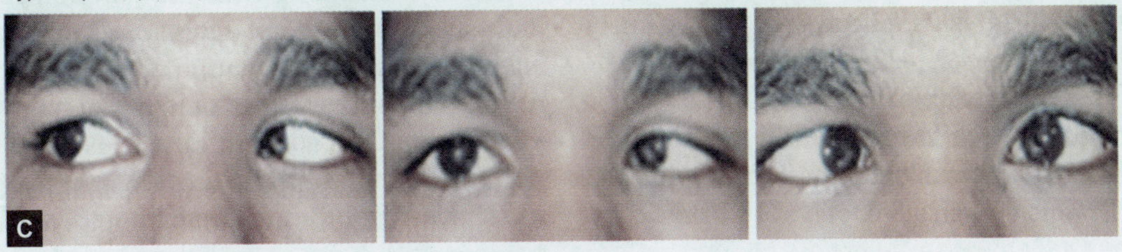

Note: Esotropia in primary position and limitation of abduction in left eye.

Figs. 2A to C

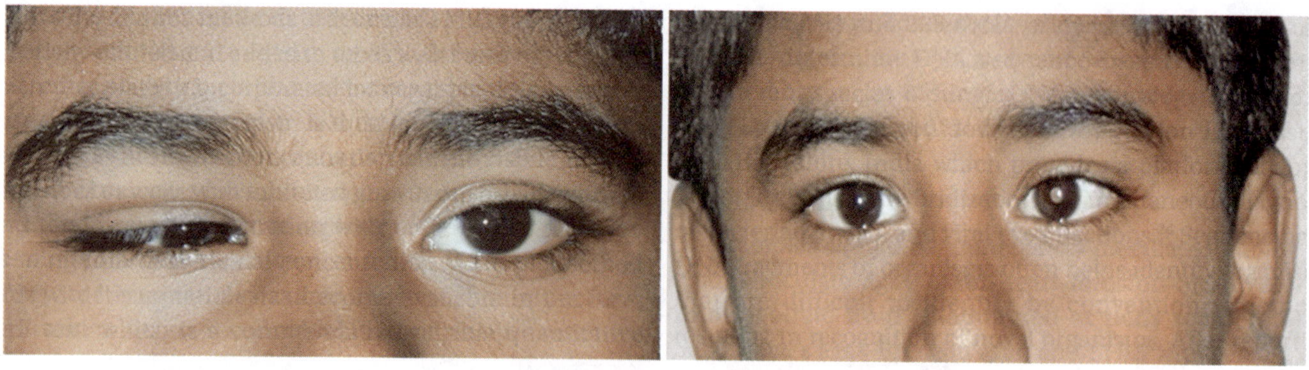

Note: Bilateral Duane's retraction syndrome: Note the esotropia in primary position, limitation of abduction on either side, change in palpebral fissure on either eye on attempted adduction.

Fig. 2D

Figs. 2A to D: *Ocular movements*: (A) Right third nerve palsy; (B) Right fourth nerve palsy; (C) Left sixth nerve palsy; (D) Bilateral Duane's retraction.

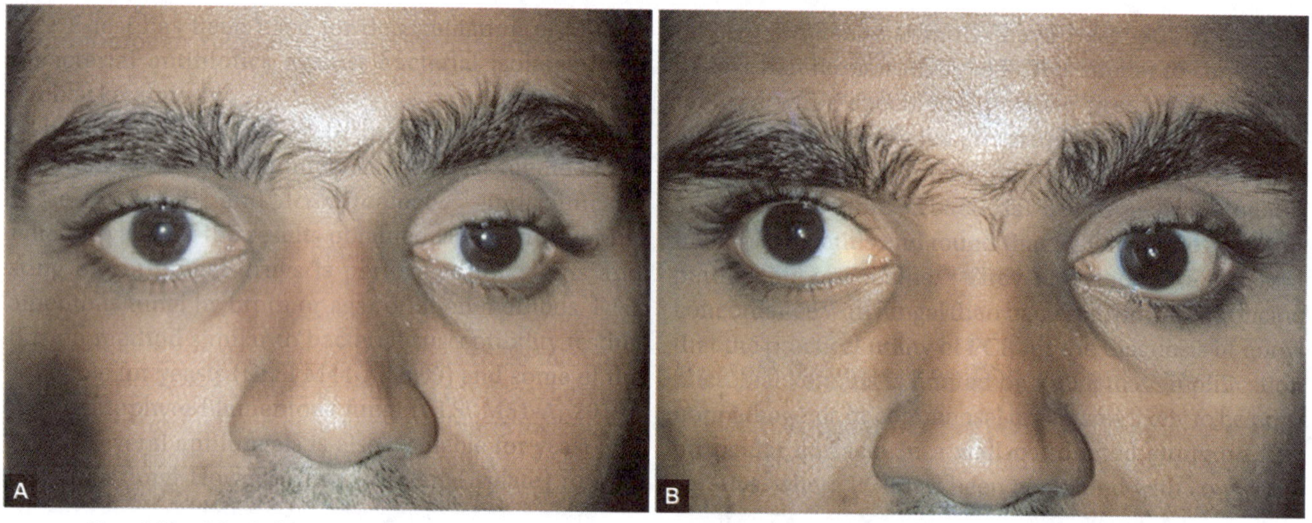

Figs. 3A and B: *Left medial rectus palsy*: (A) Fixing right (normal) eye (small primary deviation); (B) Fixing left (paretic) eye.

Cover test and the ocular deviation: Cover test will confirm the manifest squint and should be done with correction of the head posture whereas a prism cover test will measure the deviation. It may not be possible to perform the cover test if the movement is severely restricted in the direction being tested. The ocular deviation is different in different gazes and is maximal in the direction of action of the paralyzed muscle. By using prism cover test, the deviation is measured in all nine cardinal positions of gaze. The direction in which the deviation is maximal gives a clue to the paretic muscle. As an alternative, the ocular deviation can be measured in all gaze positions by using a synoptophore.

The following chart shows deviations recorded in different positions in a patient with right lateral rectus palsy.

	9 Δ BO	
Right Gaze 20 Δ BO	9 Δ BO	ORTHO
	12 Δ BO	

The deviation is maximal in right gaze: The direction of action of the paralyzed muscle.

More importantly, the cover test is to be done with either eye fixing. Placing the prism on the paretic eye measures the primary deviation and placing it on the normal eye measures the secondary deviation. In all incomitant strabismus, the ocular deviation measured with either eye fixing is different. The primary deviation is the deviation of the paretic eye on fixing with the normal eye and the secondary deviation is the deviation of the normal eye on fixing with the paretic eye. In paralytic strabismus, secondary deviation (deviation of normal eye under cover, when squinting eye is fixating) is much greater than primary deviation (deviation of squinting eye when normal eye is fixating). This is based on Herring's law of equal innervation of yoke muscles **(Figs. 3A and B)**. The strong innervation impulse required to enable the paralytic eye to fix is also transmitted to yoke muscle of sound eye resulting in greater amount of deviation.

Long-standing cases of paralytic squint develop features of comitance. When the spread of comitance is complete, the deviation becomes roughly equal in all gazes, with progressively decreasing difference between primary and secondary deviations. In cases where the inhibitional palsy giving confusion to the clinical picture, a primary paretic muscle is identified by patch test. In this test, the paretic eye is occluded (for 24 hours), and the ocular movements are recorded. In case of inhibitional palsy, this disappears with improvement of duction in that direction. For vertical deviations, perform the head tilt test also.

Bielschowsky three step test: Initially, Bielschowsky proposed a classical head tilt test **(Figs. 4A to E)** to differentiate between SO palsy in one eye and SR palsy in the other eye. But park modified it to a three step test, which is used for diagnosis of any cyclovertical muscle palsy.[2,3]

Step 1: Cover test is performed in primary position after correcting the head posture. By determining the hypertropic eye, this step reduces the number of affected muscles from eight-to-four.

Right hypertropia (RH) in primary position could be due to either of the following four muscles:

- Weakness of depressors of right eye right inferior rectus (RIR); right superior oblique (RSO)
- Weakness of elevators of left eye left superior rectus (LSR); left inferior oblique (LIO)

Step 2: Perform the cover test on both the horizontal gazes. Determine in which gaze the right hypertropia is larger. This step reduces the number of affected muscles from four to two:

- RH in left gaze implies weakness of any of the four muscles acting in left gaze: LSR, LIR; RSO, RIO.
- If RH is larger in left gaze, we are narrowed down to two muscles, i.e. RSO, LSR (these two muscles only act on the left gaze among the above four muscles).

Step 3: Perform the cover test on either side head tilt.

Determine in which head tilt the right hypertropia is larger. This step reduces two muscles to a single paralyzed muscle. When we tilt the head to one side, the intortors of the eye and the extortors of the other eye come in action. In cases of right hypertropia due to RSO palsy, when the head is tilted to left side, the intortors of the left eye (LSO, LSR) and extortors of the right eye (RIO, RIO) work together. As these four muscles are intact, the hypertropia gets either small or totally absent. If the head is tilted to the right side, intortors of the right eye (RSO, RSR) and extorters of the left eye (LIO, LIR) act together. In case of RSO palsy, the right hypertropia gets larger on right head tilt. This is because one of the right intortor (RSO) being weak, the other intortor (RSR) exerts more energy to compensate the weakness of RSO. The RSR being a strong elevator elevates the eye.

Though this test is quite useful, its value has been repeatedly questioned. The test assumes that the hypertropia can only be caused by a weakness. It is not valid in patients with contractures, absent extraocular muscles, myasthenia, patients who have had strabismus surgery in the past and paresis involving more than one extraocular muscle.

Some authors describe doing a cover test and measuring the deviation in up and down gazes after the second step. For example, as the increase in right HT is demonstrated in left gaze, the cover test done in the same direction for up and down gazes. In RSO palsy, the deviation will be larger on down gaze and in LSR palsy, the deviation will be larger in up gaze.

Binocular function test: There are various methods available for binocular vision testing. Worth's four dot test is used most commonly for near and distance. The readers are advised to refer to an appropriate section for more details.

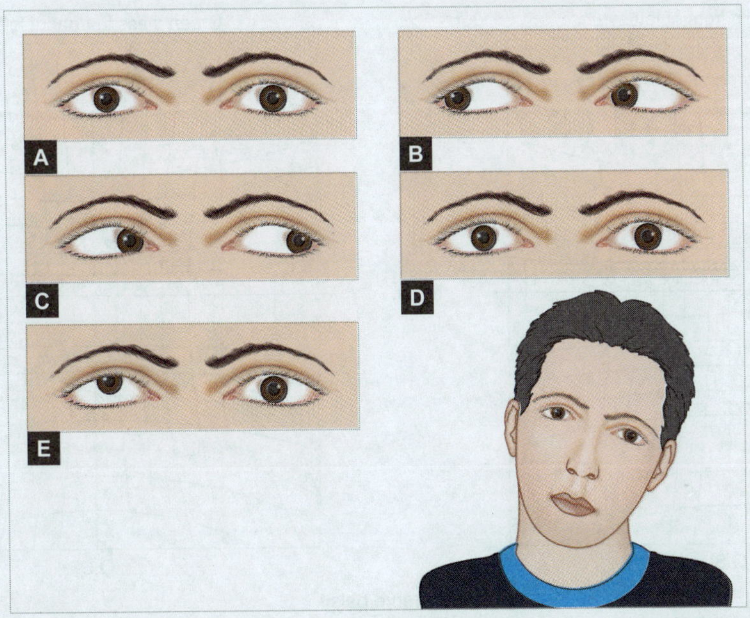

Figs. 4A to E: Three step test. (A) Note right hypertropia in primary position; (B) No hypertropia on dextroversion; (C) Right hypertropia increasing on levoversion; (D) No hypertropia on tilting the head to left; (E) Right hypertropia increasing on right head tilt.

Hess screen test: The Hess screen test is an important modality in diagnosis and prognostication of incomitant squint. It accurately determines the position of visual axis in all direction of gazes. Hess screen test has following principle:

- The screen is based on foveal projection that is both the images of the two lights fall on the foveae. This means that charts are displaced in the direction of squint.
- The screen is also based on Herring's law of equal innervation.[2,3]

Description of the test

Electrically operated Hess screen is commonly used nowadays. It has a background screen with small lights forming fixation points and a movable illuminated green indicator. A light source is present behind each red light, the illumination of which is controlled from a control unit. Each red light can be turned on, by insertion of a plug on switch board, apertures of which correspond to that of Hess screen. The patient holds a green light. Each eye is tested separately by red green glasses, which dissociate both eyes. Good binocular vision, central fixation and normal retinal correspondence are prerequisites for Hess charting.

Procedure

Patient is seated at 50 cm, with head erect and eyes in primary position **(Fig. 5)**. Patient wears red-green glasses. The head must be kept straight. The patient must have normal retinal correspondence. Instructions are given to shine green light upon each red fixation, as it is illuminated. The chart belongs to the eye over which green glasses are worn. Place indicated by patient is recorded on chart printed with similar markings. Recorded points are joined to form inner and outer square.

Interpretation of Hess chart (Figs. 6A to C)

- Central dot in each field indicates deviation in primary position
- Smaller field belongs to paretic eye
- Inward and outward displacement indicates under and over action, respectively
- Equal sized fields indicate that muscle sequelae have not developed/presence of concomitant squint
- Each small square subtends 5°. The inner and outer square hence measures 15 and 30° movement respectively from the primary position
- Relationship between inner and outer field is observed
- In larger field, position of maximum outward displacement indicates overaction of contralateral synergist
- In smaller field, outward displacement in the direction of action of ipsilateral antagonist suggests contracture

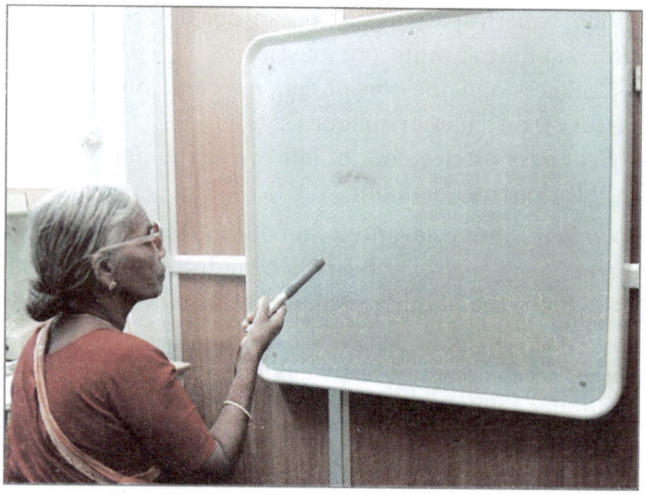

Fig. 5: Hess chart recording.

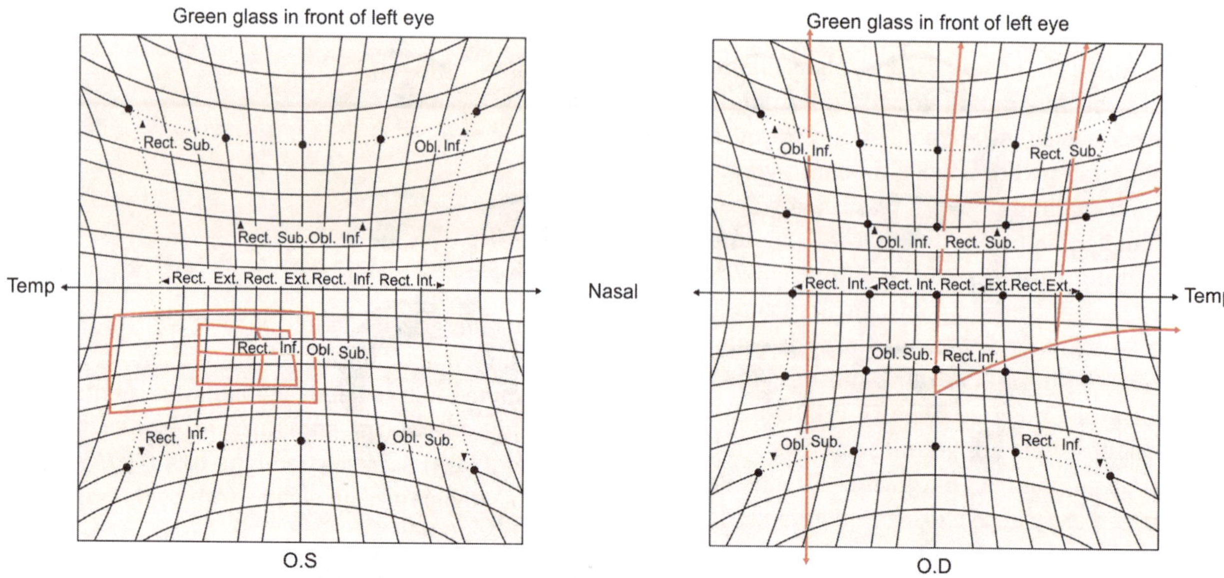

Left third nerve palsy

Fig. 6A: Left field is very small, displaced out and slightly down due to intact left lateral rectus and superior oblique. Right field is displaced up and out, very large, due to overaction of right lateral rectus, right superior oblique, right inferior oblique and right superior rectus.

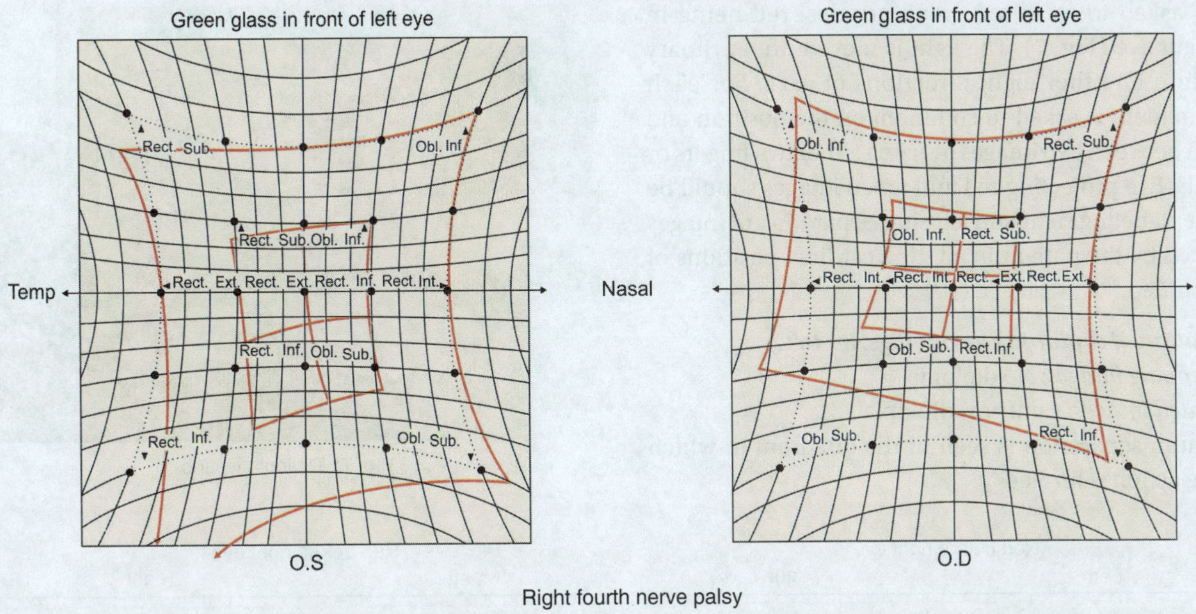

Fig. 6B: Underaction of right superior oblique in the outer field more than inner field, overaction of the contralateral synergist, left inferior rectus.

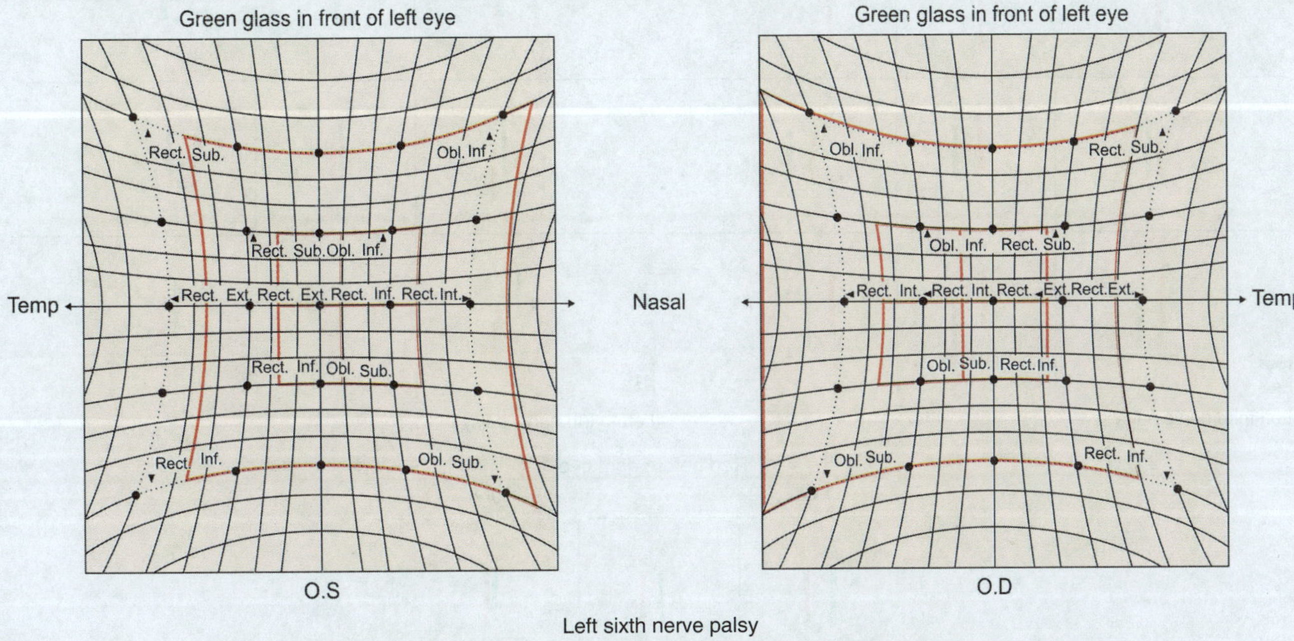

Fig. 6C: Small field left eye with underaction of lateral rectus and overaction of the right medial rectus.

- Outer field should be concentrated to look for SO muscle palsies
- Contracted fields on opposite sides imply restrictive strabismus.

Uses of Hess chart

- It is useful for diagnosis and assessing progression of incomitant squint
- It differentiates between acute onset, long-standing paralysis and restrictive strabismus
- It differentiates divergence weakness from the sixth nerve palsy
- It provides permanent and accurate record for comparison.

Diplopia charting: Diplopia charting is a useful aid in the diagnosis and follow-up of incomitant strabismus. Good visual acuity and cooperation from the patient are essential prerequisites. Following data can be derived from charting:

- Areas of single vision and diplopia
- Distance between two images in areas of diplopia
- Whether images are crossed or uncrossed
- Whether separation between images is vertical or horizontal.

Procedure

Test is explained to the patient. Patient and examiner are made to sit facing each other at 50 cm in a semi darkroom.

Patient is asked to wear red-green goggles; red being in front of right eye (**Fig. 7**). The light is moved from primary position into all other eight directions of gaze. For each direction, patient is asked to comment on the position and separation between two images by using either two fingers or two pencils. Eye projecting red and green images should be noted. After labeling right and left side, separation of images as described by the patient in all nine cardinal positions of gaze is recorded.[2,3]

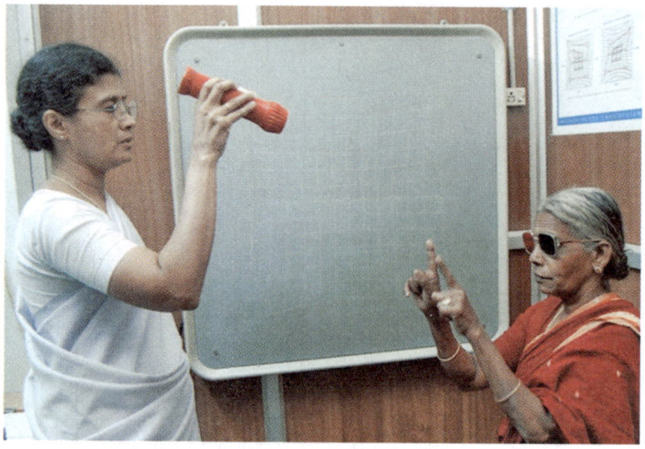

Fig. 7: Diplopia testing.

Interpretation of diplopia charts (Figs. 8A to C)

- *Overlapping images*: No diplopia
- *Separated images*: Confirms diplopia
- Maximum separation is seen in the quadrant in which muscle action is limited

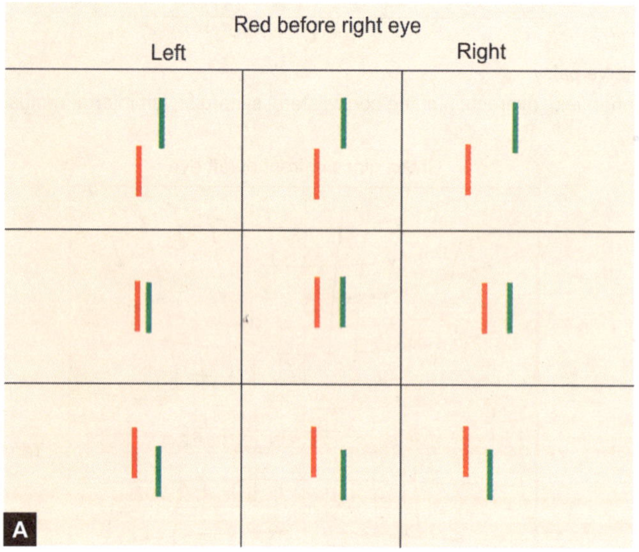

Left third nerve palsy

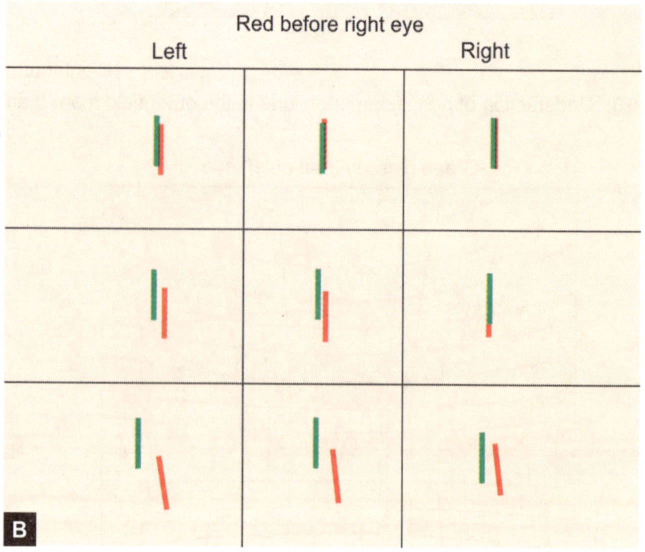

Left fourth nerve palsy

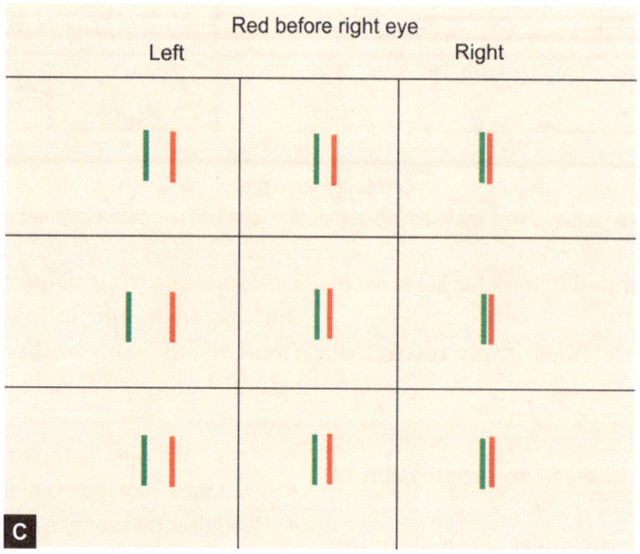

Left sixth nerve palsy

Figs. 8A to C: *Diplopia charts in oculomotor nerve palsies*: (A) Horizontal separation of images is maximum in the gaze of dextroversion (medial rectus). The vertical separation increases both in left and down gaze; (B) Maximum vertical separation and image intorsion in levodepression and binocular single vision in up gaze; (C) Binocular single vision in dextroversion, horizontal diplopia in primary position and levoversion (uncrossed) with maximum separation in levoversion.

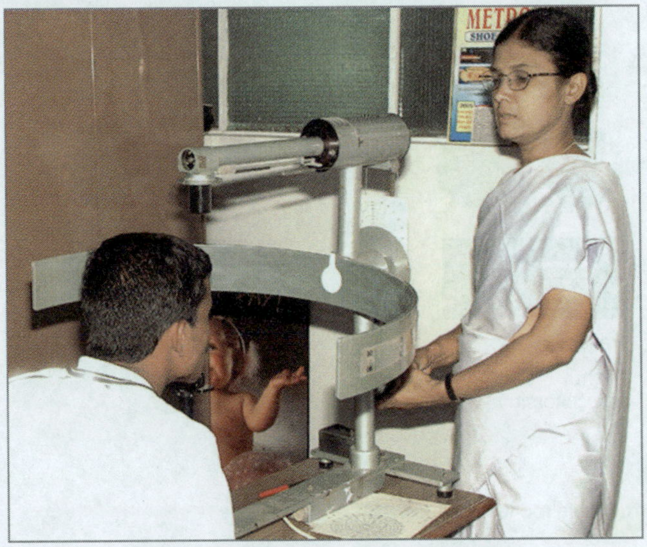

Fig. 9: Recording of binocular fields of vision.

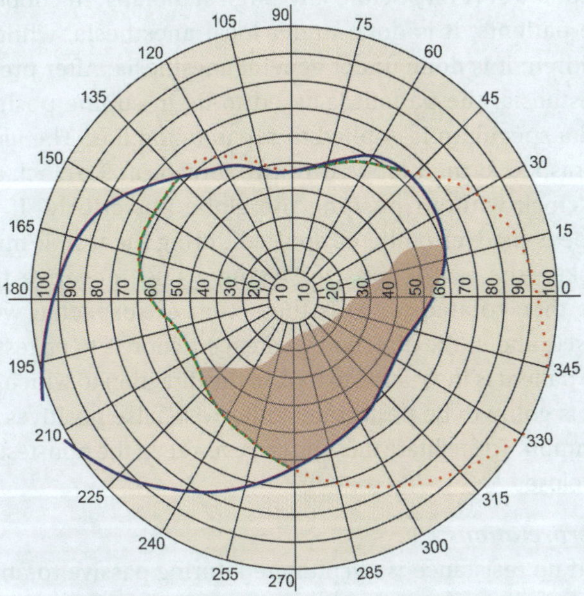

Fig. 10: Field of single and double vision.

- *Horizontal separation with uncrossed images*: Esodeviation
- *Horizontal separation with crossed images*: Exodeviation
- *Vertical separation with uncrossed images*: Oblique muscle involved
- *Vertical separation with crossed images*: Vertical recti involved.

Limitations of diplopia charting

- The test is subjective
- It needs a well-cooperative patient
- The test is not reproducible.

Binocular field of vision **(Figs. 9 and 10):** A perimeter which is used to check the peripheral field of vision is helpful to plot the fields of both eyes simultaneously ascertaining the diplopic field and diplopia free field (area of binocular single vision). The technique is same as in checking the peripheral fields, however here both eyes are kept open. The area can be plotted on, using a 2 mm white target, which can be seen easily. Red and green goggles can be used in some patients who have difficulty in seeing two white images.[4,5]

The patient is seated opposite the center of the instrument, with his head straight. The image is moved slowly along the arc in the different meridians, as it is done in peripheral field recordings. The point at which double vision occurs and single vision regained is plotted on a binocular field chart. This chart is useful when planning treatment for the palsy.

Maddox double rod test: The Maddox double rod test is a valuable qualitative test to substantiate a patient's complaint about image tilting. It is also useful to quantitatively determine the degree of tilt/torsion/cyclodeviation.

Procedure (Figs. 11A and B)

Red and white Maddox rods are placed in trial frame, the red before right eye and white before left eye. The direction of the Maddox rods is aligned with 90° marks of trial frame. The patient looks through the Maddox rods and is asked to focus at the penlight shown at 33 cm. The patient sees the images as two separate horizontal lines one red another white. If one of the lines (red) appears tilted towards the nose, excyclotropia of right eye is present. The Maddox rod is then turned until the red line is seen parallel to white line. The reading on the trial frame at this stage tells the amount of tilt or torsion of the image in degrees. In bilateral cyclotropia (excyclotropia of right and left eye in traumatic SO palsy), both red and white lines will be seen slanted towards the nose. With good observation, you can take accurate measurements. To test deviation outside the primary position, shift the penlight to the right, left, above and below, and repeat the test. Tilting of the trial frame should be avoided during the test.

Advantages of Maddox rod test

- It is easier to perform and can be completed quickly
- It provides quantitative measurement of subjective torsion.

Disadvantages of Maddox rod test

- Torsion may falsely localize in wrong eye, as ocular dominance determines the patient's response to Maddox rod test. Contradictory results with respect to the laterality of the paralyzed muscle are common.
- It presents difficulties in uncooperative and mentally challenged individuals.

Fundus examination: Fundus examination **(Fig. 12)** is a useful auxiliary method to diagnose and quantify torsion. Normally, the foveal location in relation to optic nerve head

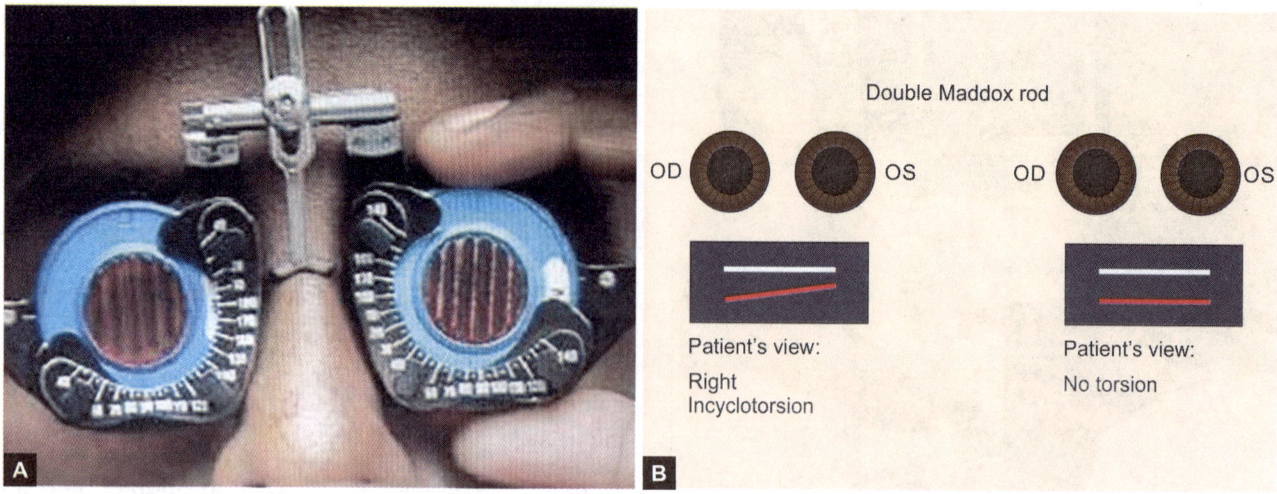

Figs. 11A and B: Maddox double rod test.

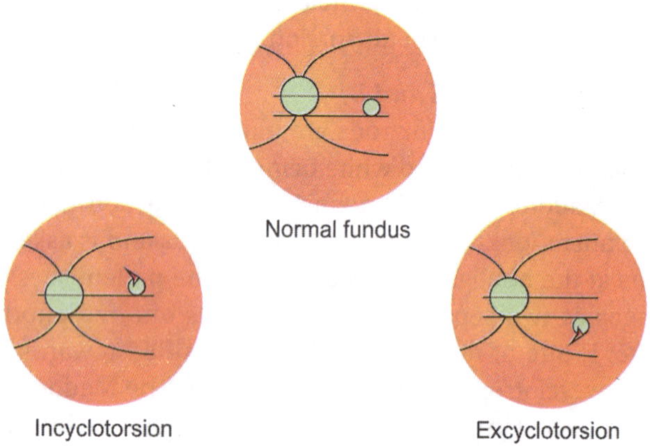

Fig. 12: Torsion in the fundus.

is 0.3 disk diameter below a horizontal line extending through the geometric center of optic disk. Incyclotropia is present when the fovea appears above the line extending horizontally from center of the optic nerve and excyclotropia is present when the fovea is below a line extending horizontally from just below the lower pole of the optic disk. The fovea's position may vary slightly in two eyes, but difference of 0.25 or more of a disk diameter in vertical position is considered significant. Precaution should be taken to avoid head tilt during the test. This is the most accurate test to measure the anatomic torsion and guides the surgeon about the selection of a muscle to be operated.

Special Tests

Some special tests, mentioned below, may be needed to correctly diagnose complicated cases of incomitant and restricted strabismus.

- Forced duction test
- Forced generation test
- Exaggerated traction test
- Saccadic velocity test
- Differential intraocular pressure (IOP) testing
- Tensilon test

Forced duction test: It is mandatory to perform forced duction test (FDT) before any surgical therapy. In cooperative patients, it is done under local anesthesia, while in children; it is done under general anesthesia. After proper anesthesia, the patient is asked to lie in supine position and a speculum is applied to separate the lids. The globe is grasped at the limbus with two forceps at 9 o'clock and 3 o'clock without pushing the globe posteriorly. If the globe is inadvertently retropulsed during the test, it might slacken the rectus muscles giving a false negative test. It is then rotated towards the action of suspected weak muscle and in the direction where restriction is to be tested. The patient is instructed to look in the direction to which the test is going to be performed, otherwise false positives are common. To facilitate this one can even keep the non-testing eye closed.[1,6,7]

Interpretations

- If no resistance is encountered during passive rotation, the test is negative. It is implied that motility defect is caused by paralysis of the weak muscle.
- If resistance is encountered during passive rotation of the globe, the test is positive. It implies a mechanical restriction.

Forced generation test: The globe is stabilized with forceps at the limbus. Patient is asked to move his both eyes in the direction of the muscle to be tested. During this movement, the force generated by contracting muscle is transmitted to the examiner's fingers. From feel of transmitted force the examiner can detect whether contracting muscle is weak or normal. For quantifying this, a calibrated forceps is available, which indicates the amount of force generated in grams (normal force generated is 60–80 g in extreme gazes). But the test can be performed only in cooperative patients.[1]

Exaggerated traction test: Exaggerated traction test is described by Guyton to test the tightness of the oblique muscle and can be done under topical anesthesia. The author commonly practices the one hand exaggerated FDT. The globe is grasped at the nasal limbus with a Lim's forceps and fully retropulsed (this is in contrast to the steps for conventional FDT, as retropulsion tightens the obliques). It is adducted and rotated superonasally to place the SO tendon on maximal stretch. The globe is then rotated into an abducted position to pluck the SO tendon. The surgeon feels a bump as the SO tendon slides into its new position. The bump can be quite subtle and considerable practice is needed before a reliable test is obtained. For the IO the globe is placed inferonasally and then rotated inferotemporally.

Another useful method to test the tightness of the obliques is to grasp the globe at the nasal and temporal limbus with a 0.5 mm toothed forceps. The globe is fully retropulsed and extorted to check the tightness of the SO muscle and intorted to check the tightness of the IO muscle.

Saccadic velocity testing: Systematic study of saccadic velocity may be useful in distinguishing between mechanical and paretic limitation of ocular motility. Useful in conjunction with other tests such as forced duction and generation test. If paralysis exists, the velocity of the paralyzed muscle will be markedly decreased, normal rapid saccades being replaced by a slow, drifting eye movement. If mechanical restriction is present, the saccadic velocity of an eye movement into the field of apparent paresis will be normal.[5]

Differential intraocular pressure testing: Intraocular pressure rises on compression of a nonrelaxing stiff muscle, when attempts are made to move the eye into the field of antagonist. Perkin's handheld tonometer can be used to measure IOP in different gazes. An increase in pressure by ≥5 mm Hg in a particular field of gaze is indicative of restriction.

Tensilon test: Tensilon test used for the diagnosis of myasthenia gravis and the test is described elsewhere.

General Examination

The patients with paralytic strabismus should have their other systems examined to pinpoint the etiology including the detection of vascular anomalies (diabetes, hypertension, etc.). The patients with restrictive strabismus should be examined for the other associated congenital abnormalities.

Neurological Examination

This becomes essential especially in cases of head trauma and in systemic vascular disorders.

Investigations

Electromyography: The electromyography (EMG) has limited value as a diagnostic tool in incomitant squints. It is of value only in conjunction with other diagnostic tests in establishing whether a paralysis of muscle is of myogenic or neurogenic origin. In the myogenic process, electromyogram is characterized by a disproportion between massive recruitment of motor units and inability to move eye. While in neurogenic processes, it will show partial or complete loss of motor units in spite of maximal volitional innervation.[1]

Orbital imaging: Magnetic resonance morphometry of muscle shows atrophy and lack of contractibility of paralyzed muscle. It is not used routinely.

Neuroimaging: The computed tomography (CT) scan and magnetic resonance imaging (MRI) are required to find out the cause of incomitant squint.

RESTRICTIVE STRABISMUS

Restrictive strabismus is a form of incomitant strabismus characterized by limitation of ocular movement, which is out of proportion to the ocular deviation in primary position. This has a mechanical or innervational restrictive element. One must differentiate restrictive strabismus from a paralytic strabismus. The differences between restrictive strabismus and paralytic strabismus are summarized in **Table 4**. Musculofacial innervational anomalies like Duane's retraction syndrome, Brown's SO tendon sheath syndrome, congenital muscle fibrosis, strabismus fixus and the acquired causes like thyroid ophthalmopathy, myositis, parasitic cysts, fibrosis secondary to orbital trauma all come under this category. Common forms of restrictive strabismus are described below.

Duane's Syndrome

To establish the diagnosis of Duane's syndrome, one should have a thorough knowledge about its clinical types along with their basic pathophysiology. There are studies to confirm that there is maldevelopment or an insult to the developing structures of 6th cranial nerve nucleus and its nerve fibers as early as 4 to 8 weeks of gestation. To compensate this, branches from 3rd nerve are then redirected to the lateral rectus. Rarely, the medial rectus may have subnormal innervations and either muscle may become fibrotic.[8] The clinical signs vary depending upon the severity of pathology. The common presentation of Duane's syndrome is esotropia of the involved eye when their head is straightened with limitation of abduction in the involved eye **(Fig. 13)**. The most comfortable head posture will be the face turn towards the involved side and the eyes directed towards the opposite side. On attempted extreme adduction enophthalmos and narrowing of palpebral fissure usually occur in the involved eye. Abduction in the involved eye is mostly just beyond the midline. A small percentage of patients present either with orthotropia or exotropia. The tighter the lateral rectus muscle, less esotropic the patient is and greater the enophthalmos on adduction.[9] These are the patients who will show up and down shoots because of the slippage of the globe from the tightened muscles. All these findings can be detected during routine examination using the examination techniques described above and the diagnosis can be confirmed by doing FDT. One should also look for other associated ocular and systemic anomalies like crocodile tears, Goldenhar syndrome, Klippel-Feil anomaly, etc.

Table 4: Differentiation between paralytic and restrictive strabismus.

Features	*Paralytic*	*Restrictive*
Deviation in primary position	Present	Little/no deviation
Head posture	All components present in vertical muscle palsy	Face turn, chin elevation/depression. No head tilt
Ocular movements	Maximum limitation of movement in field of main action of affected muscle. Duction > version	Limitation on entire gaze rather than in direction of muscle action. Duction = version
Muscle sequelae	Likely to develop	Do not develop
Retraction on ocular movements	Absent	Often present
Intraocular pressure	Same in all gazes	Rise in direction of limited movements
Pain on eye movement	None	May be present
Saccadic velocity	Decreased	Normal
Hess chart	Maximum limitation in the field of action of affected muscle	Outer and inner fields approach each other
Forced duction test	May or may not be positive	Invariably positive

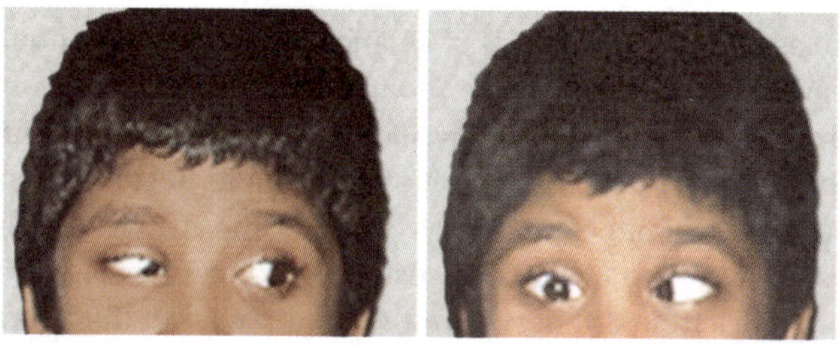

Fig. 13: Right Duane's retraction syndrome showing right abduction restriction, downshoot and globe retraction on attempted adduction.

Brown's Syndrome

In cases of Brown's syndrome, there is inability of the eye to elevate in adduction. This is caused in most cases by a restriction related to the SO tendon and/or trochlea.[9] A significant number of Brown's patients are orthotropic in primary position with good stereopsis needing no intervention. For a definitive diagnosis, Wilson and associates summarized the findings as follows:[10]

Deficient elevation in adduction, less elevation deficiency in midline, minimal or no elevation deficiency in abduction, minimal or no SO over action, "V" pattern with divergence in up gaze, and restricted forced duction **(Figs. 14A to C)**.

Less consistent findings include downshoot or hypotropia in adduction, widening of the palpebral fissure on adduction, anomalous head posture, and hypotropia in primary position. Other findings especially in acquired syndrome can be tenderness at the trochlear area and an audible or palpable click. Bilateral patients apart from the above clinical signs will exhibit an obvious "V" pattern deviation. All the examination techniques described under paretic strabismus should be followed including a detailed history to differentiate congenital from acquired causes.

Fibrosis Syndrome

Patients with generalized extraocular muscle fibrosis have blepharoptosis and a chin up posture. Ductions are severely limited. In severe drooping of the lids, patients use a finger or hand to lift the upper lid **(Fig. 15)**. Amblyopia may be present in the other eye. Unilateral fibrosis syndrome presents with enophthalmos, hypotropia apart from restricted ocular motility.

Thyroid Ophthalmopathy

Proptosis, lid retraction, conjunctival hyperemia with chemosis and restrictive motility are signs of thyroid ophthalmopathy. In thyroid eye disease, autoimmune inflammation of the extraocular muscles followed by fibrosis and deposition of glycosaminoglycans leads to stiffening of

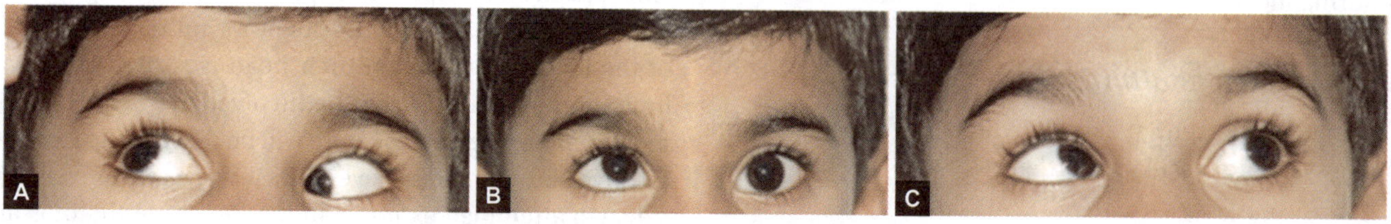

Figs. 14A to C: (A) Left Brown's syndrome showing restricted elevation of the left eye in adduction; (B) Mild restriction of elevation in primary position; (C) Elevation improves in left abduction.

the muscles and muscle belly thickening (sparing the tendon) causing restriction of motility in the opposite direction. This is in contrast to orbital pseudotumor that involves the muscle tendon as well. Medial and inferior rectus muscles are often involved though any extraocular muscle can be affected **(Fig. 16)**. Involvement of the lateral rectus is very rare in thyroid eye disease and if lateral rectus is predominantly involved, it should raise suspicion of an alternate pathology.[11] Other signs such as proptosis due to periocular soft tissue swelling and muscle thickening, lid retraction, periorbital puffiness along with systemic findings lead to the diagnosis.

Fracture Floor of the Orbit

History of orbital injury, presence of other associated signs, positive FDT with restrictive motility will confirm orbital fractures. Blow out fracture of the orbital floor can entrap the inferior rectus and the surrounding orbital fat. Entrapment of the inferior rectus anterior to the globe equator results in elevation restriction. Entrapment of the inferior rectus posterior to the globe equator results in inferior rectus paresis with depression restriction. The primary position deviation can be ortho, hypo or hypertropic **(Figs. 17A and B)**. Medial wall fracture can similarly entrap the medial rectus resulting in varying degrees of abduction restriction and medial rectus dysfunction. Infraorbital anesthesia, enophthalmos, history of trauma and orbital rim discontinuity give a clue to the diagnosis. In children the soft tissue signs may be minimal (so called white fractures) and the only clue to the diagnosis may be a history of trauma and restricted motility. Imaging of the orbit confirms the diagnosis.

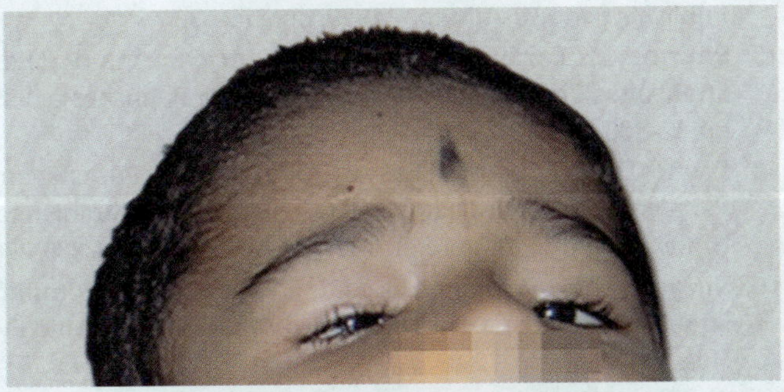

Fig. 15: Patient with congenital fibrosis of extraocular muscle and severe ptosis. Note the chin elevation because of severe ptosis and elevation restriction.

Other Causes

Restricted motility after extraocular surgeries notably pterygium excision, sclera buckling, ocular surface neoplasms are not uncommon. Conjunctival scarring and orbital fibrosis predominantly contribute **(Fig. 18)**.

To summarize, for a successful evaluation of a case of incomitant strabismus, the examiner should be aware of the various clinical signs in different entities, skilled in all the examination techniques including the Hess charting and FDT apart from being an expert in history taking. Also, should know what other ocular and systemic signs to look for. The readers are advised to read the referred books cited for more details.

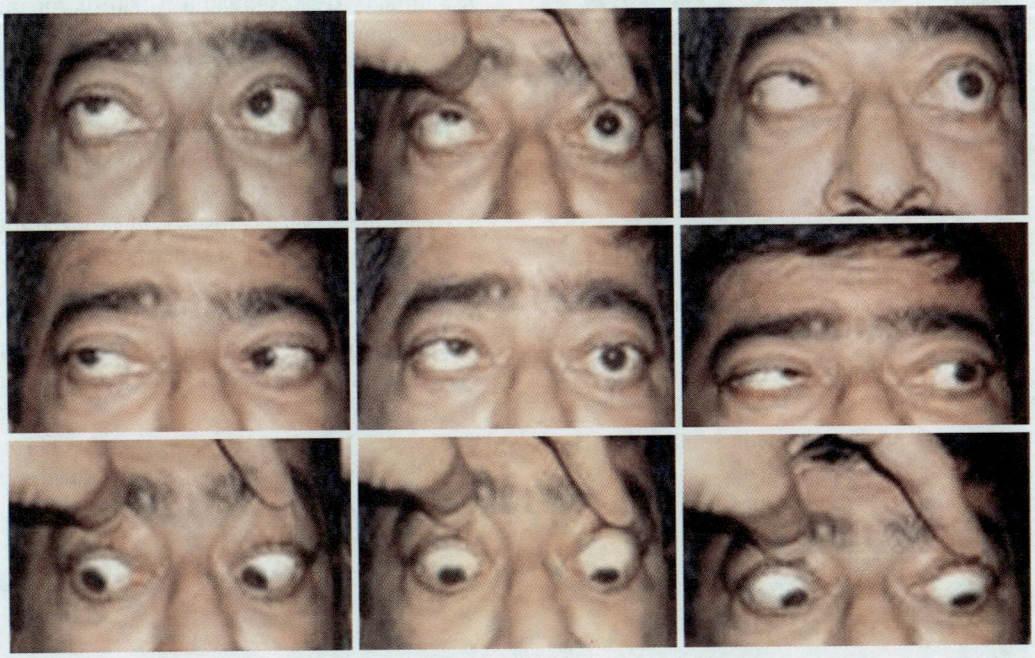

Fig. 16: Patient with thyroid ophthalmopathy. Note the proptosis and periorbital puffiness OU. Elevation is restricted in the left eye. Abduction is restricted OU. The forced duction test was noted to be positive. This is on account of tight medial and inferior recti.

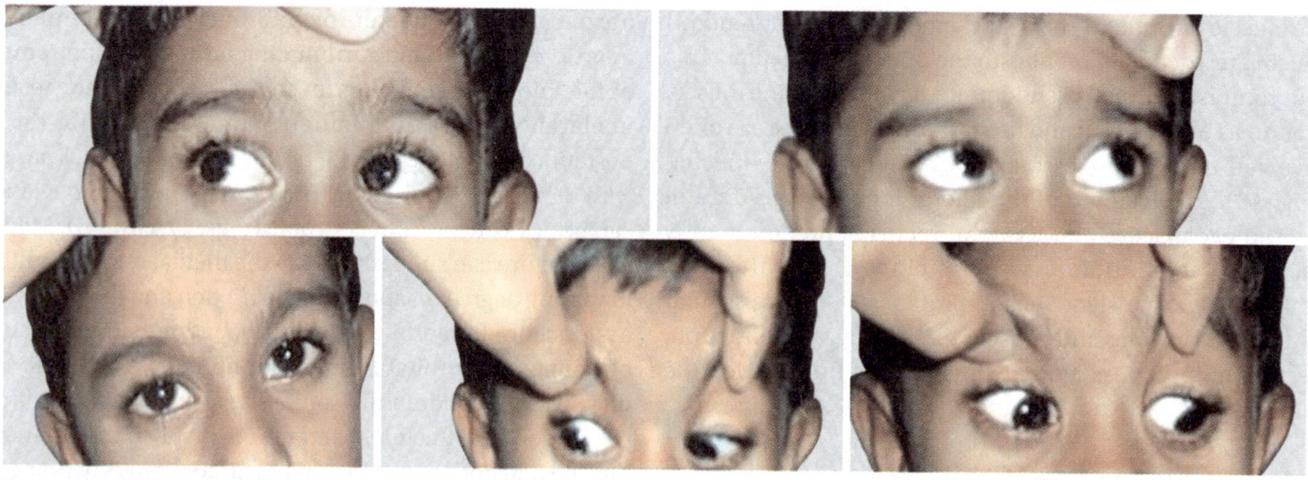

Fig. 17A: A 9-year-old patient presented with a head posture after bumping his right eye against a flowerpot. Note the depression restriction (in abduction) on the right side. Fractures in children have minimal signs of external inflammation (white fractures).

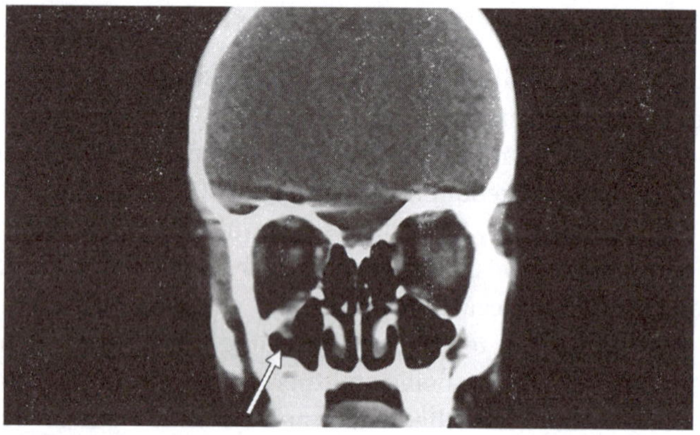

Fig. 17B: Coronal CT scan of the right orbit showing a teardrop sign. Note the entrapment of the inferior rectus behind the globe. There is minimal displacement of the bone fragments.

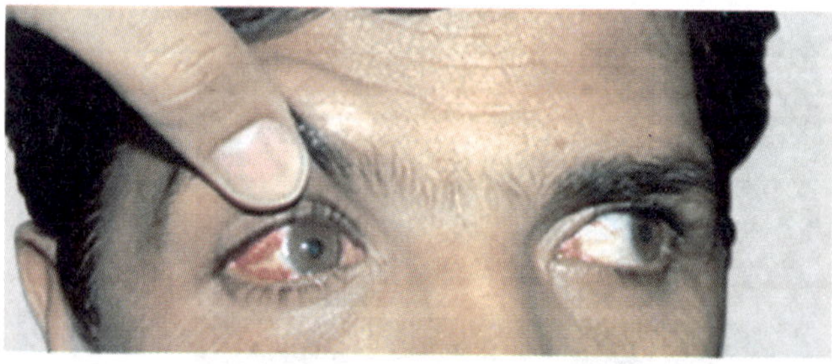

Fig. 18: Patient with right adduction restriction due to conjunctival scarring on the lateral side. The scarring is on account of extensive excision of ocular surface squamous neoplasia.

REFERENCES

1. von Noorden GK, Campos EC. Paralytic Strabismus In: von Noorden GK, Campos EC (Eds). Binocular vision and Ocular motility. United States: Mosby. 2002; pp. 414-57.
2. Khurana AK. Incomitant strabismus. In: Khurana AK (Ed). Theory and Practice of Squint and Orthoptics. New Delhi: CBS Publishers and Distributors. 1999; pp. 271-338.
3. Sharma P. Paralytic Strabismus. In: Sharma P (Ed). Strabismus Simplified. New Delhi: Modern Publishers. 1999; pp. 114-35.
4. Prieto-Díaz J, Souza-Dias C. Oculomotor Paresis and Paralysis. In: Prieto-Díaz J, Souza-Dias C (Eds). Strabismus. United Kingdom: Butterworth-Heinemann. 2000; pp. 289-358.
5. Vijayalakshmi P. Diagnosis and Treatment of Incomitant Strabismus. In: Orthoptics Simplified. New Delhi: Aravind Eye Hospital. 2007; pp. 72-89.
6. Philllips PH, Hunter DG. Evaluation of ocular torsion and principles and management. In: Rosenbaum AL, Santiago AP (Eds). Clinical Strabismus Management. United States: WB Saunders Company. 1999; pp. 52-72.
7. Santiago AP, Rosenbaum AL. Tests for muscle functions. In: Rosenbaum AL, Santiago AP (Eds). Clinical Strabismus Management. United States: WB Saunders Company. 1999; pp. 37-49.
8. Jampolsky A. Duane Syndrome. In: Rosenbaum A, Santiago AP (Eds). Clinical Strabismus Management. United States: WB Saunders Company. 1999; pp. 325-46.
9. Helveston EM. Diagnostic Categories and Classification of Strabismus. In: Surgical Management of Strabismus. Belgium: Wayenborgh Publishing. 2005; pp. 123-62.
10. Weakley DR, Stager DR, Stager DR. Brown Syndrome. In: Rosenbaum AL, Santiago AP (Eds). Clinical Strabismus Management. United States: WB Saunders Company. 1999; pp. 347-57.
11. Chen CS, Lee AW, Miller NR, et al. Double vision in a patient with thyroid disease: what's the big deal? Surv Ophthalmol. 2007;52(4):434-9.

CHAPTER

32

Diagnostic Procedures in Dry Eye Disease

Jayesh Vazirani, Virender Sangwan

"If a man's eyes are affected with dryness, he shall rub an onion, drink it in beer, and apply oil to his eyes. Thou shalt disembowel a yellow frog, mix its gall in curd, and apply to his eyes."

- Prescription from Assyro-Babylonian Ophthalmology. Krause AC. Ann Med Hist. 1934;6:42-55.

DEFINITION

Dry eye is a multifactorial disease of the ocular surface characterized by symptoms of discomfort, visual disturbance, and tear film instability with a potential damage to the ocular surface. It is accompanied by increased osmolarity of the tear film and inflammation of the ocular surface.[1]

This definition, suggested by the "international dry eye workshop", elegantly incorporates the contemporary understanding of both etiopathogenic as well as mechanistic aspects of dry eye disease. In routine clinical practice, however, it is neither feasible nor necessary to document all components of dry eye as laid down in the definition.

DRY EYE DIAGNOSIS

A considerable amount of confusion persists regarding the selection of diagnostic tests for dry eye. In an international survey of renowned practitioners in the field of tear film and dry eye, no single test emerged as the dominant first choice diagnostic tool.[2] Most practitioners reported using multiple tests, relying primarily on patient history, fluorescein break-up time, ocular surface staining and the Schirmer test.

This chapter aims to simplify the choice and order of diagnostic tests for dry eye disease in a routine clinical setting. Greater emphasis has been placed on tests that can be performed with relative ease and regularity. A brief mention has been made of other tests, which may have considerable scientific rationale and theoretical importance, but are actually impractical to perform in day-to-day clinical practice.

Symptoms: Questionnaires

Extensive symptom-based questionnaires have been developed for dry eye disease, including the ones incorporated into the European diagnostic criteria for Sjögren's syndrome.[3] A good example is the validated questionnaire developed in the USA for a large population study,[4] consisting of six questions:

1. Do your eyes ever feel dry?
2. Do you ever have a gritty or sandy sensation in your eyes?
3. Do your eyes ever have a burning sensation?
4. Are your eyes ever red?
5. Do you notice much crusting on your lashes?
6. Do your eyes ever get stuck shut in the morning?

The study found a lack of correlation between symptoms, tear deficiency (measured by the Schirmer test) and ocular surface damage (measured by rose Bengal staining). Thus, the results of diagnostic tests may not indicate the mechanisms leading to symptoms of dry eye.

SLIT-LAMP EXAMINATION

General examination of the ocular adnexa often provides vital clues towards the pathogenesis of dry eye disease. Important observations include approximation of eyelids, excursion of the upper eyelid with each blink (should cover upper two-thirds of the cornea) and interpalpebral fissure width. Trichiasis, entropion, ectropion or abnormal lid closure may interfere with tear film dynamics, and should be documented. Asking the patient to close the eye while holding the eyelid and observing the Bell's phenomenon. A deficient Bell's reflex may lead to exposure keratopathy.

Examination of the inferior marginal tear strip yields information about the volume of tears present. It is better

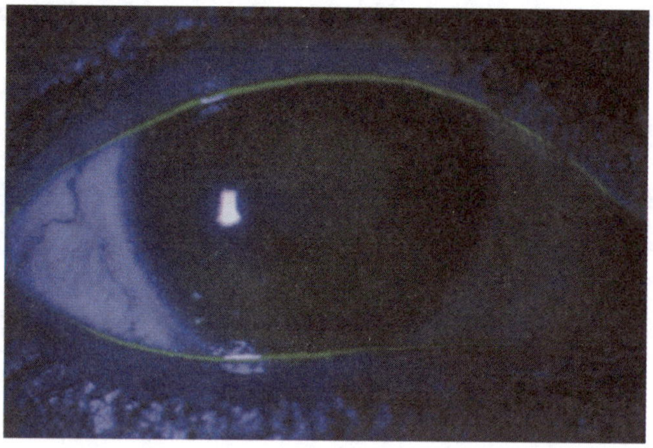

Fig. 1: Thin tear meniscus seen clearly after staining with fluorescein.

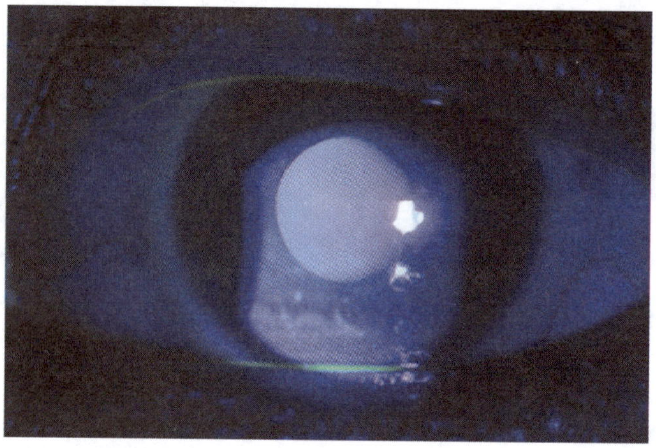

Fig. 2: Measurement of tear film breakup time is carried out by assessing time taken for appearance of first randomly distributed dry spot on the cornea after fluorescein staining.

visualized by fluorescein staining; care must be taken not to flood the surface by overwetting the fluorescein strip. It is normally about 0.5 mm in width and has a concave upper aspect. When this strip is thin or discontinuous, it presents an evidence of deficient aqueous tear volume **(Fig. 1)**. Increased tear film debris, including mucus, sloughed epithelial cells and other foreign material are suggestive of delayed tear clearance seen in dry eye.[5] Conjunctivochalasis, or redundant folds in the bulbar conjunctival epithelium, has been reported to be characteristic of dry eye.[6]

Evidence of altered meibomian gland structure includes increased vascularity of the margin, plugging of the orifices, and loss of orifices, which point towards a diagnosis of evaporative dry eye.[7] In normal subjects, it is possible to express some lipid from about two-thirds of the glands at a given time. This excretion is normally fluid and clear. Lack of expression and/or alteration in the character of the excretion (turbid or toothpaste-like), suggests the diagnosis of meibomian gland dysfunction (MGD).

Tear Film Stability

The interval between the last complete blink and the appearance of the first random dry spot in the precorneal tear film is the break-up time (BUT). This is usually measured after a slightly moistened fluorescein strip is applied to the superior bulbar conjunctiva, with the use of a cobalt blue exciter and yellow barrier filter **(Fig. 2)**. The subject is instructed to blink several times and then not to blink. The tear break-up time should be evaluated before the instillation of any eye drops and before the eyelids are manipulated in any way. In general, a break-up time of less than 10 seconds suggests an unstable tear film. Abnormally low values do not specify the type of dry eye.

The conventional test is a provocative one, as instillation of fluorescein shortens the normal break-up time.[8] In the noninvasive break-up time (NIBUT), tear break-up time is measured as the time between the last blink and the break-up of a reflected image of a target on the tear film.[9]

Tear Film Production

The Schirmer test is a widely available, low cost and commonly performed diagnostic test for aqueous tear production. A standardized size strip of filter paper is placed in the temporal part of the inferior cul-de-sac, and the extent of wetting of the strip in millimeters is noted at 5 minutes **(Fig. 3)**. If performed after the instillation of a topical anesthetic (the so-called basal secretion test), excess fluid should be gently removed from the cul-de-sac prior to insertion of the filter paper. Values of less than 6 mm are believed to indicate aqueous tear deficiency.[10] Although an isolated test may be misleading, consistently low values with repeated testing over time are highly suggestive of dry eye disease. The Schirmer-II test, which measures reflex stimulation of tears in response to vigorous stimulation of the nasal mucosa, is very uncomfortable for the patient and usually is not performed.

An alternative test uses a cotton thread treated with phenol red, which is placed in the inferior cul-de-sac. The dye is pH sensitive, and the length of wetted thread at the end of 15 seconds, indicated by change in color from yellow to orange, is noted. A cutoff value of less than 6 mm for the diagnosis of dry eye is used, and the test is reportedly more specific than the Schirmer test, with less inter-individual variability.[11]

Ocular Surface Staining

Fluorescein sodium, rose bengal, and lissamine green are the most commonly used dyes used for staining the ocular surface.

Fluorescein dye stains areas of the corneal and conjunctival epithelia where there is sufficient disruption of intercellular junctions to allow the dye to permeate into

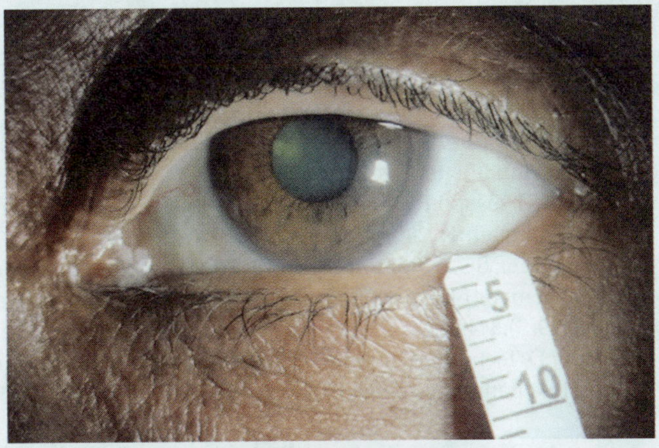

Fig. 3: Schirmer test.

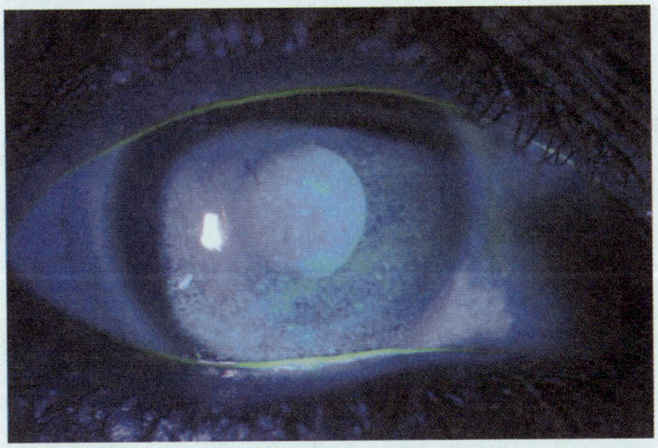

Fig. 4: Multiple punctate areas in the interpalpebral area stained with fluorescein, characteristic of dry eye disease.

the tissue.[12] A fluorescein-impregnated strip wetted with saline is applied to the eyes and the patient is asked to blink a few times to allow the dye to spread. The use of a cobalt blue exciter filter and a yellow barrier filter allows optimal visualization of staining of both the cornea and bulbar conjunctiva **(Fig. 4)**. Characteristic patterns include interpalpebral staining in aqueous tear deficiency and staining of the superior bulbar conjunctiva in superior limbic keratoconjunctivitis.[13] A number of grading scales, including the Van Bijsterveld, National Eye Institute (NEI)/Industry Workshop, and Oxford systems are available to measure the extent and intensity of staining.[14] The dye is well tolerated and causes minimal irritation.

Rose bengal staining is more intense on the conjunctiva than the cornea. The dye stains ocular surface cells that lack a mucus coating as well as debris in the tear film **(Fig. 5)**.[12] The saline drop used to moisten the strip should remain in contact with the strip for at least a minute to achieve an adequate concentration of rose bengal to stain the ocular surface. The dye causes pain on instillation, which may last for hours or days. Staining should therefore, be preceded by topical anesthesia and subsequently the dye should be washed out with sterile saline. Lissamine green produces a

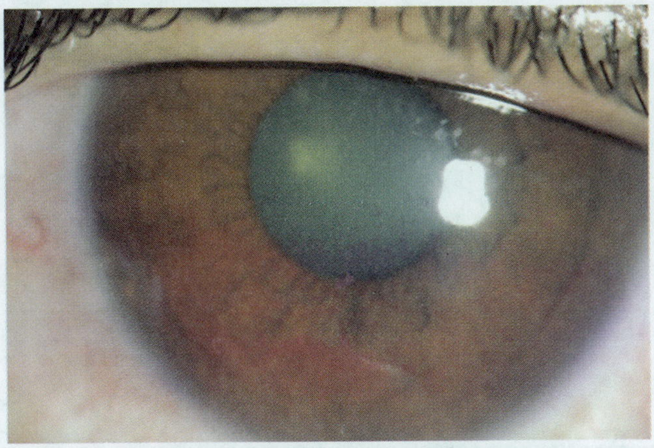

Fig. 5: Rose bengal stain taken up in inferior half of the cornea in dry eye disease.

staining pattern similar to that of rose bengal, it is distinctly visible over the bulbar conjunctiva and less so over the cornea. It causes less irritation than rose bengal, and hence is gaining wider acceptance.

Tear Film Composition and Characteristics

Decreased tear film lysozyme and lactoferrin levels have been found to be indicative of aqueous deficiency dry eye disease, amongst other conditions.[15,16] The lack of availability, cost and relatively low specificity of these tests are limiting factors for their routine use.

The tear ferning test, or a pattern resembling ferns when tear samples dried on a slide are examined under the microscope is said to be specific and sensitive for severe forms of dry eye disease, and a grading system has been developed.[17] Normally a crystalline pattern of tear mucin is observed.

Hyperosmolarity of tears is found to be a hallmark of all forms of dry eye.[18] Clinically, tear osmolarity can be measured using nanoliter samples from the lower tear meniscus, with very high sensitivity, specificity and positive predictive values. Values range from 302 ± 6.3 mOsm/L to 306 ± 7 mOsm/L in normal subjects and from 323 ± 12 mOsm/L to 343 ± 32.3 mOsm/L in eyes with keratoconjunctivitis sicca have been found in different studies. A value of 311 mOsm/L has been suggested as the upper limit of normal.

Tear Clearance Tests

Reduced tear turnover rate has been demonstrated in various forms of dry eye disease.[19] This can clinically be assessed by the fluorescein clearance test. 5 μL of fluorescein (1%) are instilled in the inferior conjunctival fornix, and serial 1-minute Schirmer tests are performed at 10-minute intervals. The strips are assessed under blue light for presence of the fluorescein, and persistence of the dye beyond 10 minutes is indicative of delayed tear clearance. Special fluorophotometers have also been built for assessment of dye clearance from tears.

Flowchart 1: Recommended sequence of tests.

Noninvasive (if available)		
Noninvasive tear break-up time	Topography	Reflective meniscometry

↓

Minimally invasive	
Tear break-up time	Ocular surface staining with fluorescein

↓

Tear secretion	
Schirmer test (without anesthesia)	Phenol red thread test

↓

Additional ocular surface staining	
Lissamine green	Rose bengal

NEWER METHODS

The quest for noninvasive methods for diagnosis of the dry eye disease has opened up multiple exciting avenues. However, most of these techniques are not currently practiced on a large scale due to issues of cost, availability of necessary equipment and feasibility of conducting tests.

Compromised visual function in dry eye can be quantified by measuring optical aberrations, serial videokeratographic/topographic analysis as well as by a functional visual acuity device which relies on rapid presentation of optotypes.[20,21]

Other noninvasive diagnostic methods include video meniscometry for demonstrating tear meniscus dysfunction, interferometry of the tear film lipid layer for assessing severity of dry eye disease and identifying candidates for puntal plugs and meibometry or laser meibometry for quantifying the amount of meibomian lipid on lid margin.[22] Anterior segment optical coherence tomography has also been demonstrated to have reasonable repeatability, sensitivity and specificity for assessing the tear meniscus height.[23]

Recommended sequence of tests are listed in **Flowchart 1**.

SYSTEMIC EVALUATION

Investigations such as anti-Sjögren's-syndrome-related antigen A (anti-SSA), anti-Sjögren's-syndrome-related antigen B (anti-SS-B), rheumatoid factor, antinuclear antibody (ANA), erythrocyte sedimentation rate (ESR) and C-reactive protein may be indicated in cases where Sjögren syndrome is suspected, in appropriate consultation with a rheumatologist.

REFERENCES

1. The definition and classification of dry eye disease: Report of the Definition and Classification Subcommittee of the International Dry Eye Work Shop. Ocul Surf. 2007;5(2):75-92.
2. Korb DR. Survey of preferred tests for diagnosis of the tear film and dry eye. Cornea. 2000;19(4):483-6.
3. Vitali C, Bombardieri S, Jonsson R, et al. Classification criteria for Sjogren's syndrome: a revised version of the European criteria proposed by the American-European Consensus Group. Ann Rheum Dis. 2002;61(6):554-8.
4. Brewitt H, Sistani F. Dry eye disease: the scale of the problem. Surv Ophthalmol. 2001;45:S199-202.
5. Pflugfelder SC, Solomon A, Stern ME. The diagnosis and management of dry eye: a twenty-five-year review. Cornea. 2000;19(5):644-9.
6. Meller D, Tseng SC. Conjunctivochalasis: Literature review and possible pathophysiology. Surv Ophthalmol. 1998;43(3):225-327.
7. Bron AJ, Benjamin L, Snibson GR. Meibomian gland disease. Classification and grading of lid changes. Eye (Lond). 1991;5(4):395-411.
8. Mengher LS, Bron AJ, Tonge SR, et al. Effect of fluorescein instillation on the pre-corneal tear film stability. Curr Eye Res. 1985;4(1):9-12.
9. Mengher LS, Bron AJ, Tonge SR, et al. A non-invasive instrument for clinical assessment of the pre-corneal tear film stability. Curr Eye Res. 1985;4(1):1-7.
10. Van Bijsterveld OP. Diagnostic tests in the Sicca syndrome. Arch Ophthalmol. 1969;82(1):10-4.
11. Bron AJ. Diagnosis of dry eye. Surv Ophthalmol. 2001;45:S221-6.
12. Feenstra RP, Tseng SC. Comparison of fluorescein and rose bengal staining. Ophthalmology. 1992;99(4):605-17.
13. Farris RL, Gilbard JP, Stuchell RN, et al. Diagnostic tests in keratoconjunctivitis sicca. CLAO J. 1983;9(1):23-8.
14. Foulks GN. Challenges and pitfalls in clinical trials of treatments for dry eye. Ocul Surf. 2003;1(1):20-30.
15. Avisar R, Menache R, Shaked P, et al. Lysozyme content of tears in patients with Sjogren's syndrome and rheumatoid arthritis. Am J Ophthalmol. 1979;87(2):148-51.
16. Van Bijsterveld OP. The Sjogren syndrome and tear function profile. Adv Exp Med Biol. 1998;438:949-52.
17. Albach KA, Lauer M, Stolze HH. Diagnosis of keratoconjunctivitis sicca in rheumatoid arthritis. The value of various tests. Ophthalmologe. 1994;91(2):229-34.
18. Gilbard JP, Farris RL. Tear osmolarity and ocular surface disease in keratoconjunctivitis sicca. Arch Ophthalmol. 1979;97(9):1642-6.
19. Pflugfelder SC, Tseng SC, Sanabria O, et al. Evaluation of subjective assessments and objective diagnostic tests for diagnosing tear-film disorders known to cause ocular irritation. Cornea. 1998;17(1):38-56.
20. Kojima T, Ishida R, Dogru M, et al. A new noninvasive tear stability analysis system for the assessment of dry eyes. Invest Ophthalmol Vis Sci. 2004;45(5):1369-74.
21. Ishida R, Kojima T, Dogru M, et al. The application of a new continuous functional visual acuity measurement system in dry eye syndromes. Am J Ophthalmol. 2005;139(2):253-8.
22. Yokoi N, Komuro A. Non-invasive methods of assessing the tear film. Exp Eye Res. 2004;78(3):399-407.
23. Ibrahim OM, Dogru M, Takano Y, et al. Application of visante optical coherence tomography tear meniscus height measurement in the diagnosis of dry eye disease. Ophthalmology. 2010;117(10):1923-9.

CHAPTER

33 Evaluation of Epiphora

AK Grover, Rituraj Baruah, Shaloo Bageja

APPLIED ANATOMY AND PHYSIOLOGY OF THE LACRIMAL APPARATUS

Lacrimal Gland

The lacrimal gland is an exocrine gland (20 × 15 × 5 mm) that lies in the lacrimal fossa formed by the frontal bone in the anterosuperior lateral orbit. It is divided into a larger orbital lobe and a smaller palpebral lobe by the fibrous extensions from the Whitnall's ligament, levator aponeurosis and its lateral horn.[1] It secretes tears through a series of ducts (10–12) into the conjunctival sac just in front of the superior fornix, 5 mm above the lateral tarsal border. Two to six ducts from the orbital portion run through and join the ducts of the palpebral lobe. Removal or damage to the palpebral lobe can thus lead to significant decrease in tear secretion.

There are accessory exocrine glands of Krause and Wolfring that are located in the superior fornix and above the superior border of the tarsus, respectively. These glands have got no apparent nerve supply.

The blood supply of the lacrimal gland is from the lacrimal branch of the ophthalmic artery. Venous blood drainage is via the ophthalmic vein.[2]

Nerve Supply

The lacrimal gland has got sensory, secretomotor and, sympathetic supply. Sensory supply comes through the lacrimal branch of the ophthalmic division of the 5th cranial nerve. Secretomotor supply is via the parasympathetic fibers. Parasympathetic preganglionic fibers arise from the lacrimal nucleus in the pons near the glossopharyngeal nucleus. Sympathetic postganglionic fibers come from superior cervical ganglion and reach the lacrimal gland via deep petrosal and also along with the sympathetic fibers around lacrimal artery and nerve.[2]

Lacrimal Excretory Apparatus (Fig. 1)

The lacrimal excretory apparatus consists of the upper and the lower puncta, canaliculi, tear sac and the nasolacrimal duct.

Puncta

These are small, round to oval orifices of about 0.2 mm in diameter on the summit of an elevation, the papilla lacrimalis that lies near the medial end of the eyelid margins at the junction of its ciliated and the nonciliated parts in line with the openings of the meibomian glands. The puncta, being relatively avascular is paler than its surrounding, serving as a guide in case of finding a stenosed punctum.

The upper punctum is slightly medial relative to the lower but when the eyelids are closed they appose each other. The medial ends of the lower lid retractors also help stabilize the puncta and prevent punctal eversion on

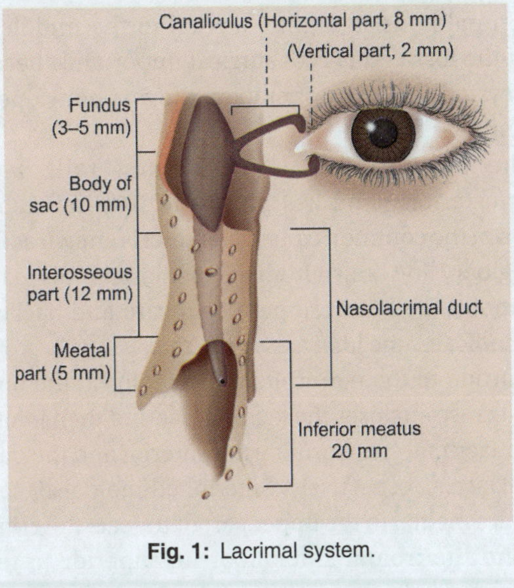

Fig. 1: Lacrimal system.

blinking. The patency of the puncta is maintained by the surrounding dense fibrous tissue continuous with the adjacent tarsal plate.

Canaliculi

The canaliculi are hollow tubes of 0.5 mm diameter connecting the puncta to the lacrimal sac. Each canaliculus has a vertical part, which is 2 mm in length and a horizontal part of 8–10 mm, which follows the eyelid margin converging towards the medial canthus. The canaliculi are enveloped by the orbicularis muscle fibers and elastic tissue, except on the posterior walls, which are covered by conjunctiva through which the probe can be easily seen. The upper is slightly shorter than the lower. There is a dilatation at the junction of these two parts, which is the ampulla. The canaliculi pierce the periorbita of the lacrimal sac separately, uniting at an angle of 25° to form a short common canaliculus (0–5 mm long). It then enters a small diverticulum of the sac, the lacrimal sinus of Maier at a point on the posterolateral surface of the sac about 2.5 mm from the apex of the sac. The common canaliculus is directed anteriorly forming an acute angle of about 45° with the sac before entering it. This acute entry into the lacrimal sac creates a potential mucosal flap or valve across the opening, the valve of Rosenmuller.[2,3]

The canaliculi are lined by stratified squamous epithelium supported with elastic tissue that can be dilated to three times the normal diameter.[2]

Lacrimal Sac

The lacrimal sac lies in the lacrimal fossa formed by the lacrimal bone and the frontal process of the maxilla in the anterior part of the medial wall of the orbit which is continuous below with the nasolacrimal duct. Vertical suture line between the frontal process of the maxilla and the lacrimal bone is slightly medial to the middle of the floor of the fossa. This is of surgical importance because in dacryocystorhinostomy operation, the first bony opening is made through this line.

The lacrimal sac is 12–15 mm tall, 4–6 mm anteroposteriorly and 2–3 mm wide. The sac above the junction of the common canalicular duct is known as fundus. An imaginary line drawn from the medial canthus to the first upper molar tooth that slopes downward and backward at 15–25° indicates the long axis of the sac.

A portion of the periorbita, which splits at the posterior lacrimal crest, encloses the lacrimal sac and then joins at the anterior lacrimal crest forming the anterior and the posterior lacrimal fascia, respectively. Anterior ethmoidal air cells and vessels are medial to the upper part of the sac; the cribriform plate and the frontal sinus floor lie superior to the sac. Between the posterior surface of the sac and the posterior lacrimal fascia there is a vascular plexus; injury to the plexus cause troublesome bleeding. Anteriorly, the upper part of the sac is in close contact with the medial palpebral ligament so much that the ligament may have to be divided near its attachment to the anterior lacrimal crest for complete mobilization of the sac. The angular vein crosses the ligament subcutaneously 8 mm from the medial canthus; however, the position of the vein is not always constant. Incision for removal of the sac should not be more that 2–3 mm medial to the medial canthus.

Nerve supply of the lacrimal sac is by the infratrochlear branch of the nasociliary nerve.

Blood supply of the lacrimal sac is via the dorsalis nasi and medial superior palpebral, both being branches of the ophthalmic artery, angular branch of the facial artery, branch of the external maxillary artery and the infraorbital branch of the internal maxillary artery. Venous drainage is through the rich venous plexus surrounding the sac into the angular vein.

Nasolacrimal Duct

The nasolacrimal duct is a continuation of the lacrimal sac. There is only a slight constriction at the junction of the nasolacrimal duct and the sac. The long axis is along the line joining the medial canthus to the first molar. It can be identified from outside by the more numerous and prominent vein surrounding the duct than the sac and from inside by the focal narrowing (valve of Krause) at the junction. The duct also has a thicker wall which becomes apparent on incision.

The nasolacrimal duct can be divided into two parts, an interosseous part (12 mm approximately) and an intermeatal part (5 mm approximately). It lies embedded in a bony canal formed medially by the maxillary bone and laterally by the lacrimal bone above and the inferior concha below. The nasolacrimal duct opens on the lateral wall of the nasal cavity about 10 mm posterior to the anterior end of the inferior concha and 30 mm from the external nares. The duct opening has a mucosal fold, the valve of Hasner, which prevents air from entering the lacrimal sac on sudden blowing the nose. The duct opening varies in size, shape and also the site of opening.

The duct is surrounded by a network of venous plexus, but a plexus of vessels exist that when engorged is sufficient to obstruct the duct.

Nerve supply to the duct is by the infratrochlear and the anterior superior alveolar nerves.

Blood supply of the nasolacrimal duct is from the palpebral branches of the ophthalmic, angular and infraorbital arteries and nasal branch of the sphenopalatine. Venous drainage is via the angular and the infraorbital vessels above and below into the nasal veins. Lymphatics of the nasolacrimal duct pass onto the submandibular and deep cervical nodes.

Orbicularis Oculi

Orbicularis oculi is the muscle that acts as the protector of the eyes through its blinking action. It has got two main parts—the orbital and the palpebral part. Our main concern here is the latter. The palpebral part is again divided into pretarsal—that part of orbicularis lying over the tarsas and the preseptal part over the orbital septum. The insertions of the orbicularis at the medial canthus around the lacrimal sac are called heads.

The *preseptal* part has its superficial head inserted into the medial canthal tendon and the deep head into the fascia on the dome of the lacrimal sac and into the upper part of the posterior lacrimal crest.

The *pretarsal* part has its circumferential fibers oriented over the superior and inferior tarsal plate. Laterally, it originates from the horizontal raphe and also from the lateral orbital tubercle. Medially, it is inserted into the anterior and posterior lacrimal crest by its two heads—the superficial and the deep head.

Two other muscle strips, the marginal preciliary and the retrociliary (muscle of Riolan) exist that are part of the pretarsal part of the orbicularis oculi.

Nerve supply to the orbicularis oculi muscle is by the facial nerve.

TEAR SECRETION AND ELIMINATION[4-6]

Tear secretions are mainly by the two sets of glands—lacrimal and the accessory glands of Wolfring and Krause. The accessory glands are the basal secretory that give a constant supply of tears as they lack any known innervations. The lacrimal gland is the reflex secretor. Autonomic stimulation, emotional stimulation, conjunctival, corneal or uveal irritation or an irritating focus in the sinus, mouth, ear, or teeth lead to reflex tearing. It can accompany yawning, laughing, sneezing and coughing.

Tears are distributed along the conjunctival fornices, precorneal tear film and the marginal tear strips. Approximately, 25% of the secreted tears are lost by evaporation. Rest are drained through the lacrimal drainage system via the punctum, the canaliculi, the sac, the nasolacrimal duct and ultimately into the inferior meatus of the nose. About 60% of the tears are drained via the lower punctum but in case of abnormalities the upper punctum can function efficiently without overflow.[6]

The blinking action of the eyelids helps in driving the tears forward into the drainage system. Jones proposed the lacrimal pump mechanism.[7] It demonstrates the blink mechanism propels tears through the lacrimal system by alternating negative and positive pressure in the lacrimal sac **(Fig. 2)**. Blinking displaces the upper as well as the lower lid medially due to the firm attachment of the orbicularis to the medial canthal tendon. Moreover, with each blink the upper and lower lid approximates at the lateral canthal area and then proceeds towards the medial canthus displacing the tear film towards the puncta.

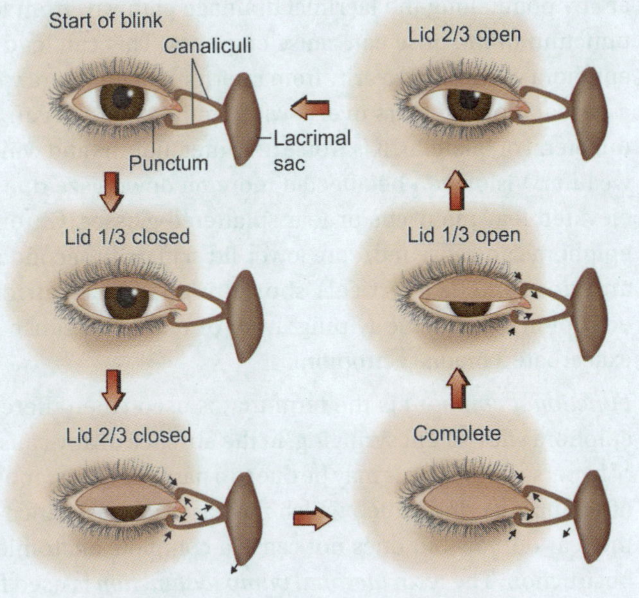

Fig. 2: Lacrimal pump mechanism.

With the start of the blink, the tears are propelled towards the puncta. As the process continues, the open puncta move towards each other and occlude. Due to the orientation of the superficial and the deep heads of the orbicularis around the canaliculi and their firm attachment to the bone, the eyelid is pulled medially on contraction, canaliculi are shortened squeezing the tear already in the ampulla and the canaliculi into the sac. The attachment of the deep head of the preseptal part of the orbicularis into the fascia on the dome of the lacrimal sac pulls the sac laterally on contraction enabling the sac filling (negative pressure). The valve of Rosenmuller reduces backflow, once the tears are in the sac.

On opening the eyes, the muscle around the canaliculi relaxes leading to the flow of tears into canaliculi again due to the reduced intracanalicular pressure. Tears can also gravitate down the nasolacrimal duct passively. But active drainage into the nose is by the complex action of the Horner's muscle.

Even in the absence of blinking, low flow of tears occurs through the puncta due to the Krehbiel's phenomenon, capillary action and the normal downhill slope of the eyelids but along with a passive reflux into the lacrimal lake.

EVALUATION OF EPIPHORA

Tearing can broadly be grouped under two main headings:

1. Epiphora (Impairment of drainage)
2. Lacrimation (Hypersecretion of tears).

It is essential to differentiate between two in planning the management.

Epiphora is a condition where there is excessive tearing due to reduced tear outflow, i.e. defective tear drainage. Obstruction at any point along the lacrimal drainage pathway, from the punctum to the nose can cause epiphora. This can lead to epiphora varying in severity from intermittent epiphora with a partial block to tears overflowing to the cheek. It can be unilateral or bilateral. It is worse in winter months and windy weather. Vision can be affected more on down gaze due to elevated tear meniscus or tear splattered glasses. Chronic epiphora can cause red, sore lower-lid skin, with secondary anterior lamella (vertical) shortening (mild cicatricial ectropion). Excessive wiping away of tears can cause or exacerbate a medial ectropion.

Functional epiphora is the term that is used when there is epiphora with patent syringing, in the absence of any causes of hypersecretion. This may be due to a narrowing or stenosis of the nasolacrimal duct, which increases the resistance to the tear outflow but does not cause a complete anatomical obstruction. The term *lacrimal pump dysfunction* is used for epiphora due to reduced tear drainage of orbicularis causes. Common causes of functional epiphora are punctal stenosis, facial palsy with paralytic ectropion, single functional canaliculus and common canalicular stenosis.

Pseudoepiphora refers to the reflex hypersecretion of aqueous tears from the main lacrimal gland due to altered production by the glands of Krause and Wolfring.[8]

Evaluating a case of epiphora needs a systematic approach, so that the causes of hypersecretion can also be ruled out.

History

A meticulous history taking is vital to the evaluation. Patient's symptoms, past ophthalmic, nasal and medical history should be elicited. A history of allergic diathesis and use of drugs should be obtained.

In case of congenital tearing, parents may complain of constant tearing with minimal or no mucopurulent discharge suggesting upper system block (punctal or canalicular dysgenesis). Constant tearing with frequent mucopurulent discharge and matting of the lashes suggest nasolacrimal duct block. Intermittent tearing with mucopurulence may suggest intermittent obstruction of the nasolacrimal duct (impaction of a swollen inferior nasal turbinate associated with an upper respiratory tract infection).

Examination

The lacrimal examination can be divided under these headings:

- *Periorbital, lid and lacrimal system assessment*:
  - General examination of the face, periorbital and medial canthal areas and eyelids is essential. It includes:
    - Slit-lamp examination of the puncta, external eye and tear meniscus
    - Syringing
    - Diagnostic probing
    - Fluorescein dye test.
- Examination of the nasal cavity
- Radiological examination
- Newer modalities.

Periorbital, Lid and Lacrimal System Assessment[9]

General Examination of the Face and Periorbital Region

Examinations of these parts with relevance to the symptoms help in establishing a diagnosis. Eyelid malposition, facial and periorbital asymmetry should be looked for.

Lacrimal Sac Swelling

A lump over the medial canthal area below the medial palpebral ligament strongly indicates to a lacrimal sac swelling **(Fig. 3)**.

Evidence of Inflammation

Fistula **(Fig. 4)** and inflammations over the sac area need to be further evaluated.

Shortening of Anterior Lamella

Vertical eyelid tightness should be checked by asking the patient to look up at the ceiling. If there is short anterior lamella, the ectropion will be exacerbated.

Assessment of Puncta

The presence of all the four puncta should be looked for the presence of any stenosis or membrane blocking it. They should face towards the lacrimal lake. The relative position

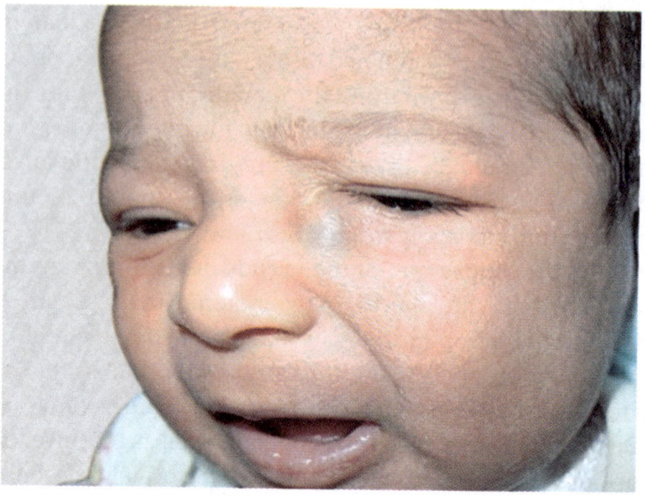

Fig. 3: Swelling over the area of the lacrimal sac in a child.

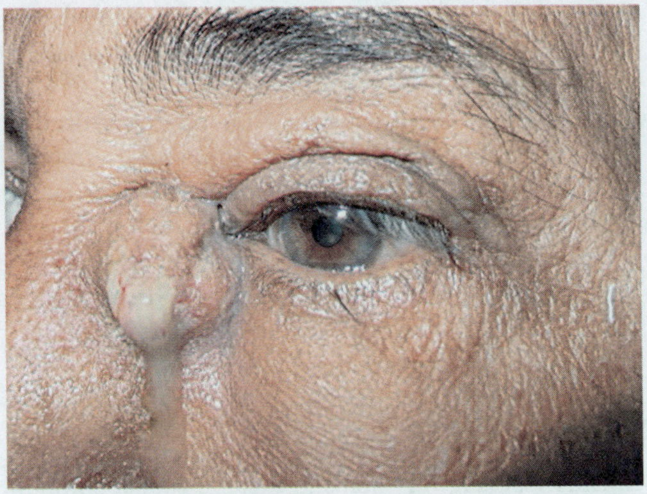

Fig. 4: Acute dacryocystitis with fistula.

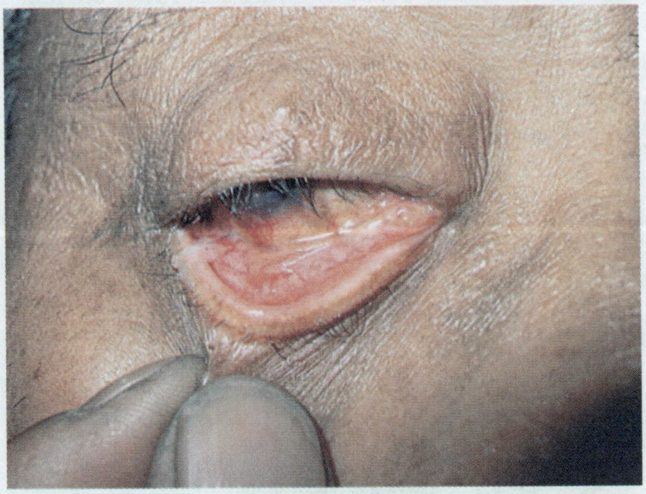

Fig. 5: Pinch test being performed to assess the eyelid laxity.

of the upper and the lower puncta to each other and to the caruncle should also be assessed.

Eyelid Laxity

The eyelid can in itself be a cause of epiphora. Involutional ectropion often progresses from punctal eversion to involve the medial third, then the medial half of the lower eyelid and eventually the entire lid. Examination of the lid with utmost care is needed to diagnose the condition.

Horizontal laxity of the eyelid can be estimated by Pinch test and snap back test:

Pinch test: Using the thumb and the index finger, the lid is pulled firmly away from the globe, the distance between the lid and the eye is measured and the laxity is documented **(Fig. 5)**.

None:	5 mm
Minimal:	5–7 mm
Mild:	8–9 mm
Moderate:	10–12 mm
Severe:	>12 mm

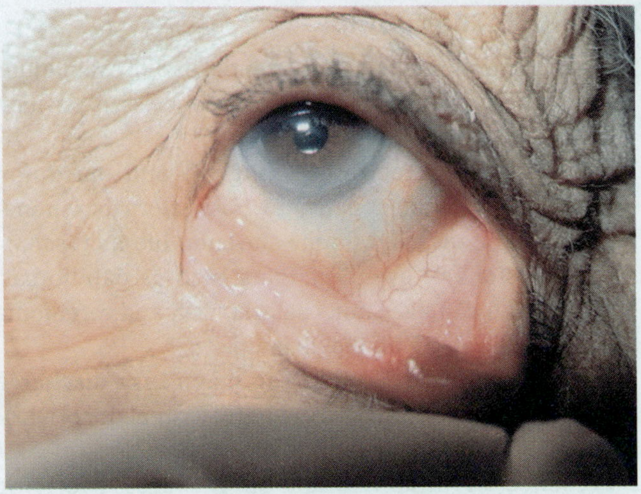

Fig. 6: Marked medial canthal tendon laxity.

Snap back test: The speed with which the lower lid settles back against the globe after being pulled down and released is to be observed, as well as whether there is a short gap between the lid and globe once settled and before the first blink.

Medial canthal tendon laxity: It is always to be assessed while evaluating a case of epiphora. It is graded with the lateral distraction test and by noting the position of the lower punctum in relation to the upper punctum. These tests depend on the fact that the lower puncta normally lies at the plica at rest and also when pulled laterally.

The patient is made to sit in front of the examiner at arm length distance with their eyes are at the same level. The patient is asked to look at the bridge of the examiner's nose and without inducing accommodative convergence by moving too close, the lower punctum position is noted relative to the upper **(Fig. 6)**.[10]

–1:	Punctal medialization
0:	Normal
+1:	Midway between the plica and the medial limbus
+2:	In line with the medial limbus
+3 ±6:	Beyond the medial limbus

Lateral distraction test: After noting the resting position of the lower punctum, the lower lid is pulled laterally, and the position of the punctum is noted again. The test is graded as:[11]

0:	No distraction at all
+1:	Punctum reaches midpoint of plica and medial limbus
+2:	Punctum reaches medial limbus
+3:	Punctum reaches midpoint of medial limbus and pupil line
+4:	Punctum reaches pupil line
+5:	Punctum reaches midpoint of pupil line and limbus line
+6:	Punctum reaches lateral limbus

Slit-lamp Examination

The slit-lamp examination is an essential part of evaluation:

- Punctum should be evaluated for patency, size, position and discharge.
- Mild degrees of ectropion **(Fig. 7)** and entropion **(Fig. 8)** that are not apparent to gross external examination may be revealed on the slit-lamp biomicroscopy. Small lesions of eyelid margins such as papillomas, molluscum contagiosum, chalazia, nevi and carcinoma are best detected with the slit lamp.
- Pressure over the lacrimal sac may cause discharge from the punctum, suggesting nasolacrimal duct (NLD) obstruction or canaliculitis.
- Presence of inflammation on the area overlying the canaliculus and discharge from the punctum on pressure over the area may suggest canaliculitis **(Figs. 9A and B)**.
- Examination for blepharitis **(Fig. 10)** should be looked for. Conjunctival lesions, particularly pingueculas and pterygia may induce tearing. The forniceal and palpebral conjunctiva should be inspected for follicles and papillae of reactive inflammatory disorders and allergic conjunctivitis.
- Cornea should be examined for any irregularities, features of dry eye syndrome or epithelial dystrophies. These examinations help us to rule out causes of hyperlacrimation.
- The vertical height of the tear meniscus should be measured prior to instillation of any eye drops. Staining the tear film with a small amount of fluorescein aids in assessing the volume of the tear lake.

Schirmer Test

Schirmer test **(Fig. 11)** helps to exclude pseudoepiphora. For this test white filter paper strips (41 Whatman) of 35 mm in length and 5 mm width are used. They are folded 5 mm at one end and inserted into the inferior fornix at the junction of the middle and lateral third of the lower lid and allowed to remain in this position for 5 minutes with the eyes open. The patient should be comfortably sitting

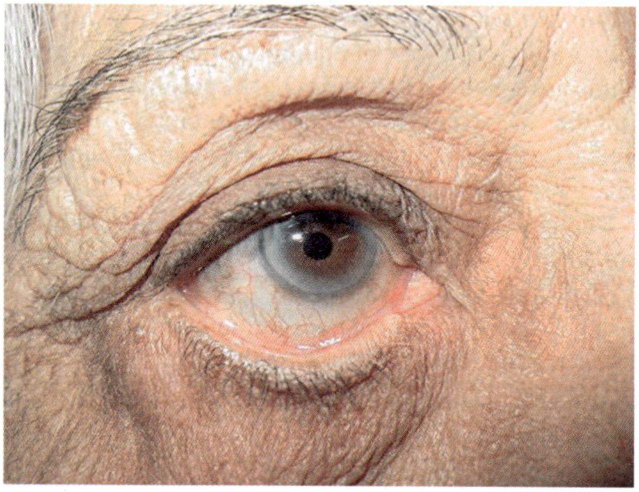

Fig. 7: Involutional ectropion.

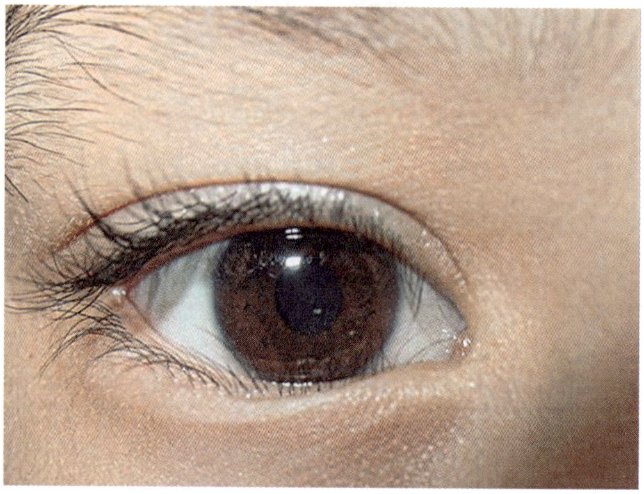

Fig. 8: Congenital entropion.

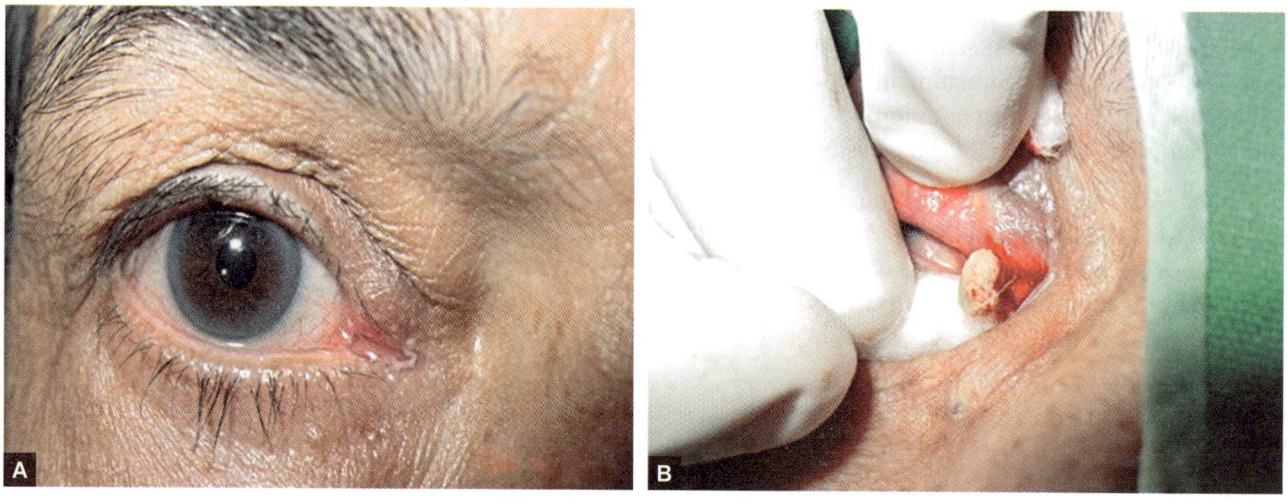

Figs. 9A and B: Canaliculitis.

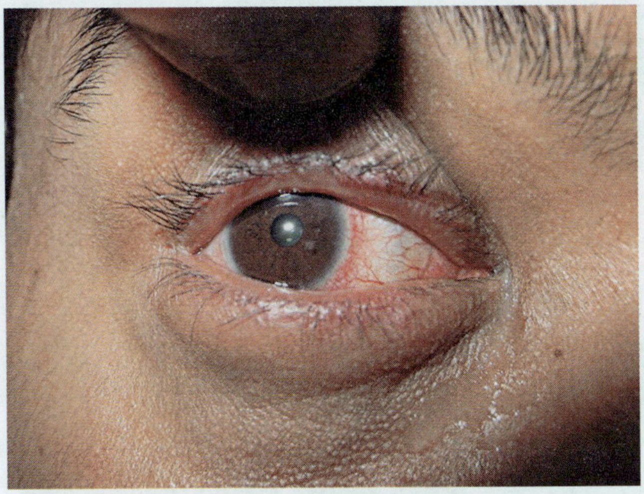

Fig. 10: Blepharitis.

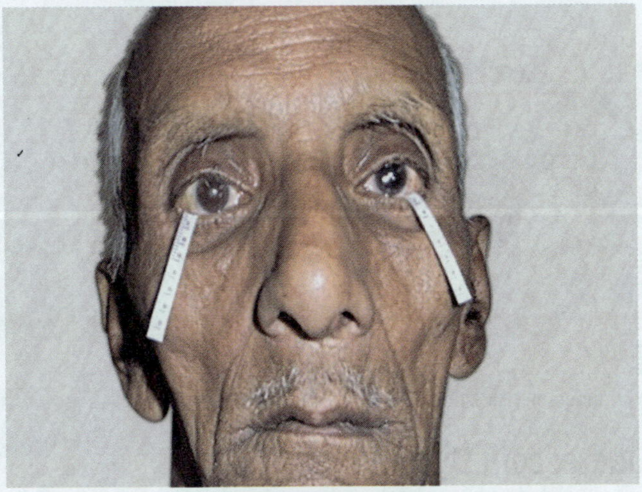

Fig. 11: Schirmer test.

in a dimly lit room away from direct air source as the fan. Moreover, there should not be any kind of verbal stimulation. After the end of the 5 minutes, the wetting of the filter paper is measured.

Schirmer test is basically of three types: Schirmer I test, basic secretion test and Schirmer II test. *Schirmer I test* is performed without topical anesthetic. 10 mm or more is taken as normal. Excessive wetting may be due to pseudoepiphora or hypersecretion.

Basic secretion test is done as the Schirmer I test but after instillation of topical anesthetic into the lower fornix. This anesthesia eliminates the local source of irritation as by the Schirmer test strips and gives an estimate of the basic tear secretion by the glands of Krause and Wolfring.[12] Wetting of less than 10 mm after 5 minutes indicates deficiency of basic tear production. A tearing patient with patent lacrimal drainage system with deficient basic tear production indicates towards reflex hypersecretion.

Schirmer II test measures the reflex tearing from the main lacrimal gland after eliminating the local causes of irritation.

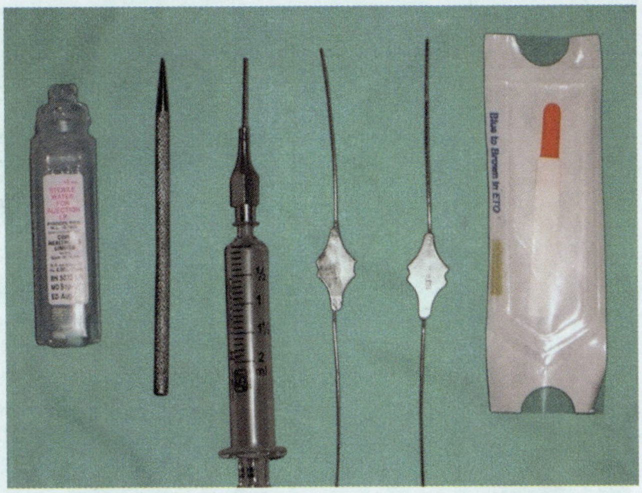

Fig. 12: Instruments used for syringing and probing.

After anesthetizing the conjunctival sac, the trigeminal nerve is stimulated either with a cotton-tipped applicator applied to the nasal mucosa or with ammonium chloride on a cotton pledget held at the external nares. The amount of excess wetting in addition to that of the basic secretion test is the reflex secretion.

Syringing

Syringing the canalicular system provides information regarding the patency status. One to two drops of topical anesthesia (proparacaine or tetracaine) is instilled into the conjunctival sac. The punctum is dilated gently by advancing the Nettleship's dilator **(Fig. 12)**, first vertically for about 2 mm and then horizontally with a twisting movement. Simultaneously, lateral traction is applied to the eyelid **(Figs. 13A and B)**. With the eyelid stretched, the dilator is withdrawn, and the lacrimal cannula attached with syringe filled with normal saline is advanced horizontally through the punctum and the canaliculus. No resistance should be felt in its entire path. Free passage of the saline into the throat indicates patency of the lacrimal passage. Regurgitation of the fluid indicates obstruction.

If there is resistance to irrigation, obstruction is present. Regurgitation of fluid from the same punctum indicates that there is a canalicular block. Regurgitation of fluid from the opposite punctum indicates blockage at the level of common canalicular duct, lacrimal sac or nasolacrimal duct. Immediate regurgitation of clear fluid usually suggests a common canalicular obstruction. Relatively delayed regurgitation of fluid mixed with mucus or pus usually indicates NLD blockage.

Diagnostic Probing

Probing the canaliculi provides information regarding the site of obstruction, which is necessary for

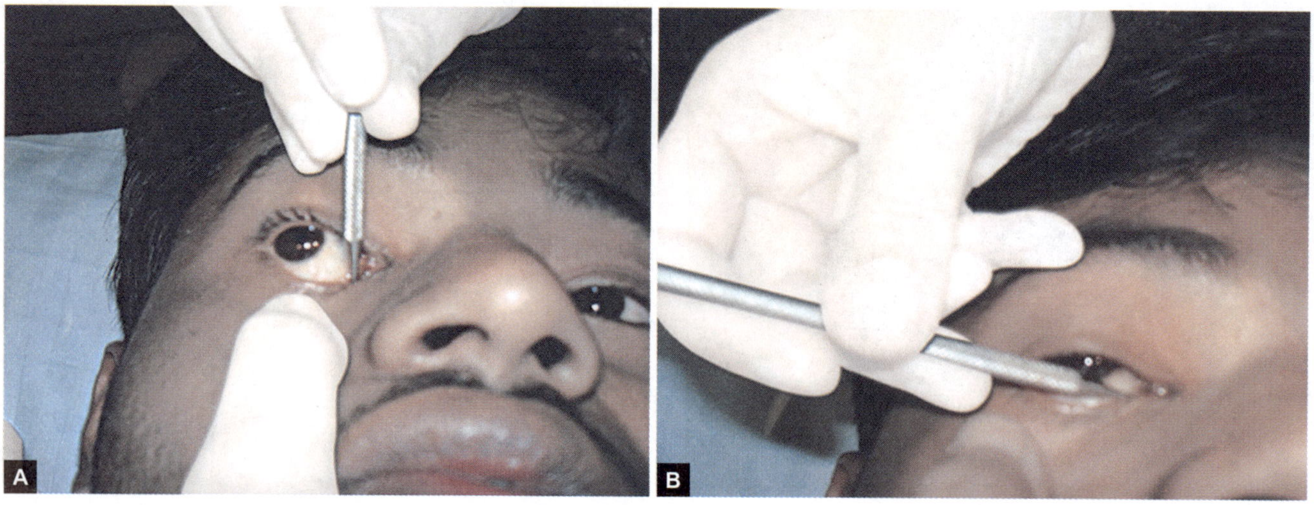

Figs. 13A and B: (A) Dilatation of punctum vertically; (B) Horizontal dilatation of canaliculus with lateral traction of the eyelid preventing the kinking of the canaliculus.

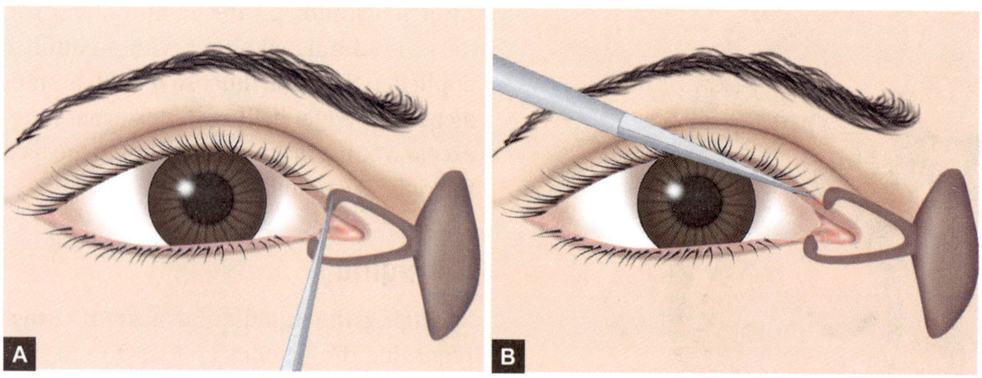

Figs. 14A and B: (A) Dilatation of punctum; (B) Probing.

decision-making. A topical anesthetic drop is instilled into the conjunctival sac. A probe of appropriate size is inserted into the punctum after dilatation. First, it is passed vertically through the punctum, turned medially and advanced until it encounters the obstruction **(Figs. 14A and B)**.

If probe enters the lacrimal sac, hard stop is felt as the probe abuts the lacrimal bone. The presence of soft stop indicates canalicular or common canalicular obstruction. One should reconfirm the soft stop as it may be felt due to kinking of the canaliculus or due to pushing of the probe into the lateral wall of the canaliculus.

The site of obstruction is determined by withdrawing the probe after grasping it with the forceps. The length of the probe is measured to assess the site of blockage. Obstruction at less than 8 mm indicates a canalicular block, 8–10 mm indicates a common canalicular obstruction and distal to that if the probe passes more than 10 mm.

While probing a child, a few considerations should be noted. Probing is usually recommended through the upper canaliculi as the lower canaliculus carries more tear flow than the upper and it is wise to avoid the possibility of injury to it. Up to 1 year of age, the distance from the punctum to the nasolacrimal duct is approximately, 12 mm, whereas, to the floor of the nose, it is approximately, 20 mm.[13]

Fluorescein Dye Test

Dye Disappearance Test or Fluorescein Dye Retention Test

This is a semiquantitative test of delayed or obstructed tear outflow. It is of particular importance for the evaluation of congenital dacryostenosis in infants and toddlers where lacrimal irrigation is impossible without anesthesia and deep sedation. One drop of 2% fluorescein is instilled into the unanesthetized conjunctival sac of both the eyes. The volume of the tear lake is then noted preferably under the cobalt blue light. The patient is instructed not to wipe the eyes. The tear lakes are examined 5 minutes later, and the relative volume is determined. Persistence of significant dye and especially asymmetric clearance of the dye from the tear meniscus over a 5 minutes period indicates a relative obstruction of the side retaining the dye.[14,15]

Jones Test[16,17]

The Jones tests are dye tests for functional epiphora where the lacrimal drainage system observed to be patent on syringing. There are two types of Jones tests.

Jones tests I: It investigates the lacrimal outflow under normal physiological conditions. Fluorescein (2%) is instilled into the conjunctival sac and presence of the dye at the inferior meatus is noted at 2 minutes and 5 minutes with the help of a cotton tip applicator. Rate of false negative is very high with this test.

Jones tests II: It is a nonphysiological test that determines the presence or absence of fluorescein in the irrigating saline fluid retrieved from the nose. Flushing of the residual dye (of the unsuccessful Jones test) from the conjunctival sac is done and after that topical anesthesia is instilled into the conjunctival sac. Patient is seated with head tilted forward and a transcanalicular irrigation with saline is done. Patient is then asked to blow or spit the fluid onto a paper tissue and fluorescein dye is looked for.

A *positive test* is with the presence of the dye on the tissue paper suggesting that the dye had reached the lacrimal sac but in the presence of a narrowed nasolacrimal duct or a nonfunctioning lacrimal pump requiring the syringing pressure to force it down.

The test is said to be *negative* when the tissue is clear of any dye indicating that it did not get into the lacrimal sac with the Jones I test as in eyelid malposition, lacrimal pump failure, punctal or canalicular stenosis.

A positive Jones test II confirms anatomical patency with a high-pressure wash out of fluorescein.

Other Tests

Taste test: One drop of saccharin is instilled into the conjunctival sac and one gets the taste of it after several minutes in case of a patent lacrimal drainage system.

Endonasal dye test: This is done as the Jones test I, except the appearance of the dye is seen through an endoscope inserted into the nares.

Oropharynx dye appearance test: Fluorescein 2% is instilled into the conjunctival sac of one side at a time and the oropharynx is checked periodically for the appearance of the dye. This test is of particular importance in infants where sedation or anesthesia is otherwise needed.

Examination of Nasal Cavity[18]

The key to success of a dacryocystorhinostomy surgery lies in the intact anatomy of the nasal cavity. Moreover, pathology of the structures around the opening of the nasolacrimal duct itself may be the cause of epiphora. Examination of the nasal cavity can be done either with a nasal speculum or more completely with a rigid nasal endoscope. One should look for abnormalities such as deviated septum, obstructed nasolacrimal duct ostium from membrane, hypertrophied turbinate, polyp, congested nasal mucosa or any mass **(Fig. 15)**. Treatment of the pathology is necessary before contemplating surgical intervention. Postoperatively, also one can visualize the opening of nasolacrimal duct under the inferior turbinate and the site of dacryocystorhinostomy ostium in anterior to the middle turbinate.

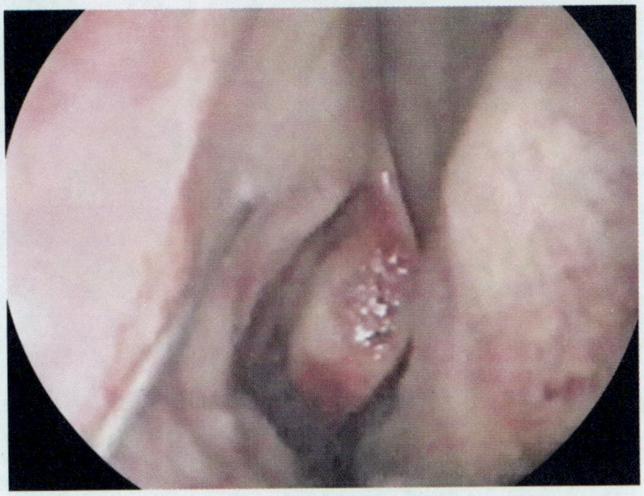

Fig. 15: Normal nasal cavity.

Visualization of Canaliculi

Canalicular mini endoscopes are now available for placement in the canaliculus to view the common canaliculus and lacrimal sac. This allows the visualization of the strictures of the canaliculus, common canaliculus and the lacrimal sac.

Ancillary Radiological Investigations

Radiological tests help in confirming the site of obstruction or stenosis in case of blocked syringing, confirm a functional cause of epiphora and delineate the anatomical as well as the pathological process pertaining to the problem.

Dacryocystography

Dacryocystography **(Figs. 16 and 17)** is of importance in case of blocked syringing to locate the site of obstruction especially in cases of incomplete obstruction where the site of stenosis cannot be localized clinically. Moreover, it gives additional information regarding any fistula or pathology inside the sac.

After instillation of local anesthesia, a fine catheter is introduced into the canaliculus (preferably the superior one) and 0.5–2 mL of water soluble iodinated contrast medium is injected continuously. Films are taken immediately in Caldwell's posteroanterior frontal projection and lateral view. The films are repeated after 5 and 15 minutes to evaluate the lacrimal drainage system. It may be combined with either conventional tomography or CT acquisition.

Distension dacryocystography is a technique in which the films are taken during the injection of the dye. This method

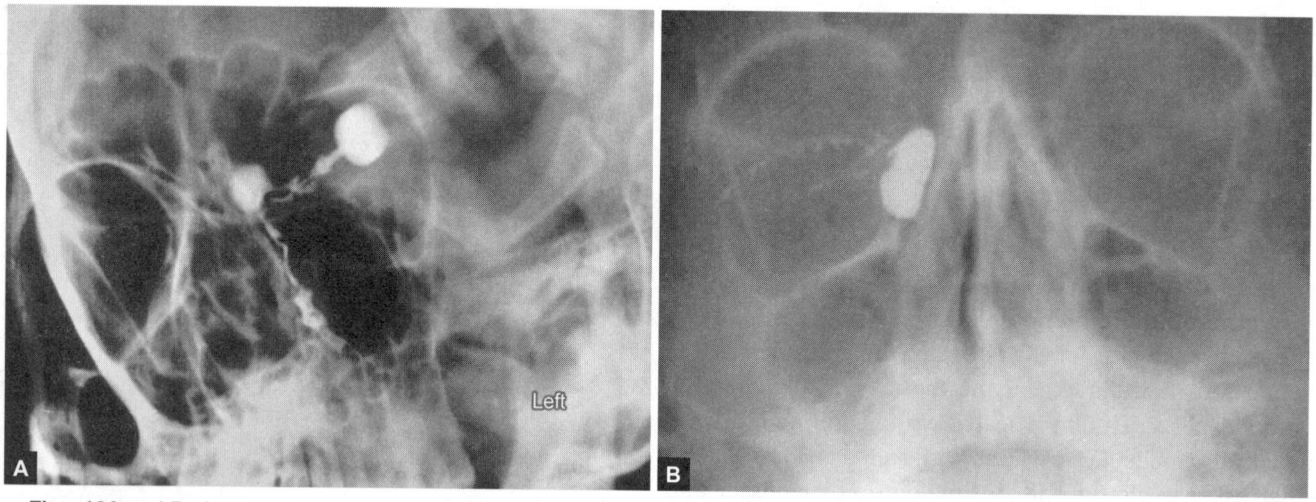

Figs. 16A and B: (A) Dacryocystography showing passage; (B) Obstruction at the sac-NLD of contrast dye into the nasal cavity junction.

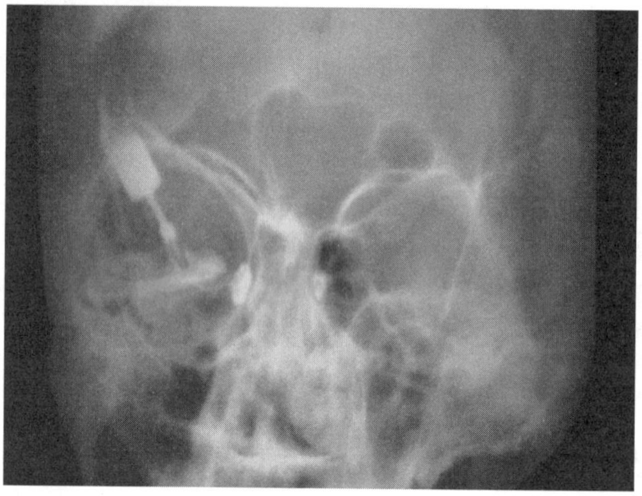

Fig. 17: Dacryocystography showing pooling of contrast dye in the lacrimal sac (NLD obstruction).

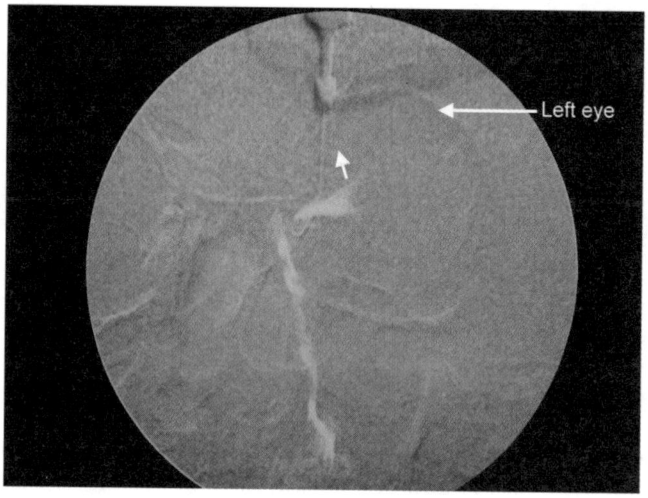

Fig. 18: Dacryocystography after digital subtraction.

provides simultaneous visualization of anatomic structures of the both lacrimal systems. It is good for demonstration of fistule, diverticulae, presence of stones and sac tumors.

Computed tomography (CT) dacryocystography is considered superior to conventional one as it provides useful anatomical information about the orbital wall, sinus as well as allowing evaluation of the nasolacrimal duct.

Magnetic resonance imaging dacryocystography provides the same information as the conventional studies, without the use of catheterization and contrast medium. Both sides are preferably done simultaneously in case of a functional epiphora. Enhancement of the film is done with digital subtraction **(Fig. 17)**.[19,20]

Subtraction dacryocystography provides improved imaging due to elimination of bony shadows. A scout film is taken before injecting contrast material and is used to produce bone free images of the dacryocystogram **(Fig. 18)**.[21]

Dacryoscintigraphy[22-24]

Functional epiphora becomes difficult to differentiate from partial block of the lacrimal drainage system. Dacryoscintigraphy assesses the lacrimal drainage system under physiological condition. Technetium-99, a gamma ray-emitting radionuclide in saline or technetium sulfur colloid are instilled into the conjunctival sac and imaged with a gamma camera at fixed interval. Delay in the passage of the dye may occur at any site as in the region of the conjunctival sac or the canaliculi, which may be due to lid or canalicular diseases. Apart from being a noninvasive technique, radiation exposure to the lens is minimal compared to that of dacryocystography. It is more sensitive for the diagnosis of incomplete blocks especially the upper system. It can be easily performed in children and both lacrimal systems can be assessed simultaneously. The disadvantage of dacryoscintigraphy (DCG) is that it lacks in showing finer anatomical detail as available with contrast DCG **(Figs. 19A and B)**.

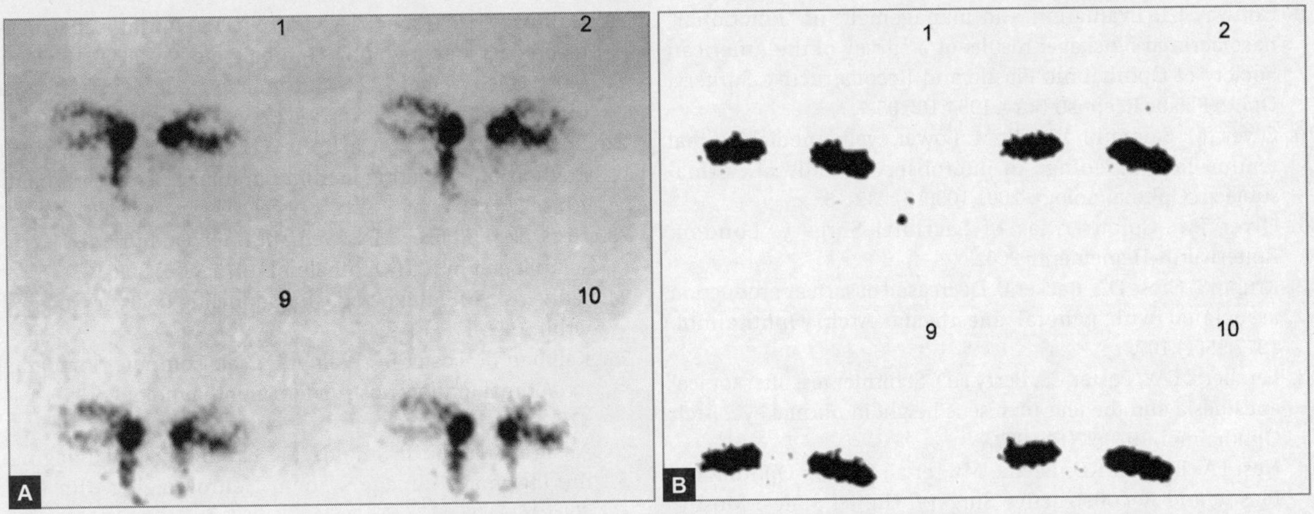

Figs. 19A and B: (A) Rapid clearance of sac; (B) Presac delay.

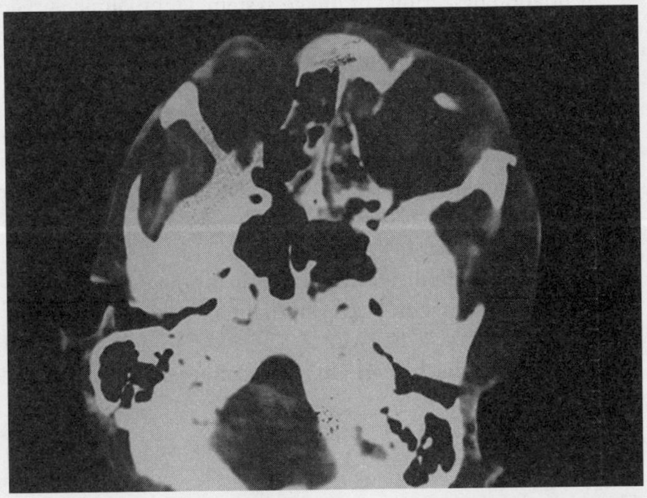

Fig. 20: Axial scan showing fractures of lamina papyracea and the adjacent nasal bones.

Computed Tomography[25,26]

High resolution CT scans in axial and coronal planes provide information about anatomical or pathological abnormalities in or around the structures adjacent to nasolacrimal system **(Fig. 20)**. The abnormalities may be due to craniofacial injury, congenital deformities or lacrimal sac neoplasia. The paranasal sinuses, especially the maxillary sinuses are imaged for any abnormalities that might be affecting the nasolacrimal duct. Preoperative assessment of the cribriform plate is noted for any abnormal position to avoid a possible cerebrospinal leak at the time of surgery.

Newer Modalities

Chemiluminescence test: It is a nonradiologic technique to demonstrate the patency of outflow passages.[27] The luminescent material, are dimethyl phthalate and tertiary butyl alcohol activated by dibutyl phthalate, which produces the cold light. When these agents are injected, the glow is visible through the skin and demonstrates the lacrimal system. However, the lower duct is not visible. It can be performed simultaneously during the surgery. The disadvantage of chemiluminescence test is that it produces the poor quality film. The extravasation of dye into surrounding tissues can produce corneal scarring and vascularization, infection, granuloma formation and fibrosis.

Dacryoscopy: It is a mini-rigid endoscope which allows the direct visualization of the interior and the lining of the lacrimal passages.[28,29]

Standardized echography: Gross anatomical structural defects can be evaluated with the standardized echography.[30]

Thermography: Lacrimal system is visualized by thermography using an infrared scanner and color monitor with a resolution of 0.5. The lacrimal passage is differentiated from surrounding tissues by lacrimal irrigation by cold water, and decreased temperature in the nose detects patency.[31]

REFERENCES

1. Jane Olver J. Colour Atlas of Lacrimal Surgery. London: Butterworth-Heinemann; 2002. pp. 11-26.
2. Bron AJ, Tripathi RC, Tripathi B. Wolff's Anatomy of the Eye and Orbit. Edinburgh: Chapman and Hall Medical Publication; 1997. pp. 72-84.
3. Tucker NA, Tucker SM, Linberg JV. The anatomy of the common canaliculus. Arch. Ophthalmol. 1996;14(10):1231-4.
4. William MH Jr. Adler's Physiology of the Eye: Clinical Application. United States: Harcourt; 1992.
5. Doane MG. Blinking and the mechanics of the lacrimal drainage system. Ophthalmology. 1981;88(8):844-50.
6. Becker BB. Tricompartmental model of the lacrimal pump mechanism. Ophthalmology. 1992;99(7):1139-45.
7. Jones LT. Epiphora II. Its relation to the anatomic structures and surgery of the medial canthal region. Am J Ophthalmol. 1957;43(2):203.
8. Evaluation and management of the tearing patient. Orbit, eyelids and the lacrimal system. United States: American Academy Ophthalmology; 2005. p. 272.

9. Conway ST. Evaluation and management of "functional" nasolacrimal blockage: results of a survey of the American Society of Ophthalmic Plastic and Reconstructive Surgery. Ophth Plastic Reconstr Surg. 1994;10:185-7.
10. Olver JM, Sathia PJ, Wright M. Lower eyelid medial canthal tendon laxity grading: an interobserver study of normal subjects. Ophthalmology. 2001;108(12):2321-5.
11. Olver JM. Colour Atlas of Lacrimal Surgery. London: Butterworth-Heinemann; 2002.
12. Krupin T, Cross DA, Becker B. Decreased basal tear production associated with general anesthesia. Arch. Ophthalmol. 1977;95(1):107.
13. Lamberts DW, Foster CS, Perry HD. Schirmer test after topical anesthesia and the tear meniscus height in normal eye. Arch Ophthalmol. 1979;97(6):1082.
14. Nesi FA, Lisman RD, Levine MR, et al. Smith's Ophthalmic Plastic and Reconstructive Surgery. United States: Mosby; 2012. pp. 649-60.
15. Flack A. The fluorescein appearance test for lacrimal obstruction. Ann Ophthalmol. 1979;11:237.
16. MacEwen CJ, Young JDH. The effect of fluorescein disappearance test (FDT): an evaluation of its uses in infants. J Paed Ophthal Strab. 1991;28:305-05.
17. Zappia RJ, Milder B. Lacrimal drainage function I. The Jones fluorescein test. Am J Ophthalmol. 1972a;74(1):154-9.
18. Zappia RJ, Milder B. Lacrimal drainage function. I. The fluorescein dye disappearance test. Am J Ophthalmol. 1972b;74(1):160-2.
19. Wobig JL, Dailey RA. Evaluation of the lacrimal system. Oculofacial Plastic Surgery: Face, Lacrimal System and Orbit. New York; Thieme Medical Publishers; 2004.
20. Galloway JE, Kavic TA, Raflo GT. Digital substraction macrodacryocystography. Ophthalmology. 1984;91(8):956-62.
21. Lloyd GAG, Welham RAN. Substraction macrodacryocystography. Br J Radiol. 1972;47:379-82.
22. Rossomondo RM, Carlton WH, Trueblood JH. A new method of evaluating lacrimal drainage. Arch Ophthalmol. 1972;88(5):523.
23. Hurwitz JJ, Maisey MN, Welham RAN. Quantitative lacrimal scintillography. Br J Ophthalmol. 1975;59(6):308-12.
24. Jedrzynski MS, Bullock JD. Radionuclide dacryocystography. Orbit. 1998;17(1):1-25.
25. Kallman JE, Foster JA, Wulc AE, et al. Computer tomography in lacrimal outflow obstruction. Ophthalmology. 1997;104(4): 676-82.
26. Ansara SA, Pak J, Shields M. Pathology and imaging of the lacrimal drainage system. Neuroimaging Clin N Am. 2005;15(1):221-37.
27. Raflo GT. Assessment of efficacy of chemiluminance evaluation of lacrimal drainage system. Ophthalmic Surgery. 1982;13(1):36.
28. Coehn SW, Prescott R, Sherman M. Dacryoscopy. Ophthalmic Surgery. 1979;10:57.
29. Sasaki T, Nagata Y, Sugiyama K. Nasolacrimal duct obstruction classified by dacryoendoscopy and treated with inferior meatal dacryorhinostomy. Part I: Positional diagnosis of primary nasolacrimal duct obstruction with dacryoendoscope. Am J Ophthalmol. 2005;140(6):1065-69.
30. Dutton JJ. Standardized echography in the diagnosis of lacrimal drainage dysfunction. Arch Ophthalmol. 1989;197(7):1010.
31. Raflo GT, Chant P, Hurwitz JJ. Thermographic evaluation of lacrimal drainage system. Ophthalmic Surgery. 1982;13(2):119.

CHAPTER

34

Diagnostic Procedures in Proptosis

AK Grover, Shaloo Bageja, Amrita Sawhney

INTRODUCTION

Proptosis is defined as forward displacement of one or both eyeballs. The term exophthalmos is synonymous but used customarily when associated with thyroid disease.

Systematic evaluation is essential to diagnose a case of proptosis as the disease process may be a part of systemic disease or have originated in the orbit itself. It can be an extension from adjacent structures like sinuses or cranial cavity.

CLINICAL EVALUATION

Clinical evaluation of proptosis includes:

- History
- General physical examination
- Systemic examination
- Ocular and orbital examination
- Investigations.

History

A detailed history is important for making a provisional diagnosis.[1] The various aspects in history taking that help in making differential diagnosis are:

- *Age of onset*: Orbital lesions seen in adults and children have a different spectrum. The age of the patient offers a clue to the possible nature of orbital pathology.
  - Orbital lesions in *infants* are:
    - Craniosynostosis **(Fig. 1)**
    - Encephalocele
    - Teratoma
    - Capillary hemangioma
    - Orbital retinoblastoma
    - Metastatic neuroblastoma.
  - The common orbital lesions in *children* are:
    - Inflammatory disorders such as preseptal cellulitis, orbital cellulitis, subperiosteal abscess **(Fig. 2)**, and fungal infections.

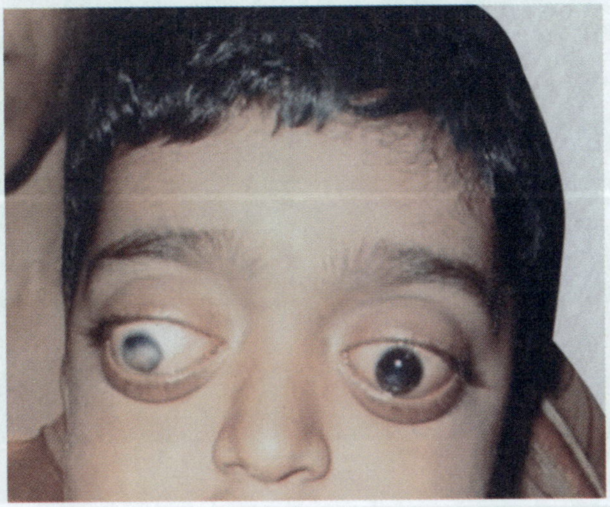

Fig. 1: Clinical picture showing proptosis in a child with craniosynostosis.

    - Parasitic infestations such as myocysticercosis
    - Orbital tumors such as dermoid, dermolipoma **(Fig. 3)**, optic nerve glioma meningioma, neurofibroma, lymphosarcoma, Rosai Dorfman syndrome, rhabdomyosarcoma, orbital extension of retinoblastoma, leukemia, etc.
    - Vascular lesions such as capillary hemangioma, lymphangioma, orbital varices **(Fig. 4)**.
  - Common orbital lesions in *adults* are:
    - Inflammatory disorders such as orbital cellulitis **(Fig. 5)**, thyroid eye disease, and fungal infections.
    - Nonspecific (idiopathic) orbital inflammatory disorder (Orbital pseudotumor); Depending upon site of involvement—diffuse, myositic, dacryoadenitis or apical **(Figs. 6A and B)**.
    - Parasitic infestations such as cysticercosis or orbital hydatid cyst.
    - Vascular lesions such as orbital varices, hamartomas, A-V malformation, caroticocavernous fistula, cavernous hemangioma **(Fig. 7)**, lymphangioma.

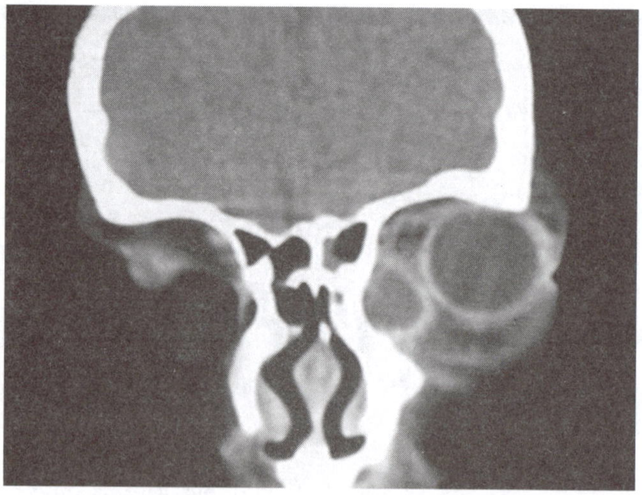

Fig. 2: CT scan showing subperiosteal abscess.

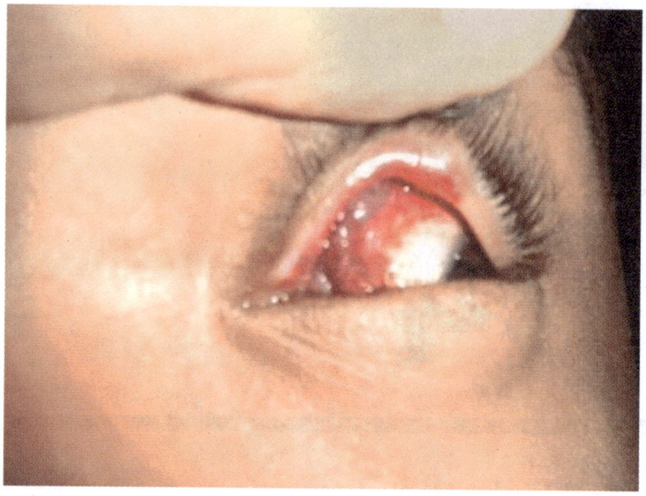

Fig. 4: Orbital varices.

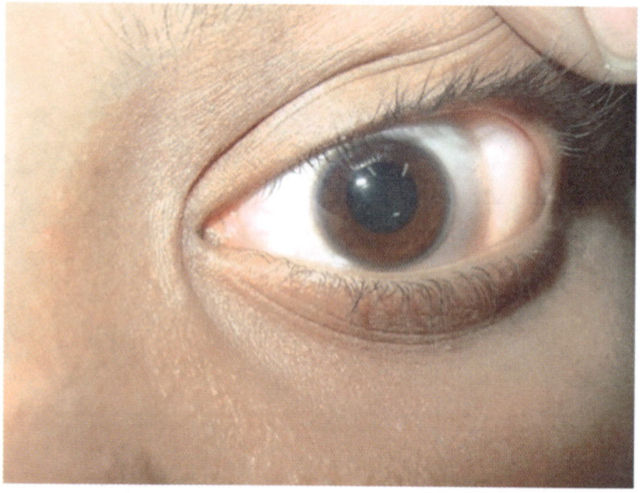

Fig. 3: Dermolipoma.

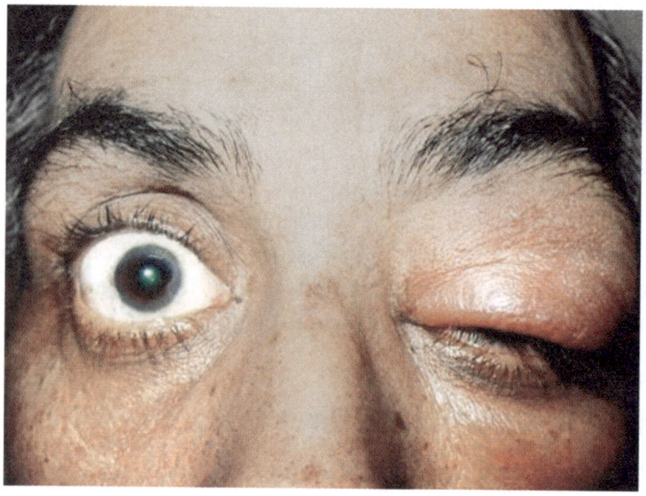

Fig. 5: Orbital cellulitis.

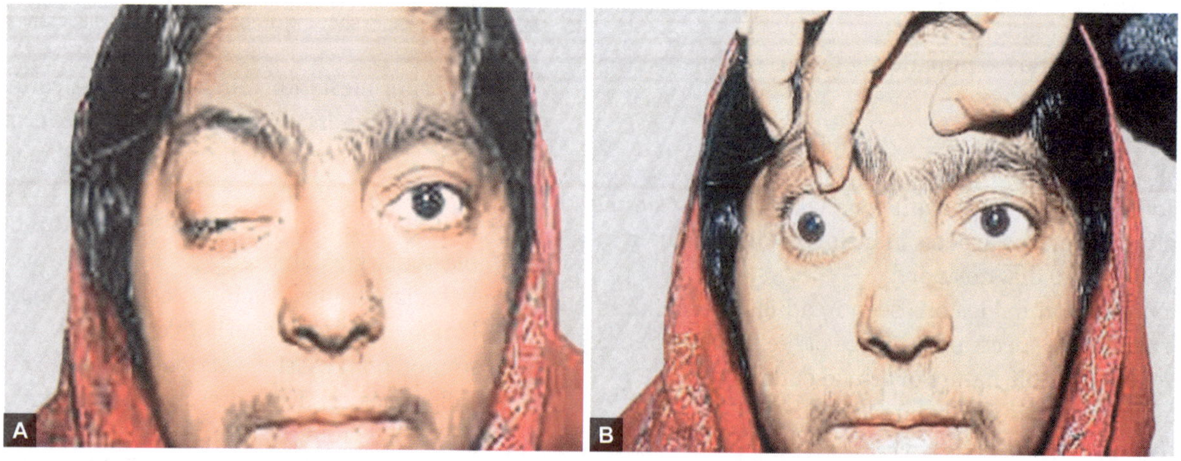

Figs. 6A and B: Clinical picture showing orbital apex syndrome due to apical pseudotumor.

    - Orbital tumors such as primary orbital tumors, lacrimal gland tumors, and secondary tumors (Extension from surrounding structures or metastasis).
    - Structural disorders like dermoid and mucocele.
- *Nature of onset, course, and duration of disease*:
  - Causes of *acute onset proptosis in children* are:
    - Retrobulbar hemorrhage
    - Orbital cellulitis
    - Rhabdomyosarcoma
    - Acute dacryoadenitis.
  - Causes of *acute proptosis in adults* are:
    - Retrobulbar hemorrhage
    - Orbital cellulitis

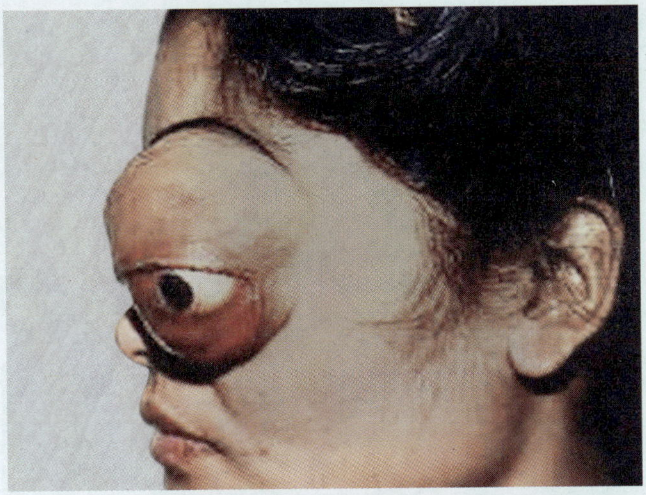

Fig. 7: Clinical picture showing cavernous hemangioma.

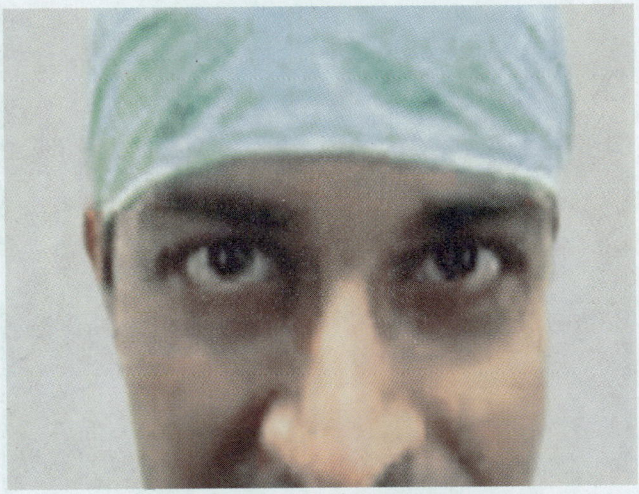

Fig. 8: Cotton wisp test for corneal sensation.

- Cavernous sinus thrombosis
- Acute dacryoadenitis.

– Causes of *gradual onset* proptosis are:
  - Thyroid eye disease
  - Orbital pseudotumor
  - Orbital parasitic infections
  - Orbital tumors
  - Orbital varices
  - Optic nerve glioma
  - Optic nerve meningioma
  - Craniosynostosis.

- History of *associated symptoms*:
  - Sensory like *pain and numbness*
  - Motor like *diplopia*
  - *Visual disturbances*
  - *Increase in proptosis* with coughing, straining or Valsalva maneuver
- *History of trauma* or *family history* must be asked for
- History regarding *systemic diseases* should be taken.

General Physical Examination and Systemic Examination

- Orientation to time, place, and person
- Lymphadenopathy
- Cranial nerves examination is essential especially corneal sensations **(Fig. 8)**
- Cutaneous lesions such as café-au-lait spots suggest neurofibromatosis and cutaneous vascular lesions are associated with hemangiomas, hence cutaneous examination is necessary **(Fig. 9)**.

Ocular and Orbital Examination

- *Visual acuity*: Uncorrected and best corrected visual acuity should be documented.

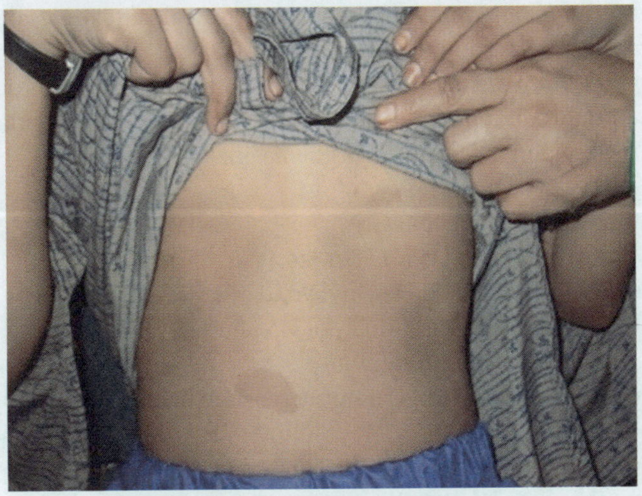

Fig. 9: Café-au-lait spots.

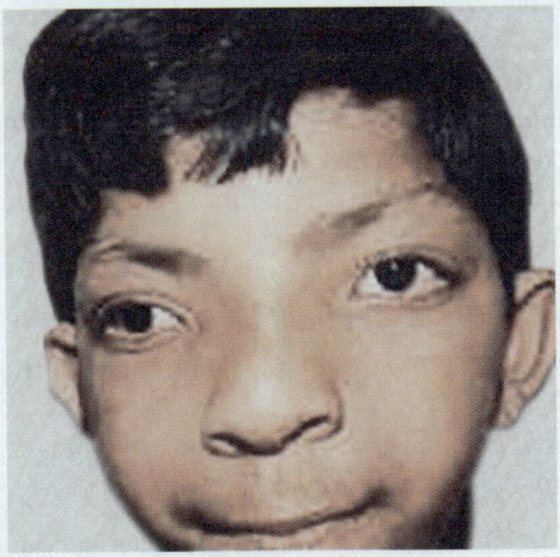

Fig. 10: Facial asymmetry.

- Color vision test
- Facial asymmetry must be noted **(Fig. 10)**
- *Pupillary reactions*: To rule out anisocoria and relative afferent pupillary defect.

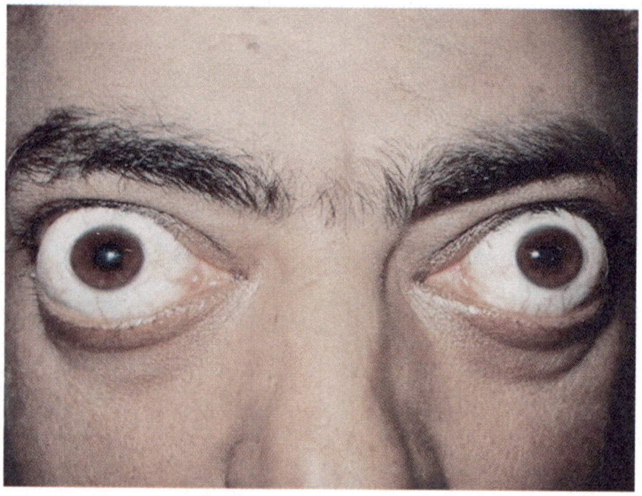

Fig. 11: Proptosis with eyelid retraction and conjunctival congestion, suggestive of thyroid orbitopathy.

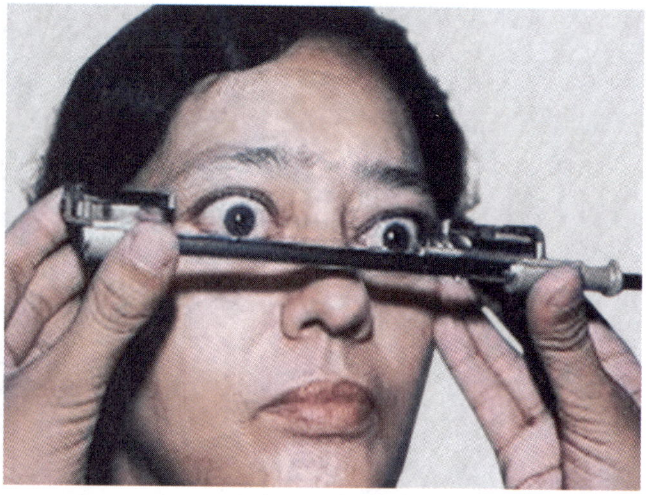

Fig. 12: Clinical photograph showing measurement using Hertel's exophthalmometer.

- *Ocular alignment*: Hirschberg corneal reflex test and cover test should be performed.
- *Ocular motility*: Restrictive motility can be due to thyroid ophthalmopathy or neurogenic due to neuromuscular junction defect like myasthenia gravis.
- *Eyelid examination*:

Palpebral fissure changes:

- Lid retraction **(Fig. 11)** or ptosis
- Eyelid fullness, lid lag in thyroid eye disease
- S-shaped deformity of eyelid in neurofibromatosis

Anterior segment examination:

- Conjunctival congestion, chemosis in thyroid eye disease **(Fig. 11)**
- Conjunctival salmon patch in orbital lymphoma
- Exposure keratopathy in severe proptosis
- Iris examination for Lisch nodules seen in neurofibromatosis

IOP measurement: Rise in intraocular pressure can be seen in restrictive orbitopathy due to thyroid eye disease.

- *Fundus examination*: It may show pressure signs such as choroidal folds, disc edema.
- Optociliary shunts can be seen in optic nerve meningioma.

Examination of Eyeball

- *Proptosis*: Forward displacement or protrusion of eyeball
- *Exophthalmos*: Forward protrusion in thyroid eye disease
- *Enophthalmos*: Shrinkage of eyeball.

Measurement: Hertel's exophthalmometer can be used to measure forward displacement or shrinkage of eye **(Fig. 12)**. The measurement is done from the lateral orbital rim to the anterior corneal surface. Proptosis of more than 21 mm or asymmetry of 2 mm or more between the two eyes is usually abnormal.

Plastic ruler, Naugle's exophthalmometer or Leudde's exopthalmometer can also be used to measure the proptosis. Leudde's exophthalmometer is better than Hertel's in cases of facial asymmetry.

Globe displacement: It can occur due to *axial or nonaxial proptosis.*

- *Axial displacement* is caused by an intraconal lesion like optic nerve glioma, optic nerve meningioma, and retrobulbar hemorrhage.
- *Nonaxial displacements*:
  - *Inferomedial* displacement can occur from mass in the superolateral quadrant like lacrimal gland tumors and dermoid cyst.
  - *Inferolateral* displacement is usually due to frontoethmoidal mucocele, any growth from frontal, sphenoid or ethmoid sinuses and dermoid **(Figs. 13A and B)**.
  - *Superior* displacement can be due to growth from maxillary sinus or orbital floor

Dystopia: This term implies displacement of globe in the coronal plane and it may coexist with proptosis.

- *Horizontal displacement is measured from midline (nose) to the center of pupil using one scale.*
- *Vertical displacement is measured using two scales. One scale is placed horizontally over the nasal bridge and the other scale is placed vertically perpendicular to the first one. Vertical dystopia is noted by reading on the vertical scale.*

Palpation

- Palpation of orbital and periorbital area **(Fig. 14)** is done to note any rise in temperature or to rule out any anterior orbital mass.
- If anterior orbital mass is located then palpation is important to note surface and hardness of the lesion.

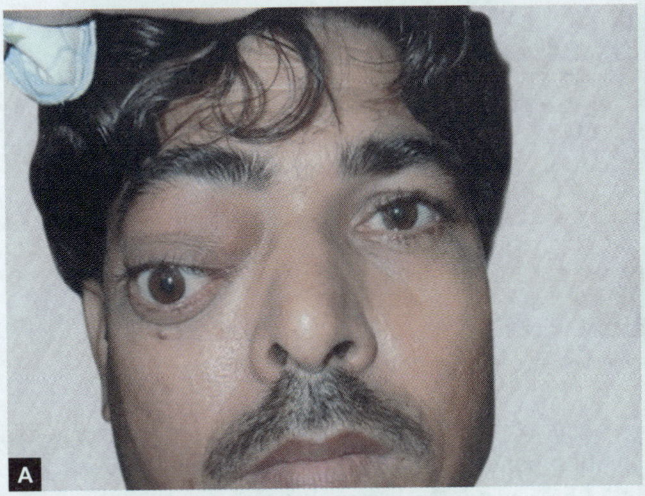

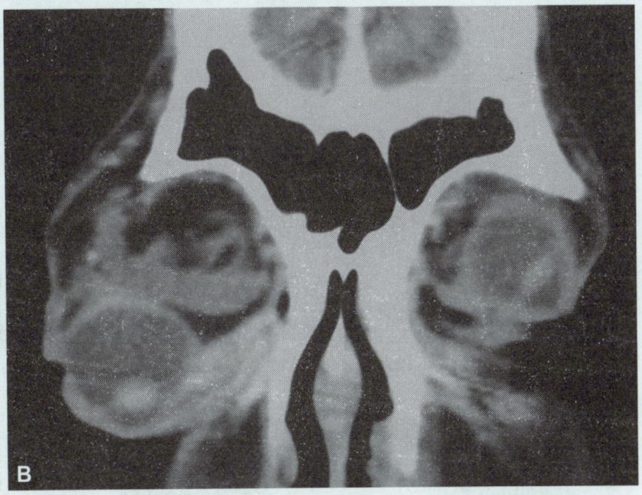

Figs. 13A and B: (A) Clinical picture showing dystopia right eye (inferolateral displacement of globe); (B) CT scan shows orbital dermoid right eye.

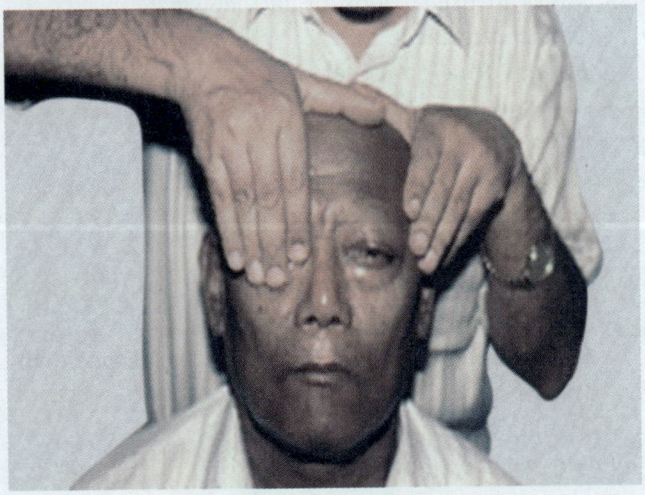

Fig. 14: Orbital palpation.

- Orbital pulsations can be present in cases of arteriovenous abnormalities like caroticocavernous fistula or defect in bony orbital walls as in meningocele, neurofibromatosis, and sinus mucocele.
- Orbital thrill can be felt in cases of AV fistulas (high flow).
- *Compressibility and reducibility* should be noted.

Retropulsion: Increased resistance to retropulsion is due to diffuse inflammation like thyroid orbitopathy.

- *Change in size of swelling or proptosis* with coughing, straining, Valsalva maneuver or bending forward. In case of orbital varices (venous orbital abnormality), swelling increases on Valsalva maneuver **(Figs. 15A and B)**.
- *Auscultation* is done for orbital bruit. This can be due to high flow AV fistulas **(Fig. 16)**.

Other tests which are relevant to a case of proptosis are:

- Diplopia charting
- Binocular vision tests in cases presenting with squint
- Forced duction test **(Fig. 17)**
- Visual field charting.

Systemic Investigations

Laboratory Diagnosis

Orbital disorders can be a manifestation of systemic disease. Hence a number of investigations should be done to establish the diagnosis.

- Thyroid function tests (T3, T4, TSH) and thyroid antibodies (antithyroglobulin and antimicrosomal antibodies) for Graves' orbitopathy
- Serum angiotensin converting enzyme (ACE) for sarcoidosis
- Complete blood count with blood picture for leukemia and lymphoma
- Antinuclear cytoplasmic antibody (c-ANCA) serum assay for Wegener's granulomatosis
- Immunology screening for systemic lupus erythematous
- Biochemical tests like Casoni's test for hydatid cyst
- Urine examination
- Stool examination.

Orbital Imaging[2]

Imaging modalities are an important tool in diagnosing orbital lesion and surgical planning. The following imaging modalities are available:

- Radiographs
- Ultrasonography (USG)
- Computed tomography (CT scan)
- Magnetic resonance imaging (MRI)
- Magnetic resonance angiography (MRA)
- Orbital venography
- Orbital arteriography
- VEP
- Orbital biopsy.

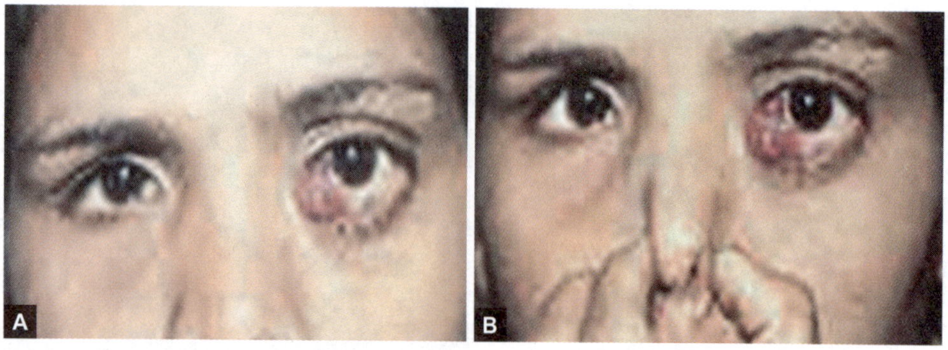

Figs. 15A and B: Clinical picture shows Valsalva maneuver causes increase in size of orbital varices.

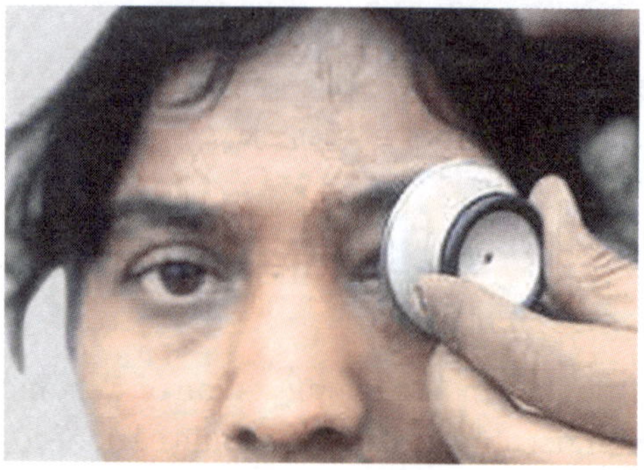

Fig. 16: Auscultation for the orbital bruit.

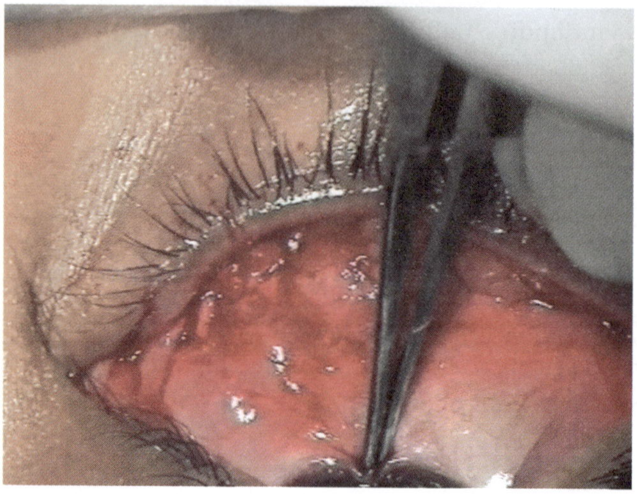

Fig. 17: Forced duction test.

Radiographs: It was the most frequently used initial radiological examination as it was easy to do and inexpensive. Commonly required views are:

- *Caldwell view*: 23° PA view with forehead and nose touching the plate.
  Useful for demonstrating: Anterior orbital rim (except inferior portion), medial wall, lacrimal fossa, lesser and greater wings of sphenoid, superior orbital fissure, and posterior part of floor.
- *Waters' view*: 37° PA view with chin and nose touching the plate.
  Useful for demonstrating: Orbital floor (blow out floor #), inferior orbital rim, maxillary sinus, infraorbital canal, and lateral orbital rim.
- *Lateral view*: Orbital roof, orbital floor, and greater wing of sphenoid.
- *Rhese view:* Optic canal diameter; 4–6 mm: normal, >7 mm: abnormal.

Plain X-rays are used to look for the following:

- *Orbital enlargement*:
  - *Symmetrical*: Intraconal masses
  - *Asymmetrical*: Extraconal masses
- *Calcification*:
  - Phlebolith
  - Optic nerve sheath meningioma
  - Retinoblastoma
- *Superior orbital fissure enlargement*:
  - Caroticocavernous fistula
  - Intracranial extension of orbital space occupying lesions
  - Meningioma
- *Enlargement of optic foramen*:
  - *Uniform widening*
    - Optic nerve glioma
    - Retinoblastoma
    - Extension of intraorbital neurofibroma
  - *Irregular widening*: Meningioma
- *Changes in bone density*:
  - *Hyperostosis*
    - Meningioma
    - Lacrimal gland carcinoma
  - *Diffuse irregular osteolysis*: Secondaries
  - *Localized osteolysis*
    - Dermoid
    - Histiocytosis X.
- *Soft tissue changes*: Clouding of PNS in infections/ malignancy
- Chest X-rays are used to diagnose systemic lesions such as sarcoidosis, Wegener's granulomatosis, and bronchogenic carcinoma. Plain film radiographs are nowadays rarely used.

Ultrasonography: USG is a rapid, noninvasive, and an inexpensive tool, providing significant dynamic information about orbital disorders. It is a better modality (as compared to CT scan and MRI) in detecting subtle soft tissue changes. It is also useful in identification and localization of the anterior orbital disease, extraocular muscles and to assess the optic nerve. USG consists of piezoelectric crystal inside the probe which vibrates and this vibration is emitted as ultrasonic waves via a transducer at the tip of the probe. These waves are absorbed, scattered as well as reflected by the media. Reflected waves are processed by the computer system to generate A scan and B scan. B scan provides two-dimensional intensity modulated images of the orbital tissue. A scan exhibits spikes of different heights suggesting the internal characteristics of the lesion. The frequency used in ocular USG is between 10 MHz and 20 MHz. Higher is the frequency, lesser is the penetration and better resolution.

Color Doppler demonstrates the vascular flow in the mass.[3]

The ultrasound features of various orbital lesions are:

- *Cavernous hemangioma*: Intraconal, well demarcated lesion with high internal reflectivity and moderate sound attenuation.
- *Capillary hemangioma*: Ill-defined lesion with irregular reflectivity.
- *Lymphangioma*: Ill-defined mass with low irregular internal reflectivity and no internal vascularity.
- *Cysticercosis*: Well-defined cystic lesion with scolex (highly reflective echo dense nodule adjacent to inner wall of the cyst).
- *Hydatid cyst*: Double-wall sign **(Fig. 18)**.

Advantages of ultrasonography (B scan):

- Quick assessment
- Kinetic properties of lesion
- Examination of pediatric cases without anesthesia
- No radiation exposure
- Ideal for serial follow-up.

Disadvantages of ultrasonography:

- Difficulty to assess diffuse lesions
- Lesions located in posterior are difficult to assess
- Inter observers variation
- Highly operator dependent.

Computed tomography (CT scan): An imaging technique where contrast differences are based on variable tissue densities obtained on the passage of X-rays through tissues. It is an important tool in delineating the shape, location, extent, and character of the lesion. A density value is assigned to each tissue proportional to their coefficient of absorption of X-rays **(Figs. 19A and B)**. A two-dimensional image is constructed from these density measurements. Two types of images can be obtained.

Orbital images can be obtained in *axial, coronal, and sagittal planes.*

- *Axial plane:* Axial scan is performed in supine position. It is especially useful for optic nerve lesions.
  It also shows horizontal recti muscles, soft tissue, both the globes and bony structures.
- *Coronal plane:* Coronal scan is done in prone position.
  - Anterior coronal cuts show relationship of recti muscles with the globe.
  - Posterior coronal cuts show all recti and oblique muscles, soft tissues and optic nerve.
  - Coronal cut at the apex shows optic foramen.
  - In blow out fractures of the orbit and thyroid ophthalmopathy 2 mm coronal cuts are required for assessment of orbital walls and extraocular muscle size **(Fig. 20)**.

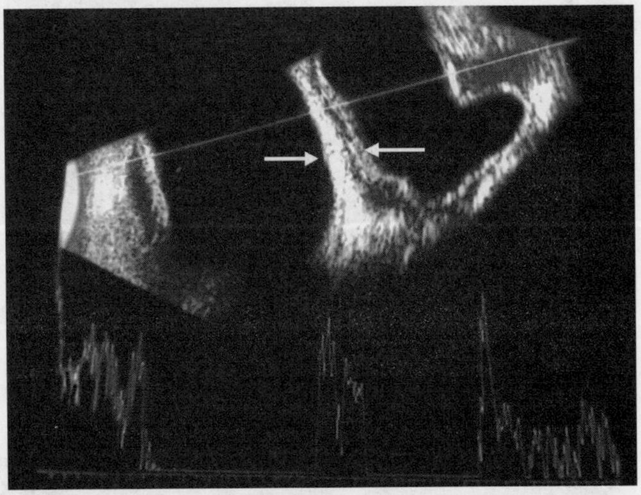

Fig. 18: USG picture showing orbital hydatid cyst with typical double wall sign.

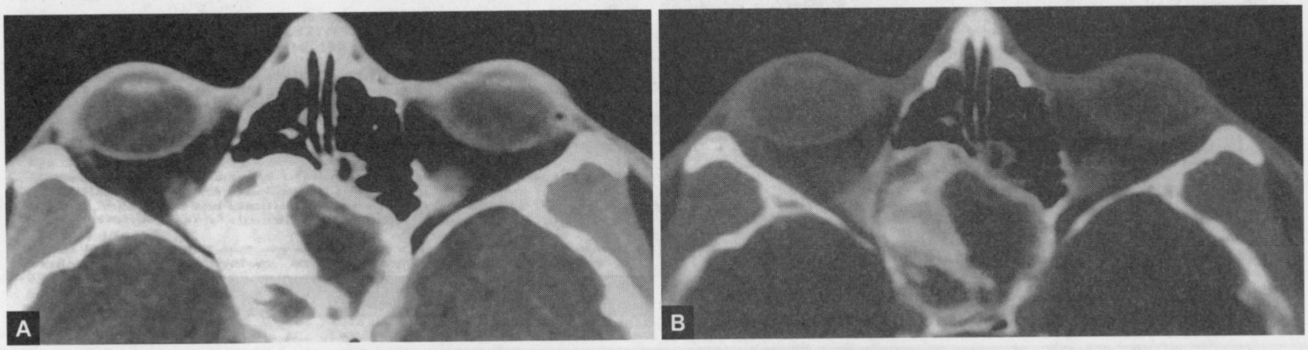

Figs. 19A and B: (A) Tissue density window; (B) Bone density window.

- *Sagittal plane*: This view cannot be taken directly it can be obtained by formatting the available images. It can be used in cases of orbital floor or roof fracture.

Simultaneous evaluation of axial and coronal views permits three-dimensional assessment of orbital tumors.

Noncontrast CT scan: It is important in cases of orbital trauma, foreign body, hemorrhage, retinoblastoma, and paranasal sinus disease.

Intravenous contrast may be useful in vascular and inflammatory tumors.

Spiral CT scan can be retrospectively reconstructed into thin sections in any required plane. It thus reduces the exposure time to radiation and is especially useful in uncooperative patients and children.

Important features of diseases on CT scan are:

- *Thyroid eye disease*: Muscle bellies are thickened with sparing of the tendons and apical crowding **(Figs. 21A and B)**.
- *Myositis:* Muscle along with its tendon is enlarged.
- *Lacrimal gland tumors:*
  - Benign tumors lead to fossa formation along the bone and push the globe
  - Malignant tumors cause bone erosions and infiltrate the globe.

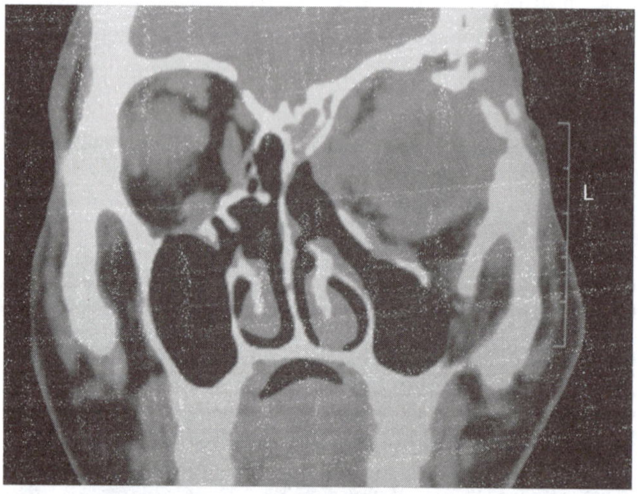

Fig. 20: CT scan showing orbital wall fracture.

Magnetic resonance imaging: The imaging is generated on the basis of the movement of protons in tissue when a patient is placed into the magnetic field. The aligned protons in the magnetic field are excited by a radiofrequency pulse emitted from a coil. These radiowaves are modified to produce T1- and T2-weighted images. These are the two methods of measuring relaxation time of excited protons when the magnetic field is switched off.

T1-weighted image: The relaxation time and echo time both are short. On imaging, vitreous is dark and fat is bright.

T2-weighted image: The relaxation time and echo time are long. Vitreous is bright and fat is dark.

Proton density imaging: Relaxation time is long but echo time is short. Fat is bright but vitreous is of intermediate density.

Fat suppression techniques such as STIR (Short T1 relaxation time by means of inversion recovery sequences): These mainly suppress adipose tissues and enhance visualization of orbital structures.

Intravenous gadolinium is used as a contrast medium. It enhances the vascular lesion.

Advantages of MRI over CT scan:

- No exposure to ionizing radiation
- It provides excellent soft tissue delineation in orbital apex, optic canal, and cavernous sinus
- It is the preferred method for imaging the optic nerve especially the intracanalicular and intracranial tract.

Disadvantages of MRI over CT scan:

- Time consuming
- Expensive
- It cannot detect calcification or bony lesions.

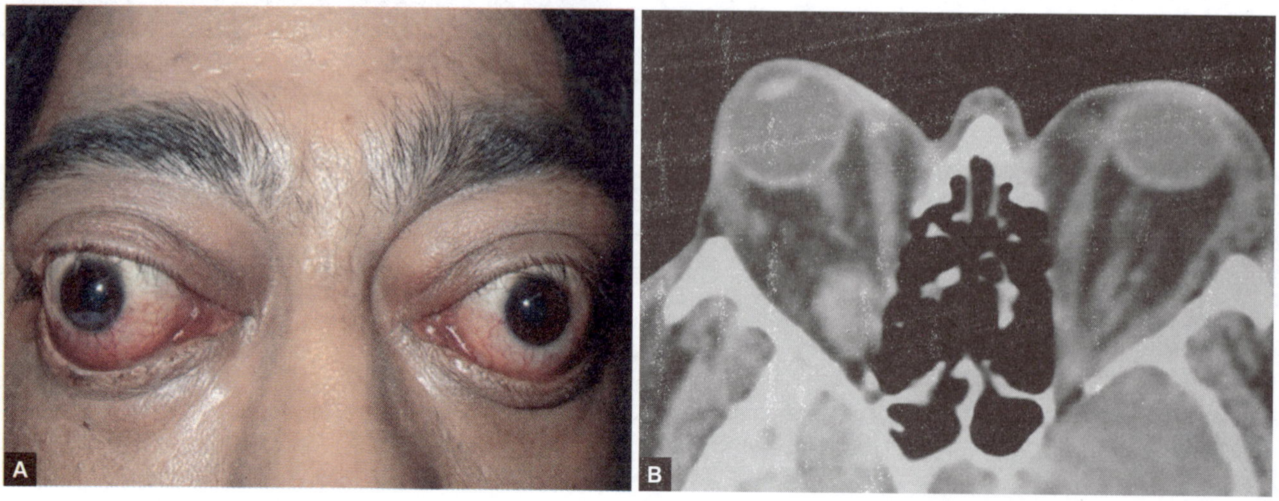

Figs. 21A and B: Clinical picture and CT scan axial view in thyroid eye disease.

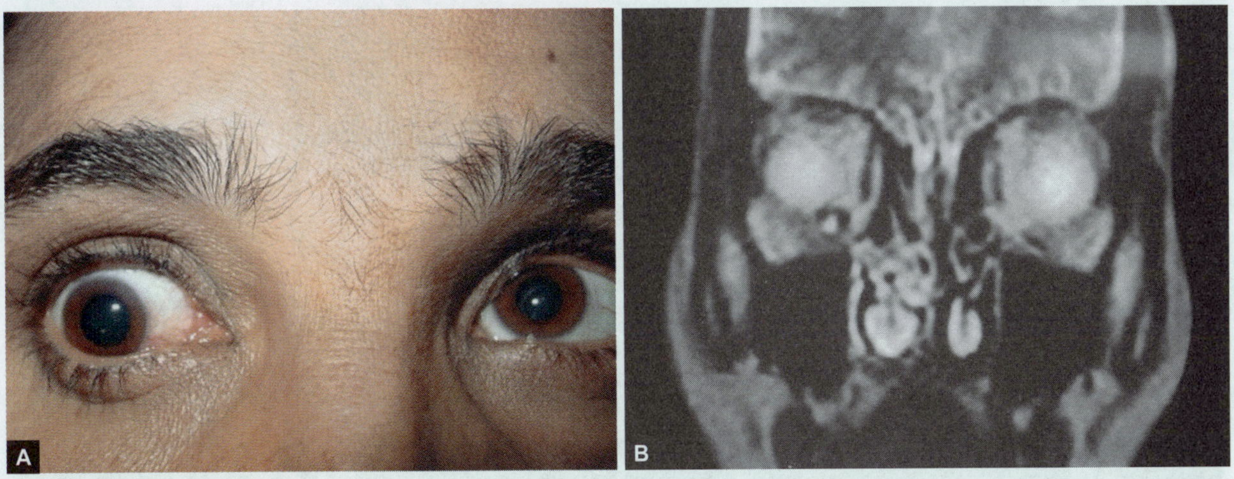

Figs. 22A and B: (A) Clinical picture showing RE ocular motility restriction in upward gaze; (B) MRI showing right eye myocysticercosis.

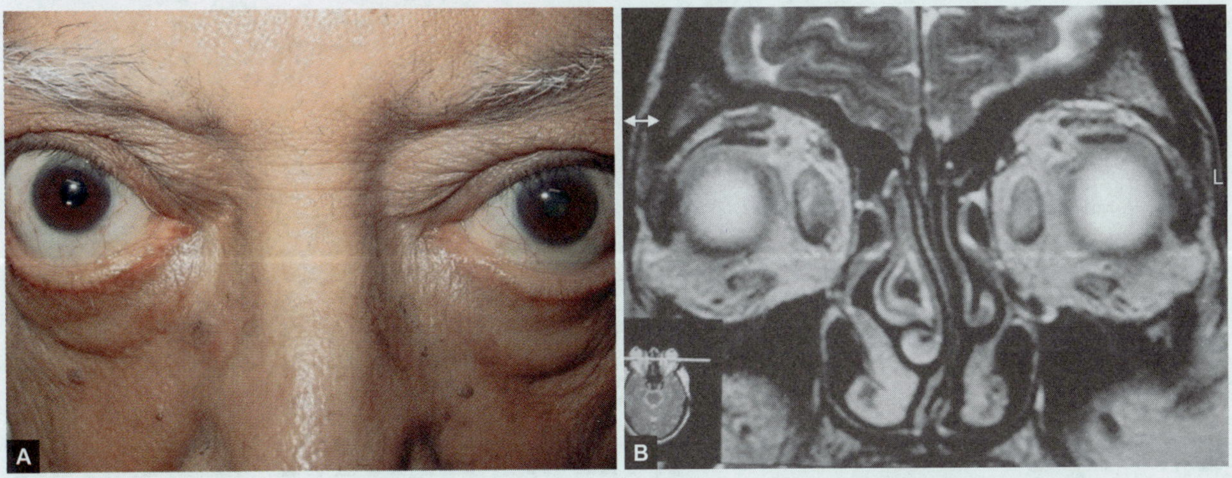

Figs. 23A and B: Clinical picture of a case of thyroid eye disease. MRI coronal view T2-weighted imaging shows extraocular muscles thickening.

Contraindications of the use of MRI:
- Pacemakers
- Cochlear implant
- Metallic foreign body
- Clips/staplers
- Claustrophobia.

Important features of few diseases on MRI:
- *Myocysticercosis*: Cyst is visible with hyperintense structure attached to the wall of cyst **(Figs. 22A and B)**.
- *Thyroid eye disease*: Muscle thickening with relative sparing of tendon. On T2-weighted imaging, the thickened muscles have high signal intensity **(Figs. 23A and B)**.

Magnetic resonance angiography: It is a noninvasive modality used in certain orbital vascular disorders. Its software suppresses normal soft tissue, thus does not utilize any contrast medium and is without any exposure to ionizing radiation. When using the arterial phase, vascular lesions and aneurysms of ophthalmic artery and cavernous sinus lesions greater than 4 mm can be diagnosed. When the venous phase is utilized, arteriovenous malformation, superior ophthalmic vein enlargement or venous thrombosis can be visualized.

Orbital venography: The procedure is not in much use nowadays. It was used earlier before the advent of CT or MRI scan to assess the extent and location of orbital masses and to diagnose orbital varices or to study the cavernous sinus. With advent of magnetic resonance angiography (MRA), this procedure has become obsolete. It had certain disadvantages such as use of contrast agent and it used to miss small lesions.

Orbital arteriography: The technique is used in patients with high suspicion of arterial disease like aneurysm or arteriovenous malformations. Some of these lesions can be treated by interventional radiologists by placing intralesional coils via the transarterial or transvenous routes.

Orbital biopsy: Biopsy is required to obtain a definitive diagnosis.

Orbital biopsy can be incisional or excisional or may be attained by fine needle aspiration.

Fine needle aspiration biopsy is mainly indicated to diagnose anterior orbital lesions or nonresectable lesions in the deep orbit. It is minimally invasive technique which can be done by just palpating the mass or under ultrasound or CT guidance.

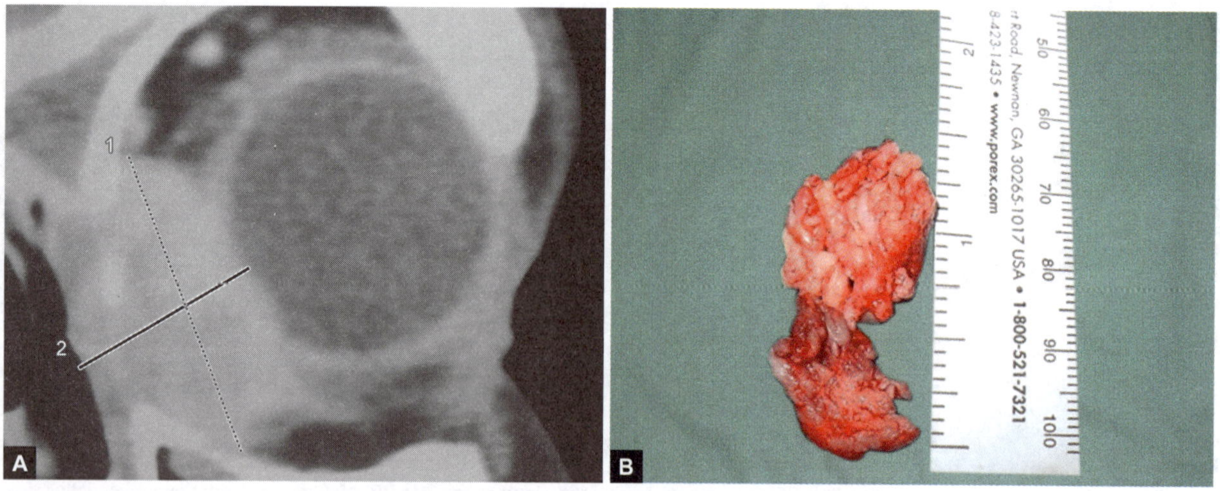

Figs. 24A and B: Excision biopsy of mass was done.

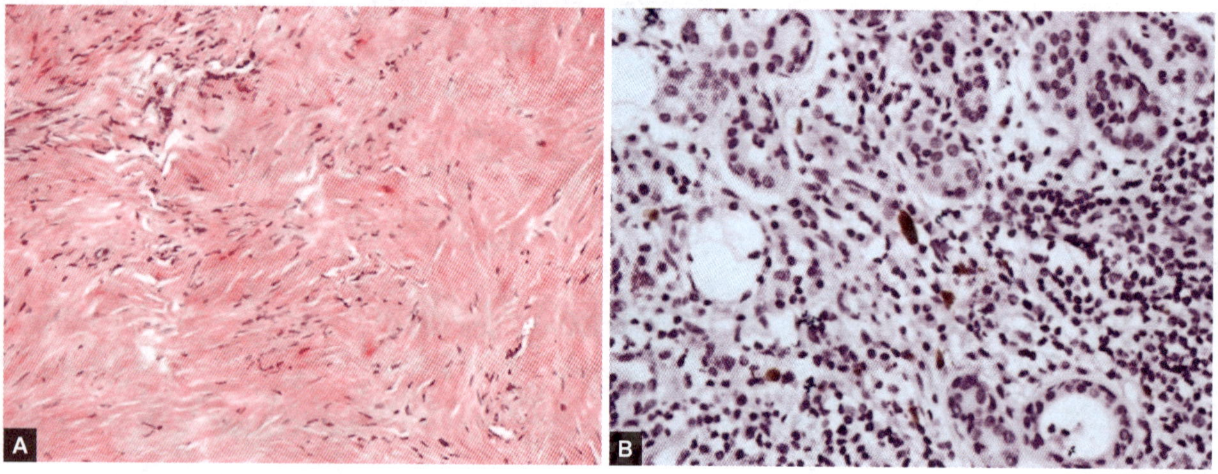

Figs. 25A and B: (A) H&E staining under 10× showing extensive fibrosis (storiform pattern); (B) Immunohistochemical staining under 40× showing IgG4 positive plasma cells.

The needle is introduced and material is aspirated by creating negative pressure, aspirate is spread over the slides which are then air dried, fixed with alcohol, and then staining is done.

The disadvantage with this technique is the availability of scanty material which is difficult to interpret.

Incisional biopsy is required for orbital lesions suggestive of malignancy or inflammation. The advantage of this technique is that good amount of tissue is available for histopathological examination.

Excisional biopsy **(Figs. 24A and B)** is required in cases of well circumscribed benign lesions or suspected pleomorphic adenoma. In this technique, entire mass is removed and subjected to histopathological examination. The added advantage with this procedure is that it is therapeutic in benign lesions.[4,5]

Pathological Investigations

- Cytology
- Gross examination of excised mass is done to note its size, shape, consistency, and surface
- Histopathological examination of the specimen is carried out **(Figs. 25A and B)**.

CONCLUSION

A case of proptosis requires a systematic approach including a good history taking, thorough clinical evaluation, and appropriate investigations to decide the strategy for management.

REFERENCES

1. Rootman J (Ed). Diseases of orbit. Multidisciplinary approach. Philadelphia: Lippincott William and Wilkins; 2003.
2. Aviv RI, Miszkiel K. Orbital imaging: Part 2. Intraorbital pathology. Clin Radiol. 2005;60:288-307.
3. Aburn NS, Sergottt RC. Orbital color Doppler imaging. Eye. 1993;7:639-47.
4. Smith BC. Orbital disease and surgery. Ophthalmic Plastic and Reconstructive Surgery. US: Mosby; 1987.
5. Leatherbarrow B. Orbital Disorders. Oculoplastic Surgery. US: Mosby; 2002.

CHAPTER 35

Diagnostic Procedures for Genetically Transmitted Eye Diseases

Sudha Dhandayuthapani, Sarangapani Sripriya, Nagasamy Soumittra, Jayamuruga Pandian Arunachalam

INTRODUCTION

In recent times, diagnostic procedures for genetic diseases has taken a new dimension not only with the advent of technologies employed in various genetic testing methodologies but also with the increasing awareness among people to comprehend the facts behind these inherited diseases. The clinical correlation of the diagnosis of genetic diseases remains crucial in terms of disease management and genetic counseling by creating cognizance among patients with respect to the inheritance pattern running through their families. Though therapeutic modalities for genetically transmitted diseases are still underway, the clinical genetics discipline is evolving and getting recognized as distinct from its strong academic and research basis. Furthermore, as of now gene replacement therapy trials are much favorable in genetically transmitted eye diseases and autoimmune diseases, hence the diagnostics procedures for those diseases have been in the limelight these days.

DNA-BASED GENE SCREENING (OR) MOLECULAR DIAGNOSTICS

Various principles and methodologies' adopted for molecular diagnostics can be listed as discussed next.

Allele-specific Mutation Detection by PCR-ARMS and PCR-ASO

The amplified refractory mutation system (ARMS) can be applied to detect known point mutations or single nucleotide polymorphisms (SNPs); that is distinguishing heterozygotes from homozygotes. PCR-ARMS is based on the principle that a mismatch between the 3' nucleotide of a polymerase chain reaction (PCR) primer and the template prevents further primer extension by *Taq* polymerase. This system involves bidirectional amplification, with the normal allele amplified using one strand as the template and the mutant allele amplified of the complementary strand. This is particularly useful for haplotyping SNPs that are located within distances that are favorable to PCR amplification. The advantage of PCR-ARMS is the ease with which multiplex assays can be developed, validated and implemented.[1]

The second approach polymerase chain reaction-allele-specific oligonucleotide probes (PCR-ASO) is based on hybridization of PCR products to allele-specific oligonucleotide probes (ASO). This method can be applied in two formats: the forward ASO approach where PCR products are immobilized on membrane and hybridized to labeled ASO probes and the reverse ASO approach where ASO probes are immobilized on the membrane and hybridized to labeled PCR products **(Fig. 1)**. The PCR-ASO method

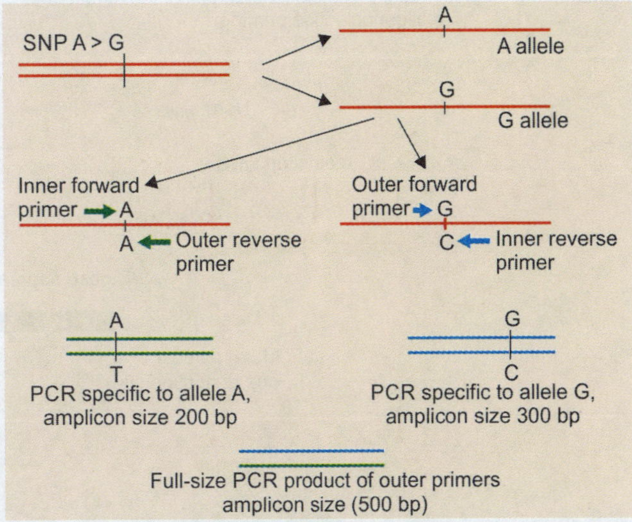

Fig. 1: Diagrammatic representation of allele-specific polymerase chain reaction (PCR) using tetraprimers.[1]
(SNP: single nucleotide polymorphisms)

particularly the reverse ASO format provides a simple approach for simultaneous genotyping of large numbers of mutations and polymorphisms.[2]

Competitive Oligopriming

Competitive oligopriming is a method with a comparably high degree of accuracy and specificity.[3] Here three primers are used in one reaction where there is one common reverse primer and two forward primers for the mutation site, one carrying the mutated sequence and the other carrying the normal counterpart, both complementary to the same template DNA strand **(Fig. 2)**. As a result, there would be three kinds of amplified DNA products:

1. Amplified product containing only normal primer which means the template DNA is wild type for the mutation
2. Amplified product containing only the mutated primer which means the DNA used is homozygous for the mutation
3. Amplified product containing both the mutated and wild type primers incorporated in equal amounts which means the DNA template is heterozygous for the mutation.

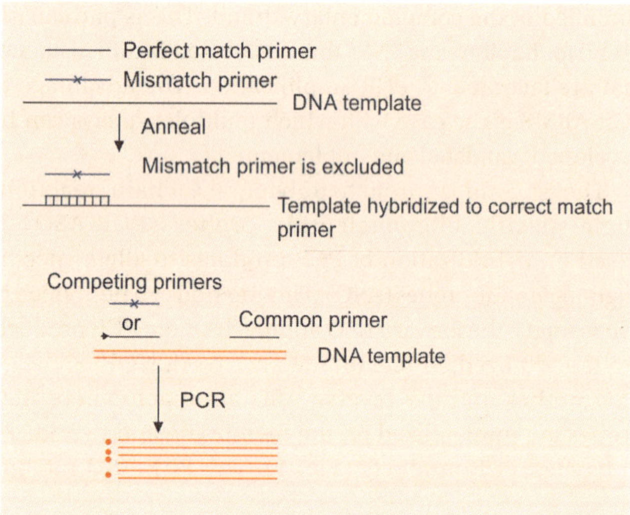

Fig. 2: Detection of single DNA base differences by competitive oligonucleotide priming.[3]

Thus, competitive oligopriming approach can be used for high throughput SNP genotyping **(Fig. 2)**.

Restriction Fragment Length Polymorphism-based Analysis

Restriction fragment length polymorphism (RFLP) is a difference in homologous DNA sequences that can be detected by the presence of fragments of different lengths through DNA electrophoresis after digestion of the DNA samples with specific restriction enzymes. RFLP is specific to a single clone/restriction enzyme combination. Most RFLP markers are codominant (both alleles in heterozygous sample will be detected) and highly locus-specific. RFLP, as a probe, is a labeled DNA sequence that hybridizes with one or more fragments of the digested DNA sample after being separated by gel electrophoresis, thus exhibiting a unique pattern characteristic to a specific genotype at a specific locus **(Fig. 3)**. The RFLP probes are frequently used in genome mapping and in variation analysis like genotyping, forensics, paternity tests, hereditary disease diagnostics, etc.[4]

Enzymatic and Chemical Cleavage Methods to Identify Genetic Variation

Although there are several methods for the high sensitivity detection of known mutations, unknown mutations are more difficult to uncover. Mutations that are not encountered by Sanger dideoxy-DNA sequencing are detected by complementary approaches that detect changes in the physical property of the DNA helix when a mismatch is present. The mutated DNA helix is first converted to mismatch heteroduplexes when the polymerase chain

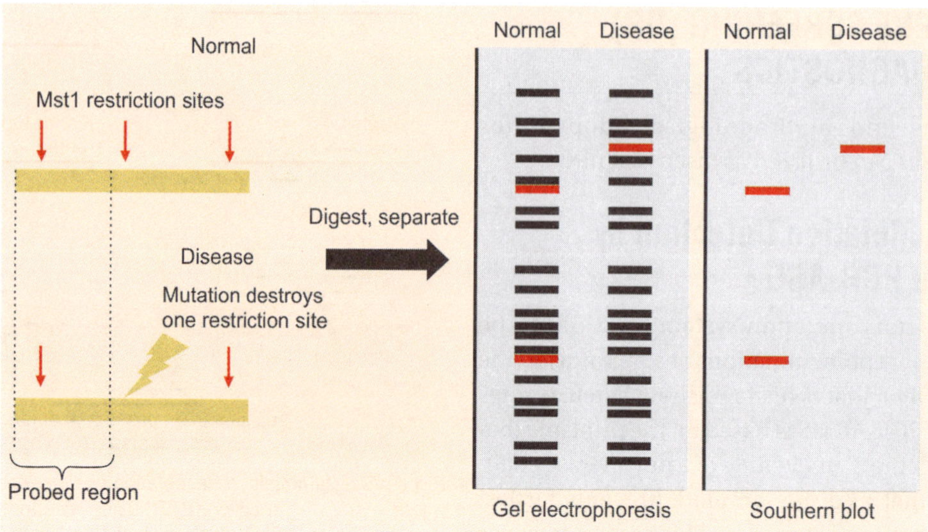

Fig. 3: Pictorial representation of restriction fragment length polymorphism.[4]

reaction products of two alleles of the gene of interest are amplified by PCR, mixed, denatured and rehybridized. Next the chemical or enzymatic properties of a mismatched base are exploited leading to a break in the DNA strand near the mismatch. Finally a suitable fragment analysis method is used to visualize the shortened DNA fragments in either single-stranded or double-stranded form that are produced by the DNA break near the mismatch residue.[5]

Mutation Detection by Single-stranded Conformation Polymorphism and Heteroduplex Analysis

The principle of single-stranded conformation polymorphism (SSCP) analysis is based on the fact that single-stranded DNA has a defined conformation. Conformational change due to a single base variation in the sequence can cause single-stranded DNA to migrate differently under nondenaturing electrophoresis conditions.[6] Therefore, wild-type and mutant DNA samples display different band patterns **(Fig. 4)**. SSCP and heteroduplex analysis (HA) are the two most popular electrophoresis-based mutation detection methods. Relatively short single-stranded DNA fragments can migrate in a nondenaturing gel not only as a function of their size but also of their sequence.[1] This property allows distinguishing wild type and mutant DNA fragment that differ even in a single base based on their migration in gel electrophoresis.[7]

Temperature and Denaturing Gradient Gel Electrophoresis

It is the most sensitive mutation detection technique and can be used for human hereditary disease diagnosis, large-scale mutation screening and predictive genetic testing, including prenatal diagnosis and counseling. They can also be used to analyze SNPs in hereditary complex traits. There are two forms of electrophoresis which either use a temperature or chemical gradient to denature the sample as it moves across a gel. In temperature gradient gel electrophoresis (TGGE) there is a temperature gradient across the gel which causes the DNA strand to separate (melt). Depending upon the specific sequence the melting point varies and they move through the gel. Thus TGGE provides a sequence dependent separation of DNA molecules and not based on size. In the case of denaturing gradient gel electrophoresis (DGGE), the gel contains a denaturing agent which is capable of inducing the DNA to melt at various stages. By comparing the melting behavior of the polymorphic DNA fragments side by side on a denaturing gel even the smallest difference in the two samples can be identified.

As it is less expensive, less labor intensive and time consuming than other point mutation detection techniques, it used widely in routine medical diagnostics.[9]

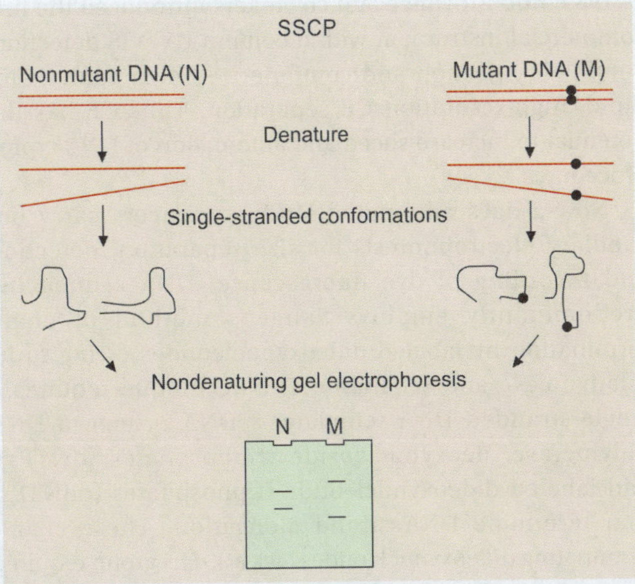

Fig. 4: The principle of polymerase chain reaction-based single-strand conformation polymorphism (SSCP) analysis.[8]

Two-dimensional Gene Scanning

Two-dimensional gene scanning (TDGS) is a method for analyzing multiple DNA fragments in parallel for all possible sequence variations, using extensive multiplex PCR and two-dimensional electrophoretic separation on the basis of size and melting temperature.[10] TDGS can be applied to find all possible sequence variation of a large number of genes using a computer program to optimally position PCR primers around the relevant target sequences (e.g. exons) and evaluating it using panels of samples with previously detected mutations **(Fig. 5)**.

Oligonucleotide Ligation Assays

Polymerase chain reaction-based oligonucleotide ligation assays (OLA) assays reliably distinguishes heterozygous and homozygous cases from normal individuals.[11,12] The ability of DNA ligases to join short oligonucleotides covalently to each other has been utilized in a number of assays where the ligation of oligonucleotides in some way reflects the genotype of the target DNA. This assay takes advantage of these events resulting in reliable, accurate and reproducible discrimination of sequence variants.[13] The reaction can be monitored by introducing a detectable function in either of the probes in the ligation reaction. Several different analytical techniques are in use, differing from each other in their detection methods and instrumentation needs. Several applications of OLA for the detection of molecular defects causing human diseases are in use in molecular diagnostic laboratories. Due to the fact that numerous mutations can contribute to inherited diseases, there is often a need to scan many loci simultaneously on the

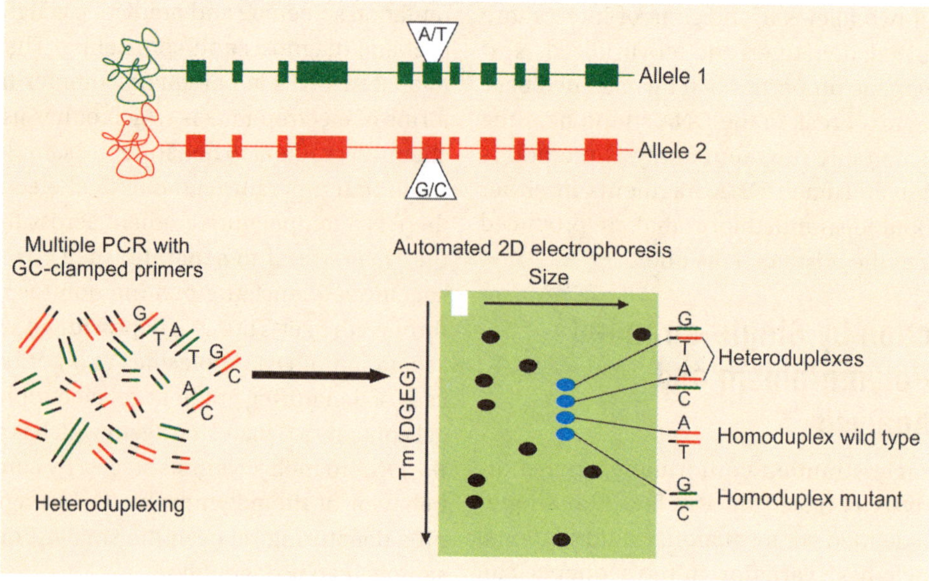

Fig. 5: Schematic representation of the different steps involved in two-dimensional gene scanning.[5]

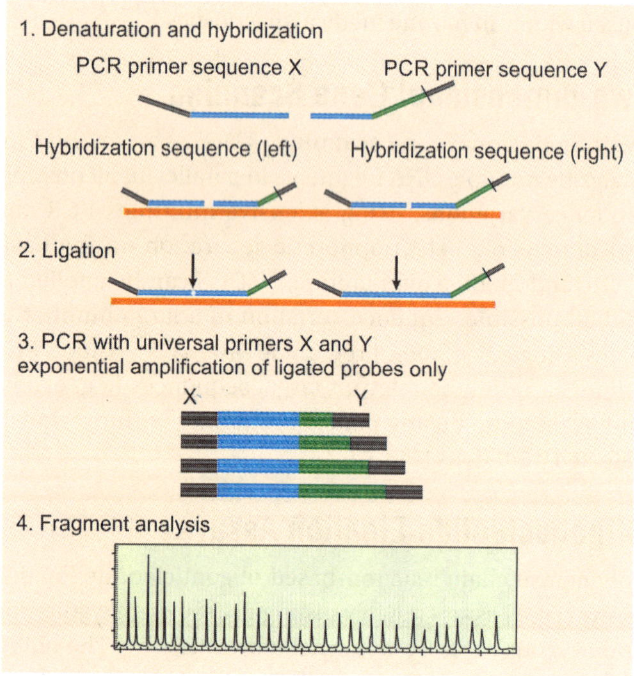

Fig. 6: Diagrammatic representation of multiplex ligation-dependent probe amplification.[23]
(PCR: polymerase chain reaction)

patient sample.[14] The best throughput of PCR-OLA has been achieved using biosensor chips enabling the detection of hundreds of sequence variants within one assay.[5,15,16] Both multiplex ligation-dependent probe amplification (MLPA) and the related oligonucleotide ligation assay (OLA) techniques[17,18] utilize DNA ligase, which is exquisitely sensitive to DNA mismatches, to obtain the target specificity and discrimination difficult to achieve by PCR alone **(Fig. 6)**. Both techniques have been used to genotype multiple single nucleotide polymorphisms (SNPs),[18-20] whereas MLPA can also be used to screen for dosage variation such as the identification of large deletions in a gene[21] and expression profiling of up to 45 signaling pathway transcripts by reverse transcription MLPA (RT-MLPA).[22] Multiplex ligation-dependent probe amplification (MLPA) has provided an efficient and reliable assay for dosage screening of multiple loci in a single reaction.

Capillary Electrophoresis

Electrophoresis is a powerful method that was developed long before molecular biology came into existence. Capillary electrophoresis (CE) was introduced almost 30 years ago as a new and automated alternative to slab gel electrophoresis. The principle behind this technique is to separate charged species based on their size to charge ratio within a small capillary filled with an electrolyte. As early as 1989, Bob Brownlee and coworkers introduced the first commercial instrument with a column UV/VIS detection, automatic injection and computerized data analysis for rapid, high-resolution CE separation. Thus CE has the potential to increase speed and automation of DNA-typing procedures.

Now-a-days automated DNA sequencers carry out capillary electrophoresis for size separation, detection and recording of dye fluorescence. DNA sequencing predominantly employs Sanger's method of chain termination by labeled dideoxynucleotides owing to its relative ease and reliability. This technique requires a single-stranded DNA template, a DNA primer, a DNA polymerase, deoxynucleoside triphosphates (dNTPs), and labeled dideoxynucleotide triphosphates (ddNTPs) that terminate DNA strand elongation. These chain-terminating dideoxynucleotides lack a 3'-OH group required for the formation of a phosphodiester bond between two nucleotides, ceasing extension of DNA. The ddNTPs may be radioactive or fluorescent labeled for its detection in automated sequencing machines.

The labeled samples are then placed in an auto sampler that brings them in contact with the cathode. During electrophoresis, a high voltage is applied between the cathode and anode. The voltage drives the movement of negatively charged DNA fragments through the polymer, towards the anode.

When the DNA fragments reach the detector window in the capillary, a laser excites the fluorescent dyes. Emitted fluorescence is collected once per second by cooled, charged-coupled device (CCD) camera at particular wavelength bands and stored as digital signals. The sequencing analysis software interprets the results, calling the bases from the fluorescence intensity at each data point.

In addition, quantitative information is available in a single step in conjunction with computer collection of data. Finally, only minute quantities of sample are consumed and very little waste is generated. These advantages make CE an efficient means of DNA analysis, particularly for DNA fragment generated by polymerase chain reaction.[24]

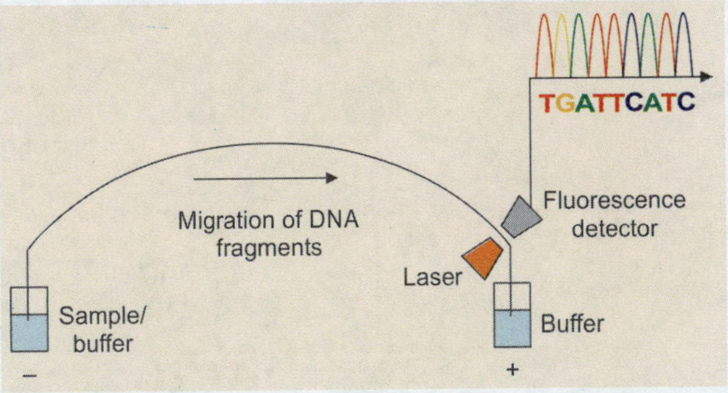

Fig. 7: Pictorial representation of DNA fragments passing through a laser beam and optical detector in capillary electrophoresis.[25]

Real Time Polymerase Chain Reaction

Real time PCRs or quantitative PCRs (qPCR) are used as powerful tool to detect small variations between sequences. SNPs are successfully identified in real-time PCR assays.[26] They have the ability to measure the PCR amplicons at early states of the reaction as they are accumulating in a real time detection mode thus measuring the amount of PCR product while the reaction is still in the exponential phase. The method is flexible, and many alternative technologies and fluorescent probe systems have been developed and are currently available.[27] They can be completed rapidly since no manipulations are required post-amplification. Identification of the amplification products by probe detection in real time is highly accurate compared with size analysis on gels. One common approach to detect sequence variations is to compare melting curves. Though the melting kinetics of PCR products is too small to be detected reliably heteroduplexes of relatively long amplicons differing by a SNP can be distinguished from the homoduplexes on the basis of their melting curves **(Fig. 7)**. This is presented as the basis of a method for mutation screening. The system could also be used to analyze copy number variations and gene expressions.

In **Figure 8**, Taqman technology has been depicted where IP indicates signal for the fluorescent reporter detected in each cycle for the target sequence. Ref indicates an analysis of the target sequence abundance in total input DNA. C_t indicates the cycle threshold number. Below the data panel is the sample calculation to determine fold difference between the IP sample and the reference sample.[29]

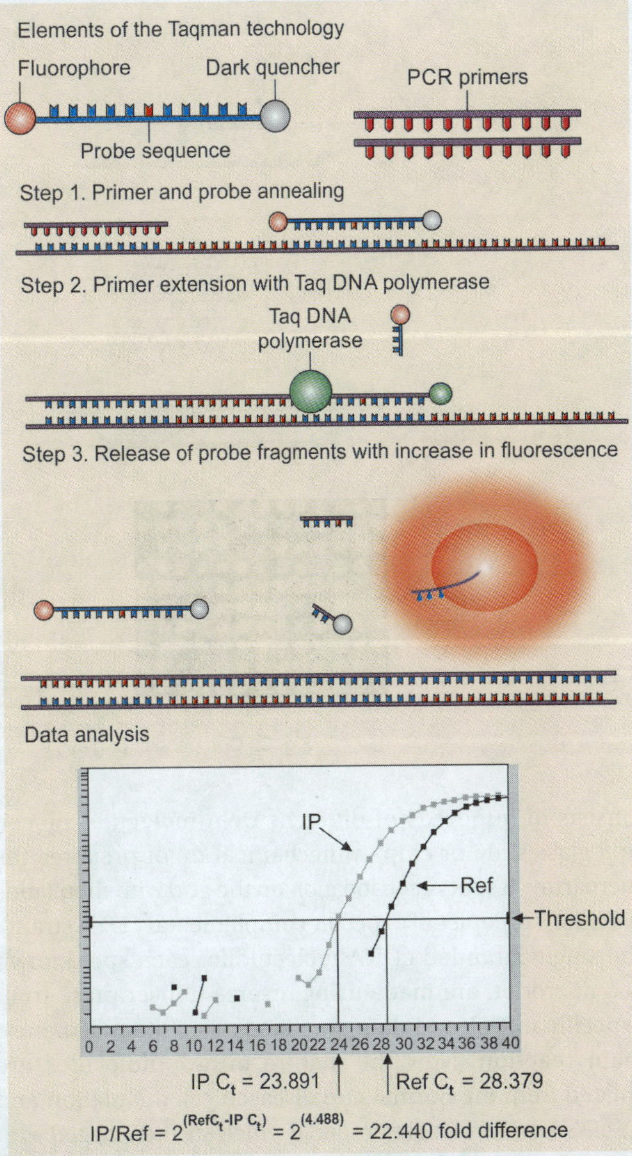

Fig. 8: Principle of Taqman assay and a representative panel of data generated by the sequence detector software for Taqman probe.[28]

DNA Microarrays and Genetic Testing

DNA microarrays provide a way to study patterns of whole genome expression and genotyping.[30,31] A DNA microarray

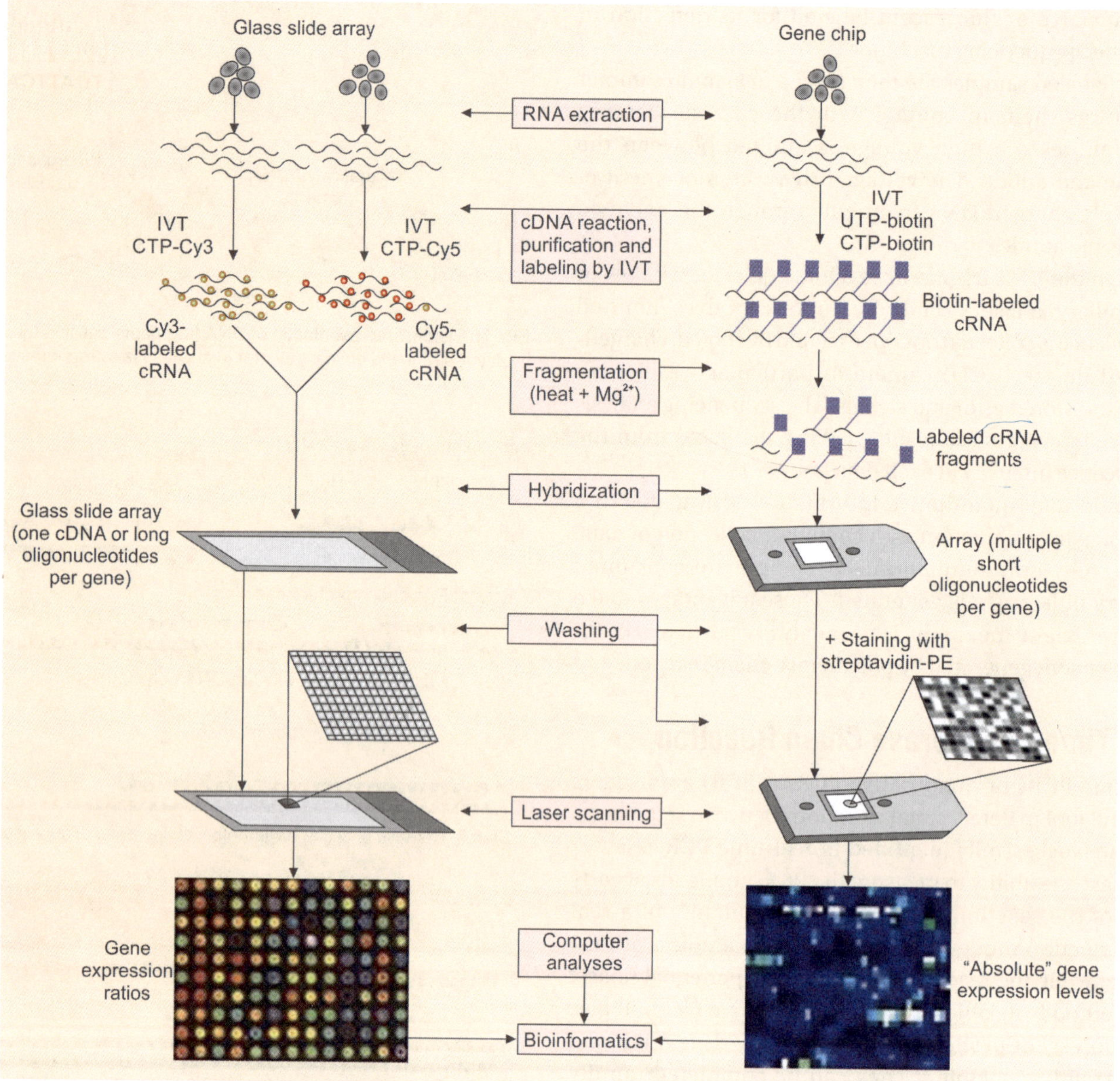

Fig. 9: Comparison of glass slide and gene chip microarray procedures.[33]

consists of hundreds of different DNA molecules placed on a glass slide or chip. A mechanical robot prepares the microarray. It spots each location on the grid with thousands to millions of copies of a specific complementary DNA strand. The single-stranded cDNA molecule for each spot known as a microdot, are made using reverse transcriptase from a specific mRNA and then amplified using the polymerase chain reaction. Now the mature mRNA molecules are isolated from the normal and diseased cell population and the cDNA molecules are prepared which are then tagged with different colored fluorescent dyes. The cDNA population is added to the array which subsequently hybridizes to its complementary strand on the array. This step is followed by washing to remove any cDNA that are not hybridized to the array. Finally the array is scanned with laser to identify the spot from which the fluorescence signal is emitted **(Fig. 9)**. Thus DNA microarrays have the potential to identify disease-causing genes or proteins they code for, which can be targeted by therapeutic drugs.[32] The technology can also be adapted for genotyping of DNA variations at whole genome level.

Next Generation Sequencing

Next generation sequencing (NGS) has fundamentally altered genomics research and allowed investigators to conduct experiments that were previously not technically feasible or affordable.

There are various next generation sequencing (NGS) platforms; however, potent technologies have been portrayed in the **Figure 10**. Although the DNA sequencing in each system is very different, all these technologies share a common technological feature; parallel sequencing of clonally amplified or single DNA molecules that are spatially

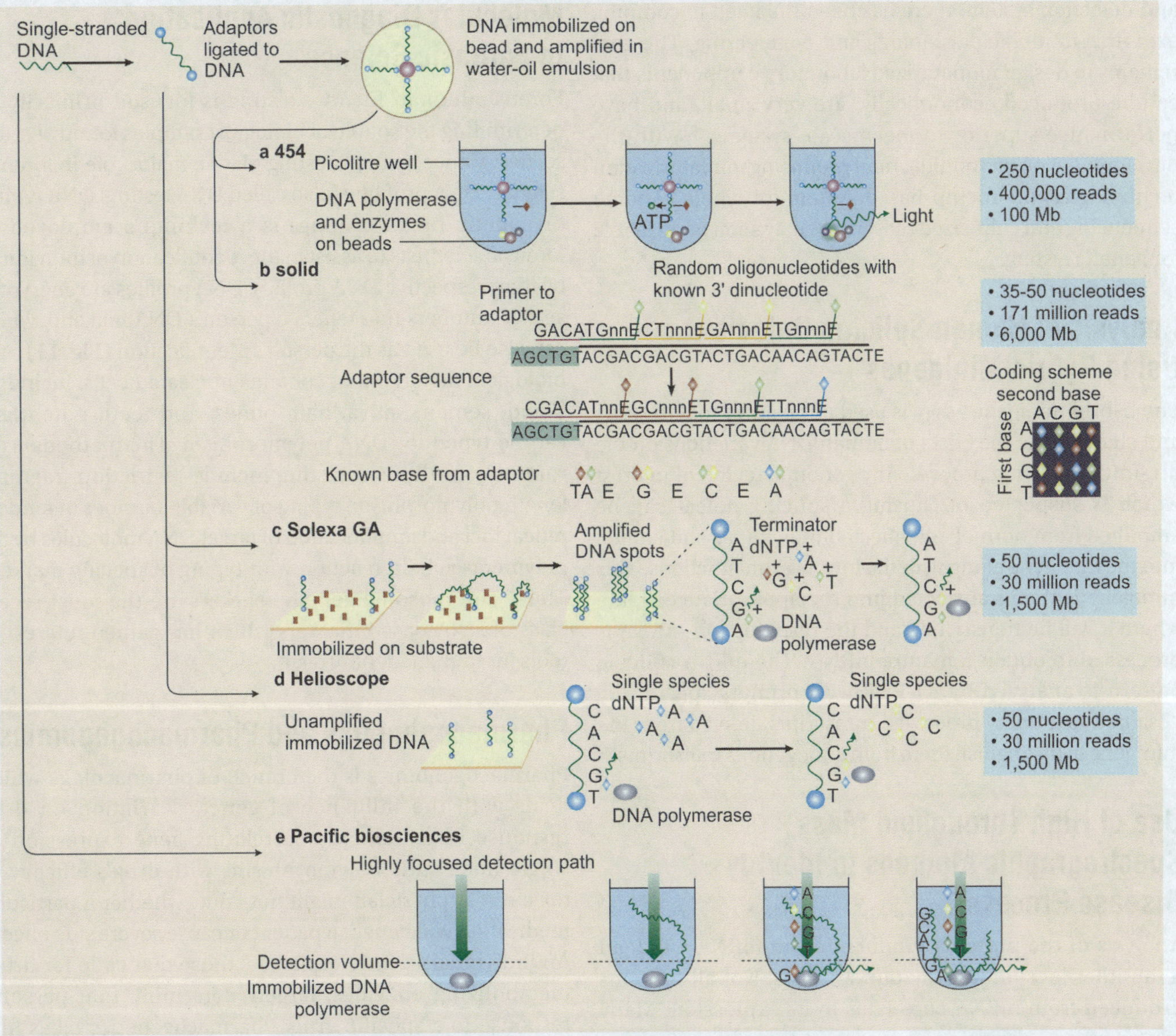

Fig. 10: Principle of various next-generation sequencing platforms.[35]

separated in a flow cell. This design is a shift from that of Sanger sequencing, which is based on the chain-termination products produced in individual sequencing reactions. In NGS, sequencing is performed by repeated cycles of PCR extensions or by continuous cycles of oligonucleotide ligation. As a parallel process, NGS generates huge nucleotide-sequence output in a single instrument run with unimaginable speed, depending on the platform.

The common applications for NGS today are sequencing of whole genomes, exomes, amplicons, transcriptomes (RNA-seq), non coding RNA discovery, mapping structural rearrangements, targeted resequencing, large scale analysis of DNA methylation and DNA: protein interactions (ChIP-seq).

Next generation sequencing experiments generate large amounts of sequence-data output which will pose a bioinformatics challenge for the clinical laboratory. In addition to data processing, the interpretation of results will require characterization of the genomic variation present in the sequences analyzed.[34]

Miniaturization Technologies for Molecular Diagnostics

Molecular diagnostics devices are getting smaller. This goal inspired many of the "miniature systems" that now include such capabilities as DNA sequencing on a chip. Performing high-throughput whole genome sequencing has been a major goal of the Human Genome Project lately. On the basis of current methods, sample collection and nucleic acid extraction are the most expensive steps involved in genetic testing. Reducing costs and developing next generation technology is a driving force in molecular diagnostics, and it is critical if this technology for testing is to compete with more conventional diagnostic methods. In the effort to create a portable and inexpensive gene amplification and detection system, there has been the need to combine expertize in molecular biology and engineering. The goal remains to design miniaturized laboratory components that can be produced economically, are very small, and have performance superior to macroscale systems.[36] With the development of microfluidics and promising miniaturization technologies, microchip-based system for whole genome sequencing and chip-sized biosensors may soon be available for genetic testing.

Analysis of Human Splicing Defects Using Hybrid Minigenes

The hybrid minigene assay is used as an assay tool to study and characterize the effect of human DNA variations on the pre-mRNA splicing process. Any genomic region of interest which is suspected of causing a splicing defect can be amplified from normal and affected individuals and cloned into the minigene along with the intron-exon junctions. This minigene is then transfected into the appropriate cell line where it will be transcribed and the resulting pre-mRNA is processed to obtain a mature mRNA. The mRNA splicing pattern is analyzed by RT-PCR with primers specifically designed to amplify processed transcripts derived from the minigene to distinguish them from endogenous transcripts.[37]

Use of High Throughput Mass Spectrographic Methods to Identify Disease Process

Analysis of the proteins produced from mRNA will lead to another level of information analysis. Not all proteins produced from mRNA correlates to its expression. Many proteins have alterations at the post-translational stage, mostly by glycosylation or phosphorylation events. It is this that may cause alteration in function of the protein product. It is therefore necessary to investigate at both gene level and at the protein level. Even when protein bands are well resolved in polyacrylamide gel electrophoresis (PAGE), the routine use of this technique for the comparison of the relative abundance of proteins in different samples is limited to the detection of big changes. Studies that require such powerful high throughput systems of analysis can be performed using mass spectrometry.[38,39] The combined use of multidimensional liquid chromatography and tandem mass spectrometry (LC-MS/MS) has made it possible to identify hundreds of proteins in the same sample containing tryptic peptides. It is a technique that combines the physical separation capabilities of liquid chromatography with the mass analysis capabilities of mass spectrometry.[40] It works by ionizing chemical compounds to generate charged molecules and then measuring their charge to mass ratios.

Molecular Diagnostic Application in Forensic Science

Forensic human identity testing is focused primarily on determining the source of biological samples found at crime scenes. Hence, genetic testing plays a major role in forensic science. DNA profiling (also called DNA testing, DNA typing, or genetic fingerprinting) is a technique employed by forensic scientists to assist in the identification of individuals by their respective DNA profiles. DNA profiles are encrypted sets of numbers that reflect a person's DNA makeup, which can also be used as the person's identification **(Fig. 11)**. Any biological material that contains nucleated cells, including blood, semen, saliva, hair, bones, and teeth potentially can be typed for DNA polymorphism. The methods used routinely for human testing include restriction fragment length polymorphism, typing of variable number of tandem repeat loci and amplification of target DNA molecules by the polymerase chain reaction with typing of specific markers. The Y chromosome genetic markers are the most recent class of DNA-based markers which has gained interest as tools for human identity testing.[41]

Pharmacogenetics and Pharmacogenomics

Pharmacogenomics is the branch of pharmacology which deals with the influence of genetic variation on drug response in patients by correlating gene expression or single-nucleotide polymorphisms with drug's efficacy or toxicity.[32] A physician might not know whether a particular medication will benefit a patient or cause severe side effects. An individual's genes, especially those that code for drug-metabolizing enzymes, largely determine that person's response to a specific drug. Pharmacogenetics takes into account the subtle genetic differences among individuals. By doing so, pharmacogenomics aims to develop rational means to optimize drug therapy with respect to the patients'

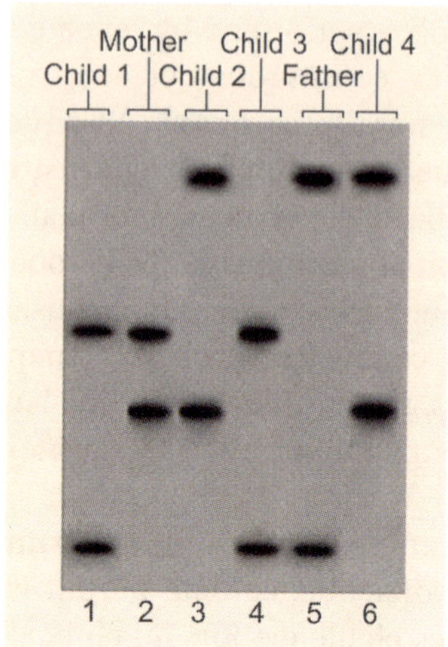

Fig. 11: Illustrative DNA fingerprinting picture.

genotype, to ensure maximum efficacy with minimum adverse effects.[42]

Positional Cloning

The strategy of positional cloning has been highly successful in identifying a number of single gene disorders that exhibit clear Mendelian patterns of inheritance. Positional cloning is a technique used to identify genes that are usually associated with diseases, based on their location in the genome. The overall strategy of positional cloning is to map the location of a human disease or trait gene by linkage analysis and to use the mapped location on the chromosome to clone the gene of interest. It is another approach to find genes involved in complex phenotypes.

Position Independent Identification of Human Disease

Prior to the advent of positional cloning, a few genes causing human disease were identified on the basis of visible cytogenetic defects or by pinpointing a biochemical pathway, which led to the identification of relevant gene. Each of this efforts required insight into the mechanism of the disease. Position independent methods include the following:

- Knowledge or identification of the dysfunctional protein and working backward toward gene identification
- Identifying a candidate gene in a mouse model, and isolating and testing the orthologous human gene
- Localizing a disease gene by a chromosomal abnormality such as inversion, translocation or monosomy
- Expression array experiments comparing the levels of mRNA in a series of patients versus control
- Knowledge of the probable mechanism of the disease.

Human Gene Patents

A gene patent refers to any patent with any claim over nucleic acid or for the purpose of diagnosing a genetic condition. The gene patent claims most relevant to genetic testing can be divided into four types: (1) Product claims to isolated DNA or RNA molecules, (2) Product claims for diagnostic kit tests, (3) Process claims for methods of diagnosis through genetic testing, and (4) Product claims to gene chips and microarrays.[43] Human gene patents were awarded by US Patent and Trademark Office right since 1982. The overriding question addressed was whether "products of nature" can be treated the same as "human-made" inventions, making them intellectual property of individuals and companies. The broader issue involved 21st century conflicts over cutting-edge medical science, the power of business and individual legal rights, and how their convergence might influence the prospect and management of certain diseases, like cancer. The issue has divided the scientific and business communities. In June 2013, a court order was issued that naturally occurring genes are no longer patentable. Whereas synthetic genes are still fair game. This decision led to a fall in costs involving testing for genetic disorders and sequencing of whole genomes have become much easier as well. Though patents for naturally occurring genes are cancelled, specific diagnostic tests, methods to isolate the gene and other trade secrets are patentable which helps in maintaining a good competition between companies.

CHROMOSOMAL STUDY/CYTOGENETICS

Cytogenetics is a branch of genetics that is concerned with the study of the structure and function of the cell, especially the chromosomes and its related abnormalities.[44] It includes routine analysis of G-banded chromosomes, other cytogenetic banding techniques, as well as molecular cytogenetics such as fluorescent in situ hybridization (FISH) and comparative genomic hybridization (CGH).

Karyotyping

Karyotyping not only helps us to study the number of chromosomes but also the structure of chromosomes. In addition to providing associations between chromosomal abnormalities and diseases, cytogenetic approaches have also allowed researchers to map genes to a particular chromosome. Shortly after the Duffy blood group locus was mapped, Maximo Drets and Margery Shaw established methods to stain metaphase chromosomes using a dye called Giemsa, which produces a signature banding pattern called as G-banding for each of the 24 different human chromosomes. The chromosomes are visualized after staining using a light microscope. They display a characteristic dark and light banding pattern according to the DNA content that is unique for individual chromosome as shown in **Figures 12 and 13**. The dark regions are the A-T rich regions (gene poor regions) and the light regions are the G-C rich regions. Based on the banding pattern obtained on the chromosomes, the phenotype of the individual can be

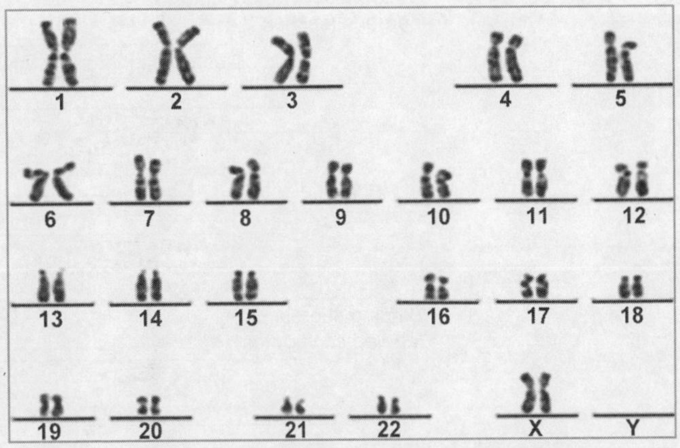

Fig. 12: Representative karyotype of a normal female.

analyzed. Geneticists use the following standardized way of describing a gene's cytogenetic location:

- The location on which the gene can be found
- The arm of the chromosome
- The position of the gene on the p or q arm.

G-banding method continues to be widely used today, though such approaches have certain drawbacks. For instance, G-banding requires metaphase chromosomes which are easily obtained from blood but are more difficult to retrieve from solid tissue samples. Moreover, metaphase chromosomes are highly condensed which can lead to lower resolution in mapping. Despite these drawbacks, G-banding serves as an important laboratory diagnostic procedure in the field of prenatal diagnosis, in patients/families with history of mental retardation, multiple birth defects, abnormal sexual development, infertility or multiple miscarriages. The technique also finds its application in malignancies and hematological disorders.[45]

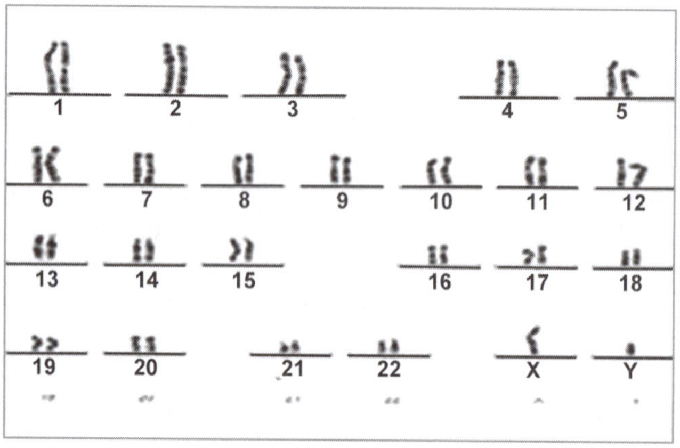

Fig. 13: Representative karyotype of a normal male.

Chromosome Analysis by Fluorescence in situ Hybridization

Another way to distinguish chromosomes in a karyotype is by FISH. It combines microscopic observation and the specificity of the hybridization. It is based on the unique ability of a portion of single stranded DNA to anneal with its complementary target sequence on a metaphase chromosome, interphase nucleus or extended chromatin fiber.[32] In FISH, the DNA probe is labeled with a fluorochrome which after hybridization with the patient's sample, allows the region where hybridization has occurred to be visualized using a fluorescence microscope **(Figs. 14 and 15)**. The sensitivity is the result of the high affinity and selectivity of DNA probes because FISH takes place under very stringent hybridization conditions.[46,1]

Fluorescence in situ hybridization image **(Fig. 15)** is showing the deletion of chromosomal region 22q11. DNA probes are used to highlight the regions of metaphase chromosome 22 in the patient sample. The white arrow indicates the area of deletion. Chromosome 22 is identified by a control probe that hybridizes to the end of long arm of chromosome 22 (blue green signals).

Comparative Genomic Hybridization

It is a molecular cytogenetic technique that can characterize excess and missing cytogenetic material often unrecognized by G-banding in a one-step procedure.[49] The advantage of comparative genomic hybridization (CGH) over conventional FISH is its ability to identify not only the chromosome from which the additional unknown

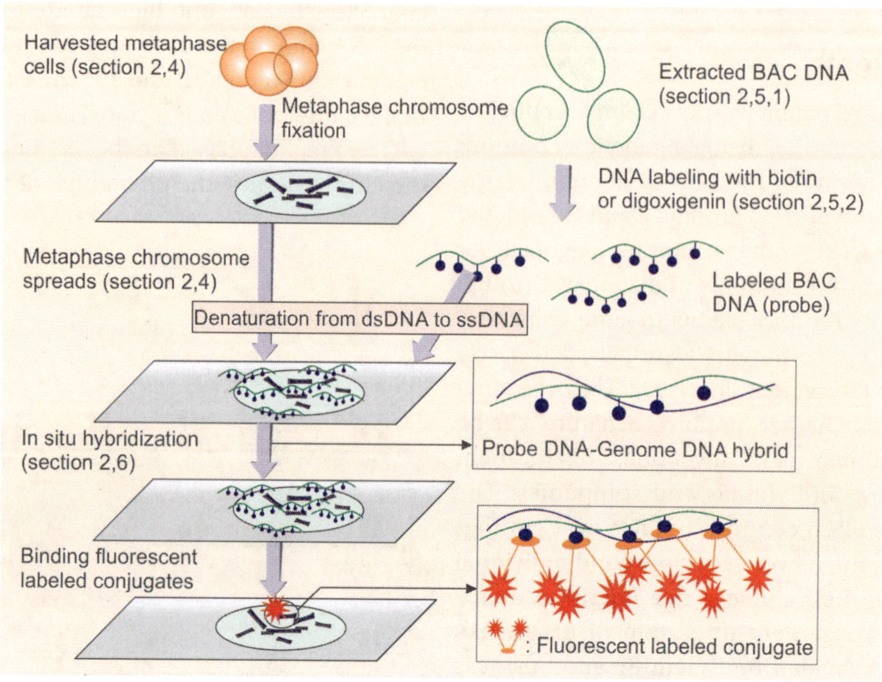

Fig. 14: Pictorial representation of fluorescent in situ hybridization.[47]

material was derived but also to map the region involved to specific bands on the source chromosome. CGH has been particularly useful in clinical cytogenetics by facilitating the identification and characterization of intrachromosomal duplications, deletions, unbalanced translocations and marker chromosomes including neocentric marker chromosomes. DNA from subject tissue and from normal control tissue is each labeled with different tags for analysis by fluorescence. After mixing subject and reference DNA, the mix is hybridized to normal metaphase chromosomes on to a slide containing hundreds or thousands of defined DNA probes. Using epifluorescence microscopy and quantitative image analysis, specific differences in the fluorescence ratio of gains/losses vs. control DNA can be detected and used for identifying abnormal regions in the genome **(Fig. 16)**.[50]

Chromosomal Array

The microarray based chromosomal analysis uses novel array CGH technology to deliver automated and objective analysis of the samples. It has average genome coverage of approximately 565 kb, with median coverage of 250 kb in sub telomeric regions and an average resolution of 100 kb in 90 known clinically relevant regions **(Fig. 17)**. Chromosomal array enables fast turn-around times, mosaic detection

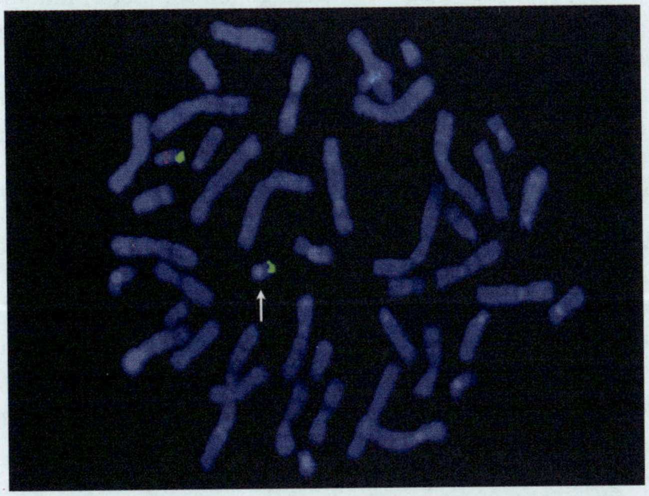

Fig. 15: Demonstrative image generated by fluorescent in situ hybridization.[48]

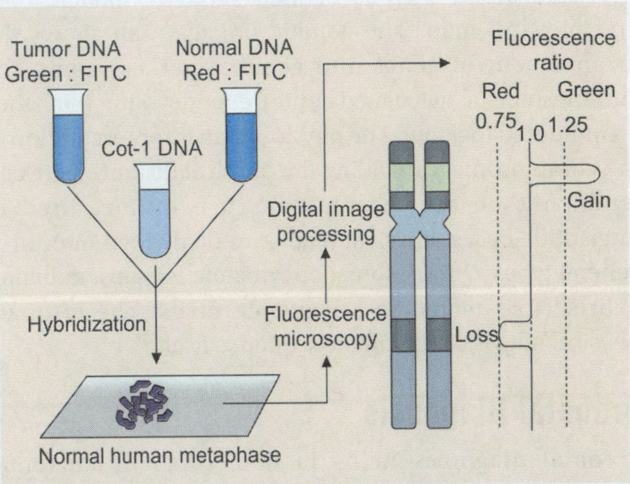

Fig. 16: Schematic representation of comparative genomic hybridization.[51]

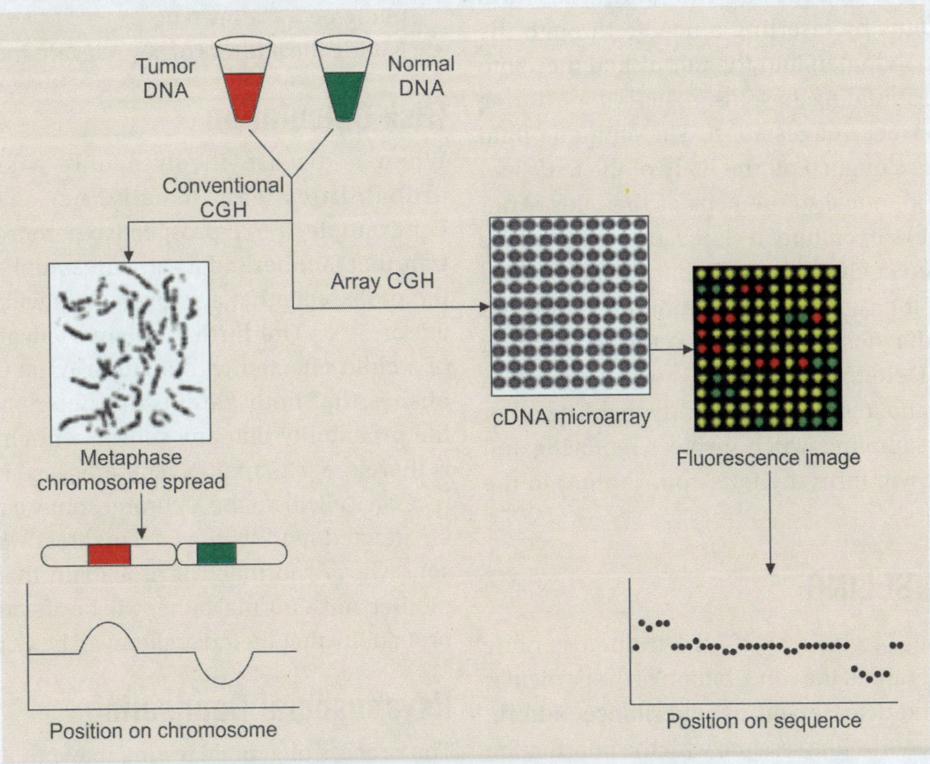

Fig. 17: Array comparative genomic hybridization.[52]

framework, reduced subjectivity, FISH follow-up and user configurable disease focused design.

Gene Mapping

Gene mapping is a graphical representation of arrangement of genes or DNA fragments on a chromosome. It offers firm evidence that a disease transmitted from parent to child is linked to one or more genes. It also helps us to identify which chromosome contains the gene and precisely where it lies on that chromosome. The central idea of gene mapping is that the frequency of recombination between two genes can be used as a measure of the actual distance between them on a chromosome.

There are two types of maps–genetic linkage map and physical map. The genetic linkage map shows the arrangement of genes and genetic markers along the chromosomes as calculated by the frequency with which they are inherited together. The physical map is representation of the chromosomes, providing the physical distance between landmarks on the chromosome, usually measured in nucleotide bases. Physical maps can be divided into three general types–chromosomal or cytogenetic maps, radiation hybrid (RH) maps, and sequence maps. The ultimate physical map is the complete sequence itself.[53]

Prenatal Diagnosis

Prenatal diagnosis helps in detecting chromosomal abnormalities and gene defects before a child is born. In the diagnostic technique called amniocentesis, a physician obtains a sample of the amniotic fluid surrounding the fetus by inserting a needle through the pregnant women's abdomen into the uterus and then into the amniotic sac surrounding the fetus.[32] This is done during the 15th and 16th weeks of gestation. The amniotic fluid contains living cells sloughed off the body of the fetus and hence genetically identical to the cells of the fetus. After cells grow for 2 weeks in culture, technicians karyotype the dividing cells to detect chromosomal abnormalities. Fetal blood sampling is the second most commonly employed invasive prenatal diagnosis procedure in the second and third trimesters.[54] Here the fetal blood is withdrawn from the umbilical cord and it is taken for karyotyping. The other is chorionic villus sampling which involves removing and studying cells that will form the fetal contribution to the placenta.[55]

GENETIC COUNSELING

Genetic counseling is given by a well-trained genetic counselor to patients about the contribution of the particular genetic defect to the disease and its inheritance pattern. During the genetic counseling session, with the information provided by the patients, a family chart (pedigree) is generated for the patients to explicate on the ways to manage the risks of inheritance of the genetic defect.[56] It is given to the patients to improve their quality of life after diagnosis of the genetic disease. A genetic counselor plays a vital role in conveying the patients about rapid advances in treatment modalities or trials available for the specified genetic disease.

Family History and Pedigree Construction

Collecting the genetic information is the first and most important step in genetic counseling and is best achieved by drawing a family tree or pedigree. A family tree that shows inheritance pattern, the transmission of genetic traits within a family over several generations, is known as a pedigree. It helps the molecular geneticists determine the exact interrelationships of the DNA molecules they analyze from related individuals.[57] Pedigrees are produced using standard symbols **(Fig. 18)**. Pedigree analysis most often identifies three modes of single locus inheritance: autosomal dominant, autosomal recessive, and X-linked recessive. A representative family pedigree is shown in **Figure 19**.

The following practical points deserve emphasis while drawing a pedigree:

- Enquiring specifically about infant deaths
- Consanguinity should be taken into account which may be a clue that suggests autosomal recessive inheritance
- Mistaken or unacknowledged paternity must be borne in mind
- Taking at least basic details about both maternal and paternal sides of the family
- Recording dates of birth and also the date when the pedigree was drawn up
- Noting the address of key relevant members.

Risk Calculation

When a disease involves only a single gene locus, probabilities can usually be easily calculated.[58] For example, if one prospective parent is affected with the trait that is inherited as an autosomal dominant disorder, the probability that any given child will have the disease is 0.5 or 50%. The birth to phenotypically normal parents of a child affected with an autosomal recessive trait establishes that both parents are heterozygous carriers and the probability that any subsequent child will be affected is therefore 0.25 or 25%. For a disease inherited through a recessive allele on the X chromosome, a normal woman and an affected man will have daughters who are carriers and sons who are normal. The probability that the son of a carrier mother and a normal father will be affected is 0.5 or 50%; the probability that their daughter will be a carrier is also 0.5.

Psychosocial Counseling

The process of genetic testing may put an individual under lot of psychological stress. Hence, counselors need to be

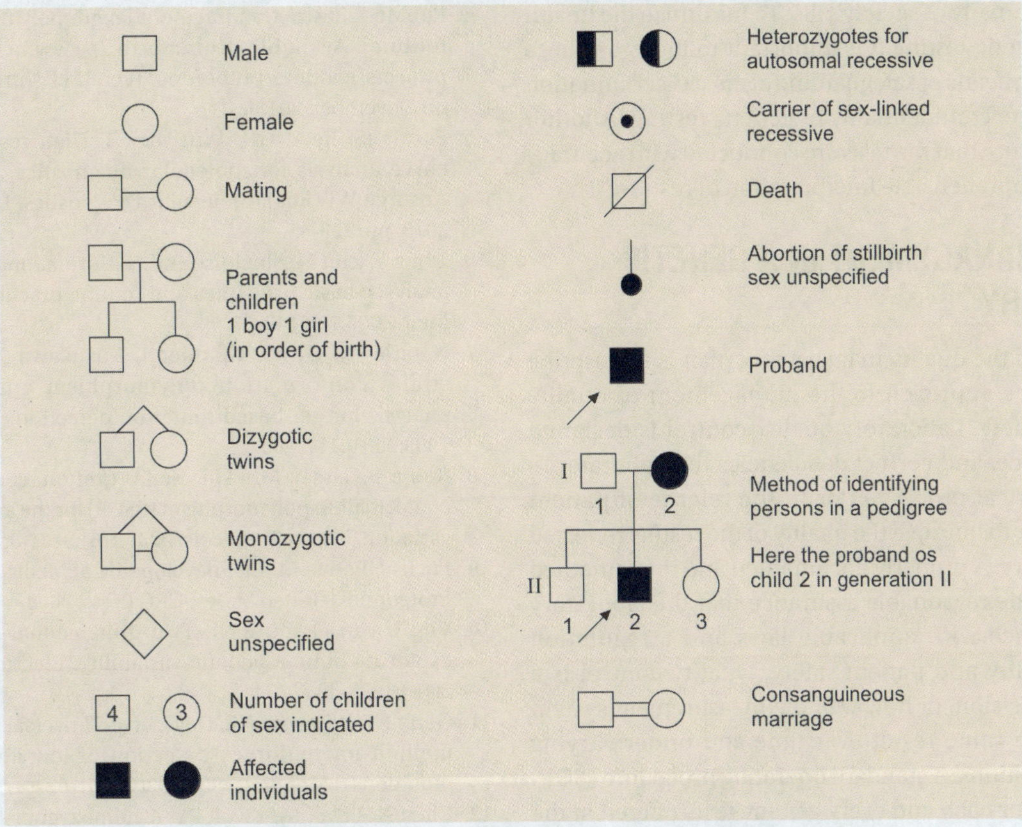

Fig. 18: Standard pedigree symbols and relationships.

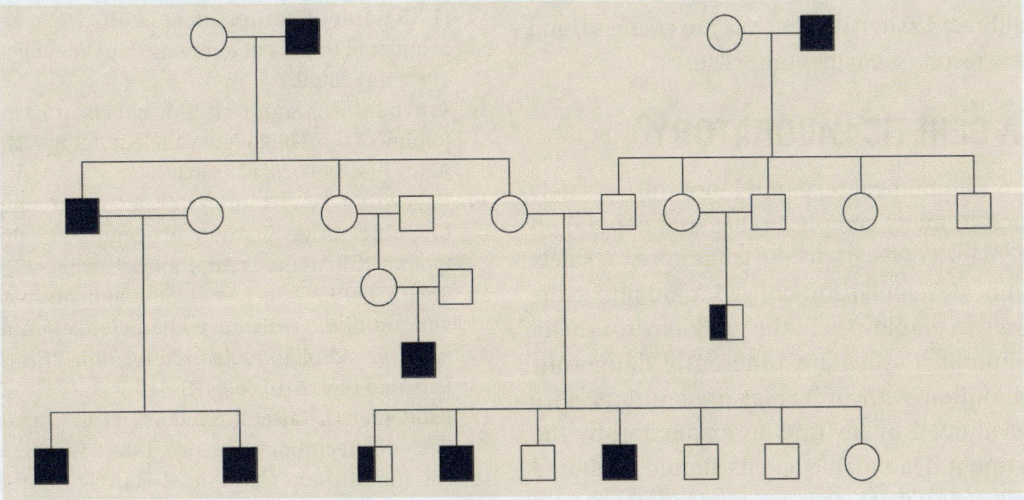

Fig. 19: A representative family pedigree.

fully in command of the psychological impact of their communications and also help the individual or the family to comprehend the medical facts of the diagnosis, the available management and to make the best possible adjustment to the disorder. Considering the individual's level of knowledge about their genetic condition is very important in reducing their anxiety and gaining a degree of control.[59]

Patient Education

Genetic counselors, who have received training in counseling medicine, and human genetics, provide people with the information they need to make reproductive decisions.[56] They offer advice, tempered with respect and sensitivity in terms of risk estimates that is the probability that any given offspring will inherit a particular condition.

Ethical and Legal Issues

There are concerns that genetic testing results may lead to discrimination by employers and society.[32] Many misconceptions exist about genetic diseases and their effects on society. Some people erroneously think of certain individuals or populations as genetically unfit and thus responsible for many of society's ills. To maximize the health benefits of genetic testing it is important to focus on these concerns. One means of safeguarding against discrimination is to address the confidentiality of genetic testing. Another means is to ensure that the tests are conducted with accuracy and offer a comprehensible interpretation of results.[60]

QUALITY MANAGEMENT IN A GENETIC LABORATORY

The purpose of the quality management plan is to describe the laboratory's approach to the management of quality and patient safety. Laboratory quality control is designed to detect, reduce, and correct deficiencies in a laboratory's internal analytical process prior to the release of patient results, in order to improve the quality of the results reported by the laboratory. A properly documented and implemented plan will provide reasonable assurance that the laboratory is in compliance with applicable laws and a regulation related to quality and patient safety. Quality control is a measure of precision, or how well the measurement system reproduces the same result over time and under varying operating conditions. A standard operating procedure (SOP) is maintained for each and every genetic tests offered at the laboratory. Laboratory quality control material is usually run at the beginning of each shift, after an instrument is serviced and calibrated, when reagent lots are changed, and whenever sample results seem inappropriate.

SAFETY IN A GENETIC LABORATORY

The operation of biomedical research laboratories safely requires attention to many complex issues that depend on the goals and activities of each specific laboratory.[5] A safety program should be developed and utilized to minimize the chance of injuries to employees in the work environment. Especially all human tissues are inherently dangerous and must be handled with universal precautions. Fire safety can be evaluated by inviting an inspection by the local fire department. Flammable agents should be stored appropriately. Electrical safety can be avoided by ensuring that all equipment is grounded.

REFERENCES

1. Mittal B. Rapid molecular diagnosis of spinal muscular atrophy. Indian J Med Res. 2012;135(1):6-8.
2. Billard A, Laval V, Fillinger S, et al. The allele-specific probe and primer amplification assay, a new real-time PCR method for fine quantification of single-nucleotide polymorphisms in pooled DNA. Appl Environ Microbiol. 2012;78(4):1063-8.
3. Gibbs RA, Nguyen PN, Caskey CT. Detection of single DNA base differences by competitive oligonucleotide priming. Nucleic Acids Res. 1989;17(7):2437-48.
4. PubMed. Restriction fragment length polymorphism (RFLP). [online] Available from: http://www.ncbi.nlm.nih.gov/projects/genome/probe/doc/TechRFLP.shtml [Last accessed on November, 2019].
5. Farrar JS, Reed GH, Wittwer CT. High resolution melting curve analysis for molecular diagnostics. In: Patrinos GP, Ansorge WJ (Eds). Molecular Diagnostics. London: Elsevier. 2010. pp. 229-45.
6. Dong Y, Zhu H. Single-strand conformational polymorphism analysis: basic principles and routine practice. Methods Mol Med. 2005;108:149-57.
7. Nataraj AJ, Olivos-Glander I, Kusukawa N, et al. Single-strand conformation polymorphism and heteroduplex analysis for gel-based mutation detection. Electrophoresis. 1999;20(6):1177-85.
8. Robin B Gasser, Min Hu, Neil B Chilton, et al. Single-strand conformation polymorphism (SSCP) for the analysis of genetic variation. Nature Protocols. 2007;1(6):3121-8.
9. Fuchs J, Podda M. In: Encyclopedia of Medical Genomics and Proteomics. United States: CRC Press. 2008.
10. Vijg J, van Orsouw NJ. Two-dimensional gene scanning: exploring human genetic variability. Electrophoresis. 1999; 20(6):1239-49.
11. Gerry NP, Witowski NE, Day J, et al. Universal DNA microarray method for multiplex detection of low abundance point mutations. J Mol Biol. 1999;292(2):251-62.
12. Chen X, Livak KJ, Kwok PY. A homozygous ligase-mediated DNA diagnostic test. Genome Res. 1998;8:549-56.
13. Wu DY, Wallace RB. The ligation amplification reaction (LAR)-amplification of specific DNA sequences using sequential rounds of template dependent ligation. Genomics. 1989;4(4):560-9.
14. Pritchard CE, Southern EM. Effects of base mismatches on joining of short oligodeoxynucleotides by DNA ligases. Nucleic Acids Res. 1997;25(17):3403-7.
15. Eggerding FA. A one-step coupled amplification and oligonucleotide ligation procedure for multiplex genetic typing. PCR Methods Appl. 1995;4(6):337-45.
16. Song J, Li PE, Gans J, et al. Simultaneous pathogen detection and antibiotic resistance characterization using SNP-based multiplexed oligonucleotide ligation-PCR (MOL-PCR). Adv Exp Med Biol. 2010;680:455-64.
17. Landegren U, Kaiser R, Sanders J, et al. A ligase-mediated gene detection technique. Science. 1988;241(4869):1077-80.
18. Nilsson M, Baner J, Mendel-Hartvig M, et al. Making ends meet in genetic analysis using padlock probes. Hum Mutat. 2002;19(4):410-5.
19. Schouten JP, McElgunn CJ, Waaijer R, et al. Relative quantification of 40 nucleic acid sequences by multiplex ligation-dependent probe amplification. Nucleic Acids Res. 2002;30(12):e57.
20. Van Eijk MJ, Broekhof JL, van der Poel HJ, et al. SNPWave™: a flexible multiplexed SNP genotyping technology. Nucleic Acids Res. 2004;32(4):e47.
21. Hogervorst FB, Nederlof PM, Gille JJ, et al. Large genomic deletions and duplications in the BRCA1 gene identified by a novel quantitative method. Cancer Res. 2004;63(7):1449-53.
22. Eldering E, Spek CA, Aberson HL, et al. Expression profiling via novel multiplex assay allows rapid assessment of gene

regulation in defined signalling pathways. Nucleic Acids Res. 2003;31(23):e153.
23. MRC-Holland. (2013). MLPA. [online] Available from: http://www.mlpa.com/WebForms/WebFormMain.aspx [Last accessed on November, 2019].
24. Gao Q, Yeung ES. High-throughput detection of unknown mutations by using multiplexed capillary electrophoresis with poly (vinylpyrrolidone) solution. Anal Chem. 2000; 72(11):2499-506.
25. Applied Biosystems. Capillary electrophoresis. [online] Available from: http://www.appliedbiosystems.com [Last accessed on November, 2019].
26. Pestana E, Belak S, Diallo A, et al. Early, rapid and sensitive veterinary molecular diagnostics - real time PCR applications. Germany: Springer. 2010. pp. 310.
27. Logan JMJ, Edwards K, Saunders NA. Real-time PCR: current technology and applications London: Caister Academic Press. 2009.
28. Neil JG. The use of real-time PCR methods in DNA sequence variation analysis. Clinica Chimica Acta. 2005;363(1-2):32-47.
29. Michael DL, Melanie S, Recillas-Targa F, et al. Transitions in histone acetylation reveal boundaries of three separately regulated neighboring loci. EMBO J. 2001;20:2224-35.
30. Naidu CK, Suneetha Y. Current knowledge on microarray technology: an overview. Trop J Pharm Res. 2012;11(1): 153-64.
31. Klopfleisch R, Gruber AD. Transcriptome and proteome research in veterinary science: what is possible and what questions can be asked? Scientific World Journal. 2012;2012:254962.
32. Solomon EP, Berg LR, Martin DW. In: Biology. Philadelphia: Saunders College Publishing. 1999.
33. Staal FJT, van der Burg M, Wessels LFA, et al. DNA microarrays for comparison of gene expression profiles between diagnosis and relapse in precursor-B acute lymphoblastic leukemia: choice of technique and purification influence the identification of potential diagnostic markers. Leukemia. 2003;17(7):1324-32.
34. Sanchez J-C, Corthals GL, Hochstrasser DF. Book Reviews: Biomedical Applications of Proteomics. WILEY-VCH. 2004;4:2512-3.
35. Voelkerding V, Dames SA, Durtschi JD. Next-generation sequencing: from basic research to diagnostics. Clinical Chemistry. 2009;55(4):641-58.
36. MacLean D, Jones JD, Studhome DJ. Application of 'next-generation' technologies to microbial genetics. Nature Reviews Microbiology. 2009;7(4):289-96.
37. McGlennen RC. Miniaturization technologies for molecular diagnostics. Clin Chem. 2001;47(3):393-402.
38. Dujardin G, Commandeur D, Le Jossic-Corcos C, et al. Splicing defects in the CFTR gene: minigene analysis of two mutations, 1811+1G>C and 1898+3A>G. J Cyst Fibros. 2011;10(3):212-6.
39. Housby JN. In: Mass Spectrometry and Genomic Analysis. Germany: Springer. 2001.
40. Cox J, Mann M. Quantitative, high-resolution proteomics for data-driven systems biology. Annu Rev Biochem. 2011;80: 273-99.
41. Roeder K. DNA fingerprinting: a review of the controversy. Statistical Science. 1994;9:222-78.
42. Relling MV, Altman RB, Goetz MP, et al. Clinical implementation of pharmacogenomics: overcoming genetic exceptionalism. Lancet Oncol. 2010;11(6):507-9
43. Hawkins N. Human Gene Patents and Genetic Testing in Europe: a Reappraisal. SCRIPTed. 2010;7(3):453.
44. Rooney DE. Human Cytogenetics: Constitutional Analysis. A Practical Approach. United Kingdom: Oxford University Press. 2001.
45. Hebrard M, Manes G, Bocquet B, et al. Combining gene mapping and phenotype assessment for fast mutation finding in non-consanguineous autosomal recessive retinitis pigmentosa families. Eur J Hum Genet. 2011;19(12):1256-63.
46. Rosie EB, Foster SJ, Monahaj BJ. Molecular diagnostic tools for detection of bacteria in dental plaque. In: Rao JR, Fleming CC, Moore JE (Eds). Molecular Diagnostics: Current Technology and Applications. United Kingdom: Horizon Scientific Press. 2006. pp. 215-42.
47. Cao Y, Kimura S, Itoi T, et al. Fluorescence in situ hybridization using bacterial artificial chromosome (BAC) clones for the analysis of chromosome rearrangement in Chinese hamster ovary cells. Methods. 2012;56(3):418-23.
48. Morris-Rosendahl DJ, Back E. The human genome: chromosome 22q11 deletion syndrome. Am J Psychiatry. 2002;159:527.
49. Fan Y-S. Molecular cytogenetics: protocols and applications. Mol Pathol. 2002;56(3):190.
50. Renn SC, Machado HE, Jones A, et al. Using comparative genomic hybridization to survey genomic sequence divergence across species: a proof-of-concept from Drosophila. BMC Genomics. 2010;11:271.
51. Weiss MM, Hermsen MA, Meijer GA, et al. Comparative genomic hybridization. Mol Pathol. 1999;52(5):243-51.
52. Bishop R. Applications of fluorescence in situ hybridization (FISH) in detecting genetic aberrations of medical significance. Bioscience Horizons. 2010;3(1):85-95.
53. Chial H. Gene mapping and disease. Nature Education. 2008;1(1):50.
54. Milunsky A, Milunsky J. In: Genetic Disorders and the Fetus: Diagnosis, Prevention and Treatment. United States: John Wiley and Sons. 2010.
55. Raymond FL, Whittaker J, Jenkins L, et al. Molecular prenatal diagnosis: the impact of modern technologies. Prenat Diagn. 2010;30(7):674-81.
56. Evans C. Genetic counseling: a psychological approach. United Kingdom: Cambridge University Press. 2006.
57. Harper P. Practical Genetic Counseling. London: Hodder Arnold Publishers. 2010.
58. Bennett RL. The Practical Guide to the Genetic Family History. New Jersey: John Wiley and Sons. 2010.
59. Baker DL, Schuette JL, Uhlmann WR. A Guide to Genetic Counseling. New York: Wiley-Liss. 1998
60. Collins RE, Wright AJ, Marteau TM. Impact of communicating personalized genetic risk information on perceived control over the risk: a systematic review. Genet Med. 2011;13(4): 273-7.

CHAPTER

36 Diagnostic Modalities in Intraocular Malignancies

Mohammad Javed Ali, Sneha Jay Shah, Santosh G Honavar

INTRODUCTION

The first step toward managing any malignancy is to diagnose it accurately. Presently, a good clinical evaluation aided with indirect ophthalmoscopy and adjunctive modalities is an established diagnostic procedure for most of the tumors. Ocular tumors are usually seen first by a general ophthalmologist and not an ocular oncologist hence the significance of detecting the tumor early with appropriate diagnostic modalities cannot be overstated. As with any other branch of medicine, diagnostic modalities in intraocular malignancies have evolved around modern techniques such as ultrasonography, fundus fluorescein angiography, fundus indocyanine green angiography, computed tomography, and tissue biopsy. In this chapter, an overview of diagnostic procedures for intraocular malignancies has been presented.

ULTRASONOGRAPHY

Ultrasonography including three-dimensional scanning is a valuable tool in aiding the diagnosis and monitoring of intraocular tumors.[1,2] Types of scanning that are frequently employed include A-scan, B-scan, ultrasound biomicroscopy, and three-dimensional imaging. Indications of ultrasonography in general for intraocular tumors are enumerated in **Box 1**. The general features of tumors that need to be assessed are enumerated in **Box 2**. Since discussing all the features for an entire spectrum of intraocular tumors is outside the purview of this chapter, only common tumors would be described.

Retinoblastoma demonstrates intraocular calcification, which manifests on A- and B-scans as multiple highly reflective echoes that persist even when the gain is reduced **(Figs. 1A and B)**. Uveal melanomas on A-scan show an initial high spike with a progressively descending slope called as angle kappa **(Fig. 2A)**. A small choroidal melanoma appears as a dome-shaped or a nodular well-circumscribed choroidal mass. As it grows, it may break through the Bruch's membrane to show the classical collar-stud appearance **(Figs. 2A and B)**. Homogeneous mass with loss of internal acoustic reflectivity can also be noted. This phenomenon is also responsible for appearance of the choroidal excavation, although it can also be partly explained when the tumor invades the sclera. Ultrasonography in melanomas is very useful technique to detect extraocular extension. Although sequential ultrasonography is more helpful in ocular metastasis for monitoring response to treatment, regular scans usually show high acoustic reflectivity throughout the tumor.[1,2]

Ultrasound B-scan with immersion technique and ultrasound biomicroscopy aid in evaluation of anterior segment especially ciliary body tumors or metastasis **(Fig. 3)**. Extraocular extension of intraocular tumors or intraocular extension of ocular surface tumors can also be detected. Ciliary body melanoma would behave similarly on ultrasonography as described for uveal melanoma.

Box 1: Indications of ultrasonography.

- Diagnosis in hazy media
- To study parameters of a mass lesion
- To aid in treatment planning and execution
- Monitor the tumor progression or regression with time and therapy
- To aid in detection of extraocular extension

Box 2: Tumor features to be assessed by ultrasonography.

- Location of the tumor
- Height or tumor thickness
- Inward extent
- Overlying retinal changes
- Largest basal diameter
- Distance from the disk
- Internal acoustic reflectivity
- Extraocular spread

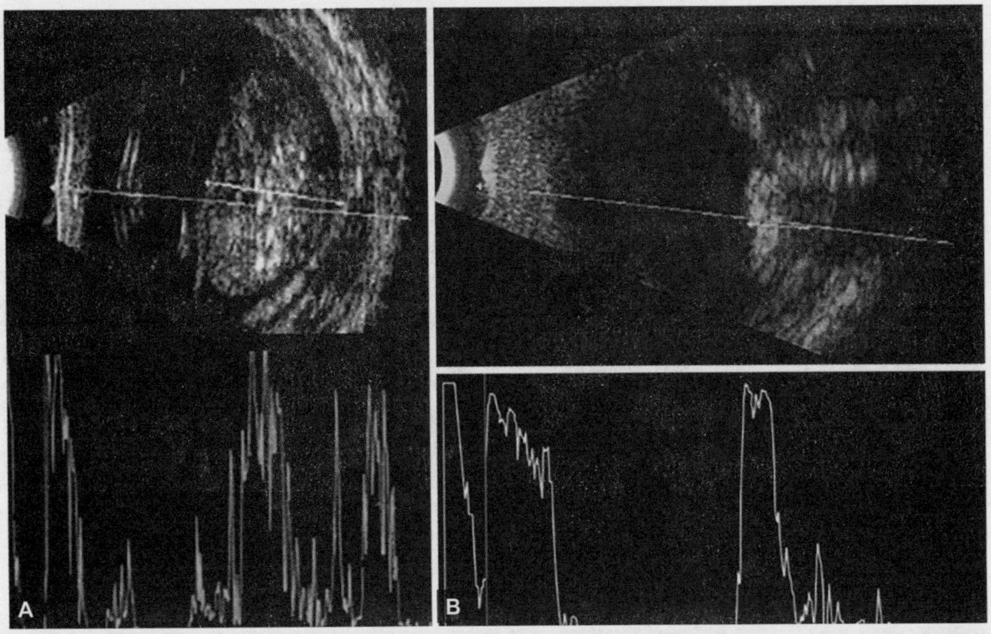

Figs. 1A and B: Ultrasound B-scan showing retinoblastoma with calcification and corresponding high reflectivity on A-scan.

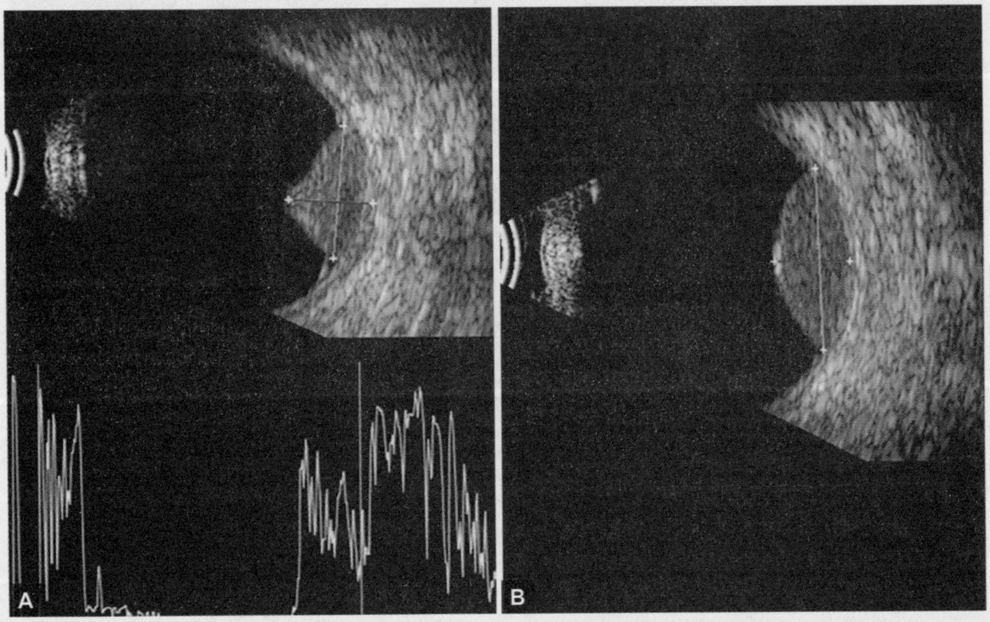

Figs. 2A and B: *Choroidal melanoma*: Presenting with typical dome-shaped elevation (right) or surface nodularity caused by break in Bruch's membrane (top left), which ultimately leads to collar-stud appearance on B-scan and A-scan shows angle kappa.

Ciliary body medulloepithelioma shows variable internal reflectivity depending on the presence or absence of heterologous elements and presence of intralesional cystic spaces[2] **(Fig. 4)**. Three-dimensional ultrasonography is an upcoming modality that is being evaluated for its role in tumor volume measurements and aiding therapeutic interventions like plaque localization for brachytherapy.[3,4]

FUNDUS FLUORESCEIN AND INDOCYANINE GREEN ANGIOGRAPHY

Fundus fluorescein angiography (FFA) and indocyanine green angiography (ICG-A) are adjunctive diagnostic tools that often provide additional information to help confirm a clinical diagnosis of intraocular tumor.[5-7]

Accurate analysis and meaningful diagnostic conclusions result from the recognition of several important events that occur during the course of an angiographic study.[6] FFA provides detailed information about intraretinal circulation and tumor vascularity arising thereof. In contrast, ICG-A is an effective method in imaging the choroidal vasculature, tumor vascularity, and circulatory alterations around the tumor.

Although there are no pathognomonic angiographic features of choroidal melanoma, large melanoma with RPE

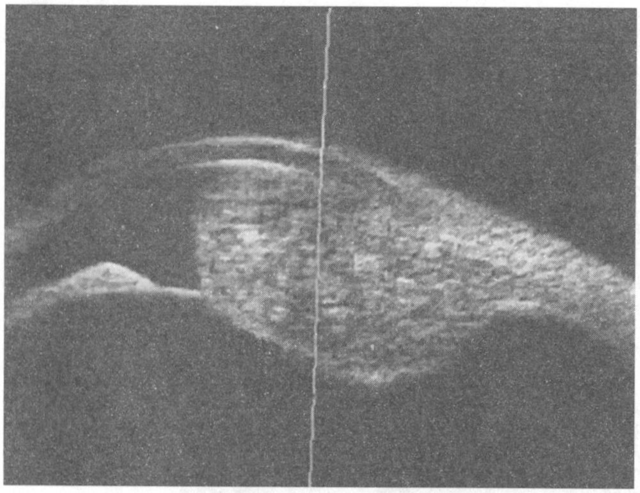

Fig. 3: Ultrasound biomicroscopy showing mass lesion arising from the ciliary body involving the iris and angle.

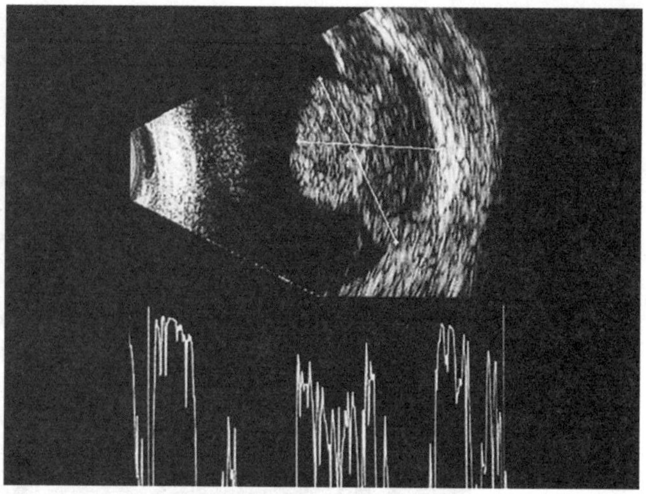

Fig. 4: Ciliary body medulloepithelioma. B-scan shows a mass filling the anterior vitreous cavity with medium to high internal reflectivity with overlying retinal detachment.

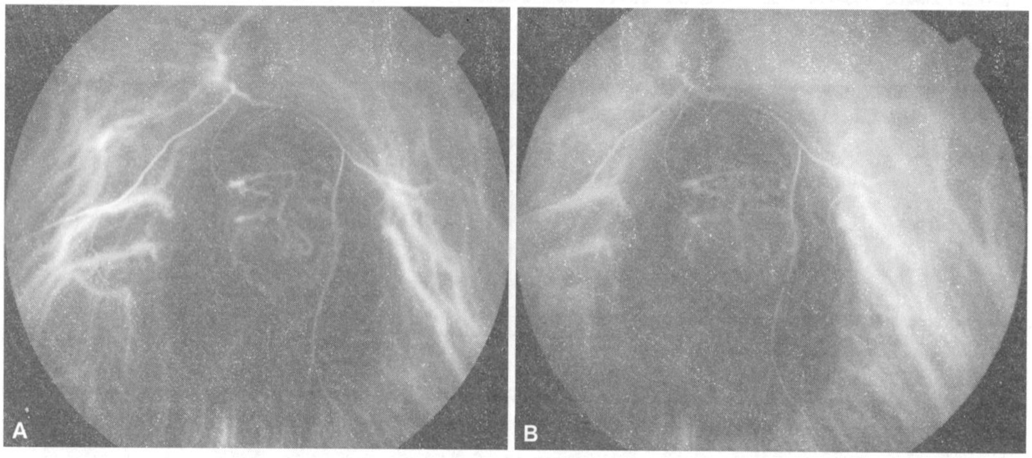

Figs. 5A and B: ICG-angiography showing intrinsic choroidal vasculature in choroidal melanoma.

disruption shows mottled hyperfluorescence in arterial phase signifying filling of tumor vessels of choroidal origin. Hyperfluorescence intensifies in the early venous phase and assumes patchy configuration with fuzzy margins due to leakage and overlying orange pigment appears hypofluorescent. Late frames show diffuse staining of the tumor and associated subretinal fluid. A mushroom-shaped melanoma that has broken through the Bruch's membrane with choroidal veins shows characteristic "double circulation" during the later arterial or early venous phase, exhibiting simultaneous fluorescence of the choroidal and retinal vasculature.[8] ICG angiography in choroidal melanoma demonstrates intrinsic choroidal vasculature **(Figs. 5A and B)**. These changes become evident in the early phase as variable caliber, irregular, randomly branching, ramifying vessels with small twig vessels arising from the main vessels and staining of vessel walls in the intermediate phase and leakage in the late phase. A mushroom-shaped choroidal melanoma shows markedly dilated tumor vessels at the apex. Hyperintensity due to choroidal vasculature may be variably masked by tumor pigmentation and tumor surface alterations.

While FFA features may not be diagnostic of circumscribed choroidal hemangiomas, ICG angiography is very characteristic in the sequence of events in various phases[9] **(Figs. 6 to 9)**. In the early phase, a network of branching, lacy, small caliber, intratumoral vessels is distinctly visualized on a hypofluorescent tumor background obscuring the normal choroidal vasculature. In the venous phase, the tumor shows heterogeneous but brilliant hyperintensity due to filling up of vascular spaces, assuming the typical mulberry pattern. Late phase shows characteristic washout, leaving the tumor hypointense in contrast to surrounding hyperintensity. Washout phenomenon is attributed to low-resistance, high-flow property of the tumor that allows emptying of the dye sooner than the surrounding normal choroid.[9]

In retinal capillary hemangioma (RCH), FFA shows rapid tumor filling and fine intrinsic vasculature in the arterial phase and helps to identify the feeder vessel. In the venous

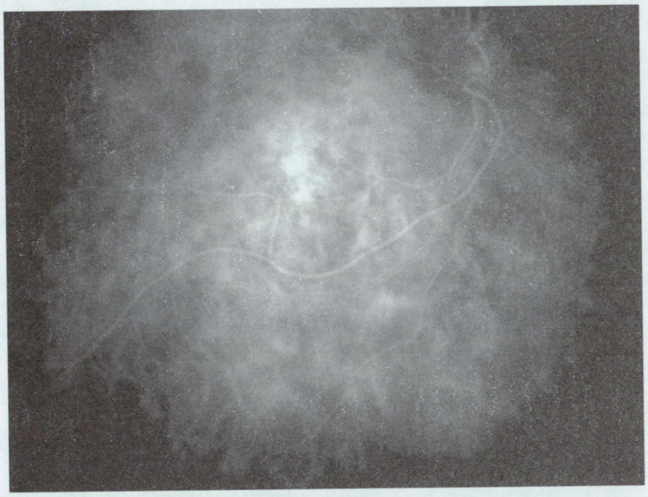

Fig. 6: Early phase shows reticular vascular pattern on hypofluorescent tumor background.

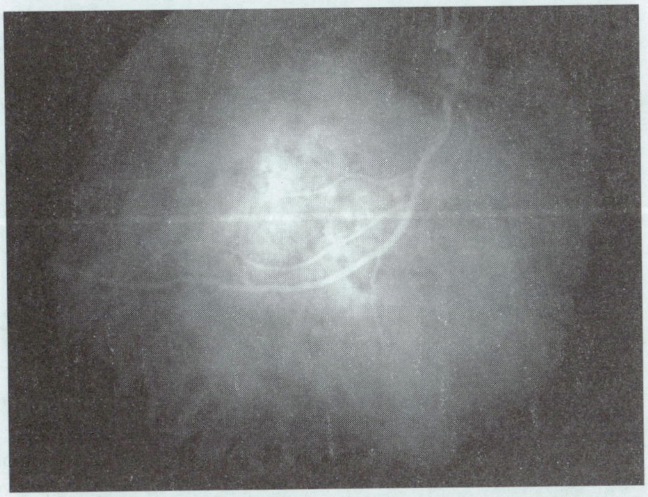

Fig. 7: Venous phase shows typical mulberry pattern.

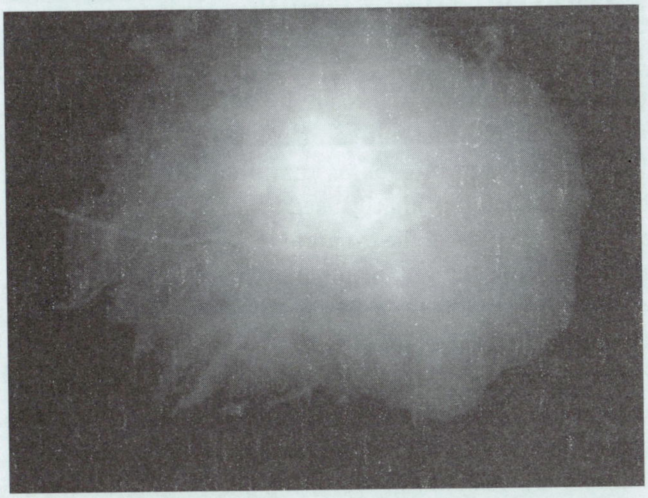

Fig. 8: Hyperintensity of the lesion due to filling of intratumoral vascular spaces.

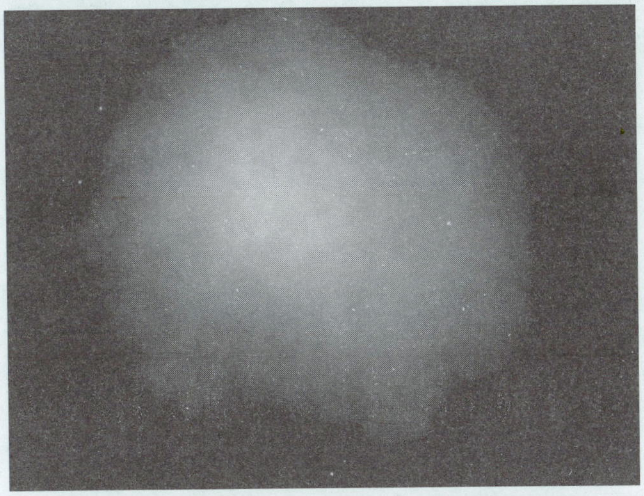

Fig. 9: Late phase shows washout of dye from tumor.

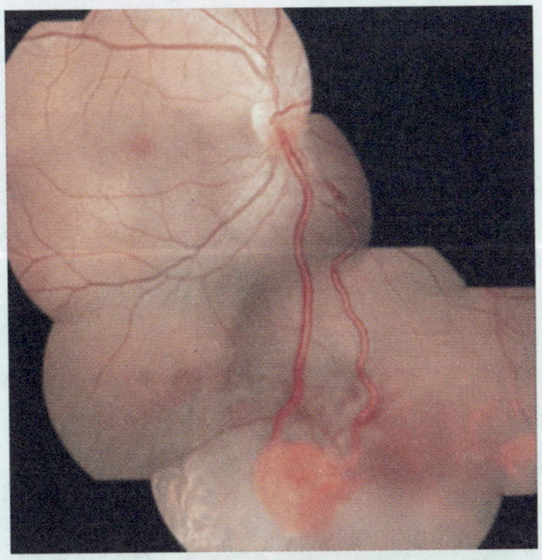

Fig. 10: Montage picture showing peripheral retinal capillary hemangioma with feeder and draining vessel.

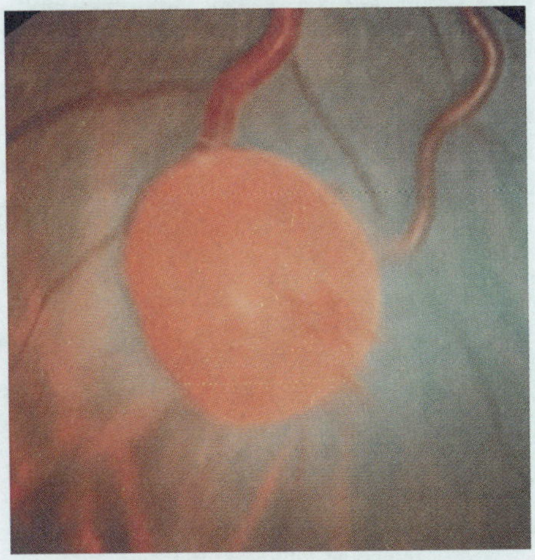

Fig. 11: *Retinal capillary hemangioma*: Orange red lesion arising from retina obscuring the choroidal vasculature with a feeding and a draining vessel.

phase, the tumor shows intense hyperfluorescence as the dye leaks from the intrinsic tumor vessels **(Figs. 10 to 14)**. Leakage continues into the overlying vitreous in late phase.[10] ICGA has no specific advantage over FFA in RCH.

Although FFA or ICGA is not routinely used for diagnosis of retinoblastoma, FFA has been found to be particularly useful to detect subtle residual tumor following treatment or subclinical tumor recurrence. While slight dilation of

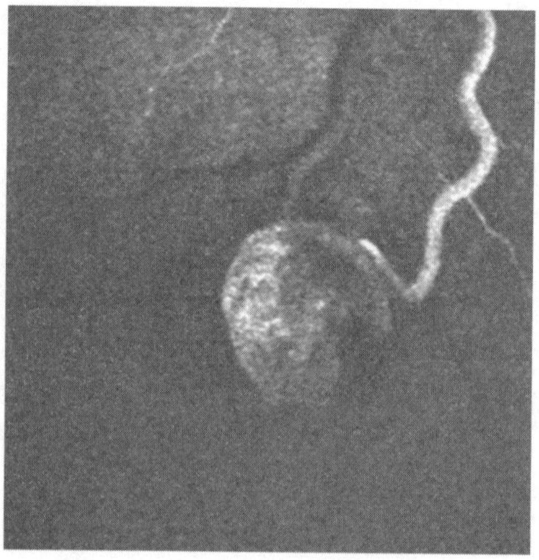

Fig. 12: Arterial phase delineating the feeder vessel.

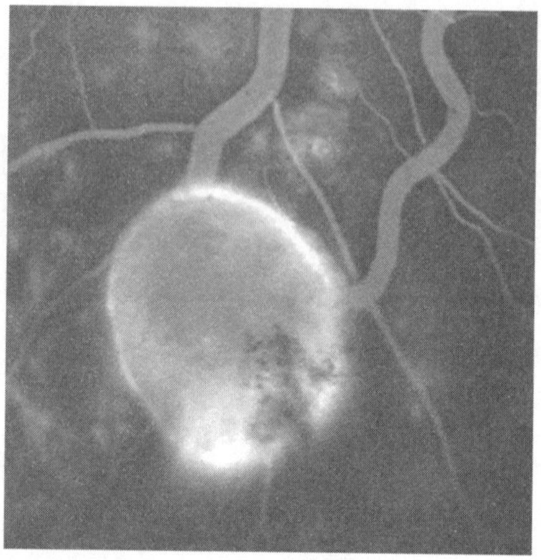

Fig. 14: Late phase showing staining of capsule with pigmentary changes on the surface.

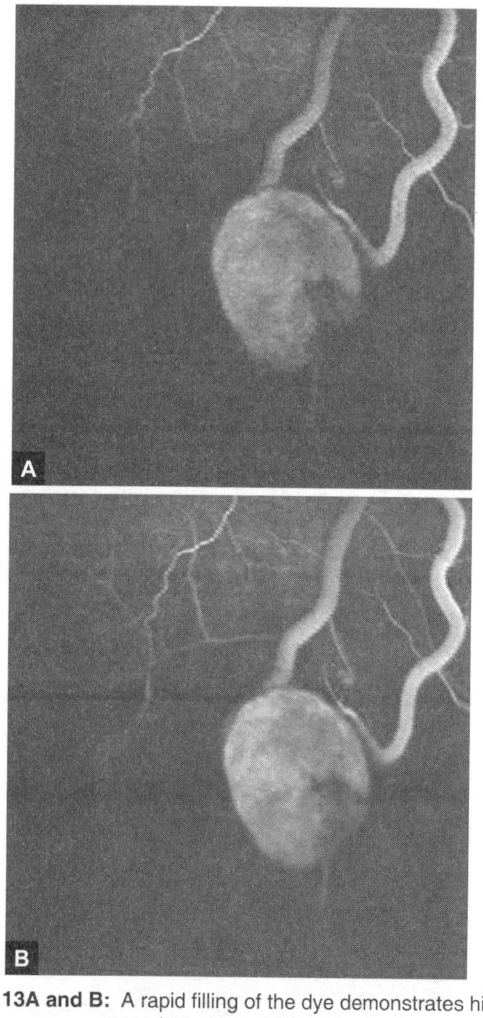

Figs. 13A and B: A rapid filling of the dye demonstrates highly vascular nature of the lesion.

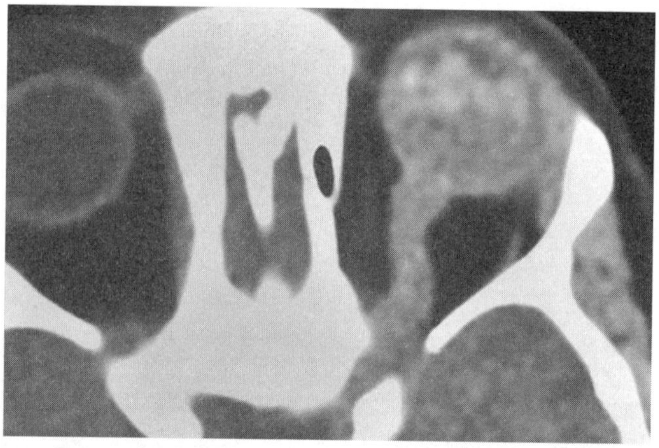

Fig. 15: CT scan—coronal section shows calcification in intraocular tumor, suggestive of retinoblastoma. Optic nerve is grossly thickened suggestive of optic nerve invasion by the tumor.

the retinal capillaries is the only significant FFA finding in a small tumor, microaneurysms become distinct in a larger tumor. As the growth of the tumor progresses, blood vessels within the tumor become thicker and permeability increases and eventually neovascularization occurs.

COMPUTED TOMOGRAPHY

Computed tomography is of limited value in diagnosis of intraocular tumors but is of immense help in the event of extraocular spread. It can demonstrate calcification in intraocular tumors such as retinoblastoma or choroidal osteoma, it is not primarily used for diagnosis. Calcification varies in each case, for example in retinoblastoma, it is in the form of specks or conglomerates in contrast to choroidal osteoma where it is like a plaque with heterogeneous areas. However, computed tomography is useful for tumors with orbital cellulitis or extraocular extension, e.g. retinoblastoma with optic nerve or intracranial extension **(Fig. 15)**, trilateral retinoblastoma or orbital masses secondary to intraocular tumors. CT scans are helpful for planning radiotherapy. Positron emission tomography (PET-CT) scans are very useful for systemic metastasis survey **(Fig. 16)**.

MAGNETIC RESONANCE IMAGING

Magnetic resonance imaging (MRI) is helpful in selected situations when dealing with intraocular tumors. Based on

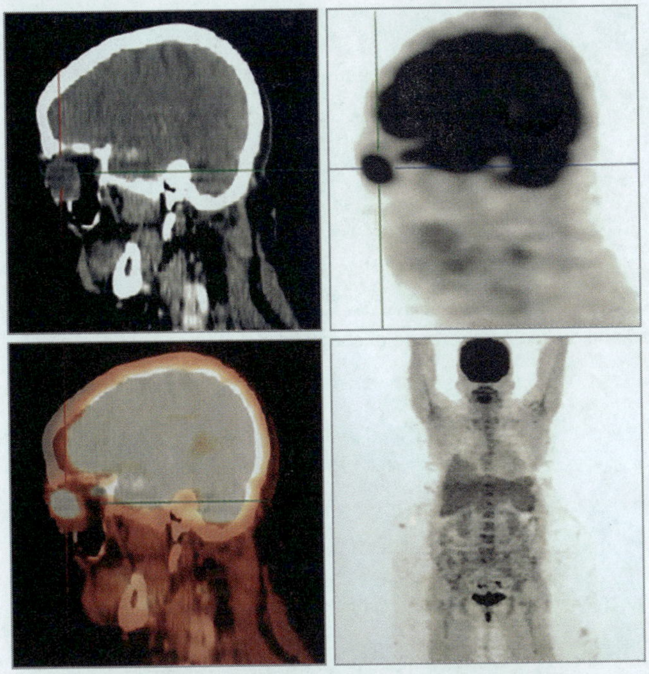

Fig. 16: Positron emission tomography scan for systemic metastatic survey.

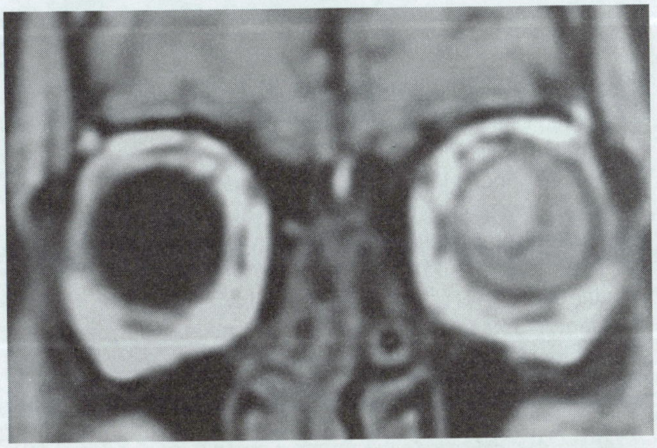

Fig. 17: *T1-weighted coronal MRI of brain and orbits*: Vitreous appears dark while orbital fat is bright, left eye shows a hyperintense mass lesion.

the behavior of hydrogen atoms, signals are classified as T1 and T2 which are further described as hyper or hypointense with respect to vitreous. In T1-weighted images, vitreous is dark whereas the orbital fat is bright and acts as a contrast **(Fig. 17)**. In T2-weighted images, the vitreous is bright **(Fig. 18)**. Most of the tumors are hypointense on T1 and hyperintense on T2 with the exception of melanomas, which are hyperintense on T1 and hypointense on T2[11] **(Figs. 19 to 21)**. MRI is also useful in studying the optic nerve or intracranial extensions in retinoblastoma as well as detecting a pinealoblastoma **(Fig. 22)**.

FINE-NEEDLE ASPIRATION BIOPSY/ CYTOLOGY

Fine-needle aspiration biopsy or cytology (FNAB/FNAC) is not a new technique. It is occasionally used to obtain

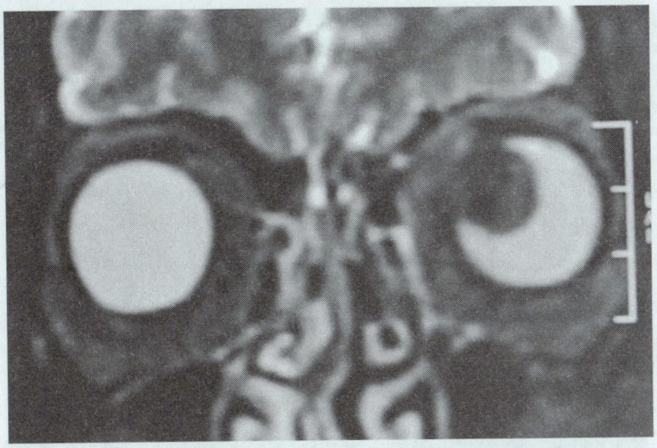

Fig. 18: T2-weighted image of same patient. Vitreous appears bright and fat appears dark. The mass lesion is now hypointense.

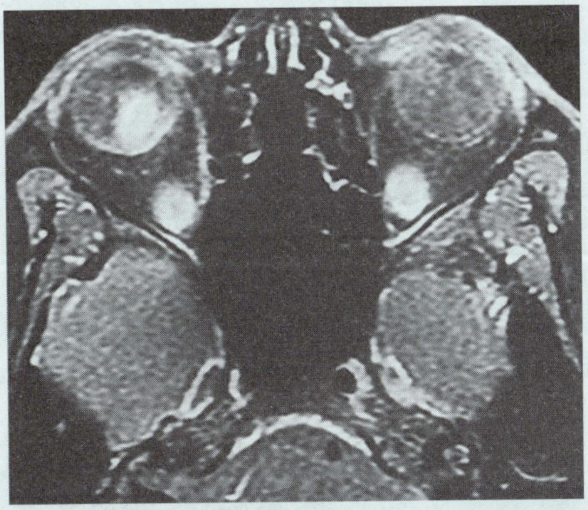

Fig. 19: T1-weighted MRI image showing intraocular tumor. Hyperintensity on T1 is suggestive of choroidal melanoma.

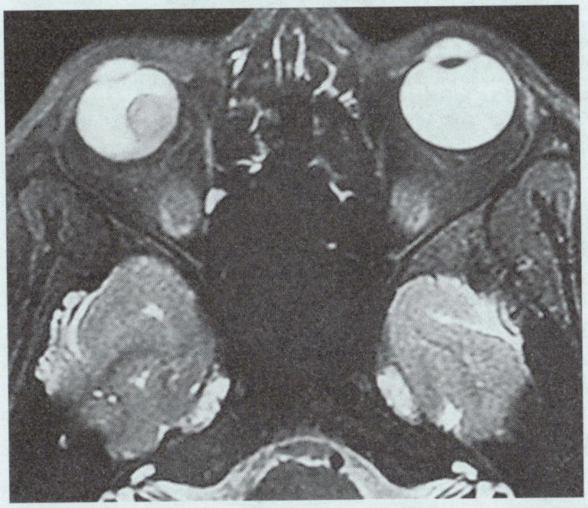

Fig. 20: Same lesion on T2-weighted image becomes hypointense.

cellular aspirates for analysis, where diagnosis becomes a dilemma.[12] FNAC has been used for both choroidal as well as retinal tumors with diagnostic difficulties. Common tumors where it has been employed include amelanotic choroidal lesions such as choroidal granulomas, lymphoma, amelanotic melanoma, schwannoma, etc. It has also been

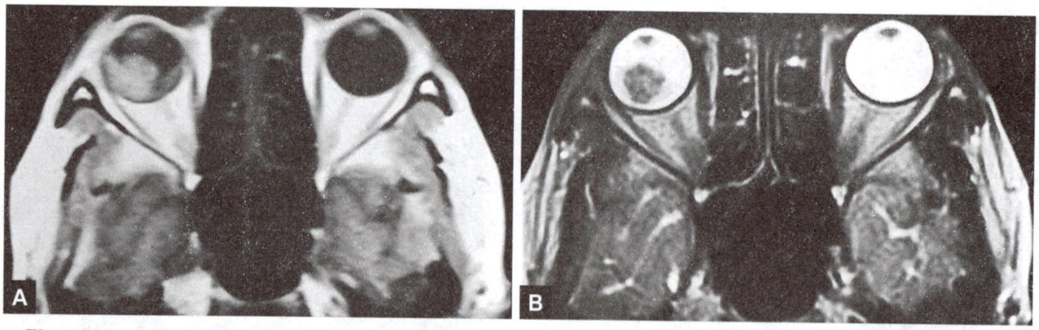

Figs. 21A and B: T1- and T2-weighted axial MRI of head and orbit in another case of choroidal melanoma.

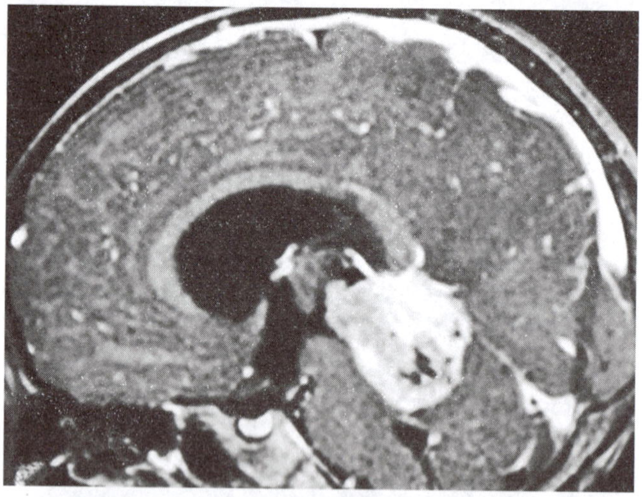

Fig. 22: MRI of brain, sagittal section shows a large pinealoblastoma.

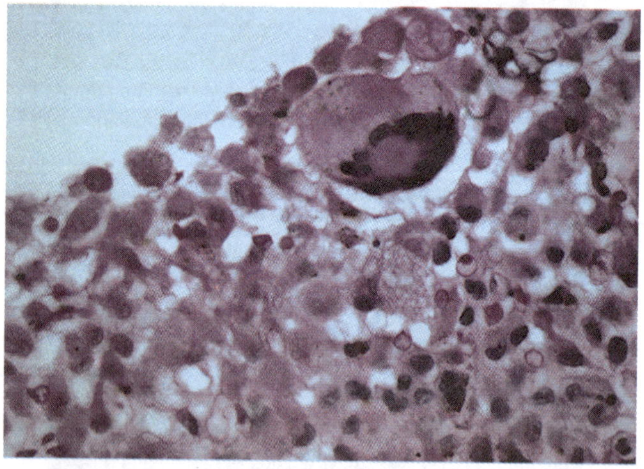

Fig. 23: *Juvenile xanthogranuloma*: Fine-needle aspiration cytology reveals cellular smears with foamy histiocytes and the typical multinucleated giant cells or Touton cells (H and E × 400).

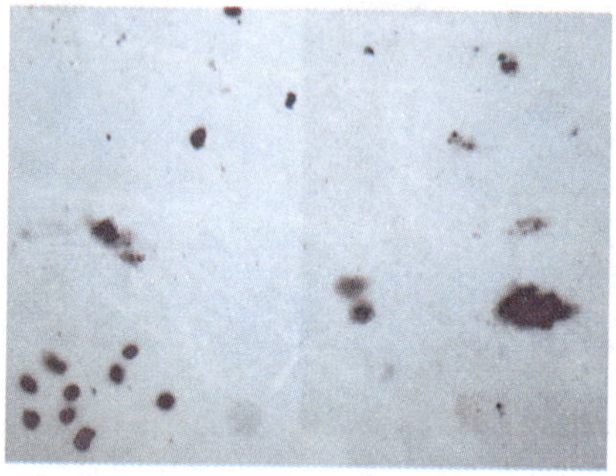

Fig. 24: *Medulloepithelioma*: Cytospin smear is highly cellular with small round cells seen singly or in clumps (H and E × 100).

Box 3: Indications for fine needle aspiration cytology.

- Major diagnostic uncertainty when there is discrepancy between clinical and noninvasive tests or discrepancy among the noninvasive tests
- An amelanotic fundus lesion in an immunosuppressed patient with diagnostic dilemma to differentiate neoplasm from opportunistic infections
- Leukocoria in a child if there is diagnostic predicament but retinoblastoma is not a strong possibility
- Patient refuses treatment until establishment of diagnosis pathologically

Box 4: Contraindications for fine-needle aspiration cytology.

- When the diagnosis is reasonably certain based on clinical and noninvasive diagnostic studies
- Diagnostic dilemma where retinoblastoma is a strong suspicion
- The procedure entails major morbidity or worsening of the outcomes

employed, but less commonly, for pigmented uveal lesions like melanoma and melanocytomas, juvenile xanthogranuloma **(Fig. 23)** and medulloepitheliomas **(Fig. 24)**.[12]

It is of utmost importance to emphasize here that FNAC should not be performed on all patients who are suspected of having retinal tumors. It is recommended only in selected cases where there is a true diagnostic dilemma.[12] In the largest published clinical experience by Shields et al., only 2.5% of the 6,500 cases of suspected intraocular tumors required FNAC because in the remaining cases, the diagnosis was reasonably certain based on the clinical features and routine noninvasive diagnostic studies.[12] Based on clinical research studies and review of literature,[12-14] indications for FNAC are tabulated in **Box 3**, and contraindications in **Box 4**. FNAC should not be seen as shortcut to diagnosis. Misuse of the modality is often seen in the diagnosis of retinoblastoma, therefore, needs elaboration.

FNAC in Retinoblastoma

Retinoblastoma is the most common intraocular malignancy of childhood and the diagnosis is usually made by observing its classical clinical features using indirect ophthalmoscopy and slit-lamp biomicroscopy aided by ultrasonography, fluorescein angiography, CT, and MRI as appropriate. FNAC in cases of retinoblastoma or suspected retinoblastoma is now generally considered to be a strong contraindication.[12-14] The risk of seeding of the tumor outside the eye is of special concern. Adhesiveness is a property of cells that allows a tissue to resist separation. Retinoblastoma is less cohesive due to large areas of necrosis within the tumor. The current understanding is that owing to poorly cohesive nature of the tumor, there is a significant possibility of dissemination of neoplastic cells through the needle track. Karcioglu et al.[15] in a well-controlled study investigated the occurrence of tumor cell seeding in needle tracks following 25-gauge FNAC. The biopsies were done immediately after enucleation and the needle-tracks from pars plana region were serially sectioned for histological examination. Clusters of tumor cells were seen in 6 of the 11 needle tracks lending support to the hypothetical risk of tumor seeding and dissemination. Such tumor seeding has also been shown in animal experiments,[16] however, it is difficult to extrapolate it to humans. Apart from the dreaded complication of tumor seeding, other possible complications such as vitreous hemorrhage can further preclude tumor assessment.[12-14]

The only possible scope for FNAC currently is in highly exceptional situations[13] of extreme diagnostic dilemma, where retinoblastoma is a consideration. If it is done in such cases, it should be performed by a modified technique.[13] Here the needle is passed parallel to the visual axis through the peripheral cornea, anterior chamber, peripheral iris, zonules (avoiding the lens), and into the suspicious area. This technique allows ocular buffer zones to prevent extraocular tumor spread, should the condition prove to be a retinoblastoma.[6]

REFERENCES

1. Damato B. Ocular tumors. Examination techniques. In: Damato B (Ed). Ocular tumors: diagnosis and treatment. Edinburgh: Butterworth-Heinemann; 2000. pp. 3-17.
2. Byrne SF, Green RL. Intraocular tumors. In: Byrne SF, Green RL (Eds). Ultrasound of the Eye and Orbit, 2nd edition. St Louis: Mosby; 2002. pp. 1-188.
3. Cusumano A, Coleman DJ, Silverman RH, et al. Three-dimensional ultrasound imaging: clinical applications. Ophthalmology. 1998;105:300-6.
4. Finger PT, Romero JM, Rosen RB, et al. Three dimensional ultrasonography of choroidal melanoma: localization of radioactive eye plaques. Arch Ophthalmol. 1998;116:305-12.
5. Rabb MF, Burton TC, Schatz H, et al. Fluorescein angiography of the fundus: a schematic approach to interpretation. Surv Ophthalmol. 1978;22:387-403.
6. Meyer K, Augsburger JJ. Independent diagnostic value of fluorescein angiography in the evaluation of intraocular tumors. Graefes Arch Clin Exp Ophthalmol. 1999;237: 489-94.
7. Shields CL, Shields JA, De Potter P. Patterns of indocyanine green videoangiography of choroidal tumours. Br J Ophthalmol. 1995;79:237-45.
8. Augsburger JJ, Golden MI, Shields JA. Fluorescein angiography of choroidal malignant melanomas with retinal invasion. Retina. 1984;4(4):232-41.
9. Schalenbourg A, Piguet B, Zografos L. Indocyanine green angiographic findings in choroidal hemangiomas: a study of 75 cases. Ophthalmologica. 2000;214:246-52.
10. Singh AD, Rundle PA, Rennie I. Retinal vascular tumors. Ophthalmol Clin North Am. 2005;18:167-76.
11. De Potter P, Shields JA, Shields CL. MRI of the Eye and Orbit. Philadelphia: JB Lippincott; 1995.
12. Ali MJ, Honavar SG, Vemuganti GK, et al. Fine needle aspiration biopsy of retinal tumors. Monograph Clin Cytol. 2012;21: 72-81.
13. Shields JA, Shields CL, Ehya H, et al. Fine needle aspiration biopsy of suspected intraocular tumors. The 1992 Urwick Lecture. Ophthalmology. 1993;100:1677-84.
14. Eide N, Walaas L. Fine needle aspiration biopsy and other biopsies in suspected intraocular malignant disease: a review. Acta Ophthalmol. 2009;83:588-601.
15. Karcioglu ZA, Gordon RA, Karcioglu GL. Tumor seeding in ocular fine needle aspiration biopsy. Ophthalmology. 1985;92:1763-7.
16. Ryd W, Hagmar B, Eriksson O. Local tumor cell seeding by fine needle aspiration biopsy: a semiquantitative study. Acta Pathol Microbiol Immunol Scan. 1983;91:17-21.

CHAPTER

37 Pupil

Navin Jayakumar

INTRODUCTION

The pupil controls retinal illumination to maximize visual perception. The dilator muscle causes pupil enlargement in dim illumination. This increases the amount of incoming light to supplement the retinal dark-adaptive mechanisms. In bright surroundings the sphincter muscle can reduce retinal illumination by as much as 1.5 log units. The pupil also controls the depth of focus of the eye (by constriction) and reduces optical aberrations.

This chapter is divided into three parts in which relevant functional anatomy of the pupil, a step-by-step method of clinical examination of the pupil, and common disorders involving the pupil are described.

FUNCTIONAL ANATOMY AND PHYSIOLOGY OF THE PUPIL REFLEXES

PUPIL LIGHT REFLEX

The pupil light reflex consists of three components **(Fig. 1)**.[1]

1. The afferent arc originates in the eye and comprises the optic nerve, optic chiasm, and anterior two-thirds of the optic tract (the lateral geniculate nucleus does not play a role in the arc).
2. The interneuron in the midbrain is the pretectal olivary nucleus.
3. The efferent arc originates in the Edinger–Westphal subnucleus of the oculomotor nuclear complex, and continues along the oculomotor nerve to the ciliary ganglion, and then along the short ciliary nerves to the pupillary sphincter muscle.

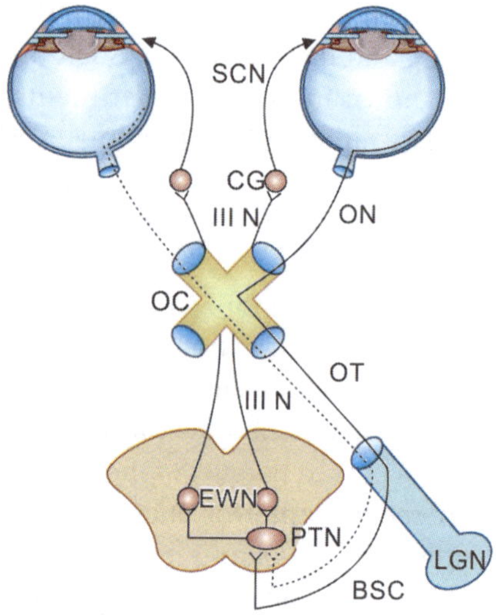

Fig. 1: The pupil light reflex pathway.
(III N: oculomotor nerve; BSC: brachium of superior colliculus; CG: ciliary ganglion; EWN: Edinger-Westphal subnucleus of oculomotor nucleus complex; LGN: lateral geniculate nucleus; OC: optic chiasm; ON: optic nerve; OT: optic tract; PTN: pretectal nucleus; SCN: short ciliary nerves)

The Afferent Arc

Photoreceptors

Both rods and cones contribute to the pupil light reflex. Under scotopic conditions, rods are far more sensitive to cones in eliciting a pupil contraction. In photopic conditions, the contribution of the cones to the pupil contraction is far more than rods. Pupil perimetry shows that the strength of pupil contraction is greatest when the central field is stimulated (where the photoreceptor and bipolar cell density is highest) and drops as the stimulus moves to the periphery.

Ganglion Cells

The retinal ganglion cells are the first neurons that give rise to action potentials that travel along their axons in the optic nerve and chiasm to cells in the lateral geniculate body and pretectal nuclei. Cells serving the afferent pupillomotor arc are most dense in the central retina. The major contribution to the pretectal olivary nucleus is from the γ ganglion cells (α- and β-cells project primarily to the lateral geniculate nucleus). The γ-cells have now been identified as the melanopsin-containing ganglion cells that play a role in other visually evoked reflexes such as the circadian rhythm.[2]

Melanopsin-containing ganglion cells are unique in that they can also be directly activated by light. Their photoreceptor-independent stimulation may explain why the pupil light reflex may be intact in patients with extensive photoreceptor damage or complete noncerebral monocular blindness. Studies comparing visual field defects with pupil perimetry (mapping of pupil sensitivity to light across the visual field) shows excellent correlation in certain diseases (e.g. anterior ischemic optic neuropathy) but large differences in other optic neuropathies (e.g. optic neuritis) where the visual field defect may be small but the defects in the "pupil field" are large.[3,4] These examples suggest that there may be relatively separate pathways for visual perception and pupillary response to light.

The Interneuron

The pretectal olivary nucleus lies in the midbrain dorsolateral to the oculomotor nuclear complex. It is the interneuron of the pupil light reflex. It receives inputs from the pupillomotor ganglion cells of the ipsilateral temporal retina and the contralateral nasal retina (via the hemidecussation in the chiasm). These fibers leave the optic tract before its culmination in the lateral geniculate nucleus and enter the midbrain via the brachium of the superior colliculus.[5] The pupillomotor output from each pretectal olivary nucleus is distributed equally to the Edinger–Westphal nuclei of both sides to produce a pupil contraction of equal amplitude.

The contralateral homonymous hemifield organization of the afferent arc explains the finding of a contralateral relative afferent pupillary defect (RAPD) in an optic tract lesion.[6] This is because the intact ipsilateral temporal field (projecting along the uninvolved contralateral optic tract) provides greater pupillomotor input owing to larger retinal area being stimulated, than the intact nasal field of the contralateral eye.

Rarely, unilateral lesions of the brachium of the superior colliculus cause a "tectal RAPD" where pupillary response to stimulation of the contralateral hemifields is affected without contralateral homonymous hemianopia as would occur if the lesion were situated in the optic tract.[5,7]

The Efferent Arc

Axons of cell bodies within the Edinger-Westphal subnucleus travel along the oculomotor nerve to synapse with the neurons in the ciliary ganglion in the orbit. The postganglionic fibers travel along with short ciliary nerves to innervate the sphincter muscle of the pupil.

Parasympathetic Oculomotor Nuclei

These subnuclei of the oculomotor nuclear complex contain cell bodies of preganglionic parasympathetic neurons that project to the ciliary ganglion and control pupil contraction to light and accommodation. Located in the dorsal midbrain they are the Edinger-Westphal nuclei, the anterior median nuclei, and the nucleus of Perlia. The Edinger-Westphal nuclei are responsible for the pupil contraction to light, while the anterior median nuclei are the primary neurons involved in producing accommodation response.

Oculomotor Nerve

The pupillomotor fibers are located superficially in the oculomotor nerve. This explains why the light reflex is "spared" in ischemic oculomotor nerve palsies, but "involved" in compressive etiologies such as aneurysms. The pupillomotor fibers are concentrated in the medial superior aspect of the oculomotor nerve as it leaves the brainstem and then gradually move medially and inferiorly as the nerve approaches the cavernous sinus.[8] These fibers are close to the posterior communicating artery. Aneurysms of this vessel compress the medial and superior aspect of the oculomotor nerve in the subarachnoid space causing a "pupil involved" oculomotor nerve palsy.

Ciliary Ganglion

The ciliary ganglion lies in the orbit 1.5–2 cm behind the globe between the optic nerve and the lateral rectus muscle, and in close association with the inferior division of the oculomotor nerve. The cell bodies are parasympathetic. Only 3% of the axons of these cell bodies project to the pupil sphincter whereas over 94% reach the ciliary muscle.[9] This correlates with the relative masses of the two muscles. Thus over 90% of the midbrain parasympathetic outflow is concerned with accommodation and not with pupil contraction.

Short Ciliary Nerves

Eight to twenty short ciliary nerves leave the ciliary ganglion in two to three bundles. Apart from postganglionic parasympathetic fibers destined for the ciliary muscle and pupil sphincter, these nerves also contain postganglionic sympathetic vasomotor fibers from the superior cervical ganglion and sensory afferents of the trigeminal nerve. The sympathetic and sensory roots to the ciliary ganglion do not synapse with its parasympathetic cell bodies. The short ciliary nerves enter the sclera at the posterior pole of the globe temporal to the optic nerve. They run anteriorly through the sclera and then in the suprachoroidal space.

THE DARK REFLEX

The pupil dilates in dim illumination and darkness. This reflex dilation is bilateral and follows a latency period that is slightly longer (about 300 ms) than the latency of the pupil light reflex. The dark reflex is mediated by the oculosympathetic pathway **(Fig. 2)**. The ocular sympathetic outflow originates at the hypothalamus and through a three-neuron pathway innervates the pupillary dilator muscle and vasomotor supply to the eye.

THE SYMPATHETIC OUTFLOW PATHWAY

First-order Neurons

The first-order neuron originates in the posterolateral hypothalamus. The axons descend in the brainstem and anterolateral columns of the spinal cord to synapse with the cell bodies of neurons of the ciliospinal center of Budge and Waller at C8 to T2 spinal cord segments.

Second-order Neurons (Preganglionic)

The cell bodies of these preganglionic neurons lie in the ciliospinal center of Budge and Waller. Their axons exit the spinal cord via the ventral root to enter the paravertebral sympathetic chain. Here they pass without synapsing through the first thoracic (or stellate) ganglion close to the pleura at the apex of the lung. The fibers proceed uninterrupted through the inferior and middle cervical ganglia to terminate by synapsing with the postganglionic neurons in the superior cervical ganglion which is located below the base of the skull between the internal jugular vein and internal carotid artery.

Two sets of branches exit from the superior cervical ganglion. The first communicates with C1 to C4 segments of the spinal cord and cranial nerves IX, X, and XII. The second set innervates the pharynx, the heart, and the sympathetic effectors in the head. This close relationship between the superior cervical ganglion and the lower cranial nerves explains their concurrent involvement in base of skull pathologies that produce a Horner's syndrome and lower cranial nerve palsies.

Third-order Neurons (Postganglionic)

The postganglionic fibers from the superior cervical ganglion accompany the internal carotid artery as a plexus surrounding the vessel. Almost immediately sudomotor and piloerector fibers destined for the face exit this plexus and follow the external carotid artery to the skin. The remaining fibers accompany the internal carotid artery intracranially through the foramen lacerum. In the cavernous sinus the oculosympathetic fibers transiently fuse with the abducens nerve before joining the ophthalmic division of the trigeminal nerve.[10] The fibers then enter the orbit with the nasociliary nerve.

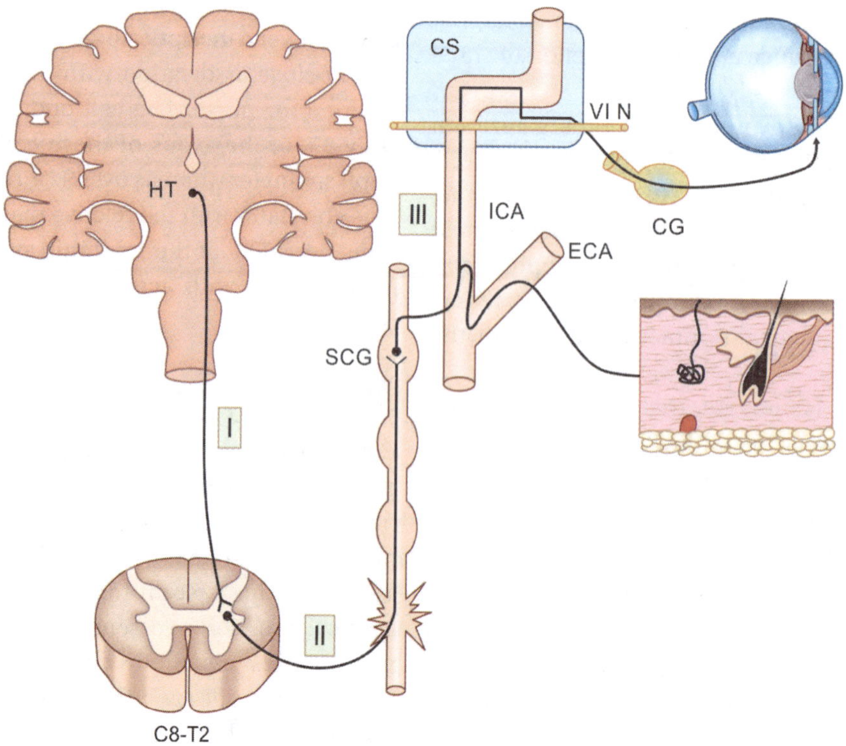

Fig. 2: The oculosympathetic pathway. I—first order neuron; C8-T2—spinal cord segments; II—second order neuron; III—third order neuron; VI N—abducens nerve. (CG: ciliary ganglion; CS: cavernous sinus; ECA: external carotid artery; HT: hypothalamus; ICA: internal carotid artery; SCG: superior cervical ganglion of the sympathetic chain)

Besides the pupil dilator muscle, other parts of the eye also receive postganglionic sympathetic innervation. These include vasomotor fibers to the orbit, fibers to the branched melanocytes of the uveal tract, fibers to the extraocular muscles, the Muller's muscle, lacrimal gland, and the retinal pigment epithelium.

Innervation of the pupil dilator muscle occurs through the long ciliary nerves that bypass the ciliary ganglion. Some sympathetic fibers enter the ciliary ganglion, but exit it without synapsing along with the short ciliary nerves. The long and short ciliary nerves pass anteriorly and blend to form a rich plexus from which the iris muscles, ciliary muscle, and the vessel walls are supplied.

THE NEAR RESPONSE

When fixation shifts from far to near, three interrelated yet distinct responses are observed: (1) the pupils contract, (2) the lens accommodates (becomes more convex), and (3) the eyes converge. This triad is described as the near response. It is not described as a near reflex because although the three occur virtually simultaneously it can be shown experimentally that each component can be selectively abolished or elicited without affecting the other two.[11]

The pupil light reflex and the near response miosis share a common final pathway from the Edinger-Westphal nucleus, along the oculomotor nerve, to the pupil sphincter muscle. The supranuclear pathways; however, are different. Visual stimuli (near-induced blur and temporal displacement of fixation on the retina) reach the visual cortex. From here impulses travel to the frontal eye fields and thereon to the Edinger-Westphal nuclei in the midbrain (causing pupil constriction and lens accommodation) and to both medial recti subnuclei (producing convergence). In the Edinger-Westphal nucleus, the cells associated with the accommodation reflex are situated more ventral to those serving the pupil response to near. This arrangement explains how dorsal midbrain lesions produce "light-near dissociation" where the light reflex is impaired but the pupil constriction to near is uninvolved.

PRINCIPLES AND TECHNIQUES OF PUPIL EXAMINATION

HISTORY

Most patients with pupillary abnormalities are unaware of it. A useful way to evaluate the duration of an abnormality in pupil size or shape is to take a magnified look the pupils in photographs of the individual taken over time. This useful method is sometimes humorously described as "family album tomography" or "FAT scanning".

Symptoms associated with pupil size and shape abnormalities include photophobia, blurring of vision, and difficulty focusing when moving between environments with very different illumination levels. A large pupil causes blur in bright environments while a small pupil causes images to look relatively dim compared to the normal eye.

PUPIL SIZE

"Are the pupils equal in size? If not, is the difference greater in darkness or in light?" This is the first question to answer in the examination of the pupil. Pupil size can be examined by simple clinical examination using a pupil gauge. A pupil gauge is a simple handheld card (as a strip or a circle) that contains a series of solid circles or semicircles of diameters that increase in 0.5 mm steps. The gauge is placed adjacent to the pupil to estimate which circle (or semicircle) size best matches the patient's pupil size.

More sophisticated instruments such as a handheld pupil camera or infrared pupillography are also used.[12,13] An infrared pupillometer allows pupil observation even in complete darkness. The iris sphincter can be transilluminated to show areas of denervation or renervation.[14] Computer-based infrared video pupillography is increasingly used clinically to study pupil related phenomena. They are used to measure pupil diameter in the planning of refractive surgical procedures, distinguish Horner's syndrome from physiological anisocoria, quantify RAPD, and for pupil perimetry.[15]

Slit-lamp biomicroscopy of the anterior segment also provides useful clues. Anterior uveitis (miotic pupil), corneal edema, and angle closure might (mid-dilated oval pupil), iris transillumination, and areas of atrophy (post-trauma) are some examples. Segmental pupil contraction (Adie's pupil or oculomotor nerve palsy) can be visualized by turning off and on the slit-lamp beam. The magnification that a slit lamp provides can be used to detect a subtle RAPD. With the patient seated at a slit lamp and the slit illumination turned off, the swinging-flashlight test is performed using a transilluminator light is swung back and forth between the eyes. The direct pupil light response and the consensual light response can be observed under slit-lamp magnification.[16]

Pupil Size Measurement

Measure and record pupil size (in mm) in both eyes: (1) In bright illumination; (2) In dim illumination; and (3) For near by using an accommodative target.

Use a scale or preferably a pupil gauge to determine pupil size. The illumination should be equal in both eyes.

It is difficult to see the pupils in dim illumination, especially in a dark iris. For practical purposes a "dim" torch or any minimal illumination is useful to visualize the pupil, for evaluation of pupil size in dim illumination in dark irides. The illumination must be just enough to allow visualization of the pupil edge.[17] Allow the illumination to fall evenly on both eyes at the same time, during measurement.

Anisocoria

Perceptible difference in pupil size between the two eyes is termed anisocoria: a difference of at least 0.4 mm between the two eyes. It is present in approximately 20% of young adults, with the prevalence increasing to 33% in the elderly.[18]

Physiological anisocoria is asymptomatic and both pupils constrict briskly to bright light and near stimulation, and dilate briskly in dim illumination. Equality of responses seen on testing for reflexes is a good indicator of "normal" pupils whatever their size.

DIRECT LIGHT REFLEX

When bright light stimulates one eye, both pupils constrict. The constriction in the ipsilateral eye is called the direct reflex while that in the opposite eye is called the consensual reflex. Provided there is no lesion in the autonomic pathways, the direct and consensual reflexes are clinically of equal magnitude.

Equipment

A good bright uniform light source is required. This is usually a pen torch or an indirect ophthalmoscope with the illumination turned to maximum. Clinically, the ideal instrument is an illuminator fitted to a direct ophthalmoscope handpiece. The light stimulus should be adequately bright. A very bright light [as seen in some light-emitting diode (LED) torches] causes discomfort. It may produce spastic miosis lasting several seconds and will make determination of the normal light reflex difficult or impossible.[19] Blinking and tearing with glaring illumination make pupil evaluation difficult. A weak light source produces a correspondingly weak pupil constriction that can be misinterpreted as being sluggish because pupil escape may occur under these conditions. Some torches have patchy uneven illumination. Do not use such torches with "central scotomas" as they may cause variable constriction of the pupils that can be misinterpreted.

Method

Keep room as dim as possible. Ask patient to look at a distant target (e.g. fixation target in mirror). Swing a bright light source in a quick motion onto the eye. Keep the eye illuminated for at least 3–4 seconds to observe events after the initial constriction. The direction of illumination should be from below and slightly temporal. This keeps the corneal images of the light source (first and second Purkinje images) outside the pupillary area allowing a good visualization the entire pupil. Keeping a light source directly in front of the eye will stimulate the near reflex that will produce a pupil constriction. Observing pupil constriction by slit-lamp biomicroscopy is not the correct method of evaluating the direct reflex.

Observation

Record the two aspects of the reaction of the pupil: (1) Speed of reaction, "brisk or sluggish?" and (2) Sustaining of pupil constriction on continued illumination, "well-sustained or ill-sustained?".

The initial pupil constriction to bright light is called "pupil capture" (or phasic response).[20] Pupillary escape is an abnormal response where the pupil after initially constricting, redilates and returns to its original size. This may happen in patients with optic nerve or severe central or widespread retinal disease and lesions of the contralateral optic tract. Occasionally, pupillary escape occurs in a normal eye if a low intensity light source is used to test the direct reflex. The latency of the pupil reflex has been shown by pupillography to be 200–280 ms and a contraction that lasts 450 ms.[21]

Consensual Light Reflex

This test evaluates the efferent pathway of the pupil light reflex of an eye by stimulating the opposite eye with a bright light **(Fig. 3)**. The consensual reflex to light is clinically equal in velocity and amplitude as the direct reflex. However, it can be shown on infrared pupillography that the consensual reflex to light is in fact slightly less than that the direct reflex. This produces about 0.1 mm or less of what is described as alternating contraction anisocoria that is not normally visible on naked eye examination.[19]

Method

Keep room as dim as possible. Ask the patient to look at a distant target (e.g. fixation target in mirror). Use a dim light source to illuminate the eye whose consensual pupil reflex

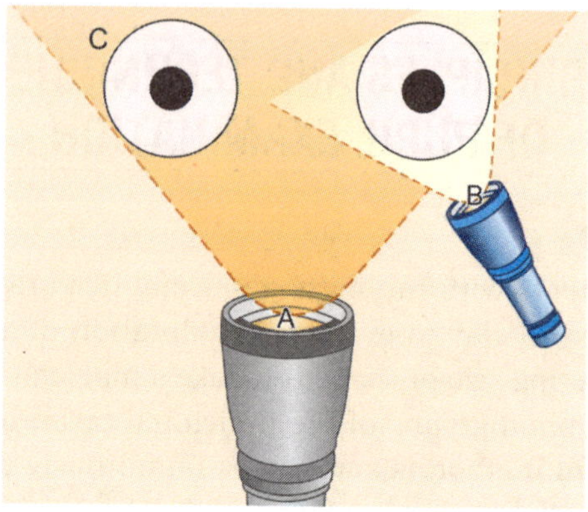

Fig. 3: The direct and consensual pupil reflex (A—dim diffuse light to illuminate both pupils equally for pupil visualization; B—bright light stimulus to elicit direct reflex in left eye; C—consensual reflex seen in right eye).

is being evaluated. This light should be dim enough not to elicit a significant direct pupil reflex. Now swing a bright light source in a quick motion onto the opposite eye. As for the direct reflex record the speed and sustaining power of the pupil constriction.

NEAR RESPONSE

The pupil constriction to a near target is a synkinesis that also involves lens accommodation and convergence. A pupil with a brisk, well-sustained direct reflex will usually have a normal near reflex. Conversely, patients may present with an impaired light reflex with good near reflex suggestive of light-near dissociation. Light-near dissociation is characterized by a near response (tested in moderate light) that exceeds the best constriction that bright light can produce. Testing for the near reflex is therefore, usually performed when the direct reflex is suspect. There is no clinical condition in which the light reflex is present and the near response is absent. A positive near reflex in a blind individual is an indication of the integrity of the efferent pathway and the pupil sphincter.

Equipment

The near response is best tested using a small accommodative target, which may sometimes include a Snellen optotype. A light source such as a pen torch should not be used. Also avoid using fingers as a near target.

Method

The ambient illumination should be moderate—sufficient enough for the patient to view the accommodative target. Ask the patient to keep his eyes focused on a distant target. Bring the near target about 30 cm in front of the patient's eyes and positioned between and slightly below them. Now instruct the patient to view the near target and observe the pupil constriction. Keeping the near target too low causes the eyes to look down making it difficult to observe the pupils. Therefore, keep the target only slightly below the level of the eyes so as not to obstruct the patient's view of the distance target. The near reflex may occur slowly in certain situations (such as in the tonic pupil). To avoid missing this finding, keep observing the pupil for at least 10 seconds.

Sources of Error

Observe the degree of convergence as an indication of patient compliance—poor convergence indicates that the patient may not be trying enough to look at the near target, or that you are not holding the target near enough. This can result in an apparently poor near reflex.

Never judge near response by adding a near stimulus to a bright light stimulus. This action almost always produces additional constriction leading to "pseudo light-near dissociation".

Testing Near Response in a Blind Individual

Observe pupil constriction while instructing patient to voluntarily cross his eyes. This action does not require vision. Alternatively, look for the eye-closure pupil reaction. This is performed by instructing the patient to close his eyes while the examiner keeps the patient's lids open. This maneuver typically produces a strong pupil constriction.

PUPIL DILATION REFLEX (DARK REFLEX)

This test evaluates the function of the pupil dilator muscle. Normal pupil dilatation is a function of sphincter relaxation plus contraction of the dilator muscle. Pupil dilation normally occurs when ambient illumination changes from bright to dim. The pupils also dilate when fixation is shifted from near to distance. Very rarely, paradoxical pupillary responses may be observed in retinal diseases where the pupil dilates in bright illumination and constricts to darkness.[22] Pupil dilation can also be elicited by sudden noise or when the back of the neck is pinched (ciliospinal reflex).

Method

Keep the ambient room illumination bright. Use minimal illumination evenly over both eyes just sufficient to keep both pupils visible in the dark. Switch off room illumination and observe dilatation of the pupils in the "dark".

Observation

Normally both pupils should dilate equally within 5 seconds and reach their widest size in 12–15 seconds. Note that the speed of the dilatation reflex is much slower than pupil constriction.

More importantly, look for a dilation lag indicating a weak dilator muscle. A dilation lag is an anisocoria developing after 2–4 seconds of dark and implies a sympathetic palsy (Horner's syndrome). Pupils that show dilation lag may take up to 25 seconds to return to their widest dilation with most of the dilation occurring about 10–12 seconds after onset of dark stimulus.

Alternative Methods

Another way to determine dilation lag is to take two sets of flash photographs of both eyes at 5 seconds (A) and 15 seconds (B) after onset of dark stimulus **(Fig. 4)**. If anisocoria (A) minus anisocoria (B) is greater than 0.4 mm, then a Horner's syndrome is confirmed.[23]

Infrared videography of the pupils demonstrates dilation lag exquisitely even in very darkly pigmented pupils. Investigators have shown that redilation lag is the most sensitive diagnostic test (70% sensitivity and 95% specificity) to detect unilateral or bilateral Horner's syndrome.[24] The test involved videographing a dilated pupil in the dark that

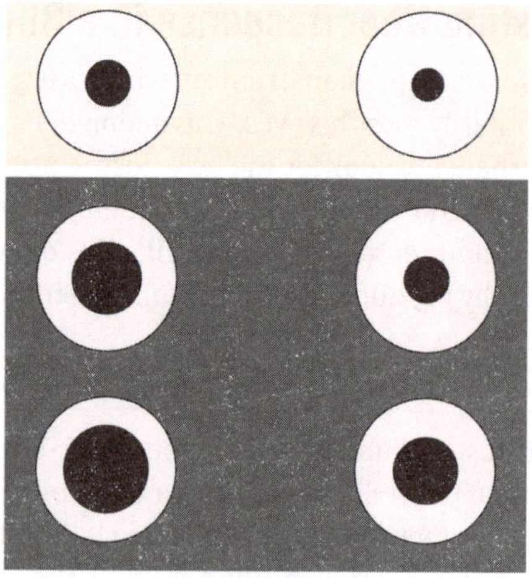

Fig. 4: Dilation lag in left Horner's syndrome. If anisocoria (at 5 seconds in dark) minus anisocoria (15 seconds after dark) is greater than 0.4 mm, then a Horner's syndrome is confirmed.

was then subjected to a bright light stimulus using a xenon arc flash. The time taken by the pupil from the peak of the light reflex to reach its baseline dilated state in the dark was measured. This is termed redilation and shows a delay in Horner's syndrome.

CILIOSPINAL REFLEX

The ciliospinal reflex induces bilateral pupillary dilation to painful stimuli applied to the skin of the neck (afferent C2 and C3). The reflex is mediated by second- and third-order sympathetic nerves to the pupil dilator muscle. Therefore, the ciliospinal reflex is a useful tool in differentiating central from peripheral sympathetic dysfunction.

Method

Pinch the side or back of the neck while observing both pupils.

Observation

Look for brisk bilateral simultaneous pupil dilation. Impaired dilatation reflex on one side suggests a lesion of the second- or third-order neurons of oculosympathetic pathway.

HIPPUS OR PHYSIOLOGICAL PUPILLARY UNREST

In ordinary illumination, healthy young pupils are in a state of almost constant motion. In the setting of prolonged illumination, both pupils constrict, then partly redilate, and begin to oscillate. In dim illumination, the pupils become larger and the oscillations are slower. In bright light they become smaller and the oscillation rate increases. This physiological unrest is termed hippus and is present in all normal individuals. It is not triggered by accommodation. Hippus is reduced or absent in impairment of the afferent or efferent arc of the pupillary light reflex and in spastic miosis.

Oscillatory pupil movements occur with reduced wakefulness. These "fatigue waves" occur when a normal patient is very drowsy and is suppressed by mental activity. This phenomenon is similar but unrelated to hippus.

RELATIVE AFFERENT PUPILLARY DEFECT

In unilateral or asymmetrical bilateral optic neuropathy, the pupils exhibit differing velocities and amplitudes of constriction when testing the direct reflex. This difference is pupil reactivity is exploited by the swinging-flashlight test that exposes this difference as a RAPD.

Hirschberg proposed the concept of RAPD while describing a case of a young woman with unilateral retrobulbar neuritis. Gunn described his ability to differentiate retrobulbar neuritis from nonorganic visual loss by observing the differences in pupil light reflex between the eyes.[25] Kestenbaum popularized the concept of RAPD and credited Gunn with its discovery. Kestenbaum's test to demonstrate RAPD was modified by Levatin who proposed the "swinging-flashlight test" to demonstrate what was he labeled the Marcus-Gunn pupil (now described as RAPD).

Kestenbaum's Pseudoanisocoria Test

This test is not commonly performed nowadays being superseded by its refinement—the swinging-flashlight test. Nevertheless, it clearly demonstrates the underlying concept of the swinging-flashlight test (and can be used in the unlikely situation of a torch being unavailable!).

Method

With the patient in bright ambient illumination, measure the pupil size of one eye, keeping opposite eye occluded. Now perform the above maneuver with the initial eye occluded and measure the pupil size of the fellow eye **(Figs. 5A and B)**.[26]

Observation

Due to unequal afferent inputs in the presence of a unilateral (or asymmetrical bilateral) optic neuropathy, the affected pupil will be larger than the normal pupil. This is a pseudoanisocoria since the occluded and therefore, unobserved pupil is actually of the same size as the unoccluded pupil. The test will be positive in unilateral or grossly asymmetric bilateral optic nerve disease. It will not be positive in normals, and cannot be detected in patients with bilateral symmetric or subtle unilateral optic nerve disease.

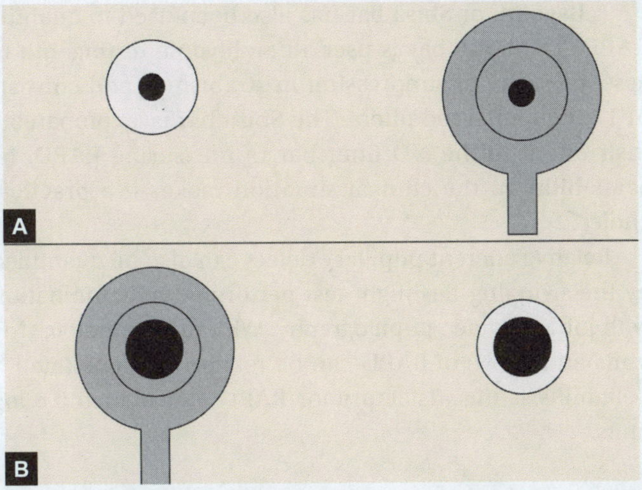

Figs. 5A and B: Kestenbaum's pseudoanisocoria test in left optic neuropathy. Measure each pupil in bright ambient illumination keeping the opposite eye occluded. Right pupil (A) measures smaller than left pupil; (B) indicating left afferent pupillary defect (note that this is a pseudoanisocoria since the occluded pupil is actually of the same size as the unoccluded pupil).

Swinging-flashlight Test

The test is named after Levatin. The pupil with the RAPD is described as a Marcus-Gunn pupil. The test compares optic nerve function between the two eyes **(Figs. 6A to D)**. It requires a normal efferent pathway (oculomotor nerve) and pupillary sphincter, on at least one side.[27]

Method

Keep ambient illumination as dim as possible. Ask the patient to look at a distant target (e.g. fixation target in mirror). Swing bright light source in a quick motion onto the eye and observe the reaction of the pupil. After about 3 seconds, rapidly swing the light source to the opposite pupil and observe its reaction. Continue swinging the light source in this manner between the two eyes to look for any relative sluggishness of the reflex or paradoxical dilation of the pupil of the illuminated eye.[26]

Observation

A paradoxical dilation of the pupil when light is directed on it signifies an optic nerve dysfunction in that eye. The pupil is called the Marcus-Gunn pupil indicating a RAPD in that eye.

It usually takes less than a second to swing the light source from one eye to another. Too great a time interval between stimulation of the eyes results in pupil dilation in the intervening "dark period" causing a false negative test in eyes with mild optic nerve disease. Therefore, the "swing" between the two eyes should be reasonably rapid. It is recommended that the light source directly swings across the bridge of the nose as it passes from one eye to the other in a straight path. This avoids "false negatives".

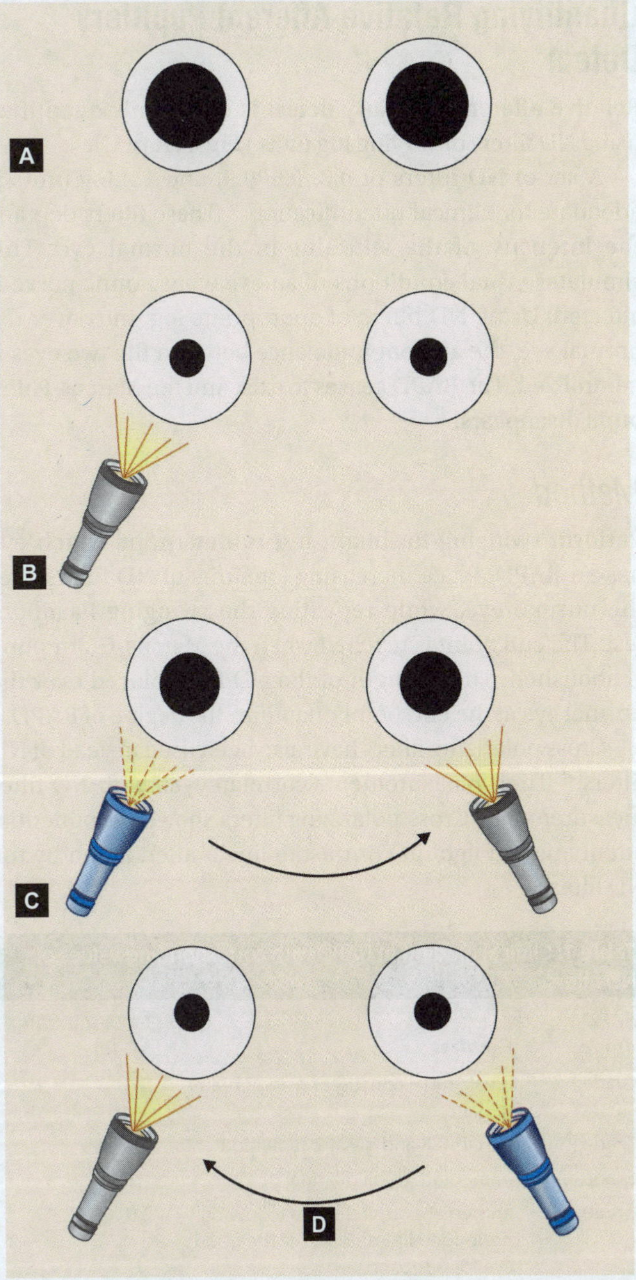

Figs. 6A to D: Swinging-flashlight test. (A) Note equal pupil size in both eyes in the dark; (B) Stimulus on right eye produces visible right pupil constriction. Note that the unobserved left pupil constricts equally; (C) When the torch swings to the left eye the left pupil paradoxically dilates. Note that the unobserved right pupil also "dilates" to the same size. Note also that compared to its size in the dark the left pupil is actually constricting to light (compare left pupil size in A and C), though not to the same degree as the right pupil in (compare right pupil size between A and B); (D) Swinging the torch back to the right eye causes normal pupil constriction. Inference—left relative afferent pupillary defect.

Clinical Grading of Relative Afferent Pupillary Defect

Relative afferent pupillary defect can be clinically graded and have been correlated with corresponding values of neutral density (ND) filter log units **(Table 1)**.[28]

Quantifying Relative Afferent Pupillary Defect

Relative afferent pupillary defect is commonly quantified using ND filters of varying log units **(Figs. 7A to C)**.

A set of ND filters of 0.3, 0.6, 0.9, and 1.2 log units is adequate for clinical quantification.[29] These filters degrade the intensity of the stimulus in the normal eye. This simulates visual conditions of an eye whose optic nerve is affected. Using ND filters of appropriate log units over the normal eye, the afferent imbalance between the two eyes is neutralized. The RAPD ceases to exist and the Marcus-Gunn pupil disappears.

Method

Perform swinging-flashlight test to determine which eye has an RAPD. Place increasing log units of ND filters over the normal eye, while repeating the swinging-flashlight test. The end point is reached when the Marcus-Gunn pupil is abolished. The strength of the ND filter placed over the normal eye at the end point quantifies the degree of RAPD.

Cross polarizing filters have also been used instead of ND filters.[30] Their measurements correlate well with ND filter measurements. Cross polarizing filters showed exponential attenuation of light in contrast to linear attenuation by the ND filters.

Table 1: Clinical grading of RAPD with corresponding values of ND filters.

RAPD grade	*Features*	*Corresponding ND filter*
Grade I	Weak initial constriction and greater redilation	0.4
Grade II	Initial stall and greater redilation	0.7
Grade III	Immediate pupil dilation	1.1
Grade IV	Immediate pupil dilation following prolonged illumination of the good eye for 6 seconds	2.0
Grade V	Immediate pupil dilation with no secondary constriction	Infinity

(ND: neutral density; RAPD: relative afferent pupillary defect)

A Bagolini or Sbisa bar has also been used to quantify RAPD. The Sbisa bar is used in amblyopia testing and to assess density of suppression in strabismus and consists of 17 sequential red filters. The Sbisa bar is a comparable instrument to the ND filter bar in measuring RAPD. Its availability in the clinical situation makes it a practical choice.[31]

Relative afferent pupillary defect can also be quantified by the swinging-flashlight test performed in combination with infrared video pupillography. With this method 0.9 log units and above of RAPD can be reliably demonstrated.[32] Reliability is unsatisfactory for RAPD of less than 0.6 log units.

Interpretation of Relative Afferent Pupillary Defect

Relative afferent pupillary defect will be present in unilateral or asymmetric bilateral optic nerve disease. RAPD will not be present in normal, and cannot be detected in patients with bilateral symmetric optic nerve disease. In unilateral optic nerve disease, the degree of RAPD is broadly proportional to the severity of visual loss caused by optic nerve dysfunction. Although the presence of RAPD usually indicates optic nerve disease, trace RAPD may be observed in dense amblyopia and significant macular disease, in these situations, the degree of visual acuity impairment will be far greater than the degree of RAPD. Significant cataract in one eye causes the stimulating light to scatter and increase the pupillomotor "effectiveness" of the stimulus in that eye. This may induce an apparent RAPD in the opposite eye.

Swinging-flashlight Test with One Normal Pupil

Common situations where this might occur include sphincter damage (e.g. post intraocular surgery, acute angle-closure glaucoma), efferent pupillary defects (e.g. oculomotor nerve palsy with internal ophthalmoplegia), or poor visualization of the pupil (e.g. corneal opacity).

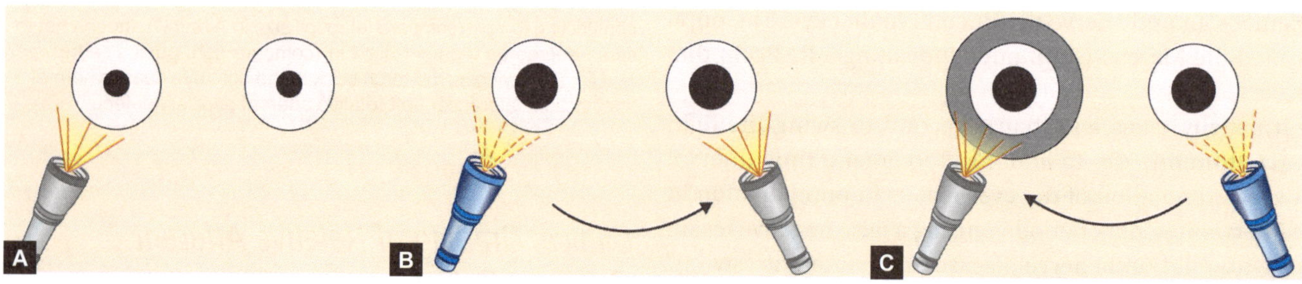

Figs. 7A to C: Quantifying RAPD with neutral density filters; (A) Bright light stimulus on right eye produces visible right pupil constriction; (B) When the torch swings over to the left eye, the left pupil paradoxically dilated indicating a left RAPD; (C) An ND filter of appropriate strength reduces the intensity of light stimulus to the normal right eye creating an artificial optic nerve dysfunction (compare direct light reflex in right eye between A and C). Since both eyes are now equally "affected", swinging the torch back to the right eye causes no pupil constriction. The left RAPD has been neutralized. (ND: neutral density; RAPD: relative afferent pupillary defect)

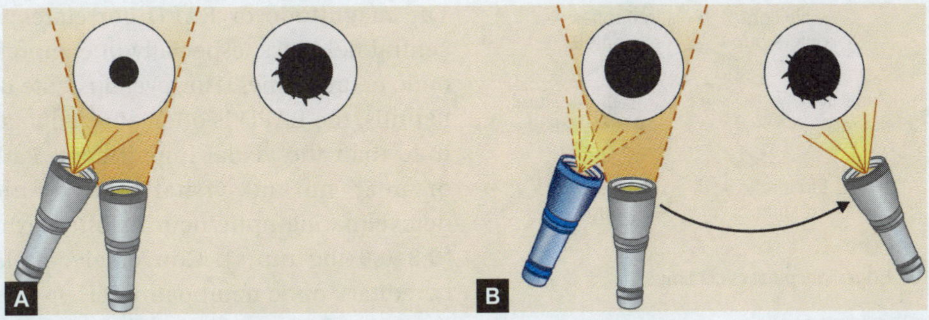

Figs. 8A and B: Testing for relative afferent pupillary defect (RAPD) with only one normal pupil in the right eye. The left pupil shows traumatic sphincter tears rendering it unreliable for pupil reflex evaluation. Dim illumination (shaded flashlight) is used to allow observation of the right pupil in the dark. (A) The right pupil shows a brisk direct reflex; (B) With the bright stimulus over the left eye, the left pupil is predictably immobile, but the right pupil dilates (by consensual reflex) indicating a left RAPD. Compare this response with the behavior of the right pupil in **Figure 6C**. The behavior is the same, the only difference being that in the present situation the right pupil (instead of the left) is being observed.

Testing in this situation is based on the principle of the consensual reflex **(Figs. 8A and B)**. The opposite pupil responds in an identical fashion to the pupil in which the light stimulus is applied.[19]

Method

Use a dim light source with just sufficient illumination to illuminate the normal pupil. Perform the swinging-flashlight test as described above, by swinging the bright stimulating light source between the two eyes but observe only the dimly illuminated normal pupil.

Observation

If there is optic nerve disease in either eye, the observed pupil will exhibit an RAPD when the affected eye (irrespective of laterality) is stimulated. Remember the eye with RAPD is the eye being stimulated by the bright light source; this may or may not be the eye whose pupil is being observed.

Swinging-flashlight Test in Ocular Misalignment

With large angle strabismus or displacement of the globe in orbital disease, an off-axis stimulation of the squinting eye may result in a suboptimal pupil response and a false positive test in that eye. This is avoided by orienting the light source along the visual axis.

Uncovering a Subtle Relative Afferent Pupillary Defect

The test is known as the "Tilt Test". This refinement of the swinging-flashlight test is useful when there is no visibly "detectable" RAPD but *clinical suspicion of unilateral optic nerve dysfunction* exists.[33] This clinical prerequisite is significant as a small percentage of normals may also demonstrate small degrees of RAPD which might also fluctuate between the eyes from time to time, a phenomenon described as an afferent equivalent of hippus.[34]

Clinical situation: 0.2 log unit clinically undetectable RAPD LE use 0.3 log unit ND filter for test			
0.3 log unit ND filter over	Total log unit defect		Observation
	RE	LE	
RE	0.3	0.2	No RAPD
LE	0.0	0.5 (0.3+0.2)	RAPD LE

Fig. 9: Tilt test for uncovering a subtle 0.2 log unit left RAPD that is clinically difficult to detect. A weak 0.3 log unit ND filter (depicted as a shaded circle) over the right eye induces a trace pseudoafferent defect rendering both eyes almost equal in terms of afferent input and no visible RAPD. However, transferring the ND filter to the left eye increases the afferent defect to 0.5 log unit (0.2 log unit afferent defect + 0.3 log unit ND filter = 0.5 log unit) rendering it clinically visible, confirming the presence of a subtle left afferent defect.

(LE: left eye; ND: neutral density; RAPD: relative afferent pupillary defect; RE: right eye)

Equipment

The test requires a weak ND filter of 0.3 log units. A 0.3 log unit ND filter placed in front of an eye with a suspect RAPD heightens the inter-eye difference in pupillomotor drive to a detectable level thus causing a Marcus-Gunn pupil to become apparent.

Method

Place 0.3 log unit ND filter in front of one eye and perform the swinging-flashlight test **(Fig. 9)**. Then repeat but with the same ND filter over fellow eye.

Observation

An eye with subtle optic nerve dysfunction will show a demonstrable RAPD in the test when the 0.3 log ND filter is placed in front of it. This occurs because the ND filter further reduces impulses along an already affected optic nerve. When the weak ND filter is placed over the normal

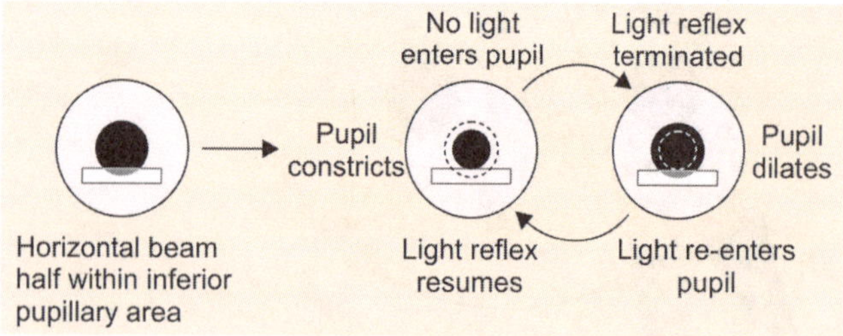

Fig. 10: Edge light pupil cycle time.

eye impulses along the normal optic nerve are slightly reduced. This would be approximately equal to the strength of impulses along the affected optic nerve in the fellow eye and thus no RAPD would be detected.

EDGE LIGHT PUPIL CYCLE TIME

This test is not a particularly sensitive indicator of optic nerve disease when compared to the swinging-flashlight test. Nevertheless, it is useful when patients have bilateral symmetrical retinal or optic nerve dysfunction or have only one eye **(Fig. 10)**.[35]

Method

The patient is seated at slit lamp in dim ambient illumination and instructed to look at an imaginary distance target. Adjust the beam of the slit lamp to make it 0.5 mm thick and horizontally oriented. The beam is now focused on the inferior edge of the pupil such that half the thickness of the beam falls into the pupillary aperture. The light entering the pupil causes it to constrict. This constriction causes the entire slit beam to fall below the inferior pupil margin. The momentary loss of stimulus causes the pupil to partly dilate. The dilation now readmits half the slit beam into the pupil. This causes reconstriction of the pupil and the cycle starts again.

Observation

Each constriction-dilation is a cycle. With a stop watch measure the time for 30 cycles. Repeat the test for five 30-cycle rounds and calculate the time taken for a single cycle. Total number of cycles = 30 × 5 = 150. Edge light pupil cycle time (ELPCT) (in ms) = Total time (in seconds) for 5 rounds × 1,000/150. The normal range of ELPCT is 850–950 ms.

DISORDERS OF PUPIL FUNCTION

AFFERENT PUPILLARY DEFECTS

Optic Nerve Disorders

Most patients with a unilateral or asymmetric bilateral optic neuropathy have an RAPD regardless of the cause. The magnitude or RAPD correlates with the extent of central field loss, especially in compressive and ischemic optic neuropathies. However, in acute demyelinating optic neuritis, the RAPD is often affected to a far greater magnitude than the visual impairment. Patients with normal or near normal visual acuity following recovered demyelinating optic neuritis often exhibit a small RAPD (0.3–0.6 log units). Conversely, patients with Leber's hereditary optic neuropathy (LHON) often have an RAPD that is much less in magnitude when compared to the extent of visual impairment.[36] It is hypothesized that there may be lower susceptibility of ganglion cells that serve the pupillary reflex in LHON.

RETINAL DISEASES

A mild RAPD is not uncommon in severe diffuse retinal disease or macular disease. Conditions such as central serous retinopathy or retinal detachments (especially if the macula is detached) can produce a 0.3–0.7 log unit RAPD.[37] In general, visual acuity is impaired to a far greater magnitude compared to the RAPD in macular disease whereas in optic neuropathy the RAPD magnitude most often correlates with the degree of visual acuity loss.

Most patients with nonischemic central retinal vein occlusion (CRVO) have a small RAPD of 0.3 log units with none exceeding 0.9 log units.[38] However, in ischemic CRVO most patients had an RAPD of 1.2 log units or more and none had an RAPD of less than 0.6 log units. A significant increase in RAPD in a patient with nonischemic CRVO is an early sign of ischemic conversion even with an unchanged fundus picture.

ASYMMETRIC RETINAL ADAPTATION WITH INDUCED RAPD

An eye patch or a ptotic lid can increase retinal sensitivity due to dark adaptation and cause a false RAPD (of up to 1.5 log units) in the uncovered eye.[39] In a patient with traumatic optic neuropathy, an RAPD of the affected eye might be masked because a patch increases retinal sensitivity to light.

In a clinically detectable anisocoria, about 0.1 log unit of RAPD is produced in the eye with the smaller pupil for every millimeter of anisocoria. This implies that a clinically significant RAPD will be induced in the smaller pupil when anisocoria is greater than 2 mm.[40]

AMBLYOPIA

A small RAPD (<0.5 log units) may be seen in an amblyopic eye and this does not correlate well with the visual acuity which is usually far more impaired.[41]

Pupillography demonstrates that RAPD is not a consistent feature of amblyopia and is present in only a small proportion of amblyopes and even these amblyopes are not necessarily associated with dense amblyopia.[42]

MEDIA OPACITIES

Dense vitreous hemorrhage that mechanically blocks light from falling on the retina can produce a small RAPD, but the visual acuity loss is far greater. Mature cataracts paradoxically may cause an RAPD to be elicited in the fellow eye. Scattering of light by the cataract with more photons hitting the macular area directly causes "supramaximal" stimulation of an already "dark adapted" retina resulting in an apparent RAPD of the fellow eye.[43]

OPTIC TRACT DISORDERS

Optic tract disorders cause a contralateral homonymous hemianopia with loss of the contralateral temporal hemifield. Since there are more afferent pupillary fibers in the nasal retina compared to the temporal retina, there are more crossed fibers than uncrossed fibers in the optic tracts. This asymmetric distribution of crossed and uncrossed fibers is the basis of the contralateral mild to moderate RAPD (of about 0.3–1.6 log units) seen in optic tract lesions.[44] The intact ipsilateral temporal field provides greater pupillomotor input owing to larger retinal area being stimulated than the intact nasal field of the contralateral eye. However, its magnitude does not correlate with the difference in the number of crossed and uncrossed axons.[45]

PRETECTAL NUCLEUS

Unilateral lesions of the brachium of the superior colliculus can produce a rare "tectal RAPD" where pupillary response to stimulation of the contralateral hemifields is affected without contralateral homonymous hemianopia as would occur if the lesion were situated in the optic tract.[46] Owing to the location of the lesion, a tectal RAPD may be associated with ipsilateral or contralateral trochlear nerve palsy.

WERNICKE PUPIL

A bitemporal hemianopia caused by an optic chiasm lesion, or a homonymous hemianopia caused by an optic tract lesion may demonstrate a Wernicke pupil. It can be demonstrated by a narrow beam of light from a slit lamp. When the beam is directed on to the retina from the affected hemifield, the pupil reaction is less. When the light is directed onto the seeing hemiretina, the pupil constricts better. This pupillary hemiakinesia is described as Wernicke pupil. It is often inconclusive and unreliable as a bedside test.

MIDBRAIN DISEASE

This can cause poorly reactive pupils to light or near stimuli or to both stimuli. Midbrain lesions can affect the pretectal afferents to the Edinger-Westphal nuclei and can cause various combinations of defects that involve the direct pupillary reflex, the pupil near response, and accommodation. The pupillographic characteristics of an RAPD resulting from a dorsal midbrain lesion resemble those of an RAPD resulting from a unilateral optic tract lesion, but without the homonymous visual field defect.[47] These defects most often occur in association with other neurological signs such as an internuclear ophthalmoplegia, vertical gaze palsies, convergence loss, convergence-retraction nystagmus, exotropia, ptosis, and other ocular motility defects.

PARADOXICAL PUPIL CONSTRICTION IN THE DARK

This uncommon finding is seen in patients with retinal conditions like congenital achromatopsia, blue cone monochromatism, and Leber's congenital amaurosis.[22] It is occasionally seen in optic nerve disorders like optic disk hypoplasia, dominant optic atrophy, and bilateral optic neuritis. It has been suggested that the cause is not due to abnormalities in the central nervous system but from selective delays in afferent signals from the retinal photoreceptors to the pupillomotor center.

EFFERENT PUPILLARY DEFECTS: ANISOCORIA

Anisocoria can also occur in the presence of a structural defect in the iris or if there is a dysfunction of either the parasympathetic or sympathetic outflow to the pupil. Anisocoria is not caused by optic nerve disease or afferent pupil pathway dysfunction.

Slit-lamp Examination

Evaluate the integrity of the pupil sphincter. Look for any iris atrophy or sphincter thinning. It is useful to examine the fellow eye pupil (if normal) for comparison. Look for segmental pupil contraction (vermiform movements) using the slit-lamp beam (diffuse illumination) as a stimulus. In cases of suspected oculomotor nerve palsy with aberrant regeneration, subtle pupil-gaze dyskinesis may be detected. This may be detected by observing the pupil in diffuse illumination while instructing patient to shift gaze (abduction-adduction and elevation-depression).

Assuming the sphincter is structurally normal on slit-lamp examination, anisocoria is a sign of autonomic (parasympathetic or sympathetic) dysfunction. The onset of anisocoria (especially if isolated and discovered as an incidental finding) can be determined by examination of pupil size in old photographs of the patient using good magnification (20 D lens of the indirect ophthalmoscope).

PUPIL SIZE AND LIGHT REFLEX

Method

Evaluate pupil size in bright and dim illumination **(Figs. 11A and B)** and then test the light reflex as described earlier. A useful pearl to remember is that in general a pupil with a brisk sustained light reflex is a normal pupil whether or not it appears larger or smaller than its fellow.

Result

If the larger pupil has an impaired light reflex, it is the likely cause of anisocoria and implies problems along the parasympathetic pathway. The anisocoria would be more in bright light and less in dim light. If both pupils have a good light reflex and the anisocoria decreases in bright light and increases in dim light then it is either a Horner's syndrome or a physiological anisocoria.

ANISOCORIA GREATER IN DARKNESS

Physiologic Anisocoria

Physiologic anisocoria is an isolated condition. There is no history of exposure of pharmacologic agents. There are no associated signs such as ptosis or dilatation lag. Slit-lamp examination shows a normal iris. Both pupils dilate equally with topical cocaine.

Lowenfeld using infrared flash photography demonstrated that pupillary inequality of less than 0.3 mm is very common but difficult to observe clinically.[48] Inequality greater than 0.3 mm may be called anisocoria and is present in 11% of normal population. The generally described incidence of 20% has been called into question because of inadequate sample sizes in studies and lack of objective records of measurement. The cause is believed to be asymmetries of supranuclear inhibitory control of the dorsal parasympathetic mesencephalic nuclei. The anisocoria always decreases in light. This decrease in light is more apparent when pupil diameters are measured. However, the ratio of the pupillary areas does not change with brighter illumination. This finding is significant as gross observation of the pupil size is related more to the ratio of pupillary areas than pupil diameters.[49]

Physiologic anisocoria has no clinical significance and should be differentiated from acquired anisocoria in the setting of ocular and head trauma. It is useful to detect preexisting asymmetries of pupil size in old photographs.

HORNER'S SYNDROME

The signs of Horner's syndrome are ptosis, apparent enophthalmos, a miotic pupil, and in certain situations ipsilateral anhidrosis. It occurs if there is an interruption of the oculosympathetic pathway. Depending on the location of the lesion, Horner's syndrome may be classified as central, preganglionic, or postganglionic.

The steps of diagnosis include:
- Recognize Horner's syndrome clinically
- Look for associated signs for localization
- Pharmacologic localization if Horner's syndrome appears isolated.

Clinical Signs of Horner's Syndrome

Ptosis: The upper lid exhibits a mild droop owing to underaction of the sympathetically innervated smooth muscle of Muller in the upper lid. Similar smooth muscle fibers in the lower lid will also be affected causing the lower lid to ride up. This is sometimes described as an "upside-down ptosis" producing a narrowing of the palpebral fissure and an apparent enophthalmos. Topical application of 2.5% phenylephrine has been shown to temporarily reverse the ptosis and may be used as a measure to defer corrective surgery.[50]

Miosis: The miosis can be reversed if the dilator muscle is stimulated directly (e.g. if an adrenergic drop is instilled in the eye). This produces "paradoxical pupillary dilation"

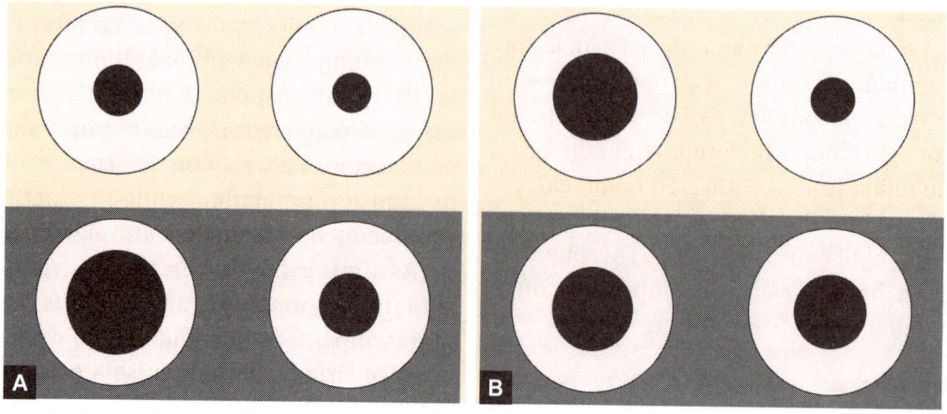

Figs. 11A and B: Anisocoria. (A) Anisocoria worse in dark. The left pupil does not dilate as well as the right pupil. This may be normal (physiological) anisocoria or a left Horner's syndrome; (B) Anisocoria worse in bright illumination. The right pupil does not contract as well as the left in bright light. This is indicative of a parasympathetic palsy (oculomotor nerve palsy or Adie's pupil) or pupil sphincter damage.

caused by denervation supersensitivity of the dilator muscle fibers to circulating and topical adrenergic molecules. This phenomenon is thus also seen when there is an increase in circulating adrenaline in the setting of intense emotional excitement.

Topical apraclonidine, an alpha-adrenergic agonist, produces dilation of a Horner pupil due to denervation supersensitivity. It has little or no effect on a normal pupil. Thus in a patient with unilateral Horner's syndrome there may be a reversal of anisocoria after apraclonidine instillation with the affected pupil more dilated than the normal pupil.[51]

Anisocoria: The anisocoria is more apparent in darkness and virtually disappears in bright light. In regular room light the degree of anisocoria is small (about 1 mm or less). This can be overlooked or mistaken for physiological anisocoria). Fatigue or drowsiness causes reduction of the normal sympathetic inhibition to the Edinger-Westphal nucleus. This will further diminish the anisocoria. If the anisocoria is greater than 2 mm, it is very unlikely to be physiological.

Dilation lag: Impaired dilation in darkness is termed dilation lag and is a feature of Horner's syndrome. One way to document this is to take flash photographs of the eyes 5 seconds and 15 seconds after onset of dark stimulus. In Horner's syndrome, there is more anisocoria in the 5-second photograph than in the 15-second photograph. This demonstrates dilation lag after 5 seconds of darkness, and also shows decreasing anisocoria in the later phase of dilation.[23] Using infrared pupillography, it has been shown that after a light flash a delay in the time needed to recover three-quarters of the baseline pupil size has a 70% sensitivity and 95% specificity in detecting unilateral Horner's syndrome.[24] This definition of dilation lag is based on a measure of time rather than the degree of anisocoria and is therefore, particularly useful in detecting bilateral Horner's syndrome. Using a commercially available camcorder to record pupillary dilation lag, it has been shown that anisocoria of 0.6 mm or more 4 seconds after switching off the illumination discriminates physiological anisocoria from Horner's syndrome with a sensitivity of 82% and a specificity of 69%. Because of the good correlation between postcocaine anisocoria and anisocoria after 4 seconds of darkness, photographic or videographic measurements of dilation lag may complete or even replace cocaine testing.[52]

Iris heterochromia: Depigmentation of the ipsilateral iris is a typical feature of congenital Horner's syndrome but is also seen in long-standing and acquired Horner's syndrome. It is never a feature of acute acquired Horner's syndrome.

Anhidrosis: In preganglionic lesions, the distribution of anhidrosis is along the entire side of the head, the face, and the neck down to the clavicle. In postganglionic lesions, it is restricted to a patch on the forehead and the medial side of the nose. Immediately following sympathetic denervation, there is flushing of the skin raised temperature, conjunctival hyperemia, and nasal stuffiness. Later the skin has lower temperature and becomes dry. This is due to denervation supersensitivity of the affected blood vessels to circulating adrenergic molecules.

Ocular hypotony and increased accommodation: These are minor effects and clinically not important. The signs reflect the sympathetic innervation of the ciliary muscle.

Clinical Localization of Horner's Syndrome

Depending on the "company it keeps" along oculosympathetic pathway, Horner's syndrome may be localized by associated signs **(Table 2)**.

Pharmacologic Localization in Horner's Syndrome

Requirement

Cocaine (5% or 10%) and hydroxyamphetamine (1%) (Paredrine). Alternatively, a combination of apraclonidine (1%) and phenylephrine (1%) may be used.

Cocaine Test

First measure pupil size in both eyes and determine pretest anisocoria. Instill the drops in the conjunctival sac in both eyes, applying in the miotic (Horner's syndrome) eye first. Wipe both eyes with a tissue. After 20–40 seconds instill a second drop of the drug to each eye (to the normal eye first and then in the affected eye to balance the dosage). Measure the size of the pupil in both the eyes 30 minutes after second instillation. This evaluation is done in dim illumination. The reason for this is that cocaine affects only the sympathetic system and if pupils are examined in bright light they will constrict and the effects of cocaine may not be appreciated.

Cocaine dilates a normal pupil but has little or no effect on a Horner pupil. Increase in post-cocaine test anisocoria by 1 mm (or at least 0.5 mm) is diagnostic of Horner's syndrome. Dark irides dilate poorly with cocaine and the test result must be interpreted with more caution.

Cocaine stings the eye and the patient may squeeze the lids during instillation of the drop in the second eye. This may result in less drug availability in that eye. Therefore, it is important to apply the drug in the apparently affected (miotic) eye first. Cocaine must be applied in eyes with intact corneal epithelium. This means that the test cannot be performed on the same day if the patient has undergone applanation tonometry, corneal sensitivity testing, or any procedure that could affect the integrity of the corneal epithelium.

Hydroxyamphetamine Test

Instillation of hydroxyamphetamine is performed in the same manner as cocaine.

Table 2: Clinical localization in Horner's syndrome.

Central	• Hypothalamic signs	• Diabetes insipidus • Disturbed temperature regulation • Altered sleep patterns
	• Brainstem signs	• Contralateral IVth cranial nerve palsy • Ipsilateral VIth cranial nerve palsy
	• Meningeal signs	• Wallenberg syndrome (other brainstem cranial nerve involvement, vertigo, sensory deficits, anhidrosis of the entire half of the body)
Preganglionic	• Pancoast syndrome (thoracic outlet)	• Ipsilateral pain or paresthesia—neck, shoulder, arm, and digits (fourth and fifth fingers—C8 and T1 roots)
	• Anhidrosis of face and neck • Brachial plexus signs	• Weakness and atrophy of hand muscles
	• Vocal cord paralysis (Rowland–Payne syndrome)	• Due to phrenic nerve (C3 to C5), vagus, and recurrent laryngeal nerve palsies
	• Chest and neck examination	• Cervicothoracic abnormalities, trauma or surgical scars, neck swellings, lung signs
Postganglionic	• Ipsilateral migraine/cluster headache	• Face pain, tearing, facial flushing, rhinorrhea
	• Cavernous sinus signs	• Associated cranial nerves palsies (III, IV, VI, V1) • Pseudopupil sparing (combined sympathetic and parasympathetic involvement (normal sized pupil that reacts poorly to light and has dilation lag in the dark) • No facial anhidrosis but anhidrosis of the forehead may be present (Reason: Sweat glands of the forehead are innervated by terminal branches of the internal carotid nerve)
	• Carotid dissection signs	• Ipsilateral pain over face, neck, or orbit • Amaurosis fugax or retinal artery occlusion • Neck swelling or bruit
	• Other CNS signs	• Dysgeusia • Tinnitus • Syncope • Cranial neuropathy (VI, IX, X, XI, XII)

(CNS: central nervous system)

A 48-hour interval between the cocaine test and the hydroxyamphetamine test is recommended. Both tests cannot be performed on the same day because cocaine inhibits the uptake of hydroxyamphetamine into the presynaptic vesicle, reducing accuracy of the hydroxyamphetamine test.

Apraclonidine and Phenylephrine Test

Both cocaine and hydroxyamphetamine are difficult to procure. Strict governmental controls surround the availability of cocaine. Paredrine is no longer produced and therefore has very limited availability.

Apraclonidine is an alternative to cocaine to differentiate a Horner pupil from physiologic anisocoria. It is an alpha-adrenergic agonist causing lowering of intraocular pressure by reducing aqueous production. A 1% solution will also dilate a Horner pupil by 1.0–1.5 mm with no change in the normal pupil. The drug might thus reverse anisocoria! A 0.5% apraclonidine solution works just as well. Apraclonidine has been shown to identify Horner's syndrome following carotid dissection as early as 3 hours after onset of symptoms.[53]

Phenylephrine 1% correlates well with the results of hydroxyamphetamine 1% in localizing the lesion to the postganglionic neuron and is a reliable alternative to hydroxyamphetamine 1% should pharmacological testing be desired and hydroxyamphetamine 1% not be available. Topical 1% phenylephrine dilates the postganglionic Horner's pupil. It has no effect on a central or preganglionic Horner pupil. It also has no effect on a normal pupil.[54]

ANISOCORIA GREATER IN LIGHT

Common causes of a dilated pupil that is poorly reactive to light reflex include iris sphincter damage due to various conditions, parasympathetic palsy (tonic pupil and oculomotor nerve palsy), and pharmacologic mydriasis.

The evaluation includes a careful slit-lamp examination and pharmacologic testing with pilocarpine.

SLIT-LAMP EXAMINATION

Examine pupil sphincter for signs of trauma or surgery. Sphincter paresis due to ischemia occurs in acute angle-closure glaucoma. Sphincter atrophy occurs following acute angle closure glaucoma. Congenital aplasia of sphincter can rarely occur.

Look for segmental pupil contraction (vermiform movement) by increasing and decreasing illumination. In the absence of sphincter damage this is a feature of tonic pupil (Adie pupil). Oculomotor nerve palsy with pupil involvement can also cause segmental paralysis of the sphincter. Look for contraction induced by ocular motility—elevation, adduction, or depression. In oculomotor nerve palsy with aberrant regeneration segmental contraction may be seen during adduction (Czarnecki sign).

PILOCARPINE TEST

Using pilocarpine of different strengths the cause of a mid-dilated pupil, whether pharmacologic, tonic pupil, or oculomotor nerve palsy, can be differentiated.

Contraindications and Precautions

The test is contraindicated in documented hypersensitivity to the drug, acute anterior uveitis, pupillary block glaucoma, and possibly in pregnancy. The test may be performed with precaution in patients with acute cardiac failure, peptic ulcer, hyperthyroidism, gastrointestinal spasm, bronchial asthma, Parkinson disease, recent myocardial infarction, urinary tract obstruction, and hypertension or hypotension. The miosis produced by the test may cause difficulty with dark adaptation and night driving.

Preparation

Pilocarpine of a weaker strength (0.125%) and stronger strength (1%) is required.

About 0.125% pilocarpine eye drops may be conveniently prepared by drawing 0.25 mL of commercially available 1% pilocarpine eye drops into a 2 mL syringe and then diluting it by drawing normal saline up to the 2 mL mark (×8 dilution). Fit a cannula to the syringe for topical instillation.

If 2% pilocarpine is available, it can first be made into a 1% solution by first drawing 0.25 mL of commercially available 2% pilocarpine eye drops into a 2 mL syringe. This is then diluted by drawing 0.25 mL (an equal amount) of normal saline (1:1 dilution). The syringe now contains 0.5 mL solution of 1% pilocarpine. Mix thoroughly and then discard 0.25 mL. What is left is 0.25 mL of 1% pilocarpine from which a 0.125% solution of pilocarpine can be prepared as described above.

Method

Measure pupil size in both eyes (in ambient or bright illumination). Photography of the pupils is useful. Instill 0.125% pilocarpine in each eye and after 30 seconds instill a second drop in each eye.[55] Make sure enough medication has been instilled equally in both eyes allowing for squeezing of the eye while applying medication in the second eye. Also ensure that the patient does not sleep and remains alert during this period (drowsiness may cause the normal pupil to constrict relatively more than an Aide pupil). Measure and document the pupil size of both eyes after 30 minutes.

Observation

In a tonic pupil a dramatic constriction of the tonic pupil occurs with no change in the size of the smaller pupil (known as denervation supersensitivity). A reversal of anisocoria may happen in some cases, as the formerly larger pupil becomes more miotic than its fellow. Pupil dilation due to oculomotor nerve palsy and a pharmacologic pupil will not show any change in anisocoria (the larger pupil remains approximately the same size). If there is little or no change in anisocoria after instillation of 0.125% pilocarpine, apply 1% pilocarpine to both eyes. A mid-dilated pupil caused by oculomotor nerve palsy will show constriction. No topical agent can overcome a pupil blockade by a pharmacologic agent.

A pilocarpine dose-dependent curve shows decreased pupil size within 15 minutes, peaking at 30–60 minutes. Infrared pupillography in the dark shows that normal pupils demonstrate some constriction to 0.125% pilocarpine but show an insignificant constriction to 0.0625% solution of the drug. Pupil constriction with 0.0625% pilocarpine more reliably distinguishes an Adie pupil from normal.[56]

Cholinergic supersensitivity of the pupil occurs frequently with nonischemic oculomotor nerve palsies and may be related to the degree of preganglionic injury to the pupillomotor fibers.[57] Cholinergic supersensitivity and a "positive" test with 0.125% pilocarpine may occasionally occur in oculomotor nerve palsy. There are two ways to clinically judge a tonic pupil from oculomotor nerve palsy in this situation. Firstly, be suspicious of "moderate" constriction of the pupil with weak pilocarpine. It could be oculomotor nerve palsy. Secondly, look for a larger pupil that becomes smaller in darkness after instillation of weak pilocarpine. It is more likely to be a tonic pupil.[49]

CAUSES OF ANISOCORIA DUE TO A DILATED PUPIL

Iris Sphincter Damage

History of trauma and a slit-lamp examination of the sphincter showing tears or iris atrophy confirm the diagnosis.

Pharmacologic Blockade with Parasympatholytic Agents

Such agents block the effect of acetylcholine on the iris sphincter and ciliary muscle. They produce cycloplegia and mydriasis. The mydriasis is often extreme (>8 mm). A pharmacologic pupil will not dilate to 1% pilocarpine.

Oculomotor Nerve Palsy

Pupillomotor fibers lie superficially in the oculomotor nerve in the subarachnoid space. Here, they are prone to compression by aneurysms, tumors, uncal herniation, basal meningitis, and rarely hemosiderin deposits from recurrent blood in the cerebrospinal fluid.

Isolated pupil sphincter palsy without any other extraocular muscle involvement in oculomotor nerve palsy is rare. If it occurs in the setting of an aneurysm, it is more likely to be due to a tip of the basilar artery aneurysm than an aneurysm of the internal carotid artery or the posterior communicating artery.

In the cavernous sinus concomitant sympathetic palsy may produce pseudo pupil sparing oculomotor nerve palsy. The pupil is normal in size (no anisocoria) but the pupil reflex will be sluggish and a dilation lag in the dark may be seen.

TONIC PUPIL

Damage to the ciliary ganglion or the short ciliary nerves produces paralysis of accommodation, a pupil that reacts poorly to light. Patients present with blurred near vision and photophobia. The pupil shows a slow tonic constriction to near and a slow dilation when the eye refixates to distance. In addition segmental contraction of the pupil (vermiform movement) is visible to bright light on slit-lamp biomicroscopy. Because of denervation supersensitivity, the pupil will constrict to weak pilocarpine (described earlier). Tonic pupils are divided into three categories: local, neuropathic, and Adie syndrome.

Local Tonic Pupils

This is due to orbital or systemic lesions that affect the ciliary ganglion or short ciliary nerves in isolation. Causes include tumors, trauma, infection (such as herpes zoster), inflammation (sarcoidosis), iatrogenic (lateral orbit exploration), and amyloid.

Neuropathic Tonic Pupils

These are usually bilateral tonic pupils. Causes include diabetes mellitus, syphilis, chronic alcoholism, and systemic lupus erythematosus (SLE). Neuropathic tonic pupils can occur as part of a paraneoplastic autonomic polyneuropathy and dysautonomic syndromes [Riley-Day, Shy-Drager, acute pandysautonomia, and human immunodeficiency virus (HIV) autonomic neuropathy].

Adie Syndrome

Adie syndrome usually presents as a unilateral tonic pupil, with approximately 4% of patients developing bilateral involvement each year. Women are more affected than men (5:1). It is often seen in early adulthood or middle age (20–50 years). Clinical signs include reduced or absent accommodation and absent deep tendon reflexes (in 50–75% of patients). The cause is thought to be viral or possibly autoimmune. Over time the pupil tends to become smaller and accommodation improves.

LIGHT-NEAR DISSOCIATION

Constriction of a pupil to near viewing that is stronger than the light response is termed light-near dissociation. It may be caused by an afferent or efferent pupillary pathway defect.

Light-near dissociation is the primary feature of Argyll-Robertson pupil. It is usually bilateral (80–90%). It occurs in neurosyphilis. The lesion is located in the rostral midbrain. A lesion along the dorsal aspect of the Edinger-Westphal nucleus damages the pretectal fibers of the pupil light reflex but spare the near response fibers that have a more ventral location.

Miosis is another characteristic of the Argyll-Robertson pupil. However, the pupil usually displays normal reflex dilation in dark and a normal ciliospinal reflex.

Irregularity of pupil shape and poor dilation to atropine are usually sequelae of syphilitic iritis and consequent structural iris damage.

Light-near dissociation can also be seen in patients with pregeniculate afferent visual pathway damage with visual impairment, compressive and infiltrative mesencephalic lesions, and damage to the parasympathetic innervation of the iris sphincter. In most dorsal midbrain syndromes, other deficits such as vertical gaze palsy, convergence-retraction nystagmus on attempted upward gaze, and lid retraction accompany light-near dissociation.

PUPILS IN TRAUMATIC BRAIN INJURY

Pupil examination is a key component in the assessment of patients with traumatic brain injury (TBI), coma, and in the certification of brain death.

Cerebral hemorrhage can cause herniation of the uncus of the hippocampus of the temporal lobe across the free edge of the tentorium causing compression of the oculomotor nerve. The pupillary sign associated with this compression is named after Hutchinson and has three stages progression as the bleeding continues and the herniation increases. *Stage 1*: Irritation of the oculomotor nerve causes ipsilateral miosis with a normal contralateral pupil. *Stage 2*: Palsy of the ipsilateral oculomotor nerve causes a dilated pupil while irritation of the contralateral oculomotor nerve causes miosis in the opposite eye. *Stage 3*: The final stage is characterized by bilateral dilated pupils and indicates a grave prognosis.

Damage to the inhibitory control of the Edinger-Westphal nucleus causes bilateral pinpoint pupils as seen in pontine hemorrhage. Under suitable magnification; however, these pupils will be seen to still retain the light reflex. Pinpoint pupils are also a feature of opiate overdose (morphine and heroin) and organophosphorous toxicity.

Investigators have shown that in TBI, fixed dilated pupils (FDPs) with a Glasgow Coma Scale (GCS) of 3 do not survive in spite resuscitation efforts.[58] This information is relevant in deciding whether or not to pursue aggressive resuscitation efforts and in discussing prognosis with family. Patients with a GCS of 3 who do not have FDPs should be aggressively resuscitated because one-third of these patients survive to discharge. Unilateral FDP patients have a relatively better chance of survival.[59] The time period between development of FDP and initiation of treatment is a significant parameter that determines survival.[60] The critical time period was determined to be 3 hours.

The pupil light reflex is an important component of the accepted brain death certification protocol.[61] It forms part of the brainstem reflex assessment along with the neurologic assessment of coma and the apnea test. The assessments are performed twice generally over a period of 6 hours to confirm irreversibility of the condition. Brain death is legally accepted as death in several countries including India, and allows the family to consider organ donation.

REFERENCES

1. Loewenfeld IE, Lowenstein O. The Pupil: Anatomy, Physiology, and Clinical Applications. Detroit: Iowa State University Press, Ames and Wayne State University Press; 1993.
2. Hattar S, Liao HW, Takao M, et al. Melanopsin-containing retinal ganglion cells: architecture, projections, and intrinsic photosensitivity. Science. 2002;295:1065-70.
3. Kardon RH, Kirkali PA, Thompson HS. Automated pupil perimetry. Ophthalmology. 1991;98:485-95.
4. Thompson HS, Montague P, Cox TA, et al. The relationship between visual acuity, pupillary defect, and visual field loss. Am J Ophthalmol. 1982;93:681-8.
5. Papageorgiou E, Wermund T, Wilhelm H. Pupil perimetry demonstrates hemifield pupillary hypokinesia in a patient with a pretectal lesion causing a relative afferent pupil defect but no visual field loss. J Neuroophthalmol. 2009; 29(1):33.
6. Newman SA, Miller NR. The optic tract syndrome: neuro-ophthalmologic considerations. Arch Ophthalmol. 1983;101:1241-50.
7. Elliott D, Cunningham ET Jr, Miller SR. Fourth nerve paresis and ispilateral relative afferent pupillary defect without visual sensory disturbance: a sign of contralateral dorsal midbrain syndrome. J Clin Neuroophthalmol. 1991;11:169-72.
8. Sunderland S, Hughes ESR. The pupillo-constrictor pathway and the nerves to the ocular muscles in man. Brain. 1946;69:301-9.
9. Warwick R. The ocular parasympathetic nerve supply and its mesencephalic sources. J Anat. 1954;88:71-93.
10. Johnston JA, Parkinson D. Intracranial sympathetic pathways associated with the sixth cranial nerve. J Neurosurg. 1974; 39:236-43.
11. Jampel RS. Representation of the near-response on the cerebral cortex of the Macaque. Am J Ophthalmol. 1959;48(5):573-82.
12. Czarnecki JSC, Pilley SFJ, Thompson HS. The analysis of anisocoria. Can J Ophthalmol. 1979;14:297-302.
13. Wachler BSB, Krueger RR. Agreement and repeatibility of infrared pupillometry and the comparison method. Ophthalmology. 1999;106:319-23.
14. Kardon RH, Corbett JJ, Thompson HS. Segmental denervation and reinnervation of the iris sphincter as shown by infrared videographic transillumination. Ophthalmology. 1998;105:313-21.
15. Wilhelm H, Wilhelm B. Clinical applications of pupillography. J Neuroophthalmol. 2003;23(1):42-9.
16. Glazer-Hockstein C, Brucker AJ. The detection of a relative afferent pupillary defect. Am J Ophthalmol. 2002;134(1):142-3.
17. Ettinger ER, Wyatt HJ, London R. Anisocoria. Variation and clinical observation with different conditions of illumination and accommodation. Invest Ophthalmol Vis Sci. 1991;32(3):501-9.
18. Thompson HS. The pupil and accommodation. In: Lessels S, van Dalen JTW (Eds). Neuro-Ophthalmology. Amsterdam: Excerpta Medica; 1980. pp. 226-40.
19. Thompson HS. The pupil. In: Hart WM (Ed). Adler's Physiology of the Eye, 9th edition. St Louis: Mosby; 1992. pp. 412-41.
20. Sun F, Stark L. Pupillary escape intensified by large pupillary size. Vision Res. 1983;23:611-5.
21. Lowenstein O, Friedman ED. Pupillographic studies. Arch Ophthalmol. 1942;27:969-93.
22. Frank JW, Kushner BJ, France TD. Paradoxical pupillary phenomenon: A review of patients with pupillary constriction to darkness. Arch Ophthalmol. 1988;106:1564-6.
23. Pilley SFJ, Thompson HS. Pupillary "dilation lag" in Horner's syndrome. Br J Ophthalmol. 1975;59:731-5.
24. Smith SA, Smith SE. Bilateral Horner's syndrome: detection and occurrance. J Neurol Neurosurg Psychiatry. 1999;66(1): 48-51.
25. Digre KB. Principles and techniques of examination of the pupils, accommodation and lacrimation. In: Miller NR, Newman NJ (Eds). Walsh and Hoyt's Clinical Neuro-ophthalmology, 6th edition. Philadelphia: Lippincott Williams & Wilkins; 2005. pp. 715-37.
26. Thompson HS. Pupillary signs in the ophthalmologic diagnosis of optic nerve disease. Trans Ophthalmol Soc UK. 1976;96: 377-81.
27. Levatin P, Prasloski PF, Collen MF. The swinging flashlight test in multiphasic screening for eye disease. Can J Ophthalmol. 1973;8:356-60.
28. Bell RA, Waggoner PM, Boyd WM, et al. Clinical grading of relative afferent pupillary defects. Arch Ophthalmol. 1993;111(7):938-42.
29. Fineberg E, Thompson HS. Quantitation of the afferent pupillary defect. In: Smith JL (Ed). Neuro-ophthalmology Focus. New York: Masson Publishers; 1979. pp. 25-30.
30. Ramsay A, Williamson TH, Parks S, et al. Crossed polarising filters to measure relative afferent pupillary defects: reproducibility, correlation with neutral density filters and use in central retinal vein occlusion. Eye (Lond). 1995;9 (Pt 5):624-8.
31. McCormick A, Bhola R, Brown L, et al. Quantifying relative afferent pupillary defects using a Sbisa bar. Br J Ophthalmol. 2002;86(9): 985-7.
32. Volpe NJ, Plotkin ES, Maguire MG, et al. Portable pupillography of the swinging flashlight test to detect afferent pupillary defects. Ophthalmology. 2000;107(10):1913-21.
33. Thompson HS. 12th Pupil Colloquium. Am J Ophthalmol. 1981;92:435-6.
34. Wilhelm H, Peters T, Lüdtke H, et al. The prevalence of relative afferent pupillary defects in normal subjects. J Neuroophthalmol. 2007;27(4):263-7.

35. Miller SD, Thompson HS. Edge-light pupil cycle time. Br J Ophthalmol. 1978;62:495-500.
36. Bremner FD, Shallo-Hoffman J, Riordan-Eva P, et al. Comparing pupil function with visual function in patients with Leber's hereditary optic neuropathy. Invest Ophthalmol Vis Sci. 1999;40:2528-34.
37. Folk JC, Thompson HS, Han D, et al. Visual function abnormalities in central serous retinopathy. Arch Ophthalmol. 1984;102:1299-302.
38. Servais GE, Thompson HS, Hayreh SS. Relative afferent pupillary defect in central retinal vein occlusion. Ophthalmology. 1986;93:301-3.
39. DuBois LG, Sadun AA. Occlusion-induced contralateral afferent pupillary defect. Am J Ophthalmol. 1989;107:306-7.
40. Lam BL, Thompson HS. An anisocoria produces a small relative afferent pupillary defect in the eye with the smaller pupil. J Neuroophthalmol. 1999;19:153-9.
41. Portnoy JZ, Thompson HS, Lennarson L, et al. Pupillary defects in amblyopia. Am J Ophthalmol. 1983;96:609-14.
42. Miki A, Iijima A, Takagi M, et al. Pupillography of automated swinging flashlight test in amblyopia. Clin Ophthalmol. 2008;2(4):781-6.
43. Lam BL, Thompson HS. A unilateral cataract produces a relative afferent pupillary defect in the contralateral eye. Ophthalmology. 1990;97:334-7.
44. Bell RA, Thompson HS. Relative afferent pupillary defect in optic tract hemianopias. Am J Ophthalmol. 1978;85:538-40.
45. Kardon R, Kawasaki A, Miller NR. Origin of the relative afferent pupillary defect in optic tract lesions. Ophthalmology. 2006;113(8):1345-53.
46. Forman S, Behrens MM, Odel J, et al. Relative afferent pupillary defect with normal visual function. Arch Ophthalmol. 1990;108:1074-5.
47. Kawasaki A, Miller NR, Kardon R. Pupillographic investigation of the relative afferent pupillary defect associated with a midbrain lesion. Ophthalmology. 2010;117(1):175-9.
48. Loewenfeld IE, Rosskothen HD. Infrared pupil camera: a new method for mass screening and clinical use. Am J Ophthalmol. 1974;78:304-13.
49. Lam BL, Thompson HS, Walls RC. Effect of light on the prevalence of simple anisocoria. Ophthalmology. 1996;103(5):790-3.
50. Parsa CF, George ND, Hoyt CS, et al. Pharmacological reversal of ptosis in a patient with acquired Horner's syndrome and heterochromia. Br J Ophthalmol. 1998;82(9):1095.
51. Brown SM, Aouchiche R, Freedman KA. The utility of 0.5% apraclonidine in the diagnosis of Horner syndrome. Arch Ophthalmol. 2003;121:1201-3.
52. Krzizok T, Gräf M, Kraus S. Photo- and videographic determination of the dilatation deficit in differential diagnosis of Horner syndrome. Ophthalmologe. 1995;92(2):125-31.
53. Cooper-Knock J, Pepper I, Hodgson T, et al. Early diagnosis of Horner syndrome using topical apraclonidine. J Neuroophthalmol. 2011;31(3):214-6.
54. Danesh-Meyer HV, Savino P, Sergott R. The correlation of phenylephrine 1% with hydroxyamphetamine 1% in Horner's syndrome. Br J Ophthalmol. 2004;88:592-3.
55. Thompson HS. Adie's syndrome: some new observations. Trans Am Ophthalmol Soc. 1977;75:587-626.
56. Leavitt JA, Wayman LL, Hodge DO, et al. Pupillary response to four concentrations of pilocarpine in normal subjects: application to testing for Adie tonic pupil. Am J Ophthalmol. 2002;133(3):333-6.
57. Jacobson DM. A prospective evaluation of cholinergic supersensitivity of the iris sphincter in patients with Oculomotor nerve palsies. Am J Ophthalmol. 1994;118:377-83.
58. Lieberman JD, Pasquale MD, Garcia R. Use of admission Glasgow Coma Score, pupil size, and pupil reactivity to determine outcome for trauma patients. J Trauma. 2003;55(3):437-42.
59. Clusmann H, Schaller C, Schramm J. Fixed and dilated pupils after trauma, stroke, and previous intracranial surgery: management and outcome. J Neurol Neurosurg Psychiatry. 2001;71:175-81.
60. Sakas DE, Bullock MR, Teasdale GM. One-year outcome following craniotomy for traumatic hematoma in patients with fixed dilated pupils. J Neurosurg. 1995;82:961-5.
61. Wijdicks EF, Varelas PN, Gronseth GS, et al. Evidence-based guideline update: determining brain death in adults: report of the Quality Standards Subcommittee of the American Academy of Neurology. Neurology. 2010;74(23):1911-8.

CHAPTER

38 Evaluation of Blepharoptosis

Shubhra Goel

INTRODUCTION

Blepharoptosis ("blephron" meaning "eyelid" and "ptosis" meaning "fall") is a common and complex eyelid anomaly seen in both genders. Although often occurring as isolated age-related change, it may sometimes signal the presence of underlying neurological or other systemic disorders. The complexity of the eyelid anatomy and the need for precise and meticulous adjustments of the eyelid position make ptosis one of the most challenging disorders to correct. Meticulous management is dependent on eliciting thorough and detailed history and clinical evaluation. This chapter gives a summary of the applied anatomy of the upper eyelid, pathophysiology of common types of ptosis, and guidelines of evaluation and diagnosing a case of blepharoptosis.

APPLIED ANATOMY OF UPPER EYELID

Every surgeon treating ptosis should have a thorough knowledge of the upper eyelid anatomy and physiology. The important structures from anterior to posterior are: the skin/subcutaneous tissue, orbicularis muscle, orbital septum, anterior extension of orbital fat, levator aponeurosis, Müller's muscle, tarsus, and conjunctiva.

- *Skin*:
  - It is the outermost and thinnest layer measuring approximately 0.6–1 mm in thickness. It extends from the eyebrow region to the upper eyelid margin, with the upper lid crease defined by the septae-like extensions of the underlying anterior levator aponeurosis to the orbicularis and skin **(Fig. 1)**.
  - The lid crease typically rests at 7–8 mm in males and 8–12 mm in females. The presence of a prominent lid crease suggests good levator action.
  - The upper lid fold is the folded layer of skin, subcutaneous tissue, and orbicularis muscle that is normally draped over the upper lid crease and is best measured in primary gaze. Excessive upper lid fold is known as dermatochalasis **(Figs. 2A and B)**.

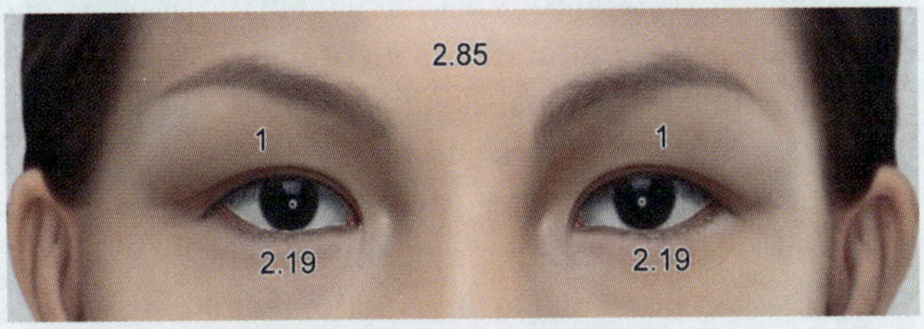

Fig. 1: Comparative measurements of periocular skin (in mm). Note the upper eyelid skin is the thinnest.

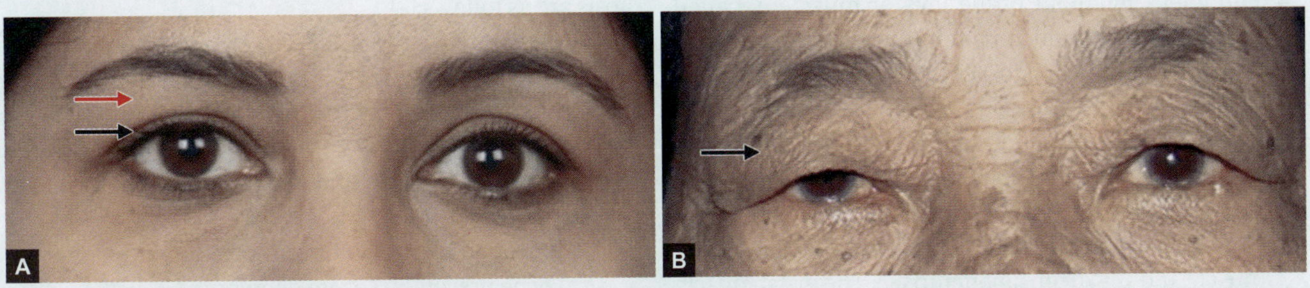

Figs. 2A and B: (A) The lid crease typically rests at 7–8 mm in males and 8–12 mm in females (black arrow). The upper lid fold is the folded layer of skin, subcutaneous tissue, and orbicularis muscle (red arrow); (B) Excessive upper lid fold known as dermatochalasis is seen as overhanging skin obscuring the visual axis (black arrow).

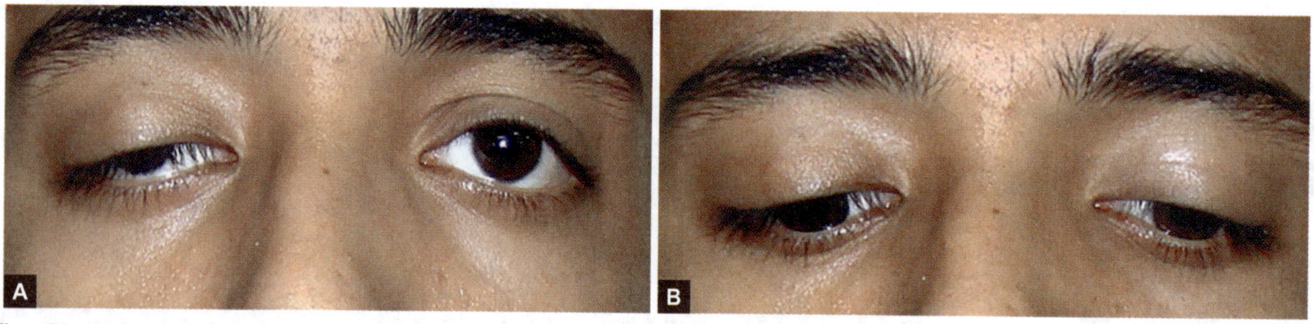

Figs. 3A and B: (A) Note the absent lid crease in the affected right upper lid; (B) Right upper lid ptosis reduces in severity (also known as lid lag) when asked to look downward, indicating a congenital type of ptosis.

- *Orbicularis oculi muscle*:
  - It is the second layer of the eyelid and is responsible for its closure and associated facial expressions.
  - The portion extending over the eyelid is the palpebral portion, and the muscle fibers overlying the orbit are called the orbital portion.
- *Orbital septum*:
  - It is a thin, translucent, white, and multilamellar fibrous layer that separates the orbit from the anterior eyelid.
  - A breach or attenuation of the orbital septum may lead to herniation of the anterior orbital fat, which manifests clinically as "puffy fat bags" in the eyelid.
  - It is an important landmark to be identified during levator surgery. Opening the orbital septum exposes the underlying preaponeurotic orbital fat, which directly overlies the levator palpebrae complex.
- *Orbital fat*:
  - Orbital fat is located between the orbital septum and the levator complex.
  - There are two pockets of orbital fat in the upper eyelid: medial, and central (preaponeurotic). Lateral fullness may indicate lacrimal gland prolapse.
- *Levator palpebrae superioris muscle*:
  - This retractor muscle complex of the upper eyelid has a muscular and aponeurotic component.
  - It lies superomedial to the superior rectus with which it shares a common sheath. Due to this common sheath, patients with congenital ptosis may have concurrent superior rectus muscle weakness.
  - The check ligament of the levator muscle is called Whitnall's ligament. It is identified as a white strip along the anterior surface of the levator muscle. The exposure of Whitnall's ligament is an important landmark, where the muscle changes to an anterior-posterior vector as it enters the orbit.
  - The total length of the levator muscle aponeurosis complex is approximately 55 mm in adults (36–40 mm muscle and 14–20 mm aponeurosis). The distal muscle and aponeurosis are the main areas of interest when performing levator surgery.
- *Müller's muscle*: It is a nonstriated upper eyelid retractor, which measures 10–12 mm long and 15 mm wide and is supplied by the sympathetic nervous system. The vascular loop overlying its surface is an important landmark while separating or dissecting along Müller's muscle.

CLASSIFICATION

In general, blepharoptosis can be classified under following categories:

- *Congenital*:
  - *Myogenic*: Levator dystrophy, myasthenia gravis, and blepharophimosis
  - *Neurogenic*: Congenital III nerve palsy, congenital Horner's syndrome, Marcus-Gunn jaw-winking ptosis.
- *Acquired*:
  - *Myogenic*: Myasthenia gravis, myotonic dystrophy, oculopharyngeal dystrophy, and chronic progressive external ophthalmoplegia (CPEO)
  - *Neurogenic*: III nerve palsy, Horner's syndrome
  - *Mechanical*: Lid masses, e.g. neurofibromatosis, tumors
  - *Traumatic*: Temporary (due to edema), or permanent (due to muscle or nerve damage)
  - Involutional (senile).
- Mixed
- Pseudoptosis.

Some of the key features of commonly encountered ptosis are as follows:

- *Congenital ptosis* ***(Figs. 3A and B)***:
  - Poor levator functions due to a dystrophic levator muscle, where muscle fibers are replaced by fat and fibrosis.
  - Present from birth, and may be unilateral or bilateral or asymmetric.
  - Associated elevated chin-up position or head posture may be present in severe degree.
  - Frontalis overaction, lid lag, and an absent or faint lid crease are also commonly seen.

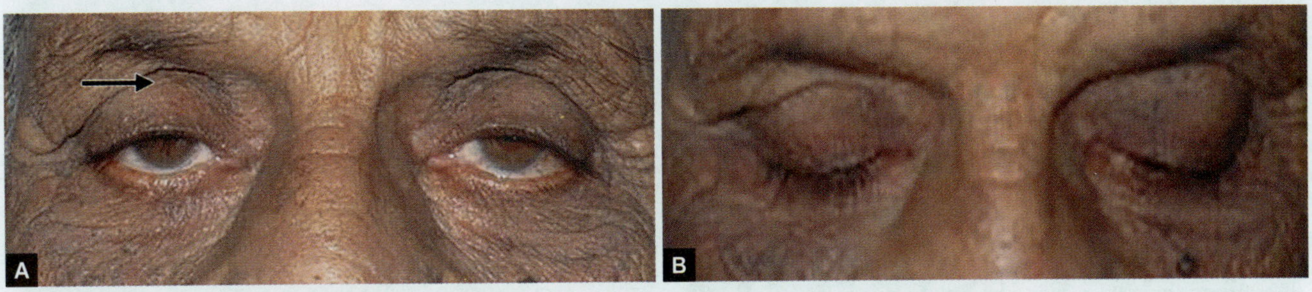

Figs. 4A and B: Right upper lid ptosis increases/worsens severity in downgaze, indicating involutional type of ptosis. Note the high riding lid crease in both upper eyelids (black arrow).

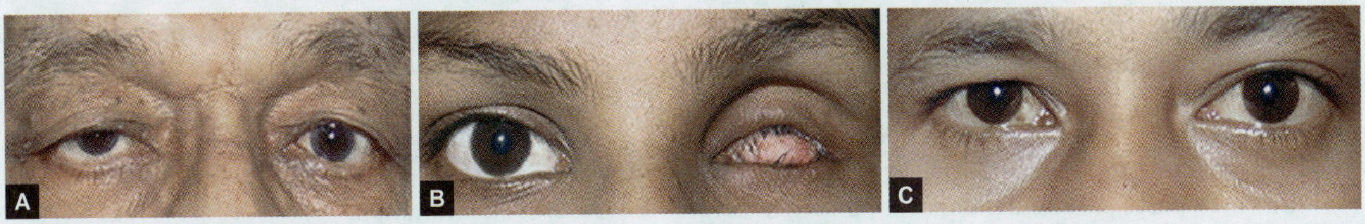

Figs. 5A to C: Different cases of pseudoptosis. (A) Right eye upper lid ptosis with dermatochalasis and brow ptosis; (B) Left upper lid ptosis due to ipsilateral enophthalmos; (C) Proptosis of left eye leading to appearance of right eyelid pseudoptosis.

- *Involutional or senile ptosis* ***(Figs. 4A and B)***:
  - Late onset of ptosis.
  - It is due to the disinsertion of the aponeurosis from the tarsus or attenuation of the aponeurosis from age-related changes.
  - Eyelid rubbing or stretching, repeated episodes of edema, or chronic ocular inflammation may similarly lead to stretching of the tissue or disinsertion/attenuation of the aponeurosis.
  - May be unilateral or bilateral, and symmetrical or asymmetrical.
  - The lid crease may be elevated, normal, or faintly seen. Ocular movements are usually normal. Associated brow ptosis, dermatochalasis, or orbital fat prolapse may be present.
- *Pseudoptosis* ***(Figs. 5A to C)***:
  - Causes include severe dermatochalasis, ipsilateral enophthalmos, contralateral exophthalmos, contralateral eyelid retraction, misdirected VII cranial nerve regeneration, oculofacial spasms, and globe malposition.
  - Hypotropia can also mimic ptosis.
- *Neurogenic ptosis*: Salient features of the most common causes of neurogenic ptosis are as follows:
  - *Horner's syndrome*:
    - Congenital or acquired
    - Unilateral
    - Nonprogressive
    - Mild ptosis
    - Good levator function
    - Normal ocular movements
    - Miotic pupil on the ptotic side, brisk constriction of pupil
    - Iris heterochromia on affected side (if congenital)
    - Lower lid ptosis may also be seen
    - Facial ipsilateral anhydrosis.
  - *Myasthenia gravis*:
    - Congenital, juvenile, or adult
    - Sudden onset
    - Variable ptosis
    - Diurnal variation
    - Associated diplopia
    - Associated intermittent phoria or tropia
    - Good to poor levator function
    - Fatigability test usually positive
    - Cogan's lid twitch
    - Decreased speed of levator excursion
    - Decreased orbicularis oculi tone
    - Asymmetrical extraocular movements (EOMs) limitation
    - Positive ice test, in which placement of ice on the ptotic lid elevates the position temporarily.
  - *Chronic progressive external ophthalmoplegia*:
    - Usually seen in young patients
    - Congenital or acquired
    - Progressive
    - Bilateral and symmetrical
    - Severe ptosis in later stages
    - Chin elevation
    - Poor levator action
    - Limited ocular movements in all gazes.

Consider retinal and cardiac abnormalities.

EVALUATION OF PTOSIS

- *History taking*: To distinguish the different types of blepharoptosis, a detailed history of the patient's symptoms must be elicited, including age of onset of symptoms, variation, and progression. The functional significance of the ptosis (i.e. interference with normal daily activities such as driving, reading) should also be documented.

- *Clinical approach for a patient presenting with ptosis*:
  - *Is it really ptosis?*: It is essential to differentiate ptosis from pseudoptosis.
  - *Age of presentation*:
    - In congenital ptosis, the age of onset is shortly after birth.
    - Chronic progressive external ophthalmoplegia is a slowly progressive paralysis of the extraocular muscles in early adulthood.
    - Myasthenia gravis can present at any age, even though it is commonly seen in middle-aged women.
    - Aponeurotic ptosis is seen in older patients. Ptosis due to III nerve palsy and trauma may present at any age.
  - *Laterality*:
    - *Unilateral*:
      - Congenital
      - Aponeurotic
      - III nerve palsy
      - Horner's syndrome
      - Trauma.
    - *Bilateral*:
      - Congenital
      - Aponeurotic
      - Chronic progressive external ophthalmoplegia
      - Myotonic dystrophy
      - Myasthenia gravis
      - Oculopharyngeal dystrophy.
  - *History of progression in the degree of ptosis*:
    - The severity of ptosis is usually of sudden onset and remains the same in congenital ptosis and Horner's syndrome.
    - Progressive worsening is seen in aponeurotic ptosis, oculopharyngeal dystrophy, and CPEO.
    - Fluctuating degrees of ptosis is seen most notably in myasthenia gravis, although sudden onset may also be reported.
  - *External examination*:
    - Abnormal head postures (head tilt, chin-up position), abnormal facies, and jaw-winking **(Figs. 6A to C)**.
    - Patient with ptosis often adopt abnormal head positions, commonly a chin elevation in order to clear the visual axis.
    - An abnormal head tilt may be seen in cases of superior rectus muscle weakness.

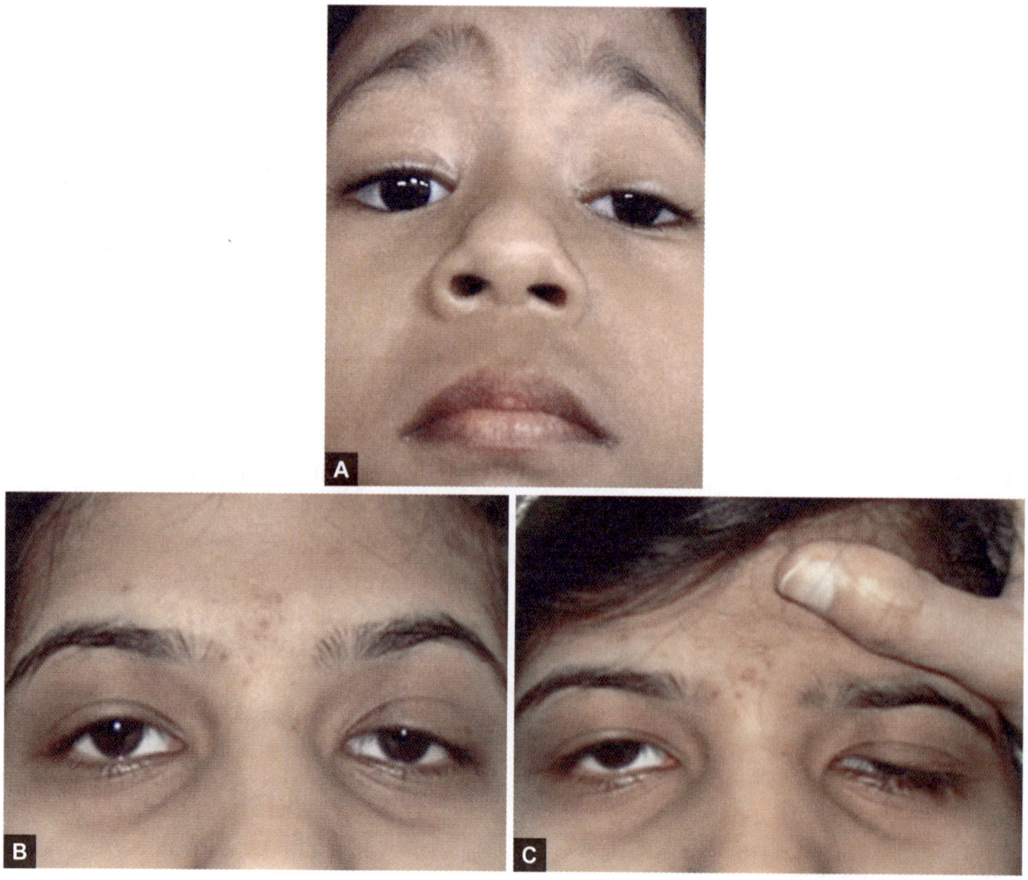

Figs. 6A to C: (A) Compensatory head elevation in a child to clear the visual axis which is obscured due to severe bilateral ptosis; (B) Left upper lid moderate amount of ptosis with obvious frontalis overaction; (C) Note the increase in ptosis once the frontalis action is negated by Berke's method.

- In severe cases, in addition to an elevated chin, the patient may compensate with the frontalis muscle to increase the visual field. Frontalis overaction can be easily identified by the elevated brows and horizontal wrinkling of the forehead.
- An associated strabismus may also lead to abnormal positions in order to maintain binocular single vision.
- *Skin scars* **(Fig. 7)**: Skin scars within the eyelid or surrounding periorbital and adnexal tissue may suggest a past surgery or trauma which could have caused the ptosis.

– *What should be evaluated in the ocular examination?*:
- *Visual acuity*:
  - The visual acuity must be documented for every patient.
  - Young children with ptosis must undergo cycloplegic refraction.
- *Pupillary evaluation*:
  - An ipsilateral miotic pupil is seen in Horner's syndrome.
  - Widely dilated, nonreactive pupil in cranial nerve III palsy.
  - A sluggish and ill-sustained pupillary reaction may be an indirect evidence of dense amblyopia.
- *Cover-uncover test*: A thorough strabismic evaluation may be helpful in all ptosis cases. As mentioned earlier, hypotropia can be mistaken for ptosis. On covering the contralateral eye, the previously hypotropic eye takes up fixation and the eyelid returns to the normal position. Intermittent phoria or tropia can also be an indicator of underlying myasthenia gravis.
- *Bell's phenomenon and corneal sensitivity*: Bell's phenomenon is the upward rolling of the eyeball on forceful closure of the lids against resistance. This would indicate that the globe would achieve lubrication if lagophthalmos occurred following surgery.

  To check for Bell's phenomenon:
  - Sit at the patient's eye level
  - Ask the patient to forcefully close the eyes
  - Try to open the eyelids with index fingers resting on the upper eyelid
  - Look for upward rolling of the eyeball.

  A weak or absent Bell's phenomenon would be a relative contraindication for corrective lid surgery. Poor corneal sensation would also carry a risk of exposure complications following surgery.
- *Dry eye evaluation*:
  - A detailed dry eye workup, including Schirmer tear secretion or measurement of the tear meniscus height, may be valuable if the history or the examination suggests baseline dry eyes.

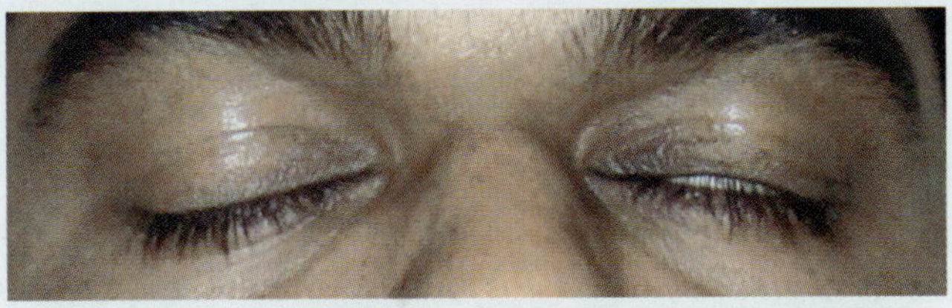

Fig. 7: Subtle scar on the left lid with lagophthalmos indicating a previous ptosis surgery.

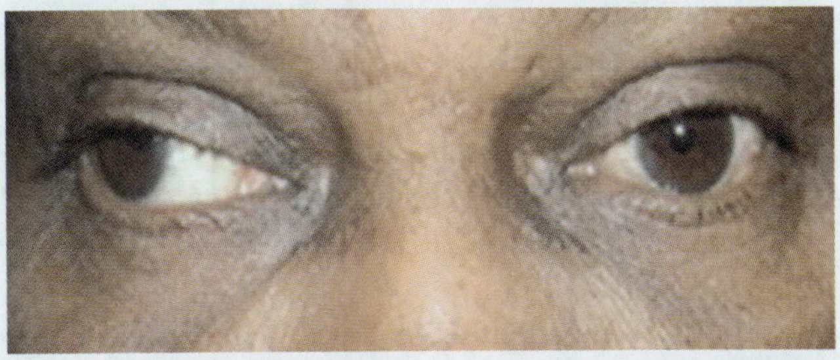

Fig. 8: Right eye exotropia. Limited movements due to right third nerve palsy.

  In older patients with marked reduction in tears, an undercorrection of the ptosis may well be indicated.
- *Ocular motility*:
  - Observe EOMs by having the patient look in all directions of gaze without moving the head. The ptotic eyelid should not be elevated by the physician while eliciting ocular motility, as this could lead to inaccurate interpretations.
  - Elevation limitation suggests superior rectus weakness seen in congenital ptosis.
  - Note the change in the degree of ptosis in association with EOMs. For example, increase in the severity of ptosis on downgaze is seen in involutional ptosis, whereas a decrease in severity of the ptosis on downgaze (i.e. lid lag) would make congenital ptosis a more likely diagnosis **(Figs. 3 and 4)**.
  - A generalized limitation in the actions of all extraocular muscles is seen in CPEO.
  - Unusual lid movements associated with ocular motility may suggest aberrant nerve regeneration.
  - In III nerve palsies, abduction is preserved, which helps confirm the diagnosis **(Fig. 8)**.
  - Myasthenia gravis should always be considered as it can present with varied ocular motility limitation.

– *What does the ptosis evaluation include?*:

A detailed examination of the ptotic eyelid would encompass the following signs:
- Margin-reflex distance (MRD)
- Palpebral fissure height (PFH) and symmetry
- Levator function
- Margin crease distance (MCD)
- Downgaze ptosis

- Hering's effect
- Brow position and dermatochalasis
- Frontalis muscle overaction
- Lagophthalmos
- Associated lid signs.
- *Margin-reflex distance*: MRD is the position of the eyelid and hence describes the degree of ptosis. It is one of the most important parameters when considering ptosis surgery. MRD1 is the distance in millimeters between the central upper lid margin and the corneal light reflex in primary gaze. MRD2 measures the distance between the central lower lid margin and the corneal light reflex. Adding both together: MRD1 + MRD2 = PFH **(Fig. 9)**. To measure the MRD:
  - Ask the patient to gently close and open the eye to relax the frontalis muscle, or negate the frontalis action by placing the thumb over the brow to immobilize it at the superior orbital rim.
  - Sit at the patient's eye level and ask the patient to look straight ahead at a distant target.
  - Hold a pen light directly in front of the patient to see the corneal reflex.
  - Measure the MRD with a millimeter scale, with 0 mm indicating the lid is located at the horizontal midpupil.
  - If the lid covers the reflex, keep the scale at the central lid, elevate the lid until the corneal reflex is seen, and measure the negative distance.

  A normal MRD is 4–4.5 mm. Measuring the MRD not only help quantify the severity of ptosis, but also helps guide the appropriate management plan for each case.

  The amount of ptosis is the difference between the MRD1 of two eyes in unilateral cases.

  The difference between the measured and the normal values gives an indication of the amount of ptosis in bilateral ptosis.

  Quantitatively, on the basis of MRD, ptosis can be classified as:
  - Mild ptosis—2 mm or less
  - Moderate ptosis—3 mm
  - Severe ptosis—4 mm or more.

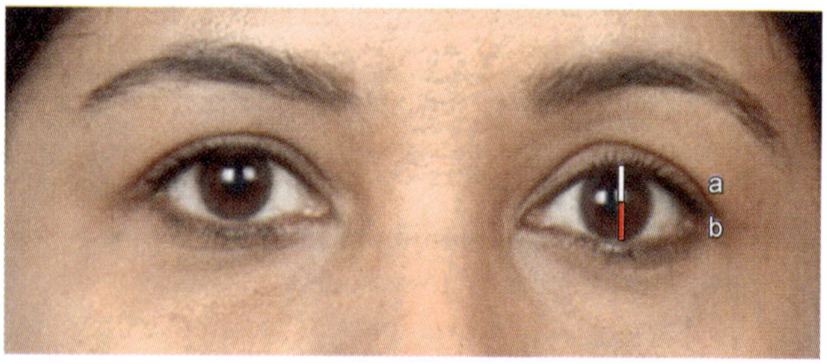

Fig. 9: White arrow—margin-reflex distance 1 (MRD1) and red arrow—MRD2. MRD1 (a) + MRD2 (b) = Palpebral fissure height.

- *Palpebral fissure height*: PFH is the vertical distance between the upper and lower lid in the pupillary plane. The normal human corneal diameter is 11 mm and the superior 1–2 mm of the cornea is normally covered by lid, therefore the normal PFH is approximately 9 mm.

  To measure PFH:
  - Follow the initial steps as for MRD
  - Place the millimeter scale at the pupillary plane
  - Measure the distance between upper and lower lid margin
  - Measure in primary, down-, and upgazes.

  Normal PFH in primary gaze is 9 mm on average (males: 7–10 mm, females: 8–12 mm).
- *Levator function* ***(Figs. 10A to C)***: Testing the levator function is important to understand the strength or health of the primary elevator muscle of the upper lid. It is assessed by the speed and amount of eyelid excursion. Berke's method of assessing levator function is as follows:
  - Follow the initial steps as for MRD
  - Negate the frontalis muscle action by pressing thumb over brow ensuring that there is no upward or downward push
  - Ask the patient to look down maximally
  - With the other hand, place the millimeter ruler with a marking resting on the lid margin in downgaze

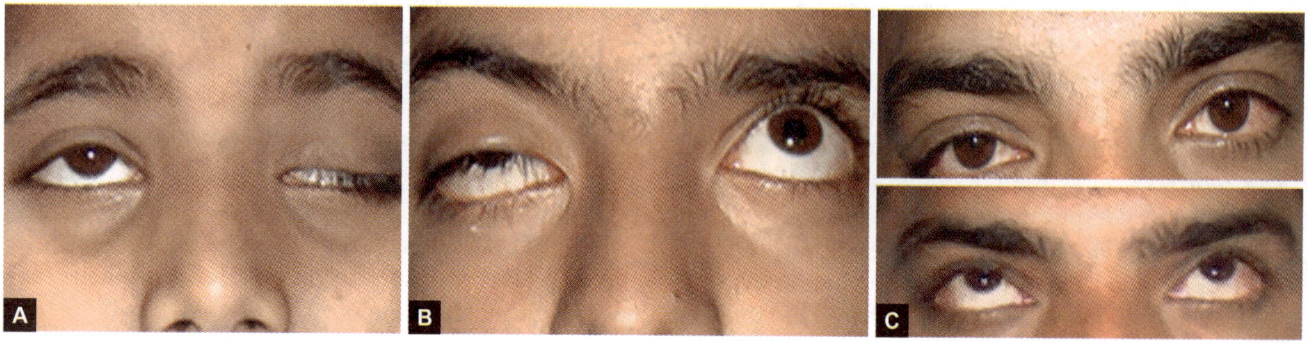

Figs. 10A to C: (A) Left eye severe ptosis with poor levator excursion; (B) Right eye moderate ptosis with fair levator excursion; (C) Right eye mild ptosis with excellent levator excursion.

- Ask the patient to look up to the ceiling while holding the ruler in position
- Measure the amount of vertical excursion of the lid
- The speed of excursion should also be examined.

Normal levator function is 15 mm or greater.

A difference between the measured and the normal levator function guides the surgical plan.

The classification of levator function is shown in **Table 1**.

- *Margin crease distance*: It measures the distance between the upper lid margin and the eyelid crease. The eyelid crease may help in the diagnosis of some types of ptosis, and is an esthetically crucial landmark for placement of the incision in ptosis surgery. The MCD is measured as follows:
  - Ask the patient to look down
  - Line up the millimeter scale at the central lid margin
  - Measure the distance between the lid margin and the most prominent skin crease
  - Measure the MCD on the opposite side for comparison
  - If there is a faint crease, accentuate its location by lifting the lid margin gently with a cotton tip or finger, and observe where are the skin folds.

  The normal MCD in males is 6–8 mm, and 8–12 mm in females.

  An abnormally elevated or asymmetric MCD should alert the physician to the presence of underlying levator disinsertion and involutional ptosis.
- *Downgaze ptosis*:
  - It is important to note the relative position of the eyelids in downgaze or reading position.
  - In severe involutional ptosis, the eyelids commonly block most of the pupils in downgaze. In another variant of involutional ptosis, the patient may have minimal ptosis in primary gaze, but exhibits severe ptosis in downgaze.
  - In levator maldevelopment ptosis, the fibrotic levator muscle prevents full downward excursion of the eyelid. This retraction in downgaze is referred to as lid lag and is a helpful sign of congenital ptosis.
- *Hering's effect*: In cases of unilateral ptosis or asymmetric ptosis, presence or absence of a Hering's effect masking a bilateral ptosis should be determined. This is done by elevating the more ptotic upper lid manually or with 2.5% phenylephrine topically **(Figs. 11A to C)**. When the more ptotic eyelid is elevated, the contralateral lid will sometimes droop more substantially. A prominent Hering's effect would indicate the need to perform bilateral ptosis correction in order to avoid contralateral ptosis postoperatively. The phenylephrine test is also helpful in predicting the result of conjunctival Müllerectomy.
- *Associated lid signs*:
  - Lid lag—the ptotic lid remains at a higher level than normal when looking down, due to failure of a fibrotic or maldeveloped levator muscle to relax in downgaze.
  - Fatigability—progressive increase in degree of ptosis of upper lid on constant focusing or inability to look upward without the eyelids gradually falling down. Ask the patient to look up without blinking at your finger for 30 seconds to observe if the elevated lid position can be sustained without dropping.
  - Cogan's lid twitch—overshoot of upper lid on rapid saccade from down to primary gaze. Ask the patient to look at your finger for several seconds in downgaze and then ask him to fixate at an object in primary gaze. Look for the lid overshooting to a higher position before settling into the normal MRD.
  - Orbicularis oculi tone—ask the patient to close the eyes forcefully and try to open them against resistance. In individuals with normal orbicularis tone, the examiner should not be able to open the lids. Ask the patient to close eyes gently. In

Table 1: The levator function.

Levator function (mm)	*Classification*
10–15	Excellent (normal)
>8	Good
5–7	Fair
<4	Poor

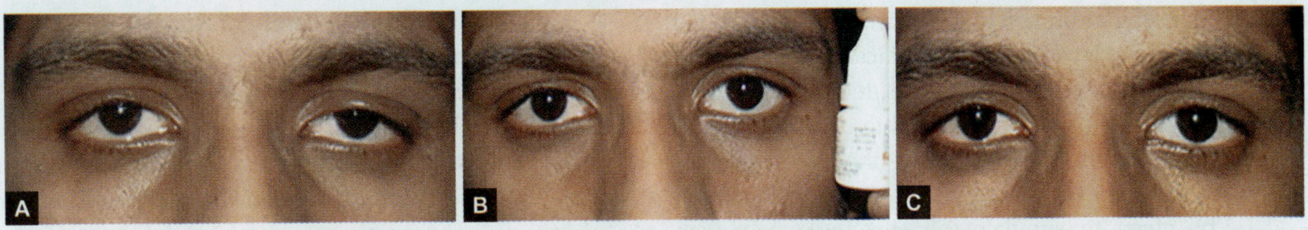

Figs. 11A to C: (A) Left upper lid mild ptosis before 2.5% phenylephrine installation; (B and C) Left improvement in ptosis after 2.5% phenylephrine installation.

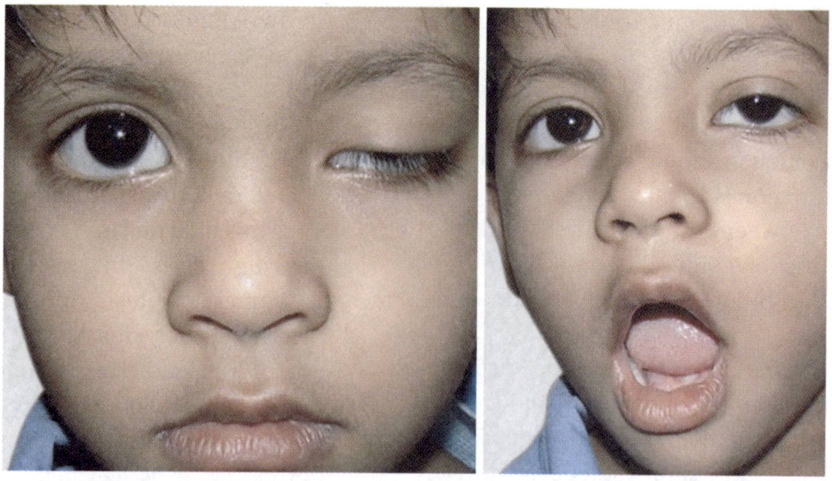

Fig. 12: Left eye severe ptosis with moderate Marcus-Gunn jaw-winking.

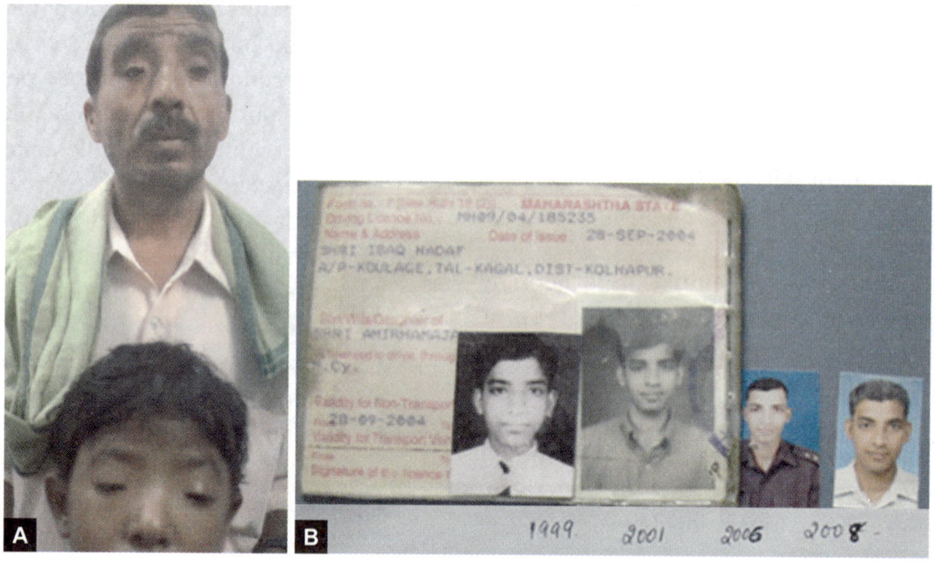

Figs. 13A and B: (A) Father and son with blepharophimosis syndrome; (B) Serial pictures of almost 10 years to note the progression and onset of the ptosis.

eyes with weak orbicularis tone, the lids may close very slowly, or the eyes may be seen through the open lids (lagophthalmos).

- Seesaw ptosis—manually lift the ptotic lid and look for droop of the contralateral eyelid. This is due to Hering's law of equal innervation, in which increased innervation to lift the ptotic lid also concurrently elevates the opposite lid leading to its retraction.
- Marcus-Gunn jaw-winking—this is a synkinetic movement that occurs due to misdirection of the mandibular branch of the trigeminal nerve to the ipsilateral levator muscle. Clinically, the upper lid elevates on wide opening or sideways movement of the mouth. Ask the patient to open the mouth wide, say the syllable "aa", or move the jaw side-to-side. In children, biscuits or chocolates can be given to simulate the chewing mechanism **(Fig. 12)**.

ANCILLARY WORKUP

- *A dilated fundus examination* is necessary prior to surgery.
- *Family photographs* **(Figs. 13A and B)** may help demonstrate the onset and progression of ptosis and also to document similar findings in family members.
- *Visual fields* are performed to document the visual fields with the lids in ptotic position, and again with the lids taped up to simulate the corrected position. The difference in improvement between the two visual fields is calculated. Insurance companies may often require this documentation.
- *Preoperative photo documentation* **(Figs. 14A to C)** should be made. Current photographs taken in primary, up- and downgazes document the ptosis severity and are helpful for comparison following surgery. Side view photos also document any associated brow ptosis or temporal skin hooding over the lid margin.

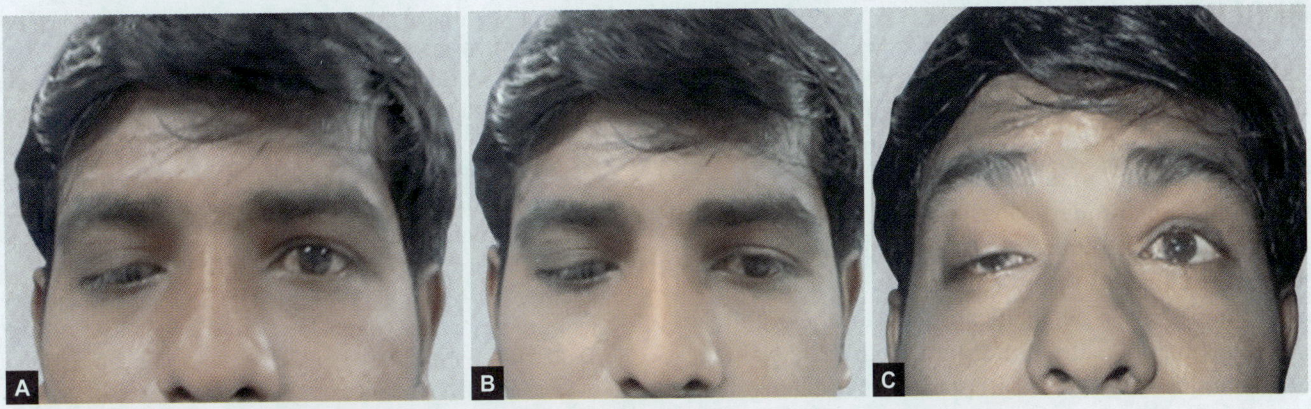

Figs. 14A to C: Ptosis photography. (A) Primary gaze; (B) Downgaze; (C) Upgaze.

Box 1: List of indications for imaging in a case of ptosis.

- History not consistent and onset not clear
- Suspected multiple sclerosis
- Other neurologic findings along with ptosis, such as nerve palsies
- New-onset diplopia or limited motility
- Orbital wall fracture suspected with history of trauma
- *Visible or palpable lid mass*: Edema, abscess, erythema, and pain
- Orbital tumors (e.g. lymphoma, leukemia, and rhabdomyosarcoma) suspected
- New onset of Horner's syndrome with or without other neurologic findings
- New onset of third cranial nerve palsy with or without other neurologic findings
- Globe displacement with either enophthalmos or proptosis
- Chest CT to locate a thymoma in case myasthenia gravis is suspected

- *Ice test* is a simple office procedure that may help confirm the diagnosis of myasthenia gravis. An icepack is placed over the closed eyelids of the affected side for 2–5 minutes (usually 2 minutes for ptosis and 5 minutes for ophthalmoparesis). The degree of ptosis should be measured before and immediately after the ice test. Although there are no strict guidelines regarding the interpretation of this test, the test is usually considered positive when the upper eyelid elevates by 2 mm or more following the application of ice. Sensitivity and specificity of this test have been reported as 76.9% and 98.3%, respectively.
- *Imaging modalities* are not routinely required in most patients with ptosis. However, if indicated, CT and MRI of the orbits and brain allow precise localization of compressive lesions that cause oculomotor nerve palsies and impairment of sympathetic input. An emergent CT angiography of brain, or MRI/MR angiogram is necessary when ptosis is accompanied by other signs of third nerve palsy and pupillary involvement **(Box 1)**.
- *Counseling*: Risks and benefits of corrective surgery should be discussed thoroughly with the patient. Potential risks of surgery include lagophthalmos, lid lag, corneal exposure leading to corneal ulcer, lid contour abnormality, infection, conjunctival prolapse, ptosis, hemorrhage, and loss of vision. Patients must be counseled regarding the possibility of undercorrection, overcorrection, and the need for additional surgery. Preoperative informed consent should be signed.

Flowchart 1: Algorithm for ptosis management based on type.

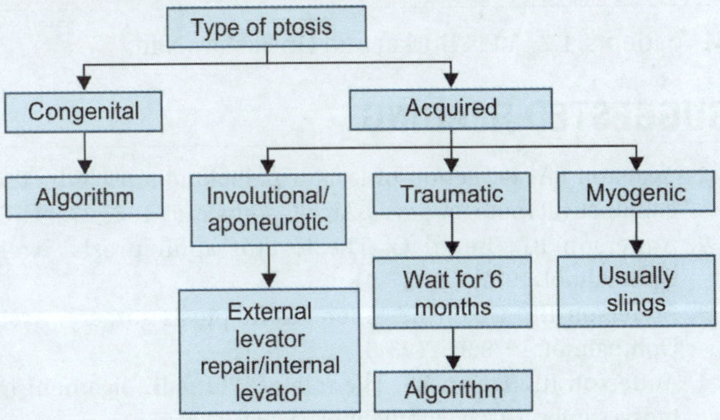

Flowchart 2: Algorithm for ptosis management based on degree.

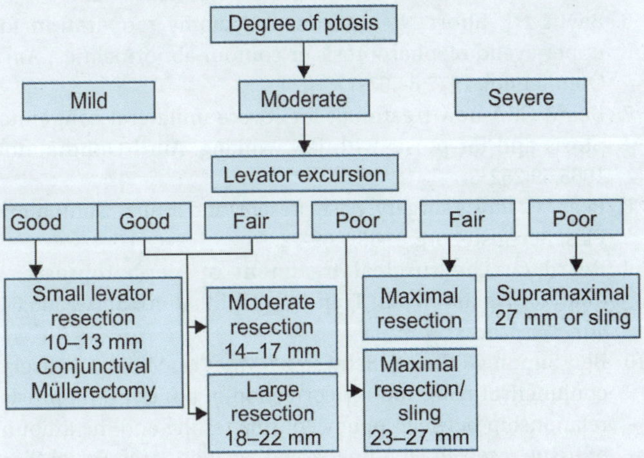

MANAGEMENT

Based on the initial evaluation as per the abovementioned parameters, a basic algorithm can be followed in management of any kind of blepharoptosis **(Flowcharts 1 and 2)**.

CONCLUSION

Blepharoptosis may impair normal visual development in children, and become visually significant to limit normal activities in adults. The etiologies of the various ptosis types and how they manifest differently are important to understand prior to undertaking surgery. Careful assessment, patient selection, and thorough preoperative evaluation are necessary to choose the most appropriate surgical plan. The surgeon must have a detailed knowledge of the eyelid and periorbital anatomy, and understand both the advantages and limitations of each surgical approach in order to provide the patient the best possible outcome.

ACKNOWLEDGMENTS

My patients, Dr Cat N Burkat and Dr Akshay Nair.

SUGGESTED READING

1. Agatston SA. Resection of levator palpebrae muscle by the conjunctival route for ptosis. Arch Ophthalmol. 1942;27:994-6.
2. Anderson RL, Beard C. The levator aponeurosis. Arch Ophthalmol. 1977;95:1437-41.
3. Anderson RL, Dixon RS. Aponeurotic ptosis surgery. Arch Ophthalmol. 1979;97:1123-8.
4. Anderson RL, Dixon RS. The role of Whitnall's ligament in ptosis surgery. Arch Ophthalmol. 1979;97:705-7.
5. Anderson RL, Jordan DR, Dutton JJ. Whitnall's sling for poor function ptosis. Arch Ophthalmol. 1990;108:1628-32.
6. Baylis HI, Shorr N. Anterior tarsectomy reoperation for upper eyelid blepharoptosis or contour abnormalities. Am J Ophthalmol. 1977;84:67-71.
7. Beard C. A new treatment for severe unilateral congenital ptosis and for ptosis with jaw winking. Am J Ophthalmol. 1965;59:252-8.
8. Beard C. Ptosis surgery: past, present, and future. Ophthalmic Plast Reconstr Surg. 1985;1:69-72.
9. Beard C. The surgical treatment of blepharoptosis: a quantitative approach. Trans Am Ophthalmol Soc. 1966;64: 401-87.
10. Ben Simon GJ, Lee S, Schwarcz RM, et al. Müller's muscle-conjunctival resection for correction of upper eyelid ptosis: relationship between phenylephrine testing and the amount of tissue resected with final eyelid position. Arch Facial Plast Surg. 2007;9:413-7.
11. Ben Simon GJ, Macedo AA, Schwarcz RM, et al. Frontalis suspension for upper eyelid ptosis: evaluation of different surgical designs and suture material. Am J Ophthalmol. 2005;140:877-85.
12. Berke RN, Wadsworth JA. Histology of levator muscle in congenital and acquired ptosis. Arch Ophthalmol. 1955;53: 413-28.
13. Berke RN. A simplified Blascovics operation for blepharoptosis: results in ninety-one operations. Arch Ophthalmol. 1952;48:460-95.
14. Berke RN. Results of resection of the levator muscle through a skin incision in congenital ptosis. AMA Arch Ophthalmol. 1959;61(2):177-201.
15. Berke RN. Surgical treatment of congenital ptosis. Pacif Med Surg. 1967;75:383-8.
16. Callahan A. Correction of unilateral blepharoptosis with bilateral eyelid suspension. Am J Ophthalmol. 1972;74:321-6.
17. Callahan MA, Beard C. Beard's Ptosis, 4th edition. Birmingham: Aesculapius Publishing Co.; 1990.
18. Carter SR, Meecham WJ, Seiff SR. Silicone frontalis slings for the correction of blepharoptosis: indications and efficacy. Ophthalmology. 1996;103:623-30.
19. Crawford JS. Repair of ptosis using frontalis muscle and fascia lata. Trans Am Acad Ophthalmol Otolaryngol. 1956;60:672-8.
20. Dailey RA, Wilson DJ, Wobig JL. Trans-conjunctival frontalis suspension. Ophthalmic Plast Reconstr Surg. 1991;7:284-97.
21. DeMartelaere SL, Blaydon SM, Cruz AA, et al. Broad fascia fixation enhances frontalis suspension. Ophthalmic Plast Reconstr Surg. 2007;23:279-84.
22. Dortzbach RK, Gausas RA, Sherman DD. Blepharoptosis. In: Dortzbach RK (Ed). Ophthalmic Plastic Surgery: Prevention and Management of Complications. New York: Raven Press; 1994.
23. Dortzbach RK, Kronish JW. Early revision in the office for adults after unsatisfactory blepharoptosis correction. Am J Ophthalmol. 1993;115:68-75.
24. Dortzbach RK, Sutula FC. Involutional blepharoptosis: a histopathologic study. Arch Ophthalmol. 1980;98:2045-9.
25. Dresner SC. Further modifications of the Müller's muscle-conjunctival resection procedure for blepharoptosis. Ophthal Plast Reconstr Surg. 1991;7:114-22.
26. Epstein GA, Putterman AM. Super-maximum levator resection for severe unilateral congenital blepharoptosis. Ophthalmic Surg. 1984;15:971-9.
27. Esmaili B, Chung H, Pashby RC. Long-term results of frontalis suspension using irradiated, banked fascia lata. Ophthalmic Plast Reconstr Surg. 1998;14:159-63.
28. Fasanella RM, Servat J. Levator resection for minimal ptosis: another simplified option. Arch Ophthalmol. 1961;65:493-6.
29. Fox SA. Congenital ptosis frontalis sling. J Pediatr Ophthalmol. 1966;3:28.
30. Frueh BR, Musch DC, McDonald HM. Efficacy and efficiency of a small-incision, minimal dissection procedure versus a traditional approach for correcting aponeurotic ptosis. Ophthalmology. 2004;111:2158-63.
31. Frueh BR. The mechanistic classification of ptosis. Ophthalmology. 1980;87:1019-21.
32. Hersh D, Martin FJ, Rowe N. Comparison of silastic and banked fascia lata in pediatric frontalis suspension. J Pediatr Ophthalmol Strabismus. 2006;43:212-8.
33. Holds JB, McLeish WM, Anderson RL. Whitnall's sling with superior tarsectomy for the correction of severe unilateral blepharoptosis. Arch Ophthalmol. 1993;111:1285-91.
34. Jones LT, Quickert MH, Wobig JL. The cure of ptosis by aponeurotic repair. Arch Ophthalmol. 1975;93:629-34.
35. Jones LT. The anatomy of the upper eyelid and its relation to ptosis surgery. Am J Ophthalmol. 1964;57:943-59.
36. Kersten RC, Bernardini FP, Khouri L, et al. Unilateral frontalis sling for the surgical correction of unilateral poor-function ptosis. Ophthalmic Plast Reconstr Surg. 2005;6:412-6.
37. Khwarg SI, Tarbet KJ, Dortzbach RK, et al. Management of moderate-to-severe Marcus-Gunn jaw-winking ptosis. Ophthalmology. 1999;106:1191-6.

38. Lemke BN, Lucarelli MJ. Anatomy of the ocular adnexa, orbit, and related facial structures. In: Nesi FA, Lisman RD, Levine MR (Eds). Smith's Ophthalmic Plastic and Reconstructive Surgery, 2nd edition. Philadelphia: Mosby; 1997. pp. 3-78.
39. Leone CR, Shore JW, Van Gemert JV. Silicone rod frontalis sling for the correction of blepharoptosis. Ophthalmic Surg. 1981;12:881-7.
40. Lucarelli MJ, Lemke BN. Small incision external levator repair: technique and early results. Am J Ophthalmol. 1999;127: 637-44.
41. Mauriello JA, Abdelsalam A. Effectiveness of homologous cadaveric fascia lata and role of suture fixation to tarsus in frontalis suspension. Ophthalmic Plast Reconstr Surg. 1998;14:99-104.
42. Meyer DR, Linberg JV, Powell SR, et al. Quantitating the superior visual field loss associated with ptosis. Arch Ophthalmol. 1989;107:840-3.
43. Naugle TC, Fry CL, Sabatier RE, et al. High leg incision fascia lata harvesting. Ophthalmology. 1997;104:1480-8.
44. O'Reilly J, Lanigan B, Bowell R, et al. Congenital ptosis: long-term results using stored fascia lata. Acta Ophthalmol Scand. 1998;76:346-8.
45. Paris GL, Quickert MH. Disinsertion of the aponeurosis of the levator palpebrae superioris muscle after cataract extraction. Am J Ophthalmol. 1976;81:337-40.
46. Patipa M. Visual field loss in primary gaze and reading gaze due to acquired blepharoptosis and visual field improvement following ptosis surgery. Arch Ophthalmol. 1992;110: 63-7.
47. Putterman AM, Fett DR. Müller's muscle in the treatment of upper eyelid ptosis: a ten-year study. Ophthalmic Surg. 1986;17(6):354-60.
48. Putterman AM, Urist MJ. Müller muscle-conjunctiva resection. Technique for treatment of blepharoptosis. Arch Ophthalmol. 1975;93:619-23.
49. Rose JG, Lemke BN, Dresner SC, et al. Blepharoptosis treatment options during upper eyelid cosmetic blepharoplasty. Am J Cosm Surg. 2003;20:73-82.
50. Stasior GO, Lemke BN, Wallow IH, et al. Levator aponeurosis elastic fiber network. Ophthalmic Plast Reconstr Surg. 1993;9:1-10.
51. Wasserman BN, Sprunger DT, Helveston EM. Comparison of materials used in frontalis suspension. Arch Ophthalmol. 2001;119:687-91.

CHAPTER

39

Cerebral Angiography in Neuro-ophthalmology

Hima Pendharkar

INTRODUCTION

Wilhelm Conrad Roentgen's discovery of X-rays in 1895 revolutionized the world of medicine. The history of angiography, which is the fluoroscopic visualization of the vascular system—arterial or venous—by the introduction of contrast medium, dates back to 1927 when Egas Moniz pioneered cerebral angiography. By the early 1950s, crude fluoroscopy was available for clinical use and two simultaneous developments gave added impetus to the refinement of diagnostic angiography. In 1952, the first synthetic vascular bypass graft was placed and in 1953 Seldinger described the use of a hollow-bore needle and guidewire system for accessing the femoral artery. Dotter percutaneously dilated a tight localized stenosis of the superficial femoral artery and thus on 16th January 1964, a new specialty was born which was formally named as "interventional radiology" by Alexander Margulis.

A thorough clinical evaluation of a patient presenting with symptoms referable to the ophthalmic system is indispensable to arrive at differential diagnoses. Cross-sectional imaging with either CT and/or MRI with dedicated protocols is then performed to localize the lesion. Contrast administration is essential for complete evaluation of the lesion. Vascular lesions form a significant part of the spectrum of lesions identified on cross-sectional imaging. CT angiogram or MR angiogram are noninvasive modalities that help characterize the lesions well. However, the role of cerebral angiography (CA) remains indispensable in certain cases. With the advent of endovascular techniques, many lesions of this spectrum can be treated completely. CA is an invasive procedure and needs careful patient selection, though the risk is significantly reduced in experienced hands. A biplane catheterization laboratory is the standard of operation presently; the importance of an equally competent radiologist to perform the procedures cannot be overlooked. The aftercare of patients plays an equally important role in obtaining good results.

INDICATIONS FOR CEREBRAL ANGIOGRAPHY

In the present times with state of art CT machines for noninvasive angiograms, the indications for a diagnostic CA are limited and include:

- To assess the hemodynamics of a given lesion.
- To study the angio-architecture of various fistulous lesions such as carotico-cavernous fistula (CCF), pail arteriovenous fistula or dural arteriovenous fistula (DAVF), and lesion such as arteriovenous malformation (AVM).
- Evaluate a vascular lesion (aneurysm), if high-end CT machine is not available.
- Evaluation of spinal vascular malformations.
- Plan therapeutic endovascular procedure for complex vascular lesions.

Review of cross-sectional imaging that the patient might have with him/her is mandatory before proceeding with the angiogram.

CONTRAINDICATIONS

- *Absolute*: Uncorrectable coagulation disorders.
- *Relative*:
  - Severe atherosclerotic disease of the access vessel
  - Local infection
  - Access site aneurysm.

PREPROCEDURAL WORKUP

- Complete hemogram
- Coagulation profile [prothrombin time (PT), activated partial thromboplastin time (APTT), international normalized ratio (INR), and platelets]

- Renal function tests
- Electrolyte status
- Human immunodeficiency virus (HIV)/hepatitis B surface antigen (HBsAg) status
- Further tests can be tailored according to the patient's condition
- The patient's drug history is required with special reference to any known drug allergies.

CONSENT

An informed consent from the immediate relatives after detailing the requirement of procedure, the technique, expected outcome, and associated complications is absolutely essential before proceeding with the CA.

ANGIOGRAPHY MACHINE

Digital subtraction angiography (DSA) is a technique for showing contrast-filled vessels without any interfering background mainly the bones. Present day, DSA systems are based on digital fluoroscopy systems, which are equipped with high-end software and display facilities. The latest machines are biplane machines with flat panel detectors.[1]

ANESTHESIA

Most diagnostic procedures are done under local anesthesia, however at times depending on the condition of the patient, sedation, or general anesthesia may be required.

PATIENT POSITION

The patient should be positioned on the table comfortably with the head secured in a special head rest. A strap should be applied if necessary to immobilize the head. The patient must be informed preprocedure about the possible sensation of the contrast including metallic taste in the mouth, warm sensation on the side of the head and face where the vessels will be injected. The patient's eyes should be covered with a blindfold to avoid apprehension that comes with seeing unfamiliar environment of the catheterization laboratory.

ARTERIAL ACCESS

Vascular access is gained from one of the arteries—mostly the femoral artery in the groin. The brachial artery route might be used rarely as in a patient with occlusion of aortic bifurcation. However, accessing the cerebral vessels via brachial route is challenging, hence alternate imaging such as CT angiography should be considered in these patients.

PROCEDURE

Once the femoral artery is punctured, a sheath is placed in situ for continued arterial access. Heparin is administered as per standard protocol. The cerebral diagnostic catheter is then passed through this sheath and navigated under fluoroscopic guidance to the area of interest. Using a nonionic contrast medium, angiography is carried out **(Figs. 1A to C)**.

The CA begins with acquiring the anteroposterior (AP) and lateral (lat) views of the right carotid bifurcation. If there are no plaques at the bifurcation, selective right external carotid artery (ECA) and internal carotid artery (ICA) are then carried out in AP and lateral views. This is followed by the injection of the left carotid system **(Figs. 2A and B)** followed by the dominant—usually left vertebral artery (VA) **(Figs. 2C to H)**. The angiogram has four phases—arterial, capillary, early venous, and late venous phase and is analyzed in both AP **(Figs. 3A to D)** and lateral views **(Figs. 4A to D)** for all arteries. The amount of contrast used is approximately 8 mL for ICA and VA and about 4 mL for ECA injections. At times, additional projections, three-dimensional (3D) acquisitions, selective arterial injections (may include microcatheter injection), and magnified views are also taken. Adequate knowledge of the catheters and wires to be used is absolutely essential, especially when accessing tortuous arteries. After the angiogram, the sheath is removed and hemostasis is achieved by manual compression of puncture site or at times by use of closure devices. Adequate measures are taken to minimize radiation exposure to all present in the catheterization laboratory.

PEDIATRIC PATIENT

The angiographic protocol *per se* remains the same. However, the choice of puncture needle, access sheath, diagnostic catheter, heparin dosage, and contrast used are all tailored as per the weight of the child.

COMPLICATIONS

The CA is an invasive procedure. The stated risk of complications associated with CA is 1.3%.[2] General complications of any angiographic procedure include:

- Puncture site hematoma
- Arterial thrombosis
- Pseudoaneurysm
- Arteriovenous fistula
- Contrast reaction
- Contrast-induced renal failure.

A WORD OF CAUTION

Clinical examination should identify markers such as abnormal facies in a given patient to identify those with a connective tissue disorder such as Ehlers-Danlos syndrome. Given the vascular fragility in these patients causing arterial dissections[3] and attendant complications, diagnostic CA

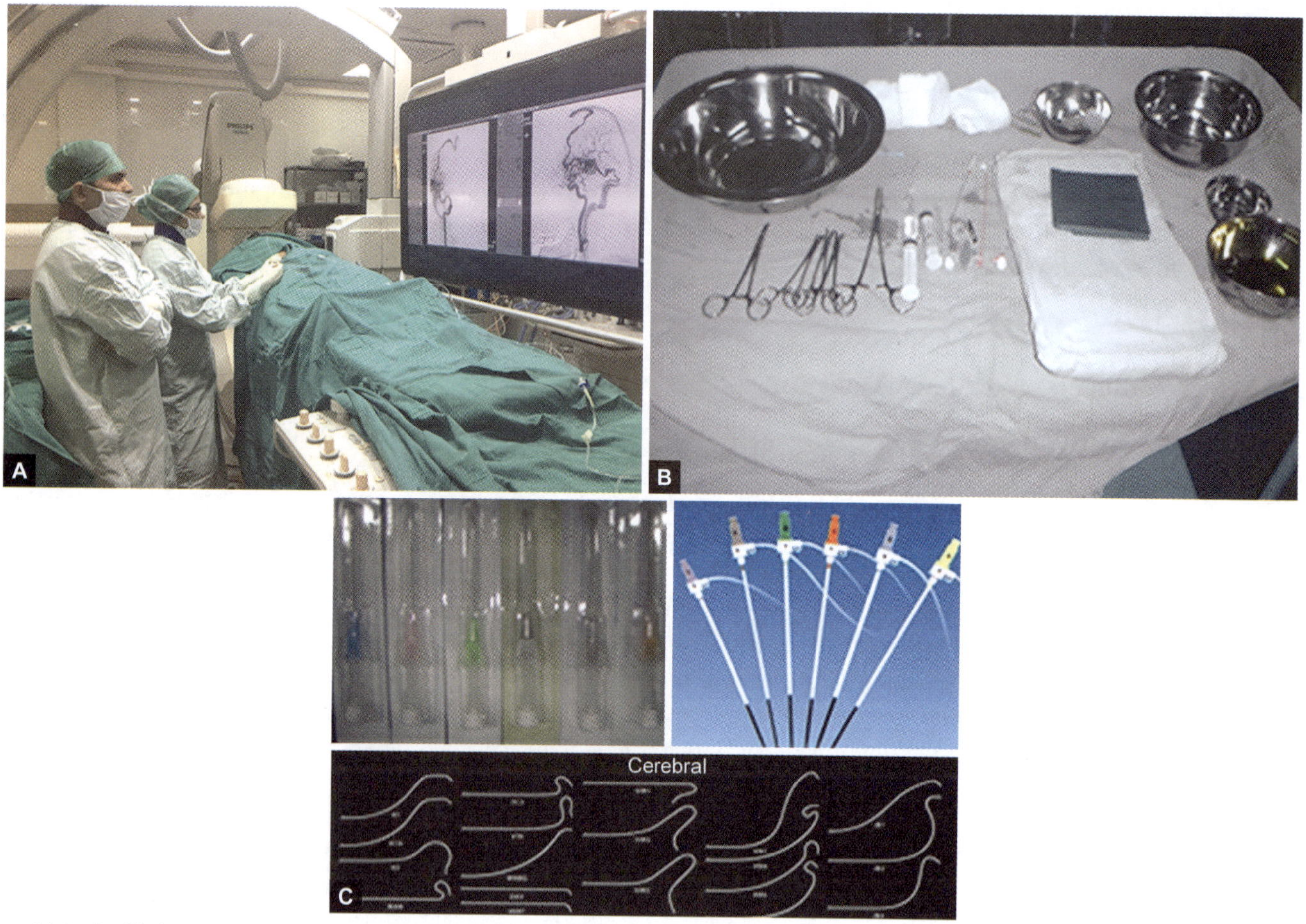

Figs. 1A to C: (A) A cerebral angiogram is in progress. The two tubes of the machine are toward the head end of the patient. A large screen with multiformatting capabilities displays angiographic images; (B) The preparation for proceeding with an angiogram; (C) *Clockwise*: The needles, sheaths, and catheters are used for a cerebral angiogram. These are color-coded for easy identification.

should never be considered as first investigation for vascular evaluation. CT angiogram provides similar necessary information.

POSTPROCEDURE CARE

A patient who has undergone an uncomplicated CA can be monitored in the ward. The leg in which the artery was accessed should be immobilized for 8 hours. Any bleeding from puncture site, change in neurological status, or absence of a peripheral pulse that was palpable preprocedure needs to be informed to the radiologist immediately. Antibiotics are not routinely administered after a diagnostic CA.

REPORT

A report detailing the findings should be provided to the patient. Relevant images depicting the lesions should also be given to the patient for reference and records.

ADVANCES IN CEREBRAL ANGIOGRAPHY: THREE-DIMENSIONAL DIGITAL SUBTRACTION ANGIOGRAPHY

With the patient supine on the table, the right femoral artery is accessed with a 6F sheath. A 5F standard angiographic catheter is navigated to the artery of interest and connected to a pressure injector. For 3D-DSA, an initial rotational acquisition (a 200° rotation of the AP X-ray tube) around the patient's head (angular velocity, 40° per second) is obtained before administration of the contrast agent and serves as a mask sequence for the subsequent subtraction process. A second identical rotational acquisition is performed as the contrast agent selectively flows through the arterial tree of interest. Volumes of contrast agent and rates for rotational acquisitions are as per standard institutional protocols. Subtracting the mask images from the contrast-enhanced images with matching angles then create rotational

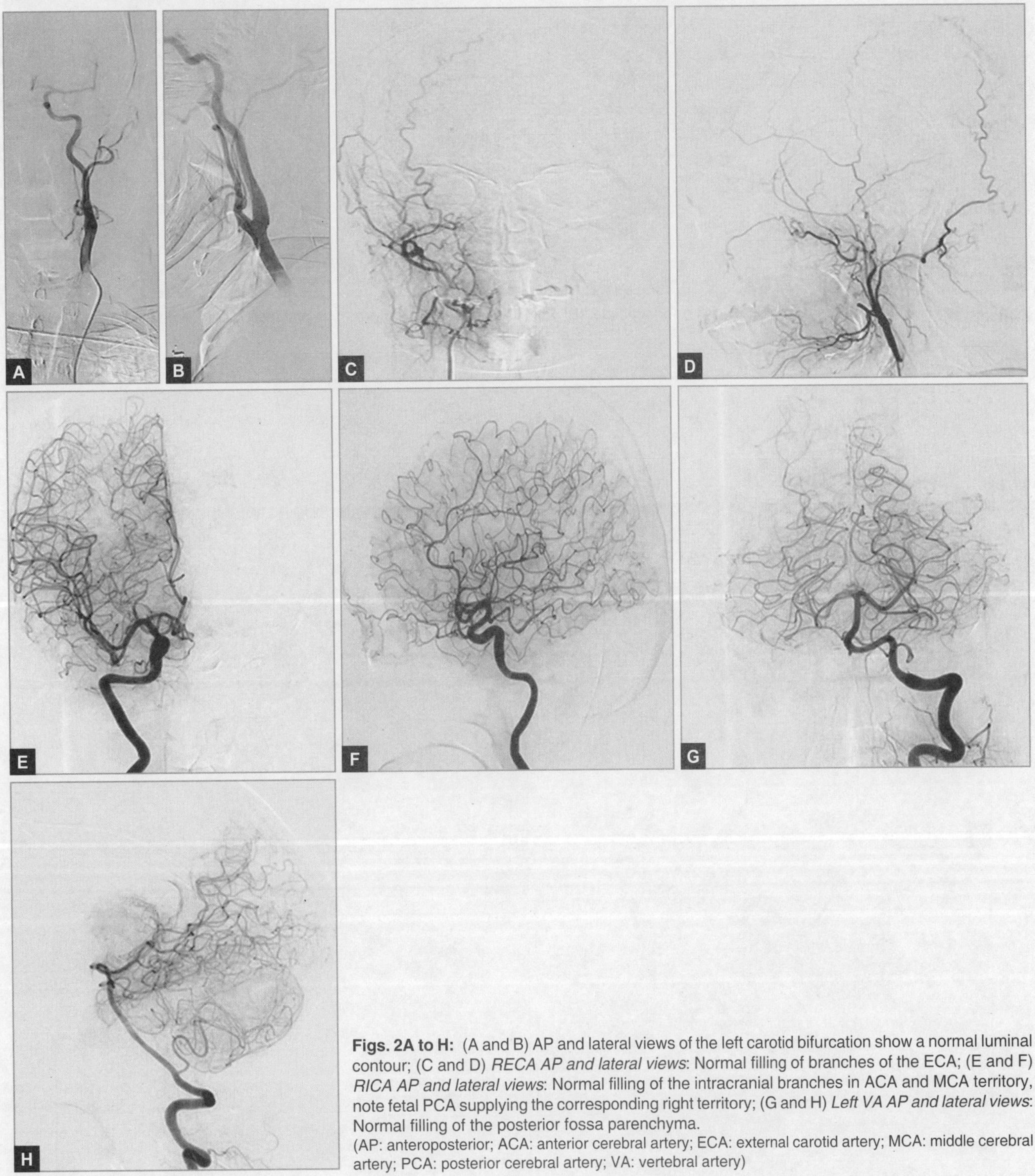

Figs. 2A to H: (A and B) AP and lateral views of the left carotid bifurcation show a normal luminal contour; (C and D) *RECA AP and lateral views*: Normal filling of branches of the ECA; (E and F) *RICA AP and lateral views*: Normal filling of the intracranial branches in ACA and MCA territory, note fetal PCA supplying the corresponding right territory; (G and H) *Left VA AP and lateral views*: Normal filling of the posterior fossa parenchyma.

(AP: anteroposterior; ACA: anterior cerebral artery; ECA: external carotid artery; MCA: middle cerebral artery; PCA: posterior cerebral artery; VA: vertebral artery)

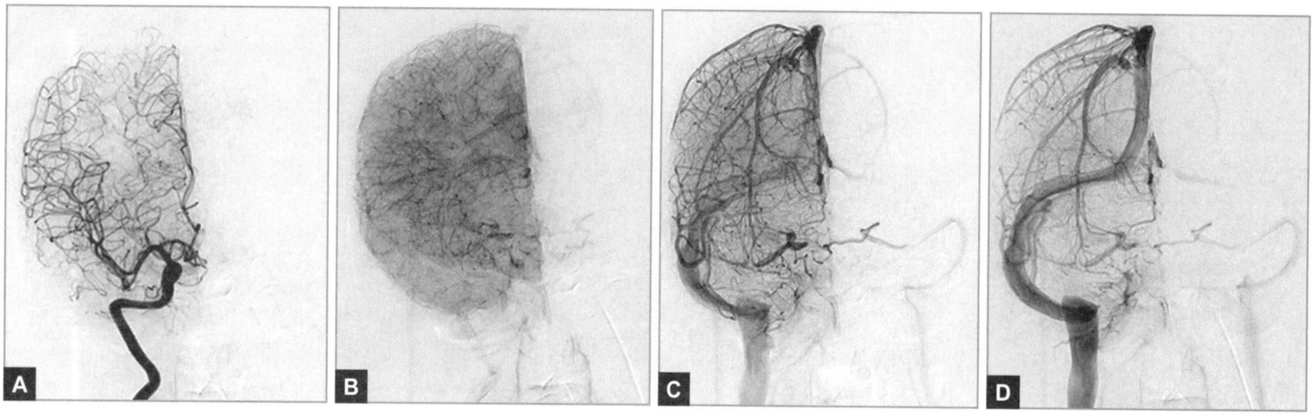

Figs. 3A to D: RICA anteroposterior view. (A) Arterial phase; (B) Capillary phase; (C) Early venous phase; (D) Late venous phase of a normal cerebral angiogram.

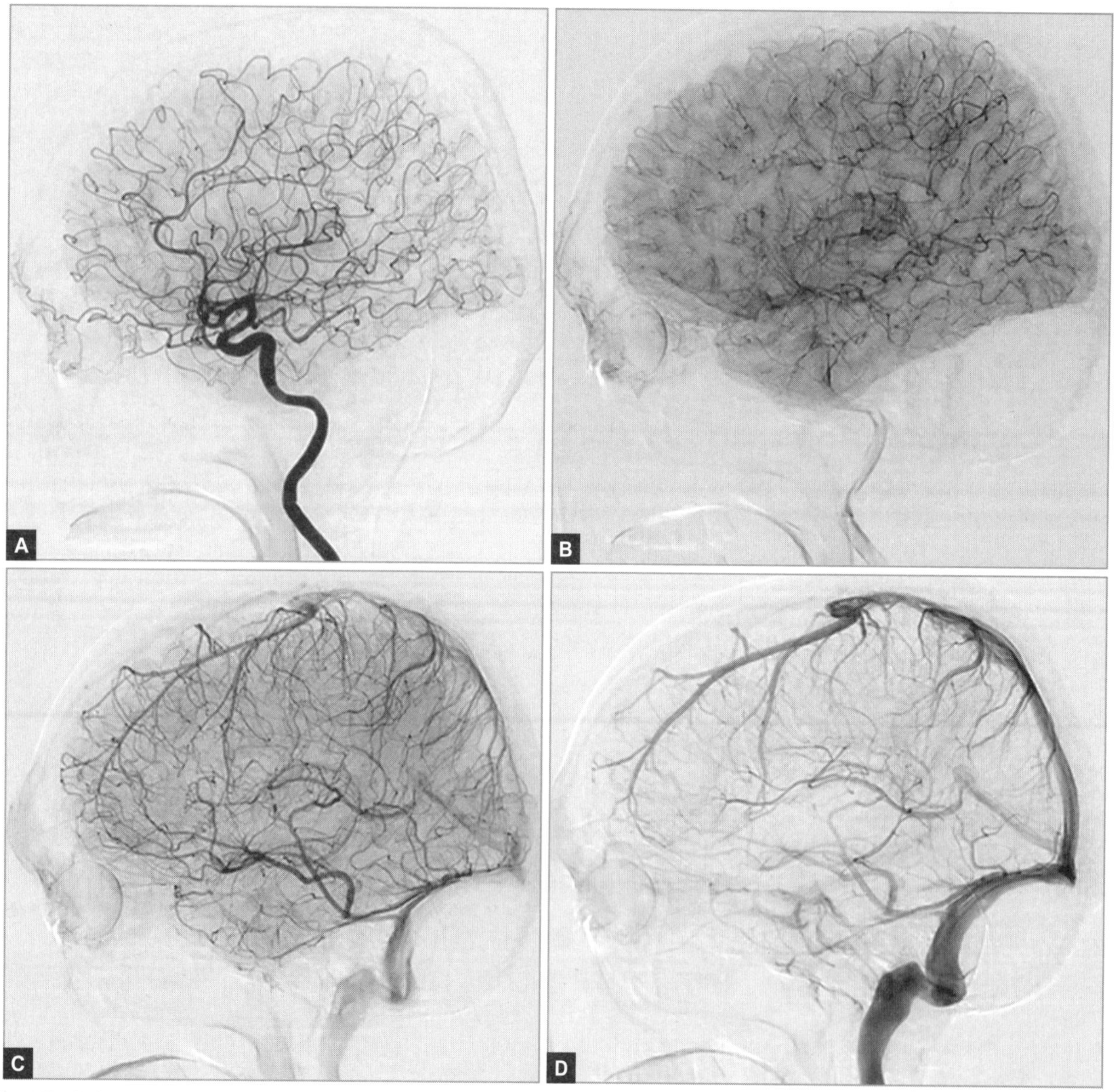

Figs. 4A to D: RICA lateral view. (A) Arterial phase; (B) Capillary phase; (C) Early venous phase; (D) Late venous phase of a normal cerebral angiogram. Note the hypoplastic anterior third of the superior sagittal sinus; the frontal lobe is drained by a prominent parietal vein which joins the sagittal sinus at its midsegment, variant anatomy.

DSA images. A detailed 3D representation of the vascular tree is finally generated from the rotational DSA dataset by using a 3D reconstruction algorithm. This mode of reconstruction produces the 3D images available on most modern angiographic units.[4]

Three-dimensional digital subtraction angiography has now become an established tool in routine cerebral angiography. It provides more detailed vascular information than standard two-dimensional (2D) angiography. It allows the possibility of free rotation of images, exquisite anatomic information, the lack of overprojecting bony structures, and extensive postprocessing capabilities all of which help in choosing the most appropriate working projection for subsequent endovascular therapy.[4-8] Postprocessing tools provide images in formats such as shaded surface display (SSD), maximum intensity projection (MIP), translucent rendering, etc. **(Figs. 5A to E)**.

However, the limitation of 2D-DSA is the inability to provide information about osseous structures surrounding the aneurysm. 3D digital angiograms (3D-DA) overcome this limitation. 3D-DA is a new reconstruction algorithm that allows simultaneous 3D display of the osseous and vascular information acquired through a rotational CA. Because 3D-DA uses a part of the dataset necessary to generate 3D-DSA images, both 3D-DA and 3D-DSA images can be reconstructed from a single rotational angiogram. The concomitant representation of vascular structures and their osseous surroundings allows 3D-DA to combine the spatial resolution of 3D-DSA with the topographic information previously offered by only CT angiography.[4]

A biplane DSA machine with features of 3D-DSA and 3D-DA eventually leads to a decrease in total number of DSA exposures in every procedure—diagnostic and during endovascular procedures which eventually reduce the number of exposures thus limiting the side effects of radiation.[8]

CASE STUDIES

Case 1

A 50-year-old male presented with sudden severe headache and transient loss of consciousness on the prior evening. He then underwent a DSA which revealed an aneurysm of the anterior communicating artery. Various reconstruction algorithms were used to demonstrate different aspects of aneurysm morphology in this patient **(Figs. 5A to E)**. He subsequently underwent surgical clipping of the aneurysm.

Case 2

A 25-year-old female presented with right-sided headache on and off for 1 year. MRI of brain revealed a large AVM in the region of the right basal ganglia, hypothalamus, and thalamus. She was subjected to a CA **(Figs. 6A to J)** which revealed multiple AVMs.

This was a case of a type 2 cerebrofacial arteriovenous metameric syndrome (CAMS). This is a condition where AVM is noted involving the lateral prosencephalic (optic) group with involvement of the optic nerve, retina, parieto-temporal-occipital lobes, thalamus, and maxilla, i.e. AVM is noted at multiple sites along this pathway. A somatic mutation developing in the region of the neural crest or adjacent cephalic mesoderm before migration causes AVM with a segmental distribution.[9] The various angiographic acquisitions in this case demonstrate the capability of the present-day technology.

Case 3

A 25-year-old male presented with left-sided proptosis, conjunctival congestion **(Fig. 7A)** and watering of eyes 3 weeks following a road traffic accident. His cerebral angiogram revealed a direct CCF **(Figs. 7B and C)**. Diagnostic CA is mandatory in patients with CCF to evaluate the anatomy and plan the access route for endovascular embolization.

Case 4

A 40-year-old female patient with a pineal mass was referred for a cerebral angiogram. Immediate postprocedure, she had aphasia. MRI revealed an acute infarct in left MCA territory **(Figs. 8A to D)**. At times, thrombus may get dislodged into the intracranial circulation during angiogram causing vascular occlusion.

CONCLUSION

Cerebral angiogram is indispensable for evaluation of vascular lesions as discussed. It is important to understand the need for dedicated neuroradiologists for best results. An integrated approach toward the diagnosis and management in these patients is absolutely essential. Equally important is the aftercare of these patients. Optimal use of the ever-advancing technology and refined human skills can be used for the advantage of the mankind.

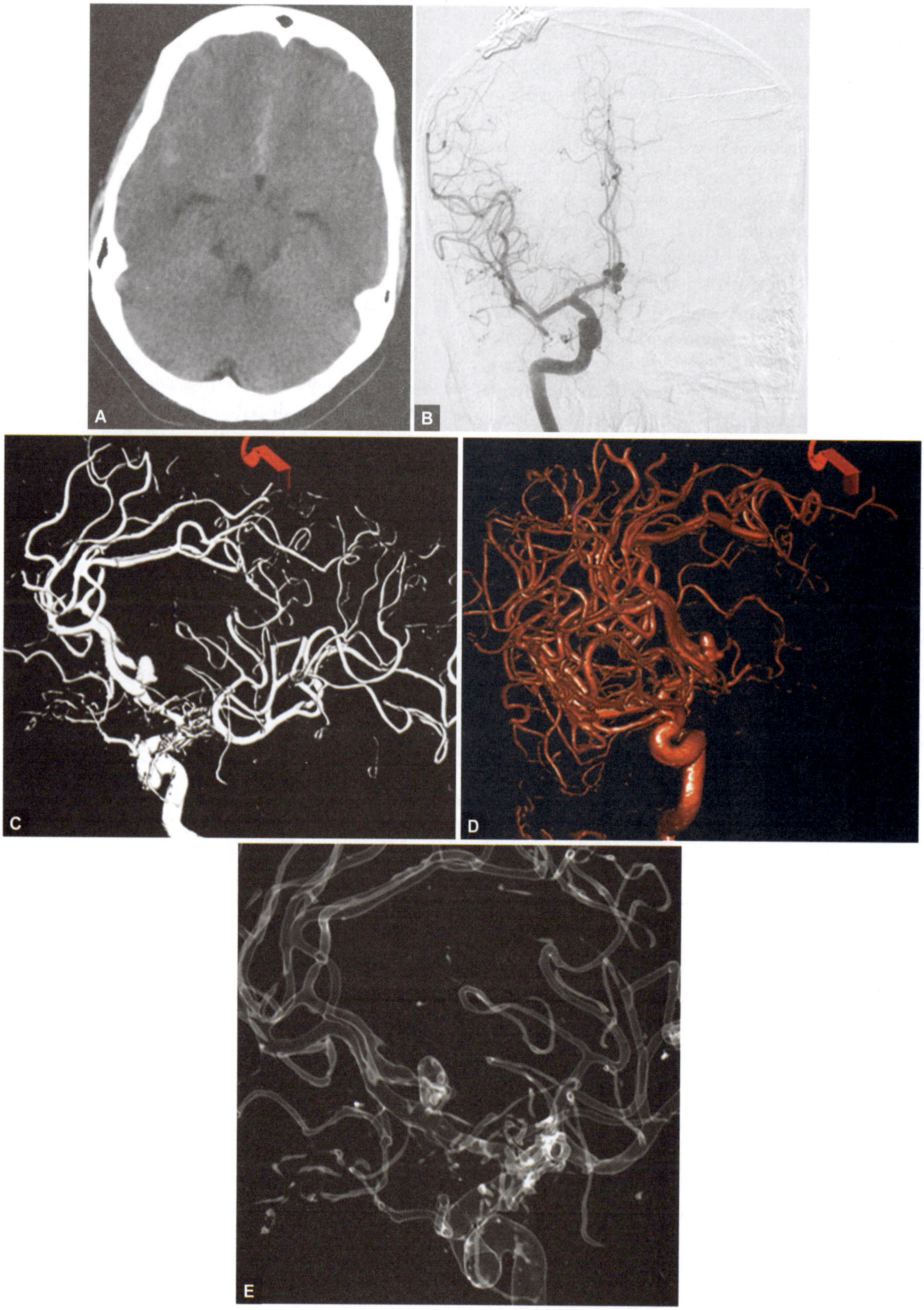

Figs. 5A to E: (A) Noncontrast CT shows diffuse subarachnoid hemorrhage (SAH) in the anterior interhemispheric fissure and the right sylvian fissure; (B) *RICA AP view*: The aneurysm was elongated, measured 6 mm × 4 mm and was directed cranially; (C) *RICA shaded surface display (SSD)*: The two daughter blebs along its posterior surface are best depicted in this figure; (D) *RICA injection*: A different colored image of the SSD in a different projection also shows relevant details of the aneurysm; (E) *RICA injection*: A transparent rendering of the 3D images can also be obtained.
(3D: three-dimensional; AP: anteroposterior)

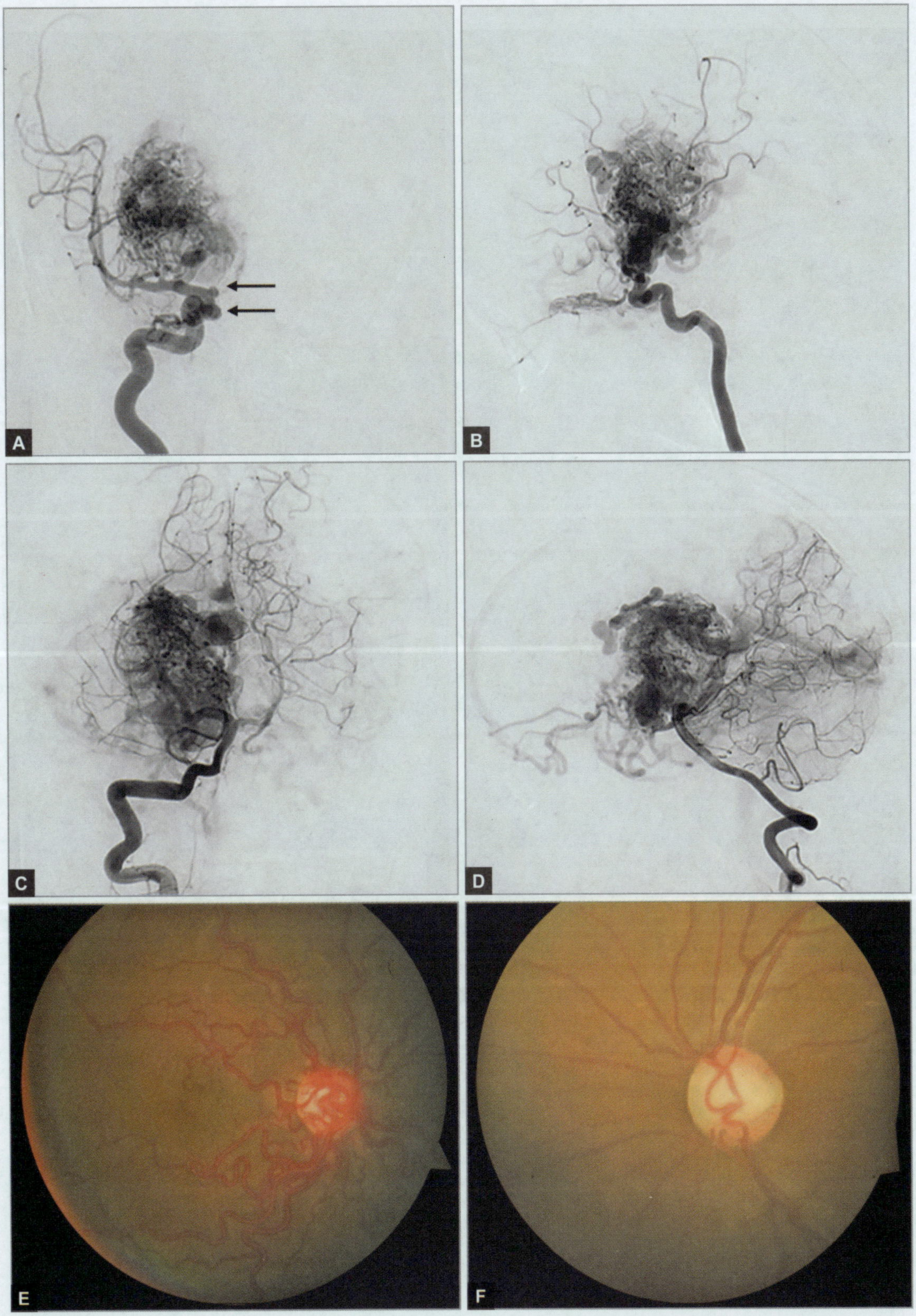

Figs. 6A to F

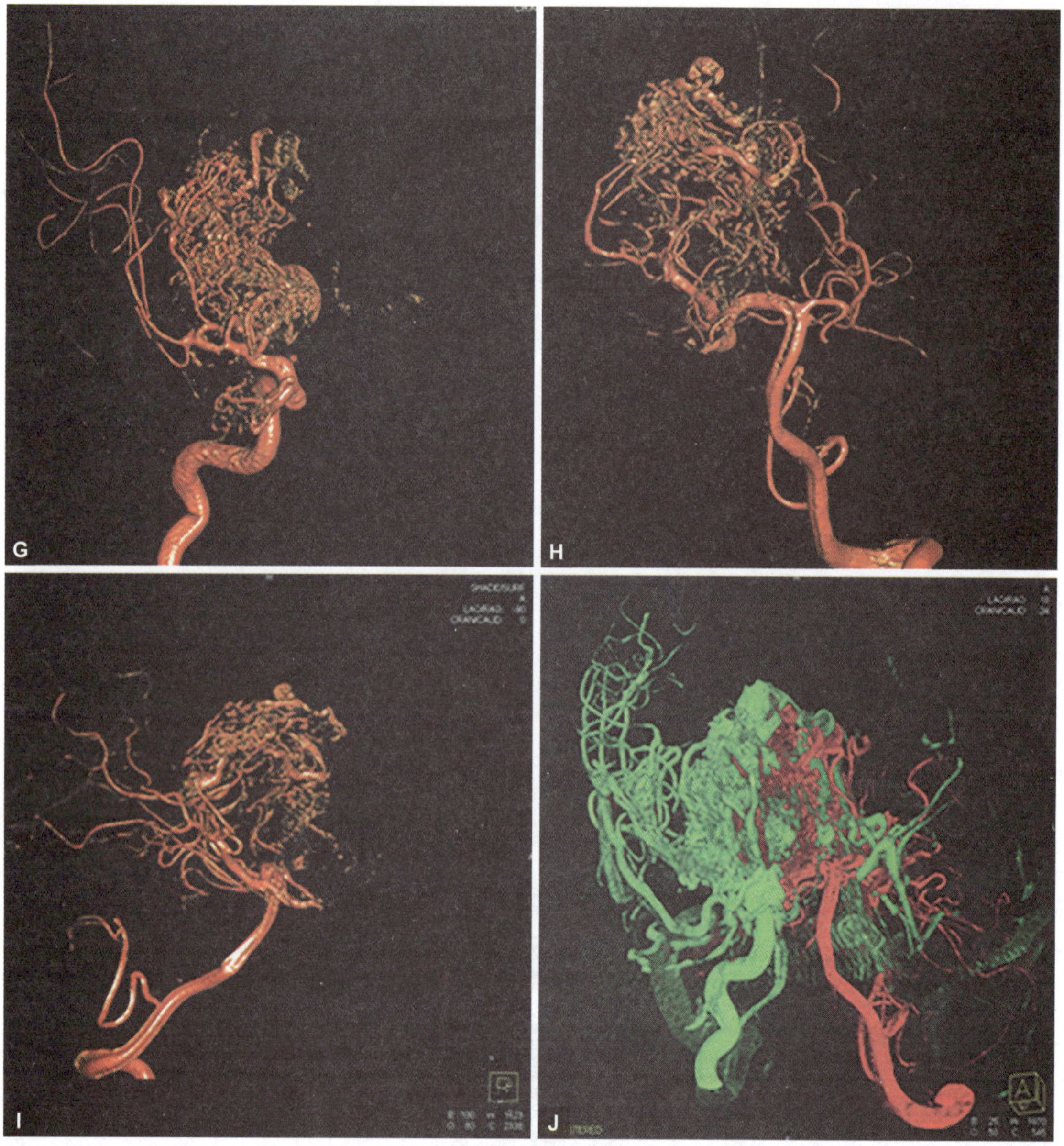

Figs. 6G to J

Figs. 6A to J: (A) *RICA AP view*: It revealed the feeders from hypertrophied lenticulostriate arteries. Aneurysms (arrows) were noted at the communicating segment of the right ICA and at right ICA bifurcation (because of increased hemodynamic flow to the AVM); (B) *RICA lateral view*: In addition to the arterial feeders, it also demonstrates abnormal vessels from the right ophthalmic artery (OA) to the right orbital region; (C) *RVA AP view*: It shows the contribution from the thalamoperforators; (D) *RVA lateral view*: It shows the arterial feeders, the AVM nidus, and the venous drainage of the AVM to the vein of Galen as also to the anterior third of the superior sagittal sinus; (E) The fundus revealed a retinal AVM on the right; (F) Note the normal vessels of the left fundus; (G) 3D reconstructed images of the angiogram of this patient demonstrate the ICA aneurysms well in addition to the details of the arterial feeders; (H and I) VA AP view and VA lateral view demonstrates exquisite detail of the anatomy of the feeding artery and the nidus. Rotation and manipulation of these images on workstation provide additional information that is required for endovascular management; (J) *Fused 3D image*: ICA (green color) and the VA (red color) acquisitions are fused on the workstation using vendor-specific software to assess the differential contribution of various arteries to AVM that involve larger anatomic regions.

(AP: anteroposterior; AVM: arteriovenous malformation; 3D: three-dimensional; ICA: internal carotid artery; VA: vertebral artery)

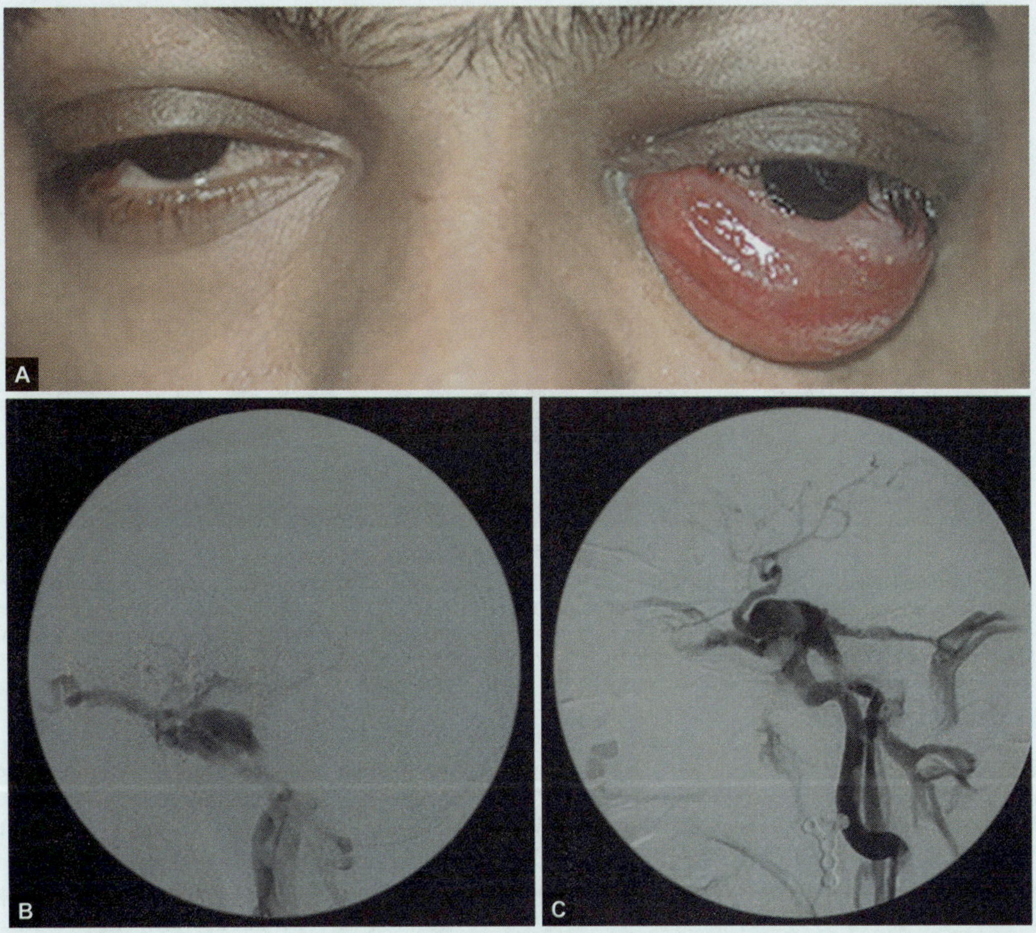

Figs. 7A to C: (A) A patient with left direct carotico-cavernous fistula (CCF) has proptosis and lower lid conjunctival congestion; (B) *LICA lateral view*: A direct CCF with venous drainage to the superior ophthalmic vein as also to the inferior petrosal sinus (IPS). Note the paucity of forward flow intracranially suggesting this to be a high flow fistula; (C) RICA lateral view in a patient with a direct CCF after placing a balloon across the rent demonstrates the venous drainage to the superior ophthalmic vein, IPS, and superior petrosal sinus (SPS). If additional balloons do not occlude the fistula, any of the venous routes demonstrated here may be used to place coils in the cavernous sinus and close the fistula.

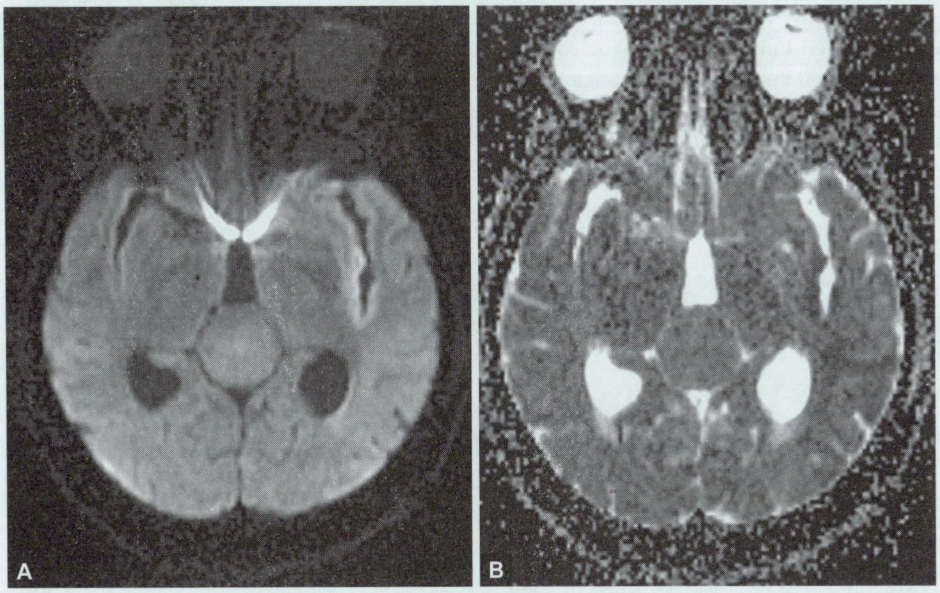

Figs. 8A and B

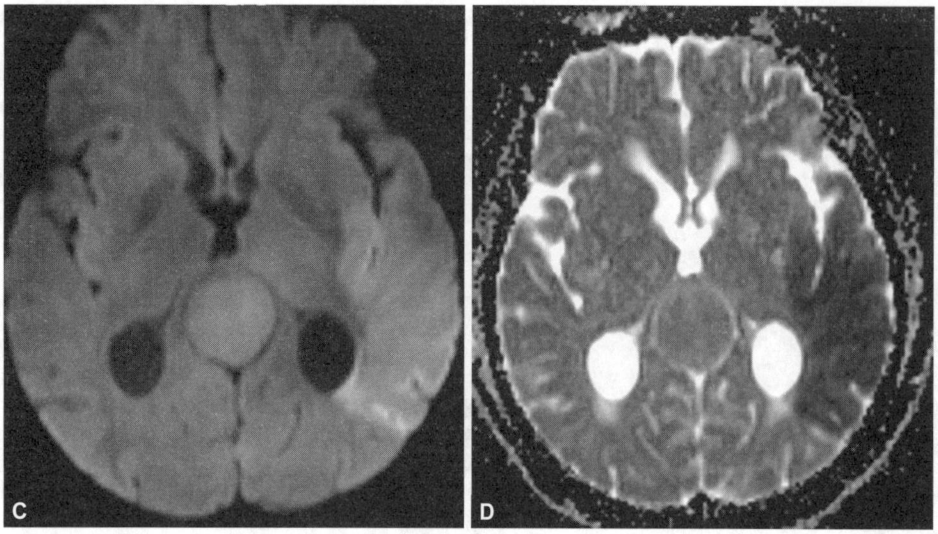

Figs. 8C and D

Figs. 8A to D: (A) Preprocedure DWI trace images; (B) Preprocedure ADC map revealed no diffusion restriction in the pineal mass and no parenchymal abnormality; (C) *Postcerebral angiogram*: DWI trace image; (D) *Postcerebral angiogram*: ADC image after aphasia was noticed, reveals hyperintensity on trace image with corresponding hypointensity on ADC maps suggesting diffusion restriction implying an acute infarct in left MCA territory.
(ADC: apparent diffusion coefficient; DWI: diffusion-weighted imaging; MCA: middle cerebral artery)

REFERENCES

1. Seibert JA. Flat-panel detectors: how much better are they? Pediatr Radiol. 2006;36(Suppl 2):173-81.
2. Willinsky RA, Taylor SM, TerBrugge K, et al. Neurologic complications of cerebral angiography: prospective analysis of 2,899 procedures and review of the literature. Radiology. 2003;227:522-8.
3. North KN, Whiteman DA, Pepin MG, et al. Cerebrovascular complications in Ehlers-Danlos syndrome type IV. Ann Neurol. 1995;38:960-4.
4. Gailloud P, Oishi S, Murphy K. Three-dimensional fusion digital subtraction angiography: new reconstruction algorithm for simultaneous three-dimensional rendering of osseous and vascular information obtained during rotational angiography. Am J Neuroradiol. 2005;26:908-11.
5. van Rooij WJ, Peluso JP, Sluzewski M, et al. Additional value of 3D rotational angiography in angiographically negative aneurysmal subarachnoid hemorrhage: how negative is negative? Am J Neuroradiol. 2008;29:962-6.
6. Hochmuth A, Spetzger U, Schumacher M. Comparison of three-dimensional rotational angiography with digital subtraction angiography in the assessment of ruptured cerebral aneurysms. Am J Neuroradiol. 2002;23: 1199-205.
7. Hirai T, Korogi Y, Suginohara K, et al. Clinical usefulness of unsubtracted 3D digital angiography compared with rotational digital angiography in the pretreatment evaluation of intracranial aneurysms. Am J Neuroradiol. 2003;24: 1067-74.
8. Abe T, Hirohata M, Tanaka N, et al. Clinical benefits of rotational 3D angiography in endovascular treatment of ruptured cerebral aneurysm. Am J Neuroradiol. 2002;23:686-8.
9. Krings TS, Geibprasert CB, Luo JJ, et al. Segmental neurovascular syndromes in children. Neuroimaging Clin N Am. 2007;17:245-58.

CHAPTER

40 Ocular Motor Nerve Palsies

Shivcharan L Chandravanshi, Nitin Nema

INTRODUCTION

Oculomotor (third cranial nerve), trochlear (fourth cranial nerve), and abducens (sixth cranial nerve) are motor cranial nerves to eyeball.[1] Paralysis of these nerves are known as ocular motor nerve palsies. Ocular motor nerve palsies may be partial or complete, congenital or acquired, isolated or associated with other neurological pathology. They can result from lesions located from the motor nerve nuclei to the termination of nerve in the extraocular muscles within the orbital cavity. The clinical presentation, diagnosis, and management of ocular motor nerve palsies depend upon type of palsy, age of the patient, etiology, and other associated neurological involvement. In this chapter, oculomotor, trochlear, and abducens nerve palsies are described with special reference to their diagnosis.

OCULOMOTOR NERVE PALSY

Applied Anatomy

The oculomotor nerve arises from medial aspect of cerebral peduncle at the level of superior colliculus.[2] The oculomotor nerve has two components: (1) general somatic efferent fibers and (2) general visceral efferent fibers. General somatic efferent fibers arise from the main oculomotor nucleus and supply extraocular muscles (including levator palpebrae superioris—LPS) except lateral rectus and superior oblique muscles. General visceral efferent fibers arise from Edinger–Westphal nucleus and supply sphincter pupillae and ciliary muscles.[2]

Etiology

Third nerve palsy can result from lesions anywhere along the anatomical pathway from the nucleus to the supplied muscles. Etiology of oculomotor nerve palsy may be divided into congenital and acquired.

Congenital Oculomotor Nerve Palsy

Congenital oculomotor nerve palsy is rare. It probably occurs due to aplasia or hypoplasia of the third nerve nucleus.[3] Intrauterine trauma, birth trauma, and intrauterine intracranial infections are other causes of congenital or neonatal third nerve palsy.[4-6]

Acquired Oculomotor Nerve Palsy

Vasculopathies: Vascular causes of third nerve palsy include diabetes, atherosclerosis, and systemic hypertension.[7]

Ophthalmoplegic migraine: It can cause partial or complete third nerve palsy.[8] It is commonly seen in pediatric patients under the age of 10 years. Other causes of acquired 3rd nerve palsy along with special features are summarized in **Table 1**.

Clinical Features

Clinical features of third nerve palsy depend on whether it is complete or incomplete and pupillary fibers are involved or not. Clinical features of isolated total third nerve palsy are as follows:[15,16,18]

- Blepharoptosis develops due to paralysis of levator palpebrae superioris (LPS) muscle
- Globe is turned down and out and slightly intorted
- Adduction, elevation, depression, and extorsion are restricted **(Figs. 1A to I)**
- Pupil may be fixed and dilated secondary to paralysis of the sphincter pupillae muscle. However, pupil sparing lesion can occur due to diabetes (ischemia)
- Accommodation is completely lost due to paralysis of the ciliary muscles. However, in pupil sparing lesions, it is intact
- A crossed horizontal diplopia is common with slight misalignment

- Abnormal head posture in third nerve palsy is characterized by face turn to opposite side, head tilted towards the affected side and chin elevation.

Incomplete third nerve palsy may manifest as external ophthalmoplegia or internal ophthalmoplegia.

Table 1: Common causes of acquired third nerve palsy.[9-22]

Level of lesion	*Common causes*	*Special features*
Nucleus	• Infarction • Demyelination • Metastatic tumor	• Bilateral ptosis • Bilateral mydriasis • Contralateral superior rectus palsy • Ipsilateral medial rectus, inferior rectus, inferior oblique palsy
Fascicular	• Infarction • Demyelination • Tumor (rare)	*Cross syndromes*: • Weber's syndrome • Benedikt's syndrome • Nothnagel's syndrome
Basilar	• Aneurysm • Raised intracranial pressure (uncal herniation)	Isolated third nerve palsy
Cavernous sinus	• Carotid-cavernous fistula • Granulomatous inflammation (Tolosa–Hunt syndrome) • Intracavernous aneurysm • Extrasellar extension of pituitary tumor • Meningioma • Sphenoidal sinus carcinoma • Metastatic tumor • Mucormycosis • Herpes zoster	*Cavernous sinus syndrome*: • Multiple cranial nerve palsies • Incomplete third nerve palsy • May be pupil sparing
Orbit	• Pseudotumor • Trauma • Tumor	• Isolated third nerve palsy • Proptosis • Visual loss

External Ophthalmoplegia

- Ocular movements are restricted in all fields except in temporal in complete paralysis, while in incomplete palsy, there is partial limitation.
- Palsy or paralysis of the superior division of the third nerve causes ptosis.

Internal Ophthalmoplegia

- Pupil is dilated and does not react to light in complete internal ophthalmoplegia.
- Pupil is semidilated and reacts sluggishly to light in incomplete internal ophthalmoplegia.
- Pupil may be spared in certain conditions.

Associated Syndromes

Syndromes[23,24] associated with oculomotor nerve palsy are described here:

- *Weber's syndrome*: Weber's syndrome is referred to an ipsilateral third nerve paralysis with a contralateral hemiplegia. It is due to a lesion in fascicular part of the oculomotor nerve, while passing through the cerebral peduncle.
- *Benedikt's syndrome*: It is characterized by ipsilateral third nerve palsy with associated contralateral hemitremors. It occurs due to involvement of fasciculus of the third nerve as it passes through the red nucleus.
- *Nothnagel's syndrome*: This syndrome is caused by a lesion at the level of the superior cerebellar peduncle and the oculomotor nucleus. It is characterized by unilateral oculomotor nerve paralysis with ipsilateral cerebellar ataxia.
- *Claude's syndrome*: This is a combination of Benedikt's and Nothnagel's syndromes.

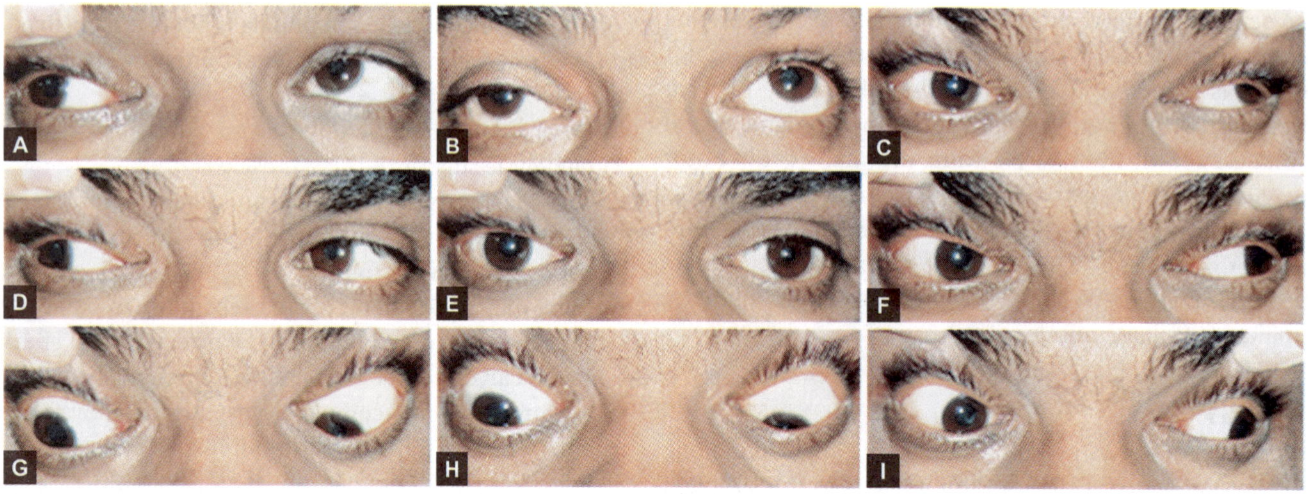

Figs. 1A to I: Right eye third nerve palsy. (A) Limitation of dextroelevation; (B) limitation in elevation; (C) limitation in levoelevation; (D) Normal abduction; (E) Right eye ptosis (eyelid elevated manually) and exotropia; (F) Limitation of adduction; (G) Limitation in dextrodepression; (H) Limitation in depression; (I) Limitation in levodepression.

Aberrant Regeneration of Third Cranial Nerve

Elevation of the eyelid and/or constriction of the pupil during adduction or depression of the eye are common signs of aberrant regeneration.

Aberrant regeneration is thought to result from a misdirection of regenerating axons, which innervate wrong extraocular muscle. If an aberrant regeneration develops following acute third nerve palsy, a compressive posterior communicating artery aneurysm or traumatic etiology should be suspected.[24] If primary aberrant regeneration occurs spontaneously without preexisting third nerve palsy, a cavernous sinus meningioma or an internal carotid artery aneurysm is a more likely possibility. An unruptured posterior communicating artery aneurysm is another alternative.

Differential Diagnosis

Differential diagnosis of oculomotor nerve palsy includes progressive external ophthalmoplegia, early thyroid eye disease, myasthenia gravis, orbital inflammatory disease, Duane's syndrome (type II), congenital blepharoptosis, generalized myopathic conditions, and other causes of anisocoria.[8]

Diagnosis

The diagnosis of oculomotor nerve palsy is mostly based on clinical features, and investigations are required only for localization of the causative lesion and determination of the underlying etiology.[25] It involves investigations like imaging, cerebrospinal fluid (CSF) examination, and blood tests.

Investigations

Imaging

Magnetic resonance imaging (MRI): MRI is a more sensitive imaging modality than computed tomography (CT) scan for detecting a small intraparenchymal brainstem lesion, such as infarction, small abscess, or tumor.[8] It is also considered the procedure of choice for demonstrating meningeal and dural inflammation and infiltration. It is also indicated, if patient has additional cranial nerve palsies or other neurological defects or the palsy does not improve within 3 months of treatment.

Magnetic resonance angiography (MRA): Magnetic resonance angiography is imaging modality of choice[26] in all patients aged 10–50 years, who have pupil-involving third nerve palsy. If MRI and MRA are normal, patients should be evaluated for diabetes and hypertension.[27]

Computed tomography scan: CT scan is more sensitive than MRI to demonstrate subarachnoid hemorrhage and calcification within lesions, as may be found in certain tumors and in large aneurysms.

Lumbar Puncture

Lumbar puncture is necessary in certain situations to demonstrate the presence of blood in CSF, malignant cells in neoplastic infiltration, an inflammatory reaction or microorganisms.[28] Bloody CSF is usually seen in third nerve palsy secondary to rupture of a posterior communicating artery berry aneurysm.

Myasthenia gravis simulates oculomotor nerve palsy therefore Tensilon or other simple and safe tests like sleep or ice tests may be performed to rule it out.

Erythrocyte Sedimentation Rate and C-reactive Protein

In patients older than 55 years of age with third nerve palsy associated with polymyalgia rheumatica, erythrocyte sedimentation rate (ESR), and C-reactive protein (CRP) should be ordered.[27] If patient is having raised ESR and CRP then temporal artery biopsy should be considered to confirm temporal arteritis.[25]

Treatment

In patient with oculomotor palsy, we should wait and watch for at least 6 months for spontaneous recovery.[25] Patient should be followed every 6 weeks and at each visit measurement of exotropia and hypotropia with prism cover test, diplopia charting, and Hess charting should be performed to assess the speed of recovery. Pediatric patients should be monitored for amblyopia. Injection of botulinum toxin into the uninvolved lateral rectus muscle is useful to prevent its contracture before the deviation improves or stabilizes. Patching therapy should be considered to prevent development of amblyopia. Treatment of diplopia is difficult in third nerve palsy. Prism or temporary occlusion therapy can be considered during wait and watch period. Surgical treatment should be considered after 6–8 months of the date of onset of palsy.[13,25,27]

Prognosis

Oculomotor palsy secondary to diabetes, herpes zoster, and acute infectious polyneuropathy has good recovery. Palsy secondary to subarachnoid hemorrhage, meningitis, and neoplasm has poor prognosis with significant mortality and morbidity.[8,21,27]

TROCHLEAR NERVE PALSY

Applied Anatomy

Trochlear nerve (fourth cranial nerve) arises from the trochlear nucleus, which is situated on the dorsal aspect of the midbrain below the inferior colliculus just lateral to the frenulum veli.[8,27] It is the only cranial nerve to arise from the dorsal aspect of the brain. It supplies to the superior oblique muscle. It is a crossed cranial nerve, which means it innervates the contralateral superior oblique muscle. Trochlear nerve is very long and slender nerve.

Etiology

Etiology of fourth nerve palsy may be congenital or acquired.

Congenital

Congenital fourth cranial nerve palsy is relatively common. It results from defect in the nucleus or motor portion of the nerve.[3] Congenital fourth nerve palsy remains compensated and unrecognized during childhood, only to become manifest later either spontaneously or following minor trauma.[8]

Acquired

Acquired causes of trochlear nerve palsy include trauma, vascular lesions (aneurysm and tumor), demyelination, ocular myasthenia, diabetic neuropathy, and herpes zoster. About 20% cases are idiopathic in nature.[20-22] Acquired causes of fourth nerve palsy are summarized in **Table 2**.

Table 2: Acquired causes of fourth nerve palsy.[8,20-22,27]

Level of lesion	*Common causes*	*Special features*
Nucleus	• Ischemia • Hemorrhage • Neoplasm • Trauma • Demyelinating diseases • Vascular malformations	Contralateral Horner's syndrome
Fascicles	• Compression • Infiltration • Demyelination • Ischemia • Hemorrhage • Infection • Trauma	Frequently bilateral in nature
Subarachnoid space	• Aneurysm • Trauma • Microvascular occlusion • Infective meningitis • Iatrogenic • Hydrocephalus • Tumors—schwannomas	May be unilateral or bilateral
Cavernous sinus	• Neoplasm • Inflammation • Microvascular occlusion • Thrombosis	Multiple cranial nerve palsies (IIIrd, VIth, V1, V2, oculosympathetic dysfunction)
Orbit	• Inflammation • Ischemia • Neoplasm • Trauma	Brown syndrome

Clinical Features

Main complaint of the patient is vertical or oblique diplopia. Patient feels difficulty in reading as letters appear tilted. Diplopia is usually worse on downgaze and gaze away from side of involved extraocular muscle.[8] The involved eye is hypertropic in primary position. Patient often adopts an abnormal head posture (chin depression, face turn toward the opposite side and the head is tilted away from the affected side) to reduce diplopia **(Figs. 2A and B)**. In case of fourth nerve palsy of the right eye, ocular movement examination may show excessive levoelevation of the right eye due to a contracture of the right inferior oblique, defective depression of the right eye in levodepression, and normal right elevation, right depression, dextroversion, dextroelevation, and dextro-depression **(Figs. 3A to I)**.

In bilateral fourth nerve palsies, both eyes show hypertropia; the right eye becomes hypertropic when patient looks to the left, and hypertropia of left eye while looking to right. Generally, hypertropia is greater in downgaze than in upgaze. Interestingly, a bilateral esotropia ("V" pattern) develops in downgaze position.

Superior Oblique Myokymia

Superior oblique myokymia is a uniocular rotatory nystagmus involving the superior oblique muscle.[29] Symptoms may be blurred vision, vertical or torsional diplopia, and oscillopsia. The etiology is unknown, but many factors such as stress, lack of sleep, fatigue, and use of alcohol may aggravate the condition.

Diagnosis

The diagnosis of unilateral fourth cranial nerve palsy is based on acute onset, vertical deviation, which increases in contralateral side gaze, downgaze, and ipsilateral head-tilt together with excyclodeviation, which also increases in

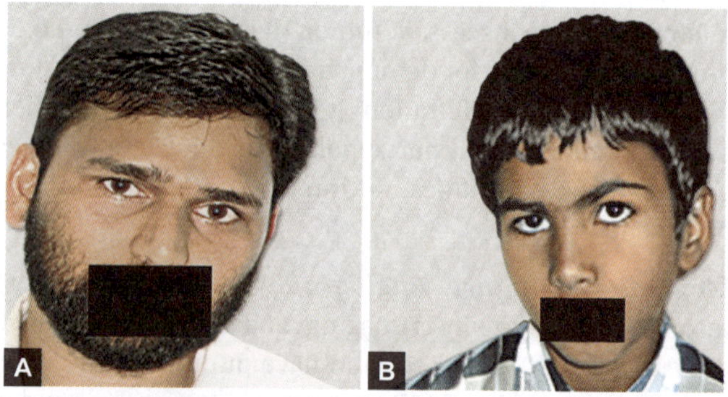

Figs. 2A and B: (A) Compensatory head posture in patient with right fourth nerve palsy; head tilted to left, face turn to left and chin depression; (B) Compensatory head posture in child with left fourth nerve palsy; head tilted to right, face turn to right and chin depression.
Courtesy: Dr Shikha Yadav, Rewa, MP; Dr Vijayalakshmi, Madurai, India

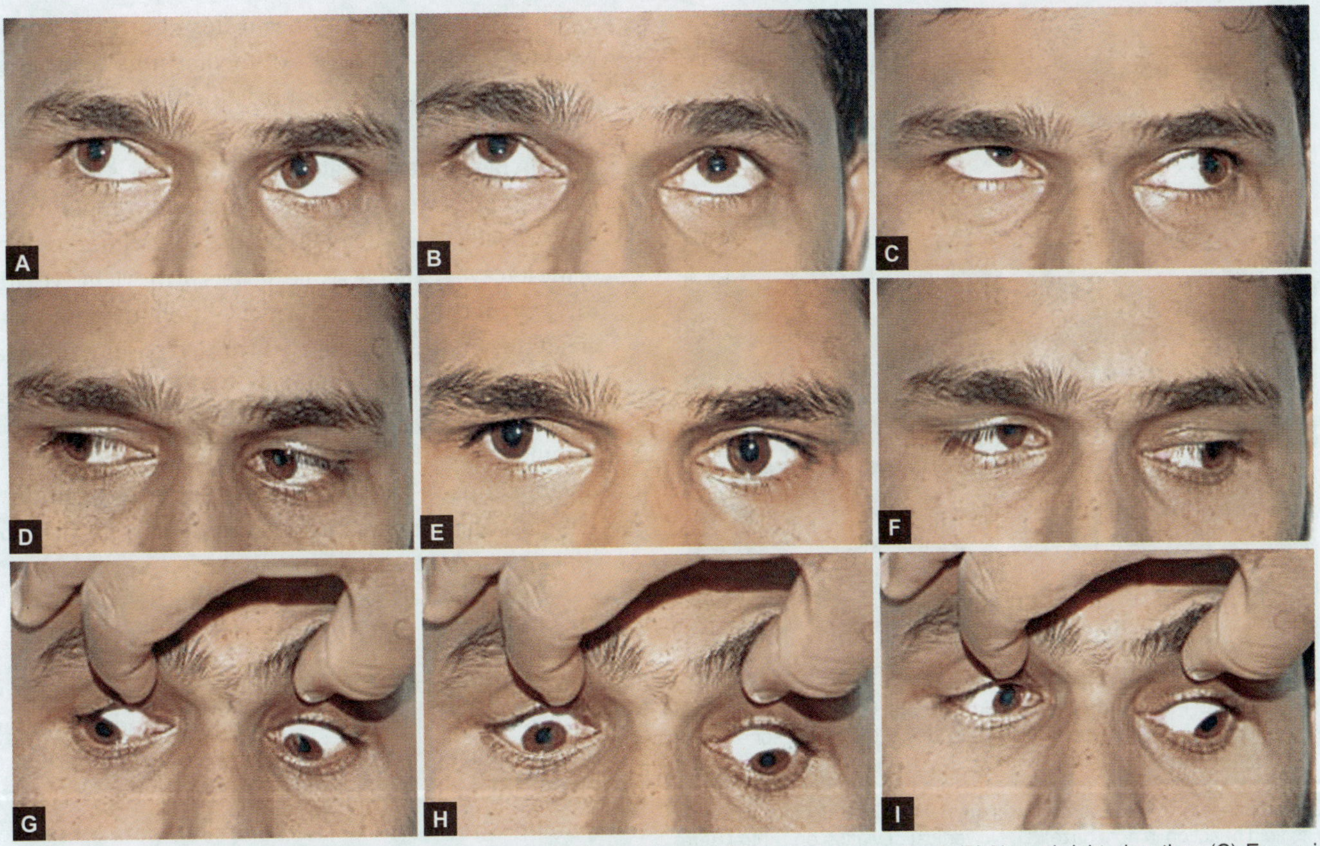

Figs. 3A to I: Extraocular movements in right eye superior oblique palsy; (A) Dextroelevation normal; (B) Normal right elevation; (C) Excessive levoelevation of the right eye due to a contracture of the right inferior oblique; (D) Visual axis is parallel in dextroversion; (E) Right hypertropia in primary position with slight extorsion of eyeball; (F) Slight updrift of right eye in levoversion; (G) Dextrodepression normal; (H) Normal right depression; (I) Defective depression of right eye in levodepression.
Courtesy: Dr Vijayalakshmi, Madurai, India

Table 3: Differentiating features of congenital versus acquired fourth nerve palsy.[8,27,32-37]

Clinical features	*Congenital fourth nerve palsy*	*Acquired fourth nerve palsy*
Occurrence/nuclear	Rare	Common
Amblyopia	Common	Uncommon
Excyclodeviation	Uncommon	Common
Abnormal head posture	Can be traced in old photographs	Cannot traced in early cases
Vertical fusional amplitude	Abnormal (3–15 prism D)	Normal (1–3 prism D)
Facial asymmetry	Present on the side of the face tilt	Not present (face normal)
Long, redundant, or floppy superior oblique tendon (during surgery)	Seen	Not seen

both downgaze and ipsilateral head tilt.[30,31] Bilateral fourth cranial nerve palsy causes a change of vertical deviation between right and left gaze and between head tilt to the right and to the left shoulder.[32-36] Differentiating features of congenital from acquired trochlear nerve palsy are summarized in **Table 3**. Differentiating features of unilateral from bilateral trochlear nerve palsy are given in **Table 4**.

Table 4: Unilateral versus bilateral fourth nerve palsy.[8,27,32-37]

Clinical features	*Unilateral fourth nerve palsy*	*Bilateral fourth nerve palsy*
Incidence	Relatively uncommon	Common
Esotropia	Less	V-shaped esotropia
Torsion	Excyclodeviation less than 10°	Excyclodeviation more than 10°
Superior oblique ductions	Normal or diminished	Usually diminished
Head tilt test	Positive for the involved eye	Positive for the both eyes

Differential Diagnosis

Differential diagnosis of trochlear nerve palsy includes thyroid eye disease, myasthenia gravis, and other causes of vertical diplopia. A fibrotic inferior rectus muscle may mimic as a contralateral superior oblique palsy.[32]

Investigations

The Bielschowsky–Parks Three-step Test

This test is useful for determining the paretic muscle by performing alternate cover test in different head positions.

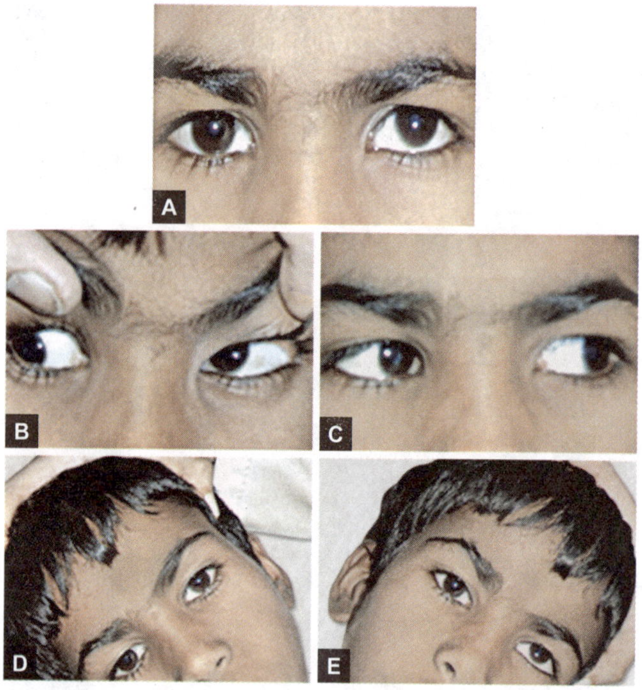

Figs. 4A to E: Park's three-step test in child with left fourth nerve palsy. (A) Primary position left hypertropia due to loss of the depressor effect of the paretic left superior oblique muscle; (B) Normal motility in left gaze, away from the fields of action of the paretic left superior oblique muscle; (C) Compensatory overaction of the antagonist left inferior oblique muscle in its field of action in right gaze; (D) No vertical deviation on contralateral head tilt; (E) Large left hypertropia on ipsilateral head tilt.
Courtesy: Dr Shikha Yadav, Rewa, Madhya Pradesh, India

It only works in cases of a single paretic muscle.[33] This test is an excellent test for diagnosis of superior oblique palsy. It involves three steps which are as follows:

- *Step 1*: This step is to determine which eye is hypertropic in the primary position **(Fig. 4A)**. The cover-uncover test can show it. Paralysis of the superior oblique muscle is one cause of hypertropia. If the right eye is hypertropic then affected muscle is either one of the right eye depressors (RSO—right superior oblique or RIR—right inferior rectus) or one of the left eye elevators (LIO—left inferior oblique or LSR—left superior rectus). If the left eye is hypertropic then affected muscle is either one of the right eye elevators (RSR—right superior rectus or RIO—right inferior oblique) or one of the left eye depressors (LIR—left inferior rectus or LSO—left superior oblique).
- *Step 2*: This step is to determine whether the hypertropia is greater in left or right gaze. If hypertropia is greater in right gaze, it implies weakness of any of the four vertically acting muscles in right gaze: RSR, LSO, LIO, and LSO. If the hypertropia is greater in left gaze, it implies weakness of any of the four vertically acting muscles in the left gaze, i.e. LSR, LIR, RIO, and RSO. Hypertropia due to superior oblique paralysis is greater on gaze to the contralateral side **(Figs. 4B and C)**.
- *Step 3*: This step is to determine whether the hypertropia is greater in left or right head tilt. If the hypertropia is greater when head is tilted to the right, this implies weakness of one of four extraocular muscles that act vertically in right head posture, i.e. either intorters of the right eye (RSR, RSO) or extorters of the left eye (LIR, LIO). If the hypertropia is greater when the head is tilted to the left, it implies weakness of one of the four muscles that act vertically in left head tilt position, i.e. either intorters of the left eye (LSR, LSO) or extorters of the right eye (RIR, RIO). Hypertropia due to superior oblique paralysis is greater when hypertropic eye is turned nasally and head tilted to the ipsilateral side **(Figs. 4D and E)**.

The Bielschowsky-Park's three-step test is very useful and simple in the diagnosis of recent onset vertically acting extraocular muscle palsies. However, it is misleading in certain situations such as long standing paresis, multiple muscle paresis and restrictive paralysis.[37]

Double Maddox Rod Test

Double Maddox rod test is useful for measurement of torsion.[34] A white Maddox rod before one eye and a red before the other is placed with the axes at 90°. Ask the patient to look at distant light source. Patient should see two horizontal and parallel streaks. If the streaks are not parallel to each other, ask the patient to rotate the Maddox rod producing a tilted streak until the streaks appear parallel to each other. If rotation is greater than 10°, it suggests the superior oblique muscle paralysis.

Vertical Fusional Amplitude

Measurement of vertical fusional amplitude with prism bar helps to differentiate between congenital and acquired fourth nerve palsies **(Table 2)**.

Other Tests

Diplopia charting and Hess screen tests are valuable for follow-up of the patients.

Certain tests are performed to determine or confirm the etiology of the palsy. These include blood sugar, glycosylated hemoglobin, ESR, CT, MRI, ice test, sleep test, and edrophonium chloride test for myasthenia gravis.

Treatment

Patients with fourth nerve palsy secondary to trauma or microvascular ischemia should be observed for 6–12 months prior to surgical intervention because of the possibility of spontaneous recovery.[30]

Prognosis

Recovery of trochlear nerve palsy ranges from no recovery to complete recovery. Complete recovery is the common in case of ischemia or trauma, or after relief of compression from tumor or aneurysm causing trochlear nerve palsy.[35]

ABDUCENS NERVE PALSY

Applied Anatomy

The abducens (sixth cranial nerve) nerve is a pure motor nerve, which supplies the lateral rectus muscle of the eyeball.[8,27,36] The abducens nucleus is situated in the lower part of pons, close to midline, beneath the floor of the fourth ventricle.[36]

Etiology

Abducens nerve palsy may be congenital or acquired.

Congenital

Congenital sixth nerve palsy is rare but may occur from injury to the abducens nerve shortly before or during birth. Congenital hypoplasia of abducens nucleus is thought to be responsible for it in some cases.[3] Unilateral agenesis of the abducens nucleus and nerve was reported in a patient with Goldenhar-Gorlin syndrome.[8]

Acquired

The sixth cranial nerve is the most commonly affected ocular motor nerve. It is vulnerable to damage due to its long course through cistern pontis and sharp bend over the superior border of the petrous part of the temporal bone. Additionally, the nerve is slender. Causes of the acquired sixth nerve palsy are summarized in **Table 5**.

Table 5: Common causes of acquired abducens palsy.[8,20-22,27]

Level of lesion	*Common causes*	*Special features*
Nucleus	• Vascular occlusion • Hemorrhage • Neoplasm • Inflammation • Metabolic disorders	• Horizontal gaze palsy • Ipsilateral lower motor neuron facial palsy
Fasciculus	• Vascular occlusion • Hemorrhage • Neoplasm (compression or infiltration) • Inflammation • Demyelinating diseases • Infections	• Raymond's syndrome • Foville's syndrome • Millard–Gubler syndrome
Subarachnoid space	• Infections (meningitis) • Increased intracranial pressure • Neoplasm • Trauma • Ischemia • Aneurysm • Dolichoectasia • Sinus infections • Rheumatoid arthritis • Carotid-cavernous sinus fistulas	Long subarachnoid course of the sixth nerve makes it prone for injuries
Petrous ridge	• Infection (mastoiditis) • Tumors (acoustic neuroma, nasopharyngeal tumors) • Trauma—fracture base of skull • Increased intracranial pressure • Thrombosis	Gradenigo syndrome
Intracavernous	• Aneurysm • Tumors (meningioma) • Ischemia (diabetes, hypertension) • Arteriovenous fistula • Inflammation • Thrombosis	• May be associated with Horner's syndrome • Cavernous sinus syndrome (multiple cranial nerve palsies)
Orbital	• Neoplasm • Inflammation • Dental anesthesia	• Isolated sixth nerve palsy • Orbital apex syndrome • Superior orbital fissure syndrome

Clinical Features

The abducens nucleus lesions do not produce ipsilateral abduction weakness but causes horizontal gaze paralysis towards the side of the lesion[37] due to involvement of horizontal centers in pontine paramedian reticular formation (PPRF). Lesions beyond the nucleus result in weakness of the nerve and esotropia in the primary position with defective abduction **(Figs. 5A to E)**. Isolated sixth nerve palsy is characterized by incomitant esotropia in the involved eye due to the unopposed action of medial rectus muscle, which increases in gaze toward action of paretic lateral rectus muscle. Face turn is common and toward the action of the paralyzed lateral rectus muscle. Diplopia is uncrossed, horizontal, and more pronounced in the direction of the paretic lateral rectus muscle. It is worse for distance than near.

Associated Syndromes

- *Möbius syndrome* is combination of congenital bilateral sixth nerve palsy associated with facial diplegia and microglossia.[38]
- *Foville's syndrome* results due to involvement of fascicular part of sixth nerve at the level of dorsal pons when it passes through PPRF. It is characterized by ipsilateral sixth and seventh nerve palsy, loss of conjugate movements, facial analgesia secondary to involvement of the sensory portion of the fifth nerve, Horner's syndrome, and deafness.[39]
- *Millard-Gubler syndrome* results from the lesions of fascicular part of sixth nerve at the level of the ventral pons when it passes through pyramidal tracts. It is characterized by a combination of ipsilateral sixth and seventh nerve palsies, and contralateral hemiparesis.[40]

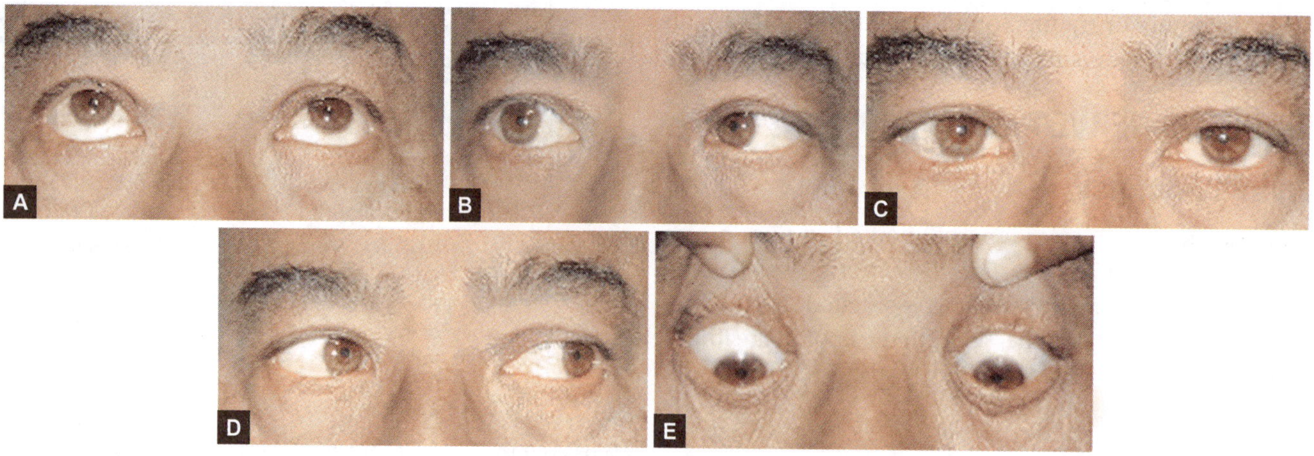

Figs. 5A to E: Right partial sixth nerve palsy. (A) Normal elevation; (B) Limitation in abduction; (C) Slight esotropia in primary position; (D) Normal adduction; (E) Normal depression.

- *Gradenigo's syndrome*: Inflammation of the petrous bone and its dura occur secondary to otitis media or chronic mastoiditis resulting in Gradenigo's syndrome. It is characterized by ipsilateral sixth nerve palsy, deafness, facial weakness, and facial pain in the distribution of first division of trigeminal nerve.[41]
- *Tolosa-Hunt syndrome (THS)* is a painful ophthalmoplegia caused by nonspecific granulomatous inflammation of the cavernous sinus. It is characterized by variable involvement of cranial nerve third, fourth, sixth, and ophthalmic division of trigeminal nerve.[42]
- *Orbital apex syndrome (Jacod syndrome)* is characterized by involvement of second, third, fourth, sixth, and ophthalmic division of trigeminal nerve.[43]
- *Superior orbital fissure syndrome* is a combination of paresis of cranial nerve third, fourth, sixth, and first division of trigeminal nerves, and sympathetic fibers following inflammation.[44]
- *Cavernous sinus syndrome* is characterized by involvement of third, fourth, sixth, and ophthalmic and maxillary divisions of trigeminal nerve (V1 and V2). It may be associated with Horner syndrome.[45]

Differential Diagnosis

Differential diagnosis of sixth nerve palsy includes restrictive thyroid orbitopathy, orbital myositis, myasthenia gravis, idiopathic orbital inflammatory syndrome, medial orbital wall blow-out fracture with medial rectus entrapment, Duane's syndrome type 1, Möbius syndrome, convergence spasm, primary divergence insufficiency, early-onset esotropia, and giant cell arteritis.[8,27,46,47]

Diagnosis

Diagnosis of sixth nerve palsy is based on clinical findings such as dysfunction of lateral rectus.[46] Imaging is necessary for identification of cause and localization of level of the lesion.

Investigations

Clinical workup to be directed toward possible etiology such as diabetes, hypertension, otitis media, giant cell arteritis, syphilis, Lyme disease, thyroid disorder, systemic and brain cancer, and myasthenia gravis.[27] Always ask about recent trauma, which is one of the major causes of sixth nerve palsy.

Laboratory Investigations

Laboratory investigations include complete blood cell (CBC) count, glucose levels, glucose tolerance test, glycosylated hemoglobin (HbA1C), erythrocyte sedimentation rate and/or C-reactive protein, rapid plasma reagin test, fluorescent Treponemal antibody-absorption test, Lyme titer, and antinuclear antibody test.[27]

Imaging

Magnetic resonance imaging is indicated in patients with sixth nerve palsy under 45 years; associated pain or other neurologic abnormality, history of malignancy, bilateral sixth nerve palsy, multiple cranial nerve palsies, and papilledema. It is also indicated, if patient does not show improvement over a period of 3–6 months or other cranial nerves become involved.[27] Lumbar puncture should be done, if MRI is unremarkable.

A temporal artery biopsy may be considered, if an imaging and laboratory finding indicates possibility of giant cell arteritis.

Treatment

Conservative Treatment

A wait and watch for a minimum period of 6 months is must when spontaneous recovery is expected.[27,48]

During this period, monocular patching may be required to avoid diplopia. Fresnel prisms are useful to correct diplopia in primary position. The injection of botulinum toxin into ipsilateral medial rectus may be helpful in better fusion.[48]

Surgical Treatment

Various muscle transposition procedures such as Jensen's procedure, Hummelsheim procedure, and Berens and Girard procedure are recommended for complete sixth nerve palsy.

Prognosis

Spontaneous recovery of sixth nerve palsies secondary to trauma occurs in 30–54% of cases, although complete recovery may not be more than 27%.[49,50]

REFERENCES

1. Nema HV, Singh VP, Nitin N. Extraocular muscles. In: Anatomy of the Eye and its Adnexa, 2nd edition. Jaypee Brothers Medical Publishers, New Delhi. 1991;77-84.
2. Nema HV, Singh VP, Nitin N. The oculomotor nerve. In: Anatomy of the Eye and its Adnexa, 2nd edition. Jaypee Brothers Medical Publishers, New Delhi. 1991;108-12.
3. Mellinger JF, Gomez MR. Agenesis of the cranial nerves. In: Vinken PJ, Bruyn GW (Eds). Handbook of Clinical Neurology. New York, Elsevier. 1977;395-414.
4. Miller NR. Solitary oculomotor nerve palsy in childhood. Am J Ophthalmol. 1977;83:106-11.
5. Victor DI. The diagnosis of congenital unilateral third-nerve palsy. Brain. 1976;99:711-8.
6. Balkan R, Hoyt CS. Associated neurologic abnormalities in congenital third nerve palsies. Am J Ophthalmol. 1984;97: 315-9.
7. Hamed LM. Associated neurologic and ophthalmologic findings in congenital oculomotor nerve palsy. Ophthalmology. 1991; 98:708-14.
8. Sargent JC. Nuclear and infranuclear ocular motility disorders. In: Walsh and Hoyt's Clinical neuroophthalmology. Miller NR, Newman NJ (Eds). Baltimore, Lippincott Williams and Wilkins. 2005;969-1040.
9. Kodsi SR, Younge BR. Acquired oculomotor, trochlear and abducent cranial nerve palsies in pediatric patients. Am J Ophthalmol. 1992;114:568-74.
10. Keane JR. Multiple cranial nerve palsies. Analysis of 979 cases. Arch Neurol. 2005;62:1714-7.
11. Tiffin PA, MacEwen CJ, Craig EA, et al. Acquired palsy of the oculomotor, trochlear and abducens nerves. Eye. 1996;10: 377-84.
12. Arroyo JG, Horton JC. Acute, painful, pupil-involving third nerve palsy in chronic inflammatory demyelinating polyneuropathy. Neurology. 1995;45:845-6.
13. Harley RD. Paralytic strabismus in children: etiologic incidence and management of the third, fourth, and sixth nerve palsies. Ophthalmology. 1980;86:24-43.
14. Keane JR. Third nerve palsy: analysis of 1400 personally-examined inpatients. Can J Neurol Sci. 2010;37:662-70.
15. Park UC, Kim SJ, Hwang JM, et al. Clinical features and natural history of acquired third, fourth, and sixth cranial nerve palsy. Eye (Lond). 2008;22:691-6.
16. Mwanza JC, Ngweme GB, Kayembe DL. Ocular motor nerve palsy: a clinical and etiological study. Indian J Ophthalmol. 2006;54:173-5.
17. Chadan N, Tamraz J, Chailloux E, et al. Etiologic diagnosis of oculomotor paralysis by computerized tomography: a statistical approach. Apropos of 472 cases. Ophtalmologie. 1989;3:114-21.
18. Gerstenblith AT, Rabinowitz MP (Eds). Wills Eye Manual, 6th edition. Philadelphia, Wolters Kluwer, 2012.
19. Leng SZ, Lü XQ, Pang SQ. Etiological analysis of 246 cases of oculomotor palsy. Zhonghua Yan Ke Za Zhi. 1994;30: 31-3.
20. Rush JA, Younge BR. Paralysis of cranial nerves III, IV, and VI. Cause and prognosis in 1,000 cases. Arch Ophthalmol. 1981;99:76-9.
21. Richards BW, Jones FR Jr, Younge BR. Causes and prognosis in 4,278 cases of paralysis of the oculomotor, trochlear, and abducens cranial nerves. Am J Ophthalmol. 1992;113: 489-96.
22. Holmes JM, Mutyala S, Maus TL, et al. Pediatric third, fourth, and sixth nerve palsies: a population-based study. Am J Ophthalmol. 1999;127:388-92.
23. Schmidt D. Classical brainstem syndrome: Definitions and history. Ophthalmologe. 2000;97:411-7.
24. Chua HC, Tan CB, Tjia H. Aberrant regeneration of the third nerve. Singapore Med J. 2000;41:458-9.
25. Yanovitch T, Buckley E. Diagnosis and management of third nerve palsy. Curr Opin Ophthalmol. 2007;18:373-8.
26. Lo CP, Huang CF, Hsu CC, et al. Neuroimaging of isolated and non-isolated third nerve palsies. Br J Radiol. 2012;85: 460-7.
27. Newman NJ. Third, fourth and sixth-nerve lesions and the cavernous sinus. In: Albert DM, Jakobiec FA (Eds). Principles and Practice of Ophthalmology. Philadelphia: WB Saunders. 2008;3:4071-100.
28. Juncos JL, Beal MF. Idiopathic cranial polyneuropathy: A fifteen-year experience. Brain. 1987;110(Pt 1):197-211.
29. Brazis PW, Miller NR, Henderer JD, et al. The natural history and results of treatment of superior oblique myokymia. Arch Ophthalmol. 1994;112:1063-7.
30. Gräf M. Diagnosis and treatment of trochlear nerve palsy. Klin Monbl Augenheilkd. 2009;226:806-11.
31. Bixenman WW. Diagnosis of superior oblique palsy. J Clin Neuroophthalmol. 1981;1:199-208.
32. Brazis PW. Palsies of the trochlear nerve: diagnosis and localization-recent concepts. Mayo Clin Proc. 1993;68: 501-9.
33. Cherednichenko VM, Martynovskaia LV. The "3-step" test in the diagnosis of vertical strabismus. Oftalmol Zh. 1990;(4): 204-6.
34. Slavin ML. Double Maddox rod test in superior oblique muscle palsy. Am J Ophthalmol. 1982;93:807-9.
35. Kobashi R, Ohtsuki H, Hasebe S. Clinical studies of ocular motility disturbances: Part 2. Ischemic ocular motor nerve palsy risk factors. Jpn J Ophthalmol. 1997;41:115-9.

36. Nema, HV, Singh VP, Nitin N. The abducent nerve. In: Anatomy of the eye and its adnexa, 2nd edition. Jaypee Brothers Medical Publishers, New Delhi. 1991;119-21.
37. Khuran AK. Incomitant strabismus. In: Theory and Practice of Squint and Orthoptics. Kurana AK (Ed). CBS Publishers, New Delhi. 1999;271-337.
38. Miller MT, Ray V, Owens P, et al. Möbius and Möbius-like syndromes (TTV-OFM, OMLH). J Pediatr Ophthalmol Strabismus. 1989;26:176-88.
39. Mutch JR. Foville's syndrome: record of a case. Br J Ophthalmol. 1939;23:225-38.
40. Gandhavadi B. Millard-Gubler syndrome: electrophysiologic findings. Arch Phys Med Rehabil. 1988;69:980-2.
41. Motamed M, Kalan A. Gradenigo's syndrome. Postgrad Med J. 2000;76:559-60.
42. Kline LB. The Tolosa-Hunt syndrome. Surv Ophthalmol. 1982;27:79-95.
43. Bray WH, Giangiacomo J, Ide CH. Orbital apex syndrome. Surv Ophthalmol. 1987;32:136-40.
44. Zachariades N, Vairaktaris E, Papavassiliou D, et al. The superior orbital fissure syndrome. J Maxillofac Surg. 1985; 13:125-8.
45. Lee JH, Lee HK, Park JK, et al. Cavernous sinus syndrome: clinical features and differential diagnosis with MR imaging. AJR Am J Roentgenol. 2003;181:583-90.
46. Prasad S, Volpe NJ. Paralytic strabismus: third, fourth, and sixth nerve palsy. Neurol Clin. 2010;28:803-33.
47. Goodwin D. Differential diagnosis and management of acquired sixth cranial nerve palsy. Optometry. 2006;77:534-9.
48. Riordan-Eva P, Lee JP. Management of VIth nerve palsy-avoiding unnecessary surgery. Eye (Lond). 1992;6 (Pt 4): 386-90.
49. Mutyala S, Holmes JM, Hodge DO, et al. Spontaneous recovery rate in traumatic sixth-nerve palsy. Am J Ophthalmol. 1996;122:898-9.
50. Holmes JM, Beck RW, Kip KE, et al. Predictors of nonrecovery in acute traumatic sixth nerve palsy and paresis. Ophthalmology. 2001;108:1457-60.

Index

Page numbers followed by *b* refer to box, *f* refer to figure, *fc* refer to flowchart, and *t* refer to table.

D

P

S

U

V